Stedman's

CARDIOVASCULAR & PULMONARY

WORDS

INCLUDES

RESPIRATORY

THIRD EDITION

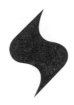

Stedman's

CARDIOVASCULAR & PULMONARY

WORDS

INCLUDES
RESPIRATORY

THIRD EDITION

LIPPINCOTT
WILLIAMS
& WILKINS

Series Editor: Beverly J. Wolpert
Associate Managing Editor: Trista A. DiPaula
Associate Managing Editor: William A. Howard
Art Director: Jennifer Clements
Production Manager: Julie K. Stegman
Production Coordinator: Kevin Iarossi
Typesetter: Peirce Graphic Services, Inc.
Printer & Binder: Victor Graphics, Inc.

Printed in the United States of America

Third Edition, 2001

Library of Congress Cataloging-in-Publication Data

Stedman's cardiovascular & pulmonary words.—3rd ed.
   p. ; cm.
Rev. ed. of: Stedman's cardiology & pulmonary words. 2nd ed.
c1997.
   ISBN 0-7817-3056-2 (alk. paper)
   1. Cardiopulmonary system—Diseases—Terminology. 2. Cardiopulmonary system—Terminology. 3. Cardiology—Terminology.

   [DNLM: 1. Cardiovascular Diseases—Terminology—English. 2. Cardiology—Terminology—English. 3. Pulmonary Disease (Specialty)—Terminology—English. WG 15 S8124 2001] 1. Title: Stedman's cardiovascular & pulmonary words.
II. Title: Cardiovascular & pulmonary words. III. Stedman, Thomas Lathrop. 1853–1938. IV. Stedman' cardiology & pulmonary words.
   RC702 .S74 2001
   616.1'001'4—dc21
2001029223

01
1 2 3 4 5 6 7 8 9 10

Contents

Acknowledgments

An important part of our editorial process is the involvement of medical transcriptionists—as advisors, reviewers, and editors.

We extend special thanks to Ellen Atwood and Shemah Fletcher for editing the manuscript, helping to resolve many difficult content questions, and contributing material for the appendix sections. We also extend special thanks to Kathryn Mason, CMT, for performing the final prepublication review.

We are grateful to our MT Editorial Advisory Board members, including Kathy Hess, CMT; Pamela Maykulsky; Velta Jo Reider; Suzanne Taubert, CMT; and Tina Whitecotton, MT. These medical transcriptionists and medical language specialists served as important editors and advisors.

Special thanks also goes to Helen-Marie Molnar, MSN, RN, ACNP-CS, CCRN, of the University of Virginia Heart Center, who provided many valuable suggestions and assisted with the appendix sections.

Other important contributors include Diana Rezac, CMT, who focused on the appendix sections; Jeanne Bock, CSR, MT; Natasha Brown; Marty Cantu, CMT; Sherry Crawford, CMT; TJ Currey; Darcy Johnson; Nancy Hill, MT; Robin Koza; Heather Little, CMT; Judy Moody; Peg Nelson, CMT; Wendy Ryan, ART; Cheri Sawyer, CMT; Jenifer Walker, MA; Judi Walls, CMT; and Mary Chiara Zaratkiewicz.

Barb Ferretti played an integral role in the process by reviewing the content files for format, updating the database, and providing a final quality check.

As with all our *Stedman's* word references, this resource incorporates the suggestions and expertise of our many contacts in the medical transcriptionist community. Thanks to all of our advisory board participants, reviewers, and editors; AAMT meeting attendees; and others who have written us with requests and comments—keep talking, and we'll keep listening.

Editor's Preface

Symbols of love, of life itself, hearts flood the stores in early February. Marketers are deliriously head-over-heels with heart-shaped candy, flowers, cookies, and cakes, mostly vibrant reds but a few whites, pinks, purples, and lavenders thrown in for variety. The actual color of the living heart would not exactly inspire romance!

These stylized love hearts are shaped nothing like the unimpressive looking chunk of specialized muscle that powers our lives. This organ begins its rhythmical contraction three weeks after conception, then beats unceasingly nearly three billion times in the average life span, resting only for a fraction of a second between beats. Its complete stillness marks the end of life, even now when there are artificial ways to start and stop it, and various other measures to legally define death.

There are so many amazing things about the heart and cardiopulmonary system, most discovered during the intense study of this past century, that it would take a separate book to list them all. Although William Harvey astonished his colleagues when he described systemic circulation 400 years ago, one aspect of the heart's function still maintains its mystery. The mechanisms by which the heart's self-generated electricity starts or stops its beating, maintains its rhythm, regulates the blood flow, and signals health or disease, when transcribed onto paper or electronic media, have yet to be fully understood.

The basic medical language describing cardiopulmonary function has not changed a great deal since the publication of *Stedman's Cardiology & Pulmonary Words, Second Edition;* what has changed is the technology used to study, understand, diagnose, and repair broken hearts. This technology has spawned a rush of new terms describing the means by which many lives have been enhanced and prolonged due to the advances in cardiopulmonary care. Babies with congenital defects, young adults stricken with an infectious cardiomyopathy, the stereotypical hard-driving male afflicted with the continuing scourge of modern civilization, and atherosclerosis leading to myocardial infarction have all benefitted from the new procedures, equipment, techniques, medications, and other treatments listed within this third edition.

With all these advances in diagnosing and treating heart disease, it still remains the major cause of death and disability in the United States. With the traditional parameters of risk factors for myocardial infarction under revision as research continues to uncover infectious, immunologic, and other factors leading to development of atherosclerotic disease, the litany of high-fat diet, high cholesterol, stress-laden sedentary lifestyle, cigarette-smoking, and overindulgence in alcohol continues to be implicated. Recognition, just recently, of the much higher than previously acknowledged incidence of heart disease in women is also triggering more research into etiology, prevention, and treatment of this indiscriminate killer.

Not to give short shrift to the other half of the cardiopulmonary system, airways diseases are increasing at an astonishing rate, with the incidence of asthma in children reflecting the largest increase. The villains underlying these increases are not yet completely understood, but indoor and outdoor pollution are the most suspect, with obesity, type II diabetes, and a dearth of exercise chiming in. On the other hand, children born with cystic fibrosis are now able to enjoy a much longer life span with appropriate antibiotic and pulmonary therapies; heart-lung transplants, no longer rare, also contribute to the survival of these children into their late teens and beyond, with near-normal quality of life. The terms describing these advances, along with the pulmonary sequelae to HIV infection and the increased incidence of drug-resistant tuberculosis, can also be found in *Stedman's Cardiovascular & Pulmonary Words, Third Edition*.

After six plus years of editing, word-finding expeditions, and other research necessary to complete several word books, I only recently came to truly appreciate and understand the complexity and teamwork necessary to bring one of these word books from concept to completion. The final product you are holding reflects the needs and input of the MT and court reporter communities; much planning and coordination of the LWW editorial staff, dedicated to reflecting current usage while maintaining strict standards; and other behind-the-scenes people who do the myriad tasks to bring a book to press. Although some do get their names printed and acknowledged in these books, there are many more who contribute valuable time, ideas, resources, and plain old hard work to ensure that you are receiving an up-to-date, usable reference. Along with many thanks to Shemah Fletcher, my co-editor, and Barb Ferretti, who makes magic with the database, I'd like to also acknowledge all the other people involved in creating *Stedman's Cardiovascular & Pulmonary Words, Third Edition*. You are all much appreciated!

Ellen Atwood

Publisher's Preface

Stedman's Cardiovascular & Pulmonary Words, Third Edition, offers an authoritative assurance of quality and exactness to the wordsmiths of the healthcare professions—medical transcriptionists, medical editors and copyeditors, health information management personnel, court reporters, and the many other users and producers of medical documentation.

We received many requests for updates to *Stedman's Cardiology & Pulmonary Words, Second Edition.* As the requests continued to accumulate, we realized that medical language professionals needed a current, comprehensive reference for these specialties.

In *Stedman's Cardiovascular & Pulmonary Words, Third Edition,* users will find thousands of words related to cardiovascular imaging, electrophysiology and pacing, invasive cardiology, heart failure, vascular medicine, bronchoscopy, pulmonary function tests, pulmonary diseases, and respiratory therapy. Included are terms for diagnostic and therapeutic procedures, new techniques, and lab tests, as well as equipment names and abbreviations with their expansions. The appendix sections provide anatomical illustrations with useful captions and labels; sample reports; common terms by procedure; and drugs listed by indication. For quick reference, we have also included listings of arterial blood gas normal lab values, as well as pulmonary function and ventilator terms.

This compilation of more than 90,000 entries, fully cross-indexed for quick access, was built from a base vocabulary of approximately 60,000 medical words, phrases, abbreviations, and acronyms. The extensive A-Z list was developed from the database of *Stedman's Medical Dictionary, 27th Edition,* and supplemented by terminology found in current medical literature (please see list of References on page xvii).

We at Lippincott Williams & Wilkins strive to provide you with the most up-to-date and accurate word references available. Your use of this word book will prompt new editions, which we will publish as often as updates and revisions justify. We welcome your suggestions for improvements, changes, corrections, and additions—whatever will make this *Stedman's* product more useful to you. Please complete the postpaid card at the back of this book, and send your recommendations care of "Stedman's" at Lippincott Williams & Wilkins.

Explanatory Notes

Medical transcription is an art as well as a science. Both approaches are needed to correctly interpret the dictation of a physician, whose language is a product of education, training, and experience. This variety in medical language means that there are several acceptable ways to express certain terms, including jargon. *Stedman's Cardiovascular & Pulmonary Words, Third Edition,* provides variant spellings and phrasings for many terms. These elements, in addition to complete cross-indexing, make *Stedman's Cardiovascular & Pulmonary Words, Third Edition,* a valuable resource for determining the validity of terms as they are encountered.

Alphabetical Organization

Alphabetization of main entries is letter by letter as spelled, ignoring punctuation, spaces, prefixed numbers, or other special characters. For example:

hydroxyproline
5-hydroxypropafenone
hydroxytoluene

Terms beginning with Greek letters show the Greek letters spelled out and listed alphabetically. For example:

alpha, α
- a. agonist
- a. blocking agent
- a. lipoprotein
- a. receptor

In subentry alphabetization, the abbreviated singular form or the spelled-out plural form of the noun main entry word is ignored.

Format and Style

All main entries are in **boldface** to expedite locating a sought-after term, to enhance distinction between main entries and subentries, and to relieve the textual density of the pages.

Irregular plurals and variant spellings are shown on the same line as the singular or preferred form of the word. For example:

scolex, pl. scoleces
curette, curet

Hyphenation
As a rule of style, multiple eponyms (e.g., Green-Kenyon corneal marker) are hyphenated. Also, hyphens have been added between a manufacturer and one or more eponyms (e.g., Vital-Metzenbaum dissecting scissors). Please note that in many cases, hyphenation is a question of style, not of accuracy, and thus is a matter of choice.

Possessives
Possessive forms have been dropped in this reference for the sake of consistency and conformance with the guidelines of the American Association for Medical Transcription (AAMT) and other groups. Please note, however, that in many cases, retaining the possessive, like hyphenating, is a question of style, not of accuracy, and thus is a matter of choice. To form the possessive of a word, simply add the apostrophe or apostrophe "s" to the end of the word.

Cross-indexing
The word list is in an index-like main entry-subentry format that contains two combined alphabetical listings:

(1) A *noun* main entry-subentry organization, which is typical of the A-Z section of medical dictionaries like *Stedman's:*

dyspnea	**endoscope**
exertional d.	Endocam e.
functional d.	lung imaging fluorescence e.
inspiratory d.	Messerklinger e.
nocturnal d.	Sine-U-View nasal e.

(2) An *adjective* main entry-subentry organization, which lists words and phrases as you hear them. The main entries are the adjectives or modifiers in a multiword term. The subentries are the nouns around which the terms are constructed and to which the adjectives or modifiers pertain:

metabolic
   m. acidosis
   m. alkalosis
   m. encephalopathy
   m. rate meter

embolic
   e. abscess
   e. aneurysm
   e. pneumonia
   e. stroke

This format provides the user with more than one way to locate and identify a multiword term. For example:

disease
   Paget d.

Paget
   P. disease

aneurysm
   cardiac a.
   fusiform aortic a.
   saccular a.

cardiac
   c. aneurysm
   c. tamponade
   c. valve prosthesis

It also allows the user to see together all terms that contain a particular descriptor, as well as all types, kinds, or variations of a noun entity. For example:

balloon
   b. laser angioplasty
   b. occlusion
   Blue Max b.
   Brandt cytology b.
   Express b.

angioplasty
   balloon laser a.
   carotid patch a.
   a. guiding catheter
   high-risk a.
   transluminal coronary a.

Wherever possible, abbreviations are separately defined and cross-referenced. For example:

AICD
   automatic implantable cardioverter-defibrillator

automatic
   a. implantable cardioverter-defibrillator (AICD)

cardioverter-defibrillator
   automatic implantable c.-d. (AICD)

Clinical Trials and Investigational Studies

Included in this edition are titles and acronyms for clinical trials and investigational studies. In some cases, the acronyms for these terms were coined from odd parts of words in the title, which were highlighted by irregular capitalization, as well as from the addition or omission of certain letters and words within the title. For *Stedman's Cardiovascular & Pulmonary Words, Third Edition*, we have standardized and simplified the respresentation of trials and studies, capitalizing only the initial letter of the words in the title. As a result, sometimes the relationship between an acronym and its expansion may not be immediately recognizable.

References

In addition to the manufacturers' literature we gather at various medical meetings, scientific reports from hospitals, and the lists created by our MT Editorial Advisory Board members from their daily transcription work, we used the following sources for new terms in *Stedman's Cardiovascular & Pulmonary Words, Third Edition:*

Books

Barnes PJ, Grunstein MM, Leff AR, Woolcock AJ, eds. Asthma. Philadelphia: Lippincott-Raven, 1997.

Baum GL, Celli BR, Crapo JD, Karlinsky JB, eds. Textbook of Pulmonary Diseases, 6th Edition. Philadelphia: Lippincott Raven, 1998.

Beyar R, Keren G, Leon M, Serruys PW, Shapiro DE, eds. Frontiers in Interventional Cardiology. London: Martin Dunitz Ltd, 1997.

Burton GG, Hodgkin JE, Ward JJ, Hess D, Pilbeam SP, Tietsort J, eds. Respiratory Care: A Guide to Clinical Practice, 4th Edition. Philadelphia: Lippincott Williams & Wilkins, 1997.

Constant J. Bedside Cardiology, 5th Edition. Philadelphia: Lippincott Williams & Wilkins, 1999.

Feigenbaum H. Echocardiography, 5th Edition. Philadelphia: Lea & Febinger, 1994.

George RB, Light RW, Matthay MA, Matthay RA, eds. Chest Medicine: Essentials of Pulmonary and Critical Care Medicine, 4th Edition. Philadelphia: Lippincott Williams & Wilkins, 2000.

Heger JW. Cardiology, 4th Edition. Philadelphia: Lippincott Williams & Wilkins, 1998.

Lance LL. Quick Look Drug Book 2000. Baltimore: Lippincott Williams & Wilkins, 2000.

Murray JF, Nadel JA, eds. Textbook of Respiratory Medicine, 3rd Edition. Philadelphia: Saunders, 2000.

Rhodes SB, ed. Dorland's Cardiology Word Book for Medical Transcriptionists. Philadelphia: Saunders, 2000.

Rosendorff C, ed. Essential Cardiology: Principles and Practice. Philadelphia: Saunders, 2000.

Serruys PW, Kutryk MJB, eds. Handbook of Coronary Stents, 3rd Edition. London: Martin Dunitz, 2000.

Stedman's Medical Dictionary, 27th Edition. Baltimore: Lippincott Williams & Wilkins, 2000.

Topol EJ, ed. Textbook of Cardiovascular Medicine. Philadelphia: Lippincott-Raven, 1997.

Vera Pyle's Current Medical Terminology, 8th Edition. Modesto, CA: Health Professions Institute, 2000.

CD

Criley JM. Physiological Origins of Heart Sounds and Murmurs: the Unique Interactive Guide to Cardiac Diagnosis. Philadelphia: Lippincott Williams & Wilkins, 1998.

Journals

ADVANCE for Managers of Respiratory Care. King of Prussia, PA: Merion, 1995, 1997–1998.

ADVANCE for Respiratory Care Practitioners. King of Prussia, PA: Merion, 1997–1999.

The American Journal of Cardiology. Belle Mead, NJ: Excerpta Medica, 1997–2000.

American Journal of Respiratory and Critical Care Medicine. New York: American Thoracic Society, 1999.

Arteriosclerosis, Thrombosis, and Vascular Biology. Baltimore: Lippincott Williams & Wilkins, 1999–2000.

ASM News. Washington, DC: American Society for Microbiology, 1996.

Cardiology in Review. Baltimore: Lippincott Williams & Wilkins, 1997–2000.

Cath-Lab Digest. Wayne, PA: Health Management Publications, 1997.

CHEST. Northbrook, IL: American College of Chest Physicians, 1995, 1999–2000.

Circulation. Baltimore: Lippincott Williams & Wilkins, 1996, 1999–2000.

Clinical Pulmonary Medicine. Baltimore: Lippincott Williams & Wilkins, 1994, 1996–2000.

The Endocrinologist. Baltimore: Lippincott Williams & Wilkins, 1988, 1996–1997, 2000.

Heart Disease. Philadelphia: Lippincott Williams & Wilkins, 1999–2000.

Hypertension. Baltimore: Lippincott Williams & Wilkins, 1999–2000.

Internal Medicine. Montvale, NJ: Medical Economics, 1996–1998.

Journal of the American College of Cardiology. New York: Elsevier Science, 1999–2000.

The Latest Word. Philadelphia: Saunders, 1999.

Pulmonary Reviews. Clifton, NJ: Clinicians Group, 1998.

Respiratory Reviews. Clifton, NJ: Clinicians Group, 1998.

Respiratory Therapy Products. Marina, CA: CurAnt Communications, 1998–1999.

RT Magazine. Marina, CA: CurAnt Communications, 1997–1998.

Stroke. Baltimore: Lippincott Williams & Williams, 1999–2000.

Websites

http://cardiology.medscape.com/Home/Topics/cardiology/cardiology.html

http://www.americanheart.org

http://www.centerwatch.com/patient/drugs/druglist.html

http://www.halcyon.com/mulder/pacemaker.html

http://www.hpisum.com

http://www.intervent.org

http://www.mtdesk.com

http://www.theheart.org

A

A band
biochanin A
A 67 lead
A point
A p value
A wave

a

a wave

A2

A2 multipurpose catheter

A$_2$

aortic second sound
A$_2$ incisural interval
A$_2$ to opening snap interval
thromboxane A$_2$

A$_{2A}$ adenosine receptor
A$_4$

leukotriene A$_4$

AA

African American
aortic arch
AA atheroma
AA cascade

A-a

alveolar-arterial

AAA

abdominal aortic aneurysm

AAASPS

African-American Antiplatelet Stroke
Prevention Study

AACD

abdominal aortic counterpulsation device

Aachener Aphasic Test
AACVPR

American Association of Cardiovascular
and Pulmonary Rehabilitation

AAD

antiarrhythmic drug

AAI

atrial demand-inhibited
AAI mode
AAI pacemaker
AAI pacing
AAI rate-responsive mode

A-A interval
A$_1$-A$_2$ interval
AAI-RR pacing
AAL

anterior axillary line

AaPO$_2$

alveolar-arterial PO$_2$ difference

AAST

American Association for the Surgery of
Trauma

AAT

alpha-1 antitrypsin
atrial demand-triggered
automatic atrial tachycardia
human pooled AAT
AAT mode
AAT pacemaker
AAT pacing

AAV

adeno-associated virus

AAV-CF

adeno-associated virus for cystic fibrosis
AAV-CF therapy

AAVNRT

atypical atrioventricular nodal reentrant
tachycardia

ABAb

anti-beta-1-adrenoreceptor antibody

ABACAS

Adjunctive Balloon Angioplasty
Following Coronary Atherectomy Study

abacavir
abacterial

a. thrombosis
a. thrombotic endocarditis

Abbe

A. flap
A. operation

Abbokinase

A. catheter
A. injection
A. Open-Cath

Abbott infusion pump
Abbreviated Injury Scale (AIS)
ABC

airway, breathing, and circulation
aspiration biopsy cytology
ABC lead
ABC protocol
ABC Study

abciximab
ABD

automated border detection
automatic boundary detection

abdomen
abdominal

a. angina
a. aorta
a. aortic aneurysm (AAA)
a. aortic aneurysmectomy
a. aortic counterpulsation device
(AACD)
a. aortic endarterectomy
a. aortography
a. asthma

abdominal (*continued*)
- a. belt
- a. bruit
- a. compartment syndrome (ACS)
- a. heart
- a. jugular test
- a. left ventricular assist device (ALVAD)
- a. paradox breathing pattern
- a. part of esophagus
- a. patch electrode
- a. pocket
- a. pulse
- a. respiration
- a. vascular retractor

abdominalis
- aorta a.
- ectopia cordis a.

abdominocardiac reflex
abdominojugular reflux
abdominothoracic
- a. arch
- a. pump

ABE
- acute bacterial endocarditis

ABECB
- acute bacterial exacerbation of chronic bronchitis

Abee support
Abelcet
Abell-Kendall equivalent
Abelson cannula
aberrancy
- acceleration-dependent a.
- atrial trigeminy with a.
- bradycardia-dependent a.
- deceleration-dependent a.
- paradoxical a.
- paroxysmal atrial tachycardia with a.
- postextrasystolic a.
- tachycardia-dependent a.

aberrant
- a. artery
- a. complex
- a. conduction
- a. QRS complex
- a. subclavian artery
- a. thyroid
- a. ventricular conduction

aberrantly conducted beat
aberration
- intraventricular a.
- nonspecific T-wave a.
- ventricular a.

abetalipoproteinemia
- Bassen-Kornzweig a.
- familial a.

ABG
- arterial blood gas
- ABG point-of-care test

ABG PCT
- arterial blood gas point-of-care test

abhesive
ABI
- ankle-brachial index
- atherothrombotic brain infarction
- ABI Vest Airway Clearance system

ability
- torquing a.

Abiomed
- A. biventricular support system
- A. Cardiac device
- A. implantable heart-replacement device

ABL
- A. 555 Analyzer
- A. 520 blood gas measurement system
- A. 625 system

ablater
- radiofrequency a.

ablation
- Ablatr temperature control device a.
- accessory conduction a. (ACA)
- alcohol a.
- atrial isthmus a.
- atrioventricular junctional a.
- atrioventricular nodal a.
- A-V junction a.
- a. catheter
- catheter a.
- catheter-induced a.
- chemical a.
- continuous-wave laser a.
- coronary rotational a.
- direct-current shock a.
- electrical catheter a.
- endocardial catheter a.
- endovascular radiofrequency catheter a.
- epicardial radiofrequency catheter a.
- fast-pathway radiofrequency a.
- fast-pathway radiofrequency catheter a.
- fluoroscopic isthmus a.
- His bundle a.
- irrigated catheter a.
- Kent bundle a.
- laser a.
- linear a.
- linear-phased radiofrequency catheter a.
- maze a.

percutaneous radiofrequency catheter a.
percutaneous transluminal septal myocardial a. (PTSMA)
pulsed laser a.
radiofrequency a. (RFA)
radiofrequency catheter a.
Revelation Tx microcatheter for RF a.
RF catheter a.
rotational a.
septal a.
slow-pathway a.
superior pulmonary vein a.
surgical a.
tissue a.
transcatheter a.
transcoronary a.
transcoronary alcohol a. (TAA)
transcoronary chemical a.
transvenous a.

ablative
a. cardiac surgery
a. device
a. laser angioplasty
a. technique

Ablatr
A. temperature control device
A. temperature control device ablation

Ablaza aortic wall retractor
Ablaza-Blanco aortic wall retractor
ABLC
amphotericin B lipid complex

abnormal
a. cleavage of cardiac valve
a. left axis deviation (ALAD)
a. right axis deviation (ARAD)
a. ST segment

abnormality
atrioventricular conduction a.
baseline ST-segment a.
brisk wall motion a.
clotting a.
electrical activation a.
figure-of-eight a.
focal motion a.
functional pacing a.
hemodynamic a.
high-risk repolarization a.
immunochemical a.
left atrial a.

left ventricular wall motion a.
lusitropic a.
neurogenic a.
nonspecific T-wave a.
pleuroparenchymal a.
regional wall motion a.
sinus node/AV conduction a.
snowman a.
transient wall motion a.
ventricular depolarization a.
wall motion a. (WMA)
white matter signal a. (WMA)

aborted
a. sudden death
a. systole

abortive pneumonia
abouchement
ABP
arterial blood pressure
automated boundary protection

ABPA
allergic bronchopulmonary aspergillosis

ABPM
ambulatory blood pressure monitoring

Abraham laryngeal cannula
Abrahams sign
Abrams
A. heart reflex
A. needle
A. pleural biopsy punch

Abrams-Lucas flap heart valve
abrasion
pleural a.

abreugraphy
abr maximal inspiratory mouth pressure
abrupt pulse
ABS
acrylonitrile-butadiene-styrene

abscess
annular a.
aortic root a.
apical a.
Brodie a.
caseous a.
cold a.
embolic a.
lung a.
myocardial a.
papillary muscle a.
periaortic a.
periprosthetic valve a.

NOTES

abscess *(continued)*
    retropharyngeal a.
    ring a.
    subphrenic a.
abscessus
    Mycobacterium a.
absent
    a. breath sounds
    a. pericardium
    a. pulmonary valve
    a. respiration
Absidia
absolute
    a. alcohol
    atmosphere a. (ATA)
    a. cardiac dullness (ACD)
    a. humidity
    a. pressure
    a. refractory period (ARP)
    a. risk reduction (ARR)
absorbable
    a. gelatin
    a. gelatin film
    a. gelatin sponge
    a. suture
absorbance
    time of flight and a. (TOFA)
absorbent vessel
absorption
    a. atelectasis
    a., distribution, metabolism, and excretion (ADME)
    fluorescent treponemal antibody a. (FTA-ABS)
    net a.
abuse
    alcohol a.
    cocaine a.
    drug a.
ABx
    antibiotic
AC
    adenylyl cyclase
    alternating current
    ante cibum
    anterior circulation
    Guaituss AC
    Mytussin AC
    Robafen AC
A-C
    A-C interval
    Robitussin A-C
AC137
ACA
    accessory conduction ablation
    anterior cerebral artery
    anticentromere antibody
    asthma care algorithm

acacia
    gum a.
ACAD
    atherosclerotic coronary artery disease
acadesine
Acanthamoeba
    A. astronyxis
    A. castellani
    A. culbertsoni
    A. glebae
    A. hatchetti
    A. palestinensis
    A. polyphaga
    A. rhysodes
acanthocytosis
acapnia
ACAPS
    Asymptomatic Carotid Artery Plaque Study
    Asymptomatic Carotid Artery Progression Study
acarbia
acarbose
acardiotrophia
Acarex test
acarian asthma
acaricidal chemical
Acarosan
acaryote
ACAS
    asymptomatic carotid atherosclerosis study
Acat 1 intraaortic balloon pump
ACB
    albumin cobalt binding
    ACB test
ACBG
    aortocoronary bypass graft
ACC
    American College of Cardiology
ACC/AHA
    American College of Cardiology/American Heart Association
    ACC/AHA pacemaker implantation guidelines
accelerated
    a. atrioventricular junctional rhythm
    a. A-V junctional rhythm
    a. A-V node conduction
    a. conduction
    a. hypertension
    a. idioventricular rhythm (AIVR)
    a. idioventricular tachycardia
    a. junctional rhythm
    a. respiration
acceleration
    flow a.
    a. time

acceleration-dependent aberrancy
acceleration-guided activity pacing
accelerator
- a. globin (AcG)
- a. globin blood coagulation factor
- a. nerve
- proconvertin prothrombin conversion a.
- serum prothrombin conversion a. (SPCA)

accelerometer
- Caltrac a.
- intracardiac a.
- Koelner Vitaport a.
- multiaxis a.
- triaxial a.
- TriTrac a.
- uniaxial a.

Accent-DG balloon
accentuated antagonism
ACCESS
- Acute Candesartan Clinical Evaluation of Stroke Survivors
- ACCESS study

access
- A-Port vascular a.
- echo record a. (ERA)
- Low Profile Port vascular a.
- A. MV system
- side-entry a. (SEA)
- venous a.
- venovenous a.

accessory
- a. arteriovenous connection
- a. artery
- a. atrium
- a. conduction ablation (ACA)
- a. cusp
- a. inspiratory muscle
- a. muscle
- a. muscles of respiration
- a. obturator artery
- a. pathway (AP)
- a. pathway effective refractory period (APERP)
- a. pathway mediated tachycardia
- a. pulmonary blood flow (APBF)
- a. saphenous vein
- a. thyroid
- a. venous vein

accident
- cardiac a.
- cardiovascular a.
- cerebrovascular a. (CVA)
- right cerebrovascular a. (RCVA)

accidental murmur
Accolate
accommodation
- period of a.

accompanying
- a. artery of ischiadic nerve
- a. artery of median nerve

accretio
- a. cordis
- a. pericardii

accrochage
Accucap CO₂/O₂ monitor
Accu-Chek
- A.-C. II Freedom
- A.-C. InstantPlus system

Accucom cardiac output monitor
Accudynamic adjustable damping
Accufix
- A. II DEC pacing lead
- A. pacemaker
- A. pacemaker lead

Accuhaler
Acculink self-expanding stent
Acculith pacemaker
AccuMark calibrated infant feeding tube
AccuMeter theophylline test
accumulation
- lipid a.
- phytanic acid a.

Accupressure infusion pump
Accupril
Accurbron
Accuretic 10/12.5
AccurOx mask
Accustaple
Accutor oscillometric device
Accutracker
- A. blood pressure device
- A. II ambulatory blood pressure monitor

ACD
- absolute cardiac dullness
- active compression-decompression
- arrhythmia control device
- Res-Q ACD
- ACD resuscitator

NOTES

ACE
  Adriamycin, cyclophosphamide,
    etoposide
  aerosol cloud enhancer
  angiotensin-converting enzyme
    ACE antisense gene therapy
    ACE balloon
    ACE Cloud Enhancer
    ACE deletion/insertion
      polymorphism
    ACE detachable mask
    ACE fixed-wire balloon catheter
    ACE I/D genotype
    ACE inhibitor
    universal ACE
acebutolol hydrochloride
acecainide hydrochloride
acedapsone
ACE-DD
  angiotensin-converting enzyme DD
    ACE-DD genotype
ACEI, ACEi
  angiotensin-converting enzyme inhibitor
ACE-ID
  angiotensin-converting enzyme ID
    ACE-ID genotype
ACE-II
  angiotensin-converting enzyme II
    ACE-II genotype
Acel-Imune
acenocoumarol
Aceon
acepifylline
ace of spades sign
acetabular artery
acetaldehyde
acetaminophen
  a. and dextromethorphan
  a., dextromethorphan, and
    pseudoephedrine
  hydrocodone and a.
acetate
  anaritide a.
  carbon-11 a.
  cortisone a.
  Cortone A.
  desmopressin a.
  Florinef A.
  fludrocortisone a.
  guanabenz a.
  guanfacine a.
  Hydrocortone A.
  leuprolide a.
  medroxyprogesterone a. (MPA)
  megestrol a.
  methylprednisolone a.
  paramethasone a.
  PET with C-11 a.

  pirbuterol a.
  sodium a.
acetazolamide
acetic acid
acetohexamide
acetonide
  triamcinolone a. (TAA)
acetoorcein stain
acetylcarnitine
acetylcholinesterase deficiency
acetylcholine test
acetyl-CoA
acetylcysteine
  N-a.
acetyldigitoxin
acetyldigoxin
acetylglucosaminyltransferase
acetylhydrolase
***N*-acetylprocainamide**
acetylsalicylate
  lysine a.
acetylsalicylic acid
acetylstrophanthidin (AcS)
acetyltransferase
ACG
  angiocardiography
  apexcardiogram
  apexcardiography
AcG
  accelerator globin
    AcG blood coagulation factor
achalasia
  esophageal a.
Aches-N-Pain
Achieve Off-Pump system
Achiever
  A. balloon dilatation catheter
  A. balloon dilator
Acholeplasma laidlawii
achromatic mass
achromatin
achromatolysis
achromin
Achromobacter xylosoxidans
Achromycin V Oral
ACI
  asymptomatic cardiac ischemia
acid
  acetic a.
  N-acetylneuraminic a.
  acetylsalicylic a.
  amino a.
  aminocaproic a.
  5-aminolevulinic a.
  aminosalicylic a.
  p-aminosalicylic a.
  amoxicillin and clavulanic a.
  arachidonic a.

ascorbic a.
aspartic a.
betamethyliodophenyl
  pentadecanoic a. (BMIPP)
carbon-11-labeled fatty a.'s
clavulanic a.
cystidine monophospho-N-
  acetylneuraminic a. (CMP-NANA)
deoxyribonucleic a. (DNA)
diethylenetriamine pentaacetic a.
  (DPTA, DTPA)
docosahexaenoic a.
EET a.
eicosapentaenoic a. (EPA)
enalaprilic a.
epoxyeicosatrienoic a.
ethacrynic a.
ethylenediaminetetraacetic a.
  (EDTA)
fatty a.
ferrous salt and ascorbic a.
ferrous sulfate, ascorbic a., vitamin
  B-complex, and folic a.
fibric a.
folic a.
fosinoprilic a.
free fatty a.'s (FFA)
fusidic a.
gadolinium-diethylenetriamine
  pentaacetic a. (gadolinium-DTPA,
  Gd-DTPA)
gamma-aminobutyric a. (GABA)
glycyrrhizinic a.
5-HPETE a.
hyaluronic a.
hydrobromic a.
hydrochloric a.
hydrocyanic a.
hydrofluoric a.
20-hydroxyeicosatetraenoic a. (20-
  HETE)
a. infusion test
inorganic a.
iodophenylpentadecanoic a.
lactic a.
linoleic a.
lysophosphatidic a.
a. maltase deficiency
mefenamic a.
messenger ribonucleic a. (mRNA)
mevalonate a.
a. mucopolysaccharide (AMP)

nalidixic a.
n-3 fatty a.
n-6 fatty a.
nicotinic a.
nonesterified fatty a. (NEFA)
omega-3 unsaturated fatty a.'s
osteopontin messenger
  ribonucleic a.
palmitic a.
paraaminobenzoic a.
paraaminosalicylic a. (PAS, PASA)
perchloric a.
a. phosphatase
phosphinic a.
polyglycolic a.
polylactic a.
poly-L-lactic a. (PLLA)
potassium citrate and citric a.
pyruvic a.
retinoic a.
ribonucleic a. (RNA)
saturated fatty a. (SFA)
sialic a.
sulfosalicylic a.
Tc-diethylenetriamine pentaacetic a.
ticarcillin and clavulanic a.
tranexamic a.
trans fatty a.'s
uric a.
urocanic a.
zofenoprilic a.
acid-base
  a.-b. determination
  a.-b. disorder
  a.-b. imbalance
acidemia
acid-fast bacillus (AFB)
acidic fibroblast growth factor (aFGF)
acidity
  total a.
acidosis
  acute respiratory a.
  hypercapnic a.
  hyperchloremic a.
  ischemia-induced intracellular a.
  lactic a.
  metabolic a.
  respiratory a.
acid-reactive
  thiobarbituric a.-r.
aciduria
Acier stainless steel suture

NOTES

acinar
> a. adenocarcinoma
> a. nodule
> a. rosette

Acinetobacter
> *A. anitratus*
> *A. baumannii*
> *A. calcoaceticus*
> *A. calcoaceticus-baumannii* complex
> *A. lwoffi*

acinus
> lung a.
> pulmonary a.

ACIP
> Asymptomatic Cardiac Ischemia Pilot
> ACIP study

acipimox
ACIT
> Asymptomatic Cardiac Ischemia Trial

acitretin
ACLA, aCLa
> anticardiolipin antibody
> ACLA IgG
> ACLA IgM

Acland-Banis arteriotomy set
Acland-Buncke counterpressor
Acland microvascular clamp
acleistocardia
ACLS
> advanced cardiac life support

ACM
> automated cardiac flow measurement

ACME
> Angioplasty Compared to Medicine
> ACME clinical trial

acnes
> *Propionibacterium a.*

ACoA
> anterior communicating arteries

ACOM
> automated cardiac output measurement

aconitine
Acorn II nebulizer
Acosta disease
Acoustascope esophageal stethoscope
acoustic
> a. densitometry
> a. imaging
> a. impedance
> a. impedance probe
> a. microscope
> a. quantification (AQ)
> a. shadow
> a. shadowing
> a. window

Acova
ACPE
> acute cardiogenic pulmonary edema

acquired
> a. atelectasis
> a. immunodeficiency syndrome (AIDS)
> a. ventricular septal defect (AVSD)

acquisition
> a. gate
> gated equilibrium ventriculography, frame-mode a.
> gated equilibrium ventriculography, list-mode a.
> multiple gated a. (MUGA)
> tagged a.
> a. time
> a. zoom (AZ)
> a. zoom technology

Acra-Cut Spiral craniotome blade
acradinium-ester-labeled nucleic acid probe
Acremonium
acrivastine and pseudoephedrine
acroasphyxia
acrocephalopolysyndactyly
acrocyanosis
acrodisc
acrohypothermy
acromegalic heart disease
acromegaly
acromelalgia
acromial
> a. articular facies of clavicle
> a. articular surface of clavicle

acromioclavicular
acrosclerosis
Acrotheca aquaspera
acrotic
acrotism
acrylate
Acrylon
acrylonitrile
acrylonitrile-butadiene-styrene (ABS)
ACS
> abdominal compartment syndrome
> acute confusional state
> acute coronary syndrome
> Advanced Cardiovascular Systems
> Advanced Catheter System
> American Cancer Society
>> ACS Alpha balloon
>> ACS Amplatz guidewire
>> ACS anchor exchange device
>> ACS Angioject
>> ACS angioplasty catheter
>> ACS angioplasty Y connector
>> ACS balloon catheter
>> ACS Concorde
>> ACS Concorde coronary dilatation catheter

ACS Concorde over-the-wire
catheter system
ACS Endura
ACS Endura coronary dilation
catheter
ACS Enhanced Torque 8/7.5-F
Taper Tip catheter
ACS exchange guidewire
ACS extra-support guidewire
ACS Gyroscan
ACS Hi-Torque Balance guidewire
ACS Hi-Torque Balance
middleweight guidewire
ACS Indeflator
ACS JL4 French catheter
ACS LIMA guide
ACS LIMA guidewire
ACS microglide wire
ACS Mini catheter
ACS Monorail catheter
ACS Multi-Link coronary stent
ACS Multi-Link coronary system
ACS Multi-Link Duet stent
ACS Multi-Link RX Ultra
coronary stent system
ACS Multi-Link RX Ultra stent
ACS Multi-Link Tristar stent
ACS OTW Lifestream coronary
dilatation catheter
ACS OTW Photon coronary
dilatation catheter
ACS OTW Photon coronary
dilation catheter
ACS OTW Solaris coronary
dilatation catheter
ACS OTW Solaris coronary
dilation catheter
ACS percutaneous introducer set
ACS Photon coronary dilatation
catheter
ACS RX Comet angioplasty
catheter
ACS RX Comet coronary dilatation
catheter
ACS RX Comet VP coronary
dilatation catheter
ACS RX Lifestream coronary
dilation catheter
ACS RX Multi-Link stent
ACS RX perfusion balloon catheter
ACS RX Rocket coronary
dilatation catheter

ACS RX Solaris coronary
dilatation catheter
ACS SULP II balloon
ACS Tourguide II guiding catheter
AcS
acetylstrophanthidin
ACSM
American College of Sports Medicine
ACSM regression equation
ACST
asymptomatic carotid surgery trial
ACST Tx2000 coronary dilatation
catheter
ACT
activated clotting time
activated coagulation time
axial computed tomography
ACT MicroCoil delivery system
act
Prescription Drug User Fee A.
(PDUFA)
Actagen
A. Syrup
A. Tablet
Actagen-C
ACTH
adrenocorticotropic hormone
Acthar
ActHIB vaccine
Actifed Allergy Tablet
Actigraph
Mini-Motionlogger A.
Actilyse
Actimmune
actin
alpha-cardiac a.
a. cytoskeleton
a. fiber
filamentous a. (F-actin)
a. gene
a. monomer
smooth muscle a. (SMA)
actin-myosin crossbridge
Actinobacillus
A. actinomycetemcomitans
A. equuli
A. hominis
A. suis
A. ureae
Actinomadura

NOTES

Actinomyces
  A. bovis
  A. israelii
actinomycetemcomitans
  Actinobacillus a.
actinomycetoma
actinomycosis
  pulmonary a.
  thoracic a.
action
  catecholamine a.
  girdle-like a.
  mechanism of a.
  A. on Secondary Prevention by
    Intervention to Reduce Events
    (ASPIRE)
  a. potential
  a. potential duration (APD)
  proepileptic a.
  purinergic a.
  A. Research Arm Test
  respiratory depressant a.
  thoracic expanding a.
Actiq Oral Transmucosal
Actis VFC
Activase injection
activated
  a. balloon expandable intravascular
    stent
  a. clotting time (ACT)
  a. coagulation time (ACT)
  a. graft
  a. partial thromboplastin time
    (aPTT, APTT)
activating transcription factor (ATF)
activation
  complement a.
  eccentric atrial a.
  endothelial a.
  endothelial cell a.
  granulocyte a.
  length-dependent a.
  a. map-guided surgical resection
  myofilament contractile a.
  platelet a.
  a. sequence
  a. sequence mapping
  thrombosis a.
activator
  Bolus Dose-Escalation Study of
    Tissue-Type Plasminogen A.
    (BEST)
  plasminogen a.
  a. protein (AP)
  recombinant tissue plasminogen a.
    (rtPA)
  recombinant tissue-type
    plasminogen a.

single chain urokinase-type
  plasminogen a.
tissue plasminogen a. (tPA)
tissue-type plasminogen a.
two-chain urokinase plasminogen a.
  (tcu-PA)
urokinase-type plasminogen a.
  (uPA)
vampire bat plasminogen a.
active
  A. Can defibrillator lead system
  a. compression-decompression
    (ACD)
  a. compression-decompression
    resuscitator
  a. congestion
  a. Doppler flow
  a. dynamic stiffness
  a. fixation lead
  a. fixation pacemaker lead
  a. hyperemia
  a. transport
  a. tuberculosis
active-site inhibited factor VIIa
Activitrax
  A. II pacemaker
  A. pacemaker
  A. single-chamber responsive
    pacemaker
  A. variable rate pacemaker
activity
  antifactor XA a.
  coagulation a.
  a.'s of daily living (ADL)
  dehydrogenase a.
  hyperadrenergic a.
  intrinsic a.
  intrinsic sympathomimetic a.
  membrane-stabilizing a.
  Motor Club Assessment test of
    motor a.
  muscle sympathetic nerve a.
    (MSNA)
  myocyte metabolic a.
  plasma renin a. (PRA)
  platelet a.
  pulseless electrical a. (PEA)
  respiratory a.
  a. scale
  a. sensor
  sinoaortic baroreflex a.
  snooze-induced excitation of
    sympathetic triggered a. (SIESTA)
  spike a.
  sympathetic a.
  sympathetic nerve a. (SNA)
  triggered a.

activity-guided
>   a.-g. pacemaker
>   a.-g. pacing

activity-sensing pacemaker

actocardiotocograph

ACT-ONE stent

Actron

Actros pacemaker

actuarial survival curve

actuation
>   direct mechanical ventricular a.
>   (DMVA)

actuator
>   dry-powder a.

AcuNav
>   A. catheter
>   A. ultrasound catheter

acupuncture

AcuSeal cardiovascular patch

Acuson
>   A. cardiovascular system
>   A. computed sonography
>   A. echocardiograph
>   A. V5M monitor
>   A. V5M multiplane transesophageal
>   echocardiographic transducer
>   A. V5M transesophageal
>   echocardiographic monitor
>   A. XP 128 echocardiographic
>   system
>   A. XP-5 ultrasonoscope
>   A. XP-10 ultrasonoscope
>   A. XP-128 ultrasonoscope

ACUTE
>   Assessment of Cardioversion Utilizing
>   Transesophageal Echocardiography
>   ACUTE clinical trial

acute
>   a. allograft rejection
>   a. bacterial endocarditis (ABE)
>   a. bacterial exacerbation of chronic
>   bronchitis (ABECB)
>   a. brain syndrome
>   A. Candesartan Clinical Evaluation
>   of Stroke Survivors (ACCESS)
>   a. cardiogenic pulmonary edema
>   (ACPE)
>   a. caudate stroke
>   a. cellular xenograft rejection
>   a. chemical injury
>   a. chest syndrome
>   a. compression triad

>   a. confusional state (ACS)
>   a. congestive heart failure
>   a. coronary care unit
>   a. coronary syndrome (ACS)
>   a. cor pulmonale
>   a. diaphragmatic myocardial
>   infarction
>   a. dissecting aneurysm
>   a. endothelial dysfunction
>   a. exacerbation of chronic
>   bronchitis (AECB)
>   a. fibrinous pericarditis
>   a. glomerulonephritis (AGN)
>   a. hemispheric stroke
>   a. hemorrhagic bronchopneumonia
>   A. Infarction Ramipril Efficacy
>   (AIRE)
>   A. Infarction Reperfusion Efficacy
>   (AIRE)
>   a. infective endocarditis (AIE)
>   a. intermittent porphyria (AIP)
>   a. interstitial pneumonia (AIP)
>   a. interstitial pneumonitis (AIP)
>   a. ischemic coronary syndrome
>   (AICS)
>   a. ischemic stroke (AIS)
>   a. isolated myocarditis
>   a. laryngotracheal bronchitis
>   a. lower respiratory tract infection
>   (ALRI)
>   a. lung injury (ALI)
>   a. lung rejection
>   a. lupus pneumonitis (ALP)
>   a. lymphocytic leukemia (ALL)
>   a. margin of heart
>   a. mediastinitis
>   a. miliary tuberculosis
>   a. multiple brain infarcts (AMBI)
>   a. myelocytic leukemia (AML)
>   a. myocardial infarction (AMI)
>   A. Myocardial Infarction
>   Angioplasty Bolus Lysis
>   Evaluation (AMIABLE)
>   a. myocardial infarction study of
>   adenosine (AMISTAD)
>   a. noncardiogenic pulmonary edema
>   a. obliterating bronchiolitis
>   a. pharyngitis
>   A. Physiology, Age, Chronic
>   Health Evaluation (APACHE)
>   a. pleurisy
>   a. preload alteration

NOTES

acute *(continued)*
    a. pulmonary alveolitis
    a. pulmonary edema (APE)
    a. pulmonary embolism
    a. radiation pneumonitis
    a. rejection (AR)
    a. renal failure
    a. respiratory acidosis
    a. respiratory distress syndrome
    (ARDS)
    a. respiratory failure (ARF)
    a. response
    a. retroviral syndrome
    a. rheumatic arthritis
    a. rheumatic fever
    a. right heart syndrome (ARHS)
    a. severe hypotension
    a. sickle cell chest syndrome
    a. sickle chest syndrome (ASCS)
    A. Stroke Study (ASS)
    a. tamponade
    a. thrombosis (AT)
    a. ventricular assist device (AVAD)
acutely decompensated cor pulmonale
acute-on-chronic status
Acutrim Precision Release
ACV
    assist/control ventilation
ACX
    A. balloon
    A. II balloon catheter
acyanotic heart disease
acyclovir
acylcarnitine
acyl-CoA, acyl-coenzyme A
acyl-CoA:cholesterol acyltransferase
  inhibitor
acyltransferase
    lecithin-cholesterol a. (LCAT)
AD
    aerodynamic mass diameter
    aerosol bolus dispersion
    aortic dissection
    autogenic drainage
Ad
    adenovirus
ADA
    adenosine deaminase
    ADA deficiency
ADAC
    ADAC/Cirrus single-headed SPECT
    camera
    ADAC single-head SPECT camera
    ADAC/Vertex dual-headed SPECT
    camera
Adagen

Adalat
    A. CC
    A. PA
ADAM
    aerosol-derived airway morphometry
Adamkiewicz artery
Adams-DeWeese
    A.-D. device
    A.-D. vena caval serrated clip
Adams disease
Adams-Stokes
    A.-S. attack
    A.-S. disease
    A.-S. syncope
    A.-S. syndrome
adaptation
    microcirculatory a.
adapter
    Bard-Tuohy-Borst a.
    Biolase laser a.
    Bodai a.
    butterfly a.
    catheter a.
    Harris a.
    Passy-Muir O2 A.
    Peep-Keep II a.
    Protex swivel a.
    Rosenblum rotating a.
    side arm a.
    Tuohy-Borst a.
    Venturi jet a.
adaptive-rate pacemaker
adaptive support ventilation (ASV)
ADC
    apparent diffusion coefficient
    ADC imaging
Adcon-C Resorbable liquid patch
Addison
    A. disease
    A. maneuver
    A. plane
adducin polymorphism
Addvent atrioventricular pacemaker
adefovir
adenine nucleotide translocator
adeno-associated
    a.-a. viral vector
    a.-a. virus (AAV)
    a.-a. virus for cystic fibrosis
    (AAV-CF)
adenocarcinoma
    acinar a.
    adenosquamous a.
    bronchiolar a.
    bronchioloalveolar a.
    bronchogenic a.
    mucinous a.
    papillary a.

Adenocard injection
adenochondroma
adenoid
    a. cystic carcinoma
    hypertrophic a.
adenoma
    adrenal a.
    bronchial a.
adenomatoid tumor
adenomatosis
    pulmonary a.
adenopathy
    hilar a.
    mediastinal a.
    perihilar a.
    retrocrural a.
Adenoscan
    A. contrast medium
    A. infusion
adenosine
    acute myocardial infarction study
      of a. (AMISTAD)
    a. deaminase (ADA)
    a. deaminase deficiency
    a. diphosphate (ADP)
    a. echocardiography
    a.-induced hyperemia
    a. monophosphate (AMP)
    a. nuclear perfusion imaging
    a. nucleotide translocator (ANT)
    a. radionuclide perfusion imaging
    a. stress
    a.-supplemented blood cardioplegia
    a. ^{99m}Tc sestamibi SPECT
    a. thallium test
    a. triphosphatase (ATPase)
    a. triphosphate (AT, ATP)
    a. triphosphate disodium
    a. triphosphate single-photon
      emission computed tomography
      (ATP-SPECT)
adenosquamous
    a. adenocarcinoma
    a. carcinoma
adenotonsillar hypertrophy
adenoviral
    a. pneumonia
    a. type 40/41 infection
    a. vector
Adenoviridae
adenovirus (Ad)

    a.-based phospholamban-antisense
      expression
    a.-mediated gene transfer
adenylate
    a. cyclase
    a. cyclase stimulator forskolin
    a. cyclase toxin
adenylyl cyclase (AC)
adequate
    a. blood flow
    a. blood supply
    a. collateral
    a. hemostasis maintained
ADH
    antidiuretic hormone
adherence assay
adherens junction
adherent
    a. leaflet
    a. mobile thrombus
    a. mural thrombus
    a. pericardium
    a. stent
adhesin
    a.-receptor interaction
adhesiolysis
adhesion
    band of a.
    chest wall a.
    fibrinous a.
    freeing up of a.
    heterotypic a.
    homotypic a.
    inflammatory a.
    pleural a.
adhesive
    Biobrane a.
    BioGlue protein-based surgical a.
    BioGlue surgical a.
    Histocryl Blue tissue a.
    a. inflammation
    a. pericarditis
    a. phlebitis
    a. pleurisy
adhesiveness
adiabatic fast passage
adiastole
adiemorrhysis
"a" dip
adipocyte

NOTES

adipose
> a. folds of the pleura
> a. tissue

adiposis
> a. cardiaca
> a. universalis

adipositas cordis

adiposum
> cor a.

adjunctive
> a. balloon angioplasty
> A. Balloon Angioplasty Following Coronary Atherectomy Study (ABACAS)
> a. measure

Adkin strut

ADL
> activities of daily living
> ADL scale

Adlone injection

ADMA
> asymmetric dimethylarginine

ADME
> absorption, distribution, metabolism, and excretion

administration
> bronchodilator a.
> closed-loop sedative a.
> sedative a.

ADMIT
> arterial disease multiple intervention trial

admixture
> venous a.

ADOPT-like software

ADP
> adenosine diphosphate

ADR-529

adrenal
> a. adenoma
> a. cortex
> a. gland
> a. hyperplasia
> a. hypertension
> a. medulla
> a. medullary implant

Adrenalin Chloride

adrenaline

adrenergic
> alpha-a.
> a. antagonist
> a. nervous system
> a. receptor (AR)
> a. receptor kinase (ARK)
> a. receptor kinase 1 (ARK-1)
> a. stimulant

β-adrenergic (*var. of* beta-adrenergic)

adrenoceptor
> alpha a.

alpha-1 a. blockade
beta a.
a. blocker

adrenocorticotropic hormone (ACTH)

adrenogenital syndrome

adrenomedullary triad

adrenomedullin (AM)
> a. infusion
> a. peptide

adrenoreceptor

Adriamycin
> A. cardiotoxicity
> A. PFS
> A. RDF

Adriamycin, cyclophosphamide, etoposide (ACE)

Adrucil injection

ADR Ultramark 4 ultrasound

Adson
> A. aneurysm needle
> A. arterial forceps
> A. forceps
> A. hemostat
> A. hook
> A. maneuver
> A. retractor
> A. test

Adson-Coffey scalenotomy

adult
> Coronary Artery Risk Development in Young A.'s (CARDIA)
> a.-onset asthma
> a. respiratory distress syndrome (ARDS)
> A. Star 1010 ultra-high-frequency ventilator
> A. Star 2000 ultra-high-frequency ventilator
> a. tuberculosis
> A. Universal bite block B116

adultorum
> scleredema a.

Advair
> A. diskus

advanced
> a. cardiac life support (ACLS)
> a. cardiac mapping
> A. Cardiovascular Systems (ACS)
> A. Cardiovascular Systems exchange guidewire
> A. Cardiovascular Systems left internal mammary artery guide
> A. Cardiovascular Systems SULP II balloon
> A. Care cholesterol test
> A. Catheter System (ACS)
> a. heart failure
> a. life support (ALS)

a. sleep phase syndrome
a. trauma life support (ATLS)
a. venous access device
advancement
genioglossal a.
maxillomandibular a. (MMA)
Advantx LC+
adventitia
aortic tunica a.
esophageal a.
adventitial
a. bed
a. cell
a. fibroblast
a. layer
adventitious
a. breath sounds
a. heart sound
a. membrane
adverse
a. event
a. ventricular remodeling
Advil Cold & Sinus Caplets
AECB
acute exacerbation of chronic bronchitis
AECD
automatic external cardioverter-
defibrillator
Powerheart AECD
AECG
ambulatory electrocardiogram
AEC pacemaker
AED
automated external defibrillator
automatic external defibrillator
FirstSave STAR biphasic AED
Aegis ICD system
Ae-H
anterograde conduction
Ae-H interval
AE-60-I-2 implantable pronged unipolar electrode
AE-85-I-2 implantable pronged unipolar electrode
AE-60-K-10 implantable unipolar endocardial electrode
AE-85-K-10 implantable unipolar endocardial electrode
AE-60-KB implantable unipolar endocardial electrode
AE-85-KB implantable unipolar endocardial electrode

AE-60-KS-10 implantable unipolar endocardial electrode
AE-85-KS-10 implantable unipolar endocardial electrode
AEM
ambulatory electrocardiographic monitoring
Aequitron
A. pacemaker
A. ventilator
aequitron
aequorin
AER
agranular endoplasmic reticulum
aerated lung
aeremia
aerendocardia
aeroallergen
Aerobacter
aerobic
a. capacity (VO_2)
a. exercise (AEX)
a. exercise stress test
a. metabolism
a. respiration
a. threshold
AerobiCycle
AeroBid
A.-M
A. Oral Aerosol Inhaler
aerocath
Simpson a.
AeroChamber
A. mask
A. Plus valved holding chamber
A. spacing device
A. VHC
AeroDose inhaler
aerodynamic
a. mass diameter (AD)
a. size
Aerodyne bicycle
AeroEclipse breath actuated nebulizer
aeroembolism
aeroemphysema
AeroGear
A. asthma action kit
A. fanny pack
aerogenes
Pasteurella a.
aerogenic tuberculosis

NOTES

aerogenosum
    sputum a.
aerogenous
aeroirritant
Aerolate
    A. III
    A. JR
    A. SR
Aerolizer
Aeromonas
    A. *caviae*
    A. *sobria*
    A. *veronii*
AeroNOx nitric oxide transport system
Aeropent
aerophagia
aerosol
    a. bolus dispersion (AD)
    Brethaire Inhalation A.
    a. challenge test
    a. cloud enhancer (ACE)
    A. Cloud Enhancer by DHD
    a. deposition
    Duo-Medihaler A.
    Flovent a.
    a. inhalation monitor (AIM)
    Maxair Inhalation A.
    Nasalide Nasal A.
    a. nebulizer
    pirbuterol acetate inhalation a.
    QVAR Inhalation A.
    respirable a.
    Sclerosol intrapleural a.
    steroid a.
    Tilade Inhalation A.
    Virazole A.
aerosol-derived airway morphometry (ADAM)
aerosolization
aerosolized
    a. antibiotic
    a. bronchodilator
    a. pentamidine
    a. pentamidine isethionate
    a. surfactant
Aerosomes
AeroSonic personal ultrasonic nebulizer
AeroTech II nebulizer
aerotherapy
aerothorax
AeroView optical intubation system
aeruginosa
    Pseudomonas a.
AerX
    A. device
    A. pulmonary drug delivery system

Aescula
    A. left ventricular IV lead
    A. left ventricular lead
AET
    atrial ectopic tachycardia
AEX
    aerobic exercise
AF
    atrial fibrillation
        nonrheumatic AF
        rheumatic AF
A-FAIR imaging
AFB
    acid-fast bacillus
AFBG
    aortofemoral bypass graft
AFCAPS/TexCAPS
    Air Force coronary/Texas atherosclerosis
      prevention study
AFCL
    atrial fibrillation cycle length
AFE
    amniotic fluid embolism
AfeCTA immunoassay
AFF
    atrial fibrillation-flutter
afferent
    a. arteriole
    a. artery
    a. impulse
    a. nerve fiber
afferentia
affinity
    A. blood pump
    a. chromatography
    a. maturation
    A. oxygenator
    A. pacemaker
AFFIRM
    atrial fibrillation followup investigation
      of rhythm management
afflux, affluxion
aFGF
    acidic fibroblast growth factor
AFO
    ankle-foot orthosis
AFORMED
    alternating, failure of response,
      mechanical, to electrical depolarization
      AFORMED phenomenon
AFP
    alpha-fetoprotein
    doxorubicin, 5-fluorouracil, cisplatin
      AFP II pacemaker
      AFP pacemaker
AFR
    atrial flutter response
      AFR algorithm

African
>A. American (AA)
>A.-American Antiplatelet Stroke Prevention Study (AAASPS)
>A. Burkitt lymphoma
>A. cardiomyopathy
>A. endomyocardial
>A. endomyocardial fibrosis
>A. histoplasmosis
>A. sleeping sickness
>A. tick typhus

africanum
>*Mycobacterium a.*

Afrin
>A. Children's Nose Drops
>A. Nasal Solution
>A. Tablet

afterdepolarization
>delayed a. (DAD)
>early a. (EAD)
>late a.

afterload
>increased a.
>a. matching
>a. mismatching
>reduced a.
>a. reduction
>a. resistance
>right-ventricle a.
>ventricular a.

afterloading catheter
afterpotential
>diastolic a.
>oscillatory a.
>a. oversensing
>pacemaker a.
>positive a.
>a. sensing

afterspike hyperpolarization (AHP)
AG
>angular gyrus

Ag
>silver

Ag-AgCl₂ electrode bipolar catheter
agalactiae
>*Streptococcus a.*

agammaglobulinemia
agar diffusion assay
agarose
>a. gel
>a. gel electrophoresis
>MetaPhor a.

Agatston score
AGE
>arterial gas embolism

age-dependent apnea
Agency for Health Care Policy and Research (AHCPR)
Agenerase
agenesis
>pulmonary a.

agent
>Albunex contrast a.
>alpha-1-adrenergic blocking a.
>alpha blocking a.
>AlphaNine clotting a.
>AngioMARK contrast a.
>antianginal a.
>antiarrhythmic a.
>anticholinergic a.
>antidiabetic a.
>antihypertensive a.
>antiinflammatory a.
>antiplatelet a.
>bacteriostatic a.
>beta-adrenergic blocking a.
>beta-adrenoreceptor blocking a.
>beta blocking a.
>blood-borne infectious a.
>BR1 contrast a.
>bronchodilating a.
>BY963 contrast a.
>calcium channel blocking a.
>chemoattracting a.
>chemotherapeutic a.
>cholinergic a.
>contrast a.
>cytoprotective a.
>diuretic a.
>dopaminergic a.
>Eaton a.
>Embolyx vascular embolizing a.
>Fibrimage diagnostic imaging a.
>fibrinolytic a.
>FS-069 contrast a.
>histocompatibility a. B27
>hydrophilic a.
>hypertensive a.
>hypoglycemic a.
>hypotensive a.
>Imagent contrast a.
>imaging a.
>inhalation a.
>inotropic a.

NOTES

agent *(continued)*
    lipid-lowering a.
    macrolide antimicrobial a.
    MRX-113 contrast a.
    MRX-408 contrast a.
    MS-325 contrast a.
    mucoregulatory a.
    neuromuscular blocking a. (NMBA)
    neuroprotective a.
    nonglycoside inotropic a.
    nonsteroidal antiinflammatory a.
    Norwalk a.
    Optison contrast a.
    Pittsburgh pneumonia a.
    progestational a.
    psychotropic a.
    Quantison contrast a.
    saluretic a.
    Schering AG Levovist echocontrast a.
    sclerosing a.
    SHU 508A contrast a.
    sonicated contrast a.
    steroid-sparing a.
    thrombolytic a.
    toxic a.
    TWAR a.
    type III antiarrhythmic a.
    ultrasound contrast a. (UCA)
    vagolytic a.
    vasodilator a.

age-related
    a.-r. apnea
    a.-r. endothelial dysfunction

age-undetermined myocardial infarction
agger valvae venae
agglutinating antibody
agglutination
agglutinative thrombus
agglutinin
    cold a.
    a. febrile

Aggrastat
aggregate
    intravascular a.
aggregation
    platelet a.
aggregometer
    Alivi a.
    NKK Hema Tracer 1 a.
aggregometry
    Born a.
    impedance a.
Aggrenox
aggrephore
aggressive platelet blockade
agitated saline solution

agitation
    echocardiogram with saline a.
    a. syndrome
aglycon
AGN
    acute glomerulonephritis
agonal
    a. clot
    a. respiration
    a. rhythm
    a. thrombosis
    a. thrombus
agonist
    alpha a.
    alpha-adrenoreceptor a.
    beta a.
    beta-adrenergic a.
    beta-adrenoreceptor a.
    calcium channel a.
    imidazoline receptor a.
    muscarinic a.
    PD 123319 AT receptor a.
agony clot
agranular endoplasmic reticulum (AER)
agranulocytosis
A greater than E
Agrelin
agricultural anthrax
Agrobacterium
AH
    artificial heart
    ataxic hemiparesis
    atrium-His bundle
    AH conduction time
    AH curve
    AH interval
AHA
    American Heart Association
    AHA type I diet
AHA.SOC
    American Heart Association Stroke Outcome Classification
AHCPR
    Agency for Health Care Policy and Research
AH:HA ratio
AHI
    apnea-hypopnea index
Ahlquist-Durham embolism clamp
AHM
    ambulatory Holter monitoring
Ahn thrombectomy catheter
AHP
    afterspike hyperpolarization
AHR
    airway hyperreactivity
    airway hyperresponsiveness
A-hydroCort Injection

3a-hydroxy-dihydroprogesterone
AI
  apical impulse
  apnea index
AIA
  aspirin-induced asthma
AICA
  anterior inferior cerebellar artery
  anterior inferior communicating artery
    AICA riboside
AICD, A-ICD
  atrial implantable cardioverter-
    defibrillator
  automatic implantable cardioverter-
    defibrillator
  automatic internal cardioverter-
    defibrillator
    AICD-B pacemaker
    AICD-BR pacemaker
    Cadence AICD
    CPI Ventak AICD
    Guardian AICD
    AICD plus Tachylog device
    Res-Q AICD
    Ventak P3 AICD
AICS
  acute ischemic coronary syndrome
AID
  automatic implantable defibrillator
AID-Check monitor
AIDS
  acquired immunodeficiency syndrome
AIDS-related
    A.-r. lymphoma (ARL)
    A.-r. lymphoma of the lung
      (ARLL)
AIE
  acute infective endocarditis
AIH
  aortic intramural hematoma
  aortic intramural hemorrhage
A-II receptor
AIM
  aerosol inhalation monitor
AIMO
  anterior inferior mandibular osteotomy
AIOD
  aortoiliac obstructive disease
AIP
  acute intermittent porphyria
  acute interstitial pneumonia
  acute interstitial pneumonitis

air
  alveolar a.
  a. bronchogram
  a. bronchogram sign
  a. cell
  a. clamp inflatable vessel occluder
  complemental a.
  complementary a.
  a. crescent sign
  a. embolism
  a. embolization
  a. embolus
  a. entry
  a. exchange
  expiratory trapping of a.
  extrapleural a.
  A. Force coronary/Texas
    atherosclerosis prevention study
    (AFCAPS/TexCAPS)
  functional residual a.
  high-efficiency particulate a.
    (HEPA)
  a. hunger
  a. medical transportation (AMT)
  a. movement
  a. pollution
  a. pulmonary embolism
  reserve a.
  residual a.
  a. sac
  a. space
  supplemental a.
  A. Supply air purifier
  tidal a.
  a. trapping
  a. trousers
  a. tube
  a. vesicle
  vitiated a.
  A. Viva
  A. Wise program
airborne
  a. allergen
  a. transmission
air-conditioner lung
air-driven artificial heart
AIRE
  Acute Infarction Ramipril Efficacy
  Acute Infarction Reperfusion Efficacy
    AIRE study
Aire-Cuf tracheostomy tube
Airet

NOTES

airflow
a. cessation
expiratory a.
inspiratory a.
a. limitation
a. obstruction
a. velocity
air-fluid level
Airlie House criteria
Air-Lon
A.-L. inhalation cannula
A.-L. tracheal tube brush
AirMax dilator
Airmed mini-Wright peak flowmeter
air-powered nebulizer
air-puff tonometer
AirSep
A. CPAP bilevel nasal mask
A. Nasal CPAP mask
A. OxiScan Oximetry Recording,
Reporting, and Archiving system
A. Ultimate Nasal mask
airspace
a. consolidation
a. disease
peripheral a.
airspace-filling pattern
air-trapping
airway, airways
anatomic a.
a. bacterial colonization
Beck mouth tube a.
Berman a.
a. branching
a., breathing, and circulation
(ABC)
a. clearance
a. closure
Combitube a.
a. conductance
conducting a.
Connell a.
a. edema
a.-esophageal balloon pressure
esophageal obturator a. (EOA)
esophagogastric tube a. (EGTA)
flabby a.
Foerger a.
Guedel a.
a. hyperreactivity (AHR)
hyperresponsive a.
a. hyperresponsiveness (AHR)
a. hypersecretion
a. hysteresis
laryngeal mask a. (LMA)
lower a.
a. lumen
a. morphometry

a. mucosa
nasal a.
a. obstruction (AO)
a. occlusion technique
a.-parenchymal dysanapsis
a. pattern
a. permeability
a. peroxidase (APO)
pharyngotracheal lumen a. (PTL,
PTLA)
a. pressure disconnect (APD)
a. pressure release ventilation
(APRV)
a. protection
a. reactivity index (ARI)
a. remodeling
a. resistance (Raw)
respiratory a.
retropalatal a.
Safar-S a.
a. secretion
a. smooth muscle (ASM)
a. stenosis
a. stenting
a. submucosa
a. tapering
upper a.
upstream a.'s
AirZone peak flowmeter
AIS
Abbreviated Injury Scale
acute ischemic stroke
AIVR
accelerated idioventricular rhythm
Ajellomyces dermatitidis
ajmaline test
Akaike information criteria
A-K diamond knife
A-kinase
akinesia
distal a.
psychic a.
septal a.
akinesic
akinesis
akinetic segment
AK-Mycin
Akron tilt table
Akt transfer
Akutsu III total artificial heart
AL
A. I catheter
A. II guiding catheter
Al
aluminum
ALAD
abnormal left axis deviation

Aladdin
 A. infant flow system
 A. nasal CPAP system
Aladdin^{II} nCPAP
ala nasi
alanine
 a. aminotransferase (ALT)
 a. exchange
alanine aminotransferase (ALT)
alanine/valine (A/V)
alar
 a. chest
 a. flaring
alaryngeal speech
AlaSTAT latex allergy test
Alatest Latex-specific IgE allergen test kit
alatrofloxacin
Alazide
Alazine Oral
alba
 pneumonia a.
albendazole sulfoxide
Albert
 A. Grass Heritage digital PSG system
 A. Grass Heritage EEG system
 A. Grass Heritage PSG system
 A. slotted bronchoscope
Albertini treatment
albicans
 Candida a.
 Monilia a.
albida
 macula a.
albidus
 Cryptococcus a.
Albini nodule
Albright syndrome
albumin
 a.-coated vascular graft
 a. cobalt binding (ACB)
 a. cobalt binding test
 macroaggregated a. (MAA)
 perfluorocarbon-exposed sonicated dextrose a. (PESDA)
 radioactive iodinated serum a. (RISA)
 a. resuscitation
 serum a.
 sonicated dextrose a.
albuminized woven Dacron tube graft

albuminoid sputum
albuminuria
Albunex contrast agent
albuterol
 a. inhaler
 ipratropium and a.
 a. nebulizer updraft
 A. Spiros
 a. sulfate inhalation solution
 a. sulfate syrup
Alcaligenes
 A. bookeri
 A. dentrificans
 A. faecalis
 A. odorans
 A. piechaudii
 A. xylosoxidans
ALCAPA
 anomalous origin of the left coronary artery from the pulmonary artery
 ALCAPA syndrome
Alcatel pacemaker
Alcian blue-PAS stain
Alcock catheter plug
alcohol
 a. ablation
 absolute a.
 a. abuse
 ethyl a.
 a. intoxication
alcoholic
 a. cardiomyopathy
 a. heart muscle disease
 a. malnutrition
 a. myocardiopathy
 a. pneumonia
alcoholism, leukopenia, pneumococcal sepsis (ALPS)
Alcon Closure System
Aldactazide
Aldactone
aldehyde-tanned bovine carotid artery graft
aldesleukin
Aldoclor
Aldomet
Aldoril
aldosterone
 a. antagonist
 a. depression
aldosterone-receptor blocker
aldosteronism

NOTES

aldosteronoma
Aldrete needle
Aldrich
    A. score
    A. ST elevation score
ALEC
    artificial lung-expanding compound
Alert catheter
alertness test
aleuronoid granule
Alexander-Farabeuf periosteotome
Alexander rib stripper
alexandrite laser
alexithymia
    A. Provoked Response Interview
alexithymic personality features
alfa
    dornase a.
alfa-2a
    interferon a.
alfa-2b
    interferon a.
alfentanil hydrochloride
Alfieri
    A. method
    A. repair
Alfred M. Large vena cava clamp
algiovascular
alglucerase
Algoform patient record
algorithm
    AFR a.
    AMC a.
    AMS a.
    ARTREK automated edge-
      detection a.
    asthma care a. (ACA)
    ATR a.
    atrial flutter response a.
    atrial tachy response a.
    automatic mode conversion a.
    automatic mode-switching a.
    detection a.
    Levenberg-Marquardt a.
    MAR a.
    mean atrial rate a.
    QuickCal a.
    SmarTracking a.
    trilinear cylindric interpolation a.
algovascular
ALI
    acute lung injury
aliasing
    a. artifact
    a. flow
    image a.
Alice4 Sleep Diagnostic system

alignment
    a. catheter
    a. mark
Alimta
A-line
    arterial line
alinidine
aliphatic amines asthma
aliquot
Alivi aggregometer
Alkaban-AQ
alkaline phosphatase (AP)
alkaloid
    ergot a.
    Rauwolfia a.
alkalosis
    altitude a.
    hypochloremic metabolic a.
    metabolic a.
    respiratory a.
alkaptonuria
Alka-Seltzer Plus Flu & Body Aches
  Non-Drowsy Liqui-Gels
Alkeran
alkylxanthine
ALL
    acute lymphocytic leukemia
    antihypertensive and lipid lowering
      ALL study
Allain method
allantoic
    a. circulation
    a. vein
Allegiance nasal prongs
Allegra
allele
    AT1 receptor C a.
    mutant a.
    prothrombin G20210A mutated a.
    S2 a.
allelic deletion
Allen
    A. and Davis classification
    A. test
Allen-Brown
    A.-B. criteria
    A.-B. shunt
Allerbiocid
Aller-Chlor Oral
Allercon Tablet
Allerdryl
Allerest
    A. 12 Hour Nasal Solution
    A. Maximum Strength
Allerfrin
    A. Syrup
    A. Tablet
    A. w/Codeine

allergen
    airborne a.
    environmental a.
    a. exposure
    HDM a.
    house dust mite a.
    Rattus norvegicus a.
allergen-induced
    a.-i. asthma
    a.-i. mediator release
allergic
    a. alveolitis
    a. angiitis and granulomatosis
    a. asthma
    a. bronchopulmonary aspergillosis
      (ABPA)
    a. bronchospasm
    a. diathesis
    a. granulomatosis
    a. granulomatous angiitis
    a. reaction
    a. rhinitis
    a. salute
    a. shiner
    a. vasculitis
allergy
    bronchial a.
    a. purpura
    seasonal a.
AllerMax Oral
Allernix
Allerphed Syrup
allescheriosis
allethrin
allethrolone
ALLHAT
    Antihypertensive and Lipid Lowering
      Treatment to Prevent Heart Attack Trial
alligator
    a. clip
    a. pacing cable
Allis clamp
Allison
    A. hiatal hernia repair
    A. lung retractor
Alliston procedure
all or none law
alloantibody
allogeneic transplant
allograft
    a. arteriosclerosis
    bovine a.

    cardiac a.
    cryopreserved heart valve a.
    cryopreserved human aortic a.
    cryopreserved valved a.
    CryoVein saphenous vein a.
    a. rejection
    a. vasculopathy
allometric
allorhythmia
allorhythmic
allosteric modification of enzyme
Allport-Babcock searcher
ALMCA
    anomalous left main coronary artery
almitrine bismesylate
almokalant
Aloka
    A. color Doppler
    A. color Doppler system for blood
      flow imaging
    A. echocardiograph machine
    A. model SSD-830 2.5- and 3.5-
      MHz transducer
    A. ultrasound
Alond
ALP
    acute lupus pneumonitis
alpha
    a.-actinin
    a. adrenoceptor
    a. agonist
    a.-alpha homodimer
    a.-B-crystallin protein
    a. blocking agent
    a.-cardiac actin
    estrogen receptor a. (ERα)
    a.-fetoprotein (AFP)
    a. Gal antibody
    a.-hydroxybutyrate dehydrogenase
    a. lipoprotein
    a.-methyldopa
    a.-MHC
        alpha-myosin heavy chain
    a.-myosin heavy chain (alpha-MHC)
    a. receptor
    A.-Tamoxifen
    a.-tocopherol
alpha-1
    a.-adrenergic blocking agent
    a.-adrenergic receptor
    a. antitrypsin (AAT)
    a. antitrypsin deficiency

NOTES

alpha-1 *(continued)*
    a. PI
    a. proteinase inhibitor
alpha-2
    a. macroglobulin
    a.-plasmin inhibitor
alpha-adrenergic
    a.-a. blocker
    a.-a. stimulation
alpha-adrenoreceptor
    a.-a. agonist
    a.-a. blocker
AlphaNine clotting agent
Alphavirus
Alport syndrome
alprazolam
alprenolol
alprostadil
ALPS
    alcoholism, leukopenia, pneumococcal
    sepsis
        ALPS syndrome
ALRI
    acute lower respiratory tract infection
ALS
    advanced life support
    amyotrophic lateral sclerosis
Alstrom syndrome
ALT
    alanine aminotransferase
Altace Oral
ALTE
    apparent life-threatening event
alteplase
    Continuous Infusion Versus Double-
    Bolus Administration of A.
    (COBALT)
    recombinant a.
alteration
    acute preload a.
    coexistent cardiac a.'s
    ST a.
altered airway secretion
alternans
    auditory a.
    auscultatory a.
    concordant a.
    cycle length a.
    discordant a.
    electrical a.
    microvolt T-wave a.
    parvus a.
    pulsus a.
    QRS a.
    respiratory a.
    ST segment a.
    systole a.
    a. test

    total a.
    T wave a. (TWA)
    U wave a.
Alternaria tenuis
alternating
    a. bidirectional tachycardia
    a. current (AC)
    a., failure of response, mechanical,
    to electrical depolarization
    (AFORMED)
    a. pulse
alternation
    cardiac a.
    concordant a.
    cycle length a.
    discordant a.
    electrical a. of heart
    mechanical a.
alternative
    Cardia Salt a.
    Citrol Smoking a.
alternobaric exposure
altitude
    a. alkalosis
    a. hypoxia
    a. simulation study
altretamine
aluminum (Al)
    a. hydroxide gel
    a. lung
    a. oxygen regulator
Alupent
ALVAD
    abdominal left ventricular assist device
    ALVAD artificial heart
Alvarez prosthesis
Alvarez-Rodriguez cardiac catheter
alvei
    Bacillus a.
alveobronchiolitis
Alveofact
alveolar
    a. air
    a.-air equation
    a.-arterial oxygen tension gradient
    a.-arterial PO_2 difference ($AaPO_2$)
    a. asthma
    a. bronchiole
    a. capillary
    a.-capillary
    a.-capillary block
    a. capillary intravascular pressure
    a.-capillary membrane
    a. carbon dioxide pressure
    a. carbon dioxide tension
    a. cell
    a. cell carcinoma
    a. dead space

A

a. destruction
a. duct emphysema
a. ectasia
a. edema
a.-filling pattern
a. flooding
a. gas
a. hyaline membrane
a. hypertension
a. hyperventilation
a. hypoventilation
a. hypoxia
a. infiltrate
a. leak
a. macrophage
a. opacification
a. overdistention
a. oxygen partial pressure (PAO_2)
a. oxygen tension
a. pattern
a. period
a. permeability (AP)
a. phospholipidosis
a. pressure (Palv)
a. proteinosis
a. recruitment
a. sac
a.-septal amyloidosis
a. ventilation
a. ventilation per minute (V_A)
a. volume (VA)
alveolar-arterial (A-a)
alveolarization
alveoli (*pl. of* alveolus)
alveolitis
　acute pulmonary a.
　allergic a.
　cryptogenic fibrosing a. (CFA)
　desquamative a.
　diffuse sclerosing a.
　extrinsic allergic a.
　fibrosing a.
　lymphoid a.
alveolocapillary
　a. membrane
　a. partial pressure gradient
alveoloclasia
alveolus, pl. **alveoli**
　pulmonary a.
　alveoli pulmonis
　ventilated alveoli
Alzate catheter

AM
　adrenomedullin
AM1 asthma monitor
AM50-1 aerosol/medication air compressor
AM-50 portable air compressor
Amadeus
AMA-Fab
　antimyosin monoclonal antibody with Fab fragment
　　AMA-Fab scintigraphy
amalonatica
　　Citrobacter a.
amantadine hydrochloride
Amapari virus
amaurosis partialis fugax
amaurotic
amazon thorax
Amazr catheter
Amba
ambasilide
Ambenyl Cough Syrup
Amberlite particles
AMBI
　acute multiple brain infarcts
Ambien
ambient pressure
ambiguus
　situs a.
AmBisome
Amblyomma americanum
Ambrose
　A. classification
　A. plaque type
ambroxol
Ambu
　A. bag
　A. CardioPump
　A. respirator
ambulatory
　a. blood pressure monitoring (ABPM)
　a. electrocardiogram (AECG)
　a. electrocardiographic monitoring (AEM)
　a. electrocardiography
　a. Holter monitor
　a. Holter monitoring (AHM)
　a. monitoring
　a. nuclear detector
　a. O_2

NOTES

ambulatory *(continued)*
  a. oximetry monitoring (AOM)
  a. ventricular function probe
ambuphylline
AmbuSPUR disposable resuscitator
AMC
  automatic mode conversion
  AMC algorithm
Amcath catheter
Amcort Injection
amdinocillin
amebiasis
  pulmonary a.
amebic
  a. pericarditis
  a. pneumonia
ameboid
  a. cell
  a. movement
ameboma
Amen Oral
Americaine
American
  African A. (AA)
  A. Association of Cardiovascular
    and Pulmonary Rehabilitation
    (AACVPR)
  A. Association for the Surgery of
    Trauma (AAST)
  A. Cancer Society (ACS)
  A. College of Cardiology (ACC)
  A. College of Cardiology/American
    Heart Association (ACC/AHA)
  A. College of Cardiology/American
    Heart Association Task Force on
    Practice guidelines
  A. College of Sports Medicine
    (ACSM)
  A. College of Sports Medicine
    regression equation
  A. Heart Association (AHA)
  A. Heart Association classification
  A. Heart Association diet
  A. Heart Association guidelines
  A. Heart Association step II diet
  A. Heart Association Stroke
    Outcome Classification
    (AHA.SOC)
  A. Heart Association type I diet
  Hispanic A. (HA)
  A. Optical Cardiocare pacemaker
  A. Optical oximeter
  A. Optical R-inhibited pacemaker
  A. Pacemaker Corporation lead
  A. Roentgen Ray Society
  A. Sleep Disorders Association
    (ASDA)

  A. Thoracic Society classification
    of dyspnea
  A. tracheotomy tube
  A. trypanosomiasis
americanum
  Amblyomma a.
americanus
  Necator a.
Amesec
A-methaPred injection
Amgenal Cough Syrup
AMI
  acute myocardial infarction
  anterior myocardial infarction
  AMI infant apnea monitor
AMIABLE
  Acute Myocardial Infarction Angioplasty
    Bolus Lysis Evaluation
Amicar
Amidate
amifloxacin
amikacin sulfate
Amikin injection
amiloride
  a. hydrochloride
  a. and hydrochlorothiazide
amine
  sympathomimetic a.
amino acid
aminocaproic acid
Amino-Cerv Vaginal Cream
aminoethyl ethanolamine
aminoglutethimide
aminoglycoside
aminoguanidine
5-aminolevulinic acid
aminopenicillin
aminophylline
  a., amobarbital, and ephedrine
Aminorex
aminosalicylate
  phenyl a.
  potassium a.
  sodium a.
  a. sodium
aminosalicylic
  a. acid
  a. acid hypersensitivity
aminoterminal propeptide
aminotransferase
  alanine a. (ALT)
  aspartate a. (AST)
amiodarone
  desethyl a.
  a. hydrochloride
  a.-induced hyperthyroidism
  a. pulmonary fibrosis
  a. therapy

A

A. Versus Implantable Defibrillators (AVID)
Amipaque contrast medium
AMIS
Aspirin in Myocardial Infarction Study
Amiscan
Amis 2000 respiratory mass spectrometer
AMISTAD
acute myocardial infarction study of adenosine
Ami-Tex LA
amitriptyline
AML
acute myelocytic leukemia
anterior mitral leaflet
amlodipine
a. and benazepril
a. besylate
ammonia
anhydrous a.
aromatic a. spirit
N-13 a.
nitrogen-13 a.
ammonium chloride
amnesia
global a.
verbal a.
visual a.
amniocentesis
amnionic
a. fluid embolism
a. fluid syndrome
amniotic
a. fluid embolism (AFE)
a. fluid syndrome
A-mode
A.-m. echocardiography
A.-m. echo-tracking device
Amorolfine
amorphous
a. hydrogenated silicon carbide (a-SiC:H)
a. parenchymal opacification
amount of use (AOU)
amoxapine
amoxicillin
a. and clavulanate potassium
a. and clavulanic acid
a. and potassium clavulanate
Amoxil

AMP
acid mucopolysaccharide
adenosine monophosphate
average mean pressure
Amp
Jaa A.
ampere
amphetamine
a. sulfate
a. toxicity
amphipathic helix
Amphojel
amphoric
a. echo
a. murmur
a. rale
a. respiration
a. voice
amphoriloquy
Amphotec
amphotericin
a. B
a. B cholesteryl sulfate complex
a. b (conventional)
a. B lipid complex (ABLC)
a. B (liposomal)
ampicillin and sulbactam
Ampicin
Amplatz
A. coronary catheter
A. dilator
A. Hi-Flo torque-control catheter
A. left I, II catheter
A. right coronary catheter
A. right I, II catheter
A. Super Stiff guidewire
A. technique
A. thrombectomy device (ATD)
A. torque wire
A. tube guide
A. ventricular septal defect device
Amplatzer
A. occluder
A. septal occluder
Amplex guidewire
Amplicor *Mycobacterium tuberculosis* **test**
amplified *Mycobacterium tuberculosis* **direct test (AMTDT)**
amplifying myocyte
amplitude
apical interventricular septal a.

NOTES

amplitude *(continued)*
 atrial pulse a.
 contractile a.
 C-to-E a.
 D-to-E a.
 a. image
 a. linearity
 a. of pulse
 pulse a.
 P wave a.
 R wave a.
 signal a.
 ventricular pulse a.
 wall a.
 wave a.
amprenavir
amprolium hydrochloride
ampulla, pl. **ampullae**
 Bryant a.
 Thoma a.
ampullary aneurysm
amrinone
 a. lactate
AMRO
 Amsterdam Rotterdam
 AMRO clinical trial
AMS
 automatic mode switching
 AMS algorithm
amsacrine
Amsterdam Rotterdam (AMRO)
AMT
 air medical transportation
AMTDT
 amplified *Mycobacterium tuberculosis*
 direct test
Amtech-Killeen pacemaker
AMV
 assisted mechanical ventilation
amygdala
amyl
 A. Nitrate Vaporole
 a. nitrite
 A. Nitrite Aspirols
 a. nitrite study
amylase
 serum a.
amyloid
 a. A protein
 a. heart disease
 a. precursor protein (APP)
amyloidoma
amyloidosis
 alveolar-septal a.
 cardiac a.
 familial a.
 mediastinal a.

 nodular pulmonary a.
 parenchymal a.
 pleural a.
 primary systemic a.
 pseudotumoral mediastinal a.
 pulmonary a.
 senile a.
 tracheobronchial a.
amyocardia
amyotrophic
 a. chorea
 a. lateral sclerosis (ALS)
AN
 A. interval
 A. region
ANA
 antinuclear antibody
anabolic steroid
Anabolin
Anacin
Anaconda
 A. delivery system
 A. device
 A. device and delivery system
anacrotic
 a. limb
 a. notch
 a. pulse
anacrotism
anadicrotic pulse
anadicrotism
anadicrotus
 pulsus a.
anaerobe
anaerobic
 a. empyema
 a. metabolism
 a. Pulsator syringe
 a. respiration
 a. threshold (AT)
anaerobiosis
Anaerobiospirillum
anaerobius
 Peptostreptococcus a.
anagrelide
analgesia
 epidural a.
 extrapleural a.
 extrapleural catheter a.
 intrapleural catheter a.
 intravenous a.
 patient-controlled a. (PCA)
 percutaneous extrapleural a.
analgesic
 a. nephropathy
 patient-controlled a. (PCA)
analog-to-digital conversion

analyser
  Oxicom-2000 a.
analysis, pl. **analyses**
  backscatter a.
  beat-to-beat a.
  body density a.
  centerline method of wall
    motion a.
  computerized texture a.
  Core Laboratory Ultrasound A.
    (CLOUT)
  Doppler flow a.
  Doppler spectral a.
  Doppler waveform a.
  electron microprobe a.
  fast Fourier spectral a.
  forced vital capacity a. (FVCA)
  Fourier series a.
  Fourier transform a.
  frequency-domain a.
  hemodynamic a.
  hydroxyproline a.
  image a.
  immunoprecipitin a.
  longitudinal a.
  microarray a.
  neutron activation a.
  Nicolet Biomedical UltraSom
    computerized sleep a.
  Northern hybridization a.
  phase image a.
  point-of-care a.
  power spectral a.
  pressure-volume a.
  quantitative coronary
    angiographic a.
  respiratory gas a.
  sensitivity a.
  Southern blot a.
  spectral a.
  sputum a.
  time-domain a.
  videodensitometric myocardial
    textural a.
  wall motion a.
  x-ray energy microprobe a.
analyzer
  ABL 555 A.
  AVL Medical Instruments model
    995-Hb arterial blood gas a.
  AVL Omni blood gas a.
  AVL OPTI Critical Care A.

  AVL OPTI 1 portable blood
    gas a.
  Beckman O_2 a.
  840 blood gas a.
  1620 blood gas a.
  BVA-100 blood volume a.
  Cat-a-Kit a.
  Cobas Fara centrifugal a.
  CO Sleuth handheld carbon
    monoxide a.
  Criticare $ETCO_2$ multigas a.
  Datex $ETCO_2$ multigas a.
  DMI a.
  Ela Medical Elatec arrhythmia a.
  V a.
  Enzymun-Test System ES22 a.
  ERA 300 dual-chamber pacing
    system a.
  $ETCO_2$ multigas a.
  Gem Premier Plus blood
    gas/electrolyte a.
  IL Synthesis a.
  i-STAT handheld a.
  Keystone PF a.
  Marquette Series 8000 Holter a.
  Medigraphics 2000 a.
  MiniOX IA oxygen a.
  MiniOX oxygen a.
  MiniOX 1000 oxygen a.
  Model O2T oxygen a.
  Nellcor N2500 $ETCO_2$ multigas a.
  New Glucorder a.
  NOA model 280 nitric oxide a.
  Novametrix $ETCO_2$ multigas a.
  Ohmeda $ETCO_2$ multigas a.
  Omni a.
  OPTI 1 pH/blood gas a.
  OPTI 1 portable blood a.
  pacing system a.
  PrinterNOx nitric oxide with
    MKII a.
  pulse-height a.
  Puritan Bennett $ETCO_2$ multigas a.
  Reynolds Pathfinder 3 a.
  Shimadzu DAR-2400 coronary
    arteriographic a.
  Sievers model 280 nitric oxide a.
  Sole Primeur 33D a.
Anamine Syrup
anandamide
Anandron
anangioplasia

NOTES

anangioplastic
anapamil
anaphylactic
    a. antibody
    a. crisis
anaphylactoid
    a. purpura
    a. reaction
    a. syndrome of pregnancy
anaphylatoxin
    chemotactic a.
anaphylaxis
    eosinophil chemotactic factors of a.
    (ECF-A)
    slow-reacting substance of a. (SRS-
    A)
anaplastic
    a. carcinoma
    a. tumor
anaplerosis
anaplerotic sequence
Anaplex liquid
anapnea
anapneic
anapnotherapy
Anaprox
anaritide acetate
anasarca
Anastaflo intravascular shunt
anastomose
anastomosis, pl. **anastomoses**
    aortic a.
    aorticopulmonary a.
    arterial a.
    arteriovenous a.
    Baffe a.
    Béclard a.
    bidirectional cavopulmonary a.
    (BCA)
    bidirectional superior
    cavopulmonary a. (BSCA)
    cavopulmonary a.
    Clado a.
    a. clamp
    cobra-head a.
    Cooley intrapericardial a.
    Cooley modification of
    Waterston a.
    cruciate a.
    distal a.
    extracardiac cavopulmonary a.
    Fontan atriopulmonary a.
    Glenn a.
    Hoyer a.
    intermesenteric arterial a.
    Kugel a.
    Nakayama a.
    portacaval a.

    portoportal a.
    portosystemic a.
    Potts a.
    Potts-Smith a.
    precapillary a.
    a. of Riolan
    Sucquet a.
    Sucquet-Hoyer a.
    systemic to pulmonary artery a.
    total cavopulmonary a.
    Waterston a.
    Waterston extrapericardial a.
anastomotica
    arteria a.
anastomotic stricture
anastrozole
anatomic
    a. airway
    a. assessment
    a. block
    a. dead space
    a. localization
    a. pulmonary atresia
anatomical
    a. dead space
    a. reentry
anatomy
    coronary a.
    designed after natural a.
    native coronary a.
anatricrotic
anatricrotism
Anatuss DM
ANCA
    antineutrophil cytoplasmic antibody
Ancef
anchor
    Harpoon suture a.
ancillary measure
Ancobon
ANCOR imaging system
Ancotil
ancrod
Ancure
    A. stent-graft
    A. system
Ancylostoma
    A. braziliense
    A. caninum
    A. duodenale
Andersen
    A. syndrome
    A. triad
Anderson
    A. phasing score
    A. procedure
    A. test
Anderson-Fabry disease

Anderson-Keys method
Anderson-Wilkins (AW)
    A.-W. acuteness score
Andes virus
Andral decubitus position
Andrews
    A. retractor
    A. suction tip
Andrews-Pynchon tube
Androcur Depot
Androderm Transdermal system
Android
Andro-L.A. Injection
Androlone
Androlone-D
Andropository Injection
Androsov vascular stapler
anechoic
Anectine Chloride
Anel operation
anemia
    aplastic a.
    chronic hemolytic a.
    Cooley a.
    hemolytic a.
    Mediterranean a.
    megaloblastic a.
    microangiopathic a.
    sickle cell a.
    splenic a.
anemic
    a. anoxia
    a. hypoxia
    a. murmur
anemometer
    hot wire a.
    mass-flow a.
anergy
    skin test a.
aneroid manometer
Anestacon Topical Solution
anesthesia
    Bier block a.
    inhalational a.
    MacIntosh blade a.
anesthetic
    inhalational a.
aneuploid
AneuRx
    A. fully supported modular system
    A. stent
    A. stent graft system

aneurysm
    abdominal aortic a. (AAA)
    acute dissecting a.
    ampullary a.
    aortic a.
    aortic sinus a.
    aortoiliac a.
    apical a.
    arterial a.
    arteriovenous pulmonary a.
    atherosclerotic a.
    atrial septal a. (ASA)
    Berard a.
    berry a.
    bilobed a.
    brain a.
    cardiac a.
    cerebral a.
    Charcot-Bouchard a.
    chronic fusiform a.
    cirsoid a.
    congenital aortic a.
    coronary a.
    Crisp a.
    cylindroid a.
    descending thoracic a.
    dissecting aortic a.
    dolichoectatic a.
    ectatic a.
    embolic a.
    embolomycotic a.
    endoluminal reconstruction of
      basilar artery fusiform a.
    false a.
    false aortic a.
    familial intracranial a.
    fusiform aortic a.
    giant a.
    infected a.
    infrarenal abdominal aortic a.
    innominate a.
    interventricular septum a.
    intracranial a.
    intracranial fusiform a.
    left ventricular a.
    luetic a.
    mitral valve a.
    mixed a.
    mouth of a.
    mural a.
    mycotic aortic a.
    Park a.

NOTES

aneurysm *(continued)*
   phantom a.
   popliteal a.
   Pott a.
   racemose a.
   Rasmussen a.
   Richet a.
   Rodriguez a.
   ruptured aortic a.
   ruptured sinus of Valsalva a.
    (RSVA)
   saccular a.
   serpentine a.
   Shekelton a.
   sinus of Valsalva a.
   spurious a.
   stent-assisted coiling of basilar
    fusiform a.
   suprasellar a.
   syphilitic a.
   syphilitic aortic a.
   thoracic aortic a.
   thoracoabdominal aortic a.
   traction a.
   traumatic aortic a.
   true aortic a.
   two-piece bifurcated intraluminal
    graft for repair of an a.
   ventricular a.
   verminous a.
   wide-necked a.
   windsock a.
   a. wrapping
   wrapping of abdominal aortic a.
aneurysmal, aneurysmatic
   a. bone cyst
   a. bruit
   a. cough
   a. dilation
   a. hematoma
   a. murmur
   a. phthisis
   a. sac
   a. thrill
aneurysmectomy
   abdominal aortic a.
   Matas a.
aneurysmography
aneurysmoplasty
aneurysmorrhaphy
aneurysmorrhectomy
Anexsia
ANF
   atrial natriuretic factor
Ang1
   angiotensin I

AngeCool
   A. RF catheter
   A. RF catheter ablation system
Angeion 2000 ICD generator
**AngeLase combined mapping-laser
  probe**
Angelchik antireflux prosthesis
Angell-Shiley
   A.-S. bioprosthetic valve
   A.-S. xenograft prosthetic valve
angel's trumpet
Angel Wings device
Anger scintillation camera
Angestat hemostasis introducer
Angetear tearaway introducer
angialgia
angiasthenia
angiectasis
angiitis
   allergic granulomatous a.
   Churg-Strauss a.
   leukocytoclastic a.
   necrotizing a.
   nonnecrotizing a.
angina
   abdominal a.
   antecedent a.
   anxiety a.
   bandlike a.
   benign croupous a.
   Bretonneau a.
   Canadian class I–IV a.
   chronic stable a.
   classic a.
   cold-induced a.
   a. cordis
   coronary spastic a.
   crescendo a.
   a. crouposa
   a. cruris
   decubitus a.
   a. decubitus
   a. dyspeptica
   a. of effort
   effort a.
   ergonovine maleate provocation a.
   esophageal a.
   exercise-induced a.
   exertional a.
   false a.
   first-effort a.
   food a.
   a. gangrenosa
   Heberden a.
   hippocratic a.
   hypercyanotic a.
   hysteric a.
   a. inversa

ischemic rest a.
lacunar a.
a. laryngea
Ludwig a.
a. membranacea
microvascular a.
mixed a.
Monotherapy Assessment of
  Ranolazine in Stable A.
  (MARISA)
neutropenic a.
nocturnal a.
nonexertional a.
a. nosocomii
a. notha
office a.
pacing-induced a.
a. pectoris
a. pectoris decubitus
a. pectoris sine dolore
a. pectoris vasomotoria
a. phlegmonosa
postinfarction a.
postprandial a.
preinfarction a.
Prinzmetal a.
Prinzmetal variant a.
pseudomembranous a.
Randomized Intervention Treatment
  of A. (RITA)
rate-dependent a.
rebound a.
reflex a.
rest a.
a. rheumatica
a. scarlatinosa
Schultz a.
sexual a.
silent a.
a. simplex
a. sine dolore
smoking-induced a.
a. spuria
stable a.
Thrombolysis and Angioplasty in
  Unstable A. (TAUSA)
toilet-seat a.
a. tonsillaris
a. trachealis
treadmill-induced a.
a. ulcerosa
unstable a.

variable threshold a.
variant a. (VA)
variant a. pectoris (VAR)
vasomotor a.
a. vasomotoria
vasospastic a. (VSA)
vasotonic a.
Vincent a.
walk-through a.
white-coat a.
anginae
  Saccharomyces a.
angina-guided therapy
anginal
  a. equivalent
  a. pain
  a. perceptual threshold
anginiform
anginoid
anginophobia
anginosa
  syncope a.
anginose, anginous
anginosus
  status a.
  Streptococcus a.
angioarchitecture
angiocardiogram
angiocardiography (ACG)
  first-pass radionuclide a.
  radionuclide a.
  transseptal a.
angiocardiokinetic
angiocardiopathy
angiocarditis
angiocatheter
  Brockenbrough a.
  Corlon a.
  Deseret a.
  Eppendorf a.
  large-bore a.
  Mikro-Tip a.
Angiocath PRN catheter
Angio-Conray contrast medium
Angiocor
  A. prosthetic valve
  A. rotational thrombolizer
angiodermatitis
angiodynagraphy
angiodynia
angiodysplasia of colon
angioedema

NOTES

Angioflow high-flow catheter
angiogenesis
    myocardial a.
    therapeutic a.
angiogenic squamous dysplasia
Angiografin
angiogram
    ECG-synchronized digital
      subtraction a.
    gated nuclear a.
    PMS Integris a.
    pulmonary a.
    Siemens biplane Neurostar digital
      subtraction a.
    venous digital a.
    wedge a.
angiograph
angiographer
angiographic
    a. assessment
    a. catheter
    a. contrast
    a. instrumentation
angiographically occult intracranial
vascular malformation (AOIVM)
angiography
    aortography a.
    balloon-occlusion pulmonary a.
    biplane orthogonal a.
    carotid a.
    cerebral a.
    color power a.
    computed tomography a. (CTA)
    contrast a.
    contrast-enhanced magnetic
      resonance a. (CEMRA)
    coronary a.
    coronary magnetic resonance a.
    CT a.
    3DFT magnetic resonance a.
    digital subtraction a. (DSA)
    digitized subtraction a.
    directional color a. (DCA)
    elective a.
    electron-beam a.
    equilibrium radionuclide a. (ERNA)
    first-pass radionuclide a.
    fluorescein a.
    FluoroPlus a.
    free-breathing coronary magnetic
      resonance a.
    gated blood-pool a.
    gated radionuclide a.
    indocyanine green a.
    internal mammary artery graft a.
    intraoperative digital subtraction a.
    intraoperative vascular a. (IVA)

    intravenous digital subtraction a.
      (IVDSA)
    left aortic a.
    left atrial a.
    left ventricular a.
    magnetic resonance a. (MRA)
    magnetic resonance coronary a.
      (MRCA)
    magnet resonance a.
    MEDIS off-line quantitative
      coronary a.
    mesenteric a.
    multigated a.
    noncardiac a.
    nonselective coronary a.
    Philips Integris 3000 biplane digital
      subtraction a.
    pulmonary a. (PA, PAG)
    pulmonary wedge a.
    quantitative coronary a. (QCA)
    quantitative edge-detection a.
    radionuclide a.
    renal a.
    renovascular a.
    rest and exercise gated nuclear a.
    rest radionuclide a.
    saphenous vein bypass graft a.
    selective a.
    subtraction a.
    surveillance a.
    synchrotron-based transvenous a.
    thermal a.
    three-dimensional time-of-flight
      magnetic resonance a.
    time-of-flight magnetic resonance a.
    total absence of circulation on
      four-vessel a.
    ultrasound a.
    ventricular a.
    A. Versus Intravascular Ultrasound-
      Directed Coronary Stent
      Placement (AVID)
    wedge pulmonary a.
Angioguard catheter device
angiohypertonia
angiohypotonia
angioid
Angioject
    ACS A.
AngioJet
    A. catheter
    A. rapid thrombectomy system
    A. rheolytic thrombectomy
    A. saline jet/vacuum device
      catheter
    A. thrombectomy catheter
angiokeratoma corporis diffusum
angiokinesis

Angio-Kit catheter
angioleiomyoma
angiologia
angiology
angioma
    cavernous a.
    cherry a.
    spider a.
AngioMARK contrast agent
angiomatosis
    bacillary a.
Angiomax
Angiomedics catheter
angiomyocardiac
angionecrosis
angioneurotic edema
Angiopac
angioparalysis
angiopathic neuropathy
angiopathy
    cerebral amyloid a. (CAA)
    microvascular a. (MVA)
angiopeptin
angiopigtail catheter
angioplasia
angioplasty
    ablative laser a.
    adjunctive balloon a.
    balloon catheter a. (BCA)
    balloon coarctation a.
    balloon coronary a.
    balloon laser a.
    bootstrap two-vessel a.
    brachiocephalic vessel a.
    carotid patch a.
    carotid stent-supported a. (CSSA)
    A. Compared to Medicine (ACME)
    complementary balloon a.
    a. complication
    coronary a.
    coronary artery a.
    culprit lesion a.
    culprit vessel a.
    cutting balloon a. (CBA)
    direct acute myocardial
      infarction a. (DAMIA)
    direct coronary a.
    directional coronary a. (DCA)
    Dotter-Judkins percutaneous
      transluminal a.

    Emergency Stenting Compared to
      Conventional Balloon A.
      (ESCOBAR)
    Enoxaparin Restenosis after A.
      (ERA)
    excimer laser-assisted a. (ELA)
    excimer laser coronary a. (ECLA,
      ELCA)
    excimer laser, rotational
      atherectomy, and balloon a.
      (ERBAC)
    facilitated a.
    failed rescue a.
    Grüntzig balloon catheter a.
    a. guiding catheter
    high-pressure adjunctive
      percutaneous transluminal
      coronary a.
    high-risk a.
    Ho:YAG laser a.
    IVUS-guided balloon a.
    Kinsey rotation atherectomy
      extrusion a.
    kissing balloon a.
    laser a.
    laser-assisted balloon a. (LABA)
    laser-balloon a.
    laser thermal a.
    multilesion a.
    new device a. (NDA)
    one-vessel a.
    Osypka rotational a.
    patch a.
    patch-graft a.
    percutaneous balloon a.
    Percutaneous Excimer Laser
      Coronary A. (PELCA)
    percutaneous laser a.
    percutaneous transluminal a. (PTA)
    percutaneous transluminal
      coronary a. (PTCA)
    percutaneous transluminal renal a.
      (PTRA)
    peripheral excimer laser a. (PELA)
    peripheral laser a. (PLA)
    precoronary a.
    primary percutaneous transluminal
      coronary a. (pPTCA)
    a.-related vessel occlusion
    rescue a.
    salvage a. (SA)
    salvage balloon a.

NOTES

angioplasty *(continued)*
    smooth excimer laser coronary a. (SELCA)
    stand-alone balloon a.
    supported a.
    Tactilaze a.
    thallium:YAG laser a.
    thermal/perfusion balloon a. (TPBA)
    Thrombolysis and A. in Myocardial Infarction (TAMI)
    thulium:YAG laser a.
    tibioperoneal vessel a.
    transluminal coronary a.
    transradial coronary a.
    vibrational a.
angiopneumography
angiopoietin-1
angiopoietin-2
AngioRad
    A. radiation for restenosis (ARREST)
    A. radiation system
angiosarcoma
angioscintigraphy
angiosclerotic gangrene
angioscope
    Coronary Imagecath a.
    Imagecath rapid exchange a.
    Masy a.
angioscopic
    a. assessment
    a. valvulotome
angioscopy
    coronary a.
    Ermenonville classification for coronary a.
    intracoronary a.
    percutaneous intracoronary a.
    percutaneous transluminal a. (PTAS)
Angio-Seal
    6-French A.-S.
    A.-S. 6 French
    A.-S. hemostatic puncture closure device
Angioskop-D
Angiosol
AngioStent
angiostomy
angiotensin
    a. I (Ang1)
    a. I-converting enzyme
    a. II
    a. II-receptor blockade
    a. II-receptor blocker (ARB)
    renin a.
angiotensinase

angiotensin-converting
    a.-c. enzyme (ACE)
    a.-c. enzyme antisense gene therapy
    a.-c. enzyme DD (ACE-DD)
    a.-c. enzyme DD genotype
    a.-c. enzyme deletion/insertion polymorphism
    a.-c. enzyme fixed-wire balloon catheter
    a.-c. enzyme ID (ACE-ID)
    a.-c. enzyme ID genotype
    a.-c. enzyme II (ACE-II)
    a.-c. enzyme II genotype
    a.-c. enzyme inhibitor (ACEI, ACEi)
angiotensinogen gene
angiotomy
Angiovist
angle
    blunted costophrenic a.
    cardiodiaphragmatic a.
    cardiophrenic a.
    costophrenic a.
    costovertebral a. (CVA)
    Ebstein a.
    flip a.
    a. of insonation
    intercept a.
    Louis a.
    Ludwig a.
    nail-to-nail bed a.
    phase a.
    Pirogoff a.
    a. port pump
    QRS-T a.
    sella nasion point A a. (SNA)
    sella nasion point B a. (SNB)
    sternoclavicular a.
    a. tipped catheter
    tracheobronchial a.
    xiphoid a.
angled
    a. balloon II catheter
    a. pigtail catheter
    a. pleural tube
angor
    a. animi
    a. pectoris
Ang-O-Span
Angstrom
    A. II ICD
    A. MD cardioverter-defibrillator
    A. MD ICD
    A. MD implantable single-lead cardioverter-defibrillator
angular gyrus (AG)

angulated
    a. coarctation
    a. multipurpose catheter
angulation
    caudal plane a.
    cranial a.
    RAO a.
angusta
    aorta a.
ANGUS technique
anhydrase
anhydride
    a. asthma
    coumaric a.
    trimellitic a.
Anhydron
anhydrous ammonia
Anichkov, Anitschkow
    A. cell
    A. myocyte
animal dander
animi
    angor a.
A-N interval
anion
    a. exchange resin
    a. gap
    superoxide a.
anisa
    Legionella a.
anisindione
anisopiesis
anisorrhythmia
anisosphygmia
anisotropic
    a. conduction
    a. reentry
anisotropy
anisoylated plasminogen streptokinase activator complex (APSAC)
anistreplase
anitratum
    Bacterium a.
anitratus
    Acinetobacter a.
Anitschkow (*var. of* Anichkov)
ankle
    a. edema
    a. exercise
ankle-arm index

ankle-brachial
    a.-b. blood pressure ratio
    a.-b. index (ABI)
ankle-foot orthosis (AFO)
ankylosing spondylitis (AS)
anlagen
annexin-V
    technetium-99m-labeled a.-V.
annihilation photon
annotation
    marker a.
annular
    a. abscess
    a. array transducer
    a. calcification
    a. constriction
    a. dehiscence
    a. dilation
    a. flow
    a. phased array system (APAS)
    a. thrombus
annuli (*pl. of* annulus)
annuloaortic ectasia
annulocuspid hinge
AnnuloFlex flexible annuloplasty ring
AnnuloFlo
    A. annuloplasty ring
    A. annuloplasty ring system
annuloplasty
    a. band implant
    Carpentier a.
    DeVega tricuspid valve a.
    Gerbode a.
    Kay a.
    prosthetic ring a.
    a. ring
    septal a.
    tricuspid a.
    tricuspid valve a.
    Wooler-type a.
annulus (*var. of* anulus), pl. **annuli**
anodal
    a. closure contraction
    a. opening contraction
anode
anomalous
    a. atrioventricular
    a. atrioventricular excitation
    a. bronchus
    a. complex
    a. conduction
    a. first rib thoracic syndrome

NOTES

anomalous *(continued)*
   a. left main coronary artery
    (ALMCA)
   a. mitral arcade
   a. movement
   a. origin
   a. origin of the left coronary
    artery from the pulmonary artery
    (ALCAPA)
   a. origin of left coronary artery
    from the pulmonary artery
    syndrome
   a. pulmonary vein
   a. pulmonary venous connection
   a. pulmonary venous drainage
    (APVD)
   a. pulmonary venous return
   a. rectification

anomaly
   atrioventricular connection a.
   coloboma, heart anomaly, choanal
    atresia, retardation, and genital
    and ear a.'s (CHARGE)
   congenital conotruncal a.
   conotruncal a.
   coronary artery a.
   Ebstein a.
   Ebstein cardiac a.
   Freund a.
   nonconotruncal a.
   pulmonary valve a.
   pulmonary venous connection a.
   pulmonary venous return a.
   Shone a.
   Taussig-Bing a.
   Uhl a.
   ventricular inflow a.
   vertebral, vascular, anal, cardiac,
    tracheoesophageal, renal, and
    limb a.'s (VACTERL)
   viscerobronchial cardiovascular a.

Anopheles
anorexia nervosa
anoxemia test
anoxia
   anemic a.
   cerebral a.
   diffusion a.
   myocardial a.
   stagnant a.

ANP
   atrial natriuretic peptide
   atrial natriuretic polypeptide

Anrep
   A. effect
   A. phenomenon

ANS
   autonomic nervous system

ansa cervicalis
ansamycin
ANT
   adenosine nucleotide translocator
antacid
antagonism
   accentuated a.
   Coronary Artery Restenosis
    Prevention on Repeated
    Thromboxane A. (CARPORT)
antagonist
   adrenergic a.
   aldosterone a.
   beta a.
   beta-1 a.
   beta-2 a.
   calcium a.
   calcium channel a.
   CVT-124 A1 receptor a.
   dihydropyridine calcium a.
   FR139317 endothelin A receptor a.
   glycoprotein IIb/IIIa a.
   glycoprotein IIb/IIIa receptor a.
   leukotriene a.
   mediator receptor a.
   IIb/IIIa receptor a.
   tachykinin receptor a.
   thromboxane receptor a.
   vitamin K a.
antasthmatic
antecedent
   a. angina
   plasma thromboplastin a.
ante cibum (AC)
antecubital
   a. approach
   a. fossa
   a. space
   a. vein
antegrade
   a. aortogram
   a. aortography
   a. approach
   a. block
   a. block cycle length
   a. collateral
   a. conduction
   a. diastolic flow
   a. double balloon/double wire
    technique
   a. internodal pathway
   a. refractory period
   a. valvulotome
**antegrade/retrograde cardioplegia
technique**
antemortem
   a. clot
   a. thrombus

A

anterior
- a. anodal patch electrode
- a. approach
- a. articular surface of dens
- a. axillary line (AAL)
- a. border of lung
- carpal arch a.
- a. cerebral artery (ACA)
- a. chamber
- a. circulation (AC)
- a. clear space
- a. communicating arteries (ACoA)
- a. dentis
- a. descending coronary artery
- a. descending segmental artery of right lung
- a. fibrous trigone
- a. flail chest
- glandula lingualis a.
- a. inferior cerebellar artery (AICA)
- a. inferior communicating artery (AICA)
- a. inferior mandibular osteotomy (AIMO)
- a. internodal pathway
- a. internodal tract of Bachmann
- a. junction line
- a. leaflet
- a. mitral leaflet (AML)
- a. mitral leaflet extension
- a. myocardial infarction (AMI)
- a. oblique projection
- a. papillary muscle (APM)
- a. papillary muscle of left ventricle
- a. projection
- a. rib fracture
- a. sandwich patch technique
- a. surface of heart
- a. table
- a. thoracic compression
- a. thoracotomy
- a. wall (AW)
- a. wall dyskinesis
- a. wall myocardial infarction

anteriores
- venae cardiacae a.

anteriorly directed jet
anteroapical dyskinesis
anterobasal wall
anterograde
- a. APERP

- a. block
- a. conduction (Ae-H)
- a. flow
- a. transseptal technique

anteroinferior myocardial infarction
anterolateral
- a. flail chest
- a. myocardial infarction
- a. segment

anteromesial hypokinesis
anteroposterior
- a. paddles
- a. projection
- a. thoracic compression
- a. thoracic diameter

anteroseptal
- a. myocardial infarction (ASMI)
- a. segment

antesystole
anthopleurin-A
anthracis
- *Bacillus a.*

anthraconecrosis
anthracosilicosis
anthracosis
anthracotic tuberculosis
anthracycline-induced cardiomyopathy
anthracycline toxicity
anthraquinone
anthrax
- agricultural a.
- industrial a.
- a. pneumonia
- pulmonary a.
- a. septicemia

Anthron
- A. II catheter
- A. heparinized antithrombogenic catheter

anthropi
- *Ochrobacterium a.*

anthropometric evaluation
antiadhesin antibody
antiadrenergic
antiaggregant therapy
antialdosterone therapy
anti-aliasing technique
antianginal
- a. agent
- a. treatment

antiarrhythmic
- a. agent

NOTES

antiarrhythmic *(continued)*
    a. challenge
    a. drug (AAD)
    a. drug classification (Ia, Ib, Ic, II, III, IV)
    a. surgery
    a. therapy
    A.'s versus Implantable Defibrillators (AVID)
antiatherogenic effect
antiatherosclerotic
antibacterial
antibasement membrane
anti-beta-1-adrenoreceptor antibody (ABAb)
antibiotic (ABx)
    aerosolized a.
    antipseudomonas a.
    azalide class of a.'s
    inhaled a.
    macrolide a.
    nonquinolone a.
    perioperative a.
    preoperative a.
    prophylactic a.
    streptogramin a.
antibody
    agglutinating a.
    alpha Gal a.
    anaphylactic a.
    antiadhesin a.
    anti-beta-1-adrenoreceptor a. (ABAb)
    anti-CagA serum a.
    anticardiolipin a. (ACLA, aCLa)
    anti-CD3 a.
    anti-CD11a a.
    anti-CD18 a.
    anti-CD31 a.
    anti-CD146 a.
    anticentromere a. (ACA)
    antidesmin a.
    anti-DNA a.
    antidystrophin a.
    antiglomerular basement membrane a.
    anti-GP Ib a.
    anti-IgE a.
    anti-La a.
    antimyocin a.
    antineutrophil cytoplasmic a. (ANCA)
    antinuclear a. (ANA)
    antiphospholipid a. (APL)
    antiphospholipid in stroke study
    antireceptor a.
    anti-Ro SSA a.
    anti-Sm a.
    anti-SSA/Ro a.

    anti-SSB/La a.
    B cell a.
    beta-adrenoceptor a.
    CD18 a.
    cross-reactive a.
    digitalis-specific a.
    direct fluorescent a. (DFA)
    7E3 glycoprotein IIb/IIIa platelet a.
    7E3 monoclonal Fab a.
    fibrin-specific a.
    fluorescent antimembrane a. (FAMA, FAMAT)
    glycolipid a.
    huN901-DM1 a.
    laminin a.
    monoclonal antimyosin a.
    monoclonal a. 3G4
    myosin-specific a.
    OKT3 a.
    panel-reactive a. (PRA)
    panel of reactive a.'s (PRA)
    platelet a.
    Rh a.
    sheep antidigoxin Fab a.
    streptococcal a.
    streptokinase a.
    teichoic acid a.
    thyroid a.
    tissue-specific a.
    treponemal a.
    TR-R9 antithrombin receptor polyclonal a.
    Y2B8 a.
antibradycardia
anti-CagA serum antibody
anticardiolipin antibody (ACLA, aCLa)
anti-CD3 antibody
anti-CD11a antibody
anti-CD18 antibody
anti-CD31 antibody
anti-CD146 antibody
anticentromere antibody (ACA)
anticholinergic
    a. agent
    a. bronchodilator
anticipated systole
anticlot therapy
anticoagulant
    lupus a.
    A.'s in Secondary Prevention of Events in Coronary Thrombosis (ASPECT)
    a. therapy
anticoagulant-related hemorrhage
anticoagulation regimen of aspirin (ASA)
antideoxyribonuclease B

antidepressant
    tricyclic a.
antidesmin antibody
antidiabetic agent
antidiuresis
    syndrome of inappropriate a.
    (SIAD)
antidiuretic hormone (ADH)
anti-DNA antibody
anti-DNase B
antidromic
    a. circus-movement tachycardia
    a. reciprocating tachycardia
antidysrhythmic
antidystrophin antibody
antielastase
antiembolism stockings
antiendotoxin therapy
antifactor XA activity
antifibrillatory
antifibrin antibody imaging
antifilarial
antifoaming inhalant
antifolate
    multitargeted a.
antifungal
antigen
    Australia a.
    avian a.
    CagA a.
    carcinoembryonic a. (CEA)
    Epstein-Barr nuclear a. (EBNA)
    heart shock protein a.
    HSP a.
    human leukocyte a. (HLA)
    inhalant a.
    KI a.
    O a.
    p24 a.
    PLA-I platelet a.
    proliferating cell nuclear a.
    (PCNA)
    recall a.
    serum cryptococcal a. (sCRAG)
    TF a.
    Thomsen-Friedenreich a.
    viral capsid a. (VCA)
antigen-binding
    a.-b. diversity
    fragment a.-b.
antigenicity

antiglomerular
    a. basement membrane antibody
    a. basement membrane disease
anti-GP Ib antibody
antigravity suit
anti-G suit
antiheart antibody titer
antihemophilic
    a. factor (human)
    a. factor (recombinant)
Antihist-1
antihistamine
antihypertensive
    a. agent
    a. diuretic therapy
    a. and lipid lowering (ALL)
    A. and Lipid Lowering Treatment
    to Prevent Heart Attack Trial
    (ALLHAT)
antihypotensive
anti-IgE antibody
antiinflammatory agent
antiinhibitor coagulant complex
antiischemic therapy
anti-La antibody
antileukotriene
antilymphocyte serum
antimalarial
    primaquine phosphate a.
antimicrobial
    a. catheter cuff
    macrolide a.
    a. therapy
Antiminth
antimitotic
antimony
    a. compound
    a. pentachloride
    a. pneumoconiosis
    a. toxicity
    a. trichloride
antimuscarinic
antimycobacterial chemotherapy
antimycotic
antimyocin antibody
antimyosin
    a. antibody imaging
    a. autoantibody
    a. Fab fragment
    a. infarct-avid scintigraphy
    a. monoclonal antibody with Fab
    fragment (AMA-Fab)

NOTES

antinatriuretic
antineutrophil cytoplasmic antibody (ANCA)
antinuclear antibody (ANA)
antionocogene
antioxidant
antioxidative
antiparasitic
antiphospholipid
    A. Antibodies in Stroke Study (APASS)
    a. antibody (APL)
    a. syndrome
antiphosphotyrosine immunoblot
antiplasmin
antiplatelet
    a. agent
    a. therapy
    A. Treatment after Intravascular Ultrasound-Guided Optimal Stent Expansion (APLAUSE)
    a. trial (APT)
antipneumococcal
antipodal
antipode
antiport
antiporter
antipressor
antiprotease
antiproteinase
antipseudomonas antibiotic
antireceptor antibody
antireflux
    a. prosthesis
    a. therapy
antirestenotic stent
antiretroviral
anti-Rho-D titer
anti-Ro SSA antibody
antisense oligodeoxynucleotide
Anti-Sept bactericidal scrub solution
antishock garment
antisialagogue
anti-Sm antibody
anti-SSA/Ro antibody
anti-SSB/La antibody
antistasin
antistreptokinase
antistreptolysin O (ASO)
antistreptozyme (AST2)
    a. test
antitachycardia
    a. pacemaker (ATP)
    a. pacing (ATP)
antitemplate
antithrombin
    a. III (AT-III)

    a. III deficiency
    recombinant human a. III
antithromboplastin
antithrombotic
    A.'s in the Prevention of Reocclusion in Coronary Thrombolysis (APRICOT)
    a. regimen
antithymocyte globulin
anti-topo I
antitopoisomerase IDCS
antitoxin
    diphtheria a.
antitrypsin
    alpha-1 a. (AAT)
    a. deficiency
    M-type alpha 1-a.
    plasma alpha 1-a. (pAAT)
    recombinant alpha-1 a. (rAAT)
antituberculin
antituberculous
    a. chemotherapy
    a. drug
    a. therapy
antitubulin
Anti-Tuss Expectorant
antitussive
antler sign
antra (*pl. of* antrum)
antrectomy
Antrin
antrum, pl. antra
    cardiac a.
Anturane
Antyllus method
anular
    a. cartilage
    a. ligament of trachea
anuloaortic ectasia
anulus, annulus
    aortic a.
    a. fibrosus
    a. fibrosus dexter/sinister cordis
    mitral valve a.
    a. ovalis
    tricuspid a.
    tricuspid valve a.
Anxanil Oral
anxiety
    a. angina
    a. attack
    a. neurosis
anxiolytic
any-plane echocardiography
AO
    airway obstruction
AoBP
    aortic blood pressure

AOD
arterial occlusive disease
AOIVM
angiographically occult intracranial
vascular malformation
A-OK ShortCut knife
AOM
ambulatory oximetry monitoring
AOO
A. pacemaker
A. pacing
aorta, gen. and pl. **aortae**
abdominal a.
a. abdominalis
a. angusta
arch of a.
arcus aortae
a. ascendens
ascending a.
bifurcation of a.
buckled a.
buckling of a.
bulb of a.
button of a.
a. chlorotica
coarctation of the a. (CoA)
cross-clamping of a.
a. descendens
descending a.
descending thoracic a. (DTA)
dextropositioned a.
dissecting a.
dissection of a.
double-barreled a.
dynamic a.
esophageal branches of the
thoracic a.
kinked a.
mediomalacia vasculativa aortae
medionecrosis aortae
medionecrosis of a.
overriding a.
porcelain a.
primitive a.
pseudocoarctation of a.
a. to pulmonary artery shunt
recoarctation of a.
retroesophageal a.
sacrococcygeal a.
straddling a.
terminal a.
a. thoracalis

thoracic a.
a. thoracica
tuberculous mycotic aneurysm of
the a.
valvula coronaria dextra valvar
aortae
aortal
aorta-left atrium ratio
aortalgia
aortarctia, aortartia
aortectasis, aortectasia
aortectomy
aortic
a. anastomosis
a. aneurysm
a. aneurysmal disease
a. aneurysm clamp
a. anulus
a. arch (AA)
a. arch arteriogram
a. arch atheroma
a. arch cannula
a. arch interruption
a. arch syndrome
a. arch vessel
a. arch vessel obstruction
a. area of auscultation
a. arteritis syndrome
a. assist balloon introducer
a. atherosclerosis
a. atresia
a. balloon pump
a. bifurcation
a. bioprosthetic valve
a. blood pressure (AoBP)
a. body
a. bulb
a. cannula
a. catheter
a. closure sound
a. coarctation
a. commissure
a. compliance
A. Connector system
a. counterpulsation
a. cross-clamp
a. cuff
a. cusp
a. cusp separation
a. dicrotic notch pressure
a. dissection (AD)
a. dissection (type A, type B)

NOTES

aortic *(continued)*
  a. distensibility
  a. ductal flow
  a. dwarfism
  a. ejection sound
  a. embolism
  a. endograft
  a. end pulmonic
  a. envelope
  a. facies
  a. flow
  a. hiatus
  a. homograft
  a. impedance
  a. incompetence
  a. injury
  a. insufficiency
  a. intramural hematoma (AIH)
  a. intramural hemorrhage (AIH)
  a. isthmus
  a. jet velocity
  a. knob
  a. knuckle
  left atrial to a. (La:A)
  a. lumen
  a. murmur
  a. nerve
  a. nipple
  a. notch
  a. obscuration
  a. obstruction
  a. orifice
  a. override
  a. perfusion cannula
  a. pressure gradient
  a. prosthesis
  a. pullback
  a. pullback pressure
  a. pulse-wave velocity
  a. reconstruction
  a. reflex
  a. regurgitation (AR)
  a. regurgitation murmur
  a. ring
  a. root
  a. root abscess
  a. root compression
  a. root dimension
  a. root ratio
  a. rupture
  a. sac (AS)
  a. sclerosis
  a. second sound (A$_2$)
  a. septal defect
  a. sinus
  a. sinus aneurysm
  a. spindle
  a. stenosis (AS)

  a. stenosis jet
  a. stenosis murmur
  a. thrill
  a. thromboembolic disease
  a. thrombosis
  a. triangle
  a. tube graft
  a. tunica adventitia
  a. tunica intima
  a. tunica media
  a. valve
  a. valve area
  a. valve disease
  a. valve gradient (AVG)
  a. valve leaflet
  a. valve prolapse
  a. valve regurgitation
  a. valve replacement (AVR)
  a. valve resistance
  a. valve restenosis
  a. valve rongeur
  a. valve vegetation
  a. valve velocity profile
  a. valvotomy
  a. valvular insufficiency
  a. valvulitis
  a. valvuloplasty
  a. vasa vasorum
  a. window
aortic-femoral-femoral
  descending thoracic a.-f.-f. (DTAF-F)
aortic-left ventricular tunnel murmur
aortic-mitral combined disease murmur
aorticopulmonary
  a. anastomosis
  a. septal defect
  a. shunt
  a. window
aorticorenal
aorticus
  hiatus a.
  torus a.
aortismus abdominalis
aortitis
  arthritis-associated a.
  Döhle-Heller a.
  giant cell a.
  luetic a.
  nummular a.
  rheumatic a.
  syphilitic a.
  Takayasu a.
aortoannular ectasia
aortoarteriopathy
  stenotic a.-a.
aortobifemoral
aortobiiliac bypass

aortocarotid bypass
aortocaval
    a. compression syndrome
    a. fistula
aortocoronary
    a. bypass
    a. bypass graft (ACBG)
    a.-saphenous vein bypass
    a. snake graft
aortofemoral
    a. arterial runoff
    a. arteriography
    a. artery shunt
    a. bypass graft (AFBG)
aortogram
    antegrade a.
    digital subtraction supravalvular a.
    end-on a.
    flush a.
    a. with distal runoff
aortography
    abdominal a.
    a. angiography
    antegrade a.
    arch a.
    ascending a.
    atherosclerotic a.
    biplane a.
    caudally angled balloon
      occlusion a.
    digital subtraction supravalvular a.
    flush a.
    laid-back balloon occlusion a.
    mycotic a.
    retrograde a.
    selective a.
    single-plane a.
    sinus of Valsalva a.
    supravalvar a.
    thoracic arch a.
    transbrachial a.
    translumbar a.
    traumatic a.
    true versus false aneurysm a.
aortoiliac
    a. aneurysm
    a. bypass
    a. bypass graft
    a. obstructive disease (AIOD)
    a. occlusive disease
    a. thrombosis

aortoiliofemoral
    a. bypass
    a. circuit
    a. endarterectomy
aortolith
aortomalacia
aortomonoiliac graft
aorto-ostial lesion
aortopathy
aortoplasty
    subclavian flap a. (SFA)
aortoptosia, aortoptosis
aortopulmonary
    a. collateral
    a. fenestration
    a. septal defect (APSD)
    a. shunt
    a. window (APW)
aortorenal bypass
aortorrhaphy
aortosclerosis
aortostenosis
aortosubclavian bypass
aortosubclavian-carotid-axilloaxillary
  bypass
aortotomy
aortovelography
    transvenous a. (TAV)
AOU
    amount of use
AP
    accessory pathway
    activator protein
    alkaline phosphatase
    alveolar permeability
AP-1 complex
APACHE
    Acute Physiology, Age, Chronic Health
    Evaluation
      APACHE II
      APACHE III
      APACHE CV Risk Predictor
      APACHE score
apallic syndrome
APAP
    self-adjusting nasal continuous positive
    airway pressure
APAS
    annular phased array system
APASS
    Antiphospholipid Antibodies in Stroke
    Study

NOTES

apathetic hyperthyroidism
APB
    atrial premature beat
APBF
    accessory pulmonary blood flow
APC
    atrial premature contraction
        blocked APC
APD
    action potential duration
    airway pressure disconnect
    atrial premature depolarization
APE
    acute pulmonary edema
A-peak velocity
APERP
    accessory pathway effective refractory
     period
        anterograde APERP
Apert syndrome
aperture
    laryngeal a.
    transducer a.
apex, pl. **apices**
    a. beat
    cardiac a.
    a. cordis
    false a.
    hypertrophied a.
    a. impulse
    left ventricular a.
    a. of lung
    a. murmur
    a. pneumonia
    a. pulmonis
    right ventricular a. (RVA)
    ventricular a.
apexcardiogram (ACG)
apexcardiography (ACG)
aphasia
    ataxic a.
    expressive a.
    global a.
    nonfluent a.
    receptive a.
    transcortical motor a.
    transcortical motor type of a.
    Wernicke a.
aphasic
apheresis
aphonic pectoriloquy
aphrophilus
    Haemophilus a.
apical
    a. abscess
    a. aneurysm
    a. blunting
    a. bronchopulmonary segment [S I]

    a. bronchus
    a. diverticulum
    a. five-chamber view
     echocardiogram
    a. four-chamber view
    a. four-chamber view
     echocardiogram
    a. hematoma
    a. hypertrophy
    a. hypoperfusion on thallium scan
    a. impulse (AI)
    a. infarction
    a. interventricular septal amplitude
    a. left ventricular puncture
    a. lordotic roentgenogram
    a. mid-diastolic heart murmur
    a. pleural bleb
    a. pneumonia
    a. scarring
    a. shelf
    a. systolic heart murmur
    a. tailoring thoracoplasty
    a. two-chamber view
    a. two-chamber view
     echocardiogram
apicale
    segmentum a.
apicalis
apices (*pl. of* apex)
apicolysis
    extrapleural a.
    Semb a.
apicoposterior
    a. branch of left
    a. bronchopulmonary segment [SI
     + SII]
    a. segment
APL
    antiphospholipid antibody
aplasia
    bone marrow a.
    focal media a.
    pulmonary a.
aplastic anemia
APLAUSE
    Antiplatelet Treatment after Intravascular
    Ultrasound-Guided Optimal Stent
    Expansion
    APLAUSE clinical trial
apleuria
Aplisol
Aplitest
APM
    anterior papillary muscle
APM-2000 vital signs monitor
apnea
    age-dependent a.
    age-related a.

A

a. alarm mattress
central a. (CA)
deglutition a.
DPAP Stealth device for sleep a.
end-expiratory a.
idiopathic central sleep a.
a. index (AI)
initial a.
late a.
mixed a. (MA)
a. monitor
a. neonatorum
obstructive sleep a. (OSA)
posthyperventilation a.
sleep a.
traumatic a.
apnea-hypopnea index (AHI)
apneic oxygenation
apneumatosis
apneumia
apneusis
apneustic
a. breathing
a. respiration
APO
airway peroxidase
Apo
A.-Amoxi
A.-Ampi
A.-ASA
A.-Atenol
A.-Capto
A.-Cephalex
A.-Chlorpromazine
A.-Chlorthalidone
A.-Clonidine
A.-Cloxi
A.-Diltiaz
A.-Dipyridamole
A.-Dipyridamole FC
A.-Dipyridamole SC
A. E3 isoform
A.-Enalapril
A.-Erythro E-C
A.-Furosemide
A.-Gain
A.-Guanethidine
A.-Hydralazine
A.-Hydro
A.-Hydroxyzine
A.-ISDN
A.-Methyldopa

A.-Metoprolol
A.-Nadol
A.-Nifed
A.-Pen VK
A.-Pindol
A.-Prazo
A.-Prednisone
A.-Procainamide
A.-Propranolol
A.-Salvent
A.-Sulfatrim
A.-Tamox
A.-Timol
A.-Timop
A.-Triazide
A.-Verap
A.-Zidovudine
ApoA-1 deficiency
apoE
apolipoprotein E
apoE test
Apogee CX 100 Interspec ultrasound machine
apolipoprotein
a. A-I
a. A-II
a. A-IV
a. B
a. B-48
a. B-100
a. C-I
a. C-II
a. C-III
a. D
a. E (apoE)
Apollo Light Systems
aponeurosis
Sibson a.
aponeurotic
apoplectic
a. coma
a. cyst
apoplexy
asthenic a.
capillary a.
cerebral a.
ingravescent a.
apoprotein A, B, C, D, E
apoptosis
cardiomyocyte a.
ischemia/reperfusion-induced a.

NOTES

apoptotic
    a. cell
    a. cell death
    a. change
    a. destruction
A-Port vascular access
aposthematosa
    pneumonia a.
APP
  amyloid precursor protein
apparatus
    Benedict-Roth a.
    Davidson pneumothorax a.
    Fell-O'Dwyer a.
    Jacquet a.
    Langendorff a.
    Nakayama anastomosis a.
    a. respiratorius
    respiratory a.
    subvalvular a.
    V-Vac suction a.
apparent
    a. diffusion coefficient (ADC)
    a. diffusion coefficient imaging
    a. life-threatening event (ALTE)
appearance
    cluster-of-grapes a.
    cottage-loaf a.
    dirty-lung a.
    finger-in-glove a.
    ground-glass a.
    hazy a.
    salt-and-pepper a.
    tree-in-winter a.
appendage
    atrial a.
    auricular a.
    left atrial a. (LAA)
    right atrial a. (RAA)
appendectomy
    atrial a.
    auricular a.
applanation tonometry
apple picker's disease
applesauce sign
appliance
    mandibular advancement a. (MAA)
    oral a. (OA)
    TheraSnore oral a.
application
    MCAS modular clip a.
apposition
    mitral-septal a.
    stent a.
approach
    antecubital a.
    antegrade a.
    anterior a.

    Bobath physiotherapy a.
    brachial artery a.
    central a.
    cephalic a.
    external jugular a.
    femoral a.
    groin a.
    Lortat-Jacob a.
    open lung a.
    percutaneous a.
    posterior a.
    radial a.
    retrograde femoral a.
    segmented K-space a.
    selective transvenous a.
    stepped bur a.
    tandem needle a.
    transradial a.
    transxiphoid a.
    trap-door a.
approximation
    Friedewald a.
approximator
    rib a.
    Wolvek sternal a.
apraxia
    buccolingual a.
    ideational a.
    ideomotor a.
    idiomotor a.
    limb-kinetic a.
Apresazide
Apresoline
    A. injection
    A. Oral
APRICOT
  Antithrombotics in the Prevention of
    Reocclusion in Coronary Thrombolysis
    Aspirin Versus Coumadin Trial
    APRICOT clinical trial
aprindine
Aprinox
Aprodine
    A. Syrup
    A. Tablet
    A. w/C
aprotinin
APRV
  airway pressure release ventilation
APSAC
  anisoylated plasminogen streptokinase
    activator complex
APSD
  aortopulmonary septal defect
APT
  antiplatelet trial
  Atherosclerosis Prevention and Treatment
    APT program

aptiganel
aPTT, APTT
    activated partial thromboplastin time
Apt test
APV
    average peak velocity
APVD
    anomalous pulmonary venous drainage
APW
    aortopulmonary window
AQ
    acoustic quantification
        Nasacort AQ
AQLQ
    Asthma Quality of Life Questionnaire
aqua
        Rhinocort A.
Aquacare topical
aquae
        Mycobacterium a.
aquagenic urticaria
AquaMEPHYTON injection
Aquaphyllin
aquaporin
AquaShield
aquaspera
        Acrotheca a.
Aquatag
Aquatensen
Aquatherm radiant heat device
Aquazide
aqueous
        a. oxygen
        penicillin G, parenteral, a.
        a. solution for nebulization
aquired ventricular septal defect
AR
        acute rejection
        adrenergic receptor
        aortic regurgitation
            beta-1 AR
            beta-2 AR
            AR jet height
βAR
        beta-adrenergic receptor
AR-1 catheter
arabinoside
        cytosine a. (CA)
Ara-C
        cytosine-arabinoside
arachidic bronchitis
arachidonate metabolism

arachidonic
        a. acid
        a. acid cascade
        a. acid metabolite
arachidonyl ethanolamide
arachnodactyly
ARAD
        abnormal right axis deviation
Araki-Sako technique
araldehyde-tanned bovine carotid artery
    graft
Aralen Phosphate
Aramine
araneus
        nevus a.
Arani double-loop guiding catheter
arantii
        ductus a.
Arantius
        A. body
        body of A.
        canal of A.
        A. nodule
ARB
        angiotensin II-receptor blocker
arborization block
arbovirus
Arbrook Hemovac
arbutamine
arc
        a. of calcium
        a. welder's pneumoconiosis
AR-C68397AA
arcade
        anomalous mitral a.
        arterial a.
        a. collateral
        polygonal a.
        septal a.
arcanobacterial pharyngitis
arch
        abdominothoracic a.
        a. of aorta
        aortic a. (AA)
        a. aortography
        a. arteriography
        axillary a.
        azygos a.
        carotid a.
        cervical aortic a.
        circumflex aortic a.
        congenital interrupted aortic a.

NOTES

arch *(continued)*
    double aortic a.
    Femo stop femoral artery
      compression a.
    interrupted aortic a. (IAA)
    jugular venous a.
    Langer axillary a.
    palmar a.
    pharyngeal a.
    pulmonary a.
    right aortic a.
    Zimmermann a.
architecture
    lung a.
    sleep a.
Arco
    A. atomic pacemaker
    A. lithium pacemaker
**Arcomax FMA cardiac angiography
system**
arcus
    a. aortae
    corneal a.
    a. cornealis
    a. costarum
    a. lipoides
    a. senilis
ardeparin sodium
ARDS
    acute respiratory distress syndrome
    adult respiratory distress syndrome
    posttraumatic ARDS
Arduan
Ardystil syndrome
area, pl. **areae, areas**
    aortic valve a.
    Bamberger a.
    body surface a. (BSA)
    a. of cardiac dullness
    cross-sectional a. (CSA)
    echo-spared a.
    EEL a.
    effective balloon-dilated a. (EBDA)
    end-diastolic a. (EDA)
    Erb a.
    external elastic lamina a.
    intrastent minimal lumen cross-
      sectional a. (ISMLCSA)
    Krönig a.
    left atrial appendage a.
    local organ procurement a.
    mitral a.
    mitral annular a.
    mitral valve a. (MVA)
    plaque a.
    proximal isovelocity surface a.
      (PISA)
    pulmonary a.

    pulmonary valve a.
    pulmonic a.
    regurgitant jet a. (RJA)
    regurgitant orifice a. (ROA)
    secondary aortic a.
    sewing ring a. (SRA)
    subxiphoid a.
    supplemental motor a. (SMA)
    tricuspid a.
    tricuspid valve a.
    truncoconal a.
    valve orifice a.
area-length
    a.-l. method
    a.-l. method for ejection
Arelix
Arenaviridae virus
AREx inhaler
ARF
    acute respiratory failure
ArF excimer laser
Arfonad injection
argatroban
Argesic-SA
arginine vasopressin (AVP)
argipressin
argon
    a. beam coagulator
    a. ion laser
    a. needle
    a. pumped tuneable dye laser
    a. vessel dilator
Argyle
    A. arterial catheter
    A. catheter
    A. CPAP nasal cannula
    A. Sentinel Seal chest tube
Argyle-Turkel
    A.-T. safety thoracentesis system
    A.-T. thoracentesis
    A.-T. thoracentesis system
Argyll Robertson pupils
ARHS
    acute right heart syndrome
ARI
    airway reactivity index
Aria
    A. coronary artery bypass graft
    A. CPAP system
    A. LX CPAP system
Arimidex
A-ring
    esophageal A.-r.
Aristocort
    A. Forte
    A. Forte Injection
    A. Intralesional Injection
    A. Intralesional Suspension

A. Oral
A. Tablet
Aristospan
A. Intra-articular Injection
A. Intralesional Injection
ARK
adrenergic receptor kinase
beta ARK
ARK-1
adrenergic receptor kinase 1
beta ARK-1
Arkin-Z
ARL
AIDS-related lymphoma
ARLL
AIDS-related lymphoma of the lung
Arloing-Courmont test
arm
chest and left a. (CL)
chest and right a. (CR)
a. cranking
a. cycle ergometry
dissected tissue a.
a. ergometry
a. ergometry treadmill
a. exercise stress test
Arm-a-Med
A.-a.-M. endotracheal tube
A.-a.-M. Isoetharine
A.-a.-M. Isoproterenol
A.-a.-M. Metaproterenol
armamentarium
arm-ankle indices
arm-leg gradient
armored heart
armor heart
Armour Thyroid
Armstrong handheld pulse oximeter
arm-tongue
a.-t. time
a.-t. time test
aromatic
A. Ammonia Aspirols
a. ammonia spirit
arousal
a. index
respiratory effort-related a.
ARP
absolute refractory period
ARR
absolute risk reduction

array
convex linear a.
multielement linear a.
PRx Endotak-Sub-Q a.
sock a.
symmetrical phased a.
ARREST
AngioRad radiation for restenosis
ARREST clinical trial
arrest
asphyxial cardiac a.
asystolic a.
blunt chest impact-induced
cardiac a.
bradyarrhythmic a.
cardiac a. (CA)
cardioplegic a.
cardiopulmonary a.
cardiorespiratory a.
chronic sinus a.
circulatory a.
cold ischemic a.
deep hypothermia circulatory a.
(DHCA)
dysrhythmic cardiac a.
heart a.
hypothermic fibrillating a.
intermittent sinus a.
respiratory a.
sinoatrial a.
sinus a.
total circulatory a.
ventricular fibrillation a.
arrest-and-reversal treatment (ART)
arrested tuberculosis
Arrhigi
point of A.
arrhythmia
atrial a.
atrioventricular junctional a.
A-V nodal Wenckebach a.
baseline a.
burst of a.
cardiac a.
a. circuit
a. circuit cryoablation
continuous a.
a. control device (ACD)
exercise-induced a.
a. focus
hypokalemia-induced a.
inducible a.

NOTES

arrhythmia *(continued)*
    inotropic a.
    juvenile a.
    lethal a.
    Lown a.
    malignant a.
    malignant ventricular a. (MVA)
    a. mapping system
    Mönckeberg a.
    A. Net
    A. Net arrhythmia monitor
    nodal a.
    nonphasic sinus a.
    nonsuppressible a.
    paroxysmal supraventricular a.
    pause-dependent a.
    perpetual a.
    phasic sinus a.
    postperfusion a.
    primary cardiac a.
    reentrant a.
    reperfusion a.
    A. Research 1200 EPX
      electrocardiograph
    respiratory a.
    respiratory sinus a.
    senile a.
    sinus a.
    stress-related a.
    suppression of a.
    supraventricular a.
    tachybrady a.
    vagus a.
    ventricular a.
    warning a.
    Xylocaine HCl I.V. Injection for
      Cardiac A.'s
arrhythmia-insensitive flow-sensitive
  alternating inversion recovery imaging
arrhythmic
arrhythmogenesis
arrhythmogenic
    a. disorder
    a. right ventricular cardiomyopathy
      (ARVC)
    a. right ventricular disease
    a. right ventricular dysplasia
      (ARVD)
    a. site
    a. substrate
    a. ventricular cardiomyopathy
arrhythmogenicity
arrhythmokinesis
arrhythmology
Arrow
    A. balloon wedge catheter
    A. Berman angiographic balloon
    A. Flex intraaortic balloon catheter

    A. Hi-flow infusion set
    A. pneumothorax kit
    A. Pullback atherectomy catheter
    A. QuadPolar electrode catheter
    A. QuadPolar pulmonary artery
      catheter
    A. sheath
    A. TwinCath multilumen peripheral
      catheter
Arrow-Clarke thoracentesis device
Arrow-Fischell EVAN needle
ArrowFlex sheath
ARROWgard
    A. Blue antiseptic-coated catheter
    A. Blue Line catheter
    A. central venous catheter
Arrow-Howes multilumen catheter
Arrow-Trerotola PTD
arsenic (As)
    a. poisoning
arsine gas poisoning
ART
    arrest-and-reversal treatment
Artegraft natural collagen vascular
  graft
artemisin
arteria, pl. **arteriae** (*See* artery)
    a. anastomotica
    a. anastomotica auricularis magna
    a. genus superior lateralis
    a. genus superior medialis
    a. glutealis inferior
    a. glutealis superior
    a. laryngea
    a. laryngea superior
    a. lingualis
    a. pericardiacophrenica
    a. pharyngea
    a. pulmonalis
    a. pulmonalis dextra
    a. pulmonalis sinistra
arterial
    a. anastomosis
    a. aneurysm
    a. arcade
    a. bleeding
    a. blood
    a. blood flow
    a. blood gas (ABG)
    a. blood gas point-of-care test
      (ABG PCT)
    a. blood pressure (ABP)
    a. calcification
    a. carbon dioxide pressure
    a. carbon dioxide tension
    a. cone
    a. coupling
    a. cutdown

a. decortication
a. desaturation
a. dicrotic notch pressure
a. disease multiple intervention trial (ADMIT)
a. dissection
a. distensibility
a. embolectomy catheter
a. embolism
a. entry site
a. filter
a. gas bubble
a. gas embolism (AGE)
a. groove
a. hyperemia
a. hypertension
a. hypotension
a. hypoxemia
a. impedance
a. insufficiency
a. line (A-line)
a. line pressure bag
a. line transducer
a. mean
a. mean line
a. media
a. mesocardium
a. murmur
a. needle
a. occlusion
a. occlusive disease (AOD)
a. oscillator endarterectomy instrument
a. oxygen partial pressure (PaO_2)
a. oxygen saturation (SaO_2)
a. partial pressure of CO_2 ($PaCO_2$)
a. pressure
a. pseudoaneurysm
a. pulse
a. pyemia
a. reconstruction
a. remodeling
a. revascularization therapy study (ARTS)
a. runoff
a. saturation
a. sclerosis
a. sheath
a. shrinkage
a. spasm
a. spider
a. stick

a. switch operation
a. switch procedure
a. thrill
a. thrombosis
a. vein of Soemmerring
a. wave
a. wedge
arterialization
arteriectasis, arteriectasia
arteries (*pl. of* artery)
arterioablation
arterioatony
arteriocapillary sclerosis
arteriogenesis
arteriogram
    aortic arch a.
    brachial a.
    runoff a.
arteriograph
    CAMAC-300 a.
arteriographic regression
arteriography
    aortofemoral a.
    arch a.
    biplane pelvic a.
    biplane quantitative coronary a.
    bronchial a.
    carotid a.
    catheter a.
    coronary a. (CAG)
    cut-film a.
    digital subtraction a.
    femoral a.
    Judkins selective coronary a.
    longitudinal a.
    quantitative a.
    quantitative coronary a. (QCA)
    renal a.
    selective a.
    Sones selective coronary a.
arteriohepatic dysplasia syndrome
arteriolar
    a. hyalinosis
    a. sclerosis
arteriole
    afferent a.
    efferent a.
    ellipsoid a.
    Isaacs-Ludwig a.
    precapillary a.
arteriolith

NOTES

arteriolitis
    necrotizing a.
arteriolonecrosis
arteriolosclerosis
arteriolovenular bridge
arteriomalacia
arteriometer
arterionecrosis
    hyaline a.
arteriopalmus
arteriopathy
    hypertensive a.
    plexogenic pulmonary a.
arterioplasty
    pulmonary a.
arteriopressor
arteriopulmonary shunt
arteriorrhexis
arteriosclerosis (*See also* atherosclerosis)
    allograft a.
    cerebral a.
    coronary a.
    decrudescent a.
    hyaline a.
    hypertensive a.
    Mönckeberg a.
    nodose a.
    nodular a.
    a. obliterans
    peripheral a.
    senile a.
arteriosclerotic
    a. cardiovascular disease (ASCVD)
    a. heart disease (ASHD)
    a. peripheral vascular disease (ASPVD)
    a. vascular disease (ASVD)
arteriospasm
arteriosum
    cor a.
    ligamentum a.
arteriosus
    conus a.
    ductus a.
    papillary muscle of conus a.
    patent ductus a. (PDA)
    persistent ductus a.
    persistent truncus a.
    pseudotruncus a.
    reversed ductus a.
    truncus a.
arteriotomy
    brachial a.
arteriotony
arteriovenosa
arteriovenous (A-V, AV)
    a. anastomosis
    a. communication

congenital pulmonary a.
    a. crossing change
    a. fistula (AVF)
    a. malformation (AVM)
    a. nicking
    a. oxygen difference (AVD O_2)
    a. pulmonary aneurysm
    a. shunt
arteritis, pl. **arteritides**
    brachiocephalic a.
    coronary a.
    cranial a.
    a. deformans
    fibrinoid a.
    giant cell a.
    granulomatous a.
    Horton a.
    a. hyperplastica
    infantile a.
    mesenteric a.
    a. nodosa
    a. obliterans
    pulmonary arteritides
    rheumatic a.
    rheumatoid a.
    syphilitic a.
    Takayasu a.
    temporal a.
    tuberculous a.
    a. umbilicalis
    a. verrucosa
artery, pl. **arteries**
    aberrant a.
    aberrant subclavian a.
    accessory a.
    accessory obturator a.
    acetabular a.
    Adamkiewicz a.
    afferent a.
    anomalous left main coronary a. (ALMCA)
    anomalous origin of the left coronary artery from the pulmonary a. (ALCAPA)
    anterior cerebral a. (ACA)
    anterior communicating arteries (ACoA)
    anterior descending coronary a.
    anterior inferior cerebellar a. (AICA)
    anterior inferior communicating a. (AICA)
    ascending ileocolic a.
    ascending pharyngeal a.
    atrioventricular node a.
    A-V nodal a.
    axillary a.
    banding of pulmonary a.

basal collateral a.
basilar a. (BA)
beading of arteries
blocked heart a.
brachial a.
brachiocephalic a.
bronchial a.
callosomarginal a.
caroticotympanic a.
carotid a.
celiac a.
cephalic a.
circumflex a.
coarctation of pulmonary a.
common carotid a.
common femoral a.
common hepatic a.
common iliac a.
complete transposition of great
  arteries
congenitally corrected transposition
  of the great arteries
copper-wire arteries
corkscrew a.
coronary a.
cricothyroid a.
crural a.
deep lingual a.
descending thoracic aorta-to-
  femoral a. (DTAFA)
diagonal a.
diagonal coronary a.
diaphragmatic a.
D-loop transposition of the great
  arteries
dorsal lingual branches of
  lingual a.
Drummond marginal a.
d-transposition of great arteries (D-
  TGA, dTGA)
a. ectasia
efferent a.
end a.
epicardial a.
epicardial coronary a.
esophageal a.
esophageal branches of the left
  gastric a.
external carotid a. (ECA)
external mammary a.
femoral a.
fetal-type posterior cerebral a.

first obtuse marginal a. (OM-1)
gastroepiploic a. (GEA)
Global Use of Strategies to Open
  Occluded Coronary Arteries
Global Utilization of Streptokinase
  and tPA for Occluded Arteries
  (GUSTO)
Global Utilization of Streptokinase
  and tPA for Occluded Coronary
  Arteries (GUSTO)
great a.
hepatic a.
Heubner recurrent a.
ileal a.
ileocolic a.
iliac a.
infarct a.
infarct-related a. (IRA)
inferior epigastric a. (IEA)
inferior laryngeal a.
inferior mesenteric a. (IMA)
inferior thyroid a.
innominate a.
intermediate circumflex a. (ICXA)
internal carotid a. (ICA)
internal mammary a. (IMA)
internal thoracic a. (ITA)
intersegmental a.
intramural coronary arteries
jejunal a.
Kugel anastomotic a.
LAD a.
LCF coronary a.
left anterior descending a. (LADA)
left circumflex a. (LCX)
left circumflex coronary a. (LCX)
left common carotid a. (LCCA)
left coronary a. (LCA)
left internal mammary a. (LIMA)
left internal thoracic a. (LITA)
left main coronary a. (LMCA)
left pulmonary a. (LPA)
left subclavian a. (LSCA)
lenticulostriate a.
lumen of a.
lysed a.
main pulmonary a. (MPA)
mainstem coronary a.
malposition of great arteries
  (MGA)
mammary a.
marginal circumflex a.

NOTES

artery *(continued)*
  medial basal branch of
    pulmonary a.
  mesenteric a.
  middle capsular a.
  middle cerebral a. (MCA)
  native coronary a.
  Neubauer a.
  nodal a.
  normal coronary arteries (NCA)
  obtuse marginal a. (OMA)
  obtuse marginal coronary a.
  occipital a. (OA)
  OM coronary a.
  parietooccipital a.
  penetrator a.
  perforating a.
  pericardiophrenic a.
  perineal a.
  peripheral a.
  peroneal a.
  pharyngeal a.
  pharyngeal branch of descending
    palatine a.
  pharyngeal branch of inferior
    thyroid a.
  phrenic a.
  popliteal a.
  posterior cerebral a. (PCA)
  posterior circumflex a. (PC)
  posterior communicating a. (PCoA)
  posterior descending a. (PDA)
  posterior inferior cerebellar a.
    (PICA)
  posterior inferior communicating a.
    (PICA)
  Pravastatin Limitation of
    Atherosclerosis in Coronary
    Arteries (PLAC)
  Pravastatin, Lipids, and
    Atherosclerosis in the Carotid
    Arteries (PLAC-2)
  profunda femoris a.
  pulmonary a. (PA)
  radial a.
  ramus intermedius a.
  ranine a.
  renal a.
  retinal a.
  right common carotid a. (RCCA)
  right coronary a. (RCA)
  right gastroepiploic a. (RGEA)
  right internal mammary a. (RIMA)
  right internal thoracic a. (RITA)
  right-middle cerebral a. (R-MCA)
  right pulmonary a. (RPA)
  second obtuse marginal a. (OM-2)
  septal perforating a.

  silver-wiring of retinal a.
  sinoatrial nodal a.
  sinuatrial nodal a.
  sinus node a.
  smooth coronary a.
  stenting in small arteries (SISA)
  sternocleidomastoid a.
  subclavian a.
  sublingual a.
  superdominant a.
  superficial external pudendal a.
  superficial femoral a. (SFA)
  superior carotid a.
  superior cerebellar a. (SCA)
  superior laryngeal a.
  superior mesenteric a. (SMA)
  superior thyroid a.
  terminal internal carotid a. (TICA)
  thoracodorsal a.
  tibial a.
  tortuous right coronary a.
  transposition of the great arteries
    (TGA)
  transverse cervical a.
  umbilical a.
  unprotected a.
Artha-G
arthritis, pl. **arthritides**
  acute rheumatic a.
  A. Foundation Ibuprofen
  A. Foundation Pain Reliever
  juvenile rheumatoid a.
  rheumatoid a. (RA)
arthritis-associated aortitis
Arthropan
arthropod venom
ArthroWand
Arthus-type reaction
articularis
  facies a.
articular surface of arytenoid cartilage
articulation
Articulose-50 injection
artifact
  aliasing a.
  bang a.
  baseline a.
  beam width a.
  blooming a.
  breast a.
  catheter impact a.
  catheter whip a.
  chemical shift a.
  coin a.
  crush a.
  cupping a.
  end-pressure a.
  flow a.

mitral regurgitation a.
muscle a.
N/2 a.
pacemaker a.
pacemaker stimulus a.
respiratory a.
reverberation a.
side lobe a.
susceptibility a.
T a.
view-aliasing a.
wrap-around ghosting a.
zebra a.

artifactual bradycardia
artificial
a. blood
a. cardiac valve
a. heart (AH)
a. larynx
a. lung
a. lung-expanding compound
  (ALEC)
a. pacemaker
a. pneumothorax
a. respiration
a. ventilation

ARTREK
A. automated edge-detection
  algorithm
A. offline 35-mm cineangiographic
  analysis system

ARTS
arterial revascularization therapy study

ARTS clinical trial
ARVC
arrhythmogenic right ventricular
cardiomyopathy

ARVD
arrhythmogenic right ventricular
dysplasia

Arvidsson dimension-length method
Arvin
arylesterase
arylsulfatase
arytenoidea cricoideae
arytenoid gland
Arzbacher pill electrode
Arzco
A. model 7 cardiac stimulator
A. pacemaker
A. preamplifier
A. TAPSUL pill electrode

AS
ankylosing spondylitis
aortic sac
aortic stenosis

AS-800
A.S.
Crysticillin A.S.

As
arsenic

ASA
anticoagulation regimen of aspirin
atrial septal aneurysm
MSD Enteric Coated ASA

asaccharolyticus
Peptostreptococcus a.

asahii
Trichosporon a.

Asaphen
Asasantine
asbestiform
asbestos
a. bodies
a. pleural effusion
a. pneumoconiosis

asbestosis
parenchymal a.

Asbron G
ASCAD
atherosclerotic coronary artery disease

A-scan echography
ascariasis
Ascaris lumbricoides
ascendens
aorta a.

ascendentis
plexus periarterialis arteriae
  pharyngeae a.

ascending
a. aorta
a. aorta to pulmonary artery shunt
a. aortic blood pressure
a. aortic pressure
a. aortography
a. ileocolic artery
a. loop of Henle
a. pharyngeal artery
a. pharyngeal plexus
a. polyneuropathy

ascent
barotrauma of a.

Ascent guiding catheter

NOTES

Aschner
    A. phenomenon
    A. reflex
    A. sign
Aschner-Dagnini reflex
Aschoff
    A. body
    A. cell
    A. nodule
Aschoff-Tawara node
ascites
    chylous a.
    a. praecox
ascorbate
    a. dilution curve
    sodium a.
ascorbic acid
Ascriptin
ASCS
    acute sickle chest syndrome
ASCVD
    arteriosclerotic cardiovascular disease
    atherosclerotic cardiovascular disease
ASD
    atrial septal defect
    ASD closure device
ASD2
    secundum atrial septal defect
ASDA
    American Sleep Disorders Association
ASDOS
    atrial septal defect occlusion system
    atrial septum defect occluder system
    ASDOS umbrella
    ASDOS umbrella occluder
asequence
ASH
    asymmetric septal hypertrophy
ash
    fly a.
ASHD
    arteriosclerotic heart disease
Asherman chest seal
Asherson syndrome
Ashley phenomenon
Ashman
    A. beat
    A. phenomenon
Ashworth Scale
Asian influenza
a-SiC:H
    amorphous hydrogenated silicon carbide
ASIST
    Atenolol Silent Ischemia Trial
Askin tumor
Ask-Upmark
    A.-U. kidney
    A.-U. syndrome

ASM
    airway smooth muscle
Asmalix
Asmanex twister
asmaPLAN+ peak flowmeter
ASMI
    anteroseptal myocardial infarction
ASO
    antistreptolysin O
asparaginase
asparagine
aspartate aminotransferase (AST)
aspartic acid
ASPECT
    Anticoagulants in Secondary Prevention
    of Events in Coronary Thrombosis
    ASPECT study
aspergilloma formation
aspergillosis
    allergic bronchopulmonary a.
    (ABPA)
    bronchopulmonary a.
    chronic necrotizing a.
    invasive pulmonary a. (IPA)
    parenchymal a.
    pleural a.
    primary pleural a.
    pseudomembranous
    tracheobronchial a.
    pulmonary a.
    semiinvasive a.
    suppurative necrotizing a.
Aspergillus
    A. *avenaceus*
    A. *caesiellus*
    A. *candidus*
    A. *carneus*
    A. *empyema*
    A. *flavus*
    A. *fumigatus*
    A. *nidulans*
    A. *niger*
    A. *oryzae*
    A. *restrictus*
    A. *sydowi*
    A. *terreus*
    A. *toxicosis*
    A. *tracheobronchitis*
    A. *ustus*
    A. *versicolor*
asphygmia
asphyxia
    blue a.
    a. carbonica
    cyanotic a.
    a. cyanotica
    a. livida
    local a.

a. neonatorum
a. pallida
secondary a.
symmetric a.
traumatic a.
white a.
asphyxial cardiac arrest
asphyxiant
asphyxiate
asphyxiating thoracic dystrophy (ATD)
asphyxiation
aspirate
bronchotracheal a.
endotracheal a. (EA)
needle a.
tracheal a.
tracheobronchial a.
aspirated and flushed
aspirating needle
aspiration
a. biopsy
a. biopsy cytology (ABC)
bronchoscopic needle a. (BNA)
diagnostic a.
endoscopic ultrasound-guided fine
needle a. (EUS-FNA)
fine-needle a. (FNA)
fluid a.
foreign body a.
a. of foreign body
gastric a.
hydrocarbon a.
intractable a.
large-volume a.
a. lung injury
massive a.
meconium a.
nosocomial a.
a. pneumonia
a. pneumonitis
small-volume a.
transbronchial needle a. (TBNA)
transthoracic needle a. (TTNA)
transtracheal a.
aspiration-induced respiratory disease
aspirator
6260 a.
Bovie ultrasound a.
bronchoscopic a.
Cavitron ultrasonic surgical a.
(CUSA)
Cook County a.

Model 6260 a.
Model 326 portable a.
Schueler Model 200 A.
Ultra-Lite portable a.
Vac-Pak-II ultra-lite portable a.
Vacu-Aide home-use a.
ASPIRE
Action on Secondary Prevention by
Intervention to Reduce Events
ASPIRE clinical trial
aspirin
anticoagulation regimen of a.
(ASA)
Bayer A.
Bayer Buffered A.
buffered a.
Carotid Artery Stenosis with
Asymptomatic Narrowing:
Operation versus A.
(CASANOVA)
dipyridamole and a.
enteric-coated a.
Extra Strength Bayer Enteric
500 A.
A. in Myocardial Infarction Study
(AMIS)
St. Joseph Adult Chewable A.
A. and Ticlid Versus
Anticoagulation for Stents
(ATLAS)
ticlopidine plus a. (T + A)
A. Versus Coumadin Trial
(APRICOT)
aspirin/extended release dipyridamole
aspirin-induced asthma (AIA)
Aspirols
Amyl Nitrite A.
Aromatic Ammonia A.
asplenia
Asprimox
ASPVD
arteriosclerotic peripheral vascular
disease
ASS
Acute Stroke Study
asthma severity score
assay
adherence a.
agar diffusion a.
Asserachrom D-DI ELISA a.
Asserachrom tPA immunologic a.
Bioclot protein S a.

NOTES

assay *(continued)*
    Cardiac T a.
    Cardiac T rapid a.
    cardiac troponin I a.
    Clauss a.
    CoA-set fibrin monomer a.
    cTnI a.
    Cushman a.
    D-dimer a.
    D-dimer enzyme-linked
      immunosorbent a.
    Enzygnost TAT ELISA a.
    enzyme-linked immunosorbent a.
      (ELISA)
    ferricytochrome a.
    Hemochron high-dose thrombin
      time a.
    hemoSTATUS a.
    Heptest clotting a.
    Hybritech immunoradiometric a.
    immune adherence
      immunosorbent a. (IAIA)
    immunoradiometric a. (IRMA)
    immunoturbidimetric a.
    MonoClone immunoenzymetric a.
    multimer a.
    myoglobin a.
    N High Sensitivity CRP a.
    Opus cardiac troponin I a.
    PCR a.
    radioligand binding a.
    sandwich enzyme-linked
      immunosorbent a.
    serum Mgb a.
    Stachrom PAI chromogenic a.
    thyrotoxin radioisotope a.
    Tina-quant immunoturbidometric a.
    TRAP a.
    TUNEL a.
    Ultegra rapid platelet function a.
      (U-RPFA)
    Velogene rapid TB a.
assembly
    Collins SurveyTach with
      MicroTach a.
    infant nasal cannula a. (INCA)
Asserachrom
    A. D-DI ELISA assay
    A. tPA immunologic assay
assessment
    anatomic a.
    angiographic a.
    angioscopic a.
    cardiovascular function a.
    A. of Cardioversion Utilizing
      Transesophageal Echocardiography
      (ACUTE)
    causality a.

    Chedoke-McMaster Stroke A.
    echocardiographic a.
    functional a.
    hemodynamic a.
    invasive a.
    jugular bulb catheter placement a.
    Multicenter Oral Carvedilol in
      Heart-Failure A. (MOCHA)
    noninvasive a.
    sequential organ failure a. (SOFA)
    transposition a.
    A. of Treatment with Lisinopril
      and Survival (ATLAS)
Assess peak flowmeter
assist
    Venturi Exhalation A.
assistance
    ventilatory a.
assist/control
    a. mode ventilation
    a. ventilation (ACV)
assisted
    a. circulation
    a. mechanical ventilation (AMV)
    a. respiration
    a. ventilation
Assmann
    A. focus
    A. tuberculous infiltrate
association
    American College of
      Cardiology/American Heart A.
      (ACC/AHA)
    American Heart A. (AHA)
    American Sleep Disorders A.
      (ASDA)
    atrioventricular a.
    CHARGE a.
    National Home Oxygen Patients A.
    New York Heart A. (NYHA)
AST
    aspartate aminotransferase
AST2
    antistreptozyme
    AST2 test
Astech peak flowmeter
Astelin nasal spray
astemizole
asterixis
asteroid body
asteroides
    Nocardia a.
asthenia
    neurocirculatory a.
    vasoregulatory a.
asthenic apoplexy
asthenicus
    thorax a.

asthma

abdominal a.
acarian a.
adult-onset a.
aliphatic amines a.
allergen-induced a.
allergic a.
alveolar a.
anhydride a.
aspirin-induced a. (AIA)
atopic a.
bacterial a.
baker's a.
benzalkonium chloride a.
brittle a.
bronchial a.
cacoon seed a.
cardiac a.
a. care algorithm (ACA)
casein a.
castor bean a.
cat a.
catarrhal a.
A. Check peak flowmeter
Cheyne-Stokes a.
chlorella a.
chronic a.
cobalt a.
cobalt-related a.
cockroach a.
coffee bean a.
cold, dry air-induced a.
cotton-dust a.
cough variant a.
a. crystal
cutaneous a.
daytime a. (DA)
diisocyanate a.
dust a.
Elsner a.
emphysematous a.
essential a.
exercise-induced a. (EIA)
extrinsic a.
factitious a.
a. flare
food a.
Global Institute for A. (GIA)
grinder's a.
Heberden a.
horse a.
humid a.

hyperventilation-induced a. (HIA)
idiosyncratic a.
infective a.
inner city a.
intrinsic a.
irritant-induced a.
isocyanate-induced a.
kapok a.
karaya a.
Kopp a.
lycopodium a.
mall a.
meat-wrapper's a.
methylene diphenyl diisocyanate a.
Mexican bean weevil a.
Millar a.
miller's a.
miner's a.
mixed a.
nacre dust a.
nasal a.
nervous a.
nocturnal a.
nonatopic a.
occupational a. (OA)
oil mist a.
osmotically induced a. (OIA)
pancreatin a.
a. paper
phthalic anhydride irrigatant-
  induced a.
pollen a.
polyether alcohol a.
poorly reversible a.
postcoital a.
potroom a.
potter's a.
prawn a.
A. Quality of Life Questionnaire
  (AQLQ)
red cedar a.
red soft coral a.
reflex a.
rose hips a.
Rostan a.
royal jelly-induced a.
a. severity score (ASS)
sexual a.
sheep blowfly a.
shellfish a.
soybean lecithin a.
spasmodic a.

NOTES

asthma (*continued*)
    steam-fitter's a.
    steroid-dependent a.
    steroid-resistant a.
    stone a.
    stone-stripper's a.
    styrene a.
    subclinical a.
    sunflower a.
    symptomatic a.
    tall oil a.
    tartrazine a.
    thymic a.
    tragacanth a.
    triad a.
    a. trigger
    trimellitic anhydride a.
    true a.
    a. Turbohaler
    tylosin tartrate a.
    Vicia sativa a.
    weeping fig a.
    Wichmann a.
    work-aggravated a.
    work-related a.
    zardaverine a.
AsthmaHaler Mist
AsthmaMentor peak flowmeter
AsthmaNefrin
Asthmanex
AsthmaPACK personal asthma care kit
Asthmastik
    Bird A.
asthmatic
    brittle a.
    a. bronchitis
    chronic stable a.
    corticosteroid-dependent a.
    steroid-dependent a.
    tight a.
asthmaticus
    status a.
asthmatiform
asthmogen
    hydrosoluble a.
    occupational a.
asthmogenic
asthmoid
    a. respiration
    a. wheeze
Astler-Coller classification
Astra
    A. profile
    A. T4, T6 pacemaker
Astrand bicycle exercise stress test
Astrand-Rhyming protocol
astrocyte

astronyxis
    Acanthamoeba a.
Astropulse cuff
Astro-Trace Universal adapter clip
Astroviridae virus
Astrup blood gas value
ASTZ test
Asuka PTA over-the-wire catheter
ASV
    adaptive support ventilation
ASVD
    arteriosclerotic vascular disease
asymmetric
    a. dimethylarginine (ADMA)
    a. septal hypertrophy (ASH)
asymptomatic
    a. cardiac ischemia (ACI)
    A. Cardiac Ischemia Pilot (ACIP)
    A. Cardiac Ischemia Trial (ACIT)
    A. Carotid Artery Plaque Study
      (ACAPS)
    A. Carotid Artery Progression
      Study (ACAPS)
    a. carotid atherosclerosis study
      (ACAS)
    a. carotid surgery trial (ACST)
    a. complex ectopy
    a. myocarditis
asynchronous
    a. pacing
    a. pulse generator
asynchrony index
asynergy
asystole
    atrial a.
    Beau a.
    transient a.
asystolia
asystolic arrest
AT
    acute thrombosis
    adenosine triphosphate
    anaerobic threshold
    atrial tachycardia
    MemoryTrace AT
AT1 receptor C allele
AT-1 three-channel resting ECG system
AT-2plusTX ECG system
ATA
    atmosphere absolute
    ATA unit
Atacand HCT
atactic hemiparesis
Atakr
    A. Ablation System clinical trial
    A. system
A-T antiembolism stockings
Atarax Oral

AT-atropine stress echocardiography
ataxia
    a. cordis
    Friedreich a.
    hereditary a.
    spinocerebellar a.
ataxia-telangiectasia
ataxic
    a. aphasia
    a. gait
    a. hemiparesis (AH)
ATD
    Amplatz thrombectomy device
    asphyxiating thoracic dystrophy
ATDR
    atrial tachycardia detection rate
atelectasia
atelectasis
    absorption a.
    acquired a.
    bibasilar a.
    compression a.
    congenital a.
    lobar a.
    obstructive a.
    patchy a.
    platelike a.
    postobstructive a.
    primary a.
    relaxation a.
    resorption a.
    rounded a.
    secondary a.
    segmental a.
    subsegmental a.
    tricuspid a.
atelectatic
    a. band
    a. rale
atelocardia
atenolol
    a. and chlorthalidone
    A. Silent Ischemia Trial (ASIST)
ATF
    activating transcription factor
Atgam
atherectomy
    Auth a.
    a. catheter
    coronary a.
    coronary rotational a. (CRA)
    directional a.

    directional coronary a. (DCA)
    excimer laser coronary a.
    excisional a.
    extraction a.
    high speed directional coronary a.
    high-speed rotational a. (HSRA)
    a. index
    Kinsey a.
    New Approaches to Coronary
      Intervention Registry Directional
      Coronary A. (NACI DCA)
    percutaneous coronary rotational a.
      (PCRA)
    percutaneous transluminal
      rotational a. (PTRA)
    rotational a. (RA)
    rotational coronary a. (RCA)
    transluminal coronary extraction a.
    transluminal extraction a. (TEA)
    transluminal extraction coronary a.
atheroablation
AtheroCath
    A. Bantam coronary atherectomy
      catheter
    A. GTO coronary atherectomy
      catheter
    Simpson peripheral A.
    A. spinning blade catheter
atheroemboli (*pl. of* atheroembolus)
atheroembolic stroke
atheroembolism
atheroembolus, pl. **atheroemboli**
atherogenesis
    monoclonal theory of a.
    response-to-injury hypothesis of a.
atherogenic
    a. dyslipidemia
    a. metabolic triad
atherogenicity index
atherolytic reperfusion guidewire
atheroma
    AA a.
    aortic arch a.
    a. burden
    complex a.
    core of a.
    coronary a.
    intimal a.
    protruding a.
atheromatous
    a. cap
    a. core

NOTES

atheromatous *(continued)*
- a. debris
- a. embolism
- a. gruel
- a. plaque

atherosclerosis *(See also* arteriosclerosis)
- aortic a.
- cardiac allograft a. (CAA)
- coronary artery a.
- de novo a.
- encrustation theory of a.
- lipogenic theory of a.
- a. obliterans
- premature a.
- A. Prevention and Treatment (APT)
- radiation-induced a.

atherosclerotic *(See also* arteriosclerosis)
- a. aneurysm
- a. aortic disease
- a. aortography
- a. cardiovascular disease (ASCVD)
- a. carotid artery disease
- a. coronary artery disease (ACAD, ASCAD)
- a. debris
- a. narrowing
- a. plaque
- a. plaque burden

atherosis
atherothrombosis
atherothrombotic
- a. brain infarction (ABI)
- a. cardiovascular disease
- a. stroke

atherotome
Athlete
- A. coronary guidewire
- A. guidewire

athlete's heart
athletic heart
AT-III
- antithrombin III

Ativan
Atkins-Cannard tracheal tube
Atkinson tube stent
ATL
- A. Ultramark 7 echocardiographic device
- A. UltraMark IV 7.5-Mhz linear array transducer
- A. Ultramark 9 ultrasound system

atlantis
- fovea articularis inferior a.
- fovea articularis superior a.
- fovea dentis a.
- A. SR IVUS catheter

ATLAS
- Aspirin and Ticlid Versus Anticoagulation for Stents
- Assessment of Treatment with Lisinopril and Survival
- ATLAS study
- ATLAS trial

atlas
- A. DG balloon angioplasty catheter
- inferior articular facet of a.
- A. LP PTCA balloon dilatation catheter
- superior articular facet of a.
- A. ULP balloon dilatation catheter

Atlee clamp
ATLS
- advanced trauma life support

atm
- atmosphere

atmosphere (atm)
- a. absolute (ATA)
- ICAO standard a.
- a.'s of pressure
- standard a.

atmospheric pressure
atmospherization
atmotherapy
ATnativ
Atolone Oral
atomic absorption spectrometry
atomizer
atopic asthma
atopy
atorvastatin calcium
atovaquone
Atozine Oral
ATP
- adenosine triphosphate
- antitachycardia pacemaker
- antitachycardia pacing
- ATP hydrolysis

ATPase
- adenosine triphosphatase
- myofibrillar ATPase
- SR calcium ATPase

ATP-SPECT
- adenosine triphosphate single-photon emission computed tomography

ATR
- atrial tachy response
- ATR algorithm

atra
- *Stachybotrys* a.

ATRAC-II double-balloon catheter
ATRAC multipurpose balloon catheter
atracurium
Atraloc needle

Atrauclip
- A. grip clamp
- A. hemostatic clip

atraumatic needle

atresia
- anatomic pulmonary a.
- aortic a.
- atrioventricular valve a.
- bronchial a.
- congenital bronchial a. (CBA)
- esophageal a.
- functional pulmonary a.
- glottic a.
- gross tracheoesophageal a.
- infundibular a.
- laryngeal a.
- membranous pulmonary a.
- mitral a.
- pulmonary a.
- tricuspid a.
- ventricular a.

atretic pulmonary valve

atria (*pl. of* atrium)

atrial
- a. activation mapping
- a. anomalous band
- a. appendage
- a. appendectomy
- a. arrhythmia
- a. asynchronous pacemaker
- a. asystole
- a.-axis discontinuity
- a. baffle operation
- a. balloon septostomy
- a.-based pacemaker
- a. beat
- a. bigeminy
- a. bolus dynamic computer tomography
- a. bradycardia
- a. capture
- a. capture beat
- a. capture threshold
- a. chaotic tachycardia
- a. complex
- a. cuff
- a. defibrillation threshold
- a. deflection
- a. demand-inhibited (AAI)
- a. demand-inhibited pacemaker
- a. demand-triggered (AAT)
- a. demand-triggered pacemaker

- a. diastole
- a. diastolic gallop
- a. disk
- a. dissociation
- a. echo
- a. ectopic beat
- a. ectopic tachycardia (AET)
- a. ectopy
- a. effective refractory period
- a. ejection force
- a. escape interval
- a. escape rhythm
- a. extrastimulus method
- a. extrasystole
- a.-femoral artery bypass
- a. fibrillation (AF)
- a. fibrillation cycle length (AFCL)
- a. fibrillation detection
- a. fibrillation-flutter (AFF)
- a. fibrillation followup investigation of rhythm management (AFFIRM)
- a. fibrillation investigators
- a. fibrillation threshold
- a. filling pressure
- a. flutter
- a. flutter response (AFR)
- a. flutter response algorithm
- a. fusion beat
- a. gallop
- a. implantable cardioverter-defibrillator (AICD, A-ICD)
- a. incremental pacing
- a. infarction
- a. isthmus ablation
- a. kick
- a. lead impedance
- a. liver pulse
- a. maze procedure
- a. myocardial infarction
- a. myocarditis
- a. myxoma
- a. natriuretic factor (ANF)
- a. natriuretic peptide (ANP)
- a. natriuretic polypeptide (ANP)
- a. non-sensing
- a. notch
- a. ostium primum defect
- a. overdrive pacing
- a.-paced cycle length
- a. pacing stress test
- a. pacing study
- a. pacing wire

NOTES

atrial *(continued)*
a. parasystole
a. paroxysmal tachycardia
a. partition
a. premature beat (APB)
a. premature complexes
a. premature contraction (APC)
a. premature depolarization (APD)
a. pressure
a. pulse amplitude
a. pulse width
a. reentry
a. reentry tachycardia
a. refractory period
a. relaxation
a. repolarization wave
a. reverse remodeling
a. rhythm
a. ring
a. sensing configuration
a. sensitivity
a. septal aneurysm (ASA)
a. septal defect (ASD)
a. septal defect occlusion system (ASDOS)
a. septal defect patch
a. septal defect single disk closure device
a. septal defect umbrella
a. septal resection
a. septectomy
a. septostomy
a. septum
a. septum defect occluder system (ASDOS)
a. septum septal pacing
a. shear
a. sound
a. spike
a. standstill
a. stasis index
a. stretch
a. synchronous noncompetitive pacemaker
a. synchronous pulse generator
a. synchronous ventricular inhibited pacemaker
a. synchrony
a. systole
a. tachycardia (AT)
a. tachycardia detection rate (ATDR)
a. tachy response (ATR)
a. tachy response algorithm
a. threshold
a. thrombus
a.-to-pulmonary venous gradient
a. tracking pacemaker

a. train pacing
a. transport function
a. trigeminy with aberrancy
a. triggered noncompetitive pacemaker
a. triggered pulse generator
a. triggered ventricular-inhibited pacemaker
a. undersensing
a. valve
a. vector loop
a. venous pulse
a. and ventricular implantable cardioverter-defibrillator (AV-ICD)
a. ventricular nodal reentry tachycardia
a. ventricular reciprocating tachycardia (AVRT)
a. ventricular shunt
a. VOO pacemaker
a.-well technique
atrialized
a. chamber
a. ventricle
Atricor Cordis pacemaker
atriocarotid interval
atriocommissuropexy
atriocyte
atriodextrofascicular tract
atriodigital dysplasia
atriofascicular
a. Mahaim reentrant tachycardia
a. tract
atriofasciculoventricular Mahaim fiber
atriography
atrio-His, atriohisian
a.-H. bypass tract
a.-H. fiber
a.-H. interval
a.-H. pathway
a.-H. tract
atrionodal bypass tract
atriopeptidase inhibitor
atriopressor reflex
atriopulmonary shunt
atrioseptal
a. defect
a. sign
atriosystolic murmur
atriotomy
atrioventricular (A-V, AV)
anomalous a.
a. association
a. block
a. bundle
a. canal
a. canal cushion
a. canal defect

complete a.
a. conduction (AVC)
a. conduction abnormality
a. conduction defect
a. conduction system
a. conduction tissue
a. connection anomaly
a. delay (AVD)
a. discordance
a. dissociation (AVD)
a. extrasystole (AVE)
a. flow rumbling murmur
a. furrow
a. gradient
a. groove
a. interval
a. junction (AVJ)
a. junctional
a. junctional ablation
a. junctional arrhythmia
a. junctional bigeminy
a. junctional escape beat
a. junctional escape complex
a. junctional escape extrasystole
a. junctional heart block
a. junctional pacemaker augmentor
a. junctional reciprocating
  tachycardia
a. junctional rhythm
a. junction motion
a. malformation (AVM)
a. nodal ablation
a. nodal bigeminy
a. nodal extrasystole
a. nodal reentrant tachycardia
  (AVNRT)
a. nodal reentry
a. nodal reentry tachycardia
  (AVNRT)
a. nodal rhythm
a. nodal tachycardia (AVNT)
a. node (AVN)
a. node artery
a. node pathway
a. orifice
a. reciprocating tachycardia
a. refractory period
a. ring
a. septal defect
a. sequential pacemaker
a. situs concordance
a. sulcus

a. synchronous pacing
a. synchrony
a. time
a. valve
a. valve atresia
a. valve insufficiency
a. valve regurgitation
a. valve ring
atrioventricularis
  crus dextrum fasciculi a.
  crus sinistrum fasciculi a.
  crux dextrum fasciculi a.
  crux sinistrum fasciculi a.
  nodus a.
Atrioverter
  A. implantable defibrillator
  A. implantable defibrillator device
  Metrix A.
**Atri-pace I bipolar flared pacing
  catheter**
atrium, pl. **atria**
  accessory a.
  auricles of atria
  A. Blood Recovery System
  common a.
  congenital single a.
  a. cordis
  a. dextrum
  Fontan right a.
  a. glottidis
  a. of heart
  high right a.
  a.-His bundle (AH)
  left a. (LA)
  low septal a.
  a. of lung
  a. pulmonale
  pulmonary venous a.
  right a. (RA)
  roof of left a.
  single a.
  a. sinistrum
  stunned a.
  systemic venous a.
Atromid-S
Atropair
atrophic
  a. cardiomyopathy
  a. catarrh
  a. emphysema
  a. laryngitis
  a. papulosis

NOTES

atrophic *(continued)*
  a. pharyngitis
  a. thrombosis
atrophy
  brown a.
  cardiac a.
  cyanotic a. of liver
  Erb a.
  multiple system a.
  olivopontocerebellar a.
  optic a.
  peroneal muscular a.
  red a.
  spinal muscular a.
atropine
  A.-Care
  Isopto A.
  a. sulfate
  a. test
Atropisol
Atrostim phrenic nerve stimulator
Atrovent
  A. Aerosol Inhalation
  A. Inhalation Solution
ATS Open Pivot bileaflet heart valve
attachment
  epithelial-mucus a.
attack
  Adams-Stokes a.
  anxiety a.
  drop a.
  heart a.
  odor-triggered panic a.
  Stokes-Adams a.
  transient ischemic a. (TIA)
  vagal a.
  vasovagal a.
attenuation
  ground-glass a. (GGA)
  heterogeneous a.
  heterogeneous parenchymal a.
  vascular a.
attenuator
attraction sphere
attrition murmur
atypical
  a. alveolar hyperplasia
  a. atrioventricular nodal reentrant
    tachycardia (AAVNRT)
  a. chest pain
  a. mycobacterial colonization
  a. pneumonia
  a. tamponade
  a. tuberculosis
  a. verrucous endocarditis
Au
  gold

auditory
  a. alternans
  a. fremitus
Auenbrugger sign
Auer body
Aufrecht sign
Aufricht elevator
auger wire
augmentation
  flow a.
  pressure a. (PA)
  a. therapy
Augmentin
augmentor
  atrioventricular junctional
    pacemaker a.
  pacemaker a.
auranofin
aureomycin sensitivity
aureus
  Staphylococcus a.
  Staphylococcus pyogenes a.
auricle
auricles of atria
auricular
  a. appendage
  a. appendectomy
  a. complex
  a. extrasystole
  a. fibrillation
  a. flutter
  a. premature beat
  a. standstill
  a. systole
  a. tachycardia
auricularis magna
Auriculin
auriculopressor reflex
auriculoventricular
  a. extrasystole
  a. groove
  a. interval
Aurora
  A. dual-chamber pacemaker
  A. pulse generator
aurothiomalate
Ausculscope
auscultation
  aortic area of a.
  cardiac a.
  Korányi a.
  percussion and a. (P&A)
auscultatory
  a. alternans
  a. gap
  a. sign
  a. sound
auscultogram

A

Austin
  A. Flint murmur
  A. Flint phenomenon
  A. Flint respiration
  A. Flint rumble
Australia antigen
Australian Q fever
australis
  Rickettsia a.
Austrian syndrome
autacoid
Auth
  A. atherectomy
  A. atherectomy catheter
Autima II dual-chamber pacemaker
auto
  a. decremental mode
  A. Suture Soft Thoracoport
  A. Suture Surgiclip
AutoAdjust CPAP device
autoanalyzer
autoantibody
  antimyosin a.
  cardiac a.
autobiotic
autobullectomy
  partial a.
autocapture
  ventricular a.
AutoCapture pacing system
AutoCat intraaortic balloon pump
Autoclix
autoclot
autocorrelation
  serial a. (SAC)
AutoCorr portable pulse oximeter
autocrine signaling
autodecremental pacing
autodigestion of connective tissue
autogamous
autogamy
autogenic
  a. drainage (AD)
  a. graft
autogenous vein
autograft
  pulmonary a. (PA)
Autohaler
  Maxair A.
autohypnosis
autoimmune disorder

autoimmunity
  cardiac a.
Auto-Injector
  LidoPen I.M. Injection A.-I.
Autolet
autologous
  a. blood
  a. blood management system
  a. blood patch
  a. clot
  a. fat graft
  a. pericardial patch
  a. transfusion
  a. vein graft-coated stent (AVGCS)
automated
  a. border detection (ABD)
  a. boundary protection (ABP)
  a. cardiac flow measurement
    (ACM)
  a. cardiac output measurement
    (ACOM)
  a. cervical cell screening system
  a. edge detection
  a. external defibrillator (AED)
automatic
  a. atrial tachycardia (AAT)
  a. beat
  a. boundary detection (ABD)
  a. capacitor formation interval
  a. cell
  a. contraction
  a. device
  a. ectopic tachycardia
  a. exposure system
  a. external cardioverter-defibrillator
    (AECD)
  a. external defibrillator (AED)
  a. implantable cardioverter-
    defibrillator (AICD, A-ICD)
  a. implantable defibrillator (AID)
  a. internal cardioverter-defibrillator
    (AICD, A-ICD)
  a. internal defibrillator
  a. intracardiac defibrillator
  a. mode conversion (AMC)
  a. mode conversion algorithm
  a. mode switching (AMS)
  a. mode-switching algorithm
  a. oscillometric blood pressure
    monitor
  a. pacemaker
  a. ventricular contraction

NOTES

automaticity
enhanced a.
pacemaker a.
sinus nodal a.
autonomic
a. dysreflexia
a. failure
a. hyperreflexia
a. modulation
a. nervous system (ANS)
pulmonary branch of a.
a. response
a. sensory innervation
autonomici
rami pulmonales systematis a.
autoperfusion
a. balloon
a. balloon catheter
Autoplex Factor VIII inhibitor bypass product
Autoplex T
autoprogramming
autoregulation
cerebrovascular a.
heterometric a.
homeometric a.
orthostasis a.
autosensing
AutoSet
A. Portable II
A. Portable II CPAP system
A. Portable II diagnosis and therapy device
autosomal-dominant familial aortic aneurysm disease
autosome
Autostat ligating and hemostatic clip
AutoSuture
A. indicator 30 Mini-CABG site stabilizer
A. Mini-CABG occlusion clamp
A. One-Shot anastomotic device
auto-threshold function
autotitrating CPAP
autotitration device
autotoxic cyanosis
Autotransfuser
Biosurge Synchronous A.
autotransfusion system
autotransplantation
Autotrans system
Autovac
A. autotransfusion system
A. LF autotransfusion system
autumnal catarrh
auxocardia
A-V, AV
arteriovenous

atrioventricular
A-V atrioventricular junctional rhythm
A-V block
A-V branch block
A-V bundle
A-V conduction
A-V conduction defect
A-V delay interval
A-V dissociation
A-V extrasystole
A-V Gore-Tex fistula
A-V groove
A-V groove block
A-V interval
A-V junction
A-V junction ablation
A-V junctional escape beat
A-V junctional escape complex
A-V junctional extrasystole
A-V junctional rhythm
A-V junctional tachycardia
A-V Miniclinic
A-V nodal artery
A-V nodal bigeminy
A-V nodal conduction
A-V nodal extrasystole
A-V nodal modification
A-V nodal reentry
A-V nodal reentry tachycardia
A-V nodal rhythm
A-V nodal tachycardia
A-V nodal Wenckebach arrhythmia
A-V node
A-V node reentrant tachycardia
A-V node Wenckebach periodicity
A-V reciprocating tachycardia
A-V sequential pacemaker
A-V synchronous pacemaker
A-V synchrony
A-V Wenckebach block
A/V
alanine/valine
AVA
A. device
A. 3Xi advanced venous access device
A. 3Xi venous access device
AVAD
acute ventricular assist device
Avalide
Avanar
A. intravascular ultrasound catheter
A. IVUS catheter
Avanti introducer
Avapro HCT
avascular necrosis

AVC
atrioventricular conduction
AVCO
A. aortic balloon
A. balloon pump
AVD
atrioventricular delay
atrioventricular dissociation
AVD O$_2$
AVE
atrioventricular extrasystole
AVE Microstent II stent
AVE S540 stent
AVE S670 stent
Avelox
avenaceus
Aspergillus a.
Avenue insertion tool
average
a. mean pressure (AMP)
a. peak velocity (APV)
a. pulse magnitude
averaging
digital a.
gated a.
signal a.
AVF
arteriovenous fistula
aVF lead
AVG
aortic valve gradient
AVGCS
autologous vein graft-coated stent
avian
a. antigen
A. transport ventilator
a. tuberculosis
aviator's disease
AV-ICD
atrial and ventricular implantable
cardioverter-defibrillator
AVID
Amiodarone Versus Implantable
Defibrillators
Angiography Versus Intravascular
Ultrasound-Directed Coronary Stent
Placement
Antiarrhythmics versus Implantable
Defibrillators
AVID clinical trial
AVID study
avidin-biotin peroxidase

Avitene
avium
Mycobacterium a.
avium-intracellulare
Mycobacterium a.-i. (MAI)
Avius sequential pacemaker
AVJ
atrioventricular junction
AVJRT
AVL
A. Medical Instruments model 995-
Hb arterial blood gas analyzer
A. Omni blood gas analyzer
A. OPTI Critical Care Analyzer
A. OPTI 1 portable blood gas
analyzer
aVL lead
Avlosulfon
AVM
arteriovenous malformation
atrioventricular malformation
AVN
atrioventricular node
AVNRT
atrioventricular nodal reentrant
tachycardia
atrioventricular nodal reentry tachycardia
AVNT
atrioventricular nodal tachycardia
AvoSure PT monitor
AVP
arginine vasopressin
AV-Paceport thermodilution catheter
AVR
aortic valve replacement
aVR lead
AVRT
atrial ventricular reciprocating
tachycardia
AVSD
acquired ventricular septal defect
AVSD defect
avulsion
AW
Anderson-Wilkins
anterior wall
AW acuteness score
A-wave spectral velocity waveform
Axcis
A. percutaneous myocardial
revascularization system
A. PMR system

NOTES

axes (*pl. of* axis)
axial
    a. computed tomography (ACT)
    a. control
    a. interstitial disease
    a. interstitium
    a. plane
axillary
    a. arch
    a. artery
    a. bifemoral bypass
    a. block
    a. lymph node
    a. nerve
    a. triangle
    a. vein
axilloaxillary bypass
axillofemoral bypass
Axiom
    A. DG balloon angioplasty catheter
    A. double sump pump
    A. thoracic trocar
Axios 04 pacemaker
axis, pl. **axes**
    clockwise rotation of electrical a.
    a. deviation
    electrical a.
    frontal a.
    horizontal long a.
    hypophyseal-pituitary adrenal a.
    hypothalamic-pituitary-adrenal a.
     (HPAA)
    instantaneous electrical a.
    J point electrical a.
    junctional a.
    long a. (LAX)
    mean electrical a.
    mean QRS a.
    normal electrical a.
    parasternal long a.
    parasternal short a.
    P wave a.
    QRS a.
    R a.
    rightward a.
    a. shift
    short a. (SAX)
    Strong unbridling of celiac
     artery a.
    superior QRS a.
    thoracic a.
    vertical long a.

    X a.
    Y a.
Ayercillin
Ayers
    A. cardiovascular needle holder
    A. sphygmomanometer
    A. T-piece
Ayerza
    A. disease
    A. syndrome
Aygestin
Ayr
    A. saline nasal drops
    A. saline nasal gel
    A. saline nasal mist
AZ
    acquisition zoom
    AZ technology
Azactam
azalide class of antibiotics
Azan-Mallory stain
azapetine phosphate
azatadine maleate
azathioprine
azidothymidine (AZT)
azimilide
    a. dihydrochloride
    a. supraventricular arrhythmia
     program
azithromycin
Azlin
azlocillin
Azmacort Oral Inhaler
azotemia
    extrarenal a.
    postrenal a.
    prerenal a.
    renal a.
AZT
    azidothymidine
aztreonam
azurophil granule
azygography
azygoportal interruption
azygos
    a. arch
    a. fissure
    a. lobe of right lung
    a. node
    a. vein
Azzopardi effect

B
  B bump
  B bump on echocardiogram
  B cell
  B cell antibody
  B cell lymphoma
  B knuckle
B₂
  11-dehydro-thromboxane B_2
B4
  leukotriene B4 (LTB4)
B6 bronchus sign
BA
  basilar artery
Babbington-type nebulizer
Babcock
  B. operation
  B. stainless steel suture wire
  B. thoracic tissue-holding forceps
Babes-Ernst body
Babesia
  B. bigemina
  B. bovis
  B. canis
  B. divergens
  B. major
  B. microti
  B. rodhaini
babesiosis
  human b.
Babinski
  downgoing B.
  B. reflex
  B. syndrome
  upgoing B.
  B.-Vasquez syndrome
baby
  blue b.
BABYbird respirator
babygram x-ray
Babyhaler spacer device
BAC
  bronchioloalveolar carcinoma
bacampicillin hydrochloride
Baccelli sign
Bachmann
  anterior internodal tract of B.
  B. bundle
  internodal tract of B.
  B. pathway
Baci-IM injection
bacillary
  b. angiomatosis
  b. embolism

  b. phthisis
  b. pneumonia
bacille
  b. Calmette-Guérin
  b. de Calmette-Guérin (BCG)
bacilli, pl. **bacilli** (*pl. of* bacilli) (*pl. of*
  bacillus)
bacilliformis
  Bartonella b.
Bacillus
  B. alvei
  B. anthracis
  B. cereus
  B. circulans
  B. funduliformis
  B. laterosporus
  B. licheniformis
  B. megaterium
  B. necroformis
  B. pneumoniae
  B. polymyxa
  B. pseudodiphtheriticum
  B. pumilus
  B. sphaericus
  B. stearothermophilus
  B. subtilis
  B. subtilis enzyme
bacillus, pl. **bacilli**
  acid-fast b. (AFB)
  Battey b.
  Bordet-Gengou b.
  Calmette-Guérin b.
  b. Calmette-Guérin Live
  b. Calmette-Guérin vaccine
  enteric Gram-negative b.
  Friedländer b.
  gram-negative b. (GNB)
  gram-positive b.
  influenza b.
  Klebs-Loeffler b.
  Koch b.
  Koch-Weeks b.
  Loeffler b.
  Much b.
  Mycobacterium intracellulare,
    Battey b.
  Warthin-Starry-staining bacillus
  Weeks b.
bacitracin
back-bleeding
backflush
background subtraction technique
back pressure
backscatter
  b. analysis

backscatter *(continued)*
    b. threshold
    two-dimensional integrated b.
backup ventilation (BUV)
backward
    b. failure
    b. heart failure
BACTEC
    B. radiometry
    B. system
bacteremia, bacteriemia
    streptococcal b.
bacteremic
bacteria (*pl. of* bacterium)
**bacteria-free stage of bacterial
  endocarditis**
bacterial
    b. asthma
    b. colonization
    b. endocarditis (BE)
    b. endotoxin
    b. infection
    b. myocarditis
    b. pericarditis
    b. pneumococcal pneumonia
    b. pneumonia
    b. respiratory tract infection
    b. superinfection
    b. vegetation
bactericidal titer
bacteriemia (*var. of* bacteremia)
bacterioid
bacteriophage
bacteriostatic
    b. agent
    b. effect
bacterium, pl. **bacteria**
    B. anitratum
    facultative bacteria
Bacteroides
    B. corrodens
    B. fragilis
    B. funduliformis
    B. furcosus
    B. melaninogenicus
    B. oralis
    B. pneumosintes
Bactocill
    B. injection
    B. Oral
Bactrim DS
Bactroban Topical
BAE
    bronchial artery embolization
Baffe anastomosis
baffle
    fabric b.
    b. fenestration

    Gore-Tex b.
    intraatrial b.
    b. leak
    manual resuscitation b.
    Mustard atrial b.
    b. obstruction
    pericardial b.
    Senning intraatrial b.
baffled jet nebulizer
bag
    Ambu b.
    arterial line pressure b.
    Douglas b.
    eXtract specimen b.
    Hope b.
    Lifesaver disposable resuscitator b.
    manual resuscitation b.
    rebreathing b.
    Sones hemostatic b.
    SureGrip breathing b.
    Tedlar b.
    Voorhees b.
bagassosis
BagEasy disposable manual resuscitator
bagged
baggy heart
bagpipe sign
bag-valve-mask (BVM)
Bahnson
    B. aortic clamp
    B. sternal retractor
BAI
    breath-actuated inhaler
Bailey
    B. aortic clamp
    B. aortic valve rongeur
    B. catheter
    B.-Gibbon rib contractor
    B.-Glover-O'Neill commissurotomy
    knife
    B. rib spreader
bailout
    b. autoperfusion balloon catheter
    emergency b.
    b. situation
    b. stent
    b. stenting
    b. valvuloplasty
Baim pacing catheter
Baim-Turi
    B.-T. cardiac device
    B.-T. monitoring/pacing catheter
Bainbridge
    B. effect
    B. reflex
Bair
    B. Hugger
    B. Hugger blanket

baker's asthma
Bakes dilator
Bakst valvulotome
BAL
    bronchoalveolar lavage
Baladi Inverter device
balance
    micronutrient b.
    sympathovagal b.
    Wilhelmy b.
balanced coronary circulation
Balectrode pacing catheter
BALF
    bronchoalveolar lavage fluid
Balke
    B. exercise stress test
    B. protocol
    B. treadmill protocol
Balke-Ware
    B.-W. test
    B.-W. treadmill protocol
ball
    carotid b.
    Esmarch b.
    fibrous b.
    fungus b.
    b. heart valve
    b. mitral commissurotomy
    NC Bandit b.
    parietal b.
    Percor DL-II intraaortic b.
    Percor dual-lumen-II intraaortic b.
    pleural fibrin b.
    b. poppet
    b. of Reil
    sinoatrial b.
    b. thrombus
    b. valve
    b. valve prosthesis
    b. valve thrombus
    b. wedge
ball-and-cage, ball-in-cage
    b.-a.-c. prosthesis
    b.-a.-c. prosthetic valve
ballerina-foot pattern
ballet
    cardiac b.
ball-in-cage (*var. of* ball-and-cage)
ballistocardiogram
ballistocardiograph (BCG)
ballistocardiography
ball-occluder valve

balloon
    Accent-DG b.
    ACE b.
    ACS Alpha b.
    ACS SULP II b.
    ACX b.
    Advanced Cardiovascular Systems SULP II b.
    b. angioplasty catheter
    B. Angioplasty Versus Rotacs for Total Chronic Coronary Occlusion (BAROCCO)
    b. aortic valvotomy (BAV)
    b. aortic valvuloplasty (BAV)
    Arrow Berman angiographic b.
    b. atrial septoplasty
    b. atrial septostomy (BAS)
    autoperfusion b.
    AVCO aortic b.
    Bandit b.
    Bandit low-profile over-the-wire b.
    Baxter Intrepid b.
    Berman angiographic b.
    bifoil b.
    Blue Max high-pressure b.
    Brandt cytology b.
    b. catheter
    b. catheter angioplasty (BCA)
    b. catheterization
    b. catheter sealing device
    b. coarctation angioplasty
    compliant b.
    Cook b.
    Cordis Powerflex angioplasty b.
    b. coronary angioplasty
    b. coronary occlusion (BCO)
    counterpulsation b.
    b. counterpulsation
    Cribier-Letac aortic valvuloplasty b.
    cutting b.
    CVD b.
    Datascope b.
    delivery b.
    b. dilation
    Dispatch b.
    b. dissector
    Distaflex b.
    b. distention test
    Dynasty b.
    Eliminator dilatation b.
    Ellswood Mylar b.
    b. embolectomy catheter

B

NOTES

balloon *(continued)*
    Epistat double b.
    Express b.
    Extractor three-lumen retrieval b.
    Falcon b.
    FasTracker b.
    fixed-wire b.
    Force b.
    Hadow b.
    Hartzler Micro II b.
    Helix b.
    Hunter b.
    Hunter-Sessions b.
    b. inflation
    Inoue b.
    Inoue self-guiding b.
    Integra II b.
    intraaortic b. (IAB)
    14K b.
    Kay b.
    Kontron b.
    b. laser angioplasty
    latex b.
    Lo-Fold b.
    low-profile, semi-compliant b.
    Mansfield b.
    Medtronic Evergreen b.
    Micross SL b.
    Microvasive Rigiflex TTS b.
    b. mitral commissurotomy (BMC)
    b. mitral valvuloplasty (BMV)
    Monorail Speedy b.
    Multi-Link Tristar b.
    NC b.
    NC Cobra b.
    noncompliant b.
    NoProfile b.
    NuMED single b.
    b. occlusion
    b. occlusive intravascular lysis
      enhanced recanalization
    Olbert b.
    Omega-NV b.
    Omniflex b.
    Omni SST b.
    Orion b.
    Owens b.
    Panther b.
    Passage exchange b.
    PE b.
    PET b.
    Piccolino b.
    pillow-shaped b.
    Pivot b.
    POC b.
    polyethylene terephthalate b.
    polyolefin copolymer b.
    polyvinyl chloride b.

    preperitoneal distention b. (PDB)
    Prime b.
    ProCross Rely b.
    b. pulmonary valvotomy
    b. pulmonary valvuloplasty (BPV)
    b. pump
    QuickFurl SL b.
    radiofrequency hot b.
    Ranger b.
    right ventricular copulsation b.
      (RVCB)
    b. rupture
    Schneider-Shiley b.
    Seajet PTCA b.
    Seloris b.
    b. septostomy
    b. septostomy catheter
    Shadow b.
    Short Speedy b.
    b. shunt
    Simpson PET b.
    Simpson positron emission
      tomography b.
    sizing b.
    Slalom b.
    Slider b.
    Slinky b.
    Solo b.
    Spears laser b.
    Speedino b.
    Stack autoperfusion b.
    Stretch b.
    Surpasse b.
    b. tamponade
    Target Therapeutics Stealth
      angioplasty b.
    Ten b.
    b. test occlusion (BTO)
    thigh b.
    Thruflex b.
    trefoil b.
    trefoil Schneider b.
    Triad PET b.
    b. tricuspid valvotomy
    Tyshak b.
    UltraFuse b.
    b. valvuloplasty (BV)
    b. valvuloplasty catheter
    b. valvuloplasty registry (BVR)
    b. versus optimal atherectomy trial
      (BOAT)
    waisting of b.
    windowed b.
    XCELON 6 b.
balloon-centered argon laser
balloon-expandable
    b.-e. flexible coil stent

b.-e. intravascular stent
b.-e. stent
balloon-flotation pacing catheter
balloon-imaging catheter
ballooning
    b. mitral cusp syndrome
    b. mitral valve syndrome
    b. posterior leaflet syndrome
balloon-occlusion pulmonary angiography
Balloon-on-a-Wire
balloon-shaped heart
balloon-tipped, balloon-tip
    b.-t. angiographic catheter
    b.-t. catheter
    b.-t. flow-directed catheter
    b.-t. thermodilution catheter
ball-wedge catheter
Balme cough
Balminil
    B.-DM
    B.-DM Children
    B. Expectorant
BALT
    bronchus-associated lymphoid tissue
Baltaxe view
Baltherm catheter
Bamberger
    B. area
    B. bulbar pulse
    B. sign
Bamberger-Marie
    B.-M. disease
    B.-M. syndrome
Bamberger-Pins-Ewart sign
bambuterol
bamiphylline
Bamyl
banana-shaped left ventricle
Bancap HC
bancrofti
    Wuchereria b.
band
    A b.
    b. of adhesion
    atelectatic b.
    atrial anomalous b.
    contraction b.
    CPK-BB b.
    CPK-MB b.
    CPK-MM b.
    I b.
    Mach b.

MB b.
moderator b.
myocardial b. (MB)
Parham b.
parietal b.
Pepper Medical tube neck b.
pulmonary artery b.
b. of Reil
b. saw effect
Vesseloops rubber b.
Z b.
bandage
    compression b.
    Esmarch b.
    b. scissors
    SteptyP hemostasis b.
    Tricodur Epi compression
      support b.
    Tricodur Omos compression
      support b.
    Tricodur Talus compression
      support b.
bandbox
    b. resonance
    b. sound
banding
    Muller b.
    PA b.
    b. of pulmonary artery
    pulmonary artery b.
    Trusler rule for pulmonary
      artery b.
Bandit
    B. balloon
    B. low-profile over-the-wire balloon
    B. PTCA catheter
bandlike
    b. angina
    b. intrapericardial echo
bandpass filter
bandwidth
bang artifact
bangungot syndrome
bank
    tissue b.
Bannister disease
Bannwarth syndrome
Banophen Oral
BAO
    basilar artery occlusion
Bapadin

NOTES

BAPV
  basal average peak velocity
  baseline average peak velocity
BAR
  beta-adrenergic receptor
Baratol
barbed
  b. epicardial pacing lead
  b. hook
Barbilixir
Barbita
barbiturate
barbourin
barb-tip lead
Bard
  B. balloon-directed pacing catheter
  B. cardiopulmonary support pump
  B. cardiopulmonary support system
  B. Clamshell septal occluder
  B. Clamshell septal umbrella
  B. Commander PTCA guidewire
  B. electrophysiology catheter
  B. guiding catheter
  B. nonsteerable bipolar electrode
  B. PDA umbrella
  B. percutaneous cardiopulmonary
    support system
  B. probe
  B. safety excaliber peripherally
    inserted central catheter
  B. sign
  B. TransAct intra-aortic balloon
    pump
  B. XT coronary stent
  B. XT stent
Bardco catheter
Bardenheurer ligation
Bardic cutdown catheter
Bard-Parker
  B.-P. blade
  B.-P. U-Mid/Lo humidifier
Bard-Tuohy-Borst adapter
bare-metal stent
BARI
  bypass angioplasty revascularization
    investigation
  BARI protocol
barium
  b. enema
  b. esophagram
  b. swallow
barium-impregnated poppet
barking cough
Barlow syndrome
Barnard
  B. mitral valve prosthesis
  B. operation

BAROCCO
  Balloon Angioplasty Versus Rotacs for
    Total Chronic Coronary Occlusion
  BAROCCO clinical trial
baroceptor
barograph
barometer-maker's disease
barometric pressure
baroreceptor
  cardiac b.
  carotid b.
  perturbed carotid b.
  b. reflex
  b. reflex sensitivity (BRS)
  b. sensitivity
  b. sensitization
baroreflex
  biochemical b.
  carotid b.
  b. sensitivity (BRS)
  sinoatrial b.
baroscope
barosinusitis
barospirator
barotaxis
barotrauma
  b. of ascent
  dental b.
  b. of descent
  facial b.
  pulmonary b.
Barraya forceps
barrel-hooping compression
barrel-shaped
  b.-s. chest
  b.-s. thorax
Barrett esophagus
barrier
  blood-air b.
  blood-brain b. (BBB)
  blood-bronchoalveolar b.
  blood-bronchus b.
  blood-gas b.
  blood-retina b.
  placental b.
Barron pump
Barrow classification
Barsony-Polgar syndrome
Barthel
  B. ADL score
  B. index
Bartholin duct
Barth syndrome
Bartonella
  B. bacilliformis
  B. elizabethae
Bartter syndrome

BAS
>balloon atrial septostomy

basal
>>B. Antiarrhythmic Study of Infarct Survival (BASIS)
>>b. average peak velocity (BAPV)
>>b. cell carcinoma
>>b. collateral artery
>>b. diastolic murmur
>>b. ganglia (BG)
>>b. part of left and right inferior pulmonary
>>b. segmental bronchus
>>b. systolic
>>b. tuberculosis

basalis communis
basaloid carcinoma
basal-septal hypertrophy
base
>>b. of lung
>>whole blood buffer b.

baseline
>>b. arrhythmia
>>b. artifact
>>b. average peak velocity (BAPV)
>>B. Dyspnea Index (BDI)
>>b. ECG
>>b. echocardiography
>>b. fetal heart rate
>>b. rhythm
>>b. shift
>>b. ST-segment abnormality
>>TP b.
>>b. variability
>>b. variability of fetal heart rate
>>wandering b.

basement membrane
baseplate
>>winged b.

basic
>>b. cardiac life support (BCLS)
>>b. cycle length (BCL)
>>b. drive cycle length
>>b. fibroblast growth factor (bFGF)
>>b. life support (BLS)

Basidiomycetes
basilar
>>b. artery (BA)
>>b. artery occlusion (BAO)
>>b. half ejection fraction
>>b. rale
>>b. sinus

basilaris ossis occipitalis
basilic vein
basipharyngeal canal
BASIS
>>Basal Antiarrhythmic Study of Infarct Survival

basis pulmonis
Basix pacemaker
basket
>>Medi-Tech multipurpose b.
>>pericardial b.
>>b. retriever

basophil
basophilic vascular streaking
Bassen-Kornzweig abetalipoproteinemia
bath
>>film fixer b.
>>film wash b.
>>fixer b.
>>Haake water b.
>>Nauheim b.
>>wash b.

Ba theorem
bathycardia
bathypnea
Batista
>>B. left ventriculectomy procedure
>>B. procedure

Bato compound
batrachotoxin
Batson plexus
battery
>>b. cell impedance
>>b. cell voltage function
>>Celsa b.
>>b. elective replacement
>>external pacemaker b.
>>LiI b.
>>lithium b.
>>lithium iodine b.
>>nickel-cadmium b.
>>b. status
>>b. voltage

battery-assisted heart assist device
Battey
>>B. bacillus
>>B. bacillus complex

bat wing shadow
Bauer syndrome
baumannii
>>*Acinetobacter b.*

NOTES

Baumanometer standard mercury sphygmomanometer
Baumes symptom
bauxite
    b. pneumoconiosis
    b. pneumonoconiosis
BAV
    balloon aortic valvotomy
    balloon aortic valvuloplasty
    bicommissural aortic valve
Baxter
    B. angioplasty catheter
    B. fiberoptic spectrophotometry catheter
    B. Flo-Gard 8200 volumetric infusion pump
    B. Health Care Continu-Flo infusion device
    B. Imagecath
    B. Intrepid balloon
    B. mechanical valve
    B. mechanical valve prosthesis
Baycol
Bayer
    B. Aspirin
    B. Buffered Aspirin
    B. Corp. Micro-Bumintest
    B. Low Adult Strength
    B. Select Chest Cold Caplets
    B. Select Pain Relief Formula
Bayes theorem
BAY K 8644
Bayle granulation
Bayliss theory
Baylor
    B. autologous transfusion system
    B. cardiovascular sump tube
    B. rapid autologous transfusion (BRAT)
    B. total artificial heart
Bayou virus
Baypress
Bazett
    B. corrected QT interval
    B. correction formula
    B. formula
Bazin disease
BBB
    blood-brain barrier
    bundle-branch block
BBBB
    bilateral bundle-branch block
BBR
    bundle-branch reentry
B&B Trachguard antidisconnection device

BCA
    balloon catheter angioplasty
    bidirectional cavopulmonary anastomosis
BCD Plus cardioplegic unit
B1 cell
BCG
    bacille de Calmette-Guérin
    ballistocardiograph
    bronchocentric granulomatosis
        Tice BCG
        BCG vaccine
BCI Capnocheck DualStream capnograph
BCKD
    branched chain alpha ketoacid dehydrogenase
BCL
    basic cycle length
Bcl-2 expression
BCLS
    basic cardiac life support
BCO
    balloon coronary occlusion
BCO$_2$
    Cardiac Stimulator BCO$_2$
B-complex
    ferrous sulfate, ascorbic acid, and vitamin B.-c.
B-D
    Becton-Dickinson
        B-D Potain thoracic trocar
BDCS
    Behavioral Dyscontrol Scale
BDG
    bidirectional Glenn procedure
BDI
    Baseline Dyspnea Index
BDT
    bronchodilator
BE
    bacterial endocarditis
bead
    Digoxin RIA B.
beading of arteries
Beall
    B. circumflex artery scissors
    B. disk valve prosthesis
    B. mitral valve
    B. mitral valve prosthesis
    B. prosthetic valve
    B. scissors
Beall-Surgitool
    B.-S. ball-cage prosthetic valve
    B.-S. disk prosthetic valve
beam
    b. splitter
    b. width artifact

bean
castor b.
green coffee b.
bean-spooning task
Bear
B. 1, 2 adult volume ventilator
B. Cub infant ventilator
B. 5 respirator
B. ventilator
B. 1000 ventilator
Beardsley aortic dilator
beat
aberrantly conducted b.
apex b.
Ashman b.
atrial b.
atrial capture b.
atrial ectopic b.
atrial fusion b.
atrial premature b. (APB)
atrioventricular junctional escape b.
auricular premature b.
automatic b.
A-V junctional escape b.
capture b.
combination b.
coupled b.
coupled premature b.
dependent b.
Dressler b.
dropped b.
echo b.
ectopic b.
ectopic Ashman b.
ectopic ventricular b.
entrained b.
escape b.
extrasystolic b.
fascicular b.
forced b.
fusion b.
heart b.
interference b.
interpolated b.
isolated ectopic b.
junctional escape b.
Lown class 4a or 4b ventricular ectopic b.
malignant b.
missed b.
mixed b.
nodal b.

paired b.'s
parasystolic b.
b.'s per minute (bpm)
postextrasystolic b.
premature b.
premature atrial b.
premature junctional b.
premature ventricular b. (PVB)
pseudofusion b.
reciprocal b.
retrograde b.
salvo of b.'s
skipped b.
summation b.
supraventricular premature b.
unifocal ventricular ectopic b. (UVEB)
ventricular captured b.
ventricular ectopic b. (VEB)
ventricular escape b.
ventricular fusion b.
ventricular premature b. (VPB)
beat-by-beat
b.-b.-b. capture
b.-b.-b. hemodynamic monitoring
beats per minute (bpm)
beat-to-beat
b.-t.-b. analysis
b.-t.-b. finger arterial pressure
b.-t.-b. variability
b.-t.-b. variability of fetal heart rate
Beatty-Bright friction sound
Beau
B. asystole
B. disease
B. lines
B. syndrome
Beaver
B. blade
B.-DeBakey blade
B. knife
BEB
blind esophageal brushing
BECAIT
Bezafibrate Coronary Atherosclerosis Intervention Trial
Beck
B. cardiopericardiopexy
B. Depression Inventory
B. epicardial poudrage
B. miniature aortic clamp

B

NOTES

Beck *(continued)*
    B. mouth tube airway
    B. I, II operation
    B. triad
Becker
    B. accelerator cannula
    B. disease
    B.-type tardive muscular dystrophy
Beckman
    B. ICS Nephelometer system
    B. O_2 analyzer
Beck-Potts aortic and pulmonic clamp
Béclard
    B. anastomosis
    B. hernia
Becloforte
beclomethasone dipropionate
Beclovent Oral Inhaler
Beconase AQ Nasal Inhaler
becquerel (Bq)
Becton-Dickinson (B-D)
    B.-D. guidewire
    B.-D. Teflon-sheathed needle
bed
    adventitial b.
    b. block
    capillary b.
    coronary b.
    cyanosis of nail b.'s
    distal b.
    myocardial b.
    nail b.
    perfusion b.
    pulmonary b.
    pulmonary vascular b.
    Sanders b.
    Stress Echo b.
    vascular b.
    venous capacitance b.
Bedfont
    B. carbon monoxide monitor
    B. EC60 Gastrolyzer hydrogen
       monitor
Bedge antireflux mattress
bedside
    b. balloon atrial septoplasty
    b. monitor
    b. transthoracic echocardiography
beef
    b. insulin
    b. Lente Iletin II
beef-lung heparin
Beepen-VK Oral
beep-o-gram
Beer
    B.-Lambert principle
    B. law

beer
    b. and cobalt syndrome
    b. heart
beer-drinker's cardiomyopathy
bee venom
beginning-of-life rate
behavior
    contractile b.
    type A, B b.
behavioral
    B. Dyscontrol Scale (BDCS)
    b. factor
    b. therapy
Behçet
    B. disease
    B. syndrome
Béhier-Hardy sign
beigelii
    Trichosporon b.
Belhaussen tachycardia
Belix Oral
bell
    b. sound
    b. stethoscope
    b. tympany
Bellavar medical support stockings
belli
    Isospora b.
bell-metal resonance
bellows
    chest b.
    b. function
    b. murmur
    b. sound
Belsey
    B. esophagoplasty
    B. Mark II, IV fundoplication
    B. two-thirds wrap fundoplication
belt
    abdominal b.
    stroke b.
Belzer solution
Bemis Air Purifier
Bena-D injection
Benadryl
    B. injection
    B. Oral
    B. Topical
benafentrine
Benahist injection
Ben-Allergin-50 Injection
benazepril
    amlodipine and b.
    b. heart failure study (BHFS)
    b. hydrochloride
    b. and hydrochlorothiazide
bendrofluazide
bendroflumethiazide

Benecol margarine
Benedict retractor
Benedict-Roth
    B.-R. apparatus
    B.-R. spirometer
Bengash needle
Bengolea forceps
benidipine
benign
    b. croupous angina
    b. early repolarization (BER)
    b. fibrous mesothelioma
    b. hypertension
    b. intracranial hypertension
benigna
    endocarditis b.
benignum
    empyema b.
Benjamin
    B. binocular slimline laryngoscope
    B. pediatric laryngoscope
Benjamin-Havas
    B.-H. fiberoptic light clip
    B.-H. light clip
Bennett
    B. Cascade II Servo Controlled
    Heated Humidifier
    B. MA-1, PR-2 ventilator
    B. monitoring spirometer
    Nellcor Puritan B. (NPB)
    B. pressure-cycled ventilator
    B. PR-2 ventilator
    B. Slip/Stream
    B. twin
Benoject injection
Bentall
    B. cardiovascular prosthesis
    inclusion technique of B.
    B. inclusion technique
    B. operation
    B. procedure
bent bronchus sign
Bentley
    B. Duraflo II
    B. Duraflo II extracorporeal
    perfusion circuit
    B. oxygenator
    B. transducer
Benton Lines Test
Bentson
    B. exchange straight guidewire
    B. floppy-tip guidewire

Bentson-Hanafee-Wilson catheter
Benylin
    B. Cough Syrup
    B. DM
    B. Expectorant
    B. Pediatric
benzalkonium chloride asthma
benzathine
    b. benzyl penicillin
    penicillin G b.
benzoate
    caffeine and sodium b.
benzocaine
    b., butyl aminobenzoate, tetracaine,
    and benzalkonium chloride
benzodiazepine
benzonatate
benzoporphyrin
benzothiadiazide
benzothiazepine
benzoylpas
    calcium b.
    b. calcium
benzthiazide
benzylpenicillin
benzyl-thiourea
bepridil hydrochloride
BER
    benign early repolarization
beractant
beraprost sodium
Berard aneurysm
Berenstein occlusion balloon catheter
Berg Balance Scale
Berger operation
Bergmeister papilla
Bergstrom needle biopsy technique
beriberi
    cerebral b.
    dry b.
    b. heart
    infantile b.
    wet b.
Berkovits-Castellanos hexapolar electrode
Berlin
    B. nosology
    B. TAH
    B. total artificial heart
Berman
    B. airway
    B. angiographic balloon

B

NOTES

Berman *(continued)*
    B. angiographic catheter
    B. balloon flotation catheter
Bernheim syndrome
Berning and Steensgaard-Hansen score
Bernoulli
    B. effect
    B. equation
    B. theorem
Bernstein
    B. procedure
    B. test
Berotec
berry aneurysm
Berry sternal needle holder
berylliosis
beryllium
    b. disease
    b.-induced lung disease
Besnier-Boeck-Schaumann
    B.-B.-S. disease
    B.-B.-S. syndrome
BEST
    beStent clinical trial
    Beta-Blocker Evaluation of Survival Trial
    Beta-Blocker Stroke Trial
    Bolus Dose-Escalation Study of Tissue-
    Type Plasminogen Activator
    Bucindolol Evaluation of Survival Trial
    BEST+ICD clinical trial
beStent
    b. clinical trial (BEST)
    b. 2 coronary stent
    b. Rival coronary stent system
    b. Rival stent
    b. stent
BEST+ICD
    beta-blocker strategy plus implantable
    cardioverter-defibrillator
BESTNEB nebulizer
besylate
    amlodipine b.
    cisatracurium b.
BETA
beta
    b. adrenoceptor
    b. adrenoceptor stimulation
    b. agonist
    b. antagonist
    b. ARK
    b. ARK-1
    b. AR kinase1 enzyme
    b. blockade
    b. blocker
    b. blocking agent
    b. carotene
    estrogen receptor b. (ERβ)
    b. lactamase

    b. lipoprotein
    b. ray
    b. receptor
    b. thromboglobulin
beta-1
    beta-1 antagonist
    beta-1 AR
    beta-1 blocker
    beta-1 receptor
beta-2
    b.-2 antagonist
    b.-2 AR
    b.-2 AR overexpression
beta-adrenergic, β-adrenergic
    b.-a. agonist
    b.-a. blockade
    b.-a. blocker
    b.-a. blocking agent
    b.-a. receptor (βAR, BAR)
    b.-a. receptor kinase
    b.-a. stimulation
beta-1-adrenergic stimulation
beta-2-adrenergic stimulation
beta-adrenoceptor antibody
beta-adrenoreceptor
    b.-a. agonist
    b.-a. blocker
    b.-a. blocking agent
beta-beta homodimer
beta blockade
beta-blocker
    B.-b. Evaluation of Survival Trial
    (BEST)
    B.-b. Heart Attack Trial (BHAT)
    b.-b. strategy plus implantable
    cardioverter-defibrillator
    (BEST+ICD)
    B.-b. Stroke Trial (BEST)
    b.-b. therapy
Beta-Cath system
Betacel-Biotronik pacemaker
Betachron ER
Betadine Helafoam solution
beta-endorphin
17-beta-estradiol
    transdermal 17-b.-e.
beta-galactosidase
betaine diet
beta-2-integrin MAC-1
beta-lactam
beta-lactamase
    CAZ b.-l.
    b.-l. inhibitor
Betaloc Durules
betamethasone
    systemic b.
**betamethyliodophenyl pentadecanoic acid
(BMIPP)**

beta-MHC gene
beta-myosin heavy-chain gene
Betapace
    B. AF tablet
    B. Oral
Betapen-VK Oral
beta-radiation
    intracoronary b.-r.
Beta-Rail catheter
beta-sitosterol
BetaStent
    P-32 BXI-15 B.
beta-thalassemia
    homozygous -t.
beta-thromboglobulin
    b.-t. level
    plasma b.-t.
Beta-Tim
Beta-Washington Radiation for In-Stent Restenosis Trial (beta-WRIST)
beta-WRIST
    Beta-Washington Radiation for In-Stent Restenosis Trial
betaxolol hydrochloride
bethanechol chloride
bethanidine
Bethea sign
Bethune
    B. Coryllosshears
    B. lobectomy tourniquet
    B. rib shears
B101 ET Tape II adhesive tape
Bettman-Fovash thoracotome
Beuren syndrome
bevantolol
beveled thin-walled needle
bezafibrate
    B. Coronary Atherosclerosis Intervention Trial (BECAIT)
Bezalip
Bezold-Jarisch reflex
BF
    breathing frequency
    BF large core bronchoscope
bFGF
    basic fibroblast growth factor
BFV
    blood flow velocity
BG
    basal ganglia
BGO
    bismuth germanate

B-H, BH
    B-H interval
BHAT
    Beta-Blocker Heart Attack Trial
BHD
    bilateral hemisphere damage
BHFS
    benazepril heart failure study
BHI
    breath-holding index
BHR
    bronchial hyperreactivity
    bronchial hyperresponsiveness
BHT
    borderline hypertension
    butylated hydroxytoluene
BI
    brain infarct
Bianchi
    B. nodules
    B. valve
biatrial
    b. enlargement
    b. pacing
biatriatum
    cor pseudotriloculare b.
Biaxin Filmtabs
bibasally
bibasilar
    b. atelectasis
    b. coarse crackle
    b. rale
Bible printer's lung
bicalutamide
BICAP
    bipolar circumactive probe
    BICAP B unit
    BICAP unit
bicarbonate (HCO_3)
    sodium b.
bicarbonaturia
Bicarbon Sorin valve
bicardiogram
bicaval
Bicer-Val prosthetic valve
Bichat tunic
Bicillin
    B. C-R
    B. C-R 900/300
    B. L-A
    B. L-A injection
Bickel ring

NOTES

BiCNU
bicommissural aortic valve (BAV)
Bicor catheter
bicuspidalis
cuspis anterior valvae b.
bicuspid aortic valve
bicuspidization
bicycle
Aerodyne b.
Collins b.
b. dynamometer
b. echocardiography
b. ergometer exercise stress test
b. ergometry
b. exercise
b. exercise test
MedGraphics CPE 2000
electronically braked b.
stationary b.
Tredex b.
Tredex powered b.
bidimensional echocardiography
bidirectional
b. block
b. cavopulmonary anastomosis
(BCA)
b. cavopulmonary shunt
b. four-pole Butterworth high-pass
digital filter
b. Glenn operation
b. Glenn procedure (BDG)
b. isthmus conduction block
b. shunt
b. shunt calculation
b. superior cavopulmonary
anastomosis (BSCA)
b. ventricular
b. ventricular tachycardia
Bier block anesthesia
Biermer sign
bifascicular
b. block
b. heart block
biferious (*var. of* bisferious)
Bifidobacterium
bifid P wave
bifocal demand DVI pacemaker
bifoil
b. balloon
b. balloon catheter
bifurcated
b. aortofemoral prosthesis
b. graft
b. J-shaped tined atrial pacing and
defibrillation lead
b. stent
b. vein graft for vascular
reconstruction

bifurcating block
bifurcatio
b. tracheae
b. trunci
bifurcation
b. of aorta
aortic b.
carotid b.
coronary b.
b. lesion (BL)
b. lymph node
b. prosthesis
b. of pulmonary trunk
b. of trachea
tracheal b.
Y-shape b.
bifurcational coronary lesion
bigemina
Babesia b.
bigeminal
b. bisferious pulse
b. pulse
b. rhythm
bigemini
bigeminus
pulsus b.
bigeminy
atrial b.
atrioventricular junctional b.
atrioventricular nodal b.
A-V nodal b.
escape-capture b.
junctional b.
nodal b.
reciprocal b.
rule of b.
ventricular b.
big endothelin
bilateral
b. adrenal hyperplasia
b. anterior flail chest
b. aortoostial coronary artery
disease
b. bundle-branch block (BBBB)
b. hemisphere damage (BHD)
b. lung transplant (BLT)
b. sagittal split ramus osteotomies
(BSSRO)
b. sequential lung transplant
b. sequential single lung transplant
bile
b. acid binding resin
b. acid sequestrant
b. solubility test
bileaflet
b. prolapse

b. prosthesis
b. tilting-disk prosthetic valve
bilevel positive airway pressure (BiPAP)
bilevel positive pressure device
Bilharzia
bilharziasis
biliary
b. cirrhosis
b. colic
b. disease
BiliBlanket phototherapy system
Bili mask
bilious pneumonia
bilirubin
bilirubinemia
billiard ball effect
Billingham criteria
billowing
cusp b.
mitral valve b.
b. mitral valve syndrome
bilobate
bilobectomy
bilobed aneurysm
bilobular
biloculare
cor b.
Biltricide
bimanual precordial palpation
Bimodality Lung Oncology Team (BLOT)
binding
albumin cobalt b. (ACB)
guanine nucleotide modulatable b.
ligand b.
table b.
Bing stylet
Bing-Taussig heart procedure
Binswanger disease
binuclear
binucleate
bioabsorbable closure device
bioassay
bioavailability
Biobrane adhesive
Biobrane/HF graft material
BioBypass, Biobypass
B. gene-based drug delivery product
Biocef
Biocell RTV implant
biochanin A

biochemical baroreflex
Bioclate
Bioclot protein S assay
biocompatibility
biocompatible stent
Biocontrol Technology/Coratomic lead
Biocor
B. 200 high performance oxygenator
B. porcine valve
B. prosthetic valve
B. softshell venous reservoir
biodegradable stent
Biodex System
BioDiamond
B. F stent
B. Micro stent
B. S rapid exchange PTCA catheter
B. stent
BiodivYsio
B. PC stent
B. stent
bioelectric
b. current
b. potential
bioelectricity
bioequivalence
biofeedback
Biofilter
B. cardiovascular hemoconcentrator
B. hemoconcentrator
biogenesis
mitochondrial b.
BioGlue
B. protein-based surgical adhesive
B. surgical adhesive
B. surgical adhesive for aortic dissection
B. surgical patch
biogold
biograft
B. bovine heterograft material
Dakin b.
Dardik B.
B. graft
bioimpedance
b. electrocardiograph
b. monitor
thoracic electrical b.
Biolase laser adapter

NOTES

87

biologic
    GenStent b.
biological
    b. aortic valve
    B. Effects of Ionizing Radiation
    b. fitness
    b. half-life
Biomatrix ocular implant
Bio-Medicus
    B.-M. arterial catheter
    B.-M. pump
Bio-Med MVP-10 pediatric ventilator
biomembrane
bio metal surface (BMS)
Biomox
biondii
    Magnolia b.
bionic baroreflex system
Bionit
    B. vascular graft
    B. vascular prosthesis
Bioplus dispersive electrode
BioPolyMeric vascular graft
Biopore TM lead
bioprosthesis
    Carpentier-Edwards Perimount RSR
     pericardial b.
    Freestyle aortic root b.
    freestyle stentless b.
    Hancock II porcine b.
    Hancock M.O. b.
    Hancock M.O. II porcine b.
    Medtronic INTACT porcine b.
    Mosaic cardiac b.
    pericarbon b.
    Perimount RSR pericardial b.
    PhotoFix alpha pericardial b.
    porcine b.
    SJM X-Cell cardiac b.
    stentless porcine b.
    Toronto SPV b.
bioprosthetic
    b. endocarditis
    b. heart valve
biopsy
    aspiration b.
    bite b.
    bronchial brush b.
    bronchoscopic needle b.
    brush b.
    catheter-guided b.
    controlled lung b.
    cytological b.
    endomyocardial b. (EMB)
    endoscopic b.
    excisional b.
    fine-needle aspiration b.
    b. forceps

    lung b.
    mediastinal lymph node b.
    mediastinal node b.
    open lung b. (OLB)
    percutaneous needle b.
    percutaneous needle aspiration b.
    percutaneous transthoracic needle b.
     (PTNB)
    pericardial b.
    pleural b.
    punch b.
    scalene fat pad b.
    scalene lymph node b.
    supraclavicular lymph node b.
    surgical lung b. (SLB)
    transbronchial b. (TBB, TBBX,
     TBBx)
    transbronchial lung b. (TBLB)
    transthoracic needle b. (TNB)
    transthoracic needle aspiration b.
    transvenous b.
    ultrasonically guided needle b.
     (UGNB)
    ventricular b.
    video-assisted thoracic surgical
     lung b.
    wedge b.
bioptic sampling
bioptome
    Bycep PC Jr b.
    cardiac b.
    Caves b.
    Caves-Schultz b.
    Cordis b.
    Kawai b.
    King b.
    Konno b.
    Mansfield b.
    Olympus b.
    Scholten endomyocardial b.
    Stanford b.
    Stanford-Caves b.
Bio-Pump
Biorate pacemaker
bioresorbable implant
Biosense
    B. left ventricular mapping
    B. mapping system
    B. NOGA catheter-based
     endocardial mapping system
    B. system
    B. Webster
**Biosense-guided laser myocardial
  revascularization**
Biosound
    B. Genesis II scanning system
    B. 2000 II s.a. high-resolution
     ultrasound

B. Phase 2 ultrasound system
B. Surgiscan echocardiograph
B. 2000 II ultrasound unit
B. 3000 ultrasound unit
B. wide-angle monoplane ultrasound scanner

BioSource Cytoscreen SAA kit
Biostent
Biosurge Synchronous Autotransfuser
biosynthesis
leukotriene b.
Biot
B. breathing
B. respiration
B. sign
Bio-Tab Oral
biotin/streptavidin system
Biotrack coagulation monitor
biotransformation
Biotronik
B. lead
B. lead connector
B. pacemaker
Bio-Vascular prosthetic valve
BI-OX III ear oximeter
BioZ
B. hemodynamic monitoring system
B. noninvasive cardiac function monitoring system
B. system
BioZ.com cardiac output monitor
BioZ.pc system
BioZtect sensor
BIP
bronchiolitis with interstitial pneumonitis
BIP study
BIP trial
BiPAP
bilevel positive airway pressure
BiPAP duet system
BiPAP S/T-D 30 system
BiPAP S/T-D ventilatory support system
BiPAP unit
BiPAP Vision system
biperiden
biphasic
b. mesothelioma
b. response
b. shock
b. stridor
b. waveform

b. waveform transthoracic defibrillation
biplanar tomography
biplane
b. aortography
b. area-length method
b. fluoroscopy
b. formula
b. imaging
b. orthogonal angiography
b. pelvic arteriography
b. quantitative coronary arteriography
b. ventriculography
bipolar
b. catheter
b. circumactive probe (BICAP)
b. coagulating forceps
b. esophageal recording
b. generator
b. lead
b. limb leads
b. myocardial electrode
b. pacemaker
BiPort hemostasis introducer sheath kit
Biquin Durules
Birbeck granules
Bird
B. Ascension ventilator
B. Asthmastik
B. low-flow blender
B. machine
B. micronebulizer
B. neonatal CPAP generator
B. sign
B. 8400STi ventilator
B. VDR ventilator
B. ventilator
bird
b. fever
bird-breeder's lung
bird-fancier's lung
bird's
b.-eye catheter
b. nest filter
b. nest lesion
b. nest vena cava filter
birefringence
birminghamensis
Legionella b.
Birtcher defibrillator
bis(chloromethyl) ether

NOTES

bisferiens
pulsus b.
bisferient
bisferious, biferious
b. pulse
bishop's
b. hat
b. nod
Bishop sphygmoscope
bishydroxycoumarin
bismesylate
almitrine b.
bismuth
b. germanate (BGO)
b. subsalicylate
Bisolvon
bisoprolol
b. fumarate
b. and hydrochlorothiazide
Bisping electrode
bistoury
Jackson b.
bisulfate
clopidogrel b.
bitartrate
hydrocodone b.
metaraminol b.
norepinephrine b.
bite
b. biopsy
b. block
bitolterol mesylate
Bitpad digitizer
BIT-Sternchen Test
BIVAD (*var. of* BVAD)
bivalirudin
bivalve
biventricular
b. assist device (BVAD, BIVAD)
b. direct cardiac compression
b. dysfunction
b. endomyocardial fibrosis
b. pacing
b. pacing wire
b. support (BVS)
Bivona
B. Fome-Cuff tube
B. TTS tracheostomy tube
Bivona-Colorado voice prosthesis
bizarre QRS complex
Bizzari-Guiffrida laryngoscope
Björk method of Fontan procedure
Björk-Shiley
B.-S. aortic valve prosthesis
B.-S. convexoconcave 60-degree
valve prosthesis
B.-S. convexoconcave disk
prosthetic valve

B.-S. floating disk prosthesis
B.-S. graft
B.-S. heart valve holder
B.-S. heart valve sizer
B.-S. mitral valve
B.-S. monostrut valve
B.-S. prosthetic valve
B.-S. valve
BL
bifurcation lesion
Blac
Linctus Codeine B.
black
B. Creek Canal virus
b. lung
b. lung disease
b. phthisis
b. pleura
b. pleura sign
b. widow spider venom
black-blood magnetic resonance imaging
Blackfan-Diamond syndrome
blackfoot disease
Blackman window
blackout
shallow water b.
b. spell
black-white interface technique
blade
Acra-Cut Spiral craniotome b.
b. atrial septostomy
Bard-Parker b.
Beaver b.
Beaver-DeBakey b.
CLM articulating laryngoscope b.
b. control wire holder
Cooley-Pontius sternal b.
DeBakey b.
electrosurgical b.
knife b.
Lite B.
RAD Airway laryngeal b.
Rosenkranz deep retractor b.
Rosenkranz small retractor b.
SCA-EX ShortCutter catheter with
rotating b.'s
b. septostomy
b. septostomy catheter
Blake exercise stress test
Blalock-Hanlon
B.-H. atrial septectomy
B.-H. operation
Blalock-Niedner pulmonic stenosis clamp
Blalock pulmonary stenosis clamp
Blalock-Taussig
B.-T. operation
B.-T. procedure
B.-T. shunt

blanche
 tache b.
blanch test
bland
 b. diet
 b. edema
 b. embolism
Bland-Altman method
Bland-Garland-White syndrome
blanket
 Bair Hugger b.
 bronchial mucus b.
 circulating water b.
 cooling b.
 hypothermia b.
blanking
 b. period
 postventricular atrial b. (PVAB)
 total atrial b. (TAB)
blast
 b. chest
 b. lung
 b. wave
blastoma
 pleuropulmonary b.
 pulmonary b.
Blastomyces dermatitidis
blastomycosis
 North American b.
BLB
 Boothby-Lovelace-Bulbulian
 BLB mask
 BLB oxygen mask
bleb
 apical pleural b.
 emphysematous b.
 pleural b.
 sarcolemmal b.
 b. stapling
bleeding
 arterial b.
 back-b.
 b. diathesis
 extraparenchymal b.
 b. globe
blender
 Bird low-flow b.
 MAXBlend oxygen/air b.
 Virtis b.
blending
 sensor b.
blennothorax

Blenoxane
bleomycin sulfate
BLES
 bovine lavage extract surfactant
blind
 b. coronary dimple
 b. cul-de-sac
 b. esophageal brushing (BEB)
 b. thoracentesis
bloater
 blue b.
bloc
 en b.
 heart-lung b.
Blocadren Oral
Bloch equation
block
 Adult Universal bite b. B116
 alveolar-capillary b.
 anatomic b.
 antegrade b.
 anterograde b.
 arborization b.
 atrioventricular b.
 atrioventricular junctional heart b.
 A-V b.
 A-V branch b.
 A-V groove b.
 A-V Wenckebach b.
 axillary b.
 bed b.
 bidirectional b.
 bidirectional isthmus conduction b.
 bifascicular b.
 bifascicular heart b.
 bifurcating b.
 bilateral bundle-branch b. (BBBB)
 bite b.
 bundle-branch b. (BBB)
 B. cardiac device
 complete A-V b.
 complete heart b. (CHB)
 conduction b.
 congenital complete heart b.
 congenital heart b.
 congenital symptomatic A-V b.
 connector b.
 b. cycle length
 diffuse intraventricular b.
 divisional b.
 divisional heart b.
 entrance b.

NOTES

block *(continued)*
    exit b.
    familial atrioventricular b.
    fascicular b.
    fascicular heart b.
    first-degree A-V b.
    first-degree heart b.
    focal b.
    functional b.
    heart b.
    3:1 heart b.
    3:2 heart b.
    heparin b.
    His bundle heart b.
    incomplete atrioventricular b.
    infrahisian b.
    interatrial b.
    intercostal nerve b.
    intraatrial b.
    intrahisian b.
    intraventricular b. (IVB)
    left bundle-branch b. (LBBB)
    Luciani-Wenckebach
      atrioventricular b.
    Mobitz b.
    Mobitz II A-V heart b.
    Mobitz second-degree b.
    Mobitz type A-V b.
    Mobitz type I A-V b.
    Mobitz type I, II
      atrioventricular b.
    Mobitz type II SA b.
    Mobitz types of atrioventricular b.
    nonspecific intraventricular b.
    paraffin b.
    partial heart b.
    Pediatric universal bite b. B117
    periinfarction b.
    Perspex b.
    protective b.
    protoplasmic b.
    pseudo-A-V b.
    rate-dependent bundle branch b.
    retrograde b.
    right bundle-branch b. (RBBB)
    B. right coronary guiding catheter
    second-degree A-V b.
    second-degree heart b.
    shock b.'s
    sinoatrial b.
    sinoatrial exit b.
    sinoauricular b.
    sinus exit b.
    subjunctional heart b.
    suprahisian b.
    suprahisian b.
    third-degree atrioventricular b.
    third-degree A-V b.

    third-degree heart b.
    transient heart b.
    trifascicular b.
    unidirectional b.
    unifascicular b.
    vagal b.
    ventricular b.
    voltage-dependent b.
    Wenckebach b.
    Wenckebach atrioventricular b.
    Wenckebach A-V b.
    Wenckebach exit b.
    Wenckebach periodicity b.
    Wilson b.

blockade
    aggressive platelet b.
    alpha-1 adrenoceptor b.
    angiotensin II-receptor b.
    beta b.
    beta-adrenergic b.
    Evaluation of PTCA to Improve
      Long-Term Outcome by c7E3
      GPIIb/IIIa Receptor B. (EPILOG)
    left stellate ganglionic b. (LSGB)
    neuromuscular b.
    platelet glycoprotein IIb/IIIa b.
    sodium channel b.
    stellate ganglion b.

blocked
    b. APC
    b. fascicle
    b. heart artery
    b. pleurisy

blocker
    adrenoceptor b.
    aldosterone-receptor b.
    alpha-adrenergic b.
    alpha-adrenoreceptor b.
    angiotensin II-receptor b. (ARB)
    beta b.
    beta-1 b.
    beta-adrenergic b.
    beta-adrenoreceptor b.
    calcium channel b.
    calcium-channel b. (CCB)
    calcium entry b.
    ganglionic b.
    integrin b.
    L-type calcium b.
    platelet glycoprotein IIb/IIIa b.
    renin-angiotensin b.
    selectin b.
    slow-channel b.
    sodium-channel b.

blocking
    b. vagal afferent fiber
    b. vagal efferent fiber

Blom-Singer
B.-S. indwelling low-pressure voice prosthesis
B.-S. valve

blood
arterial b.
artificial b.
autologous b.
b. cardioplegia
b. cast
b. clot
clot of b.
b. column
b. count
b. dyscrasia
b. expander
b. flow
b. flow measurement
b. flowmeter
b. flow reserve
b. flow velocity (BFV)
Fluosol artificial b.
frank b.
b. gas
840 b. gas analyzer
1620 b. gas analyzer
b. gas sensor
mixed venous b.
b. monocyte stimulation
b. murmur
b. oxygen
b. oxygenation level-dependent (BOLD)
b. oxygenation level-dependent technique
b. oxygen level
oxygen saturation of the hemoglobin of arterial b.
b. patch injection
b. perfusion
b. perfusion monitor (BPM)
b. platelet thrombus
b. plate thrombus
b. pool
b. pressure (BP)
b. pressure cuff
B. Pressure, Renal Effects, Insulin Control, Lipids, Lisinopril, and Nifedipine Trial (BRILLIANT)
b. pump
b. replacement
b. sampling

b. sampling instrument
shear rate of b.
shunted b.
sludged b.
tonometered whole b.
b. urea nitrogen (BUN)
venous b.
b. viscosity
b. volume
b. volume distribution
b. warmer
blood-air barrier
blood-borne infectious agent
blood-brain barrier (BBB)
blood-bronchoalveolar barrier
blood-bronchus barrier
blood-flow probe
blood-gas barrier
bloodless phlebotomy
bloodletting
blood-pool imaging
blood-retina barrier
bloodstream
blood-tinged sputum
Bloodwell forceps
bloody
b. effusion
b. sputum
b. tap
Bloom
B. programmable stimulator
B. syndrome
blooming
b. artifact
b. effect
BLOT
Bimodality Lung Oncology Team
blot
Northern b.
slot b.
Southern b.
b. test
Western b.
blow
b. bottle
diastolic b.
blow-by
b.-b. oxygen
b.-b. ventilator
blowing
b. murmur
b. wound

NOTES

blowout injury
BLS
    basic life support
BLT
    bilateral lung transplant
blubbery diastolic murmur
blue
    b. asphyxia
    b. baby
    b. bloater
    code b.
    b. Cook sheath
    b. disease
    Evans b.
    b. finger syndrome
    B. FlexTip catheter
    B. Line cuffed endotracheal tube
    B. Max high-pressure balloon
    B. Max triple-lumen catheter
    methylene b.
    b. phlebitis
    b. sclera
    Sulphan B.
    b. toe syndrome
    b. velvet syndrome
Blum arterial scissors
Blumenau test
Blumenthal lesion
blunt
    b. cardiac rupture
    b. chest impact-induced cardiac arrest
    b. chest injury
    b. chest trauma
    b. eversion
    b. eversion carotid endarterectomy
    b. injury
    b. pulmonary injury
    b. thoracic trauma
    b. torso injury
    b. trauma
blunted
    b. costophrenic angle
    b. ejection fraction
    b. exercise response
    b. flow
    b. systolic pulmonary venous flow
    b. systolic velocity
    b. waveform
blunting
    apical b.
    nocturnal cardiovascular b.
blush
    capillary b.
    myocardial b.
    b. phenomenon
    tumor b.

BMC
    balloon mitral commissurotomy
    bone mineral content
BMI
    body mass index
BMIPP
    betamethyliodophenyl pentadecanoic acid
    I-123 BMIPP
B-mode
    B.-m. echocardiography
    B.-m. ultrasonography
    B.-m. ultrasound
BMP-2
    bone morphogenetic protein type 2
BMR-4500SG sealed hard shell venous reservoir with Duraflo
BMS
    bio metal surface
BMS-186716
BMV
    balloon mitral valvuloplasty
BNA
    bronchoscopic needle aspiration
BNA-100-Behring Diagnostics immunonephelometer
BNP
    brain natriuretic peptide
    B-type natriuretic peptide
BO
    bronchiolitis obliterans
board
    SummaSketch III digitizing b.
BOAT
    balloon versus optimal atherectomy trial
boat-shaped heart
Bobath
    B. exercise
    B. physiotherapy approach
Bochdalek hernia
Bock ganglion
Bodai adapter
body
    aortic b.
    b. of Arantius
    Arantius b.
    asbestos b.'s
    Aschoff b.
    aspiration of foreign b.
    asteroid b.
    Auer b.
    Babes-Ernst b.
    b. box method
    Bracht-Wächter b.'s
    carotid b.
    central fibrous b.
    creola b.
    b. density analysis
    Döhle inclusion b.'s

b. fat
ferruginous b.
fibrous b.
foreign b.
Gamna-Gandy b.'s
gelatin compression b.
Gordon elementary b.
Heinz b.
LCL b.'s
b. mass index (BMI)
Masson b.
Medlar b.
multilamellar b.
Negri b.
neuroepithelial b.
paraaortic b.'s
b. of phalanx
b. plethysmograph
b. position
psammoma b.'s
psittacosis inclusion b.'s
b. surface area (BSA)
b. surface Laplacian mapping
  (BSLM)
thoracic vertebral b.
tracheobronchial foreign b.
vagal b.
Weibel-Palade b.'s
Zuckerkandl b.'s
**The Bodyguard emboli containment
  system**
Boeck
B. disease
B. sarcoid
Boehringer
B. Mannheim standard
B. suction regulator
Boerema hernia repair
Boerhaave
B. syndrome
B. tear
Boettcher forceps
Bogalusa criteria
boggy edema
Bogros space
Bohr
B. effect
B. equation
B. formula
B. isopleth method
bois
bruit de b.

BOLD
blood oxygenation level-dependent
BOLD technique
bolometer
bolster
Teflon felt b.
bolt
Camino microventricular b.
Boltzmann distribution
bolus
b. cardiac output calculation
B. Dose-Escalation Study of
  Tissue-Type Plasminogen Activator
  (BEST)
b. injection
b. intravenous injection
b. of medication
b. tracking
bombesin
Bonchek-Shiley
B.-S. cardiac jacket
B.-S. vein distention system
bond
soldered b.
bone
fibrous dysplasia of b.
lingual b.
b. marrow aplasia
b. marrow embolism
b. marrow transplant
b. mineral content (BMC)
b. morphogenetic protein type 2
  (BMP-2)
Paget disease of b.
pharyngeal tubercle of basilar part
  of occipital b.
Bonferroni
B. correction
B. method
boning
dog b.
bony heart
Bonzel Monorail balloon catheter
bookeri
Alcaligenes b.
Bookwalter retractor
booming rumble
BOOP
bronchiolitis obliterans with organizing
  pneumonia
booster heart

NOTES

B

95

boot
   Bunny b.
   Circulator b.
   compression b.
   Cryo/Cuff pressure b.
   gelatin compression b.
   IPC b.'s
   PNS Unna b.
   sheepskin b.
   Unna paste b.
Boothby-Lovelace-Bulbulian (BLB)
   Boothby-Lovelace-Bulbulian oxygen
   mask
boot-shaped heart
bootstrap
   b. dilation
   b. two-vessel angioplasty
   b. two-vessel technique
border
   b. of cardiac dullness
   endocardial b.
   endocardial cardiac b.
   epicardial cardiac b.
   b. rale
   sternal b.
borderline
   b. cardiomegaly
   b. ECG
   b. hypertension (BHT)
Bordetella pertussis
Bordet-Gengou
   B.-G. bacillus
   B.-G. test
Borg
   B. category-ratio
   B. dyspnea rating
   B. numerical scale
   B. Scale
   B. 6 to 20 scale
   B. treadmill exertion scale
Born aggregometry
Bornholm disease
boronic acid technetium dioxime
Boros esophagoscope
Borrelia burgdorferi
borreliosis
   Lyme b.
Borst side-arm introducer set
BOS
   bronchiolitis obliterans syndrome
Bosch ERG 500 ergometer
bosentan
Bosher commissurotomy knife
BosPac cardiopulmonary bypass system
Bostock
   B. catarrh
   B. disease

Boston Scientific Sonicath imaging
   catheter
Botallo duct
botryomycosis
   pulmonary b.
Böttcher space
bottle
   blow b.
   Castaneda b.
   Plasma-Plex b.
   b. sound
bottle-neck stenosis
botulinum
   Clostridium b.
Bouchut respiration
bougie
   bronchoscopic b.
   Celestin b.
   EndoLumina illuminated b.
bougienage
   esophageal b.
Bouillaud
   B. disease
   B. sign
   B. tinkle
bounding pulse
bouquet of vessels
Bourassa catheter
Bourdon gauge
Bourns
   B.-Bear ventilator
   B. infant respirator
   B. infant ventilator
Boutin thoracoscope
Bouveret disease
Bovie
   B. electrocautery
   B. ultrasound aspirator
bovine
   b. allograft
   b. biodegradable collagen
   b. collagen plug device
   b. heart
   b. heart valve
   b. heterograft
   b. lavage extract surfactant (BLES)
   pegademase b. (PEG-ADA)
   b. pericardial heart valve xenograft
   b. pericardial valve
   b. pericardium strip
bovinum
   cor b.
bovis
   Actinomyces b.
   Babesia b.
   Mycobacterium b.
Bowditch
   B. law

B

B. phenomenon
B. staircase effect
bowing
    leftward ventricular septal b.
      (LVSB)
    b. of mitral valve leaflet
box
    bronchoscopic battery b.
    digital constant-current pacing b.
    Elecath switch b.
    b. plot
    SunBox light b.
box-and-whisker plot
Boyce sign
Boyd
    B. perforating vein
    B. point
Boydens chamber
boydii
    Petriellidium b.
    Pseudallescheria b.
Boyle
    B. Gay-Lusac law
    B. law
bozemanii
    Legionella b.
Bozzolo sign
BP
    blood pressure
    British Pharmacopoeia
    bronchopulmonary
      BP fistula
BPD
    bronchopulmonary dysplasia
BPM
    blood perfusion monitor
bpm
    beats per minute
BPV
    balloon pulmonary valvuloplasty
BPXG body plethysmograph
BQ-123
Bq
    becquerel
BR
    breathing reserve
    bronchial responsiveness
BR1 contrast agent
brachial
    b. arteriogram
    b. arteriotomy
    b. artery

b. artery approach
b. artery cutdown
b. artery thrombosis
b. bypass
b. catheter
b. dance
b. nerve
b. plexopathy
b. plexus
b. plexus injury
b. pulse
b. syndrome
b. vein
brachial-ankle index
brachial, radial, femoral (BRAFE)
brachioaxillary bridge graft fistula
brachiocephalic
    b. arteritis
    b. artery
    b. ischemia
    b. system
    b. trunk
    b. vein
    b. vessel angioplasty
brachiogram
brachiosubclavian bridge graft fistula
Bracht-Wächter
    B.-W. bodies
    B.-W. lesion
brachycardia
brachytherapy
    endobronchial b.
Bradbury-Eggleston syndrome
Bradilan
Bradshaw-O'Neill aorta clamp
bradyarrhythmia
bradyarrhythmic arrest
bradycardia
    artifactual b.
    atrial b.
    Branham b.
    cardiomuscular b.
    central b.
    clinostatic b.
    essential b.
    fetal b.
    idiopathic b.
    idioventricular b.
    junctional b.
    nodal b.
    b. pacing support
    postinfectious b.

NOTES

bradycardia *(continued)*
    postinfective b.
    pulseless b.
    sinoatrial b.
    sinus b.
    vagal b.
    ventricular b.
bradycardiac, bradycardic
bradycardia-dependent aberrancy
bradycardia-tachycardia syndrome
bradycardic *(var. of* bradycardiac)
bradycrotic
bradydactyly
bradydiastole
brady down
bradydysrhythmia
bradykinin
    b. perfusion
    b.-stimulated cells
bradypnea
bradyrhythmia
bradysphygmia
bradytachycardia syndrome
bradytachydysrhythmia
brady-tachy syndrome
BRAFE
    brachial, radial, femoral
Bragg-Paul respirator
braid-like lesion
brain
    b. aneurysm
    b. band enzyme of CPK (CPK-BB)
    b. death
    b. infarct (BI)
    b. murmur
    b. natriuretic peptide (BNP)
    b. stem stroke
    b. wave
brain-heart infusion
branch
    descending anterior b.
    descending posterior b.
    diagonal b. #1 (D1)
    esophageal b.
    jailed side b.
    b. lesion
    lingual b.
    marginal b. #1
    obtuse marginal b. (OMB)
    pharyngeal b.
    b. pulmonary artery stenosis
    b. retinal artery occlusion (BRAO)
    b. retinal vein occlusion (BRVO)
    b.'s of segmental bronchi
    septal perforator b.
    side b.
    tracheal b.

    b. vessel occlusion
    b. vessel pruning
branched chain alpha ketoacid dehydrogenase (BCKD)
branching
    airway b.
    mirror-image brachiocephalic b.
branchiogenic
branchiomere
branchiomerism
branchiomotor
Brandt cytology balloon
Branham
    B. bradycardia
    B. sign
Branhamella catarrhalis
BRAO
    branch retinal artery occlusion
Brasdor method
Brasfield chest radiograph score
brash
    water b.
brasiliensis
    Nocardia b.
    Paracoccidioides b.
brassy cough
BRAT
    Baylor rapid autologous transfusion
    BRAT system
Brauer cardiolysis
Braunwald
    B. classification (I–IIIB)
    B. sign
Braunwald-Cutter
    B.-C. ball prosthetic valve
    B.-C. ball valve prosthesis
brawny edema
braziliense
    Ancylostoma b.
bread-and-butter
    b.-a.-b. pericardium
    b.-a.-b. textbook sign
bread knife valvulotome
breakaway splice
Breas
    B. CPAP device
    B. PV10 CPAP device
breast
    b. artifact
    b. pang
    thrush b.
breath
    b. excretion test
    exercise-induced shortness of b.
    b. marker
    b. pentane test
    shortness of b. (SOB)

B

b. sound
b. stacking
breath-actuated inhaler (BAI)
Breather
The Sports B.
Breathe Right nasal strip
breathhold
b. maneuver
b., turbo-flash tagged imaging
breath-holding
b.-h. index (BHI)
b.-h. test
breathing
apneustic b.
b. bag sign
Biot b.
bronchial b.
Cheyne-Stokes b.
controlled b.
b. exercise
b. frequency (BF)
frog b.
glossopharyngeal b.
intermittent positive pressure b. (IPPB)
Kussmaul b.
Ondine's curse b.
b. pacemaker
periodic b.
positive-negative pressure b. (PNPB)
pursed-lip b.
b. reserve (BR)
resting tidal b.
shallow b.
sign mechanism for ventilator b.
sleep-disordered b. (SDB)
b. technique
tidal b.
work of b. (WOB)
Brechenmacher fiber
Brecher and Cronkite technique
Breeze E150 ventilation system
bregmocardiac reflex
Brehmer treatment
Bremer AirFlo Vest
Brenner carotid bypass shunt
Breonesin
brequinar sodium
Brescia-Cimino A-V fistula
Breslow-Day test for homogeneity
Brethaire Inhalation Aerosol

Brethine
B. injection
B. Oral
Bretonneau angina
Bretschneider-HTK cardioplegic solution
Brett syndrome
Bretylate
bretylium
b. infusion
b. loading
b. therapy
b. tosylate
Bretylol
Breuer-Hering
B.-H. deflation index
B.-H. inflation reflex
Brevibloc injection
Brevital
Bricanyl
B. injection
B. Oral
B. Turbohaler
bridge
arteriolovenular b.
cytoplasmic b.
disulfide b.
muscle b.
myocardial b.
Wheatstone b.
B. X3 renal stent system
bridging
b. collateral
muscular b.
myocardial b. (MB)
Bright
B. disease
B. murmur
bright echo
brightness modulation
BRILLIANT
Blood Pressure, Renal Effects, Insulin Control, Lipids, Lisinopril, and Nifedipine Trial
Brilliant lead
Brill-Zinsser disease
B-ring
esophageal B.-r.
Brisbane method
brisk wall motion abnormality
Brite Tip catheter
British Pharmacopoeia (BP)

NOTES

brittle
- b. asthma
- b. asthmatic

Broadbent
- B. inverted sign
- B. sign

broad QRS complex

Brock
- B. infundibulectomy
- B. operation
- B. procedure
- B. syndrome

Brockenbrough
- B. angiocatheter
- B. atrial septoplasty
- B. atrial stenting
- B. cardiac device
- B. catheter
- B. curved needle
- B. curved-tip occluder
- B. device
- B. effect
- B. mapping catheter
- B. needle
- B. sign
- B. technique
- B. transseptal catheter
- B. transseptal commissurotomy

Brockenbrough-Braunwald-Morrow sign

Brockenbrough-Braunwald sign

brocresine

Broders index

Brodie abscess

Brodie-Trendelenburg
- B.-T. test
- B.-T. tourniquet test

Brodmann
- B. area 7
- B. area 9
- B. area 24
- B. area 40

Bromanate DC

Bromanyl Cough Syrup

bromazepam

Bromfed

bromhexine hydrochloride

bromide
- ethidium b.
- hydrogen b.
- ipratropium b.
- methyl b.
- oxitropium b.
- pancuronium b.
- pipecuronium b.
- tiotropium b.

bromocriptine

bromodiphenhydramine and codeine

Bromotuss w/Codeine Cough Syrup

Bromphen DC w/Codeine

brompheniramine
- B., phenylpropanolamine, and codeine

Brompton
- B. cocktail
- B. solution

Brom repair

Bronalide

broncatar

bronchadenitis, bronchoadenitis

bronchi (*pl. of* bronchus)

bronchia

Bronchial

bronchial
- b. adenoma
- b. allergy
- b. arteriography
- b. artery
- b. artery embolization (BAE)
- b. asthma
- b. atresia
- b. breathing
- b. breath sounds
- b. brush biopsy
- b. brushings
- b. bud
- b. calculus
- b. carcinoma
- b. challenge test
- b. collateral
- b. collateral artery murmur
- b. crisis
- b. cyst
- b. dehiscence
- b. disruption
- b. epithelial cell
- b. fremitus
- b. gland
- b. hyperreactivity (BHR)
- b. hyperresponsiveness (BHR)
- b. inflammatory polyp
- b. lavage
- b. lumen
- b. marking
- b. meniscus sign
- b. microflora
- b. mucous membrane
- b. mucus blanket
- b. mucus inhibitor
- b. pneumonia
- b. polyp
- b. provocation
- b. provocation challenge test
- b. provocation test
- b. rale
- b. respiration
- b. responsiveness (BR)

b. sarcoidosis
b. sleeve resection
b. smooth muscle
b. smooth muscle tone
b. spasm
b. stenosis
b. stump
b. stump failure
b. toilet
b. tree
b. tube
b. vein
b. washings
b. washings cytology
b. wheezing

bronchiales
rami b.
venae b.

bronchiectasia sicca
bronchiectasis
chemical b.
cylindrical b.
cystic b.
dry b.
follicular b.
fusiform b.
pseudocylindrical b.
saccular b.
suppurative b.
traction b.

bronchiectatic
b. cavity
b. rale

bronchiloquy
bronchiocele
bronchiogenic
bronchiolar
b. adenocarcinoma
b. carcinoma
b. exocrine cell
b. inflammatory infiltrate

bronchiole
alveolar b.
b.-alveolar communication
respiratory b.
terminal b.

bronchiolectasia
bronchiolectasis
traction b.

bronchioli (*pl. of* bronchiolus)
bronchiolitis
acute obliterating b.

constrictive b.
b. exudativa
exudative b.
b. fibrosa obliterans
follicular b.
infectious b.
b. obliterans (BO)
b. obliterans syndrome (BOS)
b. obliterans with organizing
pneumonia (BOOP)
obliterative b. (OB)
proliferative b.
respiratory b. (RB)
vesicular b.
viral b.
b. with interstitial pneumonitis
(BIP)

bronchioloalveolar
b. adenocarcinoma
b. carcinoma (BAC)

bronchiolocentric
bronchiolopulmonary
bronchiolus, pl. **bronchioli**
b. terminalis

bronchiomediastinalis
truncus lymphaticus b.

bronchiorum
tunica muscularis b.

bronchiostenosis
bronchitic
bronchitis
acute bacterial exacerbation of
chronic b. (ABECB)
acute exacerbation of chronic b.
(AECB)
acute laryngotracheal b.
arachidic b.
asthmatic b.
capillary b.
Castellani b.
catarrhal b.
cheesy b.
chemical b.
chronic asthmatic b.
chronic obstructive b.
croupous b.
dry b.
epidemic capillary b.
ether b.
exudative b.
fibrinous b.
hemorrhagic b.

NOTES

bronchitis *(continued)*
    infectious asthmatic b.
    mechanic's b.
    membranous b.
    nonasthmatic eosinophilic b.
    b. obliterans
    obliterative b.
    phthinoid b.
    plastic b.
    polypoid b.
    productive b.
    pseudomembranous b.
    putrid b.
    secondary b.
    b. sicca
    simple chronic b.
    smoker's b.
    staphylococcal b.
    streptococcal b.
    suffocative b.
    vegetal b.
    verminous b.
    vesicular b.
    wheezy b.
    winter b.
Bronchitrac
    B. L catheter
    B. L flexible suction catheter
bronchium
bronchoadenitis *(var. of* bronchadenitis)
bronchoalveolar
    b. carcinoma
    b. lavage (BAL)
    b. lavage fluid (BALF)
    b. washings
bronchoalveolitis
bronchoaspergillosis
bronchoblastomycosis
bronchoblennorrhea
bronchocandidiasis
Broncho-Cath double-lumen endotracheal tube
bronchocavernous respiration
bronchocele
bronchocentric granulomatosis (BCG)
bronchoconstriction
    hyperpnea-induced b. (HIB)
    reflex b.
    reflex vagal b.
bronchoconstrictive effect
bronchoconstrictor
bronchodilating agent
bronchodilation, bronchodilatation
bronchodilator (BDT)
    b. administration
    aerosolized b.
    anticholinergic b.
    b. effect

    inhaled b.
    Marax b.
    nebulized b.
    b. response
    b. therapy
bronchoedema
bronchoegophony
bronchoesophageal muscle
bronchoesophageus
    musculus b.
bronchoesophagoscopy
bronchofiberscope
bronchogenic
    b. adenocarcinoma
    b. carcinoma
    b. cyst
bronchogram
    air b.
    tantalum b.
bronchography
    Cope method b.
    inhalation b.
    percutaneous transtracheal b.
broncholith
broncholithiasis
bronchomalacia
bronchomediastinal lymphatic trunk
bronchomotor
bronchophony
    pectoriloquous b.
    sniffling b.
    whispered b.
bronchopleural fistula
bronchopleuropneumonia
bronchopneumonia
    acute hemorrhagic b.
    confluent b.
    diffuse b.
    focal b.
    hemorrhagic b.
    hypostatic b.
    necrotizing b.
    sequestration b.
    subacute b.
    tuberculous b.
    virus b.
bronchopneumonic infiltrate
bronchopneumonitis
bronchoprovocation test
bronchopulmonale
    segmentum b.
bronchopulmonales
    nodi lymphoidei b.
bronchopulmonary (BP)
    apicoposterior b. segment [SI + SII]
    b. aspergillosis
    b. carcinoid tumor

b. cyst
b. dysplasia (BPD)
b. fistula
b. lymph node
b. segment
b. spasm
b. tissue
b. tract
b. venous fistula
b. washings
bronchorrhea
Broncho Saline
bronchoscope
Albert slotted b.
BF large core b.
Broyles b.
Bruening b.
Chevalier Jackson b.
Davis b.
Dumon b.
Dumon-Harrell b.
Emerson b.
fiberoptic b.
flexible fiberoptic b.
Fujinon flexible b.
Kernan-Jackson b.
Michelson b.
Moersch b.
Negus b.
Negus-Broyles b.
Overholt-Jackson b.
Pentax b.
Pilling b.
respiration b.
Riecker respiration b.
Safar b.
Storz b.
Tucker b.
ventilation b.
Waterman b.
Yankauer b.
bronchoscopic
b. aspirator
b. battery box
b. bougie
b. brush
b. electrocautery
b. face shield
b. magnet
b. needle aspiration (BNA)
b. needle biopsy

b. smear
b. ultrasound
bronchoscopist
bronchoscopy
diagnostic b.
fiberoptic b. (FB, FOB)
flexible fiberoptic b. (FFB)
fluorescence b.
laser b.
b. quality improvement project
rigid b.
surveillance b.
therapeutic b.
ultrasound-guided b.
virtual b. (VB)
bronchospasm
allergic b.
exercise-induced b. (EIB)
paradoxical b.
reversible b.
bronchospastic component
bronchospirography
bronchospirometer
bronchospirometry
differential b.
bronchostenosis
bronchotracheal aspirate
bronchovascular bundle
bronchovenous fistula
bronchovesicular
b. breath sounds
b. marking
b. respiration
bronchus, pl. **bronchi**
anomalous b.
apical b.
basal segmental b.
branches of segmental bronchi
cardiac b.
ectopic b.
eparterial b.
hyparterial bronchi
intermediate b.
b. intermedius
left main b.
lingular b.
lobar b.
bronchi lobares
lower lobe b.
main stem b.
middle lobe b.
mucosa of b.

B

NOTES

bronchus (*continued*)
    muscular coat of b.
    primary b.
    b. principalis dexter
    b. principalis sinister
    right main b.
    secondary b.
    segmental b.
    b. segmentalis
    stem b.
    subsegmental b.
    b. suis
    supernumerary b.
    4th/5th/6th order bronchi
    tracheal b.
    tunica mucosa bronchi
    upper lobe b.
bronchus-associated lymphoid tissue (BALT)
bronchus-grasping forceps
Bronitin Mist
Bronkaid Mist
Bronkephrine injection
Bronkodyl
Bronkolid
Bronkometer
Bronkosol
Brontex
    B. Liquid
    B. Tablet
Brookfield viscometer
broth
    b. test
    Todd-Hewitt b.
Broviac atrial catheter
Brown
    B.-Adson forceps
    B.-Dodge method
    B.-McHardy pneumatic dilator
    B. and Sharp digital electronic calipers
brown
    b. atrophy
    b. edema
    b. induration of lung
    b. sputum
    b. urine
Broyles
    B. anterior commissure laryngoscope
    B. bronchoscope
Brozek formula
BRS
    baroreceptor reflex sensitivity
    baroreflex sensitivity
Bruce
    B. bundle
    B. exercise stress test

    B. protocol
    B. treadmill protocol
brucei
    Trypanosoma b.
Brucella melitensis
brucellosis
Bruening bronchoscope
Brugada syndrome
Brughleman needle
Brugia
    B. malayi
    B. timori
bruit
    abdominal b.
    aneurysmal b.
    carotid b.
    b. d'airain
    b. de bois
    b. de canon
    b. de choc
    b. de clapotement
    b. de claquement
    b. de craquement
    b. de cuir neuf
    b. de diable
    b. de drapeau
    b. de fele
    b. de froissement
    b. de frolement
    b. de frottement
    b. de galop
    b. de grelot
    b. de la roue de moulin
    b. de Leudet
    b. de lime
    b. de moulin
    b. de parchemin
    b. de piaulement
    b. de pot fele
    b. de rappel
    b. de Roger
    b. de scie
    b. de scie ou de rape
    b. de soufflet
    b. de tabourka
    b. de tambour
    b. de triolet
    epigastric b.
    false b.
    midepigastric b.
    musical b.
    Roger b.
    seagull b.
    systolic b.
    thyroid b.
    Traube b.
    Verstraeten b.
Brunelli equation

B

Brunner rib shears
Brunnstrom-Fugl-Meyer Scale for motor test
brush
    Air-Lon tracheal tube b.
    b. biopsy
    bronchoscopic b.
    b. cell
    Cragg thrombolytic b.
    Edwards-Carpentier aortic valve b.
    Mill-Rose Protected Specimen
      microbiology b.
    OTW thrombolytic b.
    protected b.
    protected specimen b. (PSB)
Brush electrocardiographic score
Brushfield spot
brushing
    blind esophageal b. (BEB)
    bronchial b.'s
    double-sheath bronchial b.'s
    microbiologic b.
    protected catheter b. (PCB)
    protected specimen b. (PSB)
    washings and b.'s
brusque dilatation of esophagus
BRVO
    branch retinal vein occlusion
Bryant
    B. ampulla
    B. mitral hook
BSA
    body surface area
BSCA
    bidirectional superior cavopulmonary
      anastomosis
B-scan frame
BSLM
    body surface Laplacian mapping
BSSRO
    bilateral sagittal split ramus osteotomies
BTF-37 arterial blood filter
BTO
    balloon test occlusion
B-type natriuretic peptide (BNP)
bubble
    arterial gas b.
    b. contrast echocardiography
    b. humidifier
    b. oxygenation
    b. oxygenator

Bubble-Jet
    Puritan B.-J.
bubbling rale
bubbly lung syndrome
bubonic plague
bucardia
buccal
    Nitrogard B.
buccalis
    Leptotrichia b.
buccolingual apraxia
buccopharyngeal
Buchbinder
    B. Omniflex catheter
    B. Thruflex over-the-wire catheter
Bucindolol Evaluation of Survival Trial (BEST)
buckled aorta
buckling
    b. of aorta
    chordal b.
    midsystolic b.
bud
    bronchial b.
    lung b.
Budd-Chiari syndrome
budesonide
    b. inhalation powder
    b. inhalation suspension
Budoxis
Bueleau empyema trocar
Buerger-Allen exercise
Buerger disease
buffer
    Krebs-Henseleit b.
buffered aspirin
Bufferin
buffy coat smear
Buhl desquamative pneumonia
buildup time (T_b)
bulb
    b. of aorta
    aortic b.
    carotid b.
    thrombosis of jugular b.
bulbar pulse
bulboventricular
    b. fold
    b. foramen
    b. groove
    b. loop

NOTES

bulboventricular *(continued)*
    b. sulcus
    b. tube
bulbus cordis
bulge
    precordial b.
    spare tire b.
bulging
    diastolic b.
    infarct b.
    systolic b.
bulla, pl. **bullae**
    emphysematous b.
    pulmonary b.
    b. resorption
Bullard intubating laryngoscope
bulldog clamp
bullectomy
    transaxillary apical b.
bullet-tip catheter
bullet wound
bullous
    b. disease
    b. emphysema
    b. lung disease
bull's-eye
    b.-e. plot
    b.-e. polar coordinate mapping
bumetanide
Bumex
bump
    B b.
    ductus b.
BUN
    blood urea nitrogen
bundle
    atrioventricular b.
    atrium-His b. (AH)
    A-V b.
    Bachmann b.
    bronchovascular b.
    Bruce b.
    central bronchovascular b.
    commissural b.
    Gantzer accessory b.
    b. of His
    His b.
    image b.
    James b.
    Keith b.
    Kent b.
    Kent-His b.
    Killian b.
    Mahaim b.
    main b.
    Marshall b.
    neurovascular b.
    b. of Stanley Kent

    Thorel b.
    vascular b.
bundle-branch
    b.-b. block (BBB)
    b.-b. fibrosis
    b.-b. reentrant tachycardia
    b.-b. reentry (BBR)
Bunnell-Howard arthrodesis clamp
Bunny boot
Bunyaviridae
bupivacaine
bupropion SR
bur
    b.-bearing catheter
    diamond-coated b.
    b. hole
burden
    atheroma b.
    atherosclerotic plaque b.
    ischemic b.
    plaque b.
Burdick
    B. ECG machine
    B. electrocardiogram
Burette multiple patient delivery system
Burford-Finochietto rib spreader
Burford rib retractor
burgdorferi
    Borrelia b.
Burger
    B. scalene triangle
    B. technique for scapulothoracic
      disarticulation
    B. triangle
Bürger-Grütz
    B.-G. disease
    B.-G. syndrome
Burghart symptom
Burhenne steerable catheter
Burinex
Burker Avance spectrometer
Burke Stroke Time-Oriented profile
    (BUSTOP)
Burkholderia cepacia
Burkitt lymphoma
burned out viral myocarditis
burnetii
    Coxiella b.
burning pain
Burns
    space of B.
Burow
    B. quantitative method
    B. solution
    B. vein
bursa
    Calori b.
    Fleischmann b.

laryngeal b.
b. subcutanea
sublingual b.
b. sublingualis
burst
b. of arrhythmia
b. atrial pacing
b. pacing
paroxysmal b.
respiratory b.
b. shock
spider b.
b. of ventricular tachycardia
Buschke
B. disease
scleredema of B.
buspirone transdermal patch
Busse-Buschke disease
buster
clot b.
BUSTOP
Burke Stroke Time-Oriented profile
busulfan lung syndrome
butanedione monoxime
butorphanol
butterfly
b. adapter
b. catheter
b. heart valve
b. needle
b. pattern
b. shadow
Butterworth bidirectional filter
buttock claudication
button
b. of aorta
cell b.
coronary artery b.
DiaTAP vascular access b.
b. electrode
Kistner tracheal b.
Moore tracheostomy b.
Panje voice b.
Perspex b.
skin b.
b. technique
tracheal b.
tracheostomy b.
buttoned device
buttonhole
b. deformity
mitral b.

b. mitral stenosis
b. stenosis
buttress
Teflon pledget suture b.
butylated hydroxytoluene (BHT)
butyrophenone
BUV
backup ventilation
BV
balloon valvuloplasty
BVA-100 blood volume analyzer
BVAD, BIVAD
biventricular assist device
BV-ara-U
BvgAS regulon
BvgS protein
BVM
bag-valve-mask
BVM device
BVR
balloon valvuloplasty registry
BVS
biventricular support
BVS pump
BVS-5000 biventricular support system
BW755C
cyclooxygenase-lipoxygenase
blocking agent B.
BX
IsoStent BX
BX IsoStent stent
BX stent
BX Velocity stent
BY963 contrast agent
Bycep
B. biopsy forceps
B. PC Jr bioptome
Bydramine Cough Syrup
bypass
b. angioplasty revascularization
investigation (BARI)
aortobiiliac b.
aortocarotid b.
aortocoronary b.
aortocoronary-saphenous vein b.
aortoiliac b.
aortoiliofemoral b.
aortorenal b.
aortosubclavian b.
aortosubclavian-carotid-
axilloaxillary b.
atrial-femoral artery b.

NOTES

bypass *(continued)*
    axillary bifemoral b.
    axilloaxillary b.
    axillofemoral b.
    brachial b.
    cardiopulmonary b. (CPB)
    carotid-axillary b.
    carotid-carotid b.
    carotid-subclavian b.
    b. circuit
    coronary artery b.
    coronary artery b. graft
    cross femoral-femoral b.
    crossover b.
    crossover femoral-femoral b.
    descending thoracic aortofemoral-
        femoral b.
    femoral-femoral b.
    femoral-popliteal b.
    femoral-tibial b.
    femoral-tibial-peroneal b.
    femoroaxillary b.
    femorofemoral crossover b.
    femoropopliteal b.
    femorotibial b.
    b. graft
    b. graft catheter
    b. graft catheterization
    heart-lung b.
    iliopopliteal b.
    infracubital b.
    internal mammary artery b.
        (IMAB)
    left heart b.
    Litwak left atrial-aortic b.

    low-flow cardiopulmonary b. (LFB)
    b. machine
    midcoronary artery b.
    minimally invasive direct coronary
        artery b.
    off-pump coronary artery b.
        (OPCAB)
    percutaneous cardiopulmonary b.
        (PCPB)
    percutaneous left heart b. (PLHB)
    perfusion-assisted direct coronary
        artery b. (PADCAB)
    peripheral artery b.
    renal artery-reverse saphenous
        vein b.
    reversed b.
    right heart b.
    subclavian-carotid b.
    subclavian-subclavian b.
    superior mesenteric artery b.
    b. surgery
    b. time
    total cardiopulmonary b.
    totally endoscopic coronary
        artery b. (TECAB)
    b. tract
bypassable
by-product
    cotinine nicotine b.-p.
    eosinophil b.-p.
Byrel
    B. SX pacemaker
    B. SX/Versatrax pacemaker
byssinosis
bystander effect

C

C oxygen cylinder
C point of cardiac apex pulse
C valvular leaflet
C wave
C wave of jugular venous

C1r deficiency

C$_4$

leukotriene C.

c4b purified human complement

C-11 palmitate

CA

cancer
carcinoma
cardiac-apnea
cardiac arrest
central apnea
croup-associated
cytosine arabinoside
CA monitor
CA virus

C3a

C4a

C5a

CAA

cardiac allograft atherosclerosis
cerebral amyloid angiopathy
CAA-related hemorrhage

CAAS

Cardiovascular Angiography Analysis
System

CABG Patch

Coronary Artery Bypass Graft Surgery
With/Without Simultaneous Epicardial
Patch for Automatic Implantable
Cardioverter-Defibrillator
CABG Patch clinical trial

cabinet respirator

cable

alligator pacing c.
OxyLead interconnect c.

Cabot-Locke murmur

Cabral coronary reconstruction

CABRI

Coronary Angioplasty versus Bypass
Revascularization Investigation
Coronary Artery Bypass
Revascularization Investigation

CAC

cold air challenge

CACh

cold air challenge

cachectic endocarditis

cachecticorum

melanoderma c.

CACHET

Comparison of Abciximab Complications
with Hirulog (and Back-Up Abciximab)
Events Trial

cachexia

cancer c.
cardiac c.
thyroid c.

cacoon seed asthma

CAD

computer-assisted diagnostics
coronary artery disease

CADASIL

cerebral autosomal dominant arteriopathy
with subcortical infarct and
leukoencephalopathy

CADD-Plus intravenous infusion pump

Cadence

C. AICD
C. biphasic ICD
C. implantable cardioverter-
defibrillator
C. tiered therapy defibrillator
system
C. TVL nonthoracotomy lead

Cadet

C. cardioverter-defibrillator
C. high voltage can implantable
cardioverter-defibrillator
C. V-115 implantable cardioverter-
defibrillator

cadherin

vascular c.

CADILLAC

Controlled Abciximab and Device
Investigation to Lower Late
Angioplasty Complications
CADILLAC clinical trial

cadmiosis

cadmium (Cd)

c. fumes
c. oxide
c. oxide fumes

CADS

Captopril and Digoxin Study

CaduCIS UMLS software

CAEP

chronotropic exercise assessment protocol

CAESAR

C. analysis system
C. system

caesiellus

Aspergillus c.

CAF
    continuous atrial fibrillation
    coronary artery fistula
Cafatine-PB
Cafcit
    C. injection
    C. oral solution
café-au-lait spot
cafe coronary
Cafergot
Cafetrate
caffeine
    c. citrate
    citrated c.
    c. citrate oral solution
    c. and sodium benzoate
CAFS
    Canadian Atrial Fibrillation Study
CAG
    coronary arteriography
CagA
    cytotoxin-associated gene product A
    CagA antigen
cage
    c. catheter device
    chest c.
    Faraday c.
    rib c.
    thoracic c.
    titanium c.
caged
    caged ball valve
    caged ball valve prosthesis
CAGEIN
    catheter-guided endoscopic intubation
CAI
    cortical arousal index
c-a interval
Caire
    C. Breeze oxygen therapy device
    C. Messenger Reporter monitor
    C. OxyMax software
    C. Sprint portable liquid oxygen device
    C. Stroller portable liquid oxygen device
caisson disease
CAL
    chronic airflow limitation
Calan SR
calcicardiogram
calcicosilicosis
calcicosis
calcific
    c. debris
    c. embolus
    c. mitral stenosis

    c. nodular aortic stenosis
    c. pericarditis
calcification
    annular c.
    arterial c.
    dystrophic c.
    dystropic c.
    eggshell c.
    metastatic c.
    mitral annular c.
    mitral annulus c. (MAC)
    napkin-ring c.
    pericardial c.
    pulmonary c.
    soft tissue c.
    c. of tips of the mitral valve
    valvular c.
calcified
    c. aortic valve
    c. lesion
    c. mitral leaflet
    c. nodule
    c. papillary muscle in the right ventricle
    c. pericardium
    c. plaque
    c. thrombus
Calcilean
calcineurin
calcinosis
    c., Raynaud phenomenon, esophageal involvement, sclerodactyly, telangiectasia (CREST)
calciphylaxis
calcitonin gene-related peptide (CGRP)
calcium
    c. antagonist
    C. Antagonist in Reperfusion (CARE)
    arc of c.
    atorvastatin c.
    benzoylpas c.
    c. benzoylpas
    c. channel
    c. channel agonist
    c. channel antagonist
    c. channel blocker
    c. channel blocking agent
    c. chloride
    coronary c.
    c. current (I_{Ca})
    c. deposit
    c. entry blocker
    fenoprofen c.
    c. gluceptate
    c. gluconate
    c. heparin (CH)

c. ion
c. ionophore A23187
mitral annular c. (MAC)
myoplasmic c.
nadroparin c.
c. oxalate
c. oxalate deposition
c. paradox
c. product
c. rigor
c. score
c. sign
spotty coronary c.
c. transient
calcium-channel blocker (CCB)
Calciviridae virus
calcoaceticus
   Acinetobacter c.
calcofluor stain
Calcort
Calculair spirometer
calculation
bidirectional shunt c.
bolus cardiac output c.
calculator
risk c.
calculosa
pericarditis c.
calculus, pl. calculi
bronchial c.
cardiac c.
pleural c.
caldesmon
calf
c. claudication
c. cramp
c. lung surfactant extract (CLSE)
c. pain
calfactant
c. intratracheal suspension
Calgary
C. SAQLI
C. Sleep Apnea Quality of Life
   Index
calibration
calibrator
Fogarty c.
Califf score
California disease
calipers
Brown and Sharp digital
   electronic c.

digital c.
electronic c.
Lange c.
Mipron digital computer-assisted c.
Tenzel c.
Tesa S.A. handheld electronic
   digital c.
callosa
pericarditis c.
callosomarginal artery
Calman
C. carotid clamp
C. ring clamp
calmers
Robitussin Cough C.
Sucrets Cough C.
Calmette-Guérin
bacille C.-G.
bacille de C.-G. (BCG)
C.-G. bacillus
C.-G. vaccine
calmodulin
Calm-X Oral
Calmylin Expectorant
Calori bursa
calorie-restricted diet
calories
ratio of ingested saturated fat and
   cholesterol to c.
calorimetry
myocardial indirect c.
Calot triangle
calphostin C
Caltrac accelerometer
Caluso PEG tube
**Calypso Rely PTCA balloon angioplasty
catheter**
CAM
cell adhesion molecule
child-adult-mist
circulating adhesion molecule
CAM tent
CAMAC-300 arteriograph
Cam-Ap-Es
Cambridge
C. defibrillator
C. electrocardiograph
C. Heart Antioxidant Study
   (CHAOS)
C. jelly electrode
**The Cambridge Heart T-Wave
Alternans Test**

NOTES

camera
ADAC/Cirrus single-headed SPECT c.
ADAC single-head SPECT c.
ADAC/Vertex dual-headed SPECT c.
Anger scintillation c.
cine c.
DSX Sopha c.
gamma scintillation c.
multicrystal gamma c.
multiwire gamma c.
scintillation c.
Siemens-Gammasonics double-head Rota gamma c.
Siemens Orbiter gamma c.
single-crystal gamma c.
Sopha Medical gamma c.
video c.
cameral fistula
Cameron-Haight elevator
CAMI
Canadian Assessment of Myocardial Infarction
CAMI clinical trial
CAMIAT
Canadian Amiodarone Myocardial Infarction Arrhythmia Trial
Canadian Myocardial Infarction Amiodarone Trial
Camino
C. intracranial catheter
C. microventricular bolt
C. microventricular bolt catheter
CAMP
cyclophosphamide, doxorubicin, methotrexate, procarbazine
CAMP test
cAMP
cyclic adenosine monophosphate
Campbell De Morgan spot
Camp-Sigvaris stockings
Camptosar
Campylobacter
camsylate
trimethaphan c.
CAN
continuous albuterol nebulization
can
high voltage c. (HVC)
pacemaker c.
C. Routine Ultrasound Improve Stent Expansion (CRUISE)
C. Routine Ultrasound Influence Stent Expansion (CRUISE)
Canada
Trial of Angioplasty and Stents in C. (TASC)

Canadian
C. Activase for Stroke Effectiveness Study (CASES)
C. American Ticlopidine Study (CATS)
C. Amiodarone Myocardial Infarction Arrhythmia Trial (CAMIAT, CAMI clinical trial)
C. Assessment of Myocardial Infarction (CAMI)
C. Atrial Fibrillation Study (CAFS)
C. Cardiovascular Coalition (CCC)
C. Cardiovascular Society (CCS)
C. Cardiovascular Society angina score (CCSAS)
C. Cardiovascular Society classification (CCSC)
C. Cardiovascular Society functional classification
C. class I–IV angina
C. Coronary Atherectomy Trial (CCAT)
C. Coronary Atherosclerosis Intervention Trial (CCAIT)
C. Digoxin Captopril (DIG-CAPTOPRIL)
C. Heart Classification (CHC)
C. Implantable Defibrillator Study (CIDS)
C. Myocardial Infarction Amiodarone Trial (CAMIAT)
C. Registry of Atrial fibrillation
canal
c. of Arantius
atrioventricular c.
basipharyngeal c.
carotid c.
common atrioventicular c.
complex atrioventricular c.
c. of Cuvier
femoral c.
hiatus of facial c.
His c.
Holmgren-Golgi c.
Hunter c.
c. of Lambert
palatovaginal c.
partial atrioventricular c.
perivascular c.
persistent atrioventricular c.
persistent common atrioventricular c.
pharyngeal c.
pleuroperitoneal c.
pulmoaortic c.
Rivinus c.'s
Van Hoorne c.
ventricular c.

Verneuil c.
Walther c.'s
canalicular period
canalization
cancer (CA)
c. cachexia
c. embolus
International Staging System for
Lung C. (ISSLC)
metachronous lung c.
non-small cell lung c. (NSCLC)
roentgenographically occult
lung c. (ROLC)
scar c.
candesartan
c. cilexetil
c., cilexetil and hydrochlorothiazide
Candida
C. albicans
C. glabrata
C. guilliermondii
C. lusitaniae
C. parapsilosis
C. pneumonia
candidemia
candidiasis
oral c.
candidum
Geotrichum c.
candidus
Aspergillus c.
Thermoactinomyces c.
candle flame pattern
candoxatril
candoxatrilat
candy wrapper edge effect
canine fossa
caninum
Ancylostoma c.
canis
Babesia c.
Toxocara c.
cannabinoid
Cann-Ease
C.-E. moisturizing nasal gel
C.-E. nasal moisturizer
Cannon
C. endarterectomy loop
C. formula
C. theory

cannon
c. sound
c. wave
cannonball
c. metastases
c. pulse
cannula
Abelson c.
Abraham laryngeal c.
Air-Lon inhalation c.
aortic c.
aortic arch c.
aortic perfusion c.
Argyle CPAP nasal c.
Becker accelerator c.
cardiovascular c.
caval c.
Churchill cardiac suction c.
Cimochowski cardiac c.
Cobe small vessel c.
c. cushion
DirectFlow arterial c.
Elecath ECMO c.
Entree thoracoscopy c.
femoral perfusion c.
Flexicath silicone subclavian c.
Floyd loop c.
Fluoro Tip c.
Gregg c.
Grinfeld c.
Grüntzig femoral stiffening c.
Heartport Endovenous Drainage c.
nasal c.
O_2 via nasal c.
Polystan perfusion c.
QuickDraw venous c.
RAP c.
remote access perfusion c.
Research Medical straight multiple-
holed aortic c.
RMI AViD dual stage venous c.
RMI dispersion aortic perfusion c.
RMI Retractaguard retrograde c.
RMI Thin-Flex 24 Fr. venous c.
RMI Trim-Flex low profile dual
drainage venous c.
Rockey mediastinal c.
Rockey ventricular c.
saphenous vein c.
Sarns aortic arch c.
Sarns soft-flow aortic c.
Sarns two-stage c.

C

NOTES

cannula *(continued)*
    Softip oxygen nasal c.
    StraightShot arterial c.
    Tibbs arterial c.
    triport c.
    two-stage c.
    vein graft c.
    vena cava c.
    venous c.
    Wallace Flexihub central venous
      pressure c.
    washout c.
cannulate
cannulated
cannulation
canola oil
canon
    bruit de c.
canrenoate potassium
canrenone
cantering rhythm
canthomeatal slice
Cantlie line
Cantrell pentalogy
CAO
    chronic airflow obstruction
CAP
    community-acquired pneumonia
    coronary artery fistula
    cyclophosphamide, doxorubicin, cisplatin
CA4P
    combretastatin A4 prodrug
cap
    atheromatous c.
    collagenous c.
    fibrous c.
    c. inflammation
    left apical c.
    pleural c.
    c. repair
    c. thickness
CAP/3SBII angiogram projection system
capacitance vessel
capacitor
    c. deformation
    c. forming time
    c. reform
capacity
    aerobic c. (VO_2)
    carbon monoxide diffusing c.
    cerebrovascular reserve c. (CRC)
    diffusing c.
    diffusion c.
    exercise c.
    forced expiratory c. (FEC)
    forced expiratory volume in 1
      second to forced vital c. ratio
      (FEV_1/FVC)

    forced inspiratory c. (FIC)
    forced inspiratory vital c. (FIVC)
    forced vital c. (FVC)
    force-generating c.
    functional reserve c. (FRC)
    functional residual c. (FRC)
    inspiratory c. (IC)
    inspiratory reserve c. (IRC)
    inspiratory vital c. (IVC)
    lung c.
    lung transfer c.
    maximal breathing c.
    maximal sustainable ventilatory c.
      (MSVC)
    maximal vital c. (MVC)
    maximum breathing c. (MBC)
    maximum expiratory flow at 50%
      vital c. (MEF_{50})
    membrane diffusing c. (Dm)
    metabolic vasodilatory c.
    normal vital c. (NVC)
    oxygen c.
    oxygen-binding c.
    oxygen-carrying c.
    oxygen-diffusing c.
    pulmonary diffusion c. (D_{CO})
    residual c.
    residual lung c.
    residual volume/total lung c.
      (RV/TLC)
    respiratory c.
    slow vital c. (SVC)
    timed vital c.
    total lung c. (TLC)
    ventilatory c.
    vital c. (VC)
    work c.
Capastat Sulfate
capecitabine
Capetown
    C. aortic prosthetic valve
    C. aortic valve prosthesis
    C. prosthetic valve
capillaries (*pl. of* capillary)
capillaritis
capillaropathy
capillary, pl. **capillaries**
    alveolar c.
    c. apoplexy
    c. bed
    c. **blood gas** (CBG)
    c. **blood sugar** (CBS)
    c. **blush**
    c. **bronchitis**
    c. **embolism**
    extraalveolar c.
    c. filling
    c. filtration **coefficient**

c. leak syndrome (CLS)
peritubular c. (PTC)
c. pulse
c. recruitment
c. thrombi
c. wedge pressure

Capintec
C. nuclear VEST monitor
C. VEST system

Capiox
C.-E bypass system oxygenator

Capiox SX oxygenation system
Capiscint
Caplan
C. nodule
C. syndrome

caplets
Advil Cold & Sinus C.
Bayer Select Chest Cold C.
Dimacol C.
Dimetapp Sinus C.
Dristan Sinus C.

Capnocheck
C. handheld capnometer
C. Plus NIPB monitor
C. quantitative capnometer

Capnocytophaga
C. canimorsus sepsis

capnogram
volumetric c.

capnograph
BCI Capnocheck DualStream c.
Clarity c.
Microcap handheld c.
Novametrix Tidal Wave
handheld c.
NPB-75 handheld c.
SC-300 portable c.
SC-210 sidestream c.
Tidal Wave handheld c.

capnography
capnometer
Capnocheck handheld c.
Capnocheck quantitative c.
Datex Oxy-cap c.
Normocap c.

capnometry
Capnostat
C. CO_2 sensor
C. Mainstream carbon dioxide
module

Capoten
Capozide
capped lead
capreomycin sulfate
CAPRIE
Clopidogrel versus Aspirin in Patients at
Risk of Ischemic Events
CAPRIE clinical trial

caprisans
pulsus c.

caprizant
caproate
hydroxyprogesterone c.

CAPS
Cardiac Arrhythmia Pilot Study

caps
Drixoral Cough & Congestion
Liquid C.
Drixoral Cough Liquid C.
Drixoral Cough & Sore Throat
Liquid C.
Sudafed Cold & Cough Liquid C.

capsaicin
capsase
CAPSO
cautery-assisted palatal stiffening
operation

capsula fibrosa glandula
capsulatum
Histoplasma c.

capsule
CellCept c.
Glisson c.
internal c.
mycophenolate mofetil c.
Neoral cyclosporine c.
Ordrine AT Extended Release C.
posterior limb of the internal c.
(PLIC)
Rescaps-D C.
Tiazac extended-release c.
TriCor c.
Tuss-Allergine Modified T.D. C.
Tussogest Extended Release C.

capsulets
Sinumist-SR C.

CapSure
C. cardiac pacing lead
C. Fix lead
C. SP lead
C. VDD lead

C

NOTES

captopril
Canadian Digoxin C. (DIG-CAPTOPRIL)
C. and Digoxin Study (CADS)
c. and hydrochlorothiazide
c. renography
C. and Thrombolysis Study (CATS)
CAPTURE
Chimeric 7E3 Antiplatelet in Unstable Angina Refractory to Standard Treatment
CAPTURE clinical trial
capture
atrial c.
c. beat
beat-by-beat c.
c. complex
failure to c.
functional failure to c.
loss of c.
pacemaker c.
retrograde arterial c.
c. threshold
ventricular c.
CAQ
Childhood Asthma Questionnaire
CAR
Cardiac Ablation Registry
Carabelli tube
Carabello sign
CARAFE
Cocktail Attenuation of Rotational Ablation Flow Effects
CARAFE study
caramiphen and phenylpropanolamine
CARAT
Coronary Angioplasty and Rotablator Atherectomy Trial
CARAT II
Coronary Angioplasty and Rotablator Atherectomy Trial II
carbachol
c. inhalation challenge (CIC)
c. provocation test
carbamazepine
carbapenem
carbazochrome salicylate
carbenicillin
indanyl c.
carbetapentane
chlorpheniramine, ephedrine, phenylephrine, and c.
carbide
amorphous hydrogenated silicon c. (a-SiC:H)
cobalt in tungsten c.
silicium c.

carbinoxamine
c. and pseudoephedrine
c., pseudoephedrine, and dextromethorphan
Carbiset-TR Tablet
Carbocaine
carbocholine
carbocysteine
Carbodec
C. DM
C. Syrup
C. TR Tablet
Carbofilm turbostatic carbon permanent coating
carbohydrate
c. intolerance
c. utilization test
Carbomedics
C. bileaflet prosthetic heart valve
C. cardiac valve prosthesis
C. prosthetic heart valve
C. top-hat supra-annular valve
C. valve device
carbomethoxyisopropyl isonitrile
carbon
c. dioxide (CO_2)
c. dioxide dissociation curve
c. dioxide pressure
c. dioxide production
c. dioxide tension
c. disulfide
c. monoxide (CO)
c. monoxide diffusing capacity
c. monoxide hemoglobin
c. monoxide oximetry (CO-oximetry)
c. monoxide sleuth
c. monoxide transfer factor (TLCO, TLco)
pyrolytic c.
carbon-11
c. acetate
c. hydroxyephedrine
c.-labeled fatty acids
c. palmitic acid radioactive tracer
carbonate
magnesium c. ($MgCO_3$)
carbonica
asphyxia c.
carbonic anhydrase inhibitor
carboplatin, etoposide (CE)
Carbo-Seal
C.-S. ascending aortic prosthesis
C.-S. cardiovascular composite graft
C.-S. graft material
carboxyhemoglobin (COHb, HbCO)
carboxyhemoglobinemia

carbuterol hydrochloride
carcinoembryonic antigen (CEA)
carcinogen
carcinogenesis
    field c.
carcinogenicity
carcinoid
    c. heart disease
    c. murmur
    c. plaque
    c. syndrome
    c. tumor
    c. valve disease
carcinoma, pl. carcinomata (CA)
    adenoid cystic c.
    adenosquamous c.
    alveolar cell c.
    anaplastic c.
    basal cell c.
    basaloid c.
    bronchial c.
    bronchiolar c.
    bronchioloalveolar c. (BAC)
    bronchoalveolar c.
    bronchogenic c.
    clear cell c.
    ductal cell c.
    epidermoid c.
    giant cell c.
    hair-matrix c.
    infiltrating lobular c.
    large cell c.
    large cell undifferentiated c.
    lung c.
    lymphangitic c.
    lymphoepithelioma-like c.
    melanotic c.
    metastatic c.
    mucinous c.
    mucoepidermoid c.
    nasopharyngeal c.
    non-small cell c.
    non-small cell lung c. (NSCLC)
    oat cell c.
    papillary c.
    poorly differentiated c.
    prickle cell c.
    primary lung c.
    reserve cell c.
    scar c.
    scirrhous c.
    signet-ring cell c.

    c. simplex
    c. in situ
    small cell c.
    small cell lung c. (SCLC)
    spindle cell c.
    squamous cell c.
    squamous cell bronchogenic c.
    transitional cell c.
    undifferentiated c.
    undifferentiated small cell c.
    verrucous c.
    well-differentiated c.
carcinomatosa
    lymphangitis c.
carcinomatosis
    lymphangitic c. (LC)
carcinomatous
    c. neuromyopathy
    c. pericarditis
carcinosarcoma
CARD
    cardiac automatic resuscitative device
card
    CardioCard optical memory c.
    FlowMinder oxygen flow and
      treatment c.
    TruZone Asthma Action Plan
      Wallet C.
Cardabid
Cardak percutaneous catheter
  introducer
Cardarelli sign
Cardec DM
Cardec-S Syrup
Carden bronchoscopy tube
Cardene SR
CARDIA
    Coronary Artery Risk Development in
      Young Adults
    CARDIA study
Cardiac
    C. Arrest in Seattle: Conventional
      versus Amiodarone Drug
      Evaluation (CASCADE)
    C. Arrhythmia Suppression Trial
      (CAST)
    C. Arrhythmia Suppression Trial II
      (CAST II)
    C. Assist intraaortic balloon
      catheter
    C. Control Systems lead
    C. Infarction Injury Score

C

NOTES

Cardiac *(continued)*
    C. STATus CK-MB/myoglobin panel test
    C. STATus rapid format troponin I panel test
    C. Stimulator BCO$_2$
    C. T assay
    C. T rapid assay

cardiac
    C. Ablation Registry (CAR)
    c. accident
    c. action potential
    c. adjustment scale
    c. allograft
    c. allograft atherosclerosis (CAA)
    c. allograft vascular disease (CAVD)
    c. allograft vasculopathy (CAV)
    c. alternation
    c. amyloidosis
    c. aneurysm
    c. antimyosin antibody uptake
    c. antrum
    c. apex
    c. apnea monitor
    c. arrest (CA)
    c. arrhythmia
    C. Arrhythmia Pilot Study (CAPS)
    c. asthma
    c. atrophy
    c. auscultation
    c. autoantibody
    c. autoimmunity
    c. automatic resuscitative device (CARD)
    c. ballet
    c. balloon pump
    c. baroreceptor
    c. bioptome
    c. blood-pool imaging
    c. border of dullness
    c. bronchus
    c. cachexia
    c. calculus
    c. catheter
    c. catheterization
    c. catheter-microphone
    c. chamber
    c. cirrhosis
    c. cocktail
    c. compensation
    c. competence
    c. compression
    c. conduction
    c. conduction system
    c. contour
    c. contraction
    c. contusion
    c. cooling jacket
    c. crisis
    c. cushion
    c. cycle
    c. death
    c. decompensation
    c. decompression
    c. defibrillation
    c. denervation
    c. depressant
    c. depressor reflex
    c. diastole
    c. diet
    c. dilation
    c. diuretic
    c. dropsy
    c. dyspnea
    c. dysrhythmia
    c. edema
    c. enlargement
    c. enzyme
    c. event
    c. examination
    c. failure
    c. fibrillation
    FluoroPlus C.
    c. function
    c. gap junction protein
    c. gating
    c. glands of esophagus
    c. glycogenosis
    c. glycoside
    c. hemoptysis
    c. hemosiderosis
    c. herniation
    c. heterotaxia
    c. hybrid revascularization procedure
    c. hypertrophy
    c. impression on lung
    c. impulse
    c. incisura
    c. incompetence
    c. index (CI)
    c. infarction
    c. infiltration
    c. insufficiency
    C. Insufficiency Bisoprolol Study (CIBIS)
    c. insult
    c. interstitium
    c. ischemia
    c. jelly
    c. lithomyxoma
    c. liver
    c. lung
    c. lymphatic ring
    c. mapping

c. mass
c. massage
c. memory
c. metastasis
c. monitor
c. monitor strip
c. murmur
c. muscle
c. muscle wrap
c. myocyte
c. myosin
c. myxoma
c. neural crest
c. neurosis
c. notch
c. notch of left lung
c. orifice
c. output (CO)
c. output demand
c. output index
c. output measurement
c. output shock
c. pacemaker
c. pacing
c. patch
c. perforation
c. performance
c. perfusion
c. polyp
c. preload
c. probe
c. rehabilitation
c. rehabilitation protocol
c. reserve
c. resuscitation
c. retraction clip
c. rhythm
c. risk factor
c. risk index
c. rotation
c. rupture
c. sarcoidosis myocarditis
c. sarcoma
c. sensory nerve
c. shadow
c. shock
c. shock wave therapy (CSWT)
c. shunt
c. silhouette
c. situs
c. skeleton
c. sling

c. sodium channel gene
c. souffle
c. sound
c. standstill
c. status
c. stretch device
c. stump
c. surgery
c. sympathetic denervation
c. symphysis
c. syncope
c. systole
c. tamponade
c. telemetry
c. thrombosis
c. thrust
c. transplant
c. troponin I (cTnI)
c. troponin I assay
c. troponin T (cTnT)
c. tumor
c. tumor plop
c. ultrasound
c. vagal tone
c. valve
c. valve prosthesis
c. valvular incompetence
c. variability
c. vasculitis
c. vein
c. vest
c. volume
c. waist
c. wall hypokinesis
c. wall thickening
c. work index (CWI)
cardiaca
    adiposis c.
    steatosis c.
cardiac-apnea (CA)
    c.-a. monitor (CA monitor)
cardiac-specific overexpression
cardial echodensity
cardialgia
Cardia Salt alternative
cardiataxia
cardiatelia
CardiData Prodigy system
cardiectasia
cardiectopia
Cardilate
Cardima Pathfinder microcatheter

C

NOTES

cardinal
    c. symptom
    c. vein
cardioacceleration
cardioaccelerator center
cardioactive
cardioangiography
cardioarterial interval
cardioauditory syndrome
Cardiobacterium hominis
cardioballistic
CardioBeeper CB 12L cardiac monitor
cardiocairograph
Cardiocap/5 monitor
CardioCard optical memory card
Cardio-Care
cardiocele
cardiocentesis
cardiochalasia
CardioCoil coronary stent
Cardio-Cool myocardial protection pouch
Cardio-Cuff
    Childs C.-C.
cardiocyte
CardioData
    C. Mark IV computer
    C. MK-3 Holter scanner
cardiodiaphragmatic angle
CardioDiary heart monitor
cardiodynamics
cardiodynia
cardioembolic stroke (CES)
cardioesophageal
    c. junction
    c. reflux
    c. sphincter
cardiofacial syndrome
CardioFix
    C. pericardium
    C. pericardium patch
Cardioflon suture
Cardiofreezer cryosurgical system
cardiogenesis
CardioGenesis PMR system
cardiogenic
    c. pulmonary edema
    c. sheath
    c. shock (CS)
    c. stroke
    c. syncope
Cardiografin
cardiogram
    esophageal c.
cardiograph
    Minnesota Impedance C.
cardiography
    Doppler c.

    echo-Doppler c.
    ultrasonic c. (UCG)
    ultrasound c.
    vector c.
Cardio-Green dye
CardioGrip handheld, battery-operated exercise device
Cardioguard 4000 electrocardiographic monitor
cardiohemothrombus
cardiohepatic triangle
cardiohepatomegaly
cardioinflammatory cytokine
cardioinhibitory
    c. carotid sinus hypersensitivity
    c. center
    c. syncope
    c. type
    c. vasovagal syncope
cardiokinetic
cardiokymogram
cardiokymograph
cardiokymography
cardiolipid
Cardiolite
    C. scan
    C. stress test
cardiolith
cardiologist
    interventional c.
cardiology
    fetal c.
    C. II stethoscope
cardiolysis
    Brauer c.
CardioMagic 2000 cardiac-monitoring software
cardiomalacia
Cardiomarker catheter
cardiomediastinal silhouette
Cardiomed thermodilution catheter
cardiomegaly
    borderline c.
    false c.
    glycogen c.
    idiopathic c.
Cardiomemo device
Cardiometrics
    C. cardiotomy reservoir
    C. Flowire Doppler echo crystal
    C. Flowire guidewire
cardiometry
cardiomotility
cardiomuscular bradycardia
cardiomyocyte apoptosis
cardiomyoliposis
cardiomyopathy
    African c.

alcoholic c.
anthracycline-induced c.
arrhythmogenic right ventricular c. (ARVC)
arrhythmogenic ventricular c.
atrophic c.
beer-drinker's c.
cobalt c.
concentric hypertrophic c.
congestive c.
diabetic c.
dilated c. (DCM)
doxorubicin c.
drug-induced c.
false c.
familial hypertrophic c.
familial hypertrophic obstructive c.
fibroplastic c.
genetic hypertrophic c.
HIV c.
hyperergopathic dilated c.
hypertensive hypertrophic c.
hypertrophic c. (HC, HCM, HCMP)
hypertrophic obstructive c. (HOCM)
idiopathic c.
idiopathic dilated c. (IDC)
idiopathic restrictive c.
infiltrative c.
inflammatory c. (InfCM)
ischemic c.
maternally inherited c.
Metoprolol in Dilated c. (MDC)
mildly dilated congestive c. (MDCM)
mitochondrial c.
Multicenter Dilated C. (MDC)
nephropathic c.
nonischemic dilated c.
obliterative c.
obstructive hypertrophic c.
parasitic c.
pediatric c.
peripartum c.
postpartum c.
primary c.
primary restrictive c.
rejection c.
restrictive c.
right ventricular c.
secondary c.
spiral hypertrophic c.
tachycardia-induced c.
valvular c.
viral c.
X-linked dilated c.
cardiomyoplasty
dynamic c.
Cardiomyostimulator SP1005
cardioneural
cardioneurogenic syncope
cardioneuropathy
cardioneurosis
cardioomentopexy
Cardio-Pace Medical Durapulse pacemaker
cardiopaludism
cardiopath
cardiopathia nigra
cardiopathy
cardiopericardiopexy
Beck c.
cardiopexy
ligamentum teres c.
cardiophobia
cardiophone
cardiophony
cardiophrenia
cardiophrenic angle
cardioplegia
adenosine-supplemented blood c.
blood c.
cold blood c.
cold crystalloid c.
cold potassium c.
c. cooling
crystalloid c.
crystalloid potassium c.
hyperkalemic c.
c. infusion
normothermic c.
nutrient c.
potassium chloride c.
St. Thomas Hospital c.
whole blood c.
cardioplegic
c. arrest
c. solution
Cardiopoint needle
cardiopressor
cardioprotection
cardioprotective role
cardioptosia

NOTES

cardiopulmonary
c. arrest
c. bypass (CPB)
c. bypass pump
c. exercise (CPX)
c. exercise test (CPET)
c. gas exchange
c. murmur
c. reserve
c. resuscitation (CPR)
c. splanchnic nerves
c. support (CPS)
c. support system
CardioPump
Ambu C.
Cardioquin Oral
cardioreparative
cardiorespiratory
c. arrest
c. depression
c. murmur
c. sign
cardiorrhaphy
cardiorrhexis
Cardioscan standardized evaluation form
cardioschisis
Cardioscint
C. ambulatory vest detector
C. nuclear detector
cardioscope
Carlen c.
Siemens BICOR c.
Siemens HICOR c.
c. U system
CardioSeal
C. occluder
C. septal occluder
cardioselectivity
Cardioserv defibrillator
Cardiosol solution
cardiosphygmograph
CardioSync cardiac synchronizer
cardiotachometer
Cardio Tactilaze peripheral angioplasty laser catheter
CardioTec scan
Cardio-Tel
Cardiotest portable electrograph
Cardiothane-51
CardioThoracic
C. Systems
C. Systems IMA Retractor wound spreader
C. Systems MV Access Platform coronary stabilizer
C. Systems Stabilizer coronary artery stabilizer

cardiothoracic
c. intensive care unit (CTICU)
c. ratio (CT, CTR)
c. surgery (CTS)
cardiothrombus
cardiothyrotoxicosis
cardiotocography
cardiotomy reservoir
cardiotonic drug
cardiotoxicity
Adriamycin c.
doxorubicin c.
cardiotoxic myolysis
cardiotoxin
Cardiotrast
cardiotrophin-1
cardiovalvotomy
cardiovalvulitis
cardiovalvulotomy
cardiovascular
c. accident
C. Angiography Analysis System (CAAS)
c. cannula
c. clamp
c. collapse
c. complication
c. disability
c. disease (CVD)
C. Disease, Hypertension and Hyperlipidemia, Adult-Onset Diabetes, Obesity, and Stroke (CHAOS)
c. excitatory center
c. fitness
c. function
c. function assessment
C. Health in Children (CHIC)
C. Information Registry (CVIR)
c. inhibitory center
C. Measurement system (CMS)
c. pressure
c. silk suture
c. steady state
c. stylet
c. syphilis
c. system
cardiovasculare
systema c.
cardioversion
chemical c.
DC c.
direct current c.
elective c.
electrical c.
external c.
external electric c.
internal c.

low-energy intracardiac c.
low-energy synchronized c.
c. paddles
pharmacological c.
synchronized DC c.
synchronized direct current c.
c. threshold
transthoracic direct current
  electrical c.
transvenous internal c.
cardioverter
  Lyra 2020 implantable c.
cardioverter-defibrillator (*See also*
defibrillator)
  Angstrom MD c.-d.
  Angstrom MD implantable single-
  lead c.-d.
  atrial implantable c.-d. (AICD, A-
  ICD)
  atrial and ventricular
  implantable c.-d. (AV-ICD)
  automatic external c.-d. (AECD)
  automatic implantable c.-d. (AICD,
  A-ICD)
  automatic internal c.-d. (AICD, A-
  ICD)
  beta-blocker strategy plus
  implantable c.-d. (BEST+ICD)
  Cadence implantable c.-d.
  Cadet c.-d.
  Cadet high voltage can
  implantable c.-d.
  Cadet V-115 implantable c.-d.
  Contour LTV-135D implantable c.-
  d.
  Contour MD implantable c.-d.
  Contour MD implantable single-
  lead c.-d.
  Contour V-145D implantable c.-d.
  Coronary Artery Bypass Graft
  Surgery With/Without
  Simultaneous Epicardial Patch for
  Automatic Implantable C.-d.
  (CABG Patch)
  CPI RPx implantable c.-d.
  CPI Ventak PRx c.-d.
  Endotak nonthoracotomy
  implantable c.-d.
  external c.-d. (ECD)
  Gem II VR implantable c.-d.
  Guardian ATP 4210 implantable c.-
  d.

implantable c.-d. (ICD)
Intermedics RES-Q implantable c.-
  d.
Jewel pacer-c.-d.
LT V-105 implantable c.-d.
Lyra 2020 implantable c.-d.
Medtronic external c.-d.
Medtronic Jewel AF 7250 dual-
  chamber implantable c.-d.
Medtronic PCD implantable c.-d.
Micron Res-Q implantable c.-d.
mycroPhylax implantable c.-d.
nonthoracotomy lead implantable c.-
  d.
pacer-c.-d.
PCD Transvene implantable c.-d.
Phylax A-V dual-chamber
  implantable c.-d.
Phylax 06 implantable c.-d.
Powerheart automatic external c.-d.
programmable c.-d. (PCD)
Res-Q ACD implantable c.-d.
Res-Q Micron implantable c.-d.
Sentinel implantable c.-d.
Sentinel 2010 implantable c.-d.
Siemens Siecure implantable c.-d.
subpectoral implantation of c.-d.
Telectronics ATP implantable c.-d.
tiered-therapy implantable c.-d.
tiered-therapy programmable c.-d.
transthoracic implantable c.-d.
Transvene nonthoracotomy
  implantable c.-d.
Ventak A-V III DR automatic
  implantable c.-d.
Ventak Mini II and III automatic
  implantable c.-d.
Ventak Prizm 2 automatic
  implantable c.-d.
ventricular implantable c.-d. (V-
  ICD)
Ventritex Angstrom MD
  implantable c.-d.
Ventritex Cadence implantable c.-d.
wearable c.-d. (WCD)
cardiovirus
Cardiovit
  C. AT-2 ECG
  C. AT-10 ECG/spirometry
  combination system
  C. AT-1 ECG system
  C. AT-10 laptop ECG

NOTES

Cardiovit *(continued)*
    C. AT-10 monitor
    C. AT-2*plus* ECG
    C. AT-10 spirometer
    C. CS-2000
    C. CS-200 ECG system
Cardiovue
    Diasonics C. 3400 and 6400
CardioWest
    C. TAH
    C. total artificial heart
carditis
    coxsackievirus c.
    rheumatic c.
    Sterges c.
    streptococcal c.
    verrucous c.
Cardizem
    C. CD
    C. Injectable
    C. Lyo-Ject
    C. Monovial
    C. Monovial delivery system
    C. SR
    C. Tablet
Cardura
CARE
    Calcium Antagonist in Reperfusion
    Cholesterol and Recurrent Events
    CARE clinical trial
care
    continuity of c.
    emergency cardiac c. (ECC)
    kangaroo c.
    long-term c. (LTC)
    subacute c.
Caregiver Strain Test
carer strain
CARET
    Carotene and Retinol Efficacy Trial
CareTone II telephonic stethoscope
Carey
    C. Coombs murmur
    C. Coombs short mid-diastolic
        murmur
Carfin
carina, pl. **carinae**
    c. not splayed
    c. sharp and mobile
    c. of trachea
    c. tracheae
carinal lymph node
carinatum
    pectus c.
carindacillin
Carinia domestica
carinii
    Pneumocystis c.

cariporide
Carity transportable monitor
Carlen
    C. cardioscope
    C. double-lumen endotracheal tube
    C. tube
C-arm
    C-arm fluoroscopy
    Siemens Hicor II C-arm
Carmalt forceps
Carmeda BioActive Surface
Carmody valvulotome
Carmol topical
carmustine
carneae
    trabeculae c.
carneus
    Aspergillus c.
Carney
    C. complex
    C. triad
carnitine deficiency
Carnoy solution
Carolina color spectrum CW Doppler
Carolon life support antiembolism
    stockings
carotene
    beta c.
    C. and Retinol Efficacy Trial
        (CARET)
carotenoid
caroticotympanic artery
caroticovertebral stenosis
carotid
    c. angiography
    c. angioplasty and stenting (CAS)
    c. angioplasty and stent placement
    c. angioplasty with stenting
    c. arch
    c. arteriography
    c. artery
    c. artery disease
    c. artery murmur
    c. artery shunt
    c. artery stenosis (CAS)
    C. Artery Stenosis with
        Asymptomatic Narrowing:
        Operation versus Aspirin
        (CASANOVA)
    c. artery stenting
    c. augmentation index
    c. ball
    c. baroreceptor
    c. baroreflex
    c. bifurcation
    c. B-mode sonography
    c. body
    c. body tumor

c. bruit
c. bulb
c. canal
c. Doppler
c. duplex scan
c. ejection time
c. endarterectomy (CE, CEA)
c. intima-media complex
c. occlusive disease
c. patch angioplasty
c. phonoangiography
c. plaque
c. pulse
c. pulse tracing
C. Revascularization Endarterectomy Versus Stenting Trial (CREST)
c. sheath
c. shudder
c. sinus
c. sinus hypersensitivity
c. sinus hypersensitivity syndrome
c. sinus massage
c. sinus nerve
c. sinus reflex
c. sinus stimulation
c. sinus syncope
c. sinus syndrome
c. sinus test
c. siphon
c. steal syndrome
c. stenosis
c. stent
c. stent-supported angioplasty (CSSA)
c. triangle
c. upstroke
c. vascular disease
C. and Vertebral Artery Transluminal Angioplasty Study (CAVATAS)
carotid-axillary bypass
carotid-carotid bypass
carotid-cavernous fistula (CCF)
carotid-subclavian bypass
carotodynia, carotidynia
carpal
c. arch anterior
c. arch dorsal
c. arch palmar
Carpenter syndrome
Carpentier
C. annuloplasty

C. annuloplasty ring prosthesis
C. pericardial valve
C. ring
C. stent
C. tricuspid valvuloplasty
Carpentier-Edwards
C.-E. aortic valve prosthesis
C.-E. glutaraldehyde-preserved porcine xenograft prosthesis
C.-E. mitral annuloplasty valve
C.-E. pericardial valve
C.-E. Perimount mitral valve
C.-E. Perimount RSR pericardial bioprosthesis
C.-E. Physio annuloplasty ring
C.-E. Physio annuloplasty ring with Duraflo
C.-E. porcine prosthetic valve
C.-E. porcine supraannular valve
Carpentier-Rhone-Poulenc mitral ring prosthesis
carpopedal spasm
CARPORT
Coronary Artery Restenosis Prevention on Repeated Thromboxane Antagonism
CARPORT study
Carrel
C. method
C. patch
Carrie coronary stent placement technique
Carrington
C. disease
C. pneumonia
Carr lobectomy tourniquet
CARS
compensatory antiinflammatory response syndrome
Carswell grapes
cart
MedGraphics CPX/D metabolic c.
metabolic c.
resuscitation c.
SensorMedics 2900 metabolic c.
Carten mitral valve retractor
carteolol hydrochloride
Carter
C. equation
C. retractor
Cartia XT
Cartilade

NOTES

cartilage
  anular c.
  articular surface of arytenoid c.
  cricoid c.
  epiglottic c.
  c.'s of larynx
  Luschka c.
  Meyer c.
  Seiler c.
  tracheal c.
  xiphoid c.
cartilagines
  c. tracheales
cartilago
  c. cricoidea
  c. laryngis
  c. sesamoidea laryngis
**CARTO-Biosense magnetic mapping
system**
CARTO-system
Cartrol Oral
Cartwright
  C. heart prosthesis
  C. valve prosthesis
carumonam
caruncula
  c. salivaris
  sublingual c.
  c. sublingualis
Carvallo sign
carvedilol
  C. Heart Attack Pilot Study
    (CHAPS)
  C. or Metoprolol European trial
  C. Prospective Randomized
    Cumulative Survival
    (COPERNICUS)
  C. Prospective Randomized
    Cumulative Survival trial
    (COPERNICUS trial)
Cary 118C spectrophotometer
CAS
  carotid angioplasty and stenting
  carotid artery stenosis
  coronary artery scan
**CAS-8000V general angiography
positioner**
Casale-Devereux criteria
CASANOVA
  Carotid Artery Stenosis with
    Asymptomatic Narrowing: Operation
    versus Aspirin
    CASANOVA study
CASCADE
  Cardiac Arrest in Seattle: Conventional
    versus Amiodarone Drug Evaluation

  Conventional Antiarrhythmic versus
    Amiodarone in Survivors of Cardiac
    Arrest Drug Evaluation
cascade
  AA c.
  arachidonic acid c.
  ischemic c.
  leukocyte-endothelial cell
    adhesion c.
  c. phenomenon
  renin-angiotensin-aldosterone c.
CASE
  C. computerized exercise ECG
    system
  C. Marquette 16 exercise system
case
  M6/C cylinder carrying c.
caseated tissue
caseating
caseation
  tuberculous c.
case-control study
casein asthma
caseous
  c. abscess
  c. osteitis
  c. pneumonia
  c. tonsillitis
CASES
  Canadian Activase for Stroke
    Effectiveness Study
casing
  Silastic electrode c.
CASL-PI MRI
  continuous arterial spin-labeled perfusion
    MRI
Casodex
Casoni test
caspase inhibitor
CASS
  continuous aspiration of subglottic
    secretions
  Coronary Artery Surgery Study
CAST
  Cardiac Arrhythmia Suppression Trial
  Chinese Acute Stroke trial
cast
  blood c.
Castaneda
  C. anastomosis clamp
  C. bottle
  C. principle
Castellani
  C. bronchitis
  C. disease
  C. point
castellani
  Acanthamoeba c.

Castellino sign
CAST II
    Cardiac Arrhythmia Suppression Trial II
Castillo catheter
Castleman disease
castor
    c. bean
    c. bean asthma
Castroviejo needle holder
CAT
    computerized axial tomography
cat
    c. asthma
    c. cry syndrome
catabolic illness
catabolism of rtPA
catacrotic
    c. pulse
    c. wave
catacrotism
catacrotus
    pulsus c.
catadicrotic
    c. pulse
    c. wave
catadicrotism
catadicrotus
    pulsus c.
Cat-a-Kit analyzer
catalase
    superoxide c.
catamenial
    c. hemoptysis
    c. hemothorax
    c. pneumothorax
cataplectic
cataplexy
Catapres Oral
Catapres-TTS Transdermal
catarrh
    atrophic c.
    autumnal c.
    Bostock c.
    hypertrophic c.
    Laënnec c.
    postnasal c.
    sinus c.
    suffocative c.
catarrhal
    c. asthma
    c. bronchitis
    c. croup

    c. laryngitis
    c. pharyngitis
    c. pneumonia
catarrhalis
    Branhamella c.
    Moraxella c.
    Neisseria c.
catastrophic hemorrhage
catatricrotic pulse
catatricrotism
Catatrol
catch 22 syndrome
catecholamine
    c. action
    plasma c.
    c. release
category-ratio
    Borg c.-r.
0 to 10 category ratio (CR-10)
catenoid
cathepsin G
catheter
    Abbokinase c.
    ablation c.
    c. ablation
    c. ablation of atrial fibrillation
    ACE fixed-wire balloon c.
    Achiever balloon dilatation c.
    ACS angioplasty c.
    ACS balloon c.
    ACS Concorde coronary
      dilatation c.
    ACS Endura coronary dilation c.
    ACS Enhanced Torque 8/7.5-F
      Taper Tip c.
    ACS JL4 French c.
    ACS Mini c.
    ACS Monorail c.
    ACS OTW Lifestream coronary
      dilatation c.
    ACS OTW Photon coronary
      dilatation c.
    ACS OTW Photon coronary
      dilation c.
    ACS OTW Solaris coronary
      dilatation c.
    ACS OTW Solaris coronary
      dilation c.
    ACS Photon coronary dilatation c.
    ACS RX Comet angioplasty c.
    ACS RX Comet coronary
      dilatation c.

C

NOTES

catheter *(continued)*
ACS RX Comet VP coronary
dilatation c.
ACS RX Lifestream coronary
dilation c.
ACS RX perfusion balloon c.
ACS RX Rocket coronary
dilatation c.
ACS RX Solaris coronary
dilatation c.
ACS Tourguide II guiding c.
ACST Tx2000 coronary
dilatation c.
AcuNav c.
AcuNav ultrasound c.
ACX II balloon c.
c. adapter
afterloading c.
Ag-AgCl$_2$ electrode bipolar c.
Ahn thrombectomy c.
Alert c.
AL I c.
alignment c.
AL II guiding c.
Alvarez-Rodriguez cardiac c.
Alzate c.
Amazr c.
Amcath c.
Amplatz coronary c.
Amplatz Hi-Flo torque-control c.
Amplatz left I, II c.
Amplatz right coronary c.
Amplatz right I, II c.
A2 multipurpose c.
AngeCool RF c.
Angiocath PRN c.
Angioflow high-flow c.
angiographic c.
AngioJet c.
AngioJet saline jet/vacuum
device c.
AngioJet thrombectomy c.
Angio-Kit c.
Angiomedics c.
angiopigtail c.
angioplasty guiding c.
angiotensin-converting enzyme
fixed-wire balloon c.
angled balloon II c.
angled pigtail c.
angle tipped c.
angulated multipurpose c.
Anthron II c.
Anthron heparinized
antithrombogenic c.
aortic c.
AR-1 c.
Arani double-loop guiding c.

Argyle c.
Argyle arterial c.
Arrow balloon wedge c.
Arrow Flex intraaortic balloon c.
ARROWgard Blue antiseptic-
coated c.
ARROWgard Blue Line c.
ARROWgard central venous c.
Arrow-Howes multilumen c.
Arrow Pullback atherectomy c.
Arrow QuadPolar electrode c.
Arrow QuadPolar pulmonary
artery c.
Arrow TwinCath multilumen
peripheral c.
arterial embolectomy c.
c. arteriography
Ascent guiding c.
Asuka PTA over-the-wire c.
atherectomy c.
AtheroCath Bantam coronary
atherectomy c.
AtheroCath GTO coronary
atherectomy c.
AtheroCath spinning blade c.
Atlantis SR IVUS c.
Atlas DG balloon angioplasty c.
Atlas LP PTCA balloon
dilatation c.
Atlas ULP balloon dilatation c.
ATRAC-II double-balloon c.
ATRAC multipurpose balloon c.
Atri-pace I bipolar flared pacing c.
Auth atherectomy c.
autoperfusion balloon c.
Avanar intravascular ultrasound c.
Avanar IVUS c.
AV-Paceport thermodilution c.
Axiom DG balloon angioplasty c.
Bailey c.
bailout autoperfusion balloon c.
Baim pacing c.
Baim-Turi monitoring/pacing c.
Balectrode pacing c.
balloon c.
balloon angioplasty c.
balloon embolectomy c.
balloon-flotation pacing c.
balloon-imaging c.
balloon septostomy c.
balloon-tipped c.
balloon-tipped angiographic c.
balloon-tipped flow-directed c.
balloon-tipped thermodilution c.
c. balloon valvuloplasty
balloon valvuloplasty c.
ball-wedge c.
Baltherm c.

Bandit PTCA c.
Bard balloon-directed pacing c.
Bardco c.
Bard electrophysiology c.
Bard guiding c.
Bardic cutdown c.
Bard safety excaliber peripherally
  inserted central c.
Baxter angioplasty c.
Baxter fiberoptic
  spectrophotometry c.
Bentson-Hanafee-Wilson c.
Berenstein occlusion balloon c.
Berman angiographic c.
Berman balloon flotation c.
Beta-Rail c.
Bicor c.
bifoil balloon c.
BioDiamond S rapid exchange
  PTCA c.
Bio-Medicus arterial c.
bipolar c.
bird's-eye c.
blade septostomy c.
Block right coronary guiding c.
Blue FlexTip c.
Blue Max triple-lumen c.
Bonzel Monorail balloon c.
Boston Scientific Sonicath
  imaging c.
Bourassa c.
brachial c.
Brite Tip c.
Brockenbrough c.
Brockenbrough mapping c.
Brockenbrough transseptal c.
Bronchitrac L c.
Bronchitrac L flexible suction c.
Broviac atrial c.
Buchbinder Omniflex c.
Buchbinder Thruflex over-the-
  wire c.
bullet-tip c.
bur-bearing c.
Burhenne steerable c.
butterfly c.
bypass graft c.
Calypso Rely PTCA balloon
  angioplasty c.
Camino intracranial c.
Camino microventricular bolt c.
cardiac c.

Cardiac Assist intraaortic balloon c.
Cardiomarker c.
Cardiomed thermodilution c.
Cardio Tactilaze peripheral
  angioplasty laser c.
Castillo c.
catheter introducing forceps c.
Cath-Finder c.
Cathlon IV c.
Cathmark suction c.
caval c.
CCOmbo c.
central venous c. (CVC)
Cerablate plus flutter ablation c.
cerebral ablation c.
Chemo-Port c.
Chilli c.
Chilli cooled-tip ablation c.
Clark expanding mesh c.
Clark helix c.
Clark rotating cutter c.
closed end-hole c.
Closer-Closure c.
Cloverleaf c.
Cobra over-the-wire balloon c.
cobra-shaped c.
coil-tipped c.
Combicath double-plugged
  telescope c.
Comet c.
conductance c.
Constellation advanced mapping c.
Cook arterial c.
Cook Cardiovascular infusion c.
Cook Spectrum c.
Cook TPN c.
Cook yellow pigtail c.
Cool Tip c.
Cordis BriteTip guiding c.
Cordis Ducor I, II, III c.
Cordis Ducor pigtail c.
Cordis guiding c.
Cordis Lumelec c.
Cordis Predator balloon c.
Cordis Predator PTCA balloon c.
Cordis Son-II c.
Cordis Titan balloon dilatation c.
Cordis Trakstar PTCA balloon c.
Cordis TransTaper tip c.
Cordis-Webster ablation c.
Cordis-Webster mapping c.
coronary angiographic c.

C

NOTES

catheter *(continued)*
    coronary angiography c.
    coronary seeking c.
    coronary sinus thermodilution c.
    corset balloon c.
    Cournand c.
    Cournand quadpolar c.
    C. R. Bard c.
    Cribier-Letac c.
    CritiCath thermodilution c.
    Critikon balloon temporary
      pacing c.
    Critikon balloon thermodilution c.
    Critikon balloon-tipped end-hole c.
    Critikon balloon wedge pressure c.
    CrossSail coronary dilatation c.
    cutdown c.
    Cynosar c.
    Dacron c.
    c. damping
    Datascope c.
    Datascope CL-II percutaneous
      translucent balloon c.
    Datascope DL-II percutaneous
      translucent balloon c.
    decapolar electrode c.
    decapolar pacing c.
    deflectable quadripolar c.
    DeKock two-way bronchial c.
    Denver Biomaterials Pleurx
      pleural c.
    Deseret flow-directed
      thermodilution c.
    diagnostic ultrasound imaging c.
    Diasonics c.
    Digiflex high flow c.
    c. dilation
    directional atherectomy c.
    Dispatch c.
    Dispatch infusion c.
    Dispatch over-the-wire c.
    dog-leg c.
    Doppler c.
    Doppler coronary c.
    Dorros brachial internal mammary
      guiding c.
    Dorros infusion/probing c.
    Dotter caged-balloon c.
    double-balloon c.
    double-chip micromanometer c.
    double-J c.
    double-lumen c.
    double-thermistor coronary sinus c.
    drill-tip c.
    D114S balloon c.
    dual balloon perfusion c. (DBPC)
    dual-sensor micromanometric high-
      fidelity c.

    Dualtherm dual thermistor
      thermodilution c.
    Ducor balloon c.
    Ducor-Cordis pigtail c.
    Ducor HF c.
    Duett c.
    duodecapolar c.
    duodecapolar Halo c.
    EAC c.
    echo c.
    EchoMark angiographic c.
    echo transponder electrode c.
    EDM infusion c.
    Edwards c.
    EID c.
    eight-lumen manometry c.
    Elecath electrophysiologic
      stimulation c.
    Elecath thermodilution c.
    electrode c.
    El Gamal coronary bypass c.
    El Gamal guiding c.
    Elite guide c.
    embolectomy c.
    c. embolectomy
    c. embolism
    c. embolus
    Encapsulon epidural c.
    Endeavor nondetachable silicone
      balloon c.
    end-hole balloon-tipped c.
    end-hole fluid-filled c.
    end-hole 7-French c.
    EndoCPB c.
    EndoSonics IVUS/balloon
      dilation c.
    Endosound endoscopic ultrasound c.
    Endotak C lead transvenous c.
    Endotak lead transvenous c.
    Enhanced Torque 8F guiding c.
    Eppendorf c.
    Erythroflex hydromer-coated central
      venous c.
    e-TRAIN 110 AngioJet c.
    c. exchange
    expandable access c. (EAC)
    Explorer 360-degree rotational
      diagnostic EP c.
    Explorer pre-curved diagnostic
      EP c.
    Express over-the-wire balloon c.
    Express PTCA c.
    Extra Back-up guiding c.
    Extreme laser c.
    8F c.
    FACT coronary balloon
      angioplasty c.
    Falcon coronary c.

Falcon single-operator exchange balloon c.
FAST balloon c.
FAST balloon flotation c.
FAST right heart cardiovascular c.
7F extended-curve thermistor c.
7F fused-tip c.
7F Hydrolyser thrombectomy c.
fiberoptic c. delivery system
fiberoptic oximeter c.
fiberoptic pressure c.
Finesse guiding c.
fixed-wire coronary balloon c.
Flexguard Tip c.
flexible balloon-tipped c.
Flexxicon Blue dialysis c.
flotation c.
flow-assisted, short-term balloon c.
flow-directed balloon cardiovascular c.
flow-directed end-hole c.
Flow Rider flow-directed c.
fluid-filled c.
fluid-filled balloon cardiovascular c.
fluid-filled balloon-tipped flow-directed c.
fluid-filled pigtail c.
7F mapping c.
2F Millar Instrument c.
focal dilatation c.
Fogarty adherent clot c.
Fogarty-Chin extrusion balloon c.
Fogarty embolectomy c.
Fogarty graft thrombectomy c.
Foltz-Overton cardiac c.
Force balloon dilatation c.
ForeRunner coronary sinus guiding c.
c. fragment
Franz monophasic action potential c.
French double-lumen c.
French JR4 Schneider c.
6-French Judkins c.
6.2-French 12.5-MHz c.
7-French 20-pole deflectable mapping c.
French SAL c.
French shaft c.
FullFlow c.
fused-tip c.
Ganz-Edwards coronary infusion c.

Gazelle balloon dilatation c.
Gensini coronary c.
Gensini coronary arteriography c.
Gensini Teflon c.
Gentle-Flo suction c.
Glidecath hydrophilic coated c.
Goeltec c.
Goodale-Lubin c.
Gorlin c.
Gould PentaCath 5-lumen thermodilution c.
graft-seeking c.
Grollman c.
Grollman pulmonary artery-seeking c.
Groshong double-lumen c.
Grüntzig c.
Grüntzig balloon c.
Grüntzig-Dilaca c.
Guardian c.
c. guide holder
c. guidewire
guiding c.
Günther c.
Hakko Dwellcath c.
Halo c.
Halo XP electrophysiology c.
Hancock embolectomy c.
Hancock fiberoptic c.
Hancock hydrogen detection c.
Hancock luminal electrophysiologic recording c.
Hancock wedge-pressure c.
Hartzler ACX II c.
Hartzler ACX-II, RX-014 balloon c.
Hartzler balloon c.
Hartzler dilatation c.
Hartzler Excel c.
Hartzler LPS dilatation c.
Hartzler Micro-600 c.
Hartzler Micro II c.
Hartzler Micro XT c.
Hartzler RX-014 balloon c.
headhunter angiography c.
Heartport Endocoronary Sinus c.
Heartport endovascular c.
helical-tip Halo c.
helium-filled balloon c.
Helix PTCA dilatation c.
hexapolar c.
Hickman c.

NOTES

catheter *(continued)*

high-density sector basket c.
high-flow c.
high-speed rotation dynamic
  angioplasty c.
Hilal modified headhunter c.
His c.
His bundle c.
hockey-stick c.
HP SONOS 30-MHz imaging c.
c. hub
HydroCath c.
Hydrogel-coated PTCA balloon c.
Hydrolyser c.
Hydrolyser hydrodynamic
  thrombectomy c.
Hydrolyser thrombectomy c.
IAB c.
Illumen-8 guiding c.
ILUS c.
Imager Torque selective c.
imaging-angioplasty balloon c.
c. impact artifact
impedance c.
indwelling central venous c.
Infiniti c.
InfusaSleeve II c.
injection c.
Inoue balloon c.
c. instability
Integra c.
Intellicath pulmonary artery c.
intercostal c.
internal mammary artery c.
Interpret ultrasound c.
Intimax vascular c.
intraaortic balloon c.
intracardiac c.
intrapleural c.
intravascular ultrasound c.
intraventricular c. (IVC)
Intrepid balloon c.
Intrepid PTCA c.
c. introduction method
irrigated coiled c.
ITC balloon c.
IVUS c.
Jackman coronary sinus
  electrode c.
Jackman orthogonal c.
JL4 c.
JL5 c.
Josephson c.
Josephson quadripolar c.
Jostra c.
JR4 c.
JR5 c.
Judkins coronary c.

Judkins curve LAD c.
Judkins curve LCX c.
Judkins curve STD c.
Judkins 4 diagnostic c.
Judkins guiding c.
Judkins pigtail left
  ventriculography c.
Judkins torque control c.
Katzen long balloon dilatation c.
Kensey atherectomy c.
King guiding c.
King multipurpose c.
Kinsey atherectomy c.
Konigsberg c.
Konton c.
Kontron balloon c.
large-bore c.
Larus high-pressure rapid exchange
  balloon c.
laser delivery c.
Laserprobe c.
Laserprobe-PLR Flex c.
latis dual-lumen graft-cleaning c.
Latson multipurpose c.
left coronary c.
left heart c.
left Judkins c.
left ventricular sump c.
Lehman ventriculography c.
lensed fiber-tip laser delivery c.
Levin c.
Leycom volume conductance c.
Lifestream coronary dilation c.
Livewire TC ablation c.
long ACE fixed-wire balloon c.
Long Brite Tip guiding c.
Longdwel Teflon c.
Long Skinny over-the-wire
  balloon c.
Long surpass 30 PTCA
  perfusion c.
Lo-Profile II c.
low-profile balloon-positioning c.
low-speed rotation angioplasty c.
LTX PTCA c.
Lumaguide c.
Lumelec pacing c.
Mallinckrodt angiographic c.
Mallinckrodt vertebral c.
c. manipulation
manometer-tipped c.
Mansfield Atri-Pace 1 c.
Mansfield orthogonal electrode c.
Mansfield Scientific dilatation
  balloon c.
Mansfield-Webster c.
mapping c.
c. mapping

mapping/ablation c.
Marathon guiding c.
marker c.
MaxForce balloon dilatation c.
Medi-Tech balloon c.
Medi-Tech steerable c.
Medtronic Transvene 6937
  electrode c.
Medtronic Zuma guiding c.
MegaSonics PTCA c.
memory c.
Mercator atrial high-density
  array c.
Metras c.
Mewi-5 sidehole infusion c.
Mewissen infusion c.
Micor c.
Micro-Guide c.
micromanometer c.
MicroMewi multiple sidehole
  infusion c.
Microsoftrac c.
Micross dilatation c.
MicroView sheath-based IVUS c.
Mikro-Tip micromanometer-tipped c.
Millar Doppler c.
Millar MPC-500 c.
Millenia balloon c.
Millenia PTCA c.
Miller septostomy c.
Mini-Profile c.
Mini-Profile dilatation c.
Mirage over-the-wire balloon c.
Molina needle c.
monofoil c.
monometer-tipped c.
Monorail angioplasty c.
Monorail imaging c.
MS Classique c.
MS Classique balloon dilatation c.
MTC c.
Mullins transseptal c.
multiaccess c. (MAC)
multielectrode basket c.
multielectrode impedance c.
multiflanged Portnoy c.
Multiflex c.
multilayer design c.
multiplex c.
multipolar c.
multipolar electrode c.
Multipurpose-SM c.

multisensor c.
MVP c.
Mylar c.
Mystic balloon c.
Namic c.
NarrowFlex intraaortic balloon c.
National Institutes of Health left
  ventriculography c.
National Institutes of Health
  marking c.
NavAblator c.
Naviport deflectable tip guiding c.
Navistar c.
NC Bandit c.
Neptune high-pressure PTCA
  balloon c.
Nestor guiding c.
NeuroVasx c.
NeuroVasx submicroinfusion c.
Newton c.
Nexus 2 linear ablation c.
NIH cardiomarker c.
NIH left ventriculography c.
NIH marking c.
nonflotation c.
nonflow-directed c.
nontraumatizing c.
NoProfile balloon c.
Norton flow-directed Swan-Ganz
  thermodilution c.
Novoste c.
Numed intracoronary Doppler c.
Nycore pigtail c.
octapolar c.
Olbert balloon c.
Olympix II PTCA dilatation c.
OmniCath atherectomy c.
Omniflex balloon c.
one-hole angiographic c.
one-hole angioplastic c.
OpenSail balloon c.
OpenSail coronary dilatation c.
Opta 5 c.
optical fiber c.
Opticath oximeter c.
Opti-Flow c.
Optiscope c.
Oracle Focus c.
Oracle Focus imaging c.
Oracle Focus PTCA c.
Oracle Micro c.

C

NOTES

catheter *(continued)*

Oracle Micro intravascular ultrasound c.
Oracle Micro Plus c.
Oracle Micro Plus PTCA c.
Oreopoulos-Zellerman c.
OTW perfusion c.
over-the-wire PTCA balloon c.
Owens balloon c.
Owens Lo-Profile dilatation c.
oximetric c.
Pace bipolar pacing c.
pacemaker c.
Paceport c.
Pacewedge dual-pressure bipolar pacing c.
pacing c.
Park blade septostomy c.
P.A.S. Port c.
c. patency
Pathfinder c.
PA Watch position-monitoring c.
Pecor intraaortic balloon c.
pediatric pigtail c.
Peel-Away c.
Peel-Away banana c.
PE-MT balloon dilatation c.
PentaCath c.
Pentalumen c.
PentaPace QRS c.
PE Plus II peripheral balloon c.
Percor DL-II intraaortic balloon c.
Percor-Stat-DL c.
percutaneous intraaortic balloon counterpulsation c.
percutaneous radiofrequency c.
percutaneous rotational thrombectomy c.
perfusion c.
perfusion balloon c. (PBC)
Periflow peripheral balloon c.
Periflow peripheral balloon angioplasty-infusion c.
peripherally inserted c. (PIC)
Per-Q-Cath percutaneously inserted central venous c.
pervenous c.
Phantom V Plus c.
Piccolino Monorail c.
Pico-ST II low-profile balloon c.
pigtail c.
pigtail rotation c.
Pilotip c.
Pinkerton .018 balloon c.
Pleurx pleural c.
plugged telescoping c.
POC Bandit c.
Polaris steerable diagnostic c.

Polystan venous return c.
Positrol II c.
Possis Medical AngioJet thrombectomy c.
Predator balloon c.
preshaped c.
Pro-Bal Protected balloon-tipped c.
probe balloon c.
probing sheath exchange c.
Procath electrophysiology c.
ProCross Rely over-the-wire balloon c.
Profile Plus balloon dilatation c.
Proflex 5 c.
Pro-Flo XT c.
Pruitt-Inahara balloon-tipped perfusion c.
pulmonary flotation c.
Q-cath c.
quadpolar w/Damato curve c.
quadripolar c.
quadripolar diagnostic c.
quadripolar electrode c.
quadripolar pacing c.
quadripolar steerable electrode c.
quadripolar steerable mapping/ablation c.
quadripolar thermocouple-equipped ablation c.
Quanticor c.
QuickFlash arterial c.
Quinton PermCath c.
Radii-T c.
radiopaque calibrated c.
radiopaque ERCP c.
Ranger over-the-wire balloon c.
Rashkind septostomy balloon c.
Rebar-18 micro c.
recessed balloon septostomy c.
Redha cut c.
RediFurl TaperSeal IAB c.
reference c.
Ref-Star EP c.
c. related peripheral vessel spasm
Rentrop c.
reperfusion c.
RF Ablatr ablation c.
RF-generated thermal balloon c.
RF Marinr c.
Rheolytic thrombectomy c.
Rhythm c.
right coronary c.
right heart c.
right Judkins c.
Rigiflex TTS balloon c.
Ritchie c.
Rivas vascular c.
RMI antegrade cardioplegia c.

Rodriguez c.
Rodriguez-Alvarez c.
Rotablator c.
rotational dynamic angioplasty c.
rove magnetic c.
Royal Flush c.
Royal Flush angiographic flush c.
R1 rapid exchange balloon
  dilatation c.
Rx perfusion c.
Rx Streak balloon c.
Sable balloon c.
Sable PTCA balloon c.
Safe-T-Coat heparin-coated
  thermodilution c.
SafTouch c.
Sarns wire-reinforced c.
SCA-EX c.
SCA-EX ShortCutter c.
Schmitz-Rode c.
Schneider c.
Schoonmaker c.
Schoonmaker multipurpose c.
Schwarten LP balloon c.
Scimed angioplasty c.
Scimed rTRA-GC guiding c.
Scoop 1, 2 c.
Selecon coronary angiography c.
self-guiding c.
self-positioning balloon c.
semirigid c.
Sensation intraaortic balloon c.
Sentron pigtail angiographic
  micromanometer c.
Sentron pigtail microtip-
  manometer c.
Seroma-Cath c.
serrated c.
S.E.T. thrombectomy system c.
Shadow over-the-wire balloon c.
shaver c.
Sherpa guiding c.
Shiley c.
SHJR4 c.
SHJR4s c.
ShortCutter c.
short monorail imaging c.
shredding embolectomy
  thrombectomy c.
side-hole Judkins right, curve 4 c.
sidewinder percutaneous intra-aortic
  balloon c.

Silastic c.
Silicore c.
Simmons II c.
Simmons III c.
Simmons-type sidewinder c.
Simplus PE/t dilatation c.
Simpson atherectomy c.
Simpson Coronary AtheroCath c.
Simpson-Robert c.
Simpson Ultra Lo-Profile II
  balloon c.
Skinny dilatation c.
Skinny over-the-wire balloon c.
Sleek c.
Slider c.
sliding rail c.
Slinky c.
Slinky balloon c.
Slinky PTCA c.
Slow-Trax perfusion balloon c.
Smart position-sensing c.
Smec balloon c.
snare c.
Softip c.
Softouch UHF cardiac pigtail c.
Softrac-PTA c.
Soft-Vu Omni flush c.
Solo c.
Sones c.
Sones Cardio-Marker c.
Sones coronary c.
Sones Hi-Flow c.
Sones Positrol c.
Sones woven Dacron c.
Sonicath imaging c.
Sorenson thermodilution c.
Spectra-Cath STP c.
Spectranetics C rapid-exchange
  laser c.
Spectranetics Extreme c.
Speedy balloon c.
Spring c.
Sprint c.
Spyglass angiography c.
Stack perfusion c.
standard Lehman c.
steerable c.
steerable decapolar electrode c.
steerable electrode c.
steerable guidewire c.
Steerocath c.
Steri-Cath c.

C

NOTES

catheter *(continued)*
 Stertzer brachial c.
 Stertzer guiding c.
 straight flush percutaneous c.
 straight tipped c.
 Sub-Microinfusion c.
 Sub-4 small vessel balloon
   dilatation c.
 SULP II balloon c.
 Superflow guiding c.
 Super-9 guiding c.
 Super Torque Plus c.
 Supreme electrophysiology c.
 Swan-Ganz c.
 Swan-Ganz balloon flotation c.
 Swan-Ganz bipolar pacing c.
 Swan-Ganz flow-directed c.
 Swan-Ganz Pacing TD c.
 Syntel latex-free embolectomy c.
 systemic arterial c.
 TAC atherectomy c.
 Tactilaze angioplasty laser c.
 TADcath temporary transvenous
   defibrillation c.
 Talon balloon dilatation c.
 TEC c.
 TEC extraction c.
 TEC-guide c.
 Teflon c.
 TEGwire balloon dilatation c.
 Tennis Racquet c.
 Tennis Racquet angiographic c.
 Ten system balloon c.
 Terumo SP coaxial c.
 tetrapolar esophageal c.
 thermistor thermodilution c.
 thermodilution c.
 thermodilution balloon c.
 thermodilution pacing c.
 thermodilution Swan-Ganz c.
 thin-walled c.
 c. thrombectomy
 Thrombektomat c.
 Thrombolizer c.
 Thruflex PTCA balloon c.
 Tidal balloon c.
 Titan mega PTCA dilatation c.
 Titan mega XL PTCA dilatation c.
 Torcon NB selective
   angiographic c.
 Torktherm torque control c.
 torque control balloon c.
 Total Cross balloon c.
 Tourguide guiding c.
 TrachCare multi-access c.
 Tracker-18 Soft Stream side-hole
   microinfusion c.
 Trac Plus c.

 Trakstar balloon c.
 transcutaneous extraction c.
 transfemoral c.
 transfemoral endoaortic occlusion c.
 transluminal angioplasty c.
 transluminal endarterectomy c.
   (TEC)
 transluminal extraction c. (TEC)
 Transport c.
 Transport dilatation balloon c.
 Transport drug delivery c.
 transseptal c.
 transtracheal oxygen c.
 trefoil balloon c.
 Triguide c.
 triple-lumen balloon flotation
   thermistor c.
 tripolar with Damato curve c.
 TTS c.
 Tyshak c.
 Tyshak balloon valvuloplasty c.
 Uldall subclavian hemodialysis c.
 ULP c.
 Ultra 8 balloon c.
 UltraCross profile imaging c.
 UltraFuse c.
 UltraFuse infusion c.
 ultra-low profile fixed-wire balloon
   dilatation c.
 ultra-low profile fixed-wire balloon
   dilation c.
 ultrasound ablation c.
 ultrasound-tipped c.
 Ultra-Thin balloon c.
 UMI c.
 Uniweave c.
 c. unstability
 Uresil embolectomy
   thrombectomy c.
 urinary c.
 USCI c.
 Van Andel c.
 Van Tassel angled pigtail c.
 Vantex central venous c.
 Variflex catheter c.
 Vas-Cath c.
 vascular access c.
 Vaxcel c.
 vector, phased-array ultrasound-
   tipped c.
 Venaport coronary sinus guiding c.
 ventriculoatrial shunt c.
 ventriculography c.
 Ventureyra ventricular c.
 Verbatim balloon c.
 vessel-sizing c.
 Viggo Spectramed c.
 Viking Bard c.

Viper PTA c.
Visa II PTCA c.
Visa II ST PTCA balloon c.
Visa ST balloon c.
Vision PTCA c.
Vitesse c.
Vitesse C c.
Vitesse Cos laser c.
Vitesse E c.
Vitesse E2 rapid-exchange c.
Vitesse PrimaFx c.
c. vitrector
Viva Primo balloon c.
V. Mueller c.
Voda c.
vortex effect c.
Vueport balloon-occlusion
  guiding c.
waist of c.
Webster halo c.
Webster orthogonal electrode c.
wedge pressure balloon c.
Wexler c.
c. whip
c. whip artifact
Wilton Webster coronary sinus
  thermodilution c.
Wilton Webster thermodilution flow
  and pacing c.
Workhorse percutaneous
  transluminal angioplasty balloon c.
woven Dacron c.
Xpeedior c.
Xpeedior 100 c.
Xtrem Medicorp c.
X-Trode electrode c.
Zavod bronchospirometry c.
Z cardiac c.
Z-Med c.
Zucker multipurpose bipolar c.
Zuma guiding c.
Zynergy Zolution
  electrophysiology c.
catheter-based
  c.-b. revascularization
  c.-b. sensor
**catheter-directed thrombolysis and
  endovascular stent placement**
catheter-guided
  c.-g. biopsy
  c.-g. endoscopic intubation
  (CAGEIN)

catheter-guide wire
catheter-induced
  c.-i. ablation
  c.-i. coronary artery spasm
  c.-i. embolus
  c.-i. spasm
  c.-i. thrombosis
catheterization
  balloon c.
  bypass graft c.
  cardiac c.
  combined heart c.
  coronary sinus c.
  hepatic vein c.
  interventional cardiac c.
  left heart c.
  Mullins modification of
    transseptal c.
  percutaneous transhepatic cardiac c.
  pulmonary artery c. (PAC)
  retrograde c.
  right heart c.
  selective cardiac c.
  subclavian approach for cardiac c.
  c. technique
  transradial cardiac c.
  transseptal c.
  transseptal left heart c.
  Y wave pressure on right atrial c.
  Z point pressure on left atrial c.
  Z point pressure on right atrial c.
catheterize
catheter-microphone
  cardiac c.-m.
catheter-snare system
catheter-tip
  c.-t. micromanometer system
  c.-t. occluder
  c.-t. spasm
Cath-Finder
  C.-F. catheter
  C.-F. catheter tracking system
CathLink
Cath-Lok catheter locking device
Cathlon IV catheter
Cathmark suction catheter
cathode
Cath-Secure tape
CATS
  Canadian American Ticlopidine Study
  Captopril and Thrombolysis Study
cat-scratch disease

C

NOTES

cattaire
    frémissement c.
cauda equina syndrome
caudally angled balloon occlusion
  aortography
caudal plane angulation
caudate
    c. hemorrhage
    c. hemorrhagic stroke
    c. infarct
    c. ischemic stroke
    c. nucleus
    c. stroke
caudocephalad
caudocranial hemiaxial view
causality assessment
cautery-assisted palatal stiffening
  operation (CAPSO)
CAV
    cardiac allograft vasculopathy
    cyclophosphamide, doxorubicin,
      vincristine
cava
    orifice of superior vena c.
    superior vena c. (SVC)
cavae
    foramen venae c.
caval
    c. cannula
    c. catheter
    c. occlusion clamp
    c. snare
    c. valve
Cavalieri method
CAVATAS
    Carotid and Vertebral Artery
    Transluminal Angioplasty Study
CAVB
    complete atrioventricular block
CAVD
    cardiac allograft vascular disease
CAVEAT
    Coronary Angioplasty versus Excisional
    Atherectomy Trial
      CAVEAT I
      CAVEAT II
caveolae
    intracellular c.
Caverject injection
cavernoma
cavernous
    c. angioma
    c. hemangioma
    c. rale
    c. respiration
    c. sinus (CS)
    c. sinus thrombosis

    c. vein of penis
    c. voice
Caves bioptome
cave sickness
Caves-Schultz bioptome
CAVH
    continuous arteriovenous hemofiltration
caviae
    Aeromonas c.
    Nocardia c.
cavitary
    c. lesion
    c. lung disease
cavitas
    c. laryngis
    c. pharyngis
    c. pleuralis
cavitation
    pulmonary c.
cavitis
Cavitron ultrasonic surgical aspirator
  (CUSA)
cavity
    bronchiectatic c.
    celomic c.
    inferior laryngeal c.
    intermediate laryngeal c.
    c. of larynx
    neoplastic c.
    pharyngonasal c.
    pleural c.
    pleuroperitoneal c.
    pulmonary c.
    superior laryngeal c.
    thrombus-filled c.
    ventricular c.
cavocaval shunt
cavopulmonary
    c. anastomosis
    c. channel
    c. connection
    c. shunt
cavotricuspid
    c. isthmus
    c. isthmus mapping
cavum
    c. laryngis
    c. pharyngis
    c. pleurae
CAZ beta-lactamase
CB
    CB lead
C4B
    human gene C.
CBA
    congenital bronchial atresia
    cutting balloon angioplasty
C-bar web-spacer

CBC
  complete blood count
CBD
  chronic beryllium disease
CBF
  cerebral blood flow
  coronary blood flow
CBFV
  cerebral blood flow velocity
  coronary blood flow velocity
CBG
  capillary blood gas
CBP
  cyclophosphamide, bleomycin, cisplatin
CBS
  capillary blood sugar
CC
    Adalat CC
    CC chemokine I-309
C-C
  convexoconcave
  C-C heart valve
CCABOT
  Cornell Coronary Artery Bypass
  Outcomes Trial
CCA-IMT
  common carotid artery intima-media
  thickness
CCAIT
  Canadian Coronary Atherosclerosis
  Intervention Trial
CCAT
  Canadian Coronary Atherectomy Trial
CCB
  calcium-channel blocker
CCC
  Canadian Cardiovascular Coalition
  common carotid compression
    CCC study
CCD
  crossed cerebellar diaschisis
CCE
  clubbing, cyanosis, and edema
CCF
  carotid-cavernous fistula
C-clamp
CCO
  continuous cardiac output
CCOmbo
  continuous cardiac output with SvO_2
    CCOmbo catheter

CCPD
  continuous cyclical peritoneal dialysis
CCS
  Canadian Cardiovascular Society
CCSAS
  Canadian Cardiovascular Society angina
  score
CCSC
  Canadian Cardiovascular Society
  classification
CCS endocardial pacing lead
CCU
  coronary care unit
CD
  conduction defect
    Cardizem CD
    Ceclor CD
CD4+
    C. cell
    C. measure
Cd
  cadmium
CD8
    C. AIS CELLector
    C. cell
CD18 antibody
CD45 cell surface protein
CD5 cell
CD62p (p-selectin) platelet activation
  marker
CD63 platelet activation marker
CD8+ T cell
CDBR
  computerized diaphragmatic breathing
  retraining
    CDBR respiratory muscle training
    RFB System-I for CDBR
CDC
  Centers for Disease Control and
  Prevention
CD3 cell
CD4 cell
CD20 cell
CD68 cell
CDE
  color Doppler energy
CDH
  congenital diaphragmatic hernia
CDI 2000 blood gas monitoring system
CDM
  change description master

NOTES

C

cDNA
    human cloned DNA
CDP
    certified distinct part
CDX Pulmoguard PFT filter
CE
    carboplatin, etoposide
    carotid endarterectomy
CEA
    carcinoembryonic antigen
    carotid endarterectomy
Ceclor CD
cedar
       Western red c.
Cedars-Sinai classification
Cedax
Cedilanid-D
Cedocard-SR
CEE
    conjugated equine estrogen
Ceelen disease
Ceelen-Gellerstedt
       C.-G. disease
       C.-G. syndrome
CeeNU Oral
c7 E3 Fab
cefaclor
cefadroxil monohydrate
Cefadyl
cefamandole nafate
Cefanex
cefazolin sodium
cefdinir
cefditoren
cefepime HCl
cefixime
Cefizox
cefmenoxine
cefmetazole sodium
Cefobid
cefonicid sodium
cefoperazone sodium
ceforanide
Cefotan
cefotaxime sodium
cefotetan disodium
cefoxitin sodium
cefpiramide
cefpodoxime proxetil
cefprozil
ceftazidime
ceftibuten
Ceftin Oral
ceftizox
ceftizoxime sodium
ceftriaxone sodium
cefuroxime
Cefzil

Cegka sign
ceiling effect in hypertension
celecoxib
celer
    pulsus c.
Celermajer method
celerrimus
    pulsus c.
Celestin
    C. bougie
    C. esophageal tube
Celestone
    C. Oral
    C. Phosphate Injection
    C. Soluspan
celiac
    c. artery
    c. disease
celiacus
    truncus c.
celiprolol
cell
    c. adhesion molecule (CAM)
    adventitial c.
    air c.
    alveolar c.
    ameboid c.
    Anichkov c.
    apoptotic c.
    Aschoff c.
    automatic c.
    B c.
    B1 c.
    bradykinin-stimulated c.
    bronchial epithelial c.
    bronchiolar exocrine c.
    brush c.
    c. button
    CD3 c.
    CD4 c.
    CD4+ c.
    CD5 c.
    CD8 c.
    CD20 c.
    CD68 c.
    CD8+ T c.
    chicken-wire myocardial c.
    ciliated epithelial c.
    clear c.
    c. cycle
    effector c.
    embryonal c.
    endodermal c.
    epithelial c.
    equator of c.
    foam c.
    foamy myocardial c.
    giant c.

goblet c.
c. granulation
great alveolar c.
heart failure c.
HeLa c.
human aortic endothelial c.
  (HAEC)
human aortic smooth muscle c.
  (HASMC)
hyperplastic mucus-secreting
  goblet c.
IgE-sensitized c.
Kulchitsky c.
Langerhans giant c.
Langhans c.
Langhans-type giant c.
mast c.
c. membrane
c. membrane-bound adenylate
  cyclase
mesangial c.
mesenchymal c.
mesenchymal intimal c.
mesothelial c.
metaplastic mucus-secreting c.
mononuclear c.
mucous c.
multinucleated giant c.
N c.
neoplastic c.
oat c.
OxyData oxygen fuel c.
P c.
Pelger-Huet c.
pi c.
prolactin-producing decidual c.
pup c.
Purkinje c.
RA c.
renal juxtaglomerular c.
c. respiration
Sala c.
C. Saver
C. Saver autologous blood recovery
  system
C. Saver Haemolite
C. Saver Haemonetics
  Autotransfusion system
sensitized c.
septal c.
smooth muscle c. (SMC)
c. sorter

squamous c.
squamous alveolar c.
stave c.
c. strain
T c.
transitional c.
c. type
typical small c.
vacuolated c.
vascular smooth muscle c. (VSMC)
vasofactive c.
whorling of myocardial c.
CellCept
  C. capsule
  C. intravenous
  C. intravenous for injection
  C. oral suspension
  C. tablet
cell-coated stent
CELLector
  CD8 AIS C.
cell-free extract
cell-mediated
  c.-m. immune response
  c.-m. immunity
Cellolite material
cellophane rale
cell-seeded stent
Celltrifuge
cellular
  c. cholesterol efflux
  c. embolism
  c. metaplasia
  c. sheets
cellulitis
cellulose
  oxidized c.
celomic cavity
celophlebitis
Celsa battery
Celsior solution
Cel-U-Jec Injection
CEMRA
  contrast-enhanced magnetic resonance
  angiography
Cenafed Plus Tablet
Cenflex central monitoring system
Cenolate
center
  cardioaccelerator c.
  cardioinhibitory c.
  cardiovascular excitatory c.

NOTES

center *(continued)*
    cardiovascular inhibitory c.
    Chemetron HR-1 Humidity C.
    chest pain c. (CPC)
    C.'s for Disease Control and
        Prevention (CDC)
    C.'s for Epidemiologic Studies
        Depression scale (CES-D)
    expiratory c.
    inspiratory c.
    Kronecker c.
    pneumotaxic c.
    respiratory c.
    vasoconstrictor c.
    vasodilator c.
    Veterans Affairs Medical C.
        (VAMC)
**centerline method of wall motion
    analysis**
Centimist nebulizer
centiMorgan (cM)
CentoRx
central
    c. apnea (CA)
    c. approach
    c. baroreflex failure
    c. bradycardia
    c. bridging strut
    c. bronchovascular bundle
    c. core wire
    c. cyanosis
    c. fibrous body
    c. hypopnea
    c. motor conduction time (CMCT)
    c. pneumonia
    c. respiration
    c. retinal artery occlusion (CRAO)
    c. sleep apnea syndrome (CSAS)
    c. splanchnic venous thrombosis
        (CSVT)
    c. tendon of diaphragm
    c. terminal electrode
    c. vein
    c. venous catheter (CVC)
    c. venous line
    c. venous oximetry
    c. venous pressure (CVP)
centriacinar emphysema
centrifugal
    c. left and right ventricular assist
        device
    c. pump
centrilobular
    c. axial interstitial disease
    c. cyst
    c. emphysema
    c. nodule

centripetal
    c. diffusion
    c. venous pulse
centroid
centronuclear myopathy
centrum tendineum diaphragmatis
Century heart-lung machine
Centyl
CEP
    chronic eosinophilic pneumonia
cepacia
    Burkholderia c.
    Pseudomonas c.
Cepacia syndrome
cephalexin monohydrate
cephalic
    c. approach
    c. artery
    c. vein
cephalization of pulmonary flow pattern
cephalocaudad
cephalometrics
cephalometry
    lateral c.
    radiographic c.
cephalopharyngeus
cephalosporin
    fourth-generation c.
    second-generation c.
    third-generation c.
cephalothin sodium
cephapirin sodium
cephradine
Ceporacin
Ceptaz
Cerablate plus flutter ablation catheter
cerebral
    c. ablation catheter
    c. air embolism
    c. amyloid angiopathy (CAA)
    c. aneurysm
    c. angiography
    c. anoxia
    c. apoplexy
    c. arteriosclerosis
    c. autosomal dominant arteriopathy
        with subcortical infarct and
        leukoencephalopathy (CADASIL)
    c. beriberi
    c. blood flow (CBF)
    c. blood flow velocity (CBFV)
    c. edema
    c. embolization
    c. embolus
    c. event
    c. HT
    c. hyperthermia
    c. infarct

c. infarction
c. ischemia
c. lupus
c. microangiopathy (CMA)
c. oximetry
c. perfusion
c. perfusion pressure (CPP)
c. pneumonia
c. protective therapy
c. rate of glucose metabolism (CMRGI$_c$)
c. rate of oxygen metabolism (CMRO$_2$)
c. red blood cell volume (CRCV)
c. respiration
c. thromboangiitis obliterans (CTAO)
c. thrombosis
c. transit time (cTT)
c. tuberculosis
c. vasculopathy
c. vasospasm (CVS)
c. venous thrombosis (CVT)
cerebritis
cerebroprotective
cerebrovascular
c. accident (CVA)
c. autoregulation
c. disease (CeVD)
c. event
c. ferrocalcinosis
c. infarction (CVI)
c. insufficiency
c. reactivity (CVR)
c. reserve capacity (CRC)
c. resistance (CVR)
c. syncope
c. thrombosis
cerebrum
Ceredase injection
cereolysin
Cerespan Oral
cereus
Bacillus c.
Cerezyme
cerivastatin
C. Gemfibrozil Hyperlipidemia Treatment (RIGHT)
c. sodium
c. sodium tablet
Cerose-DM
certified distinct part (CDP)

Certoparin
ceruleus
locus c.
Cervene
cervical
c. aortic arch
c. aortic knuckle
c. disk
c. heart
c. part of esophagus
c. pleura
c. plexus block for carotid endarterectomy surgery
c. radiculitis
c. rib syndrome
c. spine deformity
c. venous hum
cervicalis
ansa c.
cervicothoracic sympathectomy
CES
cardioembolic stroke
Cesar ventilator
CES-D
Centers for Epidemiologic Studies Depression scale
cesium chloride
cESS
circumferential end-systolic stress
cessation
airflow c.
smoking c.
cestodic tuberculosis
Cetacaine
CE-TCCS
contrast-enhanced transcranial color-coded real-time sonography
cetirizine
CETP
cholesteryl ester transfer protein
CeVD
cerebrovascular disease
CF
complex fixation
cystic fibrosis
Guiatuss CF
CF lead
Robafen CF
Synacol CF
CFA
cryptogenic fibrosing alveolitis

NOTES

CFC
chlorofluorocarbon
CFC-free product
CFM-700
Vingmed C.
CFQ
Cognitive Failures Questionnaire
CFR
coronary flow reserve
CFTR
cystic fibrosis transmembrane regulator
CFV-3000
Nihon Kohden C.
CFVR
coronary flow velocity reserve
CFZ
clofazimine
cGMP
cyclic guanosine monophosphate
CGN
compressor-generated nebulizer
CGR biplane angiographic system
CGRP
calcitonin gene-related peptide
CGVD
chronic graft vascular disease
CH
calcium heparin
CH 2000 cardiac diagnostic system
Chagas heart disease
chagasic myocardiopathy
chagoma
chain
alpha-myosin heavy c. (alpha-MHC)
imaging c.
light c.
myosin heavy c.
myosin light c.
paratracheal c.
chain-compensated spirometer
challenge
antiarrhythmic c.
carbachol inhalation c. (CIC)
cold air c. (CAC, CACh)
cold dry air c.
Desferal Mesylate c.
ergonovine c.
histamine c.
hypercapnic c.
methacholine bronchoprovocation c.
osmotic c.
challenger
Turboaire C.
chamber
AeroChamber Plus valved
holding c.
anterior c.
atrialized c.

Boydens c.
cardiac c.
c. compression
c. dilation
dual c. (DC)
EasiVent Valved Holding C.
false aneurysmal c.
Fisher-Paykel MR290 water-feed c.
HealthScan OptiChamber valved
holding c.
c.'s of the heart
hyperbaric c.
monoplace c.
MR 290 humidification c.
multiplace c.
OptiChamber valved holding c.
rudimentary c.
c. rupture
c. stiffness
valved holding c. (VHC)
Chamberlain
C. mediastinoscopy
C. procedure
Chamorro multiple-assessment scale
Champ cardiac device
Chandler V-pacing probe
change
apoptotic c.
arteriovenous crossing c.
c. description master (CDM)
E to A c.
E to I c.'s
environmental c.
fibrinoid c.
fractional area c. (FAC)
Gerhardt c.
hyaline fatty c.
ischemic ECG c.
malignancy-associated c. (MAC)
myxomatous c.
nonspecific climatic c.
obstructive sleep apnea-induced
cardiovascular c.
polyneuropathy, organomegaly,
endocrinopathothy, monoclonal
gammopathy and skin c.'s
(POEMS)
QRS c.
rheologic c.
serial c.
skin c.
ST segment c.'s
ST-T segment c.
ST-T wave c.'s
trophic c.'s
T wave c.
changer
Schonander film c.

channel
    calcium c.
    cavopulmonary c.
    collateral c.
    fast c.
    HERG potassium c.
    ion c.
    K^+ c.
    lymphatic c.
    marker c.
    membrane c.
    receptor-operated calcium c.
    sarcolemmal calcium c.
    slow c.
    sodium c.
    transmural c.
    transmyocardial laser c.
    transnexus c.
    T-type calcium c.
    voltage-dependent calcium c.
    voltage-gated c.
    voltage-sensitive calcium c. (VSCC)
    water c.
CHAOS
    Cambridge Heart Antioxidant Study
    Cardiovascular Disease, Hypertension
    and Hyperlipidemia, Adult-Onset
    Diabetes, Obesity, and Stroke
        CHAOS study
chaos theory
chaotic
    c. atrial tachycardia
    c. heart
    c. rhythm
Chapman index
CHAPS
    Carvedilol Heart Attack Pilot Study
Charcot
    C. sign
    C. syndrome
Charcot-Bouchard
    C.-B. aneurysm
    C.-B. microaneurysm
Charcot-Leyden crystal
Charcot-Marie-Tooth disease
Charcot-Neumann crystal
Charcot-Robin crystal
Charcot-Weiss-Baker syndrome
Chardack-Greatbatch
    C.-G. implantable cardiac pulse
    generator
    C.-G. pacemaker

Chardack Medtronic pacemaker
CHARGE
    coloboma, heart anomaly, choanal atresia,
    retardation, and genital and ear
    anomalies
        CHARGE association
        CHARGE syndrome
charge-coupled device transducer
charge time
Charles
    C. law
    C. procedure
Charlson comorbidity index
Charnley
    C. drain tube
    C. suction drain
Char syndrome
CHART
    continuous hyperfractionated accelerated
    radiotherapy
CHARTS
    Computerized Healthcare And Record
    Transfer System
charybotoxin
chasers
    Scot-Tussin DM Cough C.
Chassaignac axillary muscle
Chaussier tube
CHB
    complete heart block
CHC
    Canadian Heart Classification
CHD
    congenital heart disease
    coronary heart disease
Chealamide
check
    magnet c.
Check-Flo introducer
checklist
    Hopkins Symptom C.
**Checkmate gamma brachytherapy
system**
check-valve sheath
Chédiak-Higashi syndrome
Chedoke-McMaster Stroke Assessment
cheese
    c. worker's lung
    c. worker's lung disease
cheesy
    c. bronchitis
    c. pneumonia

NOTES

chelate
    gadolinium c.
chelator
    iron c.
chelonae
    Mycobacterium c.
Chemetron HR-1 Humidity Center
chemical
    c. ablation
    acaricidal c.
    c. bronchiectasis
    c. bronchitis
    c. cardioversion
    c. exposure
    c. pleurodesis
    c. pneumonitis
    c. shift artifact
    c. shift imaging (CSI)
    c. stimulus
chemiluminescence
chemoattractant
chemoattracting agent
chemodectoma
chemokine
    CXC c.
Chemo-Port
    C.-P. catheter
    C.-P. perivena catheter system
    device
chemoprophylaxis
    secondary c.
chemoreceptor
    peripheral c.
    c. reflex
    c. syndrome
chemoreflex
chemosensitivity
chemosis
chemotactic
    c. anaphylatoxin
    c. cytokine
    c. response
chemotaxis
    eosinophilic c.
chemotherapeutic
    c. agent
    c. index
chemotherapy (CMT)
    antimycobacterial c.
    antituberculous c.
    molecular c.
    neoadjuvant c.
    tuberculous c.
chemotoxin
ChemTrak AccuMeter theophylline test
Cheracol D
cherry angioma

cherry-picking procedure
chest
    alar c.
    anterior flail c.
    anterolateral flail c.
    barrel-shaped c.
    c. bellows
    bilateral anterior flail c.
    blast c.
    c. cage
    cobbler's c.
    c. compression
    c. cuirass
    dirty c.
    dropsy c.
    emphysematous c.
    empyema of c.
    flail c.
    foveated c.
    funnel c.
    c. index
    keeled c.
    lateral flail c.
    c. lead
    c. and left arm (CL)
    noisy c.
    c. pain
    c. pain center (CPC)
    paralytic c.
    c. percussion
    c. percussion and vibration
    phthinoid c.
    c. physical therapy (CPT)
    c. physiotherapy
    pigeon c.
    c. port
    pressure-like sensation in c.
    c. PT
    pterygoid c.
    quiet c.
    c. radiograph (CXR)
    c. and right arm (CR)
    c. roentgenogram
    c. shield
    sucking c.
    tetrahedon c.
    c. thump
    c. tightness
    c. tube
    c. wall
    c. wall adhesion
    c. wall compliance
    c. wall elastic recoil pressure (Pth)
    c. wall injury
    c. wall motion
    c. wall patch
    c. x-ray

Chevalier
C. Jackson bronchoscope
C. Jackson tracheal tube
chewable
E.E.S. C.
Cheyne-Stokes
C.-S. asthma
C.-S. breathing
C.-S. respiration
C.-S. sign
CHF
congestive heart failure
CHF-STAT
Congestive Heart Failure-Survival Trial
of Antiarrhythmic Therapy
Chiari
C. network
C. syndrome
Chiari-Budd syndrome
Chiba needle
CHIC
Cardiovascular Health in Children
CHIC study
chicken fat clot
chicken-wire myocardial cell
child-adult-mist (CAM)
Child classification
childhood
C. Asthma Questionnaire (CAQ)
c. tuberculosis
c.-type tuberculosis
children
Balminil-DM C.
Cardiovascular Health in C.
(CHIC)
Koffex-DM C.
Children's
C. Hold
C. Motrin Suspension
C. Silfedrine
Childs Cardio-Cuff
Chilli
C. catheter
C. cooled ablation system
C. cooled-tip ablation catheter
chimeric
C. 7E3 Antiplatelet Therapy
C. 7E3 Antiplatelet in Unstable
Angina Refractory to Standard
Treatment (CAPTURE)
c. 7E3 Fab

chimerism
hematopoietic c.
mixed hematopoietic c.
Chinese
C. Acute Stroke trial (CAST)
C. licorice
C. restaurant asthma syndrome
C. restaurant syndrome
Chlamydia
C. pecorum
C. pneumoniae
C. psittaci
C. trachomatis
Chlamydiaceae
chlamydial
Chlamydia pneumonia
Chlo-Amine Oral
Chlorafed liquid
chloral hydrate
chlorambucil
chloramine-T technique
chloramphenicol transferase
Chlorate Oral
chlordiazepoxide
chlorella asthma
chloride
Adrenalin C.
ammonium c.
Anectine C.
benzocaine, butyl aminobenzoate,
tetracaine, and benzalkonium c.
bethanechol c.
calcium c.
cesium c.
c. current (I_{Cl})
edrophonium c.
hydrogen c.
c. ion
methacholine c.
polyvinyl c. (PVC)
potassium c. (KCl)
c. secretion
c. shift
sodium c.
succinylcholine c.
sweat c.
tetraethylammonium c.
triphenyl tetrazolium c.
tubocurarine c.
vinyl c.
xenon c. (XeCl)
zinc c.

NOTES

147

chlorine dioxide
chlormethiazole
chlorofluorocarbon (CFC)
chloromethylether
Chloromycetin
chlorophenylfuranyl compound
chloroquine phosphate
chlorothiazide
 c. and methyldopa
 c. and reserpine
chlorotica
 aorta c.
chlorotic phlebitis
chlorotrianisene
Chlorphed-LA Nasal Solution
chlorpheniramine
 c., ephedrine, phenylephrine, and
  carbetapentane
 hydrocodone and c.
 hydrocodone, phenylephrine,
  pyrilamine, phenindamine, c.
 c. maleate
 c., phenylephrine, and codeine
 c., phenylephrine, and
  dextromethorphan
 c., phenylpropanolamine, and
  dextromethorphan
 c. and pseudoephedrine
 c., pseudoephedrine, and codeine
Chlor-Pro injection
Chlorprom
Chlorpromanyl
chlorpromazine hydrochloride
chlorpropamide
chlortetracycline sensitivity
chlorthalidone
 atenolol and c.
 clonidine and c.
Chlor-Trimeton
 C.-T. 4 Hour Relief Tablet
 C.-T. injection
 C.-T. Oral
choc
 bruit de c.
Choice PT plus wire
choir
 vascular c.
chokes
 the c.
cholangitis
 sclerosing c.
cholecystitis
Choledyl
cholelithiasis
cholerae
 Vibrio c.
choleraesuis
 Salmonella c.

cholera vaccine reaction
Cholestaflush
Cholestech LDX system with TC and
 Glucose Panel
cholesterol
 c. cleft
 c. embolism
 c. emboli syndrome
 c. embolization
 c. ester
 c. ester storage disease
 C. Lowering Atherosclerosis PTCA
  Trial
 C. Lowering Atherosclerosis Study
  (CLAS)
 C. Monitoring system (CMS)
 c. pericarditis
 c. pleurisy
 c. pneumonitis
 C. and Recurrent Events (CARE)
 C. Reduction in Seniors Program
  (CRISP)
 C. Reduction in Seniors Program,
  United States (CRISP-US)
 C.-Saturated Fat Index (CSFI)
 serum c.
 c. thorax
 total plasma c.
cholesteryl
 c. ester storage disease
 c. ester transfer protein (CETP)
Cholestin
Cholestron
 C. handheld diagnostic device
 C. PRO II handheld diagnostic
  device
cholestyrame
cholestyramine resin
choline
 c. magnesium trisalicylate
 c. salicylate
 c. theophyllinate
cholinergic
 c. agent
 c. receptor
 c. response
cholinesterase inhibitor
Choloxin
chondral disarticulation
chondralgia
chondrocostal disarticulation
chondroitin sulfate
chondroma
chondrosarcoma
chondrosternal
chondrosternoplasty
chondroxiphoid

chord
chorda, pl. **chordae**
    flail c.
    chordae tendineae
    chordae tendineae cordis
    chordae tendineae rupture
    c. vocalis
chordal
    c. buckling
    c. length
    c. rupture
    c. structure
    c. transfer
chordalis
    endocarditis c.
chordoplasty
chorea
    amyotrophic c.
    c. cordis
    Huntington c.
    Sydenham c.
choriocarcinoma
chorionic villus sampling
choroidopathy
    Pneumocystis c.
Chorus
    C. DDD pacemaker
    C. RM rate-responsive dual-
        chamber pacemaker
Christmas
    C. blood coagulation factor
    C. disease
    C. factor
chromaffin cell tumor
chromate
chromatin
    coarse c.
chromatography
    affinity c.
    gas c.
    high-performance liquid c. (HPLC)
    high-pressure liquid c. (HPLC)
    Sephadex G24 c.
chromic catgut suture
chromium
chromogenic method
chromosome
    5q c.
    11q c.
    c. 14q
chronic
    c. airflow limitation (CAL)

c. airflow obstruction (CAO)
c. aortic stenosis
c. asthma
c. asthmatic bronchitis
c. atrial fibrillation
c. beryllium disease (CBD)
c. catarrhal laryngitis
c. catarrhal tonsillitis
c. constrictive pericarditis
c. contractile dysfunction
c. coronary occlusions
c. cor pulmonale
c. endocarditis
c. eosinophilic pneumonia (CEP)
c. fibrous pneumonia
c. fusiform aneurysm
c. graft vascular disease (CGVD)
c. heart failure
c. hemolytic anemia
c. hypertensive disease
c. hypertrophic emphysema
c. hyperventilation syndrome
c. idiopathic orthostatic hypotension
c. inflammatory airway disease
c. interstitial lung disease
c. lunger
c. lymphocytic thyroiditis
c. mucocutaneous moniliasis
c. myocarditis
c. necrotizing aspergillosis
c. obstructive airways disease
c. obstructive bronchitis
c. obstructive lung disease (COLD)
c. obstructive pulmonary disease (COPD)
c. obstructive pulmonary emphysema (COPE)
c. obstructive respiratory disease (CORD)
c. passive congestion
c. peripheral arterial disease (CPAD)
c. pharyngitis
c. pleurisy
c. pulmonary cystic lymphangiectasis
c. pulmonary edema
c. pulmonary emphysema (CPE)
c. pulmonary insufficiency of prematurity
c. recurrent chemical injury
c. renal failure

NOTES

chronic *(continued)*
  c. respiratory failure (CRF)
  C. Respiratory Questionnaire (CRQ)
  c. sheath
  c. shock
  c. sinus arrest
  c. stable angina
  c. stable asthmatic
  c. suppurative lung disease (CSLD)
  c. tamponade
  c. thromboembolic pulmonary
    hypertension (CTEPH)
  c. total occlusion (CTO)
  c. upper respiratory obstruction
  c. valvulitis
  c. volume load
chronicity
Chronicle implantable hemodynamic
  monitor
Chronocor IV external pacemaker
chronolog
  Nebulizer C.
chronophysiology
Chronos 04 pacemaker
chronotherapeutic
chronotherapy
chronotropic
  c. effect
  c. exercise assessment protocol
    (CAEP)
  c. incompetence
  c. response
chronotropism
  negative c.
  positive c.
Church
  C. cardiovascular scissors
  C. scissors
Churchill
  C. cardiac suction cannula
  C. sucker
Churchill-Cope reflex
Churg-Strauss
  C.-S. angiitis
  C.-S. syndrome (CSS)
  C.-S. vasculitis
Chuter endovascular device
Chvostek sign
chyliform
  c. pleural effusion
  c. pleurisy
chylomicron
  c. remnant
  c. remnant receptor
chylomicronemia
chylopericarditis
chylopericardium
  primary isolated c.

chylopleura
chylopneumothorax
chylothorax, pl. chylothoraces
  traumatic c.
chylous
  c. ascites
  c. effusion
  c. hydrothorax
  c. pericardial effusion
  c. pleural effusion
  c. pleurisy
  c. spill
chymase gene locus
CI
  cardiac index
  colloidal iron
  confidence interval
  constraint-induced
    CI therapy
Ciaglia
  C. percutaneous tracheostomy
    introducer
  C. serial dilatation technique
Ciba-Corning 2500 Co-Oximeter
cibenzoline
CIBIS
  Cardiac Insufficiency Bisoprolol Study
CIC
  carbachol inhalation challenge
cicaprost
cicatricial stenosis
cicatrization
cicletanine
cidal effect
Cidecin
cidofovir
Cidomycin
CIDS
  Canadian Implantable Defibrillator Study
cifenline succinate
cigarette
  c. cough
  c. smoke (CS)
  c. smoking
cilastatin
  imipenem and c.
cilazapril
cilexetil
  candesartan c.
cilia
ciliary
  c. beat frequency
  c. dysfunction
  c. efficacy
  c. impairment
  c. movement
ciliastatic

ciliated
    c. epithelial cell
    c. epithelium
ciliocytophthoria
ciliogenesis
ciliotoxicity
cilnidipine
cilostazol
cimetidine
Cimino
    C. arteriovenous shunt
    C.-Brescia arteriovenous fistula
Cimochowski cardiac cannula
cinchonism
cincinnatiensis
    Legionella c.
cine
    c. camera
    c. computed tomography
    c. CT
    c. gradient-echo MRI
    c. loop
    c. scan
    c. view
cineangiocardiography
    radionuclide c.
cineangiogram
cineangiographic system
cineangiography
    conventional c.
cinearteriography
cinecamera
cinefilm
cinefluorography
cinefluoroscopy
cineless
cineloop recording
cine-MRI
cine-pulse system
cineventriculogram
cineventriculography
CineView Plus Freeland system
cinnarizine
Cinobac Pulvules
cinoxacin
Cin-Quin
CIPF
    classic interstitial pneumonitis with
      fibrosis
Cipralan

Cipro
    C. injection
    C. Oral
ciprofibrate
ciprofloxacin hydrochloride
ciprostene
**Circadia dual-chamber rate-adaptive
  pacemaker**
circadian
    c. blood pressure pattern
    c. disruption
    c. event recorder
    c. pacemaker
    c. pattern
    c. periodicity
    c. rhythm
    c. variation
circannual cycle
circaseptan cycle
circle
    DataVue calibrated reference c.
    c. of Vieussens
    c. of Willis (CW)
Circon videohydrothoracoscope
circuit
    aortoiliofemoral c.
    arrhythmia c.
    Bentley Duraflo II extracorporeal
     perfusion c.
    bypass c.
    FilterLine c.
    fluidic c.
    Intertech anesthesia breathing c.
    Intertech Mapleson D
     nonrebreathing c.
    Intertech nonrebreathing modified
     Jackson-Rees c.
    macroreentrant c.
    output c.
    reentrant c.
    sensing c.
    shunting c.
    timing c.
circuitry
    low-prime c.
Circulaire
    C. aerosol drug delivery device
    C. aerosol drug delivery system
    C. inhaled medication delivery
     device
circulans
    Bacillus c.

C

NOTES

circular plane
circulating
    c. adhesion molecule (CAM)
    c. bacterial endotoxin
    c. endothelin
    c. interleukin-6
    c. water blanket
circulation
    airway, breathing, and c. (ABC)
    allantoic c.
    anterior c. (AC)
    assisted c.
    balanced coronary c.
    codominant coronary c.
    collateral c.
    compensatory c.
    coronary collateral c.
    derivative c.
    extracorporeal c.
    fetal c.
    Fontan c.
    left dominant coronary c.
    lesser c.
    peripheral c.
    persistent fetal c.
    placental c.
    portal c.
    posterior c. (PC)
    pulmonary c.
    restoration of spontaneous c.
      (ROSC)
    return of spontaneous c. (ROSC)
    systemic c.
    thebesian c.
    c. time
    c. volume
circulator
    C. boot
    c. boot therapy
circulatory
    c. arrest
    c. collapse
    c. compromise
    compromise systemic c.
    c. congestion
    c. depression
    c. embarrassment
    c. failure
    c. hypoxemia
    c. hypoxia
    c. instability
    c. overload
    c. stability
    c. support system
circumaortic
    c. venous collar
    c. venous ring

circumferential
    c. end-systolic stress (cESS)
    c. ESS
    c. fiber shortening
    c. wall stress (CWS)
circumflex (CX)
    c. aortic arch
    c. artery
    left c. (LCF)
circumoral cyanosis
circumscribed
    c. edema
    c. pleurisy
circus
    c. movement
    c. senilis
circus-movement tachycardia (CMT)
CIRF
    cocaine-induced respiratory failure
CirKuit-Guard
    C.-G. device
    C.-G. pressure relief valve
cirrhosis
    biliary c.
    cardiac c.
    congestive c.
    Laënnec c.
    c. of liver
    stasis c.
cirrhotic
cirsoid
    c. aneurysm
    c. varix
CIS
    coronary implant system
cisapride
cisatracurium besylate
cisplatin
    cyclophosphamide, bleomycin, c.
      (CBP)
    cyclophosphamide, doxorubicin, c.
      (CAP)
    doxorubicin, 5-fluorouracil, c.
      (AFP)
    c., etoposide (PE)
    mitomycin, vinblastine, c. (MVP)
    c., vincristine, doxorubicin,
      etoposide (CODE)
cisterna, pl. **cisternae**
    cylindrical confronting c.
    perinuclear c.
    subsarcolemma c.
    terminal c.
CIT
    cold ischemic time
citicoline
citrate
    caffeine c.

diethylcarbamazine c.
esprolol plus sildenafil c.
c. exchange
piperazine c.
sildenafil c.
sufentanil c.

citrated caffeine
citric acid cycle
Citrobacter
    C. amalonatica
    C. freundii
Citrol
    C. Oral Spray
    C. Smoking alternative
citrovorum rescue
c-Jun
    c-J. gene
    c-J. N-terminal kinase (JNK)
CK
    color kinesis
    creatine kinase
    CK image
CK-MB
    myocardial muscle creatine kinase
      isoenzyme
    CK-MB elevation
CL
    chest and left arm
    cycle length
    CL lead
CLA
    clarithromycin
Clado anastomosis
Cladosporium
Claforan
Clagett
    C. closure
    C. procedure
clamp
    Acland microvascular c.
    Ahlquist-Durham embolism c.
    Alfred M. Large vena cava c.
    Allis c.
    anastomosis c.
    aortic aneurysm c.
    Atlee c.
    Atrauclip grip c.
    AutoSuture Mini-CABG
      occlusion c.
    Bahnson aortic c.
    Bailey aortic c.
    Beck miniature aortic c.

Beck-Potts aortic and pulmonic c.
Blalock-Niedner pulmonic
  stenosis c.
Blalock pulmonary stenosis c.
Bradshaw-O'Neill aorta c.
bulldog c.
Bunnell-Howard arthrodesis c.
Calman carotid c.
Calman ring c.
cardiovascular c.
Castaneda anastomosis c.
caval occlusion c.
Cooley anastomosis c.
Cooley aortic c.
Cooley-Beck vessel c.
Cooley bronchus c.
Cooley coarctation c.
Cooley-Derra anastomosis c.
Cooley-Satinsky c.
Cooley vena cava c.
Crafoord coarctation c.
Crile c.
Crutchfield c.
Davidson c.
DeBakey aortic aneurysm c.
DeBakey arterial c.
DeBakey-Bahnson c.
DeBakey-Bainbridge c.
DeBakey-Beck c.
DeBakey-Derra anastomosis c.
DeBakey-Harken auricle c.
DeBakey-Howard aortic
  aneurysmal c.
DeBakey-Kay aortic c.
DeBakey-McQuigg-Mixter
  bronchial c.
DeBakey patent ductus c.
DeBakey pediatric c.
DeBakey peripheral vascular c.
DeBakey-Satinsky vena cava c.
DeBakey-Semb ligature-carrier c.
Demos tibial artery c.
Derra aortic c.
Derra vena caval c.
DeWeese vena cava c.
Diethrich shunt c.
dreamer c.
C. Ease device
Edwards c.
endoaortic c.
euglycemic glucose c.
Favaloro proximal anastomosis c.

NOTES

153

clamp *(continued)*
Garcia aorta c.
Glassman c.
Glover auricular-appendage c.
Grant abdominal aortic
aneurysmal c.
Gregory baby profunda c.
Grover c.
Gutgeman auricular appendage c.
Halsted c.
Hartmann c.
Heartport Endoaortic C.
Hopkins aortic c.
Hufnagel ascending aortic c.
Hunter-Satinsky c.
Jacobson microbulldog c.
Jacobson modified vessel c.
Jacobson-Potts c.
Jahnke anastomosis c.
Javid carotid artery bypass c.
Juvenelle c.
Kantrowitz thoracic c.
Kelly c.
Kindt carotid artery c.
Koala vascular c.
Lambert aortic c.
Lambert-Kay c.
Lambert-Kay aortic c.
Liddle aorta c.
Mattox aorta c.
microvascular c.
mosquito c.
Müller vena caval c.
mush c.
myocardial c.
noncrushing vascular c.
Noon A-V fistula c.
pediatric vascular c.
Pilling microanastomosis c.
Reich-Nechtow c.
Reinhoff c.
Reinhoff swan neck c.
resection c.
Rochester-Kocher c.
Rochester-Péan c.
Roe aortic tourniquet c.
Rosenkranz universal c.
Ruel aorta c.
Rumel c.
Sarnoff aortic c.
Sarot bronchus c.
Satinsky c.
Schumacher aorta c.
side biting c.
Sideris c.
Subramanian c.
suprahepatic caval c.
VascuClamp minibulldog vessel c.

VascuClamp vascular c.
vascular c.
vessel c.
Vorse-Webster c.
Wylie carotid artery c.
Yasargil carotid c.

clamshell
c. closure of atrial septal defect
c. device
c. incision
c. septal occluder
C. septal umbrella

clandestine myocardial ischemia

clapotement
bruit de c.

claquement
bruit de c.
c. d'ouverture

Clara cell secretory protein

clarithromycin (CLA)

Claritin
C.-D 24 Hour

Clarity
C. capnograph
C. multiparameter monitoring
system
C. software

Clark
C. classification of malignant
melanoma
C. expanding mesh catheter
C. helix catheter
C. oxygen electrode
C. rotating cutter catheter

Clarke-Hadfield syndrome

CLAS
Cholesterol Lowering Atherosclerosis
Study

CLASS
Clomethiazole Acute Stroke Study

class *(var. of* classification*)*

CLASSIC
Clopidogrel Aspirin Stent International
Cooperative

classic
c. angina
c. expectorant
c. interstitial pneumonitis with
fibrosis (CIPF)
c. mucolytic
c. risk factor
C. II stethoscope

classification, class
Allen and Davis c.
Ambrose c.
American Heart Association c.
American Heart Association Stroke
Outcome C. (AHA.SOC)

antiarrhythmic drug c. (Ia, Ib, Ic, II, III, IV)
Astler-Coller c.
Barrow c.
Braunwald c. (I–IIIB)
Canadian Cardiovascular Society c. (CCSC)
Canadian Cardiovascular Society functional c.
Canadian Heart C. (CHC)
Cedars-Sinai c.
Child c.
Clark c. of malignant melanoma
Cohen-Rentrop c.
congestive heart failure c. I-IV
Croften c.
DeBakey c.
de Groot c.
Dexter-Grossman c.
Diamond c.
Dukes c.
Efron jackknife c.
Fontain c.
Forrester Therapeutic C. grades I–IV
Fredrickson c.
Fredrickson hyperlipoproteinemia c.
Fredrickson, Levy and Lees c.
Fukunaga-Hayes unbiased jackknife c.
functional capacity c.
Gray-Weale c.
Hannover c.
Heath-Edwards c.
Heitzman c.
Hinkle-Thaler c.
hip c.
Killip heart disease c.
Killip-Kimball heart failure c.
KWB c.
Lev c.
Levine-Harvey c.
Liebow c.
Loesche c.
Lown c.
Mayo c.
Minnesota ECG c.
New York Heart Association functional c. (I–IV)
NYHA functional c. I–IV
Reid c.
Rentrop c.

round-robin c.
Sellers mitral regurgitation c.
Shaher-Puddu c.
Singh-Vaughan-Williams arrhythmia c.
Stary c.
TIMI c.
Timpe and Runyon c.
TNM c.
Vaughan-Williams c.
Vaughan-Williams antiarrhythmic drug c.
Walter Reed c.
Wood c.
Yacoub and Radley-Smith c.
Classix pacemaker
claudicant limb
claudication
   buttock c.
   calf c.
   intermittent c.
   one-block c.
   three-block c.
   two-block c.
   two-flights-of-stairs c.
Claudius fossa
Clauss
   C. assay
   C. method
clavicle
   acromial articular facies of c.
   acromial articular surface of c.
   sternal extremity of c.
clavicular facet
clavipectoral triangle
clavulanic acid
Clavulin
cleaner
   VT Mercury Vac organic mercury vacuum c.
clear
   C. Advantage filter
   C. Advantage Spirometry Filter
   c. cell
   c. cell carcinoma
   c. cell tumor
   Scot-Tussin Senior c.
   C. Tussin 30
clearance
   airway c.
   c. assistive device
   creatinine c.

C

NOTES

clearance *(continued)*
  drug c.
  gas c.
  mucociliary c. (MCC)
  peripheral zone radioaerosol c.
  c. technique
  tracheobronchial c.
ClearView
  C. intracoronary shunt
  C. intravascular arteriotomy shunt
cleavage
  abnormal c. of cardiac valve
cleft
  c. anterior leaflet
  c. of aortic leaflet
  cholesterol c.
  laryngeal c.
  c. mitral valve
  Schmidt-Lanterman c.
clemastine fumarate
clenched fist sign
clentiazem
Cleocin
  C. HCl
  C. HCl Oral
  C. Pediatric
  C. Pediatric Oral
  C. Phosphate
  C. Phosphate Injection
clevidipine
click
  ejection c.
  Hamman c.
  metallic c.
  mitral c.
  c. murmur
  nonejection systolic c.
  palmar c.
  c. syndrome
  systolic c.
Clickhaler
clicking
  c. pneumothorax
  c. rale
click-murmur syndrome
clindamycin
clinical
  C. Outcomes with Ultrasound Trial (CLOUT)
  c. practice guidelines (CPG)
  c. pulmonary infection score (CPIS)
Clinitron air-fluidized therapy
clinocephaly
Clinoril
clinostatic bradycardia

clip
  Adams-DeWeese vena caval serrated c.
  alligator c.
  Astro-Trace Universal adapter c.
  Atrauclip hemostatic c.
  Autostat ligating and hemostatic c.
  Benjamin-Havas fiberoptic light c.
  Benjamin-Havas light c.
  cardiac retraction c.
  crankshaft c.
  Datex SC-103 finger c.
  Elgiloy-Heifitz aneurysm c.
  Fogarty spring c.
  Horizon surgical ligating and marking c.
  ligation c.
  microbulldog c.
  Miles vena cava c.
  Moretz c.
  nose c.
  C. On torquer
  partial occlusion inferior vena cava c.
  Smith c.
  Sugar c.
  Sugita c.
  vascular c.
  vena cava c.
ClipTip reusable sensor
clivarine
CLM articulating laryngoscope blade
cloacae
  Enterobacter c.
clockwise
  c. flutter
  c. loop
  c. rotation
  c. rotation of electrical axis
  c. torque
clofazimine (CFZ)
  c. palmitate
clofibrate
clofilium
clomethiazole
  C. Acute Stroke Study (CLASS)
clonidine
  c. and chlorthalidone
  c. hydrochloride
cloning
  DNA c.
Cloninger Temperament and Character Inventory
clonogenic technique
Clonorchis sinensis
clopidogrel
  C. Aspirin Stent International Cooperative (CLASSIC)

c. bisulfate
C. in Unstable Angina to Prevent Recurrent Ischemic Events (CURE)
C. versus Aspirin in Patients at Risk of Ischemic Events (CAPRIE)

clorprenaline hydrochloride
closed
c. chest cardiac massage
c.-chest cardiopulmonary resuscitation
c. chest commissurotomy
c. chest massage
c. chest pneumothorax
c. chest thoracostomy
c. chest water-seal drainage
c. circuit method
c.-circuit spirometer
c. end-hole catheter
c. transventricular mitral commissurotomy
c.-tube thoracostomy

closed-loop
c.-l. delivery
c.-l. device
c.-l. pacing
c.-l. sedative administration

Closer-Closure catheter
The Closer suture-mediated closure system
closing
c. slope
c. snap
c. volume

clostridial myocarditis
Clostridium
C. botulinum
C. perfringens
C. septicum
C. tetani

closure
airway c.
C. catheter/radiofrequency generator
Clagett c.
double umbrella c.
King ASD umbrella c.
nonoperative c.
patch c.
percutaneous patent ductus arteriosus c.
premature valve c.

primary c.
PTFE c.
saphenous vein patch c.
threatened c.
transcatheter c. (TCC)
umbrella c.

clot
agonal c.
agony c.
antemortem c.
autologous c.
blood c.
c. of blood
c.-bound thrombin
c. buster
C. Buster Amplatz thrombectomy device
chicken fat c.
currant jelly c.
fibrin c.
laminated c.
c. lysis
passive c.
postmortem c.
c. retraction time
C. Stop drain

cloth
Dacron c.

clotrimazole
clotted hemothorax
clotting
c. abnormality
c. disorder

cloud
signal-loss c.

clouded sensorium
clouding
hilar c.
mental c.

CLOUT
Clinical Outcomes with Ultrasound Trial
Core Laboratory Ultrasound Analysis
CLOUT study

Cloverleaf catheter
cloxacillin sodium
Cloxapen
CLS
capillary leak syndrome
CLSE
calf lung surfactant extract
clubbing
c., cyanosis, and edema (CCE)

NOTES

clubbing *(continued)*
    digital c.
    c. of fingers
    c. of toes
cluster-of-grapes appearance
cM
    centiMorgan
CM3 cocktail
CMA
    cerebral microangiopathy
CMAD
    count median aerodynamic diameter
CMAP
    compound motor action potential
CMC
    corticomedullary contrast
CMCT
    central motor conduction time
CMD
    count median diameter
CMP-NANA
    cystidine monophospho-*N*-
    acetylneuraminic acid
CMRGI$_c$
    cerebral rate of glucose metabolism
CMRO$_2$
    cerebral rate of oxygen metabolism
CMS
    Cardiovascular Measurement system
    Cholesterol Monitoring system
        CMS AccuProbe 450 system
CMT
    chemotherapy
    circus-movement tachycardia
CMV
    controlled mechanical ventilation
    cytomegalovirus
        CMV IE-2 gene expression
        CMV IE-2 riboprobe
        CMV pneumonitis
        CMV seronegative
        CMV seropositive
CMVIG
    cytomegalovirus immune globulin
cNOS
    constitutive nitric oxide synthase
CNP
    C-type natriuretic peptide
CNT
    continuous nebulization therapy
CO
    carbon monoxide
    cardiac output
        CO oximetry
        CO Sleuth
        CO Sleuth carbon monoxide
    monitor

        CO Sleuth handheld carbon
    monoxide analyzer
CO$_2$
    carbon dioxide
    arterial partial pressure of CO$_2$
    (PaCO$_2$)
    CO$_2$ oximetry
    partial pressure of end-tidal CO$_2$
    (PETCO$_2$)
    pulse oximeter/end tidal CO$_2$
    (POET)
    CO$_2$ waveform
CoA
    coarctation of the aorta
    coenzyme A
Coach incentive spirometer
coaching whistle
Coag
    Rapidpoint access/Rapidpoint C.
Coag-A-Mate coagulometer
CoaguChek
    C. aPTT testing system
    C. system
coagulation
    c. activity
    disseminated intravascular c. (DIC)
    c. factor
    c. forceps
    c. necrosis
    c. protein
    c. thrombosis
    c. time
coagulative myocytolysis
coagulator
    argon beam c.
    Concept bipolar c.
coagulometer
    Coag-A-Mate c.
coagulopathy
    consumption c.
    disseminated intravascular c. (DIC)
    hemorrhagic c.
coagulum formation
coal
    c. miner's lung
    c. tar
    c. worker's pneumoconiosis (CWP)
coalescence
coalition
    Canadian Cardiovascular C. (CCC)
Coanda effect
coapt
coarctation
    angulated c.
    c. of the aorta (CoA)
    aortic c.
    distorted c.
    juxtaductal c.

low-plaque c.
native c.
c. of pulmonary artery
reversed c.
coarctectomy
coarse
c. breath sounds
c. chromatin
c. crackle
c. murmur
c. rale
c. thrill
CoA-set fibrin monomer assay
Coat-a-Count radioimmunoassay
coating
Carbofilm turbostatic carbon
permanent c.
Hydrocoat hydrophilic c.
polylactic acid stent c.
Pro/Pel c.
Teflon c.
coaxial
c. micropuncture introducer set
c. pressure
COBALT
Continuous Infusion Versus Bolus
Alteplase Trial
Continuous Infusion Versus Double-
Bolus Administration of Alteplase
cobalt
c. asthma
c. cardiomyopathy
c. exposure
c. fumes
c.-induced airway disease
c. toxicity
c. in tungsten carbide
cobalt-related
c.-r. asthma
c.-r. disease
c.-r. lung disease
c.-r. pulmonary fibrosis
Cobas Fara centrifugal analyzer
cobbler's chest
cobblestoning
Cobe
C. cardiotomy reservoir
C. 2991 cell processor
C. double blood pump
C. gun
C. Optima hollow-fiber membrane
oxygenator

C. small vessel cannula
C. Spectra apheresis system
C.-Stockert heart-lung machine
C. Trima automated blood-
component collection system
Coblation
cobra-head anastomosis
Cobra over-the-wire balloon catheter
cobra-shaped catheter
cocaine
c. abuse
c.-induced
c.-induced myocardial infarction
c.-induced respiratory failure (CIRF)
c.-related sudden death
cocci (*pl. of* coccus)
coccidioidal
Coccidioides immitis
coccidioidin test
coccidioidoma
coccidioidomycosis
disseminated c.
meningeal c.
miliary c.
primary c.
pulmonary c.
coccobacillus
coccus, pl. **cocci**
cocci country
gram-negative cocci
gram-positive cocci
cocci granuloma
Cochrane Library
cocillana
Cockayne syndrome
Cockett procedure
cockroach asthma
cocktail
C. Attenuation of Rotational
Ablation Flow Effects (CARAFE)
Brompton c.
cardiac c.
CM3 c.
scintillation c.
coctum
sputum c.
Codafed Expectorant
Codamine Pediatric
CODE
cisplatin, vincristine, doxorubicin,
etoposide

C

NOTES

159

code
- c. blue
- ICHD pacemaker c.
- Minnesota c.
- Minnesota Q-QS c.
- pacing c.

Codehist DH

codeine
- bromodiphenhydramine and c.
- brompheniramine, phenylpropanolamine, and c.
- chlorpheniramine, phenylephrine, and c.
- chlorpheniramine, pseudoephedrine, and c.
- C. Conhn
- Deproist Expectorant With C.
- guaifenesin and c.
- guaifenesin, pseudoephedrine, and c.
- Guiatussin with C.
- Mallergan-VC with C.
- Phenergan VC With C.
- Phenergan With C.
- Pherazine VC w/ C.
- Pherazine with C.
- c. phosphate
- promethazine and c.
- promethazine, phenylephrine, and c.
- Promethist With C.
- Prometh VC With C.
- terpin hydrate and c.
- triprolidine, pseudoephedrine, and c.

Codemaster defibrillator

Codiclear DH

codominant
- c. coronary circulation
- c. system
- c. vessel

coefficient
- apparent diffusion c. (ADC)
- capillary filtration c.
- damping c.
- c. of diffusion
- fat-absorption c.
- Hill c.
- Spearman c.

coenzyme
- c. A (CoA)
- c. Q
- c. Q10

COER-24 delivery system

coeur en sabot

Coe virus

coexistent
- c. cardiac alterations
- c. pathology

coffee bean asthma

Cogan syndrome

Co-Gesic

Cognitive Failures Questionnaire (CFQ)

cogwheel respiration

COHb
- carboxyhemoglobin

Cohen-Rentrop classification

cohesiveness

Cohn cardiac stabilizer

cohort
- C. of Rescue Angioplasty in Myocardial Infarction (CORAMI)
- c. study

coil
- Cook detachable PDA c.
- Cook retrievable embolization c.
- distal shocking c.
- Duct Occluder pfm c.
- c. electrode
- elliptical end-capped quadrature radiofrequency c.
- c. embolization
- Gianturco c.
- Gianturco wool-tufted wire c.
- Guglielmi detachable c.
- Helmholtz head c.
- c. obliteration
- phased array receiver c.
- platinum c.
- prolapse c.
- quadrature birdcage c.
- quadrature head c.
- spring c.
- c. stent
- tantalum balloon-expandable stent with helical c.
- c. thrombogenicity
- c.-tipped catheter

coin
- c. artifact
- c. lesion
- c. lesion of lung
- c. percussion
- c. sound
- c. test

coincidence detection

coital hemoptysis

coitus-induced myocardial infarction

CO_2ject system

co-knitted stent

colchicine

COLD
- chronic obstructive lung disease

cold
- c. abscess
- c. agglutinin
- c. agglutinin pneumonia
- c. air challenge (CAC, CACh)
- c. blood cardioplegia

c. crystalloid cardioplegia
c. dry air challenge
c., dry air-induced asthma
c. exposure
c. gangrene
c. hemagglutinin disease
c.-induced angina
c. ischemic arrest
c. ischemic time (CIT)
c.-mist humidifier
c. nodule
c. potassium cardioplegia
c. pressor test
c. pressor testing maneuver
c. spot
Sudafed Severe C.

Coldloc
Cole
C.-Cecil murmur
C. pediatric tube
C. polyethylene vein stripper
C. uncuffed endotracheal tube
colesevelam HCl
Colestid
colestipol hydrochloride
colfosceril palmitate
coli
pneumatosis c.
colic
biliary c.
Colin
C. ambulatory BP monitor
C. Electronics BP-508 tonometry
system
colistimethate sodium
colistin
collagen
bovine biodegradable c.
c. deposition
endomysial c.
c. fatigue
fibrillar c.
c. plug
c. sponge
c. (type I–V)
c. vascular lung disease
c. vascular sealing (CVS)
collagenase
collagen-impregnated knitted Dacron velour graft
collagenolysis

collagenous
c. cap
c. pneumoconiosis
collapse
cardiovascular c.
circulatory c.
hemodynamic c.
lobar c.
massive c.
c. rale
respiratory c.
right ventricular diastolic c.
c. therapy
tracheobronchial c.
collapsed lung
collapsibility
pharyngeal c.
collapsing pulse
collar
circumaortic venous c.
c. incision
c. prosthesis
c. of Stokes
collateral
adequate c.
antegrade c.
aortopulmonary c.
arcade c.
bridging c.
bronchial c.
c. channel
c. circulation
c. filling
c. flow
c. hyperemia
perfusion via c.
reconstitution via c.
c. respiration
septal c.
systemic c.
venous c.
c. vessel
collateralization
compensatory c.
pial c.
ventilation c.
collateralizing vessel (CV)
collecting duct
collection
expired air c.

C

NOTES

collier's
    c. lung
    c. phthisis
collimation
    x-ray scatter c.
collimator
    511-keV c.
    LEAP low-energy all-purpose c.
    Picker Dyna Mo c.
    slant hole c.
    Sophy high-resolution c.
Collins
    C. bicycle
    C. bicycle ergometer
    C. chain compensated gasometer
      technique
    C. Dry spirometer
    C. Eagle I spirometry unit
    C. respiratometer
    C. solution
    C. Survey spirometer
    C. SurveyTach with MicroTach
      assembly
Collis-Nissen fundoplication
colloid
    c. oncotic pressure (COP)
    c. osmotic pressure
colloidal iron (CI)
Collostat hemostatic sponge
coloboma, heart anomaly, choanal
    atresia, retardation, and genital and
    ear anomalies (CHARGE)
Colombo inverted Y technique
colon
    angiodysplasia of c.
    marginal artery of c.
colonic ischemia
colonization
    airway bacterial c.
    atypical mycobacterial c.
    bacterial c.
colony stimulating factor (CSFs)
Coloplast wafer
color
    c. Doppler energy (CDE)
    c. Doppler flow convergence
    c. echotomography Doppler
    c. flow Doppler
    c. flow mapping
    c. kinesis (CK)
    c. kinesis echocardiographic display
    c. kinesis image
    c. kinesis imaging
    c. M-mode Doppler
      echocardiography
    c. power angiography
    c. tissue Doppler imaging
color-coded flow mapping

Colorscan II
colorvascular Doppler ultrasound
ColorZone
    C. Management system
    C. tape
Columbia S.K. virus
column
    blood c.
    plasma exchange c.
Coly-Mycin M Parenteral
coma
    apoplectic c.
    diabetic c.
Combicath
    C. double-plugged telescope
      catheter
combination beat
combined
    c. heart catheterization
    c. M-mode echophonocardiography
    penicillin G benzathine and
      procaine c.
Combipres
Combitube
    c. airway
    esophagotracheal c. (ETC)
Combivent inhaler
Combivir
combretastatin A4 prodrug (CA4P)
comet
    C. catheter
    c. sign
    c. tail sign
Comfeel Ulcus dressing
Comfit endotracheal tube holder
ComfortSeal mask
Commander
    C. angiopolasty guide wire
    C. PTCA wire line
Command PS pacemaker
commissural
    c. bundle
    c. fusion
    c. mitral regurgitation
    c. splitting
commissurales
    cuspides c.
commissure
    aortic c.
    fused c.
    scalloped c.
    split fused c.
    valve c.
commissuroplasty
commissurotomy
    ball mitral c.
    balloon mitral c. (BMC)
    Brockenbrough transseptal c.

closed chest c.
closed transventricular mitral c.
mitral c.
mitral balloon c.
mitral valve c.
percutaneous mechanical mitral c.
percutaneous mitral c. (PMC)
percutaneous mitral balloon c.
  (PMBC)
percutaneous transatrial mitral c.
percutaneous transvenous mitral c.
  (PTMC)
transventricular mitral valve c..
tricuspid c.
committed mode pacemaker
common
c. atrioventicular canal
c. atrium
c. carotid artery
c. carotid artery intima-media
  thickness (CCA-IMT)
c. carotid compression (CCC)
c. femoral artery
c. femoral vein
c. hepatic artery
c. iliac artery
commotio cordis
Commucor A+V Patient monitor
communication
arteriovenous c.
bronchiole-alveolar c.
interalveolar c.
interarterial c.
narrow c.
communis
basalis c.
community-acquired
c.-a. infection
c.-a. pneumonia (CAP)
compact
c. A-V node
C. desktop spirometer
C. II desktop spirometer
Compactin
compages thoracis
Companion 314 nasal CPAP
Comparison of Abciximab Complications
  with Hirulog (and Back-Up
  Abciximab) Events Trial (CACHET)
compartment
c. procedure
c. syndrome

Compazine
C. injection
C. Oral
compensated
c. congestive heart failure
c. edentulism
c. sheath
c. shock
compensating emphysema
compensation
cardiac c.
depth c.
electronic distance c.
time-gain c. (TGC)
compensatory
c. antiinflammatory response
  syndrome (CARS)
c. circulation
c. collateralization
c. emphysema
c. hypertrophy
c. hypertrophy of the heart
c. mechanism
c. pause
c. polycythemia
c. vessel enlargement
competence
cardiac c.
competing risks
complement
c. activation
c4b purified human c.
c. component C1r deficiency
c. inhibitor
c. system
complemental air
complementary
c. air
c. balloon angioplasty
complement-fixation test
complete
c. atrioventricular
c. atrioventricular block (CAVB)
c. atrioventricular dissociation
c. A-V block
c. A-V dissociation
c. blood count (CBC)
c. heart block (CHB)
c. pacemaker patient testing system
  (CPPTS)
C. stent delivery platform

NOTES

complete *(continued)*
  Tenax-XR C.
  c. transposition of great arteries
completed
  c. myocardial infarction
completely positive deflection flutter
complex
  aberrant c.
  aberrant QRS c.
  Acinetobacter calcoaceticus-
    baumannii c.
  amphotericin B cholesteryl
    sulfate c.
  amphotericin B lipid c. (ABLC)
  anisoylated plasminogen
    streptokinase activator c. (APSAC)
  anomalous c.
  antiinhibitor coagulant c.
  AP-1 c.
  c. atheroma
  atrial c.
  atrial premature c.'s
  c. atrioventricular canal
  atrioventricular junctional escape c.
  auricular c.
  A-V junctional escape c.
  Battey bacillus c.
  bizarre QRS c.
  broad QRS c.
  capture c.
  Carney c.
  carotid intima-media c.
  diphasic c.
  Eisenmenger c.
  electrocardiographic c.
  electrocardiographic wave c.
  equiphasic c.
  factor IX c. (human)
  far-field QRS c.
  filtered QRS c.
  c. fixation (CF)
  frequent spontaneous premature c.
  fusion c.
  Ghon c.
  Golgi c.
  HLA-DQ gene c.
  HLA-DR gene c.
  interpolated premature c.
  iron dextran c.
  isodiphasic c.
  junctional c.
  c. lesion
  LIP/PLH c.
  Lutembacher c.
  MAI c.
  membrane attack c. (MAC)
  monophasic c.
  monophasic contour of QRS c.

  multiform premature ventricular c.
  Mycobacterium avium c. (MAC)
  Mycobacterium avium-
    intracellulare c.
  nadir of QRS c.
  c. plaque
  plasminogen-streptokinase c.
  pleomorphic premature
    ventricular c.
  polymorphic premature
    ventricular c.
  polysaccharide-iron c.
  premature atrial c.
  premature atrioventricular
    junctional c.
  premature ventricular c.
  primary c.
  prothrombinase c.
  QRS c.
  QRS-T c.
  QS c.
  Ranke c.
  R-on-T premature ventricular c.
  RS c.
  Shone c.
  sling ring c.
  sodium ferric gluconate c.
  Steidele c.
  streptokinase-plasminogen c.
  Taussig-Bing c.
  thrombin-antithrombin III c.
  transposition c.
  TU c.
  VATER c.
  ventricular c.
  ventricular premature c. (VPC)
compliance
  aortic c.
  chest wall c.
  c. of heart
  left ventricular chamber c.
  left ventricular muscle c.
  lung c.
  patient c.
  c., rate, oxygenation, and pressure
  c., rate, oxygenation, and pressure
    index
  C. Related Acute Complication
    (CRAC)
  C. Related Angioplasty
    Complications (CRAC)
  specific c.
  static lung c.
  thoracic c.
  total lung c.
  ventilatory c.
Compliance-Related Angioplasty
  Complications trial

compliant balloon
complicated myocardial infarction
complication
    angioplasty c.
    cardiovascular c.
    Compliance Related Acute C.
      (CRAC)
    Compliance Related
      Angioplasty C.'s (CRAC)
    Controlled Abciximab and Device
      Investigation to Lower Late
      Angioplasty C.'s (CADILLAC)
    Evaluation of IIb/IIIa Platelet
      Receptor Antagonist c7E3 in
      Preventing Ischemic C.'s (EPIC)
    groin c.
    late angioplasty c.
    noninfectious c.
    c. rate
    thromboembolic c. (TEC)
component
    bronchospastic c.
    elastic c.
    harmonic c.
    plasma thromboplastin c.
    thrombogenic c.
composite valve graft replacement
compound
    antimony c.
    artificial lung-expanding c. (ALEC)
    Bato c.
    chlorophenylfuranyl c.
    c. cyst
    glycyl c.
    Hurler-Scheie c.
    Hycomine C.
    c. motor action potential (CMAP)
    nitinol polymeric c.
compressed-air sickness
compressed Ivalon patch graft
compressible volume
compression
    anterior thoracic c.
    anteroposterior thoracic c.
    aortic root c.
    c. atelectasis
    c. bandage
    barrel-hooping c.
    biventricular direct cardiac c.
    c. boot
    cardiac c.
    chamber c.

    chest c.
    common carotid c. (CCC)
    c. cough
    direct cardiac c. (DCC)
    dynamic tracheal c.
    extrinsic c.
    Femo stop pneumatic c.
    c. gloves
    high-frequency chest wall c.
      (HFCC)
    intermittent pneumatic c. (IPC)
    interposed abdominal c. (IAC)
    intrathoracic gas c.
    nonuniform direct cardiac c.
    sternal c.
    c. stockings
    c. thrombosis
    c. ultrasonography
compression-decompression
    active c.-d. (ACD)
compressor
    AM50-1 aerosol/medication air c.
    AM-50 portable air c.
    Deschamps c.
    DeVilbiss Pumo-Aide LT c.
    Dura-Aire c.
    Easy Air 15 c.
    Easy/Neb c.
    external inflatable c.
    Freeway Lite portable aerosol c.
    Pulmo-Mist c.
compressor-generated nebulizer (CGN)
compressor/nebulizer
    Pulmo-Aide aerosol c.
    PulmoMate aerosol c.
compromise
    circulatory c.
    respiratory c.
    side branch c.
    c. systemic circulatory
    vascular c.
Compton
    C. effect
    C. scatter
Compu-Neb ultrasonic nebulizer
Compuscan Hittman computerized
  electrocardioscanner
computed
    c. tomographic scan
    c. tomography (CT)
    c. tomography angiographic
      portography (CTAP)

C

NOTES

computed *(continued)*
  c. tomography angiography (CTA)
  c. tomography scanner
computer
  CardioData Mark IV c.
  digital c.
  Inspiron Instromedix c.
computer-assisted diagnostics (CAD)
computerized
  c. axial tomography (CAT)
  c. diaphragmatic breathing
    retraining (CDBR)
  C. Healthcare And Record Transfer
    System (CHARTS)
  c. sleep analysis system
  c. texture analysis
Comtesse medical support stockings
Comtrex Maximum Strength Non-
  Drowsy
conal
  c. septal defect
  c. septum
Concato disease
concave pattern
concealed
  c. accessory pathway
  c. bypass tract
  c. conduction
  c. entrainment
  c. retrograde conduction
  c. rhythm
Concentraid Nasal
concentration
  fractional inspired oxygen c. (FIO$_2$)
  hydrogen ion c. (pH)
  intracellular calcium c.
  lactic acid c.
  lymphocyte c.
  minimal alveolar c. (MAC)
  minimum bactericidal c.
  minimum inhibitory c. (MIC)
  plasma endothelin c.
  plasma homocysteine c.
  venous plasma norepinephrine c.
concentration-effect relation
concentrator
  NewLife Elite c.
  NewLife oxygen c.
  Puritan Bennett Aeris 590 c.
  SolAiris III oxygen c.
  SolAiris V oxygen c.
concentric
  c. hypertrophic cardiomyopathy
  c. left ventricular hypertrophy
  c. remodeling
concept
  C. bipolar coagulator
  InDirect primary stenting c.

  leading circle c.
  solid angle c.
Conchapak
concity
concordance
  atrioventricular situs c.
  ventriculoarterial c.
concordant
  c. alternans
  c. alternation
  c. changes electrocardiogram
concorde
  ACS C.
Concord line draw syringe
concretio
  c. cordis
  c. pericardii
concussion
  myocardial c.
condition
  isocapnic c.
  preexisting c.
conditio sine qua non
conductance
  airway c.
  c. catheter
  c. catheter method
  epicardial flow c.
  S-segment airway c.
  c. stroke volume
  upstream airway c.
  c. vessel
conducting airway
conduction
  aberrant c.
  aberrant ventricular c.
  accelerated c.
  accelerated A-V nodec.
  anisotropic c.
  anomalous c.
  antegrade c.
  anterograde c. (Ae-H)
  atrioventricular c. (AVC)
  A-V c.
  A-V nodal c.
  c. block
  cardiac c.
  concealed c.
  concealed retrograde c.
  decremental c.
  c. defect (CD)
  c. delay
  delayed c.
  differential transisthmus c.
  c. disorder
  c. disturbance
  electrotonic c.
  forward c.

His-Purkinje c.
c. impairment
impulse c.
internodal c.
intraatrial c.
intraventricular c.
nondecremental retrograde
  ventriculoatrial c.
orthograde c.
c. pathway
Purkinje c.
c. ratio
retrograde c.
retrograde VA c.
sinoventricular c.
c. slowing
supernormal c.
supranormal c.
c. system
c. time
transseptal c.
V-A c.
c. velocity
ventricular c.
ventriculoatrial c. (VAC, V-AC)
conductive
c. coupling
c. system
conduit
extracardiac ventriculopulmonary c.
c. lumen
Rastelli c.
respiratory syncytial virus c.
cone
arterial c.
elastic c.
pulmonary c.
coned-down view
Conex
confidence interval (CI)
configuration
atrial sensing c.
dome-and-dart c.
doughnut c.
EASI lead c.
horseshoe c.
QRS complex c.
snowman c.
spadelike c.
spike-and-dome c.
ventricular sensing c.
confirmatory evaluation

confluent bronchopneumonia
Conforma 3000 delivery system
congenita
myotonia c.
congenital
c. adrenal hyperplasia
c. anomaly of mitral valve
c. aortic aneurysm
c. aortic stenosis
c. aspiration pneumonia
c. atelectasis
c. bronchial atresia (CBA)
c. central alveolar hypoventilation
c. central hypoventilation syndrome
c. complete heart block
c. conotruncal anomaly
c. cystic adenomatoid malformation
c. diaphragmatic hernia (CDH)
c. heart block
c. heart disease (CHD)
c. interrupted aortic arch
c. laryngeal stridor
c. lobar overinflation
c. long QT interval syndrome
c. malformation
c. mitral stenosis
c. murmur
c. periobronchial myofibroblastic
  tumor
c. pseudocholinesterase deficiency
c. pulmonary arteriovenous
c. pulmonary arteriovenous fistula
c. single atrium
c. symptomatic A-V block
congenitale
P c.
congenitally
c. absent pericardium
c. corrected transposition of the
  great arteries
Congess
Congestac
congested
congestion
active c.
chronic passive c.
circulatory c.
functional c.
hypostatic c.
passive c.
physiologic c.
pulmonary c.

NOTES

congestion *(continued)*
    pulmonary venous c.
    venous c.
    Vicks 44D Cough & Head C.
Congestive
    C. Heart Failure-Survival Trial of Antiarrhythmic Therapy (CHF-STAT)
congestive
    c. cardiomyopathy
    c. cirrhosis
    c. edema
    c. heart failure (CHF)
    c. heart failure classification I-IV
    c. pulmonary disease
Conhn
    Codeine C.
coniofibrosis
conjoined cusp
conjugate
    polyribosylribitol phosphate-diphtheria toxoid c. (PRP-D)
conjugated equine estrogen (CEE)
connection
    accessory arteriovenous c.
    anomalous pulmonary venous c.
    cavopulmonary c.
    Damus-Kaye-Stansel c.
    discordant atrioventricular c.
    discordant ventriculoarterial c.
    Fontan c.
    partial anomalous pulmonary venous c. (PAPVC)
    pulmonary venous c.
    systemic to pulmonary c.
    total anomalous pulmonary venous c. (TAPVC)
    total cavopulmonary c. (TCP, TCPC)
    univentricular atrioventricular c.
connective
    c. tissue
    c. tissue growth factor (CTGF)
    c. tissue lesion
connector
    ACS angioplasty Y c.
    Biotronik lead c.
    c. block
    Cordis c.
    Luer-Lok c.
    Medtronic c.
    unipolar c.
    Y c.
Connell airway
connexin 43
connexon distribution
connori
    Nosema c.

Conn syndrome
conotruncal anomaly
conoventricular fold and groove
Conradi-Hünermann syndrome
Conradi line
Conray contrast medium
consanguineous
consanguinity
consciousness
    loss of c.
conscious sedation
consecutive vasculitis
CONSENSUS
    Cooperative North Scandinavian Enalapril Survival Study
Conservative Strategy-TIMI 18 trial
conserver, conservor
    EX-2000 DeVilbiss c.
    Hideaway oxygen c.
    high-flow oxygen c. (HFOC)
    Oxymatic c.
    Oxymatic electronic oxygen c.
    Oxymatic oxygen c.
    PulseDose EX2000D oxygen c.
    PulseDose oxygen c.
    Puritan Bennett OxiClip PC20 c.
    Walkabout oxygen c.
consolidated lung volume
consolidation
    airspace c.
    lobular c.
    c. of lung
    patchy c.
    peribronchiolar c.
    peribronchiolar airspace c.
    pulmonary c.
consolidative process
consonating rale
constant
    c. coupling
    empiric c.
    gas c. (R)
    Gorlin c.
    Hodgkin-Huxley c.
constant-flow method
Constant-T
Constellation advanced mapping catheter
constellatus
    Peptococcus c.
constitutive
    c. nitric oxide synthase (cNOS)
    c. secretion
constraint
    pericardial c.
constraint-induced (CI)
    c.-i. movement therapy

constriction
annular c.
esophageal c.
neurohormonal arterial c.
occult pericardial c.
supraannular c.
constrictive
c. bronchiolitis
c. endocarditis
c. heart disease
c. pericarditis
c. physiology
constrictor muscle of pharynx
consumption
c. coagulopathy
maximum oxygen c. (VO_2 max)
myocardial oxygen c. (MVO_2)
oxygen c. (VO_2)
peak exercise oxygen c. (VO_2)
platelet c.
volume oxygen c. (VO_2)
Contac Cough Formula Liquid
contact metastasis
contagiosum
molluscum c.
Contak CD CHF device
content
bone mineral c. (BMC)
harmonic c.
oxygen c.
contiguous ventricular septal defect
continuity
c. of care
c. equation
continuous
c. albuterol nebulization (CAN)
c. arrhythmia
c. arterial spin-labeled perfusion
MRI (CASL-PI MRI)
c. arteriovenous hemofiltration
(CAVH)
c. aspiration of subglottic
secretions (CASS)
c. atrial fibrillation (CAF)
c. cardiac output (CCO)
c. cardiac output with SvO_2
(CCOmbo)
c. cyclical peritoneal dialysis
(CCPD)
c. cyclic peritoneal
c. full-thickness linear lesion
c. heart murmur

c. hyperfractionated accelerated
radiotherapy (CHART)
C. Infusion Versus Bolus Alteplase
Trial (COBALT)
C. Infusion Versus Double-Bolus
Administration of Alteplase
(COBALT)
c. loop exercise echocardiogram
c. mandatory ventilation
c. murmur
c. nebulization therapy (CNT)
c. noninvasive monitoring of
ventilated infants
c. pericardial lavage
c. positive air pressure
c. positive airway pressure (CPAP)
c. positive pressure ventilation
c. progesterone
c. ramp protocol
c. venovenous hemofiltration
(CVVH)
c. wave Doppler echocardiogram
continuous-flow ventilation
continuous-wave
c.-w. Doppler (CWD)
c.-w. Doppler echocardiography
c.-w. Doppler imaging
c.-w. Doppler ultrasound
c.-w. laser ablation
continuum
Evolve Cardiac C.
contour
cardiac c.
c. of heart
C. High Voltage Can ICD
C. II ICD
left-heart c.
C. LT V-135D ICD
C. LTV-135D implantable
cardioverter-defibrillator
C. MD implantable cardioverter-
defibrillator
C. MD implantable single-lead
cardioverter-defibrillator
Murgo pressure c.
QRS c.
C. V-145D ICD
C. V0145D implantable
cardioverter-defibrillator
ventricular c.
Ventritex C.

NOTES

contracta
vena c.
contracted heart
contractile
c. amplitude
c. behavior
c. element
c. function
c. protein
c. reserve
c. ring dysphagia
c. work index
contractility
increased c.
isovolumetric c.
left ventricular c.
myocardial c.
ventricular c.
ventricular wall c.
contraction
anodal closure c.
anodal opening c.
atrial premature c. (APC)
automatic c.
automatic ventricular c.
c. band
c. band necrosis
cardiac c.
escape c.
escape ventricular c.
Gowers c.
isometric c.
isotonic c.
LAA c.
maximum voluntary c. (MVC)
muscular c.
nodal premature c.
c. pattern
premature c.
premature atrial c. (PAC)
premature junctional c. (PJC)
premature ventricular c. (PVC)
R on T ventricular premature c.
supraventricular premature c.
synchronous atrial c.
tertiary c.
ventricular premature c. (VPC)
volume c.
contractor
Bailey-Gibbon rib c.
Graham rib c.
contracture
ischemic c. of left ventricle
contraindication
contrast
c. agent
angiographic c.
c. angiography

c. bubble study
corticomedullary c. (CMC)
c. echocardiography
half-diluted c.
Iohexol c.
left atrial spontaneous echo c.
(LASEC)
c. left ventriculography
Levovist c.
c. material
c. medium
c. medium delivery
negative c.
Optiray c.
Optison c.
c. ratio
sonicated albumin-dextrose c.
spontaneous echo c. (SEC)
c. stagnation
time-to-peak c.
Ultravist c.
c. venography
contrast-enhanced
c.-e. CT
dynamic susceptibility c.-e. (DSC)
c.-e. echocardiogram
c.-e. magnetic resonance
angiography (CEMRA)
c.-e. transcranial color-coded real-
time sonography (CE-TCCS)
contrast-guided venipuncture
contrecoup injury
control
axial c.
CVC 123 calibration verification c.
damping c.
C. III Elite disinfectant
gain c.
pressure c. (PC)
pressure-regulated volume c.
(PRVC)
QC 253 CO-oximetry c.
quality c.
RA 523 blood gas/CO-oximetry c.
reject c.
Take C.
time-gain c. (TGC)
time-varied gain c. (TGC, TVGC)
torque c.
volume c. (VC)
c. wire
controlled
C. Abciximab and Device
Investigation to Lower Late
Angioplasty Complications
(CADILLAC)
c. breathing
c. coughing

c. diaphragmatic respiration
c. lung biopsy
c. mechanical ventilation (CMV)
C. Onset Verapamil Investigation for Cardiovascular Endpoints (CONVINCE)
c. respiration
c. ventilation
c. ventricular response

controller
DOC-2000 demand oxygen c.
flow c.
pressure c.
vacuum c.
venous flow c. (VFC)
volume c.

control-mode ventilation
ControlWire guidewire
contusion
cardiac c.
lung c.
myocardial c.
c. pneumonia
pulmonary c.

Contuss
conundrum
conus
c. arteriosus
c. cordis
c. elasticus
pulmonary c.
tendon of c.

convalescent phase
convective gas mixing
conventional
amphotericin b (c.)
C. Antiarrhythmic versus Amiodarone in Survivors of Cardiac Arrest Drug Evaluation (CASCADE)
c. cineangiography
c. ventilation (CV)

convergence
color Doppler flow c.

conversion
analog-to-digital c.
automatic mode c. (AMC)
Fontan c.
pressure c.

converter
scan c.

converting enzyme inhibitor

convex linear array
convexoconcave (C-C)
CONVINCE
Controlled Onset Verapamil Investigation for Cardiovascular Endpoints
CONVINCE clinical trial

convulsion
ConXn
cooing
c. murmur
c. sign

Cook
C. arterial catheter
C. balloon
C. Cardiovascular infusion catheter
C. County aspirator
C. deflector
C. detachable PDA coil
C. flexible biopsy forceps
C. FlexStent
C. intracoronary stent
C. locking stylet
C. multiple-assessment scale
C. pacemaker
C. retrievable embolization coil
C. Spectrum catheter
C. TPN catheter
C. yellow pigtail catheter

cookie
Gelfoam c.

Cook-Medley hostility scale
cool
c. head-warm body perfusion
c. mist

Cooley
C. anastomosis clamp
C. anemia
C. aortic clamp
C. aortic vent needle
C. atrial retractor
C.-Baumgarten aortic forceps
C.-Beck vessel clamp
C.-Bloodwell-Cutter valve
C.-Bloodwell mitral valve prosthesis
C. bronchus clamp
C. cardiac tucker
C. coarctation clamp
C.-Cutter disk prosthetic valve
C. Dacron prosthesis
C.-Derra anastomosis clamp
C. dilator
C. forceps

C

NOTES

Cooley (*continued*)
C. intrapericardial anastomosis
C.-Merz sternum retractor
C. modification of Waterston anastomosis
C. neonatal instrument
C.-Pontius sternal blade
C. retractor
C.-Satinsky clamp
C. sump tube
C. U sutures
C. vena cava clamp
C. Vital microvascular needle holder
C. woven Dacron graft

cooling
c. blanket
cardioplegia c.
core c.
topical c.

Cool Tip catheter
cool-tip laser
Cool-vapor vaporizer
Coomassie blue stain
Coombs
C. murmur
C. test

Coons Super Stiff long tip guidewire
Cooperative
C. Cardiovascular Project
Clopidogrel Aspirin Stent International C. (CLASSIC)
Echocardiography Persantine International C. (EPIC)
C. North Scandinavian Enalapril Survival Study (CONSENSUS)

Cooper ligament
Cooperman event probability
Cooper-Rand intraoral artificial larynx
coordinate system
CO-Oximeter
Ciba-Corning 2500 C.-O.
C.-O. module

CO-oximetry
carbon monoxide oximetry

COP
colloid oncotic pressure
cryptogenic organizing pneumonia
cryptogenic organizing pneumonitis

COPD
chronic obstructive pulmonary disease

COPE
chronic obstructive pulmonary emphysema

Cope
C. method bronchography
C. pleural biopsy needle
C. thoracentesis needle

Copeland technique
COPERNICUS
Carvedilol Prospective Randomized Cumulative Survival
COPERNICUS trial

Cophene XP
Coping Strategies questionnaire
copious sputum
copolymer
polyolefin c. (POC)

copper (CU)
c.-wire arteries
c.-wire effect
c. wiring

copper-62 (^{62}CU)
Co-Pyronil 2 Pulvules
cor
c. adiposum
c. arteriosum
c. biloculare
c. bovinum
c. dextrum
c. en cuirasse
c. hirsutum
c. juvenum
c. mobile
c. pendulum
c. pseudotriloculare biatriatum
c. pulmonale
c. sinistrum
c. taurinum
c. triatriatum
c. triatriatum dexter
c. triloculare
c. triloculare biatriatum
c. triloculare biventriculare
c. venosum
c. villosum

Coradur
coral thrombus
CORAMI
Cohort of Rescue Angioplasty in Myocardial Infarction
CORAMI clinical trial
CORAMI II clinical trial

Coratomic
C. implantable pulse generator
C. prosthetic valve
C. R wave inhibited pacemaker

Corazonix Predictor
CORD
chronic obstructive respiratory disease

cord
false vocal c.
true vocal c.
vocal c.

Cordarone

Cordis
- C. ablation catheter
- C. Ancar pacing lead
- C. Atricor pacemaker
- C. bioptome
- C. Bioptome sheath
- C. BriteTip guiding catheter
- C. Chronocor IV pacemaker
- C. connector
- C. coronary stent
- C. CrossFlex coronary stent
- C. Ducor I, II, III catheter
- C. Ducor pigtail catheter
- C. Ectocor pacemaker
- C. fixed-rate pacemaker
- C. Gemini cardiac pacemaker
- C. guiding catheter
- C. Hakim pump
- C.-Hakim shunt
- C. LC Multipurpose stent system
- C. lead conversion kit
- C. Lumelec catheter
- C. mapping catheter
- C. Mini stent system
- C. Multicor pacemaker
- C. Omni Stanicor Theta transvenous pacemaker
- C. Powerflex angioplasty balloon
- C. Predator balloon catheter
- C. Predator PTCA balloon catheter
- C. Sentron transducer
- C. Sequicor cardiac pacemaker
- C. sheath
- C. Son-II catheter
- C. Stabilizer marker wire
- C. Stanicor unipolar ventricular pacemaker
- C. Stockert generator
- C. Synchrocor pacemaker
- C. tantalum coil stent
- C. tantalum stent
- C. Theta Sequicor DDD pulse generator
- C. Titan balloon dilatation catheter
- C. Trakstar PTCA balloon catheter
- C. TransTaper tip catheter
- C. Ventricor pacemaker
- C.-Webster ablation catheter
- C.-Webster mapping catheter

cordis
- accretio c.
- adipositas c.
- angina c.
- anulus fibrosus dexter/sinister c.
- apex c.
- ataxia c.
- atrium c.
- bulbus c.
- chordae tendineae c.
- chorea c.
- commotio c.
- concretio c.
- conus c.
- crena c.
- delirium c.
- diastasis c.
- ectasia c.
- ectopia c.
- facies anterior c.
- facies diaphragmatica c.
- facies inferior c.
- facies pulmonalis c.
- facies pulmonalis dextra/sinistra c.
- facies sternocostalis c.
- hypodynamia c.
- ictus c.
- incisura apicis c.
- malum c.
- myasthenia c.
- myofibrosis c.
- myomalacia c.
- myopathia c.
- palpitatio cordis
- pulsus c.
- steatosis c.
- systema conducens c.
- theca c.
- trepidatio c.
- tumultus c.
- vortex c.

Cordox

cords
- Ferrein c.

cordy pulse

core
- c. of atheroma
- atheromatous c.
- c. cooling
- ischemic c.
- C. Laboratory Ultrasound Analysis (CLOUT)
- lipid c.
- c. pneumonia
- c. temperature

C

NOTES

Core Exercise Testing Laboratory
Coreg
Core-Vent implant
Cor-Flex
    C.-F. guidewire
    C.-F. wire guide
Corgard
Cori disease
Corival 400 ergometer
corkscrew artery
Corlon angiocatheter
Corlopam
Cormed ambulatory infusion pump
corneal arcus
cornealis
    arcus c.
Cornelia de Lange syndrome
Cornell
    C. Coronary Artery Bypass
       Outcomes Trial (CCABOT)
    C. exercise protocol
    C. modification of the Bruce
       protocol
    C. protocol
    C. voltage
    C. voltage-duration product criteria
corniculate tubercle
corniculum
    c. laryngis
Coroflex coronary stent system
Corometrics
    C. Doppler scanner
    C. monitor
Corometrics-Aloka echocardiograph
  machine
coronal
    c. cut
    c. plane
    c. slice
corona radiata
Coronariche
coronarism
coronaritis
coronarius
    sinus c.
coronaropathy
    dilated c.
coronary
    c. air embolism
    c. anastomotic shunt
    c. anatomy
    c. aneurysm
    c. angiographic catheter
    c. angiography
    c. angiography catheter
    c. angioplasty
    C. Angioplasty and Rotablator
       Atherectomy Trial (CARAT)

C. Angioplasty and Rotablator
   Atherectomy Trial II (CARAT II)
C. Angioplasty versus Bypass
   Revascularization Investigation
   (CABRI)
C. Angioplasty versus Excisional
   Atherectomy Trial (CAVEAT)
c. angioscopy
c. arterial reserve
c. arteriography (CAG)
c. arteriosclerosis
c. arteritis
c. artery
c. artery angioplasty
c. artery anomaly
c. artery atherosclerosis
c. artery button
c. artery bypass
c. artery bypass graft
c. artery bypass grafting surgery
C. Artery Bypass Graft Surgery
   With/Without Simultaneous
   Epicardial Patch for Automatic
   Implantable Cardioverter-
   Defibrillator (CABG Patch)
C. Artery Bypass Revascularization
   Investigation (CABRI)
c. artery disease (CAD)
c. artery dissection
c. artery distensibility
c. artery dominance
c. artery ectasia
c. artery fistula (CAF, CAP)
c. artery lesion
c. artery obstruction
c. artery occlusion
c. artery probe
C. Artery Restenosis Prevention on
   Repeated Thromboxane
   Antagonism (CARPORT)
c. artery-right ventricular fistula
C. Artery Risk Development in
   Young Adults (CARDIA)
c. artery scan (CAS)
c. artery spasm
c. artery stenosis
C. Artery Surgery Study (CASS)
c. artery thrombosis
c. atherectomy
c. atheroma
c. bed
c. bifurcation
c. blood flow (CBF)
c. blood flow measurement
c. blood flow velocity (CBFV)
c. branch occlusion
c. bypass graft patency
c. bypass surgery

cafe c.
c. calcium
C. Cardiocoil stent
c. care unit (CCU)
c. collateral circulation
c. cushion
c. cusp
c. dissection
c. embolism
c. endarterectomy
c. event
c. failure
c. flow reserve (CFR)
c. flow reserve technique
c. flow velocity
c. flow velocity reserve (CFVR, CVR)
c. heart disease (CHD)
C. Imagecath angioscope
c. implant system (CIS)
c. insufficiency
c. intravascular ultrasound
c. IVUS
c. luminal stenosis
c. luminology
c. macroangiopathy
c. magnetic resonance angiography
c. microangiopathy
c. microcirculatory vasoconstriction
c. microvascular disease
c. microvessel endothelium
c. nodal rhythm
c. occlusion
c. occlusive disease
c. ostial dimple
c. ostial stenosis
c. ostium
percutaneous transluminal c.
c. perfusion gradient
c. perfusion pressure
c. plaque regression
c. plaque rupture
C. Primary Prevention Trial (CPPT)
c. prognostic index
c. radiation therapy (CRT)
c. recanalization
c. reflex
c. remodeling
c. reserve
c. resistance vessel
c. retroperfusion

c. revascularization
C. Revascularization Ultrasound Angioplasty Device (CRUSADE)
c. ring
c. risk profile
c. roadmapping
c. rotational ablation
c. rotational atherectomy (CRA)
c. seeking catheter
c. sinus (CS)
c. sinus blood flow (CSBF)
c. sinus catheterization
c. sinus electrogram
c. sinus lead
c. sinus retroperfusion
c. sinus rhythm
c. sinus thermodilution
c. sinus thermodilution catheter
c. slow flow syndrome (CSFS)
c. spasm
c. spastic angina
c. steal
c. steal mechanism
c. steal phenomenon
c. stenting
c. sulcus
C. Syndromes trial
c. tendon
c. thrombolysis
c. thrombosis
c. tree
c. vascular reserve
c. vascular resistance
c. vascular turgor
c. vasculature
c. vasodilation
c. vasodilator reserve
c. vasomotion
c. vasospasm
c. vein
c. venous pressure
c. wire
coronary-pulmonary fistula (C-PF)
coronary-subclavian steal syndrome
Coronaviridae virus
Coronavirus
coronavirus infection
COROSCOP C cardiac imaging system
corporeal
corpus
c. linguae
c. phalangis

C

NOTES

corpuscle
>Donne c.
>Drysdale c.
>Hassall c.

corrected
>c. dextrocardia
>c. sinus node recovery time
>c. TIMI frame count (CTFC)
>c. transposition of the great
> vessels

correction
>Bonferroni c.
>metabolite c.
>Teichholz c.
>Yates c.

Correra line
corridor procedure
Corrigan
>C. disease
>C. pneumonia
>C. pulse
>C. respiration
>C. sign

corrodens
>*Bacteroides c.*
>*Eikenella c.*

corrosive esophagitis
corset balloon catheter
Cortef Oral
cortex
>adrenal c.
>premotor c. (PMC)
>primary sensorimotor c. (SM1)
>sensorimotor c. (SMC)

cortical
>c. arousal index (CAI)
>c. plasticity
>c. stroke
>c. vein thrombosis

corticomedullary contrast (CMC)
cortico-pallido-nigra-thalamo cortical
loop
corticosteroid-dependent asthmatic
corticosteroid therapy
corticosteroid-treated heart
corticostriatocerebellar loop
corticotrophin-releasing factor (CRF)
corticotropin
cortisol
>24-hour c.

cortisone acetate
Cortone
>C. Acetate
>C. Acetate injection
>C. Acetate Oral

Cortrosyn injection
Corvert injection

Corvisart
>C. disease
>C. facies

Corvita
>C. endoluminal graft
>C. endoprosthesis stent graft

Corwin
Coryllos
>C.-Bethune rib shears
>C.-Moure rib shears
>C. rib raspatory
>C.-Shoemaker rib shears
>C. thoracoscope

Corynebacterium
>*C. diphtheriae*
>*C. jeikeium*

coryza
coryzavirus
Corzide
CoSeal resorbable synthetic sealant
Cosgrove
>C. annuloplasty system
>C. annuloplasty system with
> Duraflo treatment
>C. mitral valve replacement
>C. retractor

Cosmegen
CO₂SMO
>C. capnograph/pulse oximeter
>C. Plus
>C. Plus continuous noninvasive
> respiratory profile monitor
>C. Plus monitor

Cosmos
>C. 283 DDD pacemaker
>C. II DDD pacemaker
>C. II multiprogrammable dual-
> chamber cardiac pulse generator
>C. II pacemaker
>C. II pulse generator
>C. pulse-generator pacemaker

Cosprin
cost
>oxygen c.
>Prescription Analyses and C.
> (PACT)

costal
>c. diaphragm
>c. margin
>c. part of diaphragm
>c. pit of transverse process
>c. pleura
>c. pleurisy
>c. respiration
>c. surface of lung

costalis
>pleura c.

costarum
    arcus c.
costochondral
    c. junction
    c. syndrome
costochondrectomy
costochondritis
costoclavicular
    c. ligament
    c. maneuver
    c. rib syndrome
costodiaphragmatic
    c. recess
    c. recess of pleura
costomediastinal recess of pleura
costophrenic
    c. angle
    c. septal line
    c. sinus
    c. sulci
    c. sulcus
costosternal syndrome
costotome
costoversion thoracoplasty
costovertebral angle (CVA)
cosyntropin
cotinine nicotine by-product
cotransporter
    monocarboxylate/proton c. (MCT)
Cotrim DS
co-trimoxazole
cottage-loaf appearance
cotton-dust asthma
cottonoid patty
cotton-wool
    c.-w. exudate
    c.-w. spot
Cotunnius space
couch incrementation
cough
    aneurysmal c.
    Balme c.
    barking c.
    brassy c.
    cigarette c.
    compression c.
    c. CPR
    c. CPR technique
    croupy c.
    decubitus c.
    Diphen C.
    directed c.

    dog c.
    dry c.
    c. efficiency
    extrapulmonary c.
    c. fracture
    habit c.
    habitual c.
    hacking c.
    mechanical c.
    minute-gun c.
    Morton c.
    multifactorial c.
    paroxysmal c.
    privet c.
    productive c.
    psychogenic c.
    reflex c.
    c. reflex
    c. resonance
    rhonchorous c.
    seal-bark c.
    Silphen C.
    smoker's c.
    stomach c.
    c. suppressant
    Sydenham c.
    c. syncope
    tea taster's c.
    c. threshold
    c. transportability
    trigeminal c.
    c. variant asthma
    wet c.
    whooping c.
    winter c.
coughing
    controlled c.
    expulsive c.
    Huff c.
    paroxysm of c.
    quad c.
cough-thrill
Coulter counter
CoumaCare Coumadin management
  system
Coumadin
coumadinization
coumaric anhydride
coumarin, cumarin
    c. pulsed dye laser
Coumel tachycardia
coumestan

C

NOTES

coumetarol
count
  blood c.
  complete blood c. (CBC)
  corrected TIMI frame c. (CTFC)
  differential blood c.
  double c.
  end-diastolic c.
  end-systolic c.
  first shock c.
  c. median aerodynamic diameter
    (CMAD)
  c. median diameter (CMD)
  c. rate
  relative lymphocyte c.
  second through fifth shock c.
  shock c.
  thrombolysis in myocardial
    infarction frame c.
  TIMI frame c.
  total patient shock c.
  touch shock c.
  white blood cell c.
counter
  Coulter c.
  event/episode c.
  pacing c.
  time-based c.
counterclockwise
  c. flutter
  c. rotation
counterimmunoelectrophoresis
counteroccluder
counterpressor
  Acland-Buncke c.
counterpulsation
  aortic c.
  c. balloon
  balloon c.
  enhanced external c. (EECP)
  intraaortic balloon c. (IABC)
  intraarterial c.
  percutaneous intraaortic balloon c.
countershock
  electrical c.
counting
  double c.
count-rate linearity
country
  cocci c.
coupled
  c. beat
  c. premature beat
  c. pulse
  c. rhythm
  c. suturing
couplet
  ventricular c.

coupling
  arterial c.
  conductive c.
  constant c.
  electromechanical c.
  excitation-contraction c.
  fixed c.
  intercellular c.
  c. interval
  variable c.
  vasoneuronal c.
  ventriculoarterial c.
Cournand
  C. cardiac device
  C. catheter
  C. device
  C. dip
  C.-Grino angiography needle
  C. needle
  C.-Potts needle
  C. quadpolar catheter
cove plane
cover
  OxiLink oximeter probe c.
Covera-HS
Cover-Strip wound closure strip
Coversyl
coving of ST segments
COX
  cyclooxygenase
COX-1
  cyclooxygenase-1
  COX-1 enzyme
COX-2
  cyclooxygenase-2
  COX-2 enzyme
Cox
  C. maze operation
  C. organism
Co-Xan syrup
Coxiella
  C. burnetii
coxsackie A, B, B3, B4 virus
coxsackievirus
  c. carditis
  c. myocarditis
Cozaar
CP
  Vancocin CP
CPAD
  chronic peripheral arterial disease
CPAP
  continuous positive airway pressure
    autotitrating CPAP
    Companion 314 nasal CPAP
    fixed-pressure CPAP
    intelligent CPAP

Lightweight and portable Sullivan nasal CPAP
nasal CPAP
NightBird nasal CPAP
Phantom nasal mask CPAP
Revitalizer Soft-Start nasal CPAP
Sullivan III CPAP

CPB
cardiopulmonary bypass
CPC
chest pain center
CPCA2000 counter-pulsation device
CPE
chronic pulmonary emphysema
CPET
cardiopulmonary exercise test
C-PF
coronary-pulmonary fistula
CPG
clinical practice guidelines
CPHV OptiForm mitral valve
CPI
C. Astra pacemaker
C. automatic implantable defibrillator
C. DDD pacemaker
C. endocardial defibrillation/rate-sensing/pacing lead
C. Endotak SQ electrode lead
C. Endotak transvenous electrode
C. Maxilith pacemaker
C. Microthin DI, DII lithium-powered programmable pacemaker
C. Mini device
C. Minilith pacemaker
C. pacemaker
C. porous tined-tip bipolar pacing lead
C. RPx implantable cardioverter-defibrillator
C. Sentra endocardial lead
C. Sweet Tip lead
C. tunneler
C. Ultra II pacemaker
C. Ventak AICD
C. Ventak PRx cardioverter-defibrillator
C. Vista-T pacemaker
CPI/Guidant lead
CPI-PRx pulse generator
CPIS
clinical pulmonary infection score

CPK
creatine phosphokinase
brain band enzyme of CPK (CPK-BB)
CPK isoenzyme
MB enzymes of CPK
muscle fraction enzyme of CPK (CPK-MM, CPK-3)
myocardial band enzymes of CPK (CPK-MB, CPK-2)
CPK-3 (*var. of* CPK-MM)
CPK-BB
brain band enzyme of CPK
CPK-BB band
CPK-MB, CPK-2
myocardial band enzymes of CPK
CPK-MB band
CPK-MB fraction
CPK-MM, CPK-3
muscle fraction enzyme of CPK
CPK-MM band
CPL cardiopulmonary diagnostic system
CPP
cerebral perfusion pressure
CPPT
Coronary Primary Prevention Trial
CPPTS
complete pacemaker patient testing system
CPR
cardiopulmonary resuscitation
cough CPR
four-phase Lifestick CPR
simultaneous compression-ventilation CPR (SCV-CPR)
CPS
cardiopulmonary support
CPS system
CPT
chest physical therapy
CPX
cardiopulmonary exercise
CPX test
C1qR
C-R
Bicillin C-R
CR
chest and right arm
CR lead
metoprolol CR
Norpace CR

NOTES

C

CR-10
0 to 10 category ratio
CRA
coronary rotational atherectomy
CRAC
Compliance Related Acute Complication
Compliance Related Angioplasty
Complications
CRAC study
cracked-pot
c.-p. resonance
c.-p. sound
cracking
environmental stress c.
crackle
bibasilar coarse c.
coarse c.
end-inspiratory c.
end inspiratory Velcro c.
pleural c.
crackling rale
cradle
foot c.
Crafoord
C. coarctation clamp
C.-Cooley tucker
C. lobectomy scissors
C. pulmonary forceps
C.-Sellor hemostatic forceps
C.-Senning heart-lung machine
C. tunneler
Cragg
C. Convertible wire
C. endoluminal graft
C. Endopro system
C. Endopro System I
C. Endopro System I/Passager stent
graft
C. FX wire
C. infusion wire
C. stent
C. thrombolytic brush
cramp
calf c.
cranial
c. angulation
c. arteritis
c. nerves I–XII
craniocardiac reflex
craniocaudal view
craniopharyngeal
c. duct
c. duct tumor
cranking
arm c.
crankshaft clip
Cranley-Grass phleborrheogram

CRAO
central retinal artery occlusion
craquement
bruit de c.
crash technique
crassamentum
Crawford
C. graft inclusion technique
C. suture ring
C. R. Bard catheter
CRC
cerebrovascular reserve capacity
CRCV
cerebral red blood cell volume
C-reactive protein (CRP)
cream, creme
Amino-Cerv Vaginal C.
Gormel c.
Medrol Veriderm C.
Synapse electrocardiographic c.
crease
ear lobe c. (ELC)
creatine
c. kinase (CK)
c. phosphokinase (CPK)
creatinine clearance
Creech
C. aortoiliac graft
manner of C.
C. manner
C. technique
creep
stent c.
creeping thrombosis
Crego traction
creme (var. of cream)
crena cordis
crenulated tantalum wire
creola
c. body
Creo-Terpin
crepitance
crepitant rale
crepitation
crepitus
crescendo
c. angina
c. murmur
c. sleep
c. TIA
crescendo-decrescendo murmur
crescent
sublingual c.
crescentic glomerulonephritis
CREST
calcinosis, Raynaud phenomenon,
esophageal involvement, sclerodactyly,
telangiectasia

Carotid Revascularization
Endarterectomy Versus Stenting Trial
CREST syndrome

crest
cardiac neural c.
supraventricular c.
vagal neural c.

CRF
chronic respiratory failure
corticotrophin-releasing factor

Cribier-Letac
C.-L. aortic valvuloplasty balloon
C.-L. catheter

Cribier method

Cricket
C. pulse oximeter
C. pulse oximetry monitor
C. recording pulse oximeter

cricoesophageal tendon

cricoesophageus
tendo c.

cricoid
c. cartilage
c. pressure

cricoidea
cartilago c.

cricoideae
arytenoidea c.

cricopharyngeal achalasia syndrome

cricothyroid
c. artery
c. membrane

cricotracheotomy

cri du chat syndrome

Crile
C. clamp
C.-Duval lung-grasping forceps
C. tip occluder

crimper

crimping

Crinone

crinophagy

crisis, pl. **crises**
anaphylactic c.
bronchial c.
cardiac c.
hypertensive c.
laryngeal c.
myasthenic c.
pharyngeal c.
sickle cell c.
thoracic c.

CRISP
Cholesterol Reduction in Seniors
Program

Crisp aneurysm

CRISP-US
Cholesterol Reduction in Seniors
Program, United States

crisscross
c. atrioventricular valve
c. fashion
c. heart
c. heart malposition

crista
c. supraventricularis
c. terminalis

criteria, sing. **criterion**
Airlie House c.
Akaike information c.
Allen-Brown c.
Billingham c.
Bogalusa c.
Casale-Devereux c.
Cornell voltage-duration product c.
Dallas c.
Duke c.
Eagle c.
Estes ECG c.
exclusion c.
Framingham heart failure c.
Gubner-Ungerleider voltage c.
Heath-Edwards c.
Jones c.
Krichenko c.
12-lead voltage-duration product c.
Light c.
Penn Convention c.
pseudodisappearance criterion
Rand appropriateness selection c.
Rautaharju ECG c.
Romhilt-Estes point score c.
Saccomanno morphologic c.
Sellers c.
Sokolow-Lyon voltage c.
TIMI c.
voltage c.
von Reyn c.
Wilks lambda criterion

critical
c. aortic stenosis
c. care unit
C. Care Ventilator
c. coronary stenosis

NOTES

C

critical *(continued)*
    c. coupling interval
    c. flicker frequency
    c. flicker fusion
    c. rate
    c. valvular stenosis
Criticare
    C. $ETCO_2$ multigas analyzer
    C. $ETCO_2/SpO_2$ monitor
    C. pulse oximeter
CritiCath thermodilution catheter
Critikon
    C. automated blood pressure cuff
    C. balloon temporary pacing
      catheter
    C. balloon thermodilution catheter
    C. balloon-tipped end-hole catheter
    C. balloon wedge pressure catheter
    C. guidewire
    C. pressure infuser
Crixivan
crochetage pattern
Crocq disease
Croften classification
Crolom Ophthalmic Solution
cromafiban
cromakalim
cromoglycate
    disodium c. (DSCG)
    PMS-Sodium C.
    sodium c.
cromolyn
    c. sodium
    c. sodium inhalation solution
Cronassial
cross
    c. femoral-femoral bypass
    yellow c.
crossbridge
    actin-myosin c.
cross-checking
    sensory c.-c.
cross-clamp
    aortic c.-c.
    c.-c. time
cross-clamping of aorta
crossed
    c. cerebellar diaschisis (CCD)
    c. embolism
CrossFlex
    C. coil stent
    C. LC coronary stent
    C. LC-stainless steel, laser-cut
      coronary stent
    C. stent
Cross-Jones
    C.-J. disk prosthetic valve

    C.-J. disk valve prosthesis
    C.-J. mitral valve
cross-linkage theory
crosslinked D fragment
crossover
    c. bypass
    femoral-femoral c.
    c. femoral-femoral bypass
cross-reactive antibody
CrossSail coronary dilatation catheter
cross-sectional
    c.-s. area (CSA)
    c.-s. echocardiography (CSE)
    c.-s. two-dimensional
      echocardiogram
    c.-s. ventilatory functional study
crosstalk pacemaker
Cross Top replacement oxygen sensor
Crosswire nitinol hydrophilic guidewire
Crotalus
croup
    catarrhal c.
    diphtheritic c.
    false c.
    membranous c.
    pseudomembranous c.
    spasmodic c.
    c. tent
croup-associated (CA)
Croupette child tent
crouposa
    angina c.
croupous
    c. bronchitis
    c. laryngitis
    c. pharyngitis
    c. pneumonia
croupy cough
crowded oropharynx
Crow-Fukase syndrome
crowing
    c. breath sounds
    c. inspiration
Crown
    C.-Crisp index
    C. needle
    C. stent
CRP
    C-reactive protein
CRQ
    Chronic Respiratory Questionnaire
CRT
    coronary radiation therapy
cruces *(pl. of crux)*
cruciate anastomosis
crude stroke
crudum
    sputum c.

cruentum
> sputum c.

CRUISE
> Can Routine Ultrasound Improve Stent Expansion
> Can Routine Ultrasound Influence Stent Expansion
>> CRUISE study

Crump vessel dilator

crunch
>> Hamman c.
>> Means-Lernan mediastinal c.
>> mediastinal c.

crunching sound

crural
>> c. artery
>> c. diaphragm

cruris
> angina c.

crus
>> c. dextrum fasciculi atrioventricularis
>> c. sinistrum diaphragmatis
>> c. sinistrum fasciculi atrioventricularis

CRUSADE
> Coronary Revascularization Ultrasound Angioplasty Device
>> CRUSADE clinical trial

crush artifact

crushing chest pain

Crutchfield clamp

Cruveilhier
>> C. murmur
>> C. nodes
>> C. sign
>> C. sign

Cruveilhier-Baumgarten

crux, pl. **cruces**
>> c. dextrum fasciculi atrioventricularis
>> c. of heart
>> c. sinistrum fasciculi atrioventricularis

cruzi
> *Trypanosoma c.*

cryoablation
>> arrhythmia circuit c.
>> encircling c.
>> c. lesion

cryocardioplegia

cryocatheter
> Freezor c.

cryocrit

Cryo/Cuff pressure boot

Cryo-Cut microtome

cryofrigitronics

cryoglobulinemia

CryoLife
>> C. Single Step dilution method
>> C. valve graft

CryoLife-O'Brien
>> C.-O. stentless valve
>> C.-O. valve

cryoprecipitate

cryopreservation

cryopreserved
>> c. heart valve allograft
>> c. homograft valve
>> c. human aortic allograft
>> c. valved allograft
>> c. vein

cryoprobe
>> ERBE c.
>> MST c.
>> Spembly c.

cryoprotectant

cryosurgical technique

cryotherapy
> endobronchial c.

CryoValve-SG human allograft heart valve

CryoVein saphenous vein allograft

cryptococcal
>> c. myocarditis
>> c. pulmonary disease

cryptococcoma

cryptococcosis
> disseminated c.
> pulmonary c.

Cryptococcus
>> *C. albidus*
>> *C. histolyticus*
>> *C. laurentii*
>> *C. neoformans*

cryptogenic
>> c. fibrosing alveolitis (CFA)
>> c. organizing pneumonia (COP)
>> c. organizing pneumonitis (COP)
>> c. stroke

cryptophthalmos syndrome

cryptosporidiosis

Cryptosporidium

NOTES

C

crystal
asthma c.
Cardiometrics Flowire Doppler echo c.
Charcot-Leyden c.
Charcot-Neumann c.
Charcot-Robin c.
Leyden c.
LZT c.
piezoelectric c.
sonomicrometer piezoelectric c.
crystalline nicotine
crystalloid
c. cardioplegia
c. cardioplegic solution
c. fluid
c. potassium cardioplegia
c. prime
c. resuscitation
Crysticillin
C. A.S.
C. A.S. injection
Crystodigin
CS
cardiogenic shock
cavernous sinus
cigarette smoke
coronary sinus
cycloserine
Pertussin CS
Poly-Histine CS
CS-2000
Cardiovit C.
CSA
cross-sectional area
CSAS
central sleep apnea syndrome
CSBF
coronary sinus blood flow
CSE
cross-sectional echocardiography
CSFI
Cholesterol-Saturated Fat Index
CSFS
coronary slow flow syndrome
CSFs
colony stimulating factor
CSI
chemical shift imaging
CSLD
chronic suppurative lung disease
CSS
Churg-Strauss syndrome
CSSA
carotid stent-supported angioplasty
CSSA clinical trial
CSVT
central splanchnic venous thrombosis

CSWT
cardiac shock wave therapy
CT
cardiothoracic ratio
computed tomography
CT angiography
cine CT
contrast-enhanced CT
helical CT
high-resolution CT (HRCT)
reference phantom CT
CT scan
Siemens Evolution electron beam CT
Technicare Omega 500 CT
thin-section CT
CTA
computed tomography angiography
CTAO
cerebral thromboangiitis obliterans
isolated CTAO
CTAP
computed tomography angiographic portography
CTB
cytotrophoblast
CTEPH
chronic thromboembolic pulmonary hypertension
CTFC
corrected TIMI frame count
CTGF
connective tissue growth factor
CT-guided stereotaxic technique
CTICU
cardiothoracic intensive care unit
CTLA4Ig protein
cTnI
cardiac troponin I
cTnI assay
cTnT
cardiac troponin T
CTO
chronic total occlusion
C-to-E amplitude
CTR
cardiothoracic ratio
CTS
cardiothoracic surgery
CTS Voyager Aortic IntraClusion device
cTT
cerebral transit time
C-type natriuretic peptide (CNP)
CU
copper
⁶²CU
copper-62

cubitus valgus
cuff
    antimicrobial catheter c.
    aortic c.
    Astropulse c.
    atrial c.
    blood pressure c.
    Critikon automated blood
        pressure c.
    Dinamap blood pressure c.
    endotracheal tube c.
    Finapres finger c.
    finger c.
    c. plethysmography
    pneumatic c.
    c. sign
    c. suctioning
    c. test
    tracheostomy c.
cuffed
    c. endotracheal tube
    c. hypertension
    c. tracheostomy tube
cuffing
    peribronchial c.
cuff-leak test
Cuidant system
cuirass
    chest c.
    c. jacket
    c. respirator
    tabetic c.
    c. ventilator
cuirasse
    cor en c.
culbertsoni
    Acanthamoeba c.
cul-de-sac
    blind c.-d.-s.
culotte
    c. coronary stenting technique
    c. fashion
culprit
    c. lesion
    c. lesion angioplasty
    c. vessel angioplasty
culture-negative endocarditis
cumarin (var. of coumarin)
cumetharol
cumethoxaethane
cuneiform tubercle
Cunninghamella

cup
    Ster-O_2-Mist ultrasonic c.
cupping artifact
cuprophane membrane
cupula
    c. of pleura
    c. pleurae
    pleural c.
curare
curd
    soap c.
CURE
    Clopidogrel in Unstable Angina to
        Prevent Recurrent Ischemic Events
        CURE clinical trial
curette
Curosurf intratracheal suspension
Curracino-Silverman syndrome
currant
    c. jelly clot
    c. jelly sputum
    c. jelly thrombus
current
    alternating c. (AC)
    bioelectric c.
    calcium c. (I_{Ca})
    chloride c. (I_{Cl})
    diastolic c.
    direct c. (DC)
    fast sodium c.
    K c.
    low energy direct c. (LEDC)
    membrane c.
    pacemaker c. (I_F)
    pseudoalternating c.
    pump c.
    radiofrequency c. (RFC)
    range-alternating c.
    sodium c. (I_{Na})
    systolic c.
    toxin-insensitive c.
    transient inward c.
    transsarcolemmal calcium c.
Curretab Oral
Curry needle
Curschmann spiral
curve
    actuarial survival c.
    AH c.
    ascorbate dilution c.
    carbon dioxide dissociation c.
    dissociation c.

NOTES

C

curve *(continued)*
    dose-effect curve dose-response c.
    dye-dilution c.
    flow volume c.
    Frank-Starling c.
    function c.
    green dye c.
    hemoglobin-oxygen dissociation c.
    indocyanine dilution c.
    intracardiac pressure c.
    isovolume pressure-flow c.
    J c.
    Kaplan-Meier event-free survival c.
    left ventricular pressure-volume c.
    length-active tension c.
    length-tension c. (LT)
    mitral E velocity c.
    nitrogen c.
    oxygen dissociation c.
    oxyhemoglobin dissociation c.
    pressure-natriuresis c.
    pressure-volume c.
    pulse c.
    single-breath nitrogen c.
    Starling c.
    thermal dilution c.
    thermodilution c.
    time-activity c.
    Traube c.
    venous return c.
    venovenous dye dilution c.
    ventricular function c.
    volume-time c.
curved J-exchange wire
Curvularia lunata
CUSA
    Cavitron ultrasonic surgical aspirator
CUSALap device
Cushing
    C. forceps
    C. pressure response
    C. reflex
    C. syndrome
    C. triad
cushingoid facies
cushion
    atrioventricular canal c.
    cannula c.
    cardiac c.
    coronary c.
    endocardial c.
    pharyngoesophageal c.'s
    Sullivan bubble c.
Cushman assay
cusp
    accessory c.
    aortic c.
    c. billowing

    conjoined c.
    coronary c.
    c. degeneration
    c. eversion
    c. excursion
    c. fenestration
    fish-mouth c.
    c. motion
    noncoronary c.
cuspis, pl. cuspides
    c. anterior valvae bicuspidalis
    c. anterior valvae tricuspidalis
    cuspides commissurales
CustomPac custom tubing back with Duraflo treatment
cut
    coronal c.
    DCA c.
    c. point
    sagittal c.
cutaneous
    c. asthma
    c. hyperesthesia
    c. malignancy
    c. necrotizing venulitis
    c. thoracic patch electrode
cutdown
    arterial c.
    brachial artery c.
    c. catheter
    c. technique
    venous c.
cut-film arteriography
Cutinova Hydro dressing
cutis
    c. laxa
    c. laxa syndrome
    c. marmorata
Cutler-Ederer method
cutpoint
cutter
    Endopath ETS-FLEX endoscopic articulating linear c.
    EZ45 thoracic linear c.
    rib c.
Cutter aortic valve prosthesis
Cutter-Smeloff
    C.-S. aortic valve prosthesis
    C.-S. disk valve
    C.-S. mitral valve
cutting
    c. balloon
    c. balloon angioplasty (CBA)
    c. balloon before stent
    c. balloon device
    C. Balloon Randomized Clinical Trial
    c. balloon RCT

cuvette
    dye c.
Cuvier
    canal of C.
    duct of C.
Cu/Zn superoxide dismutase
CV
    collateralizing vessel
    conventional ventilation
        CV wave of jugular venous pulse
CVA
    cerebrovascular accident
    costovertebral angle
CVC
    central venous catheter
        CVC 123 calibration verification
        control
CVD
    cardiovascular disease
    CVD balloon
    CVD Focustent Enforcer
C-VEST
        C.-V. ambulatory radionuclide
        detector
        C.-V. radiation detector system
CVI
    cerebrovascular infarction
        multiple CVIs
CVIR
    Cardiovascular Information Registry
CVIS imaging device
CVIS/InterTherapy intravascular
ultrasound system
CVP
    central venous pressure
        CVP line
CVR
    cerebrovascular reactivity
    cerebrovascular resistance
    coronary flow velocity reserve
CVS
    cerebral vasospasm
    collagen vascular sealing
c-v systolic wave
CVT
    cerebral venous thrombosis
CVT-124 A1 receptor antagonist
CVVH
    continuous venovenous hemofiltration
CVX-300 XeCl excimer laser
CW
    circle of Willis

CWD
    continuous-wave Doppler
CWI
    cardiac work index
CWP
    coal worker's pneumoconiosis
CWS
    circumferential wall stress
CX
    circumflex
CXC chemokine
CXR
    chest radiograph
cyanide
    c. antidote kit
    hydrogen c. (HCN)
cyanmethemoglobin method
cyanoacrylate
    n-butyl c. (n-BCA)
2-cyanoacrylate
    isobutyl 2-c.
cyanochroic, cyanochrous
cyanogen bromide method
cyanosed
cyanosis
    autotoxic c.
    central c.
    circumoral c.
    edema, clubbing, and c. (ECC)
    false c.
    hereditary methemoglobinemic c.
    late c.
    c. of nail beds
    peripheral c.
    pulmonary c.
    c. retinae
    reverse differential c.
    shunt c.
    tardive c.
cyanotic
    c. asphyxia
    c. atrophy of liver
    c. congenital heart disease
    c. heart defect
cyanotica
    asphyxia c.
Cyberlith
    C. multiprogrammable pulse
    generator
    C. pacemaker

C

NOTES

Cybertach
>C. automatic-burst atrial pacemaker
>C. 60 bipolar pacemaker

Cybex isokinetic dynamometer
Cyclan
cyclandelate
cyclase
>adenylate c.
>adenylyl c. (AC)
>cell membrane-bound adenylate c.
>guanylate c.
>guanylyl c.

cycle
>cardiac c.
>cell c.
>circannual c.
>circaseptan c.
>citric acid c.
>c. ergometer
>c. ergometry
>forced c.
>isometric period of cardiac c.
>Krebs c.
>c. length (CL)
>c. length alternans
>c. length alternation
>moiety-conserved c.
>ratio of expiration time and total time of breathing c. (tE/tTOT)
>ratio of inspiration time and total time of breathing c. (tI/tTOT)
>respiratory c.
>restored c.
>returning c.
>RR c.
>short-long-short c.
>sound wave c.
>Wenckebach c.

cycle-length window
cyclic
>c. adenosine monophosphate (cAMP)
>c. guanosine monophosphate (cGMP)
>c. nucleotide adenosine monophosphate
>c. progesterone
>c. respiration

cyclin A gene
cyclocumarol
cycloergometer
>Mijnhard electrical c.

cycloheximide
cyclohexylamine

Cyclomen
cyclooxygenase (COX)
>c.-o. inhibitor

cyclooxygenase-1 (COX-1)
cyclooxygenase-2 (COX-2)
cyclooxygenase-lipoxygenase blocking agent BW755C
cyclopentamine hydrochloride
cyclopenthiazide
cyclopentylpropionate
>hydrocortisone c.

cyclophosphamide
>c., bleomycin, cisplatin (CBP)
>c., doxorubicin, cisplatin (CAP)
>c., doxorubicin, methotrexate, procarbazine (CAMP)
>c., doxorubicin, vincristine (CAV)
>vindesine, cisplatin, lomustine, c. (VCPC)

cyclopropane
cycloserine (CS)
Cyclospasmol
cyclosporin A
cyclosporine
cyclothiazide
cyclotron
>c.-produced F-18 fluorodeoxyglucose

Cycofed Pediatric
Cycrin
>C. Oral

CYFRA 21-1 tumor marker
Cyklokapron
>C. injection
>C. Oral

Cylexin
cylinder
>C oxygen c.
>M6 oxygen c.

cylindrical
>c. bronchiectasis
>c. confronting cisterna

cylindroadenoma
cylindroid aneurysm
cylindroma
cylindruria
Cynosar catheter
CYP1A2 isoform
CYP2C9 isoform
CYP2D6 isoform
CYP3A isoform
CYP2C19 isoform
cypionate
>hydrocortisone c.

cyproheptadine hydrochloride
cyproterone
Cyriax syndrome
cys-LT
>cysteinyl leukotriene

cyst
>   aneurysmal bone c.
>   apoplectic c.
>   bronchial c.
>   bronchogenic c.
>   bronchopulmonary c.
>   centrilobular c.
>   compound c.
>   echinococcal c.
>   hemorrhagic c.
>   hepatic hydatid c.
>   honeycomb c.
>   honeycombing c.
>   hydatid c.
>   locular c.
>   loculated c.
>   mucoretention c.
>   multilocular c.
>   necrotic c.
>   neurenteric c.
>   pericardial c.
>   pleuropericardial c.
>   renal c.
>   springwater c.
>   thymic c.
>   Tornwaldt c.
>   true c.
>   unilocular c.

cystathionine
>   c. synthase deficiency

cystatin C
cysteine
cysteinyl leukotriene (cys-LT)
cystic
>   c. adenomatoid malformation
>   c. bronchiectasis
>   c. disease of lung
>   c. emphysema
>   c. fibrosis (CF)
>   c. fibrosis transmembrane
>   conductance regulator
>   c. fibrosis transmembrane regulator
>   (CFTR)
>   c. lesion
>   c. medial necrosis
>   c. space

cystica
>   Erdheim medionecrosis aortae
>   idiopathica c.
>   medionecrosis aortae idiopathica c.
>   osteitis tuberculosa multiplex c.

cysticercosis

cystidine monophospho-*N*-acetylneuraminic acid (CMP-NANA)
Cytadren
cytarabine hydrochloride
cytobrush
cytocentrifugation
cytochalasin B
cytochrome
>   c. c oxidase
>   c. P450 system

CytoGam
cytokine
>   cardioinflammatory c.
>   chemotactic c.
>   c. expression
>   c.-induced endothelial synthesis
>   inflammatory c.
>   pleiotropic c.
>   proinflammatory c.

cytological biopsy
cytology
>   aspiration biopsy c. (ABC)
>   bronchial washings c.
>   sputum c.

cytomegalic inclusion disease
cytomegalovirus (CMV)
>   c. encephalitis
>   human c. (HCMV)
>   c. immune globulin (CMVIG)
>   c. immune globulin intravenous,
>   human
>   c. pneumonitis

Cytomel Oral
cytometer
>   Ortho Cytofluorograf 50-H flow c.

cytometric indirect immunofluorescence
cytomitome
cytomorphology
cytomorphosis
cytoplasmic bridge
cytoprotective
>   c. agent
>   c. effect

Cytosar-U
cytosine-arabinoside, cytosine arabinoside (Ara-C)
cytosine-thymine-guanine trinucleotide
cytoskeleton
>   actin c.

cytosolic protein
cytosome

NOTES

cytotoxic
- c. edema
- c. gene therapy
- c. singlet oxygen

cytotoxicity

cytotoxin-associated gene product A (CagA)

cytotrophoblast (CTB)

Cytovene

Cytoxan
- C. injection
- C. Oral

Czaja-McCaffrey rigid stent introducer/endoscope

D

    2D echocardiography
    D gate
    D loop
    D point
    D sleep
    D wave

D1

    diagonal branch #1

D2

    prostaglandin D2

2D

    two-dimensional
    2D echocardiogram
    2D gradient-echo sequence
    2D TEE system Ultra-Neb 99

3D

    3D IVUS
    3D segmented-FLASH imaging sequence
    3D SPGR image
    3D tagged magnetic resonance imaging
    3D time-of-flight magnetic resonance angiographic sequence
    3D TOF MRA

D_4

    leukotriene D.

D_{CO}

    pulmonary diffusion capacity

Do_2

    oxygen delivery

D114S balloon catheter

D1790G mutant gene

DA

    daytime asthma

Da

    dalton

Daae disease

DAC

    Guiatuss DAC
    Guiatussin DAC
    Halotussin DAC
    Mytussin DAC

dacarbazine

DaCosta syndrome

Dacron

    D. catheter
    D. cloth
    D.-covered Delerin frame of valve prosthesis
    D. fiber
    D. intracardiac patch
    D. onlay patch-graft
    D. pledget

    D. Sauvage graft
    D. tube graft

dactinomycin

DAD

    delayed afterdepolarization
    diffuse alveolar damage

dagger-shaped aortic envelope

DAH

    diffuse alveolar hemorrhage
    disordered action of heart

daidzein

Daig

    D. Corporation lead
    D. ESI-II or DSI-III screw-in lead pacemaker
    D./Medcor lead
    D. sheath

Daiichi Radioisotope Labs. Techne MAA kit

d'airain

    bruit d.

DAIS

    Diabetes Atherosclerosis Intervention Study

Dakin

    D. biograft
    D. solution

Dalalone

Dale

    D.-Schwartz tube
    D. tracheostomy tube holder

dalfopristin

Dallas

    D. Classification System
    D. criteria

dalteparin

    d. sodium
    d. sodium injection

Dalton

    D.-Henry law
    D. law

dalton (Da)

damage

    bilateral hemisphere d. (BHD)
    diffuse alveolar d. (DAD)
    enzyme-induced d.
    left brain d. (LBD)
    left hemisphere d. (LHD)
    parietal pleural d.
    regional alveolar d. (RAD)
    right brain d. (RBD)
    right hemisphere d. (RHD)
    silent ischemic brain d. (SIBD)

D'Amato sign

D

DAMIA
   direct acute myocardial infarction angioplasty
Damian graft procedure
dampened waveform
damping
   Accudynamic adjustable d.
   catheter d.
   d. coefficient
   d. control
Damus-Kaye-Stansel (DKS)
   D.-K.-S. connection
   D.-K.-S. operation
   D.-K.-S. procedure
   D.-K.-S. procedure for single ventricle physiology
Damus-Stansel-Kaye procedure
DAN
   diabetic autonomic neuropathy
danaparoid sodium
danazol
dance
   brachial d.
   hilar d.
   St. Vitus d.
dander
   animal d.
Dane particle
Danielson method
Danocrine
Dantrium
dantrolene sodium
dapsone (DDS)
daptomycin for injection
Daranide
Daraprim
DAR breathing system
Dardik Biograft
darkfield microscopy
Darling disease
Darox cutaneous thoracic patch electrode
DART
   Dilation versus Ablation Revascularization trial
Dart
   D. coronary stent
   D. pacemaker
Das Angel Wings atrial septal defect closure device
DASE
   dobutamine atropine stress echocardiography
DASH
   Delay in Accessing Stroke Healthcare
   Dietary Approach to Prevent Hypertension

   DASH clinical trial
   DASH study
Dash
   D. pacemaker
   D. single-chamber rate-adaptic pacemaker
DASI
   Duke Activity Status Index
DAT
   direct amplification test
data
   d. base management
   measured d.
   nonparametric d.
   pressure-volume d.
database
   Duke Carcinoid D.
DataCare ABG Data Management system
Datascope
   D. Accutor bedside monitor
   D. balloon
   D. catheter
   D. CL-II percutaneous translucent balloon catheter
   D. DL-II percutaneous translucent balloon catheter
   D. intraaortic balloon pump
   D. pulse oximeter
   D. System 90 balloon pump
   D. System 90 intraaortic balloon pump
DataVue calibrated reference circle
Datex
   D. ETCO$_2$ multigas analyzer
   D. Oxy-cap capnometer
   D. SC-103 finger clip
Datex-Ohmeda pulse oximeter
DATI
   diastolic amplitude time index
DaunoXome
DAVID
   Dual-Chamber and VVI Implantable Defibrillator
   DAVID multicenter comparative study
Davidson
   D. clamp
   D. pneumothorax apparatus
   D. protocol exercise test
   D. retractor
   D. scapular retractor
   D. thoracic trocar
Davies
   D. disease
   D. endomyocardial fibrosis
   D. myocardial fibrosis
   D. technique

daVinci surgical system
Davis
    D. bronchoscope
    D. rib spreader
    D. sign
Davol pacemaker introducer
day
    mg/kg per d.
    milligrams per kilograms per d.
daytime asthma (DA)
Dazamide
dazoxiben
DBP
    diastolic blood pressure
DBPC
    dual balloon perfusion catheter
DC
    direct current
    dual chamber
        Bromanate DC
        DC cardioversion
        DC electric shock
        Myphetane DC
DCA
    dichloroacetate
    directional color angiography
    directional coronary angioplasty
    directional coronary atherectomy
        DCA cut
        DCA debulking technique
DCC
    direct cardiac compression
DCFM
    Doppler color flow mapping
DCHS
    dysarthria-clumsy hand syndrome
DCI
    delayed cerebral ischemia
DCI-S automated coronary analysis system
DCLHb
    diaspirin cross-linked hemoglobin
DCM
    dilated cardiomyopathy
DCMAG-1 gene
DCS
    decompression sickness
    distal coronary sinus
        neurologic DCS
        pulmonary DCS
DCV
    delayed cerebral vasoconstriction

DDAVP
    D. injection
    D. Nasal
ddC
DDD
    dual-mode, dual-pacing, dual-sensing
        DDD pacemaker
        DDD pacing
DDDR pacing
DDFP
    dodecafluoropentane
DD genotype
DDI
    D. mode pacemaker
    D. pacing
ddI
    didanosine
D-dimer
    D.-d. assay
    D.-d. enzyme-linked immunosorbent assay
    fibrin D.-d.
    D.-d. test
DDIR pacing
DD2R
    dopamine D2 receptor
DDS
    dapsone
DE
    dobutamine echocardiography
2DE
    two-dimensional echocardiography
3DE
    three-dimensional echocardiography
De
    D. Martel scissors
    D. Morgan spots
    D. Vega prosthesis
de
    d. Groot classification
    d. la Camp sign
    d. Lange syndrome
    d. Musset sign (aortic aneurysm)
    d. Mussy point
    d. Mussy sign (pleurisy)
    d. novo
    d. novo atherosclerosis
    d. novo coronary lesion
    d. novo malignancy
    d. Quervain thyroiditis
dead
    d. space

NOTES

D

dead (*continued*)
    d. space:tidal volume ratio
    d. space ventilation
    d. time
deadly quartet syndrome
dead-space gas volume to tidal gas volume ratio (V_{DS}/V_T)
deaired
deairing procedure
deaminase
    adenosine d. (ADA)
Deane tube
dearterialization
    hepatic d.
death
    aborted sudden d.
    apoptotic cell d.
    brain d.
    cardiac d.
    cocaine-related sudden d.
    ischemic sudden d.
    late d.
    late sudden d.
    out-of-hospital sudden cardiac d. (OOH-SCD)
    postresuscitative d.
    pump failure d.
    sudden d.
    sudden cardiac d. (SCD)
    sudden unexplained d. (SUND)
    vascular d.
    voodoo d.
DeBakey
    D. anastomosis clamp
    D. anastomosis forceps
    D. aneurysm repair
    D. aortic aneurysm clamp
    D. arterial clamp
    D. arterial forceps
    D. Atraugrip forceps
    D.-Bahnson clamp
    D.-Bainbridge clamp
    D. ball valve prosthesis
    D.-Beck clamp
    D. blade
    D. chest retractor
    D. classification
    D.-Colovira-Rumel thoracic forceps
    D.-Creech aneurysm repair
    D.-Creech manner
    D.-Derra anastomosis clamp
    D.-Derra anastomosis forceps
    D.-Diethrich coronary artery forceps
    D.-Harken auricle clamp
    D. heart pump oxygenator
    D.-Howard aortic aneurysmal clamp
    D.-Kay aortic clamp
    manner of D.

    D. manner
    D.-McQuigg-Mixter bronchial clamp
    D.-Mixter thoracic forceps
    D.-NASA axial-flow ventricular-assist device
    D. patent ductus clamp
    D.-Péan cardiovascular forceps
    D. pediatric clamp
    D. peripheral vascular clamp
    D. rib spreader
    D.-Satinsky vena cava clamp
    D.-Semb ligature-carrier clamp
    D.-Surgitool prosthetic valve
    D. tissue forceps
    D.-type aortic dissection
    D. VAD
    D. VAD continuous-axial-flow pump
    D. Vasculour-II vascular prosthesis
    D. Vital needle holder
debilis
    pulsus d.
debility
DeBove
    D. membrane
    D. treatment
debris
    atheromatous d.
    atherosclerotic d.
    calcific d.
    grumous d.
    pultaceous d.
    valve d.
debrisoquine sulfate
debt
    oxygen d.
debubbling procedure
debulking
    d. device
    mechanical d.
    d. procedure
Decabid
Decadron
    D. Injection
    D. Oral
    D. Phosphate
Decadron-LA
Deca-Durabolin
Decaject
Decaject-LA
decamethonium
decanoate
    Hybolin d.
    nandrolone d.
decapolar
    d. electrode catheter
    d. pacing catheter

decarboxylase
    histidine d.
decay
    isovolumic pressure d.
    pressure d.
deceleration
    d.-dependent aberrancy
    early d.
    horizontal d.
    horizontal anteroposterior d.
    late d.
    d. time
    variable d.
    vertical d.
decerebrate posturing
Decholin
declamping
    d. shock
    d. shock syndrome
Declomycin
Decofed Syrup
Decohistine
    D. DH
    D. Expectorant
décollement
decompensate
decompensated shock
decompensation
    cardiac d.
decompression
    cardiac d.
    d. disorder
    d. illness
    microvascular d. (MVD)
    d. sickness (DCS)
    d. table
decompressive chest tube
Deconamine
    D. SR
    D. Syrup
    D. Tablet
deconditioning
Deconsal II
decortication
    arterial d.
    d. of heart
    d. of lung
decreased
    d. breath sounds
    d. respiration
    d. valve excursion
decrement

decremental
    d. atrial pacing
    d. conduction
decrescendo murmur
decrudescence
decrudescent arteriosclerosis
decubitus
    d. angina
    angina d.
    angina pectoris d.
    d. cough
    d. ulcer
dedicated bipolar lead
Dedo-Jako microlaryngoscope
Dedo-Pilling laryngoscope
deductive echocardiography
deendothelialization
deenergization
    myocyte d.
deep
    d. chest therapy
    d. Doppler velocity interrogation
    d. hypothermia circulatory arrest (DHCA)
    d. lingual artery
    d. lingual vein
    d. pathologic Q wave
    d. sleep
    d. venous insufficiency (DVI)
    d. venous thrombosis (DVT)
    d. white matter hyperintensity (DWMHI)
    d. white matter lesion (DWML)
de-epicardialization, deepicardialization
deer-antler vascular pattern
Defares rebreathing method
defecation syncope
defect
    acquired ventricular septal d. (AVSD)
    aorticopulmonary septal d.
    aortic septal d.
    aortopulmonary septal d. (APSD)
    aquired ventricular septal d.
    atrial ostium primum d.
    atrial septal d. (ASD)
    atrioseptal d.
    atrioventricular canal d.
    atrioventricular conduction d.
    atrioventricular septal d.
    A-V conduction d.
    AVSD d.

D

NOTES

defect *(continued)*
clamshell closure of atrial septal d.
conal septal d.
conduction d. (CD)
contiguous ventricular septal d.
cyanotic heart d.
Eisenmenger reaction with septal d.
endocardial cushion d. (ECD)
extrafusion d.
factor V Leiden coagulation d.
filling d.
fixed perfusion d.
fixed-rate perfusion d.
Gerbode d.
humoral immune d.
iatrogenic atrial septal d.
infundibular septal d.
intimal d.
lucent d.
match d.
muscular ventricular septal d.
  (MVSD)
myocardial long-chain fatty acid
  uptake d.
napkin-ring d.
nonsegmental perfusion d.
nonuniform rotational d. (NURD)
obstructive ventilatory d.
ostium primum d.
ostium secundum d.
panconduction d.
partial A-V canal d.
perfusion d.
periinfarction conduction d. (PICD)
perimembranous ventricular
  septal d.
primum atrial septal d.
pulmonary atresia with ventricular
  septal d. (PAVSD)
restrictive airways d.
restrictive ventilatory d.
reversible ischemic neurologic d.
  (RIND)
scintigraphic perfusion d.
secundum atrial septal d. (ASD2)
secundum-type atrial septal d.
septal d.
sinus venosus atrial septal d.
supracristal d.
supracristal ventricular septal d.
Swiss cheese d.
T cell d.
thallium uptake d.
transcatheter closure of atrial d.
transcatheter occlusion of atrial
  septal d.
ventilation/perfusion d.
ventricular septal d. (VSD)

ventriculoseptal d. (VSD)
V̇/Q̇ d.
defects syndrome
Defen-LA
defensiveness
emotional d. (ED)
deferoxamine mesylate
defervesce
defervescence
defibrillation
biphasic waveform transthoracic d.
cardiac d.
Moe multiple wavelet hypothesis
  of atrial d.
d. paddles
d. patch
public access d. (PAD)
d. shock
d. threshold (DFT)
defibrillator
Amiodarone Versus
  Implantable D.'s (AVID)
Antiarrhythmics versus
  Implantable D.'s (AVID)
Atrioverter implantable d.
automated external d. (AED)
automatic external d. (AED)
automatic implantable d. (AID)
automatic internal d.
automatic intracardiac d.
Birtcher d.
Cambridge d.
Cardioserv d.
Codemaster d.
CPI automatic implantable d.
Dual-Chamber and VVI
  Implantable D. (DAVID)
Endotak lead d.
external d.
FirstSave automated external d.
ForeRunner d.
Gem d.
Gem II DR dual-chamber d.
Gem DR implantable d.
Guidant d.
Heart Aid 80 d.
Heartstream ForeRunner automatic
  external d.
Hewlett-Packard d.
d. implant
implantable atrial d. (IAD)
Intec implantable d.
IPCO-Partridge d.
Jewel AF implantable d.
Lifepak d.
Marquette Responder 1500
  multifunctional d.

Medtronic Gem automatic implantable d.
Medtronic Micro Jewel II d.
Medtronic Micro Jewel II implantable d.
Metrix implantable atrial d.
Odam d.
d. paddles
PD 2000 d.
Porta Pulse 3 d.
public access d. (PAD)
smart d.
transvenous implantable d.
d. unit
Ventak d.
Ventak Prizm d.
Ventak Prizm dual-chamber implantable d.
Zoll d.
Zoll PD1200 external d.

deficiency
acetylcholinesterase d.
acid maltase d.
ADA d.
adenosine deaminase d.
alpha-1 antitrypsin d.
antithrombin III d.
antitrypsin d.
ApoA-1 d.
carnitine d.
complement component C1r d.
congenital pseudocholinesterase d.
C1r d.
cystathionine synthase d.
dopamine beta-hydroxylase d.
enzymatic d.
factor III d.
familial apoA-I d.
familial HDL d.
familial high-density-lipoprotein d.
galactosidase d.
glucosidase d.
hemostatic d.
hexosaminidase d.
homogentisic acid oxidase d.
HRF d.
hydroxylase d.
17-hydroxylase d.
magnesium d.
maltase d.
Owren factor V d.
Pax3 d.

protein C d.
protein-calorie d.
protein S d.
pseudocholinesterase d.
selenium d.
surfactant d.
thiamine d.
vasopressor d.

deficit
neurologic d.
pulse d.
spectacular shrinking d.

Definity perflutren
deflated profile
deflation
deflazacort
deflectable
7-French 20-pole d. mapping catheter
d. quadripolar catheter

deflection
atrial d.
delta d.
His d.
His bundle d.
intrinsic d.
intrinsicoid d.
QS d.
RS d.

deflector
Cook d.

deformans
arteritis d.
endarteritis d.
osteitis d.

deformation
capacitor d.

deformity
buttonhole d.
cervical spine d.
gooseneck d.
gooseneck outflow tract d.
hockey-stick d.
joint d.
parachute d.
pectus d.
pigeon-breast d.
shepherd's crook d.

deftitox
denileukin d.

degeneration
cusp d.

D

NOTES

degeneration *(continued)*
    fibrinoid d.
    glassy d.
    Mönckeberg d.
    mucoid medial d.
    myxomatous d.
    Quain fatty d.
    spinocerebellar d.
    Wallerian d. (WD)
de Gimard syndrome
deglutition
    d. apnea
    d. mechanism
    d. murmur
    d. pneumonia
    d. syncope
Degos disease
degranulation
    goblet cell d.
Dehio test
dehiscence
    annular d.
    bronchial d.
    sternal d.
dehydroemetine
dehydrogenase
    d. activity
    alpha-hydroxybutyrate d.
    11-beta-hydroxysteroid d.
    branched chain alpha ketoacid d.
      (BCKD)
    glucose-6-phosphate d. (G6PD)
    hydroxybutyrate d. (HBDH)
    lactate d.
    lactic d. (LDH)
    lactic acid d.
    pyruvate d. (PDH)
dehydromonocrotaline
11-dehydro-thromboxane B$_2$
Deklene II cardiovascular suture
DeKock two-way bronchial catheter
Del
    D. Mar Avionics Scanner
    D. Mar Avionics three-channel
      recorder
Delaborde tracheal dilator
Delalande Spectradop 2 4-MHz probe
Delatest Injection
Delatestryl Injection
delavirdine
delay
    D. in Accessing Stroke Healthcare
      (DASH)
    atrioventricular d. (AVD)
    conduction d.
    electromechanical d.
    intramyocardial conduction d.
    intraventricular conduction d.

    ischemia-induced intramyocardial
      conduction d.
delayed
    d. afterdepolarization (DAD)
    d. cerebral ischemia (DCI)
    d. cerebral vasoconstriction (DCV)
    d. conduction
    d. depolarization
    d. pulmonary toxicity syndrome
      (DPTS)
    d. xenograft rejection (DXR)
Delbet sign
deletion
    allelic d.
    22q11 d.
delimitation
delineation
    endocardial border d.
delirium
    d. cordis
    toxic d.
Delirium Rating Scale of Trzepacz
delivery
    d. balloon
    closed-loop d.
    contrast medium d.
    MSI pulmonary drug d.
    oxygen d. (Do$_2$)
    d. wire
Delmege sign
Delorme thoracoplasty
Delphian node
Delrin
    D. frame of valve prosthesis
    D. heart valve
Delsym
delta
    d. deflection
    D. pacemaker
    D. TRS pacemaker
    d. wave
Delta-Cortef Oral
Deltasone Oral
DeltaTrac II metabolic monitor
deltopectoral groove
Deltran disposable transducer
Demadex
    D. injection
    D. Oral
demand
    cardiac output d.
    d. hypoxia
    d. mode
    myocardial oxygen d.
    d. oxygen delivery system (DODS)
    d. pacemaker
    d. pacing
    d. pulse generator

Demarquay sign
demeclocycline hydrochloride
dementia
    multiinfarct d.
    thalamic d.
    vascular d.
Demerol
Demos tibial artery clamp
Demser
denatured homograft
dendritic lesion
dendroaspis natriuretic peptide (DNP)
denervated
denervation
    cardiac d.
    cardiac sympathetic d.
    d. supersensitivity
dengue fever
Denhardt solution
denileukin deftitox
denivelation
Dennis dissecting scissors
dens
    anterior articular surface of d.
    facet of atlas for d.
dense
    d. hemiplegia
    d. thrill
densitogram
    ear d.
densitometry
    acoustic d.
    video d.
density
    dependent d.
    echo d.
    full caloric d.
    hydrogen d.
    lipid core d.
    power spectral d. (PSD)
    proton d.
    spin d.
density-exposure relationship of film
dental barotrauma
dentis
    anterior d.
dentocariosa
    Rothia d.
dentrificans
    Alcaligenes d.
Denucath

denudation
    endothelial d.
Denver
    D. Biomaterials Pleurx pleural catheter
    D. PAK
    D. pleuroperitoneal shunt
    D. Pleurx pleural catheter/home drainage kit
deoxycorticosterone
deoxygenated hemoglobin
2-deoxyglucose
    2-d. F-18 2-d
deoxyhemoglobin
deoxyribonuclease (DNase)
    human recombinant d.
deoxyribonucleic acid (DNA)
15-deoxyspergualin
depAndro Injection
dependence
    use d.
dependency
    ventilator d.
dependent
    d. beat
    d. density
    d. edema
    d. rubor
dephosphorylation
deplasmolysis
deplasmolyze
depletion
    glycogen d.
    volume d.
deployment
    high-pressure stent d.
    stent d.
depMedalone injection
Depoject
    D. injection
depolarization
    alternating, failure of response, mechanical, to electrical d. (AFORMED)
    atrial premature d. (APD)
    delayed d.
    diastolic d.
    His bundle d.
    intrinsic d.
    myocardial d.
    rapid d.

NOTES

199

depolarization *(continued)*
    transient d.
    ventricular premature d. (VPD)
depolarizing drug
depolymerization
depolymerized porcine mucosal heparin
Depo-Medrol injection
Deponit Patch
Depopred injection
Depo-Provera injection
deposit
    calcium d.
    intraalveolar d.
deposition
    aerosol d.
    calcium oxalate d.
    collagen d.
    mitochondrial calcium d.
depot
    Androcur D.
    Lupron D.
Depot-Ped
    Lupron D.-P.
depreotide
    technetium d.
depressant
    cardiac d.
depressed ventricular function
depression
    aldosterone d.
    cardiorespiratory d.
    circulatory d.
    downhill ST segment d.
    downsloping ST segment d.
    horizontal d.
    horizontal ST segment d.
    Hospital Anxiety and D. (HAD)
    junctional d.
    myocardial d.
    postdrive d.
    P-Q segment d.
    precordial ST d.
    reciprocal ST d.
    rectilinear ST-segment d.
    respiratory d.
    spreading d. (SD)
    ST segment d. (STD)
    upsloping ST segment d.
    vascular d.
    x d.
depressor reflex
deprivation
    sleep d.
Deproist Expectorant With Codeine
depth
    d. compensation
    volumetric lung d. (Vp)
Depthalon

DEQ
    digital echo quantification
derivative
    d. circulation
    ergotamine d.'s
    hematoporphyrin d. (HPD)
    JTV519 1,4-benzothiazepine d.
    methanesulfonanilide d.
    purified protein d. (PPD)
    quaternary ammonium atropine d.
    thiazolidinedione d.
derived 12-lead electrocardiogram
Dermaflex Gel
Dermalon suture
dermatan sulfate
dermatitidis
    Ajellomyces d.
    Blastomyces d.
dermatitis, pl. **dermatitides**
    exfoliative d.
    livedoid d.
    stasis d.
    weeping d.
dermatomyositis
Dermatophagoides pteronyssimus
dermonecrotic
Derra
    D. aortic clamp
    D. commissurotomy knife
    D. knife
    D. valve dilator
    D. vena caval clamp
DES
    diethylstilbestrol
desaturation
    arterial d.
descendens
    aorta d.
    ramus anterior d.
    ramus posterior d.
descending
    d. anterior branch
    d. aorta
    left anterior d. (LAD)
    d. necrotizing mediastinitis (DNM)
    d. phlebitis
    d. posterior branch
    d. thoracic aneurysm
    d. thoracic aorta (DTA)
    d. thoracic aorta-to-femoral artery (DTAFA)
    d. thoracic aorta-to-femoral artery bypass graft
    d. thoracic aortic-femoral-femoral (DTAF-F)
    d. thoracic aortofemoral-femoral bypass

descent
>barotrauma of d.
>rapid y d.
>x d.
>y d.

Deschamps compressor

Deseret
>D. angiocatheter
>D. flow-directed thermodilution catheter
>D. sump drain

deserpidine
>methyclothiazide and d.

desert fever

desethylamiodarone, desethyl amiodarone

Desferal
>D. Mesylate
>D. Mesylate challenge

desferrioxamine

desflurane

desiccation
>mucous d.

designed after natural anatomy

Desilets
>D.-Hoffman catheter introducer
>D.-Hoffman sheath
>D. introducer
>D. introducer system
>D. system

desipramine hydrochloride

desirudin

deslanoside

desloratadine

desmethyldiazepam

desmin gene

desmoplastic
>d. mesothelioma
>d. small round cell tumor

desmopressin acetate

desmosine

desmosome

Desnos
>D. disease
>D. pneumonia

desoxycorticosterone

Desoxyn

d'Espine sign

desquamation
>peribronchial d.

desquamative
>d. alveolitis

>d. interstitial pneumonia (DIP)
>d. interstitial pneumonitis (DIP)

DESTINI-CFR
>Doppler Endpoints Stenting International Investigation: Coronary Flow Reserve
>DESTINI clinical trial

destruction
>alveolar d.
>apoptotic d.
>lung tissue d.
>plasmatic vascular d.

desulfatohirudin
>recombinant d.

desynchronized sleep

Desyrel

detachment velocity

detection
>d. algorithm
>atrial fibrillation d.
>automated border d. (ABD)
>automated edge d.
>automatic boundary d. (ABD)
>coincidence d.
>echocardiographic automated border d.
>edge d.
>d. enhancement
>manual edge d.
>molecular coincidence d. (MCD)
>shunt d.
>single-photon d.

detective quantum efficiency

detector
>ambulatory nuclear d.
>Cardioscint ambulatory vest d.
>Cardioscint nuclear d.
>C-VEST ambulatory radionuclide d.
>Doppler blood flow d.
>multihead d.
>TubeChek esophageal intubation d.
>vest ambulatory nuclear d.
>VEST left ventricular function d.

detect time

Detensol

detergent worker's lung

deterioration
>d. following improvement (DFI)
>structural valve d. (SVD)

Determann syndrome

determination
>acid-base d.
>metabolic parameter d.

D

NOTES

detrusor-sphincter dyssynergia
Detsky
>D. modified risk index
>D. score

Detussin
>D. Expectorant
>D. liquid

deuterosome
devascularization
DeVega tricuspid valve annuloplasty
Devereux formula
Devereux-Reichek method
deviation
>abnormal left axis d. (ALAD)
>abnormal right axis d. (ARAD)
>axis d.
>left axis d. (LAD)
>right axis d. (RAD)
>ST d.
>standard d.
>ST-T d.
>tracheal d.

device
>abdominal aortic counterpulsation d. (AACD)
>abdominal left ventricular assist d. (ALVAD)
>Abiomed Cardiac d.
>Abiomed implantable heart-replacement d.
>ablative d.
>Ablatr temperature control d.
>Accutor oscillometric d.
>Accutracker blood pressure d.
>ACS anchor exchange d.
>acute ventricular assist d. (AVAD)
>Adams-DeWeese d.
>advanced venous access d.
>AeroChamber spacing d.
>AerX d.
>AICD plus Tachylog d.
>A-mode echo-tracking d.
>Amplatz thrombectomy d. (ATD)
>Amplatz ventricular septal defect d.
>Anaconda d.
>Angel Wings d.
>Angioguard catheter d.
>Angio-Seal hemostatic puncture closure d.
>Aquatherm radiant heat d.
>arrhythmia control d. (ACD)
>Arrow-Clarke thoracentesis d.
>ASD closure d.
>ATL Ultramark 7 echocardiographic d.
>atrial septal defect single disk closure d.

>Atrioverter implantable defibrillator d.
>AutoAdjust CPAP d.
>automatic d.
>AutoSet Portable II diagnosis and therapy d.
>AutoSuture One-Shot anastomotic d.
>autotitration d.
>AVA d.
>AVA 3Xi advanced venous access d.
>AVA 3Xi venous access d.
>Babyhaler spacer d.
>Baim-Turi cardiac d.
>Baladi Inverter d.
>balloon catheter sealing d.
>battery-assisted heart assist d.
>Baxter Health Care Continu-Flo infusion d.
>B&B Trachguard antidisconnection d.
>bilevel positive pressure d.
>bioabsorbable closure d.
>biventricular assist d. (BVAD, BIVAD)
>Block cardiac d.
>bovine collagen plug d.
>Breas CPAP d.
>Breas PV10 CPAP d.
>Brockenbrough d.
>Brockenbrough cardiac d.
>buttoned d.
>BVM d.
>cage catheter d.
>Caire Breeze oxygen therapy d.
>Caire Sprint portable liquid oxygen d.
>Caire Stroller portable liquid oxygen d.
>Carbomedics valve d.
>cardiac automatic resuscitative d. (CARD)
>cardiac stretch d.
>CardioGrip handheld, battery-operated exercise d.
>Cardiomemo d.
>Cath-Lok catheter locking d.
>centrifugal left and right ventricular assist d.
>Champ cardiac d.
>Chemo-Port perivena catheter system d.
>Cholestron handheld diagnostic d.
>Cholestron PRO II handheld diagnostic d.
>Chuter endovascular d.
>Circulaire aerosol drug delivery d.

Circulaire inhaled medication
delivery d.
CirKuit-Guard d.
Clamp Ease d.
clamshell d.
clearance assistive d.
closed-loop d.
Clot Buster Amplatz
thrombectomy d.
Contak CD CHF d.
Coronary Revascularization
Ultrasound Angioplasty D.
(CRUSADE)
Cournand d.
Cournand cardiac d.
CPCA2000 counter-pulsation d.
CPI Mini d.
CTS Voyager Aortic
IntraClusion d.
CUSALap d.
cutting balloon d.
CVIS imaging d.
Das Angel Wings atrial septal
defect closure d.
DeBakey-NASA axial-flow
ventricular-assist d.
debulking d.
DIASYS Novacor cardiac d.
Digiflator digital inflation d.
Digitrapper MkIII reflux testing d.
Dinamap automated blood
pressure d.
directional atherectomy d.
displacement sensing d.
Doppler d.
double-disk ASD closure d.
double-umbrella d.
DPAP Stealth d.
Duett arterial closure d.
Duett sealing d.
Duett vascular sealing d.
Durathane cardiac d.
Elecath circulatory support d.
El Gamal d.
El Gamal cardiac d.
emergency infusion d. (EID)
Encore inflation d.
Endo Grasp d.
Equinox EEG acquisition d.
esophageal detection d. (EDD)
extended collection d.
extraction atherectomy d.

ExtreSafe phlebotomy d.
Femo stop inflatable pneumatic
compression d.
fiberoptic delivery d.
Finesse cardiac d.
finger photoplethysmographic d.
flutter d.
flutter chest percussion d.
Flutter mucus clearance d.
Flutter therapeutic d.
ForeRunner automatic external
defibrillator d.
Gensini d.
Gensini cardiac d.
Goetz d.
Goetz cardiac d.
Goodale-Lubin d.
Goodale-Lubin cardiac d.
grip torque d.
Guidant-CPI d.
HeartMate implantable ventricular
assist d.
hemostatic occlusive leverage d.
(HOLD)
hemostatic puncture closure d.
(HPCD)
Hi-Per d.
Hi-Per cardiac d.
Horizon CPAP d.
HSRA d.
ICD-ATP d.
Ideal d.
Ideal cardiac d.
IMED infusion d.
ImPulse electronic oxygen
conserving d.
ImPulse Oxygen Conserving D.
In-Exsufflator respiratory d.
Infiltrator local drug delivery d.
Innervase dilatable percutaneous
vascular access d.
InspirEase d.
Inspiron d.
Insuflon d.
InSync cardiac resynchronization d.
interrogation d.
intraaortic balloon d.
intracaval d.
inverted buttoned d.
I-STATE bedside blood testing d.
Jewel AF · implantable arrhythmia
management d.

NOTES

203

device *(continued)*
Jewel atrial fibrillation dual
chamber d.
Kendall Sequential Compression d.
King cardiac d.
King interlocking d.
lead locking D. (LDD)
left ventricular assist d. (LVAD)
Lehman d.
Lehman cardiac d.
LifeStick CPR d.
LifeStick resuscitation d.
Light Talker d.
Linx-EZ cardiac d.
Linx guidewire extension cardiac d.
Lock Clamshell d.
locking d.
mandibular advancement d. (MAD)
MDILog therapy monitoring d.
Mediflex-Bookler d.
Medtronic defibrillator implant
support d.
Medtronic external tachyarrhythmia
control D.
Medtronic-Hall d.
Medtronic-Hancock d.
Medtronic Hemopump cardiac
assist d.
Medtronic Inspire implantable d.
Medtronic Jewel AF arrhythmia
management d.
Medtronic Jewel AF implantable
arrhythmia management d.
Medtronic Jewel 7219D and C d.
Medtronic Octopus tissue
stabilizing d.
Medtronic tremor control
therapy d.
MicroDigitrapper-S apnea
screening d.
Microsampler d.
Miltner constraint compliance d.
21 Mini d.
26 Mini II d.
motorized transducer pullback d.
Mullins cardiac d.
Multileaf collimator d.
NBIH cardiac d.
Needle-Pro needle protection d.
Nicolet/EME Muller and Moll
probe fixation d.
nonthoracotomy system
antitachycardia d. (NTS-AICD)
Novacor DIASYS cardiac d.
Novacor left ventricular assist d.
Nycore d.
Nycore cardiac d.
O2 Advantage conserving d.

Omniscience valve d.
Oxymizer d.
Passager d.
Pavenik monodisk d.
Penn State ventricular assist d.
Perclose/Prostar d.
Perclose vascular closure d.
percutaneous thrombolytic d. (PTD)
PerDUCER percutaneous
pericardial d.
PerDUCER pericardial access d.
personal heart d. (PHD)
PET balloon atherectomy d.
phased array ultrasonographic d.
PhotoDerm VL d.
Pierce-Donachy Thoratec ventricular
assist d.
Pleur-evac d.
PlexiPulse d.
PlexiPulse compression d.
POCT d.
point-of-care testing d.
POMS 20/50 oxygen
conservation d.
portable aerosol delivery d.
portable monitoring d.
Port-A-Cath d.
Portex Neo-Vac meconium
suction d.
Positrol cardiac d.
Presto cardiac d.
Prima Total Occlusion D.
Probe cardiac d.
Pro/Pel coating cardiac d.
Prostar XL hemostatic puncture
closure d.
35-PRXIII d.
pullback atherectomy d.
pulsatile assist d. (PAD)
pulse oximetry d.
radiant heat d. (RHD)
Rashkind cardiac d.
Rashkind double umbrella d.
Rashkind hooked d.
Rashkind umbrella d.
rate-adaptive d.
Resistex PEP therapy d.
Respiradyne pulmonary function d.
Res-Q arrhythmia control d.
right ventricular assist d. (RVAD)
Rotablator atherectomy d.
Rotablator RotaLink Plus rotational
atherectomy d.
Rotablator RotaLink rotational
atherectomy d.
Rotacs d.
rotary atherectomy d.
rotational atherectomy d.

Sarns ventricular assist d.
Selute Picotip steroid-eluting d.
Selute steroid-eluting d.
Sentinel ICD d.
Sequential Compression D.
Servo Screen 390 ventilator
  monitoring d.
Sideris adjustable buttoned d.
Sideris buttoned d.
Silent Night diagnostic and
  screening d.
snare d.
SomaSensor d.
SomnoStar apnea testing d.
stent-anchoring d.
St. Jude cardiac d.
subcutaneous tunneling d.
Sub-Q-Set subcutaneous continuous
  infusion d.
Sullivan III nasal continuous
  positive air pressure d.
Super-9 guiding cardiac d.
Surveyor recording d.
Swiss Kiss intrastent balloon
  inflation d.
Symbion cardiac d.
Tandem cardiac d.
Taperseal hemostatic d.
TEC atherectomy d.
Techstar d.
Techstar suturing closure d.
tedding d.
Telectronics Guardian ATP 4210 d.
d. therapy
Thermedics cardiac d.
Thermedics HeartMate 10001P left
  anterior assist d.
Thermocardiosystems left ventricular
  assist d.
Thermo-STAT armcuff heat d.
Thoratec biventricular assist d.
Thoratec cardiac d.
Thoratec right ventricular assist d.
Thoratec ventricular assist d.
Threshold PEP d.
tiered-therapy antiarrhythmic d.
tongue-retaining d.
Trak Back pullback d.
Tranquility BiLevel airway patency
  maintenance d.
Tranquility BiLevel positive airway
  pressure therapy d.

Tranquility Quest CPAP d.
transcatheter d.
transvenous d.
Trapper catheter exchange d.
Unilink anastomotic d.
Valleylab Force 2 electrosurgical d.
Vanguard d.
Vascugel d.
vascular hemostatic d. (VHD)
vascular sealing d.
VasoSeal vascular hemostasis d.
VasoView balloon dissection d.
ventricular assist d. (VAD)
Ventritex Cadence d.
Venture demand oxygen delivery d.
Veriflex cardiac d.
Viringe vascular access flush d.
Vita-Stat automatic d.
Voyager Aortic IntraClusion d.
wearable cardioverter-defibrillator d.
Williams cardiac d.
Wizard cardiac d.
Wizard disposable inflation d.
XT cardiac d.
Zipper antidisconnect d.
Zucker-Myler cardiac d.

Devices, Ltd. pacemaker
DeVilbiss
  D. nebulizer
  D. Pumo-Aide LT compressor
devil's grip
Devon-Pura stent
DeWeese vena cava clamp
Dew sign
Dexacort Phosphate in Respihaler
dexamethasone
  oral-inhalation d.
  d. sodium phosphate (DSP)
  d. suppression test
  d. systemic
Dexasone L.A.
Dexatrim
Dexchlor
dexchlorpheniramine maleate
Dexedrine
dexfenfluramine (dFEN)
dexiocardia (*var. of* dextrocardia)
dexmedetomidine HCl
Dexon
  D. Plus suture
  D. suture

D

NOTES

Dexone
    D. LA
dexrazoxane
dexter
    bronchus principalis d.
    cor triatriatum d.
    lobus d.
    pulmo d.
Dexter-Grossman classification
dextorphan
dextra
    arteria pulmonalis d.
    valvula semilunaris d.
    vena pulmonalis inferior d.
    vena pulmonalis superior d.
dextrae
    ramus lobi medii arteriae
      pulmonalis d.
dextran
    d. 1, 70
    high molecular weight d.
    low molecular weight d. (LMD)
    molecular-weight d.
    d. solution
    d. sulfate
dextri
    fissura horizontalis pulmonis d.
    foramen venarum minimarum
      atria d.
    lobus azygos pulmonis d.
    lobus medius pulmonis d.
    pars intralobaris intersegmentalis
      venae posterioris lobi superioris
      pulmonis d.
dextroamphetamine
    d. sulfate
    d. toxicity
dextrocardia, dexiocardia
    corrected d.
    false d.
    isolated d.
    mirror image d.
    secondary d.
    type 1, 2, 3, 4 d.
    d. with situs inversus
dextrocardiogram
dextrogastria
dextrogram
dextro isomer
dextroisomerism
dextromethorphan
    acetaminophen and d.
    carbinoxamine, pseudoephedrine,
      and d.
    chlorpheniramine, phenylephrine,
      and d.
    chlorpheniramine,
      phenylpropanolamine, and d.

guaifenesin and d.
guaifenesin, phenylpropanolamine,
    and d.
guaifenesin, pseudoephedrine,
    and d.
promethazine and d.
pseudoephedrine and d.
dextropositioned aorta
dextroposition of heart
dextropropoxyphene
dextrorotation
Dextrostat
Dextrostix
dextrothyroxine
    d. sodium
dextrotransposition
dextroversion of heart
dextrum
    atrium d.
    cor d.
Dey-Dose
    D.-D. Isoproterenol
    D.-D. Metaproterenol
Dey-Lute Isoetharine
Dey-Pak
DFA
    direct fluorescent antibody
dFEN
    dexfenfluramine
DFI
    deterioration following improvement
D/Flex filter
DFP
    diastolic filling pressure
DFT
    defibrillation threshold
3DFT
    three-dimensional Fourier transform
      3DFT magnetic resonance
      angiography
DGS
    DiGeorge syndrome
DH
    Codehist DH
    Codiclear DH
    Decohistine DH
    Dihistine DH
DHBP
    direct His bundle pacing
DHCA
    deep hypothermia circulatory arrest
DHD
    Aerosol Cloud Enhancer by D.
D.H.E. 45 injection
DHPG
DiaBeta

diabetes
> D. Atherosclerosis Intervention Study (DAIS)
> d. mellitus (DM)

diabetic
> d. autonomic neuropathy (DAN)
> d. cardiomyopathy
> d. coma
> d. diet
> d. gangrene
> d. nephropathy
> d. neuropathy
> d. phthisis
> d. retinopathy
> D. Tussin DM
> D. Tussin EX
> d. ulcer

diabeticorum
> necrobiosis lipoidica d.

Diabinese

diable
> bruit de d.

diacetate
> triamcinolone d.

diacylglycerate pathway

diacylglycerol lipase

diadzein

diagnosis
> Prospective Investigation of Pulmonary Embolism D. (PIOPED)

diagnostic
> d. aspiration
> d. bronchoscopy
> computer-assisted d.'s (CAD)
> d. HRCT
> Mogul 3F steerable decapolar electrophysiology d.
> d. peritoneal lavage (DPL)
> sleep d.'s
> d. ultrasound imaging catheter

diagnostic-related group (DRG)

diagonal
> d. artery
> d. branch #1 (D1)
> d. coronary artery

diagram
> Dieuaide d.
> ladder d.
> pressure-volume d.

Dialog pacemaker

dialysis
> continuous cyclical peritoneal d. (CCPD)
> peritoneal d.
> renal d.

dialyzer
> Terumo d.

diameter
> aerodynamic mass d. (AD)
> anteroposterior thoracic d.
> count median d. (CMD)
> count median aerodynamic d. (CMAD)
> end-diastolic d. (EDD)
> geometric mean d. (GMD)
> internal d.
> left atrial d.
> left ventricular internal diastolic d. (LVIDD)
> luminal d.
> LV end-diastolic d.
> mass median aerodynamic d. (MMAD)
> mean reference d. (MRD)
> minimal luminal d. (MLD)
> minimum lumen d. (MLD)
> outer d. (OD)
> reference vessel d. (RVD)
> stretched d.
> total end-diastolic d. (TEDD)
> total end-systolic d. (TESD)

Diameter Index Safety system (DISS)

diaminobenzidine tetrahydrochloride

Diamond
> D. classification
> D.-Forrester table

diamond-coated bur

diamond ejection murmur

Diamond-Lite titanium instrument

diamond-shaped
> d.-s. murmur
> d.-s. tracing

Diamox

diaphanoscopy

diaphoresis

diaphragm
> central tendon of d.
> costal d.
> costal part of d.
> crural d.
> dome of d.
> eventrated d.

D

NOTES

diaphragm *(continued)*
    eventration of d.
    left crus of d.
    lumbar part of d.
    d. phenomenon
    right crus of d.
    d. of stent
    sternal part of d.
    d. transducer
    vertebral part of d.
diaphragma
    musculus d.
diaphragmalgia
diaphragmatic
    d. artery
    d. dysfunction
    d. excursion
    d. flutter
    d. hernia
    d. myocardial infarction
    d. pacing
    d. paralysis
    d. pericardium
    d. phenomenon
    d. pleura
    d. pleurisy
    d. respiration
    d. rupture
    d. surface
    d. surface of heart
diaphragmatica
    facies d.
    pleura d.
diaphragmatis
    centrum tendineum d.
    crus sinistrum d.
    pars costalis d.
    pars lumbalis d.
Diaqua
diary
    event d.
    Holter d.
    sleep d.
DiaryCard
    2110 PEF/FEV$_1$ D.
diaschisis
    crossed cerebellar d. (CCD)
Diasonics
    D. Cardiovue 3400 and 6400
    D. Cardiovue SectOR scanner
    D. catheter
    D. Gateway2D duplex sonography
    D.-Sonotron Vingmed CFM 800
      imaging system
    D. transducer
diaspirin cross-linked hemoglobin
  (DCLHb)
diastasis cordis

diastatic
Diastat vascular access graft
diastema
diaster
diastole
    atrial d.
    cardiac d.
    electrical d.
    late d.
    ventricular d.
diastolic
    d. afterpotential
    d. amplitude time index (DATI)
    d. blood pressure (DBP)
    d. blow
    d. bulging
    d. closing velocity
    d. current
    d. current of injury
    d. decrescendo murmur
    d. depolarization
    d. doming
    d. dysfunction
    d. filling
    d. filling pattern
    d. filling period
    d. filling pressure (DFP)
    d. fluttering
    d. fluttering aortic valve
    d. function
    d. gallop
    d. gradient
    d. grunt
    d. heart disease
    d. heart failure
    d. hump
    d. hypertension
    d. motion
    d. murmur
    d. overload
    d. pressure
    d. pressure-time index (DPTI)
    d. pressure-volume relation
    d. relaxation
    d. reserve
    d. rumble
    d. shock
    d. stiffness
    d. suction
    d. thrill
    d. upstroke
    d. ventricular dysfunction
diastology
DIASYS Novacor cardiac device
DiaTAP vascular access button
diathermy
diathesis, pl. **diatheses**

allergic d.
bleeding d.
diatrizoate
sodium meglumine d.
diazepam
diazine
diazoxide
Dibenzyline
DIC
disseminated intravascular coagulation
disseminated intravascular coagulopathy
DIC tracheostomy tube
dichloroacetate (DCA)
sodium d.
dichloroisoprenaline
dichloroisoproterenol
dichlorphenamide
dichotomization
dichotomy
Dick cardiac valve dilator
diclofenac
dicloxacillin sodium
DICOM
digital imaging and communications in medicine
dicrotic
d. notch
d. pulse
d. wave
dicrotism
dicumarol
dicumylperoxide
didanosine (ddI)
didehydrodideoxythymidine
dideoxycytidine
dideoxyinosine
dideoxynucleoside
dielectrography
dielthylamine
diesel exhaust
diet
AHA type I d.
American Heart Association d.
American Heart Association step II d.
American Heart Association type I d.
betaine d.
bland d.
calorie-restricted d.
cardiac d.
diabetic d.

Feed or Ordinary D. (FOOD)
high-fiber d.
Karell d.
Kempner d.
low-fat d.
low-methionine d.
low-salt d.
low-sodium d.
NCEP Step-One d.
Ornish d.
Portagen d.
prudent d.
renal d.
salt-free d.
Sauerbruch-Herrmannsdorfer-Gerson d.
Step-One D.
Step-Two D.
dietary
D. Approach to Prevent Hypertension (DASH)
d. fat
d. salt
d. sodium
Dieterle stain
Diethrich
D. coronary artery set
D. shunt clamp
diethylcarbamazine citrate
diethylenetriamine
d. pentaacetate (DTPA)
d. pentaacetate aerosol inhalation lung scintigraphy
d. pentaacetic acid (DPTA, DTPA)
diethylstilbestrol (DES)
Dieuaide
D. diagram
D. sign
difference
alveolar-arterial PO_2 d. ($AaPO_2$)
arterial-venous oxygen content d.
arteriovenous oxygen d. ($AVD\ O_2$)
pulmonary A-V O_2 d.
differens
pulsus d.
differential
d. blood count
d. blood pressure
d. bronchospirometry
d. pressure transducer
d. stethoscope
d. transisthmus conduction

D

NOTES

differentiation
   echocardiographic d.
   pressure pulse d.
difficulty
   rating of perceived breathing d.
      (RPBD)
Diff-Quik stain
diffuse
   d. airways disease
   d. alveolar damage (DAD)
   d. alveolar hemorrhage (DAH)
   d. arterial ectasia
   d. bronchopneumonia
   d. cutaneous scleroderma (IDCS)
   d. emphysema
   d. esophageal spasm
   d. infiltrative lung disease (DILD)
   d. in-stent restenosis
   d. interstitial infiltrate
   d. interstitial lung disease (DILD)
   d. interstitial pulmonary fibrosis
   d. intimal thickening
   d. intraventricular block
   d. lung injury
   d. malignant pleural mesothelioma
      (DMPM)
   d. panbronchiolitis (DPB)
   d. parenchymal disease
   d. paroxysmal slowing
   d. pleurisy
   d. pulmonary lymphangiomatosis
   d. sclerosing alveolitis
   d. vasospasm
diffusing
   d. capacity
   d. capacity of lung for carbon
      monoxide (DLCO)
diffusion
   d. anoxia
   d. capacity
   centripetal d.
   coefficient of d.
   d. hypoxia
   lung d.
   d. MRI
   d. respiration
   single-breath d.
   d. tensor imaging (DTI)
diffusion-weighted
   d.-w. imaging (DWI)
   d.-w. MRI
diffusometry
   NMR d.
diffusum
   angiokeratoma corporis d.
Diflucan
   D. injection
   D. Oral

diflunisal
DIG
   Digitalis Investigation Group
   digoxin investigators group
   DIG study
DIG-CAPTOPRIL
   Canadian Digoxin Captopril
   DIG-CAPTOPRIL study
DiGeorge syndrome (DGS)
digestive system vascular disease
Digibind
   D. digoxin immune Fab fragments
   D. pneumatonometer
Digidote digoxin immune Fab fragments
Digiflator digital inflation device
Digiflex high flow catheter
Digipate
digital
   d. averaging
   d. calipers
   D. Cardiac Imaging system
   d. clubbing
   d. color Doppler velocity
      integration method
   d. color Doppler velocity profile
      integration
   d. computer
   d. constant-current pacing box
   d. echocardiography
   d. echo quantification (DEQ)
   d. endarteropathy
   d. fluoroscopic unit
   d. imaging and communications in
      medicine (DICOM)
   d. necrosis
   d. phase mapping (DPM)
   d. radiography
   d. runoff
   d. smoothing
   d. subtraction
   d. subtraction angiography (DSA)
   d. subtraction arteriography
   d. subtraction echocardiography
      (DSE)
   d. subtraction imaging
   d. subtraction supravalvular
      aortogram
   d. subtraction supravalvular
      aortography
   d. subtraction technique
   d. vascular imaging
   d. videoangiography
digitalate pulse
Digitaline
digitalis
   d. effect
   d. glycoside
   d. intoxication

D. Investigation Group (DIG, DIG study)
D. lanata
D. purpurea
d. sensitivity
d. toxicity
digitalis-specific antibody
digitalization
digitalize
Digitek
digitization
digitized
d. caliper method
d. subtraction angiography
digitizer
Bitpad d.
digitizing pad
digitoxicity
digitoxin
Digitrapper
D. MkIII reflux testing device
D. MkIII sleep monitor
Digit Span test for short-time memory
digoxigenin-labeled DNA probe
digoxin
d. effect
d. immune fab
d. investigators group (DIG)
d. level
D. RIA Bead
d. toxicity
digoxin-immune Fab
digoxin-specific Fab
Dihistine
D. DH
D. Expectorant
dihydralazine
dihydrochloride
azimilide d.
dihydrocodeine
dihydroergotamine mesylate
dihydropyridine calcium antagonist
dihydroxyphenylalanine
dihydroxypropyltheophylline
Dihyrex Injection
diisocyanate
d. asthma
methylene diphenyl d. (MDI)
toluene d. (TDI)
Dilacor XR
Dilantin
dilatable lesion

dilatancy
dilated
d. cardiomyopathy (DCM)
d. coronaropathy
dilation, dilatation
aneurysmal d.
annular d.
balloon d.
bootstrap d.
cardiac d.
catheter d.
chamber d.
esophageal d.
finger d.
flow-mediated d. (FMD)
d. of heart
idiopathic d.
idiopathic right atrial d.
intrapulmonary vascular d.
left ventricular cavity d.
lymphatic d.
nitroglycerin-induced d.
onion-bulb d.
oscillating d.
poststenotic d.
reactive d.
sequential d.
serial d.
d. thrombosis
transient ischemic d. (TID)
ventricular d.
D. versus Ablation Revascularization trial (DART)
Wirsung d.
dilator
Achiever balloon d.
AirMax d.
Amplatz d.
argon vessel d.
Bakes d.
Beardsley aortic d.
Brown-McHardy pneumatic d.
Cooley d.
Crump vessel d.
Delaborde tracheal d.
Derra valve d.
Dick cardiac valve d.
Einhorn esophageal d.
Encapsulon vessel d.
Garrett d.
Gohrbrand cardiac d.
Hohn vessel d.

D

NOTES

dilator *(continued)*
    Jackson-Trousseau d.
    Lucchese mitral valve d.
    Maloney mercury-filled
      esophageal d.
    mitral valve d.
    Mullins d.
    Nozovent nasal-valve d.
    Parsonnet d.
    Plummer water-filled pneumatic
      esophageal d.
    Quantum TTC balloon d.
    Savary-Gilliard esophageal d.
    Scanlan vessel d.
    d. and sheath technique
    Sippy esophageal d.
    Steele bronchial d.
    Tubbs d.
    vessel d.
    wire-guided oval intracostal d.
dilator-sheath system
Dilatrate-SR
DILD
    diffuse infiltrative lung disease
    diffuse interstitial lung disease
DILE
    drug-induced lupus erythematosus
dilevalol
Dilocaine Injection
Dilor
Diltia XT
diltiazem
    enalapril and d.
    D. HCl extended-release tablet
    d. hydrochloride
dilution
    gas d.
    helium d.
    transpulmonary thermal-dye d.
      (TDD)
Dimacol Caplets
dimenhydrinate
dimension
    aortic root d.
    effective airspace d. (EAD)
    end-diastolic d. (EDD)
    end-systolic d. (ESD)
    left atrial d. (LAD)
    left ventricular end-diastolic d.
      (LVEDD)
    left ventricular end-systolic d.
      (LVESD)
    left ventricular internal diastolic d.
      (LVIDD)
    left ventricular systolic d. (LVSD)
    right ventricular d. (RVD)
dimer
    excited d.'s

Dimetabs Oral
Dimetane-DC
Dimetapp Sinus Caplets
dimethyl
    d. hydrazine
    d. sulfate
    d. sulfoxide
dimethylarginine
    asymmetric d. (ADMA)
1,1-dimethylbiguanide
dimethyl-L-arginine
dimorphism
dimple
    blind coronary d.
    coronary ostial d.
Dinamap
    D. Accutorr A1, 3 blood pressure
      monitor
    D. automated blood pressure device
    D. blood pressure cuff
    D. blood pressure monitor
    D. monitor
    D. pulse oximeter
    D. system
    D. ultrasound blood pressure
      manometer
dinitrate
    isosorbide d. (ISDN)
dinitrile
    pyridazinone d.
dinucleotide
    nicotinamide adenine d. (NAD)
diode
    light-emitting d. (LED)
    Zener d.
Diomycin
DIOS
    distal intestinal obstruction syndrome
Diovan HCT
dioxide
    carbon d. (CO_2)
    chlorine d.
    end-tidal carbon d. ($ETCO_2$)
    fraction of expired carbon d.
      ($FECO_2$)
    fraction of inspired carbon d.
      ($FICO_2$)
    nitrogen d. (NO_2)
    partial pressure of carbon d.
      (PCO_2)
    selenium d.
    sulfur d. (SO_2)
dioxime
    boronic acid technetium d.
DIP
    desquamative interstitial pneumonia
    desquamative interstitial pneumonitis

dip
"a" d.
Cournand d.
midsystolic d.
d. phenomenon
septal d.
type I, II d.
dipalmitoyl
d. phosphatidylcholine (DPPC)
d. phosphatidylcholine test
dip-and-plateau pattern
diphasic
d. complex
d. P wave
d. T wave
Diphen Cough
Diphenhist
diphenhydramine (DPHM)
d. hydrochloride
Diphenylan Sodium
diphenylhydantoin
diphosphate
adenosine d. (ADP)
histamine d.
5′-diphosphate
2,3-diphosphoglycerate
diphosphonate
methylene d. (MDP)
technetium-99m methylene d.
diphtheria
d. antitoxin
d. and tetanus toxoid
d. tetanus toxoids, and acellular
pertussis vaccine
d. tetanus toxoids, and whole-cell
pertussis vaccine
d. tetanus toxoids, and whole-cell
pertussis vaccine and *Haemophilus*
b conjugate vaccine
diphtheriae
Corynebacterium d.
diphtherial tonsillitis
diphtheric
d. paralysis
d. pharyngitis
diphtherin
diphtheritic
d. croup
d. laryngitis
d. myocarditis
d. paralysis
d. pharyngitis

diphtheroid
diplegia
facial d.
diplocardia
diplococci
Diplococcus pneumoniae
diplodiotoxicosis
Diplos M 05 pacemaker
dipole theory
Diprivan injection
dipropionate
beclomethasone d.
dipyridamole
d. and aspirin
aspirin/extended release d.
d. echocardiography
d. echocardiography test
d. handgrip test
d. stress
d. stress echocardiography
d. thallium-201 cardiac perfusion
study
d. thallium-201 scan
d. thallium-201 scintigraphy
d. thallium stress test
dipyridamole-thallium imaging
dipyrine
direct
d. acute myocardial infarction
angioplasty (DAMIA)
d. amplification test (DAT)
d. cardiac compression (DCC)
d. cardiac massage
d. cardiac puncture
d. coronary angioplasty
d. current (DC)
d. current cardioversion
d. current electric shock
d. embolism
d. excitation
d. fluorescent antibody (DFA)
d. Fourier transformation imaging
d. His bundle pacing (DHBP)
d. immunofluorescent stain
d. insertion technique
d. laryngoscopy
d. lead
d. mapping sequence
d. mechanical ventricular actuation
(DMVA)
d. murmur

D

NOTES

direct *(continued)*
    d. myocardial revascularization
      (DMR)
    d. respiration
    d. stimulation
    d. thrombin inhibitor
direct-current
    d.-c. shock ablation
directed cough
DirectFlow arterial cannula
directional
    d. atherectomy
    d. atherectomy catheter
    d. atherectomy debulking technique
    d. atherectomy device
    d. color angiography (DCA)
    d. coronary angioplasty (DCA)
    d. coronary atherectomy (DCA)
directly
    d. observed therapy (DOT)
    d. observed treatment (DOT)
dirithromycin
Dirofilaria immitis
dirofilariasis
dirty
    d. chest
    d. film
    d. necrosis
dirty-lung appearance
Dirythmin
disability
    cardiovascular d.
Disalcid
disappearance slope
disarray
    myocardial d.
    myofibrillar d.
disarticulation
    Burger technique for
      scapulothoracic d.
    chondral d.
    chondrocostal d.
DISA-SPECT
    dual-isotope simultaneous acquisition
    single-photon emission computed
    tomography
disc *(var. of* disk)
discission of pleura
discoid
disconnect
    airway pressure d. (APD)
discontinuity
    atrial-axis d.
**discontinuous incremental threshold
loading**
discordance
    atrioventricular d.
    ventriculoarterial d.

discordant
    d. alternans
    d. alternation
    d. atrioventricular connection
    d. changes electrocardiogram
    d. ventriculoarterial connection
discovery
    D. DDDR pacemaker
    D. handheld spirometer
discrete
    d. coronary lesion
    d. subaortic stenosis (DSS)
    d. subvalvular aortic stenosis
      (DSAS)
disease
    Acosta d.
    acromegalic heart d.
    acyanotic heart d.
    Adams d.
    Adams-Stokes d.
    Addison d.
    airspace d.
    alcoholic heart muscle d.
    amyloid heart d.
    Anderson-Fabry d.
    antiglomerular basement
      membrane d.
    aortic aneurysmal d.
    aortic thromboembolic d.
    aortic valve d.
    aortoiliac obstructive d. (AIOD)
    aortoiliac occlusive d.
    apple picker's d.
    arrhythmogenic right ventricular d.
    arterial occlusive d. (AOD)
    arteriosclerotic cardiovascular d.
      (ASCVD)
    arteriosclerotic heart d. (ASHD)
    arteriosclerotic peripheral
      vascular d. (ASPVD)
    arteriosclerotic vascular d. (ASVD)
    aspiration-induced respiratory d.
    atherosclerotic aortic d.
    atherosclerotic cardiovascular d.
      (ASCVD)
    atherosclerotic carotid artery d.
    atherosclerotic coronary artery d.
      (ACAD, ASCAD)
    atherothrombotic cardiovascular d.
    autosomal-dominant familial aortic
      aneurysm d.
    aviator's d.
    axial interstitial d.
    Ayerza d.
    Bamberger-Marie d.
    Bannister d.
    barometer-maker's d.
    Bazin d.

Beau d.
Becker d.
Behçet d.
beryllium d.
beryllium-induced lung d.
Besnier-Boeck-Schaumann d.
bilateral aortoostial coronary
  artery d.
biliary d.
Binswanger d.
blackfoot d.
black lung d.
blue d.
Boeck d.
Bornholm d.
Bostock d.
Bouillaud d.
Bouveret d.
Bright d.
Brill-Zinsser d.
Buerger d.
bullous d.
bullous lung d.
Bürger-Grütz d.
Buschke d.
Busse-Buschke d.
caisson d.
California d.
carcinoid heart d.
carcinoid valve d.
cardiac allograft vascular d.
  (CAVD)
cardiovascular d. (CVD)
carotid artery d.
carotid occlusive d.
carotid vascular d.
Carrington d.
Castellani d.
Castleman d.
cat-scratch d.
cavitary lung d.
Ceelen d.
Ceelen-Gellerstedt d.
celiac d.
centrilobular axial interstitial d.
cerebrovascular d. (CeVD)
Chagas heart d.
Charcot-Marie-Tooth d.
cheese worker's lung d.
cholesterol ester storage d.
cholesteryl ester storage d.
Christmas d.

chronic beryllium d. (CBD)
chronic graft vascular d. (CGVD)
chronic hypertensive d.
chronic inflammatory airway d.
chronic interstitial lung d.
chronic obstructive airways d.
chronic obstructive lung d. (COLD)
chronic obstructive pulmonary d.
  (COPD)
chronic obstructive respiratory d.
  (CORD)
chronic peripheral arterial d.
  (CPAD)
chronic suppurative lung d.
  (CSLD)
cobalt-induced airway d.
cobalt-related d.
cobalt-related lung d.
cold hemagglutinin d.
collagen vascular lung d.
Concato d.
congenital heart d. (CHD)
congestive pulmonary d.
constrictive heart d.
Cori d.
coronary artery d. (CAD)
coronary heart d. (CHD)
coronary microvascular d.
coronary occlusive d.
Corrigan d.
Corvisart d.
Crocq d.
cryptococcal pulmonary d.
cyanotic congenital heart d.
cytomegalic inclusion d.
Daae d.
Darling d.
Davies d.
Degos d.
Desnos d.
diastolic heart d.
diffuse airways d.
diffuse infiltrative lung d. (DILD)
diffuse interstitial lung d. (DILD)
diffuse parenchymal d.
digestive system vascular d.
Döhle d.
Duroziez d.
dust d.
Ebstein d.
effusive-constrictive d.
Eisenmenger d.

D

NOTES

disease *(continued)*
  electrical d.
  elevator d.
  Emery-Dreifuss d.
  endomyocardial d.
  end-stage liver d. (ESLD)
  end-stage renal d. (ESRD)
  environmental lung d.
  eosinophilic endomyocardial d.
  epicardial coronary artery d.
  Epstein d.
  Erb-Goldflam d.
  Erdheim d.
  extracranial carotid d. (ECD)
  extracranial carotid arterial d. (ECAD)
  extracranial internal carotid d.
  Fabry d.
  Fahr d.
  family history of heart d.
  Fast Revascularization During Instability in Coronary Artery D. (FRISC)
  fibroplastic d.
  fibroproliferative d.
  fish-meal worker's lung d.
  flax-dresser's d.
  flint d.
  Fothergill d.
  Fragmin During Instability in Coronary Artery D. (FRISC)
  Friedländer d.
  Friedreich d.
  functional cardiovascular d.
  furrier's lung d.
  Gairdner d.
  gallbladder d.
  gannister's d.
  gastroesophageal reflux d. (GERD)
  Gaucher d.
  giant bullous d.
  Gilchrist d.
  global cardiac d.
  glycogen storage d.
  glycogen storage d. type III
  Goldflam d.
  Goldflam-Erb d.
  gonadal d.
  graft-versus-host d. (GVHD)
  grain handler's d.
  granulomatous d.
  Graves d.
  Hamman d.
  hand-foot-and-mouth d.
  Hand-Schüller-Christian d.
  hard metal d.
  heart d.
  Heller-Döhle d.

  hematologic d.
  hepatic d.
  Hodgkin d.
  Hodgson d.
  Horton d.
  Huchard d.
  humeroperoneal neuromuscular d.
  Hutinel d.
  hyaline membrane d.
  hypereosinophilic heart d.
  hypertensive arteriosclerotic heart d. (HASHD)
  hypertensive cardiovascular d. (HCVD)
  hypertensive heart d.
  hypertensive pulmonary vascular d.
  iatrogenic d.
  idiopathic venoocclusive d.
  immune-mediated d.
  inflammatory airway d.
  inorganic dust d.
  interstitial d.
  interstitial lung d. (ILD)
  intracranial atherosclerotic d. (IAD)
  intrastent recurrent d.
  intrinsic d.
  iron storage d.
  Isambert d.
  ischemic heart d. (IHD)
  isolated cerebral thromboangiitis obliterans d.
  Kawasaki d.
  Keshan d.
  Kikuchi d.
  kinky-hair d.
  Krishaber d.
  Kugelberg-Welander d.
  Kussmaul d.
  Kussmaul-Maier d.
  large-vessel d.
  Leaman classification of coronary d.
  left main d. (LMD)
  left main coronary d. (LMC)
  left main coronary artery d.
  left main stem coronary artery d. (LMS-CAD)
  Legionnaire d.
  Lemierre d.
  Lenègre d.
  Letterer-Siwe d.
  leukoencephalopathy d.
  Lev d.
  Lewis upper limb cardiovascular d.
  Libman-Sacks d.
  Little d.
  Löffler d.

Long-Term Intervention with Pravastatin in Ischemic D. (LIPID)
lower extremity arterial d. (LEAD)
Lucas-Championnière d.
luetic d.
lupus-associated valve d.
Lutz-Splendore-Almeida d.
Lyme d.
macrovascular artery d.
maple bark d.
Marek d.
McArdle d.
metastatic d.
microvascular artery d.
Mikity-Wilson d.
Mondor d.
Monge d.
Morgagni d.
Morquio-Brailsford d.
Moschcowitz d.
moyamoya d.
Multicenter Ultrasound Stent in Coronary Artery D. (MUSIC)
multilobar d.
multivalvular d.
multivessel d. (MVD)
multivessel coronary artery d.
mushroom worker's d.
mycobacterial d.
myocardial d.
myxomatous valve d.
nail-patella d.
necrotizing arterial d.
neoplastic d.
neurodegenerative d.
neuromuscular d.
Niemann-Pick d.
nonsegmental d.
nosocomial d.
obliterative vascular d.
obstructive airway d. (OAD)
obstructive lung d. (OLD)
occlusive d.
occupational lung d.
oculocraniosomatic d.
organic heart d. (OHD)
Osler-Weber-Rendu d.
Owren d.
Paget d. of bone
parenchymal d.
peribronchovascular d.

pericardial d.
peripartal heart d.
peripheral d.
peripheral arterial d. (PAD)
peripheral arterial occlusive d. (PAOD)
peripheral atherosclerotic d.
peripheral interstitial d.
peripheral vascular d. (PVD)
pigeon-breeder's d.
pleural d.
Plummer d.
pneumatic hammer d.
polycystic kidney d.
polysaccharide storage d.
Pompe d.
Posadas-Wernicke d.
primary electrical d.
primary pleuropulmonary d.
primary pulmonary parenchymal d.
pulmonary valve d.
pulmonary vascular obstructive d.
pulmonary venoocclusive d. (PVOD)
pulseless d.
Purkinje d.
Quincke d.
radiation lung d.
ragpicker's d.
ragsorter's d.
Raynaud d.
reactive airways d. (RAD)
recalcitrant obstructive airways d.
Refsum d.
Reiter d.
renal artery d.
renal parenchymal d.
Rendu-Osler-Weber d.
Research on Instability in Coronary Artery D. (RISC)
restrictive airways d.
restrictive heart d.
restrictive lung d.
reversible obstructive airways d. (ROAD)
rheumatic heart d. (RHD)
Roger d.
Rokitansky d.
Rosai-Dorfman d.
Rougnon-Heberden d.
Roussy-Lévy d.
Sandhoff d.

D

NOTES

disease *(continued)*
San Joaquin Valley d.
Schaumann d.
Second Manifestations of Arterial D. (SMART)
Shaver d.
Shoshin d.
shuttlemaker's d.
sickle cell d.
silo-filler's d.
single-vessel d. (SVD)
sinus node d.
slim d.
Sly d.
small airways d.
Spatz-Lindenberg d. (SLD)
spirochetal d.
Steinert d.
stenotic valvular heart d.
stentable d.
Still d.
Stokes-Adams d.
structural heart d. (SHD)
Surveillance of Work-related and Occupational Respiratory D. (SWORD)
Sylvest d.
synchronous endobronchial d.
Takayasu d.
Takayasu-Onishi d.
Tangier d.
Taussig-Bing d.
Tay-Sachs d.
Thomsen d.
three-vessel coronary d.
thromboembolic d. (TED)
thyrocardiac d.
thyroid d.
thyrotoxic heart d.
transplant coronary artery d. (TCAD, TxCAD)
traumatic heart d.
tricuspid valve d.
TWAR d.
type I glycogen storage d.
Uhl d.
unstable coronary artery d. (UCAD)
valvular heart d.
van den Bergh d.
Vaquez d.
vasospastic d.
venoocclusive d.
vertebrobasilar occlusive d.
vibration d.
von Recklinghausen d.
von Willebrand d.

Warfarin-Aspirin Symptomatic Intracranial D. (WASID)
Weber-Christian d.
Weil d.
Wenckebach d.
Werlhof d.
wheat weevil d.
Whipple d.
Wilkie d.
Wilson d.
Wilson-Kimmelsteil d.
Winiwarter-Buerger d.
winter vomiting d.
Wolman d.
wood pulp worker's lung d.
woven coronary artery d.
Yamaguchi d.

disinfectant
Control III Elite d.

disintegration rate

disk, disc
atrial d.
cervical d.
Eigon d.
HCH d.
intervertebral d.
Molnar d.
open atrial d.
optic d.
d. oxygenation
d. oxygenator
Simpson Method of D.'s
d. spring

disk-cage valve

Diskhaler

diskus
Advair d.
Flovent d.
D. inhaler
Serevent D.

dislodgment, dislodgement
lead d.

dismutase
Cu/Zn superoxide d.
manganese superoxide d. (Mn-SOD)
superoxide d.

disodium
adenosine triphosphate d.
cefotetan d.
d. cromoglycate (DSCG)
edetate d.
ticarcillin d.

disopyramide phosphate

disorder
acid-base d.
arrhythmogenic d.
autoimmune d.
clotting d.

conduction d.
decompression d.
dysbaric d.
endocrine d.
genetic d.
glycosphingolipid d.
iatrogenic d.
International Classification of
  Sleep D.'s (ICSD)
lupus anticoagulant d.
lymphocytic infiltrative d.
mendelian d.
movement d.
neurological d.
neuromuscular d.
neuromyopathic d.
panic d.
periodic limb movement d.
  (PLMD)
posttransplantation
  lymphoproliferative d. (PTLPD,
  PTLD)
Sheffield Screening Test for
  Acquired Language D.'s (STALD)
single-gene d.
disordered action of heart (DAH)
disorganization
segmental arterial d.
Disotate
dispar
  Entamoeba d.
Dispatch
D. balloon
D. catheter
D. infusion catheter
D. over-the-wire catheter
D. Urokinase Efficacy Trial
  (DUET)
dispersing electrode
dispersion
aerosol bolus d. (AD)
interlead QT d.
QT d. (QTd)
QT interval d.
QT/QTc d.
d. of refractoriness
Taylor d.
temporal d.
dispersive electrode
displacement
d. sensing device
d. waveform

display
color kinesis echocardiographic d.
liquid crystal d. (LCD)
PerfTrak d.
PerfTrak perfusion waveform d.
disposable
Metaplus arterial pump with d.
disposable aortic rotating punch
Dispos-a-Med Isoproterenol
Disprin
disrupted plaque
disruption
bronchial d.
circadian d.
great vessel d.
plaque d.
traumatic aortic d.
DISS
Diameter Index Safety system
dissecans
pneumonia d.
dissected tissue arm
dissecting
d. aorta
d. aortic aneurysm
d. hematoma
dissection
d. of aorta
aortic d. (AD)
aortic d. (type A, type B)
arterial d.
BioGlue surgical adhesive for
  aortic d.
coronary d.
coronary artery d.
DeBakey-type aortic d.
epiphenomena of d.
intraluminal d.
long d.
spiral d.
spontaneous cervical artery d.
  (sCAD)
spontaneous coronary artery d.
  (SCAD, sCAD)
Stanford aortic d.
Stanford type B aortic d.
therapeutic d.
thoracic aortic d.
type A aortic d.
type B aortic d.
dissector
balloon d.

D

NOTES

dissector *(continued)*
    Holinger d.
    SAPH Finder surgical balloon d.
    SAPHtrak balloon d.
    Spacemaker balloon d.

disseminated
    d. coccidioidomycosis
    d. cryptococcosis
    d. intravascular coagulation (DIC)
    d. intravascular coagulopathy (DIC)
    d. lupus erythematosus
    d. polyarteritis
    d. tuberculosis

dissemination
    hematogenous bacterial d.
    micronodular d.

dissociation
    atrial d.
    atrioventricular d. (AVD)
    A-V d.
    complete atrioventricular d.
    complete A-V d.
    d. curve
    electromechanical d. (EMD)
    electromyocardial d.
    incomplete atrioventricular d.
    incomplete A-V d.
    d. by interference
    interference d.
    intracavitary pressure-electrogram d.
    isorhythmic d.
    longitudinal d.

dissolution

Distaflex balloon

distal
    d. akinesia
    d. anastomosis
    d. bed
    d. convoluted tubule
    d. coronary perfusion pressure
    d. coronary sinus (DCS)
    d. ectasia
    d. intestinal obstruction syndrome (DIOS)
    d. perfusion system (DPS)
    d. runoff
    d. shocking coil
    d. splenorenal shunt
    d. stenosis
    d. vascular insufficiency
    d. vessel embolization

distance
    half-power d.
    interelectrode d.
    Mahalanobis d.

distant
    d. breath sounds
    d. heart sounds

distensibility
    aortic d.
    arterial d.
    coronary artery d.
    ventricular d.

distention, distension
    jugular venous d. (JVD)
    premature diastolic d.
    d. waveform

distorted coarctation

distortion
    peribronchovascular d.
    pincushion d.

distress
    respiratory d.

distribution
    blood volume d.
    Boltzmann d.
    connexon d.
    interstitial d.
    microvascular flow d.
    nonhomogeneous pulmonary time-constant d.
    perilymphatic d.
    stocking-glove d.
    tracer d.
    volume of d.

distributive shock

disturbance
    conduction d.
    electrolytic d.
    rhythm d.
    sleep d.

disturbed
    d. circadian blood pressure pattern
    d. flow

disulfide
    d. bridge
    carbon d.
    glutathione d.

Dittrich
    D. plug
    D. stenosis

Diucardin

Diuchlor

Diulo

Diupres

diurese

diuresis
    loop d.

diuretic
    d. agent
    cardiac d.
    high-ceiling d.
    indirect d.
    loop d.
    osmotic d.
    potassium-sparing d.

potassium-wasting d.
d. therapy
thiazide d.
Diurexan
Diurigen
Diuril
diurnal
d. peak flow variability
d. rhythm
d. sleep
d. variation
Diutensin
divalinil
divarication
divergens
Babesia d.
diversity
antigen-binding d.
diver's syncope
diverticulectomy
Harrington esophageal d.
diverticulum, pl. **diverticula**
apical d.
Heister d.
laryngotracheal d.
tracheobronchial d.
Zenker d.
divided respiration
diving
d. air embolism
d. goiter
d. reflex
division
vascular ring d.
divisional
d. block
d. heart block
DivYsio
D. PC-coated stent
D. stent
Dixarit
dizziness
DKS
Damus-Kaye-Stansel
DKS operation
DL
double lumen
QuickFurl DL
DLCO
diffusing capacity of lung for carbon
monoxide
D-looping

D-loop transposition of the great arteries
DLP cardioplegic needle
d,l-**sotalol**
DLT
double lung transplant
DM
diabetes mellitus
Anatuss DM
Benylin DM
Carbodec DM
Cardec DM
Diabetic Tussin DM
Fenesin DM
Genatuss DM
Halotussin DM
Hold DM
Humibid DM
Iobid DM
Monafed DM
Mytussin DM
Phenameth DM
Profen II DM
Pseudo-Car DM
Robafen DM
Silphen DM
Siltussin DM
Tolu-Sed DM
Triaminic DM
Uni-tussin DM
Dm
membrane diffusing capacity
DM-400 Holter ECG cassette recorder
D-Med Injection
DMI analyzer
DMP-444
^{99m}Tc D.
DMPM
diffuse malignant pleural mesothelioma
DMR
direct myocardial revascularization
DMVA
direct mechanical ventricular actuation
DNA
deoxyribonucleic acid
DNA cloning
DNA-coated stent
DNA histogram
human cloned DNA (cDNA)
DNA probe
DNA sequencing
DNA switch

D

NOTES

DNase
deoxyribonuclease
DNM
descending necrotizing mediastinitis
DNP
dendroaspis natriuretic peptide
DNR
do not resuscitate
Doan's
Extra Strength D.
D. Original
dobutamine
d. atropine stress echocardiography (DASE)
d. echocardiography (DE)
d. holiday
d. hydrochloride
d.-induced ischemia
d. perfusion scintigraphy
d. stress echocardiography (DSE)
d. stress test
Dobutrex injection
DOC
D. exchange technique
D. guidewire extension
DOC-2000 demand oxygen controller
docetaxel
Docke murmur
docking wire
dock wire
docosahexaenoic acid
Dodd perforating vein
dodecafluoropentane (DDFP)
dodecapeptide
Dodge area-length method
DODS
demand oxygen delivery system
DOE
dyspnea on exertion
Doesel-Huzly bronchoscopic tube
dofetilide
dog
d. boning
d. cough
d.-leg catheter
Döhle
D. disease
D.-Heller aortitis
D. inclusion bodies
Dolacet
Dolastatin
dolens
phlegmasia alba d.
phlegmasia cerulea d.
dolichoectatic aneurysm
dolichol
dolichostenomelia
Dolobid

dolore
angina pectoris sine d.
angina sine d.
domain
time d.
dome
d.-and-dart configuration
d. of diaphragm
d. excursion
d.-shaped
domestica
Carinia d.
dominance
coronary artery d.
dominant positive deflection flutter
doming
diastolic d.
d. of leaflet
systolic d.
tricuspid valve d.
domino procedure
domperidone
donation
predeposit autologous d.
Donders pressure
Donne corpuscle
donor
d. heart
d. organ ischemic time
d.-specific transfusion
do not resuscitate (DNR)
door-to-needle time
L-**dopa**
Dopamet
dopamine
d. beta-hydroxylase deficiency
d. D2 receptor (DD2R)
d. hydrochloride
dopaminergic
d. agent
d. function
Dopastat
dopexamine
Doplette monitor
Doppler
Aloka color D.
D. auto-correlation technique
D. blood flow detector
D. cardiography
Carolina color spectrum CW D.
carotid D.
D. catheter
D.-Cavin monitor
color echotomography D.
color flow D.
D. color flow
D. color flow mapping (DCFM)
D. color jet

D. continuity equation
continuous-wave D. (CWD)
D. coronary catheter
D.-derived index
D. device
D. echocardiography
D. effect
D. Endpoints Stenting International Investigation: Coronary Flow Reserve (DESTINI-CFR)
D. fetal heart monitor
D. fetal stethoscope
D. flow analysis
D. FloWire
D. Flowire guidewire
D. flow mapping
D. flow probe
FreeDop cordless D.
D. gradient
D. interrogation
intravascular D.
D. measurement
D. pressure
D. pressure gradient
pulsed D. echocardiography
pulsed-wave D. (PWD)
pulsed-wave tissue D. (PWTD)
quantitative D.
D. recording
D. shift
D. signal
D. sonography (DS)
D. speckle
spectral D.
D. spectral analysis
steady D.
D. study
D.-tipped angioplasty guidewire
D. tissue imaging (DTI)
transcranial D. (TCD)
D. transducer
D. transesophageal color flow imaging
D. ultrasonic flowmeter
D. ultrasonography
D. ultrasound
D. velocimetry
D. velocity probe
D. velocity wire
D. waveform analysis
dopplered
dopplergram

dopplergraphy
Dopplette
Dopram
D. injection
Doptone monitoring
d'orange
peau d.
Dorendorf sign
Dorian rib stripper
Dormarex 2 Oral
dormescent jerk
Dormin Oral
dornase
d. alfa
pancreatic d.
Dorros
D. brachial internal mammary guiding catheter
D. infusion/probing catheter
dorsal
carpal arch d.
d. lingual branches of lingual artery
d. mesocardium
dorsalis pedis pulse
dorsi
latissimus d.
dorsum linguae
DORV
double-outlet right ventricle
Doryx Oral
dosage regimen
dose
maximum tolerated d. (MTD)
nonpressor d.
priming d.
radiation absorbed d. (rad)
threshold d.
dose-effect curve dose-response curve
Dosepak
Medrol D.
dosimetry
dosing
trough d.
Dos Santos needle
DOT
directly observed therapy
directly observed treatment
Dotter
D. caged-balloon catheter
D. effect
D. Intravascular Retrieval Set

NOTES

Dotter *(continued)*
    D.-Judkins percutaneous transluminal angioplasty
    D.-Judkins technique
    D. percutaneous transluminal angioplasty
    D. technique
dottering
    d. effect
    d. of lesion
Dotter-Judkins
DOUBLE
    Double Bolus Lytic Efficacy
    DOUBLE trial
double
    d. aortic arch
    d. aortic stenosis
    D. Bolus Lytic Efficacy (DOUBLE)
    d. bubble flushing reservoir
    d. count
    d. counting
    d. ectopic tachyarrhythmia
    d. external direct current shock
    d. extrastimulus
    d. lumen (DL)
    d. lung transplant (DLT)
    d. pleurisy
    d. pneumonia
    d. product
    d. simultaneous stimulation test
    d. switch procedure
    d. tachycardia
    d. umbrella
    d. umbrella closure
    d. ventricular extrastimulus
    d. voice
double-balloon
    d.-b. catheter
    d.-b. (9-11) technique
    d.-b. technique
    d.-b. valvotomy
    d.-b. valvuloplasty
double-barreled aorta
double-chain rtPA
double-chip micromanometer catheter
double-disk
    d.-d. ASD closure device
    d.-d. occluder
double-dummy technique
double-flanged valve sewing ring
double-headed stethoscope
double-inlet left ventricle
double-J
    d.-J. catheter
    d.-J. stent
double-lumen
    d.-l. catheter

    d.-l. endobronchial tube
    d.-l. sign
double-oblique imaging
double-outlet
    d.-o. left ventricle
    d.-o. left ventricle malposition
    d.-o. right ventricle (DORV)
    d.-o. right ventricle malposition
double-rib fracture
double-sandwich IgM ELISA
double-sheath bronchial brushings
double-shock sound
double-syringe technique
doublet
double-thermistor coronary sinus catheter
double-umbrella device
double-wire technique
doubling time
doughnut
    d. configuration
    d. sign
Douglas
    D. bag
    D. bag collection method
    D. bag spirometer
    D. bag technique
d'ouverture
    claquement d.
dove coo musical murmur
Dow
    D. Corning tube
    D. method
down
    brady d.
    D. syndrome
downgoing Babinski
downhill
    d. esophageal varix
    d. ST segment depression
down-regulation
Down's Flow Generator
downsloping
    d. ST segment
    d. ST segment depression
downstream
    d. sampling method
    d. segment
    d. venous pressure
doxacurium
doxapram hydrochloride
doxazosin mesylate
doxepin hydrochloride
doxofylline
doxophylline
doxorubicin
    d. cardiomyopathy

d. cardiotoxicity
d. hydrochloride
doxorubicin, 5-fluorouracil, cisplatin (AFP)
doxorubicin-induced cardiac toxicity
Doxychel
D. injection
D. Oral
doxycycline pleurodesis
Doxy Oral
Doyen
D. elevator
D. rib hook
Doyle vein stripper
DPAP
D. interactive airway management system
D. Stealth device
D. Stealth device for sleep apnea
DPB
diffuse panbronchiolitis
dP/dt$_{MAX}$ end-diastolic volume
D-penicillamine
D-Phe-L-Pro-L-Arg-chloromethyl ketone (PPACK)
DPHM
diphenhydramine
DPI
dry powder inhaler
DPL
diagnostic peritoneal lavage
DPM
digital phase mapping
DPPC
dipalmitoyl phosphatidylcholine
DPPC test
DPS
distal perfusion system
QuickFlow DPS
DPTA
diethylenetriamine pentaacetic acid
DPTI
diastolic pressure-time index
DPTS
delayed pulmonary toxicity syndrome
DR-70 tumor marker test
Dräger
D. respirometer
D. ventilator
D. Volumeter
drag force

drain
Charnley suction d.
Clot Stop d.
Deseret sump d.
Relia-Vac d.
drainage
anomalous pulmonary venous d. (APVD)
autogenic d. (AD)
closed chest water-seal d.
external ventricular d. (EVD)
partial anomalous pulmonary venous d. (PAPVD)
percussion and postural d. (P&PD)
postural d. (PD)
pulmonary venous d.
Snyder Surgivac d.
thoracic duct d. (TDD)
Thoracoseal d.
Thora-Drain III chest d.
total anomalous pulmonary venous d. (TAPVD)
underwater seal d.
water-seal d.
Dramamine Oral
Drapanas mesocaval shunt
drapeau
bruit de d.
dreamer clamp
dreaming sleep
dream pain
Drechslera hawaiiensis
dressing
Comfeel Ulcus d.
Cutinova Hydro d.
jacket-type chest d.
Kaltostat wound packing d.
stent d.
Veingard d.
Vigilon d.
wet-to-dry d.
Dressler
D. beat
D. syndrome
DRG
diagnostic-related group
Dr. Gibaud thermal health support
drill-tip catheter
Drinker respirator
drip
heparin d.
postnasal d. (PND)

D

NOTES

Dripps-American Surgical Association
  score
Dristan
  D. Long Lasting Nasal Solution
  D. Sinus Caplets
drive
  d. cycle length
  respiratory d.
  d. train
  ventricular d.
driver
  TLC-II portable VAD d.
Drixoral
  D. Cough & Congestion Liquid
    Caps
  D. Cough Liquid Caps
  D. Cough & Sore Throat Liquid
    Caps
  D. Nasal
  D. Non-Drowsy
Dromos pacemaker
dromotropic effect
dronabinol
droop
  facial d.
drop
  Afrin Children's Nose d.'s
  d. attack
  Ayr saline nasal d.'s
  falling d.
  d. heart
  Rondamine-DM d.'s
  Rondec D.'s
  Tussafed d.'s
droperidol
drophonium
dropout
  septal d.
dropped beat
dropsy
  cardiac d.
  d. chest
  d. of pericardium
drowned
  d. lung
  d. newborn syndrome
drowsiness
  Tylenol Cold No D.
Droxia
drug
  d. abuse
  antiarrhythmic d. (AAD)
  antituberculous d.
  cardiotonic d.
  d. clearance
  depolarizing d.
  hydrophobic d.
  hypnotic d.

investigational new d. (IND)
lipophilic d.
neuroprotective d.
nondepolarizing d.
nonsteroidal antiinflammatory d.
  (NSAID)
pressor d.
sedative-hypnotic d.
sympathomimetic d.
vasoactive d.
drug-associated pericarditis
drug-induced
  d.-i. cardiomyopathy
  d.-i. lupus erythematosus (DILE)
  d.-i. lupus syndrome
  d.-i. pericarditis
  d.-i. thrombocytopenia
drug-loaded biodegradable polymer stent
drug-refractory tachycardia
Drummond
  marginal artery of D.
  D. marginal artery
  D. sign
dry
  d. beriberi
  d. bronchiectasis
  d. bronchitis
  d. cough
  d. gangrene
  d. pericarditis
  d. pleurisy
  d. powder inhaler (DPI)
  d. rale
dry-powder actuator
Drysdale corpuscle
DS
  Doppler sonography
  Bactrim DS
  Cotrim DS
  Septra DS
  Sulfatrim DS
  Uroplus DS
DSA
  digital subtraction angiography
DSAS
  discrete subvalvular aortic stenosis
DSC
  dynamic susceptibility contrast-enhanced
    DSC MRI
DSCG
  disodium cromoglycate
DSE
  digital subtraction echocardiography
  dobutamine stress echocardiography
DSI-III screw-in lead pacemaker
D-Sotalol
  D-Sotalol block of HERG

Survival with Oral D-Sotalol
(SWORD)
DSP
dexamethasone sodium phosphate
DSS
discrete subaortic stenosis
DSX Sopha camera
DTA
descending thoracic aorta
DTAFA
descending thoracic aorta-to-femoral
artery
DTAFA bypass graft
DTAF-F
descending thoracic aortic-femoral-
femoral
2D-TCCS
two-dimensional transcranial color-coded
sonography
D-TGA, dTGA
d-transposition of great arteries
DTI
diffusion tensor imaging
Doppler tissue imaging
DTIC-Dome
D-to-E
D-t.-E amplitude
D-t.-E slope
DTPA
diethylenetriamine pentaacetate
diethylenetriamine pentaacetic acid
DTPA aerosol inhalation lung
scintigraphy
**d-transposition of great arteries (D-
TGA, dTGA)**
dual
d. atrioventricular node
d. balloon perfusion catheter
(DBPC)
d. chamber (DC)
d. echophonocardiography
d. marker
dual-chamber
d.-c. ICD
d.-c. Medtronic Kappa 400
pacemaker
d.-c. pacemaker
d.-c. pacing
d.-c. rate-responsive
d.-c. and VVI Implantable
Defibrillator (DAVID)
dual-coil transvenous lead

dual-demand pacemaker
dual-energy digital radiography
**dual-isotope simultaneous acquisition
single-photon emission computed
tomography (DISA-SPECT)**
duality
dual-lead electrocardiogram
dual-loop intraatrial reentry
**dual-mode, dual-pacing, dual-sensing
(DDD)**
**dual-sensor micromanometric high-
fidelity catheter**
dual-site right atrial pacing
**Dualtherm dual thermistor
thermodilution catheter**
Dubois index
Du Bois-Reymond law
Duchenne
D. muscular dystrophy
D. sign
duckbill voice prosthesis
Duckworth phenomenon
Ducor
D. balloon catheter
D.-Cordis pigtail catheter
D. HF catheter
D. tip
duct
Bartholin d.
Botallo d.
collecting d.
craniopharyngeal d.
d. of Cuvier
medullary collecting d.
D. Occluder pfm coil
omphalomesenteric d.
pharyngobranchial d.
thoracic d.
thyrolingual d.
ductal cell carcinoma
ductus
d. arantii
d. arteriosus
d. bump
percutaneous occlusion of d.
d. sublinguales minores
d. sublingualis major
d. thoracicus
d. venosus
DUET
Dispatch Urokinase Efficacy Trial

D

NOTES

Duett
  D. arterial closure device
  D. catheter
  D. sealing device
  D. vascular sealing device
Duffield cardiovascular scissors
Duguet siphon
Duke
  D. Activity Status Index (DASI)
  D. bleeding time
  D. Carcinoid Database
  D. criteria
  D. treadmill exercise score
  D. treadmill prognostic score
  D. treadmill score
Dukes classification
dullness
  absolute cardiac d. (ACD)
  area of cardiac d.
  border of cardiac d.
  cardiac border of d.
  percussion d.
  tympanic d.
dull pain
dumoffii
  Legionella d.
Dumon
  D. bronchoscope
  D. endobronchial silicone stent
  D.-Harrell bronchoscope
  D. tracheobronchial stent
Dumont thoracic scissors
Duncan syndrome
Dunham fan
Dunlop thrombus stripper
DuoCet
duodecapolar
  d. catheter
  d. Halo catheter
duodenale
  Ancylostoma d.
duodenal string test
Duo-Medihaler Aerosol
Duostat rotating hemostatic valve
Duo-Trach Injection
Duotrate
DUPEL drug delivery system
duplex
  d. Doppler scan
  d. imaging
  d. pulsed-Doppler ultrasonography
  pulsus d.
  d. scan
  d. scanning
  d. ultrasound
Dura-Aire compressor
Duracep biopsy forceps
Duraclon Injection

Duraflo
  BMR-4500SG sealed hard shell
    venous reservoir with D.
  Carpentier-Edwards Physio
    annuloplasty ring with D.
Duraflow heart valve
Duragesic Transdermal
Dura-Gest
Duralone injection
Duralutin injection
Duralyn
Duramax
Duramist Plus
Duran annuloplasty ring
Durapulse pacemaker
Duraquin
Dura-Tabs
  Quinaglute D.-T.
Duratest injection
Durathane cardiac device
Durathate Injection
duration
  action potential d. (APD)
  d. of ECG wave
  d. of exercise
  d. of expiration (T_E)
  half amplitude pulse d.
  d. of inspiration (T_I)
  monophasic action potential d.
    (MAPD)
  D. Nasal Solution
  P d.
  pacing d.
  pulse d.
  pulse wave d.
  d. of P wave
  P-wave d.
  QRS complex d.
  QT interval d.
  signal-averaged P-wave d. (SAPD)
  sustained rate d.
Duratuss
Duratuss-G
Dura-Vent
Durham tube
Duricef
Duromedics
  D. mitral valve
  D. valve prosthesis
Duroziez
  D. disease
  D. murmur
  D. sign
  D. symptom
Durrax Oral
Durules
  Betaloc D.
  Biquin D.

durus
    pulsus d.
duskiness
dusky
dust
    d. asthma
    d. disease
    grain d.
    inorganic d.
    mushroom d.
    organic d.
Dutch
duteplase
duty factor
Duval
    D.-Coryllos rib shears
    D.-Crile lung forceps
    D. lung-grasping forceps
DVI
    deep venous insufficiency
    DVI pacemaker
    DVI pacing
DVT
    deep venous thrombosis
    residual DVT
D-5-W, D$_5$W
dwarfism
    aortic d.
DWI
    diffusion-weighted imaging
DWL Multidop X 4-channel TCD scanner
DWMHI
    deep white matter hyperintensity
DWML
    deep white matter lesion
DX-Portable spirometry
DXR
    delayed xenograft rejection
Dyazide
Dycill
dyclonine
dye
    Cardio-Green d.
    d. cuvette
    d. dilution technique
    flashlamp excited pulsed d.
    Fox green d.
    indocyanine green d.
    d. injection
    d. laser

    radiocontrast d.
    Unisperse blue d.
dye-dilution
    d.-d. curve
    d.-d. method
Dymedix sleep sensor
Dymelor
Dymer
    D. excimer delivery probe
    D. excimer delivery system
Dynabac
Dynacin Oral
DynaCirc
dynamic
    d. aorta
    d. cardiomyoplasty
    d. compliance of lung
    d. CT scan
    d. exercise
    fluid d.'s
    d. frequency response
    funnel d.'s
    d. hyperinflation
    d. intracavitary obstruction
    left ventricular-left atrial crossover d.'s
    d. method
    d. murmur
    d. pressure
    d. range
    d. relaxation
    RR interval d.'s
    d. stenosis
    d. susceptibility contrast-enhanced (DSC)
    d. susceptibility contrast-enhanced MRI
    d. tracheal compression
    D. Y stent
dynamite heart
dynamometer
    bicycle d.
    Cybex isokinetic d.
    Jamar hand d.
    Jamar model 0030J4 d.
Dynapen
DynaPulse 5000A blood pressure monitor
Dynasty
    D. balloon
    D. delivery system

D

NOTES

dyne
    d. seconds
dynein
Dynepo
dynorphin
dyphylline
Dyrenium
dysanapsis
    airway-parenchymal d.
dysanaptic growth
dysarteriotony
dysarthria
    isolated d.
    pure d. (PD)
dysarthria-clumsy hand syndrome (DCHS)
dysautonomia
    familial d.
dysbaric
    d. disorder
    d. osteonecrosis
dysbarism
dysbetalipoproteinemia
    familial d.
dyscontrol
dyscrasia
    blood d.
dysfibrinogenemia
dysfunction
    acute endothelial d.
    age-related endothelial d.
    biventricular d.
    chronic contractile d.
    ciliary d.
    diaphragmatic d.
    diastolic d.
    diastolic ventricular d.
    endothelial d.
    extrathoracic airway d.
    focal ventricular d.
    global ventricular d.
    intellectual d.
    irritant-associated vocal cord d.
    left ventricular d. (LVD)
    left ventricular systolic d.
    lung d.
    microvascular d.
    multiple-organ d.
    obstructive ventilatory d.
    papillary muscle d.
    postischemic d.
    restrictive ventilatory d.
    reversible left ventricular d.
    sinoatrial node d.
    sinus node d.
    Studies of Left Ventricular D. (SOLVD)

valvular d.
    ventricular d.
    vocal cord d. (VCD)
dysfunctional
    d. airway immune response
    d. myocardium
dysgenesis
    gonadal d.
dysgeusia
dyskinesia
    d. intermittens
    primary ciliary d. (PCD)
    d. syndrome
    tracheobronchial d.
dyskinesis
    anterior wall d.
    anteroapical d.
    left ventricular d.
    posteroinferior d.
dyskinetic segment
dyslipidemia
    atherogenic d.
    Fredrickson d.
dyslipidemic hypertension syndrome
dyslipoproteinemia
dysmetria
dysmodulation
dysmotility
    esophageal d.
dysnystaxis
dyspeptica
    angina d.
dysphagia, dysphagy
    contractile ring d.
    d. inflammatoria
    d. lusoria
    d. nervosa
    d. paralytica
    sideropenic d.
    d. spastica
    vallecular d.
    d. valsalviana
dysphasia
dysphasic
dysplasia
    angiogenic squamous d.
    arrhythmogenic right ventricular d. (ARVD)
    atriodigital d.
    bronchopulmonary d. (BPD)
    ectodermal d.
    fibromuscular d.
    fibrous d.
    mucoepithelial d.
    polyostotic fibrous d.
    right ventricular d.
    ventriculoradial d.

dysplastic
  d. mitral valvar leaflet
  d. valve

dyspnea
  American Thoracic Society
   classification of d.
  cardiac d.
  effort d.
  episodic d.
  exercise-induced d.
  exertional d.
  expiratory d.
  functional d.
  inspiratory d.
  Monday d.
  nocturnal d.
  nonexpansional d.
  one-flight exertional d.
  d. on exertion (DOE)
  orthostatic d.
  paroxysmal nocturnal d. (PND)
  progressive d.
  psychogenic d.
  pulmonary d.
  renal d.
  rest d.
  d. scale
  D. Scale questionnaire
  sighing d.
  d. target
  Traube d.
  two-flight d.
  two-flight exertional d.

dyspneic
dysreflexia
  autonomic d.

The entry preceding dysplastic:
  vertebral defects, imperforate anus,
  transesophageal fistula, and radial
  and renal d. (VATER)

dysrhythmia
  cardiac d.
dysrhythmic cardiac arrest
dysrhythmogenic
dyssynchronization
**dyssynchronous thoracoabdominal
  excursion**
dyssynchrony
  mechanical d.
  thoracoabdominal d.
dyssynergia
  detrusor-sphincter d.
dyssynergic
  d. myocardial segment
  d. myocardium
dyssynergy
  regional d.
  ventricular d.
dystrophic calcification
dystrophin
dystrophinopathy
dystrophy
  asphyxiating thoracic d. (ATD)
  Becker-type tardive muscular d.
  Duchenne muscular d.
  Emery-Dreifuss muscular d.
  facioscapulohumeral d.
  familial asphyxiant thoracic d.
  Landouzy-Dejerine d.
  limb-girdle muscular d.
  muscular d.
  myotonic muscular d.
  reflex sympathetic d.
  Steinert myotonic d.
  thoracic asphyxiant d.
  thoracic-pelvic-phalangeal d.
dystropic calcification
dysvascular
dZ/dt

D

NOTES

E

    E to A change
    E to F slope
    E greater than A
    E to I changes
    E point
    E point on echocardiogram
    E point to septal separation
    (EPSS)
    E sign
    E wave
    E wave to A wave (E/A, E:A)

E_4

    leukotriene E_4

7E3

    7E3 glycoprotein IIb/IIIa platelet
    antibody
    7E3 monoclonal Fab antibody

44E

    Vicks 44E
    Vicks Pediatric Formula 44E

E-150 Breeze ventilator

E-4031

EA

    endotracheal aspirate

E/A, E:A

    E wave to A wave

EAC

    expandable access catheter
    EAC catheter

EAD

    early afterdepolarization
    effective airspace dimension

EAE

    effective arterial elastance

EAG

    endovascular aortic graft

Eagle

    E. criteria
    E. equation
    E. medium
    E. portable ventilation system
    E. risk score index
    E. spirometer

ear

    e. densitogram
    e. lobe crease (ELC)
    e. oximeter

earclip

    Satlite pulse oximeter with e.

early

    e. afterdepolarization (EAD)
    e. deceleration
    e. diastolic murmur

    Intravenous tPA for Treatment of
    Infarcting Myocardium E.
    (INTIME)
    e. ischemic recurrence (EIR)
    e. lung injury
    e. opening valve
    e. progressing stroke (EPS)
    e. pulmonary injury
    e. rapid repolarization
    e. repolarization (ER)
    e. repolarization syndrome

early-peaking systolic murmur

EasiVent Valved Holding Chamber

Easprin

EAST

    Emory Angioplasty versus Surgery Trial
    external rotation, abduction, stress test

Easy

    E. Air 15 compressor
    E. Analysis system

Easy-Breathe

Easy/Dial Reg oxygen regulator

Easyhaler

Easy/Neb compressor

EASYTRAK coronary venous lead

EAT

    ectopic atrial tachycardia

Eaton

    E. agent
    E. agent pneumonia

Eaton-Lambert syndrome

E/A wave ratio

EBCT

    electron beam computed tomography

EBDA

    effective balloon-dilated area

Eberth perithelium

EBM

    evidence-based medicine

EBNA

    Epstein-Barr nuclear antigen

Ebola virus

EBR

    embolus-to-blood ratio

Ebrantil

Ebstein

    E. angle
    E. anomaly
    E. cardiac anomaly
    E. disease
    E. malformation
    E. malformed valve
    E. sign

EBV

    Epstein-Barr virus

E

EC50 TOXCO breath carbon monoxide monitor
ECA
    external carotid artery
E-CABG
    endarterectomy and coronary artery bypass grafting
    endoscopic coronary artery bypass graft
ECAD
    extracranial carotid arterial disease
ecadotril
ECAT III positron tomograph
ECBV
    effective circulating blood volume
ECC
    edema, clubbing, and cyanosis
    emergency cardiac care
eccentric
    e. atrial activation
    e. hypertrophy
    e. ledge
    e. lesion
    E. locked rib shears
    e. monocuspid tilting-disk prosthetic valve
    e. narrowing
    e. stenosis
    e. stenotic jet
eccentricity index
ecchymosis, pl. **ecchymoses**
ecchymotic
    e. facies
    e. mask
Eccovision acoustic pharyngometer
ECD
    endocardial cushion defect
    external cardioverter-defibrillator
    extracranial carotid disease
    extracranial Doppler sonography
    Ventak ECD
ECF-A
    eosinophil chemotactic factors of anaphylaxis
ECG, EKG
    electrocardiogram
    electrocardiograph
    electrocardiography (*See also* EKG)
      baseline ECG
      borderline ECG
      Cardiovit AT-2 ECG
      Cardiovit AT-10 laptop ECG
      Cardiovit AT-2*plus* ECG
      esophageal ECG
      intracardiac ECG
      KoKo rhythm ECG
      KoKo rhythm PC-based ECG
      ECG leads I, II, III; V1 through V6; aVF, aVL, aVR

    Micro-Tracer portable ECG
    Minnesota classification of ECG
    ECG monitor strip
    Mortara Instruments ELI-100XR 12-lead ECG
    ECG signal-averaging technique
    ECG silence
    straight-line ECG
    ECG triggering unit
    Welch Allyn/Shiller AT-2 full-size ECG
    Welch Allyn/Shiller AT-10 hospital grade ECG
    Welch Allyn/Shiller AT-2*plus* full-size ECG
    Welch Allyn/Shiller AT-1 three channel ECG
    Welch Allyn/Shiller MS-3 pocket size ECG
ECG-synchronized digital subtraction angiogram
echinococcal cyst
echinococcosis
Echinococcus
    E. granulosus
    E. multilocularis
ECHO
    enteric cytopathogenic human orphan
    enterocytopathogenic human orphan
    ECHO virus
echo, pl. **echoes**
    amphoric e.
    atrial e.
    bandlike intrapericardial e.
    e. beat
    bright e.
    e. catheter
    e. delay time (TE)
    e.-dense valve
    e. density
    gradient recall e. (GRE)
    e. guidance
    high density e.
    e. intensity
    linear e.
    metallic e.
    motion display e.
    nodus sinuatrialis e.
    NS e.
    pericardial e.
    e. planar imaging (EPI)
    e. probe
    e. ranging
    e. record access (ERA)
    e. reverberation
    RT3D e.
    scattered e.
    e. score

smokelike echoes
specular e.
Stroke Prevention in Atrial
  Fibrillation III Transesophageal E.
  (SPAF TEE)
transcutaneous e.
transesophageal e.
e. transponder electrode catheter
ventricular e.
e. zone

echoaortography
echo-bright endocardium
echocardiogram
apical five-chamber view e.
apical four-chamber view e.
apical two-chamber view e.
B bump on e.
continuous loop exercise e.
continuous wave Doppler e.
contrast-enhanced e.
cross-sectional two-dimensional e.
2D e.
E point on e.
exercise e. (EE)
Feigenbaum e.
12-lead e.
15-lead e.
long-axis parasternal view e.
meridian e.
M-mode e.
Ochsner-Mahorner e.
parasternal long-axis view e.
parasternal short-axis view e.
postcontrast e.
posterior left ventricular wall
  motion on e.
postexercise e.
signal-averaged e.
transthoracic e. (TTE)
e. with saline agitation
W wave on e.

echocardiograph
Acuson e.
Biosound Surgiscan e.
Ultramark 9 e.

echocardiographic
e. assessment
e. automated border detection
e. automated boundary detection
  system
e. differentiation
e. scoring system

e. smoke
e. strain rate imaging
e. transducer

echocardiography
adenosine e.
A-mode e.
any-plane e.
Assessment of Cardioversion
  Utilizing Transesophageal E.
  (ACUTE)
AT-atropine stress e.
baseline e.
bedside transthoracic e.
bicycle e.
bidimensional e.
B-mode e.
bubble contrast e.
color M-mode Doppler e.
continuous-wave Doppler e.
contrast e.
cross-sectional e. (CSE)
2 D e.
deductive e.
digital e.
digital subtraction e. (DSE)
dipyridamole e.
dipyridamole stress e.
dobutamine e. (DE)
dobutamine atropine stress e.
  (DASE)
dobutamine stress e. (DSE)
Doppler e.
epiaortic e.
ergonovine e.
esophageal e.
exercise e.
exercise stress e. (Ex-Echo)
high-frequency epicardial e. (HFEE)
interventional e.
intracardiac e. (ICE)
intraoperative e. (IOE)
meridian e.
mitral valve e.
M-mode e.
multiplane e.
multiplane transesophageal e.
myocardial contrast e. (MCE)
paraplane e.
E. Persantine International
  Cooperative (EPIC)
pharmacologic stress e.
pulmonary valve e.

E

NOTES

echocardiography *(continued)*
    pulsed Doppler e.
    quantitative two-dimensional e.
    real-time e.
    real-time three-dimensional e.
    sector scan e.
    signal-averaged e.
    SonoHeart hand-carried e.
    stress e.
    stress-injected sestamibi-gated
     SPECT with e.
    supine bicycle stress e. (SBSE)
    TDI M-mode e.
    three-dimensional e. (3DE)
    transesophageal e. (TEE)
    transesophageal contrast e.
    transesophageal dobutamine stress e.
    transesophageal echocardiography-
     dobutamine stress e. (TEE-DSE)
    transthoracic e. (TTE)
    transthoracic color Doppler e.
    transthoracic contract e.
    treadmill e.
    two-dimensional e. (2DE)
    Value of Transesophageal E.
    (VOTE)
echodense
    e. mass
    e. structure
echodensity
    cardial e.
    linear e.
    superimposed e.
echo-Doppler cardiography
echoendoscope
    Olympus GIF-EUM2 e.
echoes (*pl. of* echo)
EchoFlow blood velocity meter system
echo-free space
EchoGen
    E. emulsion
    E. injectable emulsion
echogenic
    e. mass
    e. plaque
echogenicity
    end-diastolic wall e.
echogram
echograph
    Siemens Sonoline CD e.
echography
    A-scan e.
echo-guided
    e.-g. pericardiocentesis
    e.-g. ultrasound
echolucent plaque
EchoMark
    E. angiographic catheter

echophonocardiography
    combined M-mode e.
    dual e.
echophony
EchoQuant acoustic quantification system
echoreflective
echoreflectivity
echoscanner
echoscope
echo-signal shape
echo-spared area
Echovar Doppler system
echovirus
    e. myocarditis
Echovist
EC/IC
    extracranial/intracranial
    EC/IC arterial bypass study
Eck fistula
ECLA
    excimer laser coronary angioplasty
eclampsia
Eclipse
    E. holmium laser
    E. PTMR system
    E. TMR laser
ECLS
    extracorporeal life support
ECM
    extracellular matrix
ECMO
    extracorporeal membrane oxygenation
    ECMO pump
    ECMO therapy
ecNOS
    endothelial constitutive nitric oxide
    synthase
    endothelial nitric oxide
EcoCheck oxygen monitor
ECOM
    endotracheal cardiac output monitor
    endotracheal cardiac output monitoring
Economics and Quality of Life Substudy of GUSTO (EQOL)
Eco-Oxymax
Ecotrin
ECP
    effective conduction period
    eosinophil cationic protein
ECS
    extracellular-like, calcium-free solution
    ECS cardioplegic solution
ectasia, ectasis
    alveolar e.
    annuloaortic e.
    anuloaortic e.
    aortoannular e.

artery e.
e. cordis
coronary artery e.
diffuse arterial e.
distal e.
vascular e.
Ectasule
ectatic
e. aneurysm
e. emphysema
ecto-ADPase
ectocardia
ectocardiac, ectocardial
Ectocor pacemaker
ectodermal dysplasia
ectopia
e. cordis
e. cordis abdominalis
e. cordis pectoral
e. lentis
ectopic
e. Ashman beat
e. atrial pacemaker
e. atrial tachycardia (EAT)
e. beat
e. bronchus
e. impulse
e. junctional tachycardia
e. pacemaker
e. rhythm
e. tachycardia
e. ventricular beat
ectopy
asymptomatic complex e.
atrial e.
supraventricular e.
ventricular e.
ECT pacemaker
ED
emotional defensiveness
EDA
end-diastolic area
EDD
end-diastolic diameter
end-diastolic dimension
esophageal detection device
eddy sound
Edecrin
E. Oral
E. Sodium injection

edema
acute cardiogenic pulmonary e.
(ACPE)
acute noncardiogenic pulmonary e.
acute pulmonary e. (APE)
airway e.
alveolar e.
angioneurotic e.
ankle e.
bland e.
boggy e.
brawny e.
brown e.
cardiac e.
cardiogenic pulmonary e.
cerebral e.
chronic pulmonary e.
circumscribed e.
clubbing, cyanosis, and e. (CCE)
congestive e.
cytotoxic e.
dependent e.
fingerprint e.
flash pulmonary e.
florid pulmonary e.
focal e.
hereditary angioneurotic e. (HANE)
high-altitude pulmonary e. (HAPE)
high-pressure e.
high-pressure cardiogenic
pulmonary e.
hydrostatic e.
idiopathic cyclic e.
increased-permeability pulmonary e.
interstitial e.
interstitial pulmonary e.
e. of lung
lung e.
lymphatic e.
Milton e.
mucosal e.
myocardial e.
neurogenic pulmonary e.
noncardiogenic pulmonary e.
nonpitting e.
obstructive e.
paroxysmal pulmonary e.
passive e.
pedal e.
periodic e.
periorbital e.
peripheral e.

E

NOTES

edema *(continued)*

    perivascular e.
    pitting e.
    postanesthesia pulmonary e.
    postcardioversion pulmonary e.
    presacral e.
    pretibial e.
    pulmonary e.
    pulmonary interstitial e.
    Quincke e.
    reperfusion e.
    reperfusion pulmonary e.
    sacral e.
    stasis e.
    subpleural e.
    tense e.
    terminal e.
    vasogenic e.
    woody e.

edema, clubbing, and cyanosis (ECC)
edematous
edentulism

    compensated e.

Eder-Hufford esophagoscope
Eder-Puestow wire
edetate disodium
edge

    e. detection
    leading e.
    shelving e.
    trailing e.

edge-detection

    e.-d. method
    e.-d. system

EDHF

    endothelium-derived hyperpolarizing
    factor

Edinburgh Handedness Inventory (EHI)
Edmark

    E. mitral valve
    E. monophasic waveform

EDM infusion catheter
EDNO

    endothelium-derived nitric oxide

EDP

    end-diastolic pressure

EDPS

    esophageal-directed pressure support

EDRF

    endothelium-derived relaxing factor

edrophonium chloride
EDS

    excessive daytime sleepiness

EDTA

    ethylenediaminetetraacetic acid

EDV

    end-diastolic volume

EDVI

    end-diastolic volume index

Edwards

    E.-Carpentier aortic valve brush
    E. catheter
    E. clamp
    E.-Duromedics bileaflet heart valve
    E. heart valve
    E. septectomy
    E.-Tapp arterial graft
    E. Teflon intracardiac patch
     prosthesis
    E. woven Teflon aortic bifurcation
     graft

EE

    exercise echocardiogram

EECP

    enhanced external counterpulsation

EEG

    electroencephalogram
    electroencephalograph
    electroencephalography
    Equinox digital EEG
    Neurotrac II EEG
    EEG and PSG instrumentation

EEL

    external elastic lamina
    EEL area

EELV

    end-expiratory lung volume

EEM

    external elastic membrane

E.E.S.

    E. Chewable
    E. Granules
    E. Oral

EET

    epoxyeicosatrienoic
    EET acid

EEV

    elastic equilibrium volume

EF

    ejection fraction

efaroxan
efavirenz
EFE

    endocardial fibroelastosis

Efedron
efegatran
effect

    Anrep e.
    antiatherogenic e.
    Azzopardi e.
    bacteriostatic e.
    Bainbridge e.
    band saw e.
    Bernoulli e.
    billiard ball e.

blooming e.
Bohr e.
Bowditch staircase e.
Brockenbrough e.
bronchoconstrictive e.
bronchodilator e.
bystander e.
candy wrapper edge e.
chronotropic e.
cidal e.
Coanda e.
Cocktail Attenuation of Rotational Ablation Flow E.'s (CARAFE)
Compton e.
copper-wire e.
cytoprotective e.
digitalis e.
digoxin e.
Doppler e.
Dotter e.
dottering e.
dromotropic e.
erectile e.
extrapyramidal side e.
Fahraeus e.
first-night e.
fish-scaling e.
founder e.
Haldane e.
Hawthorne e.
horse-race e.
implosion e.
inertial e.
inotropic e.
jet e.
late proarrhythmic e.
Mach e.
mass e.
mille-feuilles e.
neurotoxic e.
nonhemodynamic e.
peripheral vasodilator e.
postantibiotic e. (PAE)
pressor e.
Prinzmetal e.
proarrhythmic e.
protooncogenic e.
Rivero-Carvallo e.
second gas e.
silver-wire e.
snare-drum e.
snowplow e.

space-occupying e.
spalling e.
squeeze e.
time-of-flight e.
tongue-rolling e.
training e.
vasodilator e.
Vaughan-Williams class e.
Venturi e.
volume of distribution e.
Vroman e.
waterfall e.
Wedensky e.
windkessel e.
work e.
wrecking ball e.

effective
    e. airspace dimension (EAD)
    e. arterial elastance (EAE)
    e. balloon-dilated area (EBDA)
    e. circulating blood volume (ECBV)
    e. conduction period (ECP)
    e. refractory period (ERP)
    e. regurgitant orifice (ERO)
    e. renal blood flow (ERBF)

effector cell

efferent
    e. arteriole
    e. artery

efficacious

Efficacy
    E. and Safety of Subcutaneous Enoxaparin in Non-Q-Wave Coronary Events (ESSENCE)

efficacy
    Acute Infarction Ramipril E. (AIRE)
    Acute Infarction Reperfusion E. (AIRE)
    ciliary e.
    Double Bolus Lytic E. (DOUBLE)
    e. of drug therapy
    Late Assessment of Thrombolytic E. (LATE)
    therapeutic e.
    e. of treatment

efficiency
    cough e.
    detective quantum e.
    mucociliary e.

E

NOTES

Effler
> E.-Groves mode of Allison procedure
> E. hiatal hernia repair
> E. tack

efflux
> cellular cholesterol e.

effort
> angina of e.
> e. angina
> e. dyspnea
> first e.
> e.-independent lung volume
> e.-induced thrombosis
> poor expiratory e.
> relative inspiratory e. (RIE)
> e. syndrome

effusion
> asbestos pleural e.
> bloody e.
> chyliform pleural e.
> chylous e.
> chylous pericardial e.
> chylous pleural e.
> eosinophilic e.
> exudative e.
> exudative pleural e.
> hemorrhagic e.
> interlobar e.
> loculated e.
> malignant pleural e.
> parapneumonic e.
> partially coagulated e.
> pericardial e.
> pericarditis with e.
> pleural e.
> pleurisy with e.
> pulmonary e.
> purulent e.
> serosanguineous e.
> serous e.
> silent pericardial e.
> stranding e.
> subpulmonic e.
> transudative pleural e.

effusive-constrictive
> e.-c. disease
> e.-c. pericarditis

Efidac/24
eflornithine
efonidipine
EFR
> extended field radiation

Efron jackknife classification
Efudex Topical
EG
> eosinophilic granuloma

eGFP
> enhanced green fluorescent protein

eggcrate mattress
Eggleston method
egg-shaped heart
eggshell
> e. calcification
> e. friability
> e. pattern

egg-yellow reaction
egg-yolk sputum
EGM
> electrogram

egobronchophony
egophony
EGT
> exuberant granulation tissue

EGTA
> esophagogastric tube airway

EHI
> Edinburgh Handedness Inventory

Ehlers-Danlos syndrome
Ehrenritter ganglion
Ehret phenomenon
ehrlichiosis
EI
> endovascular irradiation

EIA
> enzyme immunoassay
> exercise-induced asthma

EIB
> exercise-induced bronchospasm

Eicken method
eicosanoid excretion
eicosapentaenoic acid (EPA)
EID
> emergency infusion device
> EID catheter

Eidemiller tunneler
eight-lumen manometry catheter
Eigon
> E. CardioLoop recorder
> E. disk

Eikenella corrodens
EILV
> end-inspiratory lung volume

Einhorn esophageal dilator
Einthoven
> E. equation
> E. law
> E. lead
> E. string galvanometer
> E. triangle

EIR
> early ischemic recurrence

E:I ratio
Eis
> Eisenmenger syndrome

Eisenmenger
    E. complex
    E. disease
    E. physiology
    E. reaction
    E. reaction with septal defect
    E. syndrome (Eis)
    E. tetralogy
    E. VSD
EIT
    electrical impedance tomography
ejection
    area-length method for e.
    e. click
    e. fraction (EF)
    e. murmur
    e. period
    e. phase
    e. phase index
    e. rate
    e. shell image
    e. sounds (ES)
    e. time
    e. velocity
ejection-fraction image
Ejrup maneuver
EKG (*var. of* ECG)
    electrocardiogram
    electrocardiograph
    electrocardiography (*See also* ECG)
EKY
    electrokymogram
El
    E. Gamal cardiac device
    E. Gamal coronary bypass catheter
    E. Gamal device
    E. Gamal guiding catheter
ELA
    excimer laser-assisted angioplasty
Ela
    E. Chorus DDD pacemaker
    E. Medical Elatec arrhythmia
    analyzer V 3.03A
    E. ventricular pacing lead
E-LAM
    endothelium-leukocyte adhesion molecule
Elantan
**Elastalloy Ultraflex Strecker nitinol
stent**
elastance
    effective arterial e. (EAE)

    end-systolic e.
    maximum ventricular e. (Emax)
elastase
    leukocyte e.
    neutrophil e.
    Pseudomonas e.
    sputum e.
elastic
    e. component
    e. cone
    e. equilibrium volume (EEV)
    e. fibers in sputum
    e. lamella
    e. lamina
    e. load
    e. pressure-volume (Pel-V)
    e. pulse
    e. recoil
    e. recoil pressure
    e. resistance
    e. stiffness
    e. stockings
    e. tissue hyperplasia
elasticity
    lung e.
    sputum viscosity and e.
elasticum
    pseudoxanthoma e.
elasticus
    conus e.
elastin
elastogram
    intravascular e.
elastography
Elastorc catheter guidewire
Elavil
elbow flexion
ELC
    ear lobe crease
ELCA
    excimer laser coronary angioplasty
    ELCA laser
    ELCA registry
elderly
    Evaluation of Losartan in the E.
    (ELITE)
    Hospital Outcomes Reversibility for
    the E. (HOPE)
    Pacemaker Selection in the E.
    (PASE)
Elecath
    E. circulatory support device

E

NOTES

241

Elecath *(continued)*
- E. ECMO cannula
- E. electrophysiologic stimulation catheter
- E. pacemaker
- E. switch box
- E. thermodilution catheter

Elecsys troponin T immunoassay system

elective
- e. angiography
- e. cardioversion
- e. replacement indicator (ERI)

electric
- e. cardiac pacemaker
- e. replacement indicator (ERI)
- e. storm

electrical
- e. activation abnormality
- e. alternans
- e. alternation of heart
- e. axis
- e. cardioversion
- e. catheter ablation
- e. countershock
- e. diastole
- e. disease
- e. failure
- e. fulguration
- e. heart position
- e. impedance tomography (EIT)
- e. injury
- e. potential
- e. sector scanner
- e. systole

electroacuscope

electroanatomical
- e. map
- e. mapping system

electrocardiogram (ECG, EKG)
- ambulatory e. (AECG)
- Burdick e.
- concordant changes e.
- derived 12-lead e.
- discordant changes e.
- dual-lead e.
- exercise e.
- Fourier analysis of e.
- His bundle e.
- 3-lead e.
- 6-lead e.
- 12-lead e.
- 16-lead e.
- orthogonal e.
- scalar e.
- signal-averaged e. (SAECG)
- stored e.
- stress MUGA e.
- thallium e.

- three-channel e.
- time domain signal-averaged e.
- treadmill e.
- unipolar e.
- vector e.
- Wedensky modulated signal-averaged e.

electrocardiograph (ECG, EKG)
- Arrhythmia Research 1200 EPX e.
- bioimpedance e.
- Cambridge e.
- MAC-VU e.
- Marquette e.
- Megacart e.
- Mingograf 62 6-channel e.

electrocardiographic
- e. complex
- e. gated SPECT myocardial perfusion imaging
- e. gating
- e. lead
- e. transtelephonic monitor
- e. wave
- e. wave complex

electrocardiography (ECG, EKG)
- ambulatory e.
- endocoronary e. (endo-ECG)
- esophageal e.
- exercise e.
- exercise stress e. (Ex-ECG)
- fetal e.
- intracardiac e.
- intracavitary e.
- 12-lead e.
- precordial e.
- signal-averaged e. (SAECG)
- time domain signal-averaged e.

electrocardiophonogram

electrocardiophonography

electrocardioscanner
- Compuscan Hittman computerized e.

electrocautery
- Bovie e.
- bronchoscopic e.
- needlepoint e.

electrochemical
- e. gradient
- e. polarization

electroconvulsive therapy

electrode
- abdominal patch e.
- AE-60-I-2 implantable pronged unipolar e.
- AE-85-I-2 implantable pronged unipolar e.
- AE-60-KB implantable unipolar endocardial e.

AE-85-KB implantable unipolar endocardial e.
AE-60-K-10 implantable unipolar endocardial e.
AE-85-K-10 implantable unipolar endocardial e.
AE-60-KS-10 implantable unipolar endocardial e.
AE-85-KS-10 implantable unipolar endocardial e.
anterior anodal patch e.
Arzbacher pill e.
Arzco TAPSUL pill e.
Bard nonsteerable bipolar e.
Berkovits-Castellanos hexapolar e.
Bioplus dispersive e.
bipolar myocardial e.
Bisping e.
button e.
Cambridge jelly e.
e. catheter
e. catheter ablation operation
central terminal e.
Clark oxygen e.
coil e.
CPI Endotak transvenous e.
cutaneous thoracic patch e.
Darox cutaneous thoracic patch e.
dispersing e.
dispersive e.
EnGuard PFX lead e.
epicardial e.
epicardial sock e.
esophageal pill e.
exploring e.
Fast-Patch disposable defibrillation/electrocardiographic e.
e. gel
Goetz bipolar e.
hydrogen e.'s
implantable cardioverter e.
indifferent e.
intravascular catheter e.
ion-selective e. (ISE)
e. jelly
J orthogonal e.
Josephson quadpolar mapping e.
J-shaped pacemaker e.
large-tip e.
Laserdish e.
Lifeline e.
Mansfield Polaris e.

Medtronic Transvene e.
monopolar temporary e.
multiple point e.
multipolar catheter e.
MVE-50 implantable myocardial e.
myocardial e.
Myowire II cardiac e.
Nyboer esophageal e.
Osypka Cereblate e.
pacemaker e.
e. pad
e. paddles
e. paste
PE-60-I-2 implantable pronged unipolar e.
PE-85-I-2 implantable pronged unipolar e.
PE-60-K-10 implantable unipolar endocardial e.
PE-85-K-10 implantable unipolar endocardial e.
PE-60-KB implantable unipolar endocardial e.
PE-85-KB implantable unipolar endocardial e.
PE-85-KS-10 implantable unipolar endocardial e.
platinum-iridium e.
Polaris e.
PORT e.
QuadPolar e.
quadripolar Quad e.
reference e.
ring e.
Rychener-Weve e.
scalp e.
screw-in epicardial e.
screw-in sutureless myocardial e.
Severinghaus e.
sew-on e.
silent e.
silver bead e.
silver-silver chloride e.
Skylark surface e.
Soft-EZ reusable e.
stab e.
stab-in epicardial e.
steroid-eluting e.
Stockert cardiac pacing e.
subcutaneous patch e.
Surgicraft pacemaker e.
sutured plaque e.

NOTES

E

electrode (*continued*)
   e. system
   Tapcath esophageal e.
   Tapsul pill e.
   tined ventricular e.
   Transvene tripolar e.
   transvenous e.
   tripolar defibrillation coil e.
   unipolar defibrillation coil e.
   USCI Goetz bipolar e.
   USCI NBIH bipolar e.
   Vitatron catheter e.
electrodesiccation
electrode-skin interface
electrodispersive skin patch
Electrodyne pacemaker
electrodynogram
electroencephalogram (EEG)
electroencephalograph (EEG)
electroencephalography (EEG)
electrofluoroscopy
electrogenic
electrogram (EGM)
   coronary sinus e.
   evoked endocardial e.
   evoked ventricular e.
   far-field e.
   e. fractionation
   Furman Type II e.
   His bundle e. (HBE)
   intracardiac e.
electrograph
   Cardiotest portable e.
electrokymogram (EKY)
electrokymograph
electrokymography
electrolyte imbalance
electrolytic disturbance
electromagnetic
   e. interference/radiofrequency
    interference (EMI/RFI)
   e. mapping
electromanometer
electromechanical
   e. artificial heart
   e. coupling
   e. delay
   e. dissociation (EMD)
   e. interval
   e. left ventricular mapping
   e. mapping
   e. systole
electromyocardial dissociation
electromyogram (EMG)
   kinesiological e.
electromyograph (EMG)
electromyography (EMG)

electron
   e. beam computed tomography
    (EBCT)
   e. microprobe analysis
   e. microscope
   e. microscopy
   e. paramagnetic resonance
    spectroscopy
   e. volt (eV)
electron-beam
   e.-b. angiography
   e.-b. fence
electronic
   e. calipers
   e. distance compensation
   e. fetal monitor
   E. HouseCall system
   e. pacemaker
   e. pacemaker load
   refractory period of e.
   e. scanning
electrooculogram (EOG)
electrooculograph (EOG)
electrooculography (EOG)
electropharmacology
electrophoresis
   agarose gel e.
   gradient gel e.
   polyacrylamide gel e.
   protein e.
   sodium dodecylsulfate
    polyacrylamide gel e. (SDS-
    PAGE)
electrophrenic respiration
electrophysiologic
   e. mapping
   e. study (EPS)
   e. test
electrophysiologist
electrophysiology (EP)
   intracardiac e.
   e. study
electrostethograph
electrosurgery
electrosurgical blade
electrotonic
   e. conduction
   e. transmission
electrovectorcardiogram
electroversion
Elema
   E. lead
   E. pacemaker
   E.-Schonander pacemaker
element
   contractile e.
   length contraction compensation e.
    (LCCE)

peroxisome proliferator response e. (PPRE)
   series elastic e.

elephantiasis
elephant-on-the-chest sensation
elevated gradient
Elevath pacemaker
elevation
   CK-MB e.
   e. of enzyme
   e. MI
   1-natural-log-unit e.
   e. pallor of extremity
   ST e.
   ST segment e.
   transient ST segment e.
   upsloping ST e.

elevator
   Aufricht e.
   Cameron-Haight e.
   e. disease
   Doyen e.
   Friedrich rib e.
   Lemmon sternal e.
   Matson rib e.
   Phemister e.
   rib e.

ELF
   epithelial lining fluid
   ELF levels

elfin
   e. facies
   e. facies syndrome

Elgiloy
   E. frame
   E.-Heifitz aneurysm clip

elimination
   e. half-life
   single-breath nitrogen e.

Eliminator dilatation balloon
eliprodil
ELISA
   enzyme-linked immunosorbent assay
   double-sandwich IgM ELISA

Elispot test
ELITE
   Evaluation of Losartan in the Elderly
   ELITE study

Elite
   E. dual-chamber rate-responsive pacemaker

E. guide catheter
E. pacemaker

Elixicon
Elixomin
Elixophyllin
elizabethae
   Bartonella e.

Ellence
Ellestad
   E. exercise stress test
   E. protocol

ellipse
   E. compact spacer
   prolate e.

ellipsoid arteriole
elliptical
   e. end-capped quadrature radiofrequency coil
   e. loop

Ellis sign
Ellis-van Creveld syndrome
Ellswood Mylar balloon
Eloesser flap
Elscint tomography system
Elsner asthma
ELSO
   Extracorporeal Life Support Organization
   ELSO registry

Elspar
Eltroxin
eluting stent
elution
   isocratic e.
   steroid e.

ELWRITE
   E. lead
   E. pediatric lead

Emax
   maximum ventricular elastance

EMB
   endomyocardial biopsy

embarrassment
   circulatory e.
   respiratory e.

embolectomy
   catheter e.
   e. catheter
   femoral e.
   pulmonary e.
   surgical e.

emboli (*pl. of* embolus)

E

NOTES

embolic
- e. abscess
- e. aneurysm
- e. event
- e. gangrene
- e. infarct
- e. necrosis
- e. obstruction
- e. phenomenon
- e. pneumonia
- e. shower
- e. stroke
- e. thrombosis

embolism
- acute pulmonary e.
- air e.
- air pulmonary e.
- amnionic fluid e.
- amniotic fluid e. (AFE)
- aortic e.
- arterial e.
- arterial gas e. (AGE)
- atheromatous e.
- bacillary e.
- bland e.
- bone marrow e.
- capillary e.
- catheter e.
- cellular e.
- cerebral air e.
- cholesterol e.
- coronary e.
- coronary air e.
- crossed e.
- direct e.
- diving air e.
- fat e.
- gas e.
- hematogenous e.
- infective e.
- miliary e.
- multiple e.
- myxomatous pulmonary e.
- obturating e.
- oil e.
- pantaloon e.
- paradoxic e.
- paradoxical e.
- paradoxical cerebral e.
- *Plasmodium* e.
- pulmonary e. (PE)
- pulmonary air e.
- pyemic e.
- retrograde e.
- riding e.
- saddle e.
- silent e.
- spinal e.

- straddling e.
- submassive pulmonary e.
- systemic arterial air e.
- trichinous e.
- tumor e.
- venous e.
- venous air e.

embolization
- air e.
- bronchial artery e. (BAE)
- cerebral e.
- cholesterol e.
- coil e.
- distal vessel e.
- paradoxical e.
- plaque e.
- pulmonary e.
- septal artery e.
- septic e.
- Silastic bead e.
- stent e.
- subsegmental transcatheter arterial e. (STAE)
- e. therapy
- transcatheter e.
- transcatheter arterial e. (TAE)

embolized foreign material

embolomycotic aneurysm

embolotherapy
- transcatheter e.

embolus, pl. **emboli**
- air e.
- calcific e.
- cancer e.
- catheter e.
- catheter-induced e.
- cerebral e.
- femoral e.
- paradoxic e.
- paradoxical e.
- polyurethane foam e.
- pulmonary e.
- riding e.
- saddle e.
- threw an e.

embolus-to-blood ratio (EBR)

Embol-X arterial cannula and filter system

Embolyx
- E. liquid embolic system
- E. vascular embolizing agent

embryocardia
- jugular e.
- e. rhythm

embryologic

embryology

embryoma

embryonal cell

embryonic phenotype pattern
EMC
    encephalomyocarditis
      EMC virus
Emcyt
EMD
    electromechanical dissociation
EMD-57033
emergency
    e. bailout
    e. bailout stent
    e. cardiac care (ECC)
    hypertensive e.
    e. infusion device (EID)
    e. reperfusion
    E. Room Assessment of Sestamibi
      for Evaluation of Chest Pain
      (ERASE)
    E. Stenting Compared to
      Conventional Balloon Angioplasty
      (ESCOBAR)
emergent thoracotomy
Emerson
    E. bronchoscope
    E. cuirass respirator
    E. Post-Op
    E. postoperative ventilator
    E. pump
    E. vein stripper
Emery-Dreifuss
    E.-D. disease
    E.-D. muscular dystrophy
emesis
    posttussive e.
emetine toxicity
EMF
    endomyocardial fibrosis
EMG
    electromyogram
    electromyograph
    electromyography
EMIAT
    European Myocardial Infarct Amiodarone
    Trial
Eminase
EMI/RFI
    electromagnetic
    interference/radiofrequency interference
emission
    e. flame photometry
    single-photon e.

    stimulated acoustic e.
    vascular acoustic e.
Emory
    E. Angioplasty versus Surgery
    Trial (EAST)
emotional
    e. defensiveness (ED)
    e. stress
emphysema
    alveolar duct e.
    atrophic e.
    bullous e.
    centriacinar e.
    centrilobular e.
    chronic hypertrophic e.
    chronic obstructive pulmonary e.
      (COPE)
    chronic pulmonary e. (CPE)
    compensating e.
    compensatory e.
    cystic e.
    diffuse e.
    ectatic e.
    false e.
    familial e.
    focal e.
    focal-dust e.
    gangrenous e.
    glass blower's e.
    heterogenous e.
    hypertrophic e.
    hypoplastic e.
    idiopathic unilobar e.
    infantile lobar e.
    interlobular e.
    interstitial e.
    Jenner e.
    lobar e.
    localized obstructive e.
    loculated e.
    mediastinal e.
    obstructive e.
    panacinar e.
    panlobular e.
    paracicatricial e.
    paraseptal e.
    perinodular e.
    peripheral paracicatricial e.
    predominant e.
    pulmonary e. (PE)
    pulmonary interstitial e. (PIE)
    scar e.

E

NOTES

emphysema *(continued)*
    senile e.
    small-lung e.
    subcutaneous e.
    surgical e.
    traumatic e.
    unilateral e.
    vesicular e.
emphysematous
    e. asthma
    e. bleb
    e. bulla
    e. chest
    e. gangrene
empiric
    e. constant
    e. therapy
Empirin
empyema
    anaerobic e.
    Aspergillus e.
    e. benignum
    e. of chest
    exudative e.
    fibrinopurulent e.
    free-flowing e.
    interlobar e.
    latent e.
    loculated e.
    metapneumonic e.
    e. necessitatis
    organizing e.
    e. of pericardium
    pleural e.
    pneumococcal e.
    postinjury e.
    postpneumonectomy tuberculous e.
    pulsating e.
    putrid e.
    sacculated e.
    streptococcal e.
    synpneumonic e.
    thoracic e.
    e. thoracis
    tuberculous e.
empyesis
    tuberculous e.
EMS
    eosinophilia-myalgia syndrome
emulation
    pectoral e.
emulsion
    EchoGen e.
    EchoGen injectable e.
    fat e.
    intravascular perfluorochemical e.
    perflenapent e.
    perflenapent injectable e.

emu oil
E-Mycin-E
E-Mycin Oral
en
    e. bloc
    e. bloc bilateral lung transplant
    e. bloc, no-touch technique
    e. face
    e. face view
enalapril
    e. and diltiazem
    e. and felodipine
    e. and hydrochlorothiazide
    e. maleate
enalaprilat
enalaprilic acid
enantiomer
Enbrel
encainide hydrochloride
Encap
    Novo-Rythro E.
encapsulated organism
Encapsulon
    E. epidural catheter
    E. sheath introducer
    E. vessel dilator
encarditis
encased heart
encephalitis
    cytomegalovirus e.
Encephalitozoon
encephalomyelitis
encephalomyocarditis (EMC)
    e. virus
encephalopathy
    hypertensive e.
    metabolic e.
    subcortical vascular e. (SVE)
encircling
    e. cryoablation
    e. endocardial ventriculotomy
    e. endocardial ventriculotomy operation
encode
encoding
    respiratory ordered phase e. (ROPE)
    velocity e.
Encor
    E. lead
    E. pacemaker
Encore inflation device
encroachment
    luminal e.
encrustation theory of atherosclerosis
encysted pleurisy

end
    e. artery
    e. inspiratory Velcro crackle
Endal
endangiitis
Endantadine
endaortitis
endarterectomy
    abdominal aortic e.
    aortoiliofemoral e.
    blunt eversion carotid e.
    carotid e. (CE, CEA)
    coronary e.
    e. and coronary artery bypass
      grafting (E-CABG)
    femoral e.
    gas e.
    Mayo Asymptomatic Carotid E.
      (MACE)
    transluminal e.
    vertebral e.
endarterial
endarteritis
    e. deformans
    Heubner specific e.
    e. obliterans
    e. proliferans
    syphilitic e.
endarteropathy
    digital e.
end-diastole
end-diastolic
    e.-d. area (EDA)
    e.-d. count
    e.-d. diameter (EDD)
    e.-d. dimension (EDD)
    e.-d. left ventricular pressure
    e.-d. murmur
    e.-d. pressure (EDP)
    e.-d. velocity
    e.-d. volume (EDV)
    e.-d. volume index (EDVI)
    e.-d. wall echogenicity
    e.-d. wall enlargement
Endeavor nondetachable silicone balloon
  catheter
endemic
    e. fungal infection
    e. influenza
end-expiratory
    e.-e. apnea
    e.-e. esophageal pressure (Pesend)

    e.-e. film
    e.-e. lung volume (EELV)
end-hole
    e.-h. balloon-tipped catheter
    e.-h. fluid-filled catheter
    e.-h. 7-French catheter
    e.-h. Tracker microcatheter
end-inspiratory
    e.-i. crackle
    e.-i. film
    e.-i. lung volume (EILV)
endless-loop tachycardia
endoaneurysmorrhaphy
    ventricular e.
endoaortic clamp
endoaortitis
endoauscultation
Endo-Avitene
endobronchial
    e. brachytherapy
    e. cryotherapy
    e. infection
    e. laser therapy
    e. obstruction
    e. tree
    e. tube
    e. tuberculosis
endobronchially
Endocam endoscope
endocannabinoid
endocardiac
endocardial
    e. balloon lead
    e. bipolar lead
    e. border
    e. border delineation
    e. cardiac border
    e. catheter ablation
    e. cushion
    e. cushion defect (ECD)
    e. to epicardial resection operation
    e. excursion
    e. fibroelastosis (EFE)
    e. fibrosis
    e. flow
    e. lead
    e. mapping
    e. mapping of ventricular
      tachycardia
    e. motion
    e. murmur
    e. pacing

E

NOTES

endocardial *(continued)*
    e. pressure
    e. resection
    e. sclerosis
    e. shortening
    e. stain
    e. thickening
    e. triangle
    e. tube
    e. vegetation
    e. wire

endocardial-to-endocardial resection
endocardiography
endocarditic
endocarditis
    abacterial thrombotic e.
    acute bacterial e. (ABE)
    acute infective e. (AIE)
    atypical verrucous e.
    bacteria-free stage of bacterial e.
    bacterial e. (BE)
    e. benigna
    bioprosthetic e.
    cachectic e.
    e. chordalis
    chronic e.
    constrictive e.
    culture-negative e.
    enterococcal e.
    experimental enterococcal e.
    fungal e.
    gonococcal e.
    gram-negative e.
    green strep e.
    Haemophilus e.
    infectious e.
    infective e. (IE)
    isolated parietal e.
    e. lenta
    Libman-Sacks e.
    Löffler e.
    Löffler parietal fibroplastic e.
    malignant e.
    marantic e.
    methicillin-sensitive right-sided e.
    mitral valve e.
    mural e.
    mycotic e.
    native valve e. (NVE)
    native valve fibroplastic e.
    nonbacterial thrombotic e. (NBTE)
    nonbacterial verrucous e.
    noninfective valve e.
    nosocomial e.
    pacemaker e.
    parietal e.
    e. parietalis fibroplastica
    plastic e.

    polypous e.
    postoperative e.
    prosthetic valve e. (PVE)
    pulmonic e.
    rheumatic e.
    rickettsial e.
    septic e.
    staphylococcal e.
    streptococcal e.
    subacute bacterial e. (SBE)
    subacute infective e.
    syphilitic e.
    terminal e.
    thrombotic e.
    tricuspid valve e.
    tuberculous e.
    ulcerative e.
    valvular e.
    vegetative e.
    verrucous e.

endocardium
    echo-bright e.
    mural e.

endocoronary electrocardiography (endo-ECG)
EndoCPB catheter
endocrine
    e. disorder
    e. system

endocytosis
endoderm
endodermal cell
endo-ECG
    endocoronary electrocardiography
endofibrosis
end-of-life
    e.-o.-l. pacemaker
    e.-o.-l. rate (EOL)

endogenous
    e. fibrinolysis
    e. kinin
    e. lipid

endograft
    aortic e.
    Prograft bifurcated e.
    Talent bifurcated e.
    Vanguard e.

Endo Grasp device
Endoknot suture
endolaryngeal
endoleak
    e., type I–IV
EndoLoc lead
endolumen enlargement
EndoLumina illuminated bougie
endoluminal
    e. reconstruction of basilar artery fusiform aneurysm

e. stent graft
e. stenting
endolymphatic sac
endolymphaticus
sacculus e.
saccus e.
endolysosome
endomyocardial
African e.
e. biopsy (EMB)
e. disease
e. fibroelastosis
e. fibrosis (EMF)
endomyocarditis
endomysial
e. collagen
e. fibrosis
endomysium
end-on aortogram
endonuclease
restriction e.
EndoOctopus
Endopath ETS-FLEX endoscopic articulating linear cutter
endopeptidase
e. inhibitor
neutral e. (NEP)
endopericarditis
endoperimyocarditis
endoperimysial interstitial fibrosis
endoperoxide steal
endophthalmitis
endoplasmic reticulum
endopolyploidy
EndoPro
E. prosthesis
E. stent
E. system I
endoprosthesis
Passager e.
Wallgraft e.
endorphin
Endosaph
E. saphenous vein harvesting system
E. vein harvest system
endoscope
Endocam e.
lung imaging fluorescence e. (LIFE)
Messerklinger e.
Sine-U-View nasal e.

velolaryngeal e.
Visicath e.
endoscopic
e. biopsy
e. coronary artery bypass graft (E-CABG)
e. ultrasound-guided fine needle aspiration (EUS-FNA)
EndoSonics IVUS/balloon dilation catheter
Endosound endoscopic ultrasound catheter
Endotak
E. C lead transvenous catheter
E. C transvenous lead
E. C tripolar pacing/sensing/defibrillation lead
E. C tripolar transvenous lead
E. DSP lead
E. lead defibrillator
E. lead system
E. lead transvenous catheter
E. nonthoracotomy implantable cardioverter-defibrillator
E. pacemaker
E. Picotip defibrillation lead
endothelial
e. activation
e. cell activation
e. constitutive nitric oxide synthase (ecNOS)
e. denudation
e. derived relaxation factor
e. dysfunction
e. nitric oxide (ecNOS)
e. nitric oxide synthase (eNOS)
e. permeability
e. purinoceptors
endothelialization
endothelin (ET)
e. A, B receptor
big e.
circulating e.
myocardial e.
endothelin-1 (ET-1)
e. immunoreactivity
endothelin-2 (ET-2)
plasma e.
endothelin-3 (ET-3)
endothelin-converting enzyme
endothelioma

NOTES

E

endothelium
> coronary microvessel e.
> nonfenestrated e.

endothelium-dependent
> e.-d. dilator response to substance P
> e.-d. vascular relaxation
> e.-d. vasodilation

endothelium-derived
> e.-d. hyperpolarizing factor (EDHF)
> e.-d. nitric oxide (EDNO)
> e.-d. relaxing factor (EDRF)

endothelium-independent vascular relaxation

endothelium-leukocyte adhesion molecule (E-LAM)

endothelium-mediated relaxation

endotoxemia

endotoxic sepsis

endotoxin
> bacterial e.
> circulating bacterial e.
> e. shock

endotracheal
> e. aspirate (EA)
> e. cardiac output monitor (ECOM)
> e. cardiac output monitoring (ECOM)
> e. intubation
> e. tube (ETT)
> e. tube cuff

Endotrol
> E. endotracheal tube
> E. tracheal tube

endovascular
> e. aortic graft (EAG)
> e. graft
> e. irradiation (EI)
> e. radiation therapy
> e. radiofrequency catheter ablation
> e. repair (EVR)
> e. stent grafting

endoventricular circular patch plasty

EndoWrist instrument

endpoint
> Controlled Onset Verapamil Investigation for Cardiovascular E.'s (CONVINCE)
> Guidance by Ultrasound Imaging for Decision E.'s (GUIDE)
> Guidance by Ultrasound Imaging for Decision E.'s II (GUIDE II)
> hemodynamic e.
> Randomized Evaluation of Salvage Angioplasty with Combined Utilization of E.'s (RESCUE)
> therapeutic e.

end-pressure artifact

endralazine

Endrate

end-stage
> e.-s. heart failure
> e.-s. liver disease (ESLD)
> e.-s. lung
> e.-s. renal disease (ESRD)

end-systole

end-systolic
> e.-s. circumferential wall stress
> e.-s. count
> e.-s. dimension (ESD)
> e.-s. elastance
> e.-s. force-velocity index
> e.-s. left ventricular pressure
> e.-s. left ventricular stress (ESS)
> e.-s. murmur
> e.-s. pressure-volume relation
> e.-s. stress (ESS)
> e.-s. stress-dimension relation
> e.-s. volume (ESV)
> e.-s. volume index (ESVI)
> e.-s. volume ratio
> e.-s. wall stress

end-tidal
> e.-t. carbon dioxide (ETCO$_2$)
> e.-t. sample

end-to-end

end-to-side suture

Endura
> ACS E.

Enduron

Enduronyl Forte

enema
> barium e.
> Kayexalate e.
> sodium polystyrene sulfonate e.

Enemol

energometer

energy
> color Doppler e. (CDE)
> e. expenditure
> myocardial e.
> e. production
> radiofrequency e.
> e. resolution
> e. supply

Enertrax 7100 pacemaker

e-Net headpiece

enflurane

enforcer
> CVD Focustent E.

Enforcer SDS coronary stent

Englert forceps

engorgement
> venous e.

Engstrom respirator

EnGuard
- E. double-lead ICD system
- E. pacing and defibrillation lead system
- E. PFX lead electrode

enhanced
- e. automaticity
- e. external counterpulsation (EECP)
- e. external counterpulsation unit
- e. green fluorescent protein (*eGFP*)

Enhanced Torque 8F guiding catheter
enhancement
- detection e.
- leading edge e.
- mean contrast e.

enhancer
- ACE Cloud e.
- aerosol cloud e. (ACE)
- universal aerosol cloud e.

enhancing lesion
Enkaid
enlargement
- biatrial e.
- cardiac e.
- compensatory vessel e.
- end-diastolic wall e.
- endolumen e.
- left atrial e. (LAF)
- panchamber e.
- right atrial e.
- right ventricular e. (RVE)
- Survival and Ventricular E. (SAVE)

Enlon injection
eNO, ENO
- exhaled nitric oxide
- expired nitric oxide

enolase
- neuron-specific e. (NSE)

Enomine
eNOS
- endothelial nitric oxide synthase
- eNOS gene expression

enoxacin
enoxaparin
- e. bridge therapy
- E. in Non-Q-wave Coronary Events trial
- E. Restenosis after Angioplasty (ERA)

- e. sodium
- E. and Ticlopidine after Elective Stenting (ENTICES)
- E. and TNK-tPA with/without GP IIb/IIIa Inhibitor as Reperfusion Strategy in ST Elevation MI (ENTIRE)

enoximone
Enseals
- Potassium Iodide E.

Ensite 3000 system
Entamoeba
- *E. dispar*
- *E. histolytica*

entangling technique
enteral
- e. nutrition
- e. tube feeding

enteric
- e. cytopathogenic human orphan (ECHO)
- e. cytopathogenic human orphan virus
- e. fistula
- e. Gram-negative bacillus

enteric-coated aspirin
enteroadherent
enteroaggregative
Enterobacter
- *E. cloacae*
- *E.* pneumonia

Enterobacteriaceae
enterococcal endocarditis
enterococci
- vancomycin-resistant e.

Enterococcus
- *E. faecalis*
- *E. faecium*

enterocolitica
- *Yersinia e.*

enterocolitis
enterocytopathogenic human orphan (ECHO)
enterohemorrhagic
enteroinvasive
enterotoxin
- *Escherichia coli* e.

enteroviral
enterovirus
Entex

E

NOTES

ENTICES
Enoxaparin and Ticlopidine after Elective Stenting
ENTICES clinical trial
ENTIRE
Enoxaparin and TNK-tPA with/without GP IIb/IIIa Inhibitor as Reperfusion Strategy in ST Elevation MI
ENTIRE study
Entity pacemaker
entocyte
entoplasm
entoptic pulse
entrained beat
entrainment
concealed e.
epicardial e.
high air flow with oxygen e. (HAFOE)
e. mapping
oxygen e.
e. of tachycardia
transient e.
e. with concealed fusion
entrance
e. block
e. wound
entrapment
lung e.
Entree
E. thoracoscopy cannula
E. thoracoscopy trocar
EnTre guidewire
Entrophen
entropy
entry
air e.
e. site
Entuss-D Liquid
ENT wash
enucleation of subaortic stenosis
envelope
aortic e.
dagger-shaped aortic e.
flow e.
maximal flow-volume e. (MFVL)
spectral e.
env gene
environment
normobaric e.
pharmacologic e.
environmental
e. allergen
e. change
e. lung disease
e. stress cracking
e. survey
e. tobacco smoke (ETS)

EnviroNOx surveillance system
Enzygnost
E. F1+2 ELISA kit
E. TAT complex kit
E. TAT ELISA assay
enzymatic
e. deficiency
e. infarct size
enzyme
allosteric modification of e.
angiotensin-converting e. (ACE)
angiotensin-converting e. DD (ACE-DD)
angiotensin-converting e. ID (ACE-ID)
angiotensin-converting e. II (ACE-II)
angiotensin I-converting e.
Bacillus subtilis e.
beta AR kinase1 e.
cardiac e.
COX-1 e.
COX-2 e.
elevation of e.
endothelin-converting e.
fibrinolytic e.
glycolytic e.
e. immunoassay (EIA)
lysosomal e.
mitochondrial e.
pancreatic e.
phosphodiesterase e.
proteolytic e.
Randomized Assessment of Digoxin on Inhibitors of the Angiotensin Converting E. (RADIANCE)
sarcoplasmic reticulum-associated glycolytic e.'s
enzyme-induced damage
enzyme-linked immunosorbent assay (ELISA)
Enzymun-Test System ES22 analyzer
EOA
esophageal obturator airway
EOG
electrooculogram
electrooculograph
electrooculography
EOL
end-of-life rate
eosin
hematoxylin and e. (H&E)
eosinophil
e. by-product
e. cationic protein (ECP)
e. chemotactic factors of anaphylaxis (ECF-A)

eosinophilia
  nonallergic rhinitis with e.
    (NARES)
  peripheral blood e.
  prolonged pulmonary e.
  pulmonary infiltrate with e. (PIE)
  pulmonary infiltration with e. (PIE)
  tropical pulmonary e.
eosinophilia-myalgia syndrome (EMS)
eosinophilic
  e. chemotaxis
  e. effusion
  e. endomyocardial disease
  e. granuloma (EG)
  e. granulomatosis
  e. lung
  e. lung syndrome
  e. pneumonia
  e. pneumonitis
  e. pneumonopathy
  e. pulmonary syndrome
EP
  electrophysiology
  HearTwave EP
  EP mapping
EPA
  eicosapentaenoic acid
Epanutin
EPAP
  expiratory positive airway pressure
eparterial bronchus
EPC
  extent of pleural carcinomatosis score
E-peak velocity
ephedrine
  aminophylline, amobarbital, and e.
  e. sulfate
Ephedsol
ephelis, pl. ephelides
  nevi, atrial myxoma, myxoid
    neurofibromas, and ephelides
    (NAME)
ephemeral pneumonia
EPI
  echo planar imaging
epiaortic echocardiography
**epibronchial right pulmonary artery
  syndrome**
EPIC
  Echocardiography Persantine
  International Cooperative

Evaluation of IIb/IIIa Platelet Receptor
  Antagonist c7E3 in Preventing Ischemic
  Complications
  EPIC clinical trial
  EPIC study
epicardial
  e. arterial spasm
  e. artery
  e. artery patency
  e. cardiac border
  e. coronary artery
  e. coronary artery disease
  e. defibrillator patch
  e. electrode
  e. entrainment
  e. fat
  e. fat pad sign
  e. fat tag
  e. flow
  e. flow conductance
  e. lead
  e. pacing
  e. patch
  e. radiofrequency atrial lesion
  e. radiofrequency catheter ablation
  e. sock electrode
  e. vessel patency
epicardial-mesenchymal transformation
epicardin gene
epicardium
  left ventricular e.
Epicoccum nigrum
epidemic capillary bronchitis
epidermal growth factor
epidermidis
  Staphylococcus e.
epidermoid carcinoma
epidural analgesia
EpiE-ZPen
Epifrin
epigastric bruit
epiglottic cartilage
epiglottiditis
  petiolous e.
epiglottitis
epiglottoplasty
epi illuminated microscope
epilepsy
epilepticus
  status e.

NOTES

EPILOG
Evaluation of PTCA to Improve Long-Term Outcome by c7E3 GPIIb/IIIa Receptor Blockade
EPILOG study
epimyocarditis
epimysium
epinephrine
high-dose e.
racemic e.
EpiPen
epiphenomena of dissection
epirubicin
episode
presyncopal e.
vasovagal e.
ventilation e.
episodic
e. dyspnea
e. hypertension
Epistat double balloon
epistaxis
epistenocardiac pericarditis
epistenocardica
pericarditis e.
EPISTENT
Evaluation of Platelet IIb/IIIa Inhibitor for Stenting Trial
epithelial
e. cell
e. lining fluid (ELF)
e. mucin
e. 5'-nucleotide receptor
epithelial-mucus attachment
epithelioid
e. hemangioendothelioma
e. mesothelioma
epithelium
ciliated e.
pulmonary e.
sloughed bronchial e.
epitope
epituberculous infiltration
Epivir
Epivir-HBV
eplerenone
EPMSystems piezoelectric strain gauge
Epogen
epoprostenol
e. sodium
e. sodium for injection
epoxyeicosatrienoic (EET)
e. acid
epoxy resin
EPP
equal-pressure point
extrapleural pneumonectomy

Eppendorf
E. angiocatheter
E. catheter
eprosartan
EPS
early progressing stroke
electrophysiologic study
EPS-410
Venodyne external pneumatic compression System E.
epsilon wave
EPSS
E point to septal separation
Epstein-Barr
E.-B. nuclear antigen (EBNA)
E.-B. virus (EBV)
Epstein disease
EPT-1000 cardiac ablation system
EPTFE
expanded polytetrafluoroethylene
EPTFE graft
EPTFE vascular suture
eptifibatide
Epworth sleepiness scale (ESS)
EQOL
Economics and Quality of Life Substudy of GUSTO
equal-pressure point (EPP)
equation
ACSM regression e.
alveolar-air e.
American College of Sports Medicine regression e.
Bernoulli e.
Bloch e.
Bohr e.
Brunelli e.
Carter e.
continuity e.
Doppler continuity e.
Eagle e.
Einthoven e.
Fick e.
Ford e.
Framingham e.
Friedewald e.
Gorlin e.
Gorlin and Gorlin e.
Hagenbach extension of Poiseuille e.
Harris-Benedict e.
Henderson-Hasselbalch e.
Holen-Hatle e.
Krovetz-Gessner e.
Navier-Stokes e.
Nernst e.
Poiseuille e.
regression e.

Riley-Cournand e.
Rodrigo e.
Rohrer e.
Siri e.
Starling e.
Teichoiz e.
Torricelli orifice e.
equator of cell
Equen magnet
equi
Rhodococcus e.
equilibrate
equilibration
equilibrium
e. image
e. multigated radionuclide
ventriculography
e. radionuclide angiography
(ERNA)
voltage e.
equilibrium-gated blood pool study
Equinox
E. digital EEG
E. digital EEG system
E. EEG acquisition device
E. occlusion balloon system
equiphasic complex
equipment
equipotency
equipotent
equistenotic plaque
equivalency
left main e.
equivalent
Abell-Kendall e.
anginal e.
metabolic e.
right anterior oblique e.
ventilation e.
ventilatory e.
equol
equuli
Actinobacillus e.
ER
early repolarization
ERα
estrogen receptor alpha
ERβ
estrogen receptor beta
ERA
echo record access
Enoxaparin Restenosis after Angioplasty

ERA clinical trial
ERA study
ERA 300 dual-chamber pacing system analyzer
ERASE
Emergency Room Assessment of
Sestamibi for Evaluation of Chest Pain
ERASE study
Erb
E. area
E. atrophy
limb-girdle dystrophy of E.
E. point
ERBAC
excimer laser, rotational atherectomy, and
balloon angioplasty
ERBAC study
ERBE cryoprobe
Erben reflex
ERBF
effective renal blood flow
Erb-Goldflam disease
erbium:YAG laser
erbumine
perindopril e.
Ercaf
Erdheim
E. cystic medial necrosis
E. disease
E. medionecrosis aortae
idiopathica E.
erectile effect
Ergamisol
Ergoline bicycle ergometer
Ergomar
ergometer
Bosch ERG 500 e.
Collins bicycle e.
Corival 400 e.
cycle e.
Ergoline bicycle e.
Gauthier bicycle e.
Gould-Godart type 18070 e.
Jaeger ER 900 electromagnetically
braked cycle e.
Load model WLP-450
electromagnetically braked
cycle e.
Lode BV Excalibur braked
cycle e.
MGC Cardi-O2 cycle e.
Monark bicycle e.

E

NOTES

ergometer *(continued)*
    pedal-mode e.
    Siemens-Albis bicycle e.
    Siemens-Elema AG bicycle e.
    Tunturi EL400 bicycle e.
ergometry
    arm e.
    arm cycle e.
    bicycle e.
    cycle e.
    supine bicycle e.
ergonomic vascular access needle (EVAN)
ergonovine
    e. challenge
    e. echocardiography
    e. infusion
    e. injection
    e. maleate
    e. maleate provocation angina
    e. provocation test
ergonovine-induced
    e.-i. coronary vasospasm
    e.-i. spasm
    e.-i. vasospasm
ergoreceptor
    muscle e.
ergoreflex
Ergos O$_2$ dual-chamber rate-responsive pacemaker
Ergostat
ergot alkaloid
ergotamine
    e. derivative
    Medihaler E.
ERI
    elective replacement indicator
    electric replacement indicator
Erie System
ERIG serum
ERK
    extracellularly responsive kinase
    extracellular-regulated kinase
Erlanger sphygmomanometer
Ermenonville classification for coronary angioscopy
ERNA
    equilibrium radionuclide angiography
Erni sign
ERO
    effective regurgitant orifice
erosion
    intimal e.
    spark e.
erosive
    e. esophagitis
    e. reflux

ERP
    effective refractory period
ERT
    estrogen replacement therapy
eruptive xanthoma
ERV
    expiratory reserve volume
Erwinia
Erwiniar
Erybid
Eryc Oral
EryPed Oral
Erysipelothrix
Ery-Tab Oral
erythema
    e. marginatum
    e. migrans
    e. multiforme
    e. nodosum
    palmar e.
erythematosus
    disseminated lupus e.
    drug-induced lupus e. (DILE)
    lupus e. (LE)
    systemic lupus e. (SLE)
erythematous maculopapular rash
erythrityl tetranitrate
Erythro-Base
erythroblastosis fetalis
Erythrocin Oral
erythrocyte sedimentation rate (ESR)
erythrocytosis
erythroderma
Erythroflex hydromer-coated central venous catheter
erythrogenin
erythromelalgia
erythromycin
    e. and sulfisoxazole
    systemic e.
erythropheresis
erythropoiesis
erythropoietin
    gene-activated e.
    plasma e.
Eryzole Oral
ES
    ejection sounds
    ES 300-Cardiac T ELISA troponin T immunoassay system
    Pertussin ES
ESAT-6 protein
escalator
    mucociliary e.
escape
    e. beat
    e. contraction
    e. impulse

e. interval
junctional e.
nodal e.
e. pacemaker
e. rhythm
vagal e.
ventricular e.
e. ventricular contraction
escape-capture bigeminy
Escherichia coli **enterotoxin**
Escherich test
ESCOBAR
Emergency Stenting Compared to
Conventional Balloon Angioplasty
ESCOBAR clinical trial
E-Scope
ESD
end-systolic dimension
E-selectin
E.-s. cell adhesion molecule
Esidrix
Esimil
ESLD
end-stage liver disease
Esmarch
E. ball
E. bandage
E. tourniquet
esmolol
e. hydrochloride
Esophacoil self-expanding esophageal stent
esophagagram
esophagalgia
esophageae
glandulae e.
venae e.
esophageal
e. achalasia
e. adventitia
e. angina
e. A-ring
e. artery
e. atresia
e. bougienage
e. branch
e. branches of the left gastric artery
e. branches of the thoracic aorta
e. branches of the vagus nerve
e. B-ring
e. cardiogram

e. constriction
e. contraction ring
e. detection device (EDD)
e. dilation
e. dysmotility
e. ECG
e. echocardiography
e. electrocardiography
e. gland
e. hiatus
e. lead
e. lumen
e. lung
e. manometry
e. motility
e. mucosa
e. nervous plexus
e. obturator airway (EOA)
e. opening
e. perforation
e. pill electrode
e. prosthesis
e. reflux
e. rupture
e. sling procedure
e. sound
e. spasm
e. speech
e. sphincter
e. stricture
e. tamponade
e. temperature
e. temperature probe
e. transit time
e. varices
e. vein
e. web
esophageal-directed pressure support (EDPS)
esophageales
rami e.
vena obliqua atrial sinistra venae e.
esophagectomy
esophagei
rami e.
esophageus
hiatus e.
plexus nervosus e.
esophagi
pars abdominalis e.
pars cervicalis e.

NOTES

E

esophagi *(continued)*
    pars thoracica e.
    tunica mucosa e.
    tunica muscularis e.
esophagism
    hiatal e.
esophagismus
esophagitis
    corrosive e.
    e. dissecans superficialis
    erosive e.
    infectious e.
    monilial e.
    peptic e.
    reflux e.
esophagogastric
    e. junction
    e. orifice
    e. tamponade
    e. tube airway (EGTA)
    e. vestibule
esophagomyotomy
    Heller e.
esophagoplasty
    Belsey e.
    Grondahl e.
esophagoplication
esophagorespiratory fistulae
esophagosalivary reflex
esophagoscope
    Boros e.
    Eder-Hufford e.
    Foregger rigid e.
    Jesberg e.
    Lell e.
    Moure e.
    Schindler e.
esophagoscopy
    fiberoptic e.
esophagospasm
esophagotracheal
    e. combitube (ETC)
esophagram
    barium e.
esophagus
    abdominal part of e.
    Barrett e.
    brusque dilatation of e.
    cardiac glands of e.
    cervical part of e.
    muscular coat of e.
    nutcracker e.
    suspensory ligament of e.
    thoracic e.
    thoracic part of e.
ESP radiation reduction examination gloves
Esprit ventilator

esprolol
    e. hydrochloride
    e. plus sildenafil citrate
ESR
    erythrocyte sedimentation rate
ESRD
    end-stage renal disease
ESS
    end-systolic left ventricular stress
    end-systolic stress
    Epworth sleepiness scale
    European Stroke Scale
        circumferential ESS
        meridional ESS (mESS)
ESSENCE
    Efficacy and Safety of Subcutaneous Enoxaparin in Non-Q-Wave Coronary Events
        ESSENCE clinical trial
essential
    e. asthma
    e. bradycardia
    e. brown induration of lung
    e. hemoptysis
    e. hypertension
    e. pulmonary hemosiderosis
    e. tachycardia
    e. thrombocytopenia
EST
    exercise stress test
    expression sequence tagged
EST40 stethoscope
estazolam
ester
    cholesterol e.
    N^G-nitro-L-arginine methyl e. (L-NAME)
Estes
    E. ECG criteria
    E. point system
    E.-Romhilt ECG point-score system
    E. score
estimated
    e. Fick method
    e. MET
Estlander operation
estradiol
estramustine
Estratest H.S.
estrogen
    conjugated equine e. (CEE)
    e., medroxyprogesterone
    e., methyltestosterone
    e. receptor alpha (ERα)
    e. receptor beta (ERβ)
    e. replacement therapy (ERT)
estrone
Estrovis

ESV
end-systolic volume
ESVI
end-systolic volume index
ET
endothelin
ET-1
endothelin-1
ET-2
endothelin-2
ET-3
endothelin-3
ETA
ethionamide
etanercept
ETC
esophagotracheal combitube
Etch-on-a-Tube
Photo-Mask-and E.-o.-a.-T.
(PMEOAT)
ETCO$_2$
end-tidal carbon dioxide
ETCO$_2$ multigas analyzer
sidestream ETCO$_2$
E-test
ETFE
ethylene tetrafluor ethylene
ETFVL
exercise tidal flow-volume loop
ethacrynic acid
Ethalloy needle
ethambutol hydrochloride
ethamivan
Ethamolin injection
ethane
exhaled e.
ethanol (EtOH)
selective septal branch injection
of e.
ethanolamide
arachidonyl e.
ethanolamine
aminoethyl e.
e. oleate
Ethaquin
Ethatab
ethaverine hydrochloride
Ethavex-100
ether
bis(chloromethyl) e.
e. bronchitis

e. pneumonia
e. test
Ethibond suture
Ethicon Endopath EZ45 and TL60
stapler
ethidium bromide
ethionamide (ETA)
ethmozin
Ethmozine
ethoxysclerol
ethyl alcohol
ethylene
ethylene tetrafluor e. (ETFE)
ethylenediamine
theophylline e.
ethylenediaminetetraacetic
e. acid (EDTA)
e. acid disodium salt
ethylnorepinephrine hydrochloride
Etibi
etiennei
Octomyces e.
etilefrine
etiopathogenesis
EtOH
ethanol
etomidate
Etopophos
etoposide
Adriamycin, cyclophosphamide, e.
(ACE)
carboplatin, e. (CE)
cisplatin, e. (PE)
cisplatin, vincristine, doxorubicin, e.
(CODE)
e. phosphate
ETO Sleuth
e-TRAIN 110 AngioJet catheter
ETS
environmental tobacco smoke
ETT
endotracheal tube
exercise tolerance test
exercise treadmill test
eucapneic voluntary hyperventilation
Eudal-SR
Euflex
euglobulin clot lysis time
euglycemia
euglycemic
e. glucose clamp

E

NOTES

261

euglycemic *(continued)*
  e. hyperinsulinemic glucose clamp test
eugonic
eukaryon
eukaryosis
eukaryote
Eulexin
eunuchoid voice
eupaverin
eupnea
Euro-Collins
  E.-C. multiorgan perfusion kit
  E.-C. solution
European
  E. Myocardial Infarct Amiodarone Trial (EMIAT)
  E. Stroke Scale (ESS)
EUS-FNA
  endoscopic ultrasound-guided fine needle aspiration
Eustace Smith murmur
eustachian
  e. ridge
  e. valve
eusystole
eusystolic
euthyroid sick syndrome
Eutron
euvolemic
eV
  electron volt
evacuation
  pleural space e.
evagination
evaluation
  Acute Myocardial Infarction Angioplasty Bolus Lysis E. (AMIABLE)
  Acute Physiology, Age, Chronic Health E. (APACHE)
  anthropometric e.
  Cardiac Arrest in Seattle: Conventional versus Amiodarone Drug E. (CASCADE)
  confirmatory e.
  Conventional Antiarrhythmic versus Amiodarone in Survivors of Cardiac Arrest Drug E. (CASCADE)
  Gianturco-Roubin Stent Acute Closure E. (GRACE)
  Heart Outcomes Prevention E. (HOPE)
  E. of IIb/IIIa Platelet Inhibitor for Stenting

  E. of IIb/IIIa Platelet Receptor Antagonist c7E3 in Preventing Ischemic Complications (EPIC)
  E. of Losartan in the Elderly (ELITE)
  medication-use e. (MUE)
  noninvasive e.
  Physical Activity Scale for the Elderly E. (PASE)
  E. of Platelet IIb/IIIa Inhibitor for Stenting Trial (EPISTENT)
  Post Intracoronary Treatment Ultrasound Result E. (PICTURE)
  Prospective Randomized Amlodipine Survival E. (PRAISE)
  E. of PTCA to Improve Long-Term Outcome by c7E3 GPIIb/IIIa Receptor Blockade (EPILOG)
  Survival of Myocardial Infarction: Long-Term E. (SMILE)
  Ticlopidine Aspirin Stent E. (TASTE)
  Trandolapril Cardiac E. (TRACE)
  valsartan antihypertensive long-term e.
  Valsartan Antihypertensive Long-Term Use E. (VALUE)
EVAN
  ergonomic vascular access needle
Evans blue
EVD
  external ventricular drainage
Eve method
even-echo rephasing
event
  Action on Secondary Prevention by Intervention to Reduce E.'s (ASPIRE)
  adverse e.
  apparent life-threatening e. (ALTE)
  cardiac e.
  cerebral e.
  cerebrovascular e.
  Cholesterol and Recurrent E.'s (CARE)
  Clopidogrel in Unstable Angina to Prevent Recurrent Ischemic E.'s (CURE)
  Clopidogrel versus Aspirin in Patients at Risk of Ischemic E.'s (CAPRIE)
  coronary e.
  e. diary
  Efficacy and Safety of Subcutaneous Enoxaparin in Non-Q-Wave Coronary E.'s (ESSENCE)

embolic e.
Family Index of Life E.'s (FILE)
hard cardiac e.
intracardiac e.
ischemic e.
major adverse cardiac e. (MACE)
e. monitor
nonfatal cardiac e.
Omapatrilat in Persons with
Enhanced Risk of
Atherosclerotic E.'s (OPERA)
e. recorder
e. recorder monitor
reducing e.
respiratory e.
sleep-disordered breathing e.
soft e.
transient ischemic e. (TIE)
wave coronary e.
event/episode counter
event-link data system
eventrated diaphragm
eventration of diaphragm
EverGrip clamp insert
Everone Injection
eversion
blunt e.
cusp e.
everting mattress suture
evidence-based medicine (EBM)
EvitaMobil universal trolley
EVLW
extravascular lung water
evoked
e. endocardial electrogram
e. ventricular electrogram
evolution
R-Test E.
Evolution scanner
evolutus
Peptostreptococcus e.
Evolve Cardiac Continuum
evolving myocardial infarction
EVR
endovascular repair
Ewald tube
Ewart sign
E-wave
E.-w. spectral velocity waveform
E.-w. velocity
Ewing sign

EX
Diabetic Tussin E.
Naldecon Senior E.
Ex
Touro E.
ex
e. vivo
e. vivo gene transfer
EX-2000 DeVilbiss conserver
exacerbation
infective e.
recurrent infective e.
ExacTech blood glucose meter
EXACTO
Excimer Laser Angioplasty in Coronary
Total Occlusion
EXACTO clinical trial
examination
cardiac e.
funduscopic e.
limited Doppler e.
Mini Mental State E. (MMSE)
neurologic e.
parasternal e.
supraclavicular e.
suprasternal e.
excavatum
pectus e.
Excedrin IB
EXCEL
Expanded Clinical Evaluation of
Lovastatin
EXCEL trial
Excelsior 1018 microcatheter
excessive daytime sleepiness (EDS)
exchange
air e.
alanine e.
cardiopulmonary gas e.
catheter e.
citrate e.
FFA e.
gas e.
glucose e.
glutamate e.
e. guidewire
oxygen e.
perfluorocarbon-associated gas e.
(PAGE)
pulmonary gas e.
respiratory e.
sodium-potassium e.

E

NOTES

exchange *(continued)*
    e. technique
    e. transfusion
exchanger
    heat/moisture e. (HME)
    Hygrobac-Dar heat-moisture e.
    Na^+/H^+ e. (NHE)
    Portex ThermoVent heat and
      moisture e.
    ThermoVent heat and moisture e.
excimer
    e. cool laser
    e. gas laser
    E. Laser Angioplasty in Coronary
      Total Occlusion (EXACTO)
    e. laser-assisted angioplasty (ELA)
    e. laser coronary angioplasty
      (ECLA, ELCA)
    e. laser coronary atherectomy
    e. laser, rotational atherectomy, and
      balloon angioplasty (ERBAC)
    e. sheath
    e. vascular recanalization
excision
    wedge e.
excisional
    e. atherectomy
    e. biopsy
    e. cardiac surgery
excitability
    supranormal e.
excitable gap
excitation
    anomalous atrioventricular e.
    direct e.
    premature e.
    reentrant e.
    supranormal e.
    e. wave
excitation-contraction coupling
excited dimers
excitotoxic
exclusion
    e. criteria
    Medicine versus Angioplasty for
      Thrombolytic E.'s (MATE)
excrescence
    Lambl e.
excretion
    absorption, distribution, metabolism,
      and e. (ADME)
    eicosanoid e.
excursion
    cusp e.
    decreased valve e.
    diaphragmatic e.
    dome e.
    dyssynchronous thoracoabdominal e.

    endocardial e.
    phasic e.
    respiratory e.
Ex-ECG
    exercise stress electrocardiography
Ex-Echo
    exercise stress echocardiography
exercise
    aerobic e. (AEX)
    ankle e.
    bicycle e.
    Bobath e.
    breathing e.
    Buerger-Allen e.
    e. capacity
    cardiopulmonary e. (CPX)
    duration of e.
    dynamic e.
    e. echocardiogram (EE)
    e. echocardiography
    e. electrocardiogram
    e. electrocardiography
    e. factor
    e. hyperpnea
    e. hypertension
    e. imaging
    e. index
    e. intolerance
    isometric e.
    isotonic e.
    e. load
    e. LV function
    mild-intensity e.
    peak e.
    e. prescription
    e. pressor reflex
    Prospective Randomized Evaluation
      of Carvedilol in Symptoms
      and E. (PRECISE)
    e. regimen
    rehabilitation e.
    So Much Improvement with a
      Little E. (SMILE)
    strenuous e.
    e. stress echocardiography (Ex-
      Echo)
    e. stress electrocardiography (Ex-
      ECG)
    e. stress test (EST)
    e. study
    supine e.
    e. termination
    e. test
    e. thallium scintigraphy
    e. thallium-201 scintigraphy
    e. tidal flow-volume loop (ETFVL)
    e. tolerance
    e. tolerance test (ETT)

e. tomographic TI-201 imaging
e. treadmill
e. treadmill test (ETT)
unsupported arm e. (UAE)
upright e.

exercise-induced
e.-i. angina
e.-i. arrhythmia
e.-i. asthma (EIA)
e.-i. bronchospasm (EIB)
e.-i. dyspnea
e.-i. fatigue
e.-i. ischemia
e.-i. shortness of breath
e.-i. silent myocardial ischemia
e.-i. ventricular tachycardia

exerciser
Resistex expiratory resistance e.

exertion
dyspnea on e. (DOE)
perceived e.
rating of perceived e. (RPE)

exertional
e. angina
e. dyspnea
e. hypotension
e. syncope

exfoliative dermatitis
exhalation
exhale
exhaled
e. ethane
e. nitric oxide (eNO, ENO)

exhaust
diesel e.

exhaustion
vital e.

Exirel
exit
e. block
e. block murmur
e. point
e. site
e. surgical osteosynthesis
e. wound

Exna
exocardia
exocardial murmur
exogenous
e. lipid
e. lipid pneumonia

e. obesity
e. substrate

exon
exophthalmica
tachycardia e.
tachycardia traumosa e.

exophthalmos
exophytic
exopneumopexy
exopolysaccharide
mucoid e.

Exorcist technique
Exosurf
E. Neonatal
E. Pediatric

exotoxin
Pseudomonas e.

expandable access catheter (EAC)
expanded
E. Clinical Evaluation of
Lovastatin (EXCEL)
e. polytetrafluoroethylene (EPTFE)
e. polytetrafluoroethylene vascular
graft

expander
blood e.
Hespan plasma volume e.
hetastarch plasma e.
plasma volume e.
PMT AccuSpan tissue e.
Ruiz-Cohen round e.
E. stent

expansion
Antiplatelet Treatment after
Intravascular Ultrasound-Guided
Optimal Stent E. (APLAUSE)
Can Routine Ultrasound Improve
Stent E. (CRUISE)
Can Routine Ultrasound Influence
Stent E. (CRUISE)
infarct e.
ProWrap e.
stent e.
volume e.

expectorant
Anti-Tuss E.
Balminil E.
Benylin E.
Calmylin E.
classic e.
Codafed E.
Decohistine E.

NOTES

E

265

expectorant *(continued)*
    Detussin E.
    Dihistine E.
    Fedahist E.
    Genamin E.
    GuiaCough E.
    Isoclor E.
    liquifying e.
    Myminic E.
    Nucofed Pediatric E.
    Phenhist E.
    Ru-Tuss E.
    Silaminic E.
    SRC E.
    Stokes e.
    Theramin E.
    Triaminic E.
    Tri-Clear E.
    Triphenyl E.
    Tussafin E.
expectorated sputum volume
expectoration
    prune juice e.
    sputum e.
expedited recovery program
expenditure
    energy e.
    resting energy e. (REE)
experiment
    Müller e.
    Weber e.
experimental enterococcal endocarditis
expiration
    duration of e. (T_E)
    prolongation of e.
expiratory
    e. airflow
    e. center
    e. dyspnea
    e. flow rate
    e. grunt
    e. murmur
    e. positive airway pressure (EPAP)
    e. reserve volume (ERV)
    e. resistance
    e. retard
    e. rhonchi
    e. tidal flow
    e. time (T_E)
    e. trapping of air
    e. view
    e. wheezing
expired
    e. air collection
    e. gas
    e. nitric oxide (eNO, ENO)
expirograph
    Godart e.

explant
explanted heart
Explorer
    E. 360-degree rotational diagnostic EP catheter
    E. pre-curved diagnostic EP catheter
exploring electrode
exposure
    allergen e.
    alternobaric e.
    chemical e.
    cobalt e.
    cold e.
    hyperbaric e.
    hypobaric e.
    toxin e.
    workplace e.
Express
    E. balloon
    E. over-the-wire balloon catheter
    E. PTCA catheter
expression
    adenovirus-based phospholamban-antisense e.
    Bcl-2 e.
    CMV IE-2 gene e.
    cytokine e.
    eNOS gene e.
    fibroblast growth factor e.
    gene e.
    P-selectin e.
    e. sequence tagged (EST)
expressive aphasia
expulsive coughing
exsanguinate
exsanguination protocol
exsanguinotransfusion
EXS femoropopliteal bypass graft
exsorption
extended
    e. collection device
    e. field radiation (EFR)
extended-release niacin/lovastatin
extender
    Taq e.
extension
    anterior mitral leaflet e.
    DOC guidewire e.
    infarct e.
    knee e.
    Linx guidewire e.
    LOC guidewire e.
Extentabs
    Quinidex E.
extent of pleural carcinomatosis score (EPC)

external
    e. branch of superior laryngeal nerve
    e. cardiac massage
    e. cardioversion
    e. cardioverter-defibrillator (ECD)
    e. carotid artery (ECA)
    e. chest wall oscillation
    e. defibrillator
    e. elastic lamina (EEL)
    e. elastic lamina area
    e. elastic membrane (EEM)
    e. electric cardioversion
    e. grid
    e. high-output ramp pacing
    e. inflatable compressor
    e. intercostal
    e. jugular approach
    e. jugular vein
    e. mammary artery
    e. pacemaker
    e. pacemaker battery
    e. pudendal vein
    e. respiration
    e. rotation, abduction, stress test (EAST)
    e. ventricular drainage (EVD)

externum
    pericardium e.

Extra
    E. Action Cough Syrup
    E. Back-up guiding catheter
    E. Sport coronary guidewire
    E. Strength Bayer Enteric 500 Aspirin
    E. Strength Doan's

extraalveolar capillary
extracardiac
    e. cavopulmonary anastomosis
    e. murmur
    e. shunt
    e. ventriculopulmonary conduit

extracelluar matrix metabolism
extracellular
    e. F-actin
    e. lipid
    e. matrix (ECM)
    e. signal-regulated kinase

extracellular-like, calcium-free solution (ECS)
extracellularly responsive kinase (ERK)
extracellular-regulated kinase (ERK)

extracoronary
extracorporeal
    e. carbon dioxide removal
    e. cardiac shock wave therapy
    e. circulation
    e. exchange hypothermia
    e. heart
    e. life support (ECLS)
    E. Life Support Organization (ELSO)
    e. membrane differential filtration
    e. membrane oxygenation (ECMO)
    e. membrane oxygenation therapy
    e. membrane oxygenator
    e. pump oxygenator
    e. rheopheresis

extracranial
    e. carotid arterial disease (ECAD)
    e. carotid disease (ECD)
    e. carotid obstruction
    e. Doppler sonography (ECD)
    e. internal carotid disease

extracranial/intracranial (EC/IC)
    e./i. bypass surgery

extract
    calf lung surfactant e. (CLSE)
    cell-free e.
    pancreatic e.
    Rauwolfia e.
    shiitake mushroom e.
    thyroid e.

extraction
    e. atherectomy
    e. atherectomy device
    lactate e.
    myocardial lactate e.
    oxygen e.
    e. reserve
    transvenous catheter e.

Extractor three-lumen retrieval balloon
eXtract specimen bag
extraesophageal reflux
extraflexible wire
extrafusion defect
extralobar
extranuclear
extraparenchymal bleeding
extrapericardial patch
extrapleural
    e. air
    e. analgesia
    e. apicolysis

E

NOTES

extrapleural *(continued)*
   e. catheter analgesia
   e. pneumonectomy (EPP)
   e. pneumothorax
   e. space
extrapulmonary
   e. cough
   e. site
   e. tuberculosis
extrapyramidal side effect
extrarenal azotemia
extrastimulation
   single premature e.
extrastimulus, pl. **extrastimuli**
   double e.
   double ventricular e.
   premature atrial e.
   single e.
   e. test
   triple e.
extra-support guidewire
extrasystole
   atrial e.
   atrioventricular e. (AVE)
   atrioventricular junctional escape e.
   atrioventricular nodal e.
   auricular e.
   auriculoventricular e.
   A-V e.
   A-V junctional e.
   A-V nodal e.
   infranodal e.
   interpolated e.
   junctional e.
   lower nodal e.
   midnodal e.
   nodal e.
   return e.
   spontaneous e.
   supraventricular e.
   tip e.
   upper nodal e.
   ventricular e.
extrasystolic beat
extrathoracic
   e. airway dysfunction
   e. airway obstruction
   e. neoplasm
   e. rale

   e. soft tissue
   e. tumor
extratracheal
extravasation
   plasma e.
extravascular
   e. granulomatous feature
   e. lung water (EVLW)
Extreme laser catheter
extremitas
extremity
   elevation pallor of e.
   e. ischemia
   mottling of e.'s
ExtreSafe phlebotomy device
extrinsic
   e. allergic alveolitis
   e. asthma
   e. compression
   e. factor
   e. force
extrusion
   Kensey rotation atherectomy e.
extubation time
exuberant granulation tissue (EGT)
exudate
   cotton-wool e.
   fibrinous e.
   fluffy cotton-wool e.
exudation
   plasma e.
   plasma protein e.
exudativa
   bronchiolitis e.
exudative
   e. bronchiolitis
   e. bronchitis
   e. effusion
   e. empyema
   e. pleural effusion
   e. pleurisy
   e. tuberculosis
eyeball
   e. compression reflex
   e.-heart reflex
eyeless needle
EZ-3
EZ45 thoracic linear cutter
Ezide

F

French

F gate

F point of cardiac apex pulse

F wave

f

respiratory frequency

f wave

f wave of jugular venous pulse

F$_{2alpha}$

8-iso-prostaglandin F. (8-iso-PGF$_{2alpha}$)

6F

6F delivery system

7F

7F extended-curve thermistor catheter

7F fused-tip catheter

7F Hydrolyser thrombectomy catheter

7F mapping catheter

Fab

c7 E3 Fab

chimeric 7E3 Fab

digoxin-immune Fab

digoxin-specific Fab

Fab fragment

m7E3 Fab

fab

digoxin immune f.

fabric baffle

Fabry disease

FAC

fractional area change

face

en f.

moon f.

f. shield

f. squeeze

transverse artery of f.

FACET

Flosequinan ACE Inhibitor Trial

Fosinopril Versus Amlodipine Cardiovascular Events Randomized Trial

facet

f. of atlas for dens

clavicular f.

inferior costal f.

superior costal f.

transverse costal f.

facial

f. barotrauma

f. diplegia

f. droop

f. vein

facies, pl. **facies**

f. anterior cordis

aortic f.

f. articularis

Corvisart f.

f. costalis pulmonis

cushingoid f.

f. diaphragmatica

f. diaphragmatica cordis

ecchymotic f.

elfin f.

f. inferior cordis

f. interlobares pulmonis

f. medialis pulmonis

f. mediastinalis pulmonis

mitral f.

f. mitralis

mitrotricuspid f.

f. pulmonalis cordis

f. pulmonalis dextra/sinistra cordis

f. sternocostalis cordis

facilitated angioplasty

facility

long-term care f.

LTC f.

skilled nursing f. (SNF)

faciobrachiocrural paresis

facioscapulohumeral

f. dystrophy

f. dystrophy of Landouzy-Déjérine

FACS

fluorescence-activated cell sorter

FACT-22

Focus Angioplasty Catheter Technology

FACT coronary balloon angioplasty catheter

F-actin

filamentous actin

extracellular F-actin

factitious asthma

Factive

factor

f. I (fibrinogen)

f. II (prothrombin)

f. III deficiency

f. III (thromboplastin)

f. IV (calcium ions)

f. V Leiden coagulation defect

f. V Leiden mutation

f. V (proaccelerin)

f. VI (factor VI - cannot be identified)

f. VII

F

factor *(continued)*
  f. VII (proconvertin)
  f. VIII (antihemophilic f.)
  f. viii:c (porcine)
  f. VIII:C (von Willebrand f.)
  f. IX complex (human)
  f. Xa
  f. X (Stuart f. or Stuart-Prower f.)
  f. XI (plasma thromboplastin
    antecedent f.)
  f. XII (Hageman f.)
  f. XII-kallikrein-kinin system
  f. XIII (fibrin stabilizing f.)
  accelerator globin blood
    coagulation f.
  AcG blood coagulation f.
  acidic fibroblast growth f. (aFGF)
  activating transcription f. (ATF)
  active-site inhibited f. VIIa
  antihemophilic f. (recombinant)
  atrial natriuretic f. (ANF)
  f. B
  basic fibroblast growth f. (bFGF)
  behavioral f.
  carbon monoxide transfer f.
    (TLCO, TLco)
  cardiac risk f.
  Christmas f.
  Christmas blood coagulation f.
  classic risk f.
  coagulation f.
  colony stimulating f. (CSFs)
  connective tissue growth f. (CTGF)
  corticotrophin-releasing f. (CRF)
  f. D
  duty f.
  endothelial derived relaxation f.
  endothelium-derived
    hyperpolarizing f. (EDHF)
  endothelium-derived relaxing f.
    (EDRF)
  epidermal growth f.
  exercise f.
  extrinsic f.
  fibrin-stabilizing blood
    coagulation f.
  fibroblast growth f. (FGF)
  Fletcher f.
  granulocyte/macrophage colony-
    stimulating f. (GM-CSF)
  gravitation f.
  growth f.
  f. H
  Hageman f.
  heparin-binding epidermal growth f.
  histamine release inhibitory f.
    (HRIF)
  histamine-releasing f. (HRF)

  insulin-like growth f. (IGF)
  intravascular procoagulant f.
  lipid risk f.
  lymphocyte chemoattractant f.
    (LCF)
  monocyte chemotactic and
    activating f. (MCAF)
  Moody friction f.
  myocardial depressant f. (MDF)
  necrosis f.
  neurohumoral f.'s
  N-terminal proatrial natriuretic f.
  f. P
  paracrine f.
  platelet f. 4
  platelet activating f. (PAF)
  platelet-aggregating f.
  platelet-derived growth f. (PDGF)
  platelet-derived histamine-
    releasing f. (PDHRF)
  proatherosclerotic f.
  proatrial natriuretic f. (proANF)
  proconvertin blood coagulation f.
  psychological f.
  psychosocial f.
  recombinant human vascular
    endothelial growth f. (rhVEGF)
  Rh f.
  rheumatoid f.
  risk f.
  stem cell f. (SCF)
  Stuart-Prower f.
  tissue f.
  transforming growth f. (TGF)
  transfusion f.
  tumor necrosis f. (TNF)
  vascular endothelial growth f.
    (VEGF)
  vascular permeability f. (VPF)
  von Willebrand f. (vWP)
factor-alpha
  tumor necrosis f. (TNF-alpha)
factor-κB
  nuclear f. (NF-kappa-B)
factor-beta
  transforming growth f.
facultative bacteria
faecalis
  Alcaligenes f.
  Enterococcus f.
  Streptococcus f.
faecium
  Enterococcus f.
faeni
  Micropolyspora f.
Fagerstrom
  F. tolerance questionnaire (FTQ)
  F. tolerance scale

Faget sign
Fahraeus effect
Fahr disease
FAI
> functional aerobic impairment

failed rescue angioplasty
failing lung sign
failure
> acute congestive heart f.
> acute renal f.
> acute respiratory f. (ARF)
> advanced heart f.
> autonomic f.
> backward f.
> backward heart f.
> bronchial stump f.
> f. to capture
> cardiac f.
> central baroreflex f.
> chronic heart f.
> chronic renal f.
> chronic respiratory f. (CRF)
> circulatory f.
> cocaine-induced respiratory f.
> (CIRF)
> compensated congestive heart f.
> congestive heart f. (CHF)
> coronary f.
> diastolic heart f.
> electrical f.
> end-stage heart f.
> florid congestive heart f.
> forward heart f.
> heart f. (HF)
> hepatic f.
> high output f.
> high-output heart f.
> hypercapnic respiratory f.
> impending respiratory f.
> insulation f.
> left-sided heart f.
> left ventricular f.
> Living with Heart F.
> low-output f.
> low-output heart f.
> multiple-organ f.
> multisystem organ f. (MSOF)
> myocardial f.
> nonhypercapnic respiratory f.
> Outcomes of a Prospective Trial
> of Intravenous Milrinone for

> Exacerbations of Chronic
> Heart F. (OPTIME-CHF)
> pacemaker f.
> pacing-induced heart f.
> power f.
> primary graft f. (PGF)
> progressive pump f.
> pulmonary f.
> pump f.
> refractory congestive heart f.
> renal f.
> respiratory f.
> right heart f.
> right-sided heart f.
> right ventricular f.
> systolic heart f.
> tachycardia-induced heart f.
> ventilatory f.
> ventricular f.

faint
> f. flow
> f. opacification
> f. pulmonary regurgitation

fainting
> hysterical f.

faintness
FAK
> focal adhesion kinase

falciparum
> *Plasmodium f.*

Falcon
> F. balloon
> F. coronary catheter
> F. single-operator exchange balloon
> catheter

fallen lung sign
falling drop
Fallot
> F. pentalogy
> pentalogy of F.
> pink tetralogy of F.
> F. pink tetralogy
> F. tetrad
> tetralogy of F. (TOF)
> total repair of tetralogy of F.
> F. triad
> trilogy of F.
> F. trilogy

false
> f. aneurysm
> f. aneurysmal chamber
> f. angina

F

NOTES

false *(continued)*
    f. aortic aneurysm
    f. apex
    f. bruit
    f. cardiomegaly
    f. cardiomyopathy
    f. combined hyperlipidemia
    f. croup
    f. cyanosis
    f. dextrocardia
    f. emphysema
    f. hypercholesterolemia
    f. lumen
    f. mass
    f. tendon
    f. vocal cord
false-negative
false-positive
FAMA, FAMAT
    fluorescent antimembrane antibody
    fluorescence antimembrane antibody
famciclovir
familial
    f. abetalipoproteinemia
    f. amyloidosis
    f. apoA-I deficiency
    f. asphyxiant thoracic dystrophy
    F. Atherosclerosis Treatment Study
      (FATS)
    f. atrial myxoma
    f. atrial myxoma syndrome
    f. atrioventricular block
    f. cholestasis syndrome
    f. chylomicronemia syndrome
    f. combined hyperlipidemia (FCHL)
    f. dysautonomia
    f. dysbetalipoproteinemia
    f. dyslipidemic hypertension
    f. emphysema
    f. HDL deficiency
    f. high-density-lipoprotein deficiency
    f. hypercholesterolemia (FH)
    f. hyperchylomicronemia
    f. hypertrophic cardiomyopathy
    f. hypertrophic obstructive
      cardiomyopathy
    f. hypobetalipoproteinemia (FHBL)
    f. hypocalciuric hypercalcemia
    f. intracranial aneurysm
    f. Mediterranean fever
    f. multifocal fibrosclerosis
    f. nephritis
    f. paroxysmal polyserositis
    f. pulmonary fibrosis
    f. recurrence
    f. tachycardia
family
    f. history of heart disease

    f. history of myocardial infarction
    signal transducer and activator of
      transcription protein f.
    STAT protein f.
    trefoil factor f. (TFF)
Family Index of Life Events (FILE)
Famvir
fan
    Dunham f.
Fansidar
Fansimef
Faraday cage
Fareston
far-field
    f.-f. electrogram
    f.-f. QRS complex
    f.-f. R-wave sensing
    f.-f. visualization
FARI
    filtered atrial rate interval
farmer's lung
Farr test
FAS
    fetal alcohol syndrome
Fas
    F. ligand (FasL)
    F. receptor
fascia
    pectoral f.
    pectoralis f.
    Scarpa f.
fascial layer
fascicle
    blocked f.
fascicular
    f. beat
    f. block
    f. heart block
    f. tachycardia
fasciculation
fasciculoventricular Mahaim fiber
fasciotomy
Fas-Fas ligand pathway
fashion
    crisscross f.
    culotte f.
    stoichiometric f.
FasL
    Fas ligand
    FasL pathway
    soluble FasL (sFasL)
FAST
    flow-assisted, short-term
    Fourier-acquired steady-state technique
    Frenchay Aphasia Screening Test
    FAST balloon catheter
    FAST balloon flotation catheter

FAST right heart cardiovascular catheter

fast
- f. channel
- f. Fourier
- f. Fourier spectral analysis
- f. Fourier transform (FFT)
- f. low-angle shot
- f. pathway
- F. Revascularization During Instability in Coronary Artery Disease (FRISC)
- f. sodium current
- f. tissue
- f. wave sleep

Fast-Cath Duo introducer
FASTER
    Fibrinolytic and Aggrastat ST Elevation Resolution
    FASTER study
Fast-Fit vascular stockings
fasting
- f. blood sugar
- f. plasma norepinephrine
Fast-Pass endocardial lead
Fast-Patch disposable defibrillation/electrocardiographic electrode
fast-pathway
- f.-p. radiofrequency ablation
- f.-p. radiofrequency catheter ablation
FasTrac
- F. guidewire
- F. hydrophilic-coated guidewire
- F. introducer
FasTracker balloon
fat
- body f.
- dietary f.
- f. embolism
- f. embolism syndrome (FES)
- f. emulsion
- epicardial f.
- monosaturated f.
- polyunsaturated f.
- preperitoneal f.
- trans f.
- truncal distribution of body f.
fat-absorption coefficient
fat-free mass (FFM)

fatigue
- collagen f.
- exercise-induced f.
- inspiratory muscle f.
- respiratory muscle f.
fat-laden microphages
FATS
    Familial Atherosclerosis Treatment Study
fatty
- f. acid
- f. degeneration of heart
- f. heart
- f. streak
faucial branches of lingual nerve
faucium
    Mycoplasma f.
Faught sphygmomanometer
Fauvel granules
Favaloro
- F.-Morse rib spreader
- F. proximal anastomosis clamp
- F. saphenous vein bypass graft
FB
    fiberoptic bronchoscopy
FBN1 gene
FC
    Apo-Dipyridamole F.
FCHL
    familial combined hyperlipidemia
FCP
    functional conduction period
Fc receptor
FDG
    fluorodeoxyglucose
FE
    Slow FE
feature
    alexithymic personality f.'s
    extravascular granulomatous f.
    RapidScore software f.
febrile
    agglutinin f.
FEC
    forced expiratory capacity
FECO$_2$
    fraction of expired carbon dioxide
Fedahist
- F. Expectorant
- F. Expectorant Pediatric
- F. Tablet
Federici sign

F

NOTES

feedback
 mechanoelectrical f.
 respiratory f. (RFb)
feeder vessel
feeding
 enteral tube f.
 nasogastric tube f. (NTF)
Feed or Ordinary Diet (FOOD)
feeleii
 Legionella f.
feet of sea water (fsw)
FEF
 forced expiratory flow
FEF$_{25-75\%}$
 mean midexpiratory flow rate
FEFmax
 maximal forced expiratory flow
Feiba VH Immuno
Feigenbaum echocardiogram
Feinstein methodologic standard
fele
 bruit de f.
 bruit de pot f.
Fell-O'Dwyer apparatus
felodipine
 enalapril and f.
Felson
 silhouette sign of F.
felt strip
female hormone
Femara
Femiron
Femo
 F. stop femoral artery compression arch
 F. stop inflatable pneumatic compression device
 F. stop pneumatic compression
femoral
 f. approach
 f. arteriography
 f. artery
 f. artery occlusion
 f. artery pressure
 f. artery thrombosis
 brachial, radial, f. (BRAFE)
 f. canal
 f. embolectomy
 f. embolus
 f. endarterectomy
 percutaneous f.
 f. perfusion cannula
 f. pseudoaneurysm
 f. vascular injury
 f. vein
 f. vein occlusion
 f. venous sheath

 f. venous thrombosis
 f. vessel
femoral-femoral
 f.-f. bypass
 f.-f. crossover
femoral-popliteal bypass
femoral-tibial bypass
femoral-tibial-peroneal bypass
femoris
 venae circumflexae laterales f.
femoroaxillary bypass
femorofemoral crossover bypass
femoropopliteal
 f. bypass
 f. stenting
femorotibial
 f. bypass
FemoStop
femtoliter (fL)
fenbufen
fence
 electron-beam f.
 Kirklin f.
Fenesin DM
fenestrated
 f. Fontan operation
 f. Fontan procedure
 f. tracheostomy tube
fenestration
 aortopulmonary f.
 baffle f.
 cusp f.
fenfluramine
 f. hydrochloride
 phentermine and f. (phen-fen)
Fenico
fenofibrate
fenoldopam mesylate
fenoprofen calcium
fenoterol
fentanyl
 F. Oralet
Feosol
Feostat
FEP-ringed Gore-Tex vascular graft
Ferancee
Feratab
Fergie needle
Fergon
Ferguson needle
Fergus percutaneous introducer kit
Fer-In-Sol
Fer-Iron
Fernandez reaction
Fero-Grad 500
Fero-Gradumet
Ferospace
Ferralet

Ferralyn Lanacaps
Ferra-TD
Ferrein cords
ferricytochrome assay
ferritin
Ferrlecit
ferrocalcinosis
    cerebrovascular f.
Ferromar
Ferro-Sequels
ferrous
    f. fumarate
    f. gluconate
    f. salt and ascorbic acid
    f. sulfate
    f. sulfate, ascorbic acid, and
      vitamin B-complex
    f. sulfate, ascorbic acid, vitamin
      B-complex, and folic acid
ferruginous
    f. body
FES
    fat embolism syndrome
    flame emission spectroscopy
    forced expiratory spirogram
FET
    forced expiratory time
fetal
    f. alcohol syndrome (FAS)
    f. aspiration syndrome
    f. atrial wall motion
    f. bradycardia
    f. cardiology
    f. circulation
    f. electrocardiography
    f. heart monitor tracing
    f. heart rate
    f. heart rhythm
    f. origins hypothesis
    f. PR interval
    f. souffle
    f. tachycardia
    f. ventricular myocyte proliferative
      response
    f. ventricular wall motion
fetalis
    erythroblastosis f.
    hydrops f.
fetal-type
    f.-t. PCA
    f.-t. posterior cerebral artery

fetocardia
FEV
    forced expiratory volume
FEV_1
    forced expiratory volume in 1 second
fever
    acute rheumatic f.
    Australian Q f.
    bird f.
    dengue f.
    desert f.
    familial Mediterranean f.
    hay f.
    hemorrhagic f.
    Jaccoud dissociated f.
    Katayama f.
    Korean hemorrhagic f.
    Lassa f.
    lung f.
    Mediterranean f.
    metal fume f. (MFF)
    Monday f.
    Omsk hemorrhagic f.
    parrot f.
    pharyngoconjunctival f.
    pneumonic f.
    polymer fume f. (PFF)
    Pontiac f.
    pulmonary f.
    Q f.
    Queensland f.
    query f.
    rabbit f.
    relapsing f.
    rheumatic f. (RF)
    Rocky Mountain spotted f.
    San Joaquin f.
    San Joaquin Valley f.
    scarlet f.
    septic f.
    shoddy f.
    sthenic f.
    thermic f.
    threshing f.
    typhoid f.
    Valley f.
    yellow f.
    zinc fume f.
FEV/FVC
    forced expiratory volume timed to forced
    vital capacity ratio

F

NOTES

FEV$_1$/FVC
> forced expiratory volume in 1 second to forced vital capacity ratio

fexofenadine hydrochloride

FF
> fibrillation-flutter

FFA
> free fatty acids
> > FFA exchange

FFB
> flexible fiberoptic bronchoscopy

F-18 FDG
> fluorine-18 fluorodeoxyglucose

f-f interval

FFM
> fat-free mass

FFP
> fresh frozen plasma

FFR
> fractional flow reserve

FFR$_{myo}$
> myocardial fractional flow reserve

FFT
> fast Fourier transform
> free-floating thrombus

FGF
> fibroblast growth factor

FH
> familial hypercholesterolemia

FHBL
> familial hypobetalipoproteinemia

FHS
> Framingham Heart Study

FI
> fundamental imaging

fib

fiber
> actin f.
> afferent nerve f.'s
> atriofasciculoventricular Mahaim f.
> atrio-His f.
> blocking vagal afferent f.'s
> blocking vagal efferent f.'s
> Brechenmacher f.
> Dacron f.
> fasciculoventricular Mahaim f.
> His-Purkinje f.'s
> James f.'s
> Kent f.'s
> laser f.
> Mahaim f.'s
> manmade vitreous f. (MMVF)
> nodoventricular f.
> parasympathetic nerve f.'s
> pseudo-Mahaim f.
> Purkinje f.'s
> f. shortening
> f. shortening velocity (V$_{cf}$)

> sinospiral f.
> sinuspiral f.
> spindle f.
> terminal Purkinje f.'s
> wavy f.

Fiberlase system

fiberoptic
> f. bronchoscope
> f. bronchoscopy (FB, FOB)
> f. catheter delivery system
> f. delivery device
> f. delivery system
> f. esophagoscopy
> f. oximeter catheter
> f. pressure catheter
> f. rhinoscopy (RHINOS)

fibrate

fibremia

fibric acid

fibrillar
> f. collagen
> f. collagen network
> f. mass of Fleming

fibrillary wave

fibrillation
> atrial f. (AF)
> auricular f.
> Canadian Registry of Atrial f.
> cardiac f.
> catheter ablation of atrial f.
> chronic atrial f.
> continuous atrial f. (CAF)
> focal atrial f.
> Guiaraudon corridor operation for atrial f.
> idiopathic ventricular f.
> inducible polymorphic ventricular f.
> lone atrial f.
> nonprimary ventricular f.
> nonvalvular atrial f. (NVAF)
> paroxysmal atrial f. (PAF)
> f. potential
> primary ventricular f.
> f. rhythm
> Stroke Prevention in Atrial F. (SPAF)
> Stroke Prevention in Nonrheumatic Atrial F. (SPINAF)
> Systemic Trial of Pacing to Prevent Atrial F. (STOP-AF)
> f. threshold
> vagal atrial f.
> ventricular f. (VF)
> ventricular tachycardia/ventricular f. (VT/VF)

fibrillation-flutter (FF)
> atrial f.-f. (AFF)

fibrillatory wave

fibrillin-1
fibrilloflutter
Fibrimage diagnostic imaging agent
fibrin
    f. bodies of pleura
    f. clot
    f. D-dimer
    f. degradation product
    f. formation
    f. gel
    f. glue
    f. monomer (FM)
    f. split product
    f. thrombus
fibrinogen
    f. degradation product
    plasma f.
    radiolabeled f.
fibrinogen-fibrin
    f.-f. conversion syndrome
    f.-f. degradation product
fibrinogenolysis
fibrinohematic material
fibrinoid
    f. arteritis
    f. change
    f. degeneration
    f. necrosis
fibrinolysis
    endogenous f.
fibrinolytic
    f. agent
    F. and Aggrastat ST Elevation
    Resolution (FASTER)
    f. enzyme
    f. medium
    f. reaction
    f. system
    f. therapy
fibrinopeptide
    f. A
    f. B
fibrinopurulent
    f. empyema
    f. phase
fibrinous
    f. acute lobar pneumonia
    f. acute pleuritis
    f. adhesion
    f. bronchitis
    f. exudate

    f. pericarditis
    f. pleurisy
fibrin-specific antibody
fibrin-stabilizing blood coagulation
    factor
Fibriscint
fibroatheroma
fibroblast
    adventitial f.
    f. growth factor (FGF)
    f. growth factor expression
    human fetal lung f. (HFL)
fibrobronchoscope
fibrobullous
fibrocalcification
fibrocalcific lesion
fibrocystic
    f. lung
    f. sarcoidosis
fibroelastoma
    papillary f. (PES)
fibroelastosis
    endocardial f. (EFE)
    endomyocardial f.
    primary endocardial f.
fibrofatty plaque
fibrogenesis
fibroid
    f. heart
    f. lung
    f. phthisis
fibrolipoid plaque
fibroma
fibromuscular dysplasia
fibromusculoelastic lesion
fibronectin
fibroplastic
    f. cardiomyopathy
    f. disease
fibroplastica
    endocarditis parietalis f.
fibroproliferative disease
fibrosa
    intervalvular f.
fibrosarcoma
fibrosclerosis
    familial multifocal f.
fibrosing
    f. alveolitis
    f. mediastinitis

F

NOTES

fibrosis
  adeno-associated virus for cystic f. (AAV-CF)
  African endomyocardial f.
  amiodarone pulmonary f.
  biventricular endomyocardial f.
  bundle-branch f.
  classic interstitial pneumonitis with f. (CIPF)
  cobalt-related pulmonary f.
  cystic f. (CF)
  Davies endomyocardial f.
  Davies myocardial f.
  diffuse interstitial pulmonary f.
  endocardial f.
  endomyocardial f. (EMF)
  endomysial f.
  endoperimysial interstitial f.
  familial pulmonary f.
  focal f.
  hard metal-related lung f.
  idiopathic alveolar f. (IAF)
  idiopathic interstitial f.
  idiopathic pulmonary f. (IPF)
  interstitial f.
  interstitial pulmonary f. (IPF)
  Löffler endocardial f.
  lung f.
  mediastinal f.
  myocardial f.
  nonspecific idiopathic pulmonary f.
  nonspecific lung f.
  parahilar f.
  parenchymal f.
  partial intermixed f.
  periarteriolar f.
  peribronchial f.
  perielectrode f.
  perimyocytic f.
  perimysial f.
  perivascular f.
  progressive interstitial pulmonary f.
  progressive massive f. (PMF)
  pulmonary f.
  radiation f.
  rejection-associated pulmonary f.
  subendocardial f.
  tropical endomyocardial f.
fibrosum
  pericardium f.
fibrosus
  anulus a.
fibrothorax
fibrotic
  f. mass
  f. scar
fibrous
  f. ball

f. body
f. cap
f. cap lesion
f. capsule of thyroid gland
f. dysplasia
f. dysplasia of bone
f. infiltrate
f. mediastinitis
f. pericarditis
f. pericardium
f. plaque
f. pneumonia
f. ring
f. skeleton
f. subaortic stenosis
FIC
  forced inspiratory capacity
Fick
  F. cardiac output
  F. equation
  F. method
  F. oxygen method
  F. principle
  F. relationship
  F. technique
FICO$_2$
  fraction of inspired carbon dioxide
Fiedler myocarditis
field
  f. carcinogenesis
  f. flow velocity
  near f.
  stippling of lung f.
  f. of view (FOV)
FIF
  forced inspiratory flow
fighter
  Flimm F.
fight-or-flight
  f.-o.-f. reaction
  f.-o.-f. response
figure-of-eight
  f.-o.-e. abnormality
  f.-o.-e. heart
  f.-o.-e. intraatrial reentry
  f.-o.-e. suture
filamentous actin (F-actin)
filariasis
Filcard vena cava filter
FILE
  Family Index of Life Events
filiform
  f. pulse
  f. stenosis
filiformis
  pulsus f.
filling
  capillary f.

collateral f.
f. defect
diastolic f.
f. fraction
f. gallop
LAA f.
period of ventricular f.
f. pressure
rapid f.
retrograde f.
f. rumble
ventricular f.

film

absorbable gelatin f.
density-exposure relationship of f.
dirty f.
end-expiratory f.
end-inspiratory f.
f. fixer bath
f. oxygenation
f. processing
Repel-CV bioresorbable adhesion-
barrier f.
scout f.
serial cut f.'s
f. wash bath

filming

serialographic f.

Filmtab

Biaxin F.'s
Rondec F.

Filoviridae virus
filter

arterial f.
bandpass f.
bidirectional four-pole Butterworth
high-pass digital f.
bird's nest f.
bird's nest vena cava f.
BTF-37 arterial blood f.
Butterworth bidirectional f.
CDX Pulmoguard PFT f.
Clear Advantage f.
Clear Advantage Spirometry F.
D/Flex f.
Filcard vena cava f.
Gianturco-Roehm bird's nest vena
cava f.
Greenfield f.
Greenfield IVC f.
Greenfield vena cava f.
Hamming-Hahn f.

heparin arterial f.
Interface arterial blood f.
Jostra arterial blood f.
Kim-Ray Greenfield antiembolus f.
Kim-Ray Greenfield caval f.
KoKo Moe PF/spirometry f.
K-37 pediatric arterial blood f.
LeukoNet F.
low-pass f.
mediastinal sump f.
Millipore f.
Mobin-Uddin vena cava f.
MultiSPIRO Clear Advantage
pulmonary function f.
nitinol f.
Re/Flex f.
Simon nitinol f.
Simon nitinol inferior vena cava f.
Simon nitinol IVC f.
Swank high-flow arterial blood f.
temporary f.
third-order Butterworth f.
triple-bandpass f.
umbrella f.
vena cava f.
Vena Tech LGM f.
Vitalograph Bacterial/Viral F.
Wiener f.
William Harvey arterial blood f.

filtered

f. atrial rate interval (FARI)
f. QRS complex

filtering

four-pole Butterworth f.

FilterLine circuit
FilterWatch Sensor
filtragometry
filtration

extracorporeal membrane
differential f.
x-ray beam f.

FIM

functional independence measure

final

f. common pathway
f. rapid repolarization

Finapres

F. blood pressure monitor
F. finger cuff
F. technique

finder

lumen f.

F

NOTES

fine-needle
>f.-n. aspiration (FNA)
>f.-n. aspiration biopsy

Finesse
>F. cardiac device
>F. guiding catheter

finger
>clubbing of f.'s
>f. cuff
>f. dilation
>f. oximetry
>F. Phantom pulse oximeter testing system
>f. photoplethysmographic device

finger-in-glove appearance
fingernail
>watch-crystal f.

fingerprint
>f. edema

FingerPrint handheld pulse oximeter
finned pacemaker lead
Finney mask
Finochietto
>F. forceps
>F. retractor
>F. rib spreader

Finochietto-Geissendorfer rib retractor
FIO$_2$
>fractional inspired oxygen concentration
>fraction of inspired oxygen

firing
>laser f.

first
>f. effort
>f. heart sound (S$_1$)
>f. obtuse marginal artery (OM-1)
>f. pass view
>f. Response manual resuscitator
>f. shock count

first-degree
>f.-d. A-V block
>f.-d. heart block

first-effort angina
first-line therapy
first-night effect
first-order kinetics
first-pass
>f.-p. radionuclide angiocardiography
>f.-p. radionuclide angiography
>f.-p. technique

first-phase tilt
FirstSave
>F. automated external defibrillator
>F. STAR biphasic AED

first-third filling fraction
Fischer
>F. & Paykel HC100 heated humidifier

>F. pneumothoracic needle
>F. sign
>F. symptom

Fischl index
FISH
>fluorescence in situ hybridization
>fluorescent in situ hybridization

fish
>f. meal lung
>f. oil

Fisher
>F. Micro-capillary Tube Reader
>F. murmur

Fisher-Paykel MR290 water-feed chamber
fishhook lead
fish-meal worker's lung disease
fish-mouth
>f.-m. cusp
>f.-m. incision
>f.-m. mitral stenosis

fishnet pattern
fish-scaling effect
F$_2$-isoprostane
fissura
>f. horizontalis pulmonis dextri
>f. obliqua pulmonis

fissure
>azygos f.
>horizontal f.
>inferior accessory f.
>f. of lung
>major f.
>minor f.
>oblique f.
>plaque f.
>f. sign
>sphenoidal f.
>Sylvian f.
>tissue f.

fissuring
>plaque f.

fist percussion
fistula, pl. **fistulae, fistulas**
>aortocaval f.
>arteriovenous f. (AVF)
>A-V Gore-Tex f.
>BP f.
>brachioaxillary bridge graft f.
>brachiosubclavian bridge graft f.
>Brescia-Cimino A-V f.
>bronchopleural f.
>bronchopulmonary f.
>bronchopulmonary venous f.
>bronchovenous f.
>cameral f.
>carotid-cavernous f. (CCF)
>Cimino-Brescia arteriovenous f.

congenital pulmonary
arteriovenous f.
coronary artery f. (CAF, CAP)
coronary artery-right ventricular f.
coronary-pulmonary f. (C-PF)
Eck f.
enteric f.
Gore-Tex AF f.
gross tracheoesophageal f.
H-type tracheoesophageal f.
pancreaticopleural f.
pancreatopleural f.
pleurodural f.
pleuroesophageal f.
pulmonary arteriovenous f.
renal f.
silent coronary artery f.
solitary pulmonary arteriovenous f.
spontaneous closure of f.
subclavian arteriovenous f.
T-E f.
tracheoesophageal f. (TEF)
traumatic f.

fistulae
esophagorespiratory f.
fistulous opening
Fitch obturator
fitness
biological f.
cardiovascular f.
Fitzgerald forceps
FIVC
forced inspiratory vital capacity
five-chamber view
fixation
complex f. (CF)
f. mechanism
fixative
Saccomanno f.
fixed
f. airflow obstruction
f. coupling
f. orifice resistor
f. perfusion defect
f. rate pulse generator
fixed-pressure CPAP
fixed-rate
f.-r. mode
f.-r. pacemaker
f.-r. perfusion defect
f.-r. pulse generator

fixed-wire
f.-w. balloon
f.-w. balloon dilatation system
f.-w. coronary balloon catheter
fixer bath
FK-506
FL
flow limitation
fL
femtoliter
FL4 guide
flabby airway
Flack node
flagella
flagellar
Flagyl Oral
flail
f. chest
f. chorda
f. leaflet
f. mitral valve
f. segment
FLAIR
fluid-attenuated inversion recovery
FLAIR image
flame emission spectroscopy (FES)
flame-shaped hemorrhage
Flantadin
flap
Abbe f.
Eloesser f.
intimal f.
intraluminal f.
Linton f.
liver f.
microvascular free f.
pericardial f.
subclavian f.
f. tracheostomy
flapping
f. sound
f. tremor
f. valve syndrome
flare
asthma f.
wheal and f.
flaring
alar f.
nasal f.
flash
f. MRI
F. portable spirometer

NOTES

F

flash *(continued)*
  f. pulmonary edema
  f. sequence
flashlamp excited pulsed dye
flashlamp-pulsed Nd:YAG laser
flask-shaped heart
flat
  f. diastolic slope
  f. wire coil stent
flattening
  T wave f.
flavonoid
flavus
  Aspergillus f.
flax-dresser's disease
Flaxedil
flea-bitten kidney
flecainide
fleeting infiltrate
Fleet Phospho-Soda
Fleischmann bursa
Fleischner
  F. lines
  F. syndrome
Fleisch pneumotachograph
Fleming
  fibrillar mass of F.
Fletcher factor
Flex
  F. stent
  F. Tip guidewire
Flexguard Tip catheter
Flexguide intubation guide
flexibility
flexible
  f. balloon-tipped catheter
  f. coil stent
  f. fiberoptic bronchoscope
  f. fiberoptic bronchoscopy (FFB)
  f. guidewire
  f. stent
Flexicath silicone subclavian cannula
flexion
  elbow f.
  hip f.
  shoulder horizontal f.
  trunk forward f.
FlexStent
  Cook F.
Flexxicon Blue dialysis catheter
flicker fusion threshold
flight
  time of f. (TOF)
Flimm Fighter
flint disease
Flint murmur

flip
  f. angle
  LDH f.
flipped T wave
flitter
floating
  f. lead
  f. wall motion study
flock-worker's lung
Flolan injection
FloMap
  F. guidewire
  F. velocimeter
Flonase
flooding
  alveolar f.
floppy
  f. guidewire
  f. mitral valve (FMV)
  f. valve syndrome
floppy-tipped guidewire
flora
  gastrointestinal f.
  mixed f.
  oral f.
  respiratory f.
  tracheobronchial f.
Flo-Rester vascular occluder
Florex medical compression stockings
florid
  f. congestive heart failure
  f. pulmonary edema
Florinef Acetate
FloSeal Matrix hemostatic sealant
flosequinan
  F. ACE Inhibitor Trial (FACET)
flotation catheter
Flo-Thru shunt
flour
  refined f.
Flovent
  F. aerosol
  F. diskus
  F. Rotadisk
flow
  f. acceleration
  accessory pulmonary blood f.
    (APBF)
  f. across orifice
  active Doppler f.
  adequate blood f.
  aliasing f.
  annular f.
  antegrade diastolic f.
  anterograde f.
  aortic f.
  aortic ductal f.
  arterial blood f.

f. artifact
f. augmentation
blood f.
blunted f.
blunted systolic pulmonary
 venous f.
cerebral blood f. (CBF)
collateral f.
f. controller
f. convergence method
coronary blood f. (CBF)
coronary sinus blood f. (CSBF)
disturbed f.
Doppler color f.
effective renal blood f. (ERBF)
endocardial f.
f. envelope
epicardial f.
expiratory tidal f.
faint f.
forced expiratory f. (FEF)
forced inspiratory f. (FIF)
forced midexpiratory f. (FMF)
forearm blood f.
great cardiac vein f. (GCVF)
hepatofugal f.
hepatopetal f.
high f. (HF)
holodiastolic f.
infradiaphragmatic venous f.
f. injector
isovolume f.
laminar blood f.
limb blood f.
f. limitation (FL)
f. mapping
f. mapping technique
maximal forced expiratory f.
 (FEFmax)
maximal midexpiratory f. (MMEF,
 MMF)
mean forced midexpiratory f.
mean inspiratory f. (MIF)
myocardial blood f. (MBF)
pansystolic f.
peak cough f. (PCF)
peak expiratory f. (PEF)
peak inspiratory f. (PIF)
peak tidal expiratory f. (PTEF)
peak tidal inspiratory f. (PTIF)
percent predicted peak expiratory f.
 (%PEF)

perigraft f.
petal-fugal f.
pressure-compensated f.
f. profile
pulmonary blood f.
pulmonary venous f. (PVF)
pulsatile f.
f. rate
f. ratio (Qp/Qs)
ratio of tidal expiratory flow at
 25% of tidal volume and peak
 tidal expiratory f. (TEF_{25}/PTEF)
regional cerebral blood f. (rCBF)
regional myocardial blood f.
 (RMBF)
renal cortical blood f. (RCBF)
renal plasma f. (RPF)
f. reserve
F. Rider flow-directed catheter
splanchnic blood f.
systemic blood f. (SBF)
thrombolysis in myocardial
 infarction f.
tidal f.
time to peak expiratory f. (tPTEF)
time to peak inspiratory f. (tPTIF)
TIMI f.
transvalvular f.
tricuspid valve f.
f. velocity
f. volume curve
f. volume loop
vortex f.
f. wire
Wright peak f.
flow-assisted
 f.-a., short-term (FAST)
 f.-a., short-term balloon catheter
flow-directed
 f.-d. balloon cardiovascular catheter
 f.-d. end-hole catheter
FloWire
 Doppler F.
 F. Doppler guidewire
 F. guidewire
flow-limiting stenosis
flow-mediated
 f.-m. dilation (FMD)
 f.-m. vasodilation
flowmeter (*See also* meter)
 Airmed mini-Wright peak f.
 AirZone peak f.

F

NOTES

flowmeter *(continued)*
    asmaPLAN+ peak f.
    Assess peak f.
    Astech peak f.
    Asthma Check peak f.
    AsthmaMentor peak f.
    blood f.
    Doppler ultrasonic f.
    FM color-coded f.
    FME color-coded f.
    Gould electromagnetic f.
    laser Doppler f.
    MultiSPIRO The Peak peak f.
    Narcomatic f.
    Parks 800 bidirectional Doppler f.
    peak f. (PFM)
    Periflux PF 1 D blood-f.
    Personal Best peak f.
    PocketPeak peak f.
    SensorMedics Mass Flow Sensor
      heated wire f.
    SPIR-O-FLOW peak f.
    The PEAK peak f.
    Thorpe f.
    Transonic f.
    TruZone peak f.
    Wright peak f.
    Youlten nasal inspiratory peak f.
flowmetry
    laser-Doppler f.
    magnetic resonance f. (MRF)
    pulsed Doppler f.
**FlowMinder oxygen flow and treatment
card**
flow-responsive remodeling
flow-sensing
    f.-s. pneumotachograph
    f.-s. spirometer
flow-time registration
Flowtron
    F. DVT pump
    F. DVT pump system
flow-volume
    tidal breathing f.-v. (TBFV)
Floxin
    F. injection
    F. Oral
floxuridine
Floyd loop cannula
FLU
    flunisolide
flucloxacillin
fluconazole
flucytosine
Fludara
fludrocortisone acetate
fluens
    pulsus f.

FLUENT
    Fluvastatin Long-Term Extension Trial
fluffy
    f. alveolar infiltrate
    f. cotton-wool exudate
fluffy-cuffed tube
Flu-Glow strip
fluid
    f. aspiration
    bronchoalveolar lavage f. (BALF)
    crystalloid f.
    f. dynamics
    epithelial lining f. (ELF)
    interstitial f.
    f. mechanics
    pericardial f.
    periciliary f.
    pleural f.
    respiratory tract lining f. (RTLF)
    retained lung f. (RLF)
    f. shift
    f. therapy
    vesicular f.
    viscoelastic f.
fluid-attenuated
    f.-a. inversion recovery (FLAIR)
    f.-a. inversion recovery image
fluid-filled
    f.-f. balloon cardiovascular catheter
    f.-f. balloon-tipped flow-directed
      catheter
    f.-f. catheter
    f.-f. pigtail catheter
    f.-f. pressure monitoring guidewire
fluidic circuit
Flu-Imune
fluindione
Fluitran
fluke
    lung f.
Flumadine Oral
flumazenil
FluMist
flunarizine
flunisolide (FLU)
flunitrazepam
Fluogen
fluorescein angiography
fluorescence
    f. antimembrane antibody (FAMA,
      FAMAT)
    f. bronchoscopy
    laser-induced arterial f. (LIAF)
    f. polarization
    f. in situ hybridization (FISH)
    f. spectroscopy
    f. treponemal antibody absorption
      (FTA-ABS)

f. treponemal antibody absorption test
fluorescence-activated cell sorter (FACS)
fluorescence-guided smart laser
fluoride
hydrogen f.
f. toxicity
fluorine-18
f. fluorodeoxyglucose (F-18 FDG)
fluorocarbon poisoning
5-fluorocytosine
fluorodeoxyglucose (FDG)
cyclotron-produced F-18 f.
fluorine-18 f. (F-18 FDG)
fluoro-2-deoxyglucose
2-fluoro-2-deoxyglucose
18-fluorodeoxyglucose
technetium-99-m-tetrofosmin/fluorine 18-f.
fluorodeoxyuridine (FUDR)
fluorodopamine positron emission tomographic scanning
Fluoro-Free
P.A.S. Port F.-F.
fluorogenic
fluorography
spot-film f.
fluorohydrocortisone
fluorometry
Fluoropassiv thin-wall carotid patch
Fluoroplex Topical
FluoroPlus
F. angiography
F. Cardiac
F. Roadmapper
fluoroquinolone
fluoroscopic
f. guidance
f. isthmus ablation
f. visualization
fluoroscopy
biplane f.
C-arm f.
kV f.
Fluoro Tip cannula
fluorouracil
5-fluorouracil (5-FU)
Fluosol artificial blood
Fluotec vaporizer
fluoxetine hydrochloride
fluoxymesterone
flurazepam

flush
f. aortogram
f. aortography
f. and bathe technique
heparin f.
mahogany f.
malar f.
f. technique
warm heparinized saline f.
flushed
aspirated and f.
flushing time
flutamide
fluticasone
f. propionate (FP)
f. propionate inhalation powder
f. propionate and salmeterol inhalation powder
Flutter
flutter
atrial f.
auricular f.
f. chest percussion device
clockwise f.
completely positive deflection f.
counterclockwise f.
f. cycle length
f. device
diaphragmatic f.
dominant positive deflection f.
impure f.
inferior-axis f.
isthmus-dependent atrial f.
mediastinal f.
F. mucus clearance device
pure f.
f. R interval
F. therapeutic device
ventricular f.
f. wave
flutter-fibrillation
f.-f. waves
fluvastatin
F. Long-Term Extension Trial (FLUENT)
f. sodium
f. sodium 80 mg
Fluviral
flux
soldering f.
transmembrane calcium f.
fluxionary hyperemia

NOTES

F

Fluzone
fly ash
flying W sign
Flynt needle
FM
  fibrin monomer
    FM color-coded flowmeter
FMA cardiovascular imaging system
FMD
  flow-mediated dilation
FME color-coded flowmeter
FMF
  forced midexpiratory flow
FMIV
  forced mandatory intermittent ventilation
fMRI
  functional magnetic resonance imaging
FMV
  floppy mitral valve
FNA
  fine-needle aspiration
FO
  forced oscillation
foam
  f. cell
  polyurethane f.
  f. stability test
foamy
  f. macrophage
  f. myocardial cell
FOB
  fiberoptic bronchoscopy
focal
  f. adhesion kinase (FAK)
  f. atrial fibrillation
  f. block
  f. bronchopneumonia
  f. dilatation catheter
  f. eccentric stenosis
  f. edema
  f. emphysema
  f. fibrosis
  f. media aplasia
  f. motion abnormality
  f. myocytosis of heart
  f. vasospasm
  f. ventricular dysfunction
focal-dust emphysema
FocalSeal
  F. liquid sealant
  F. surgical sealant
FocalSeal-L surgical sealant
focus, pl. foci
  arrhythmia f.
  Assmann f.
  Ghon f.

Kampmeier foci
Simon foci
Focus Angioplasty Catheter Technology (FACT-22)
Focustent coronary stent
Foerger airway
Foerster forceps
Fogarty
  F. adherent clot catheter
  F. calibrator
  F. embolectomy catheter
  F. forceps
  F. graft thrombectomy catheter
  F. spring clip
Fogarty-Chin extrusion balloon catheter
Foix-Cavany-Marie syndrome
fold
  bulboventricular f.
  Marshall f.
  pleuroperitoneal f.
  Rindfleisch f.
  vestibular f.
  vestigial f.
folded-lung syndrome
Folex PFS
folic acid
follicular
  f. bronchiectasis
  f. bronchiolitis
  f. pharyngitis
Foltz-Overton cardiac catheter
Fome-Cuf tracheostomy tube
fomivirsen
Fontain classification
Fontan
  F. atriopulmonary anastomosis
  F.-Baudet procedure
  F. circulation
  F. connection
  F. conversion
  F.-Kreutzer procedure
  F. modification of Norwood procedure
  F. operation
  F. procedure
  F. repair
  F. right atrium
FOOD
  Feed or Ordinary Diet
  FOOD clinical trial
food
  f. angina
  f. asthma
  sodium content of f.
  whole-grain f.
foot
  f. cradle
  superficial medial artery of f.

trash f.
f. ulcer
footprint of transducer
Foradil
foramen, pl. **foramina**
bulboventricular f.
f. diaphragmatis sellae
Galen f.
interventricular f.
Lannelongue f.
f. of Luschka
f. of Monro
f. of Morgagni
oval f.
f. ovale
f. quadratum
f. rotundum
round f.
f. secundum
thebesian foramina
f. of veins of heart
vena caval f.
f. venae cavae
f. venarum minimarum atria dextri
force
atrial ejection f.
F. balloon
F. balloon dilatation catheter
drag f.
extrinsic f.
left ventricular f.
life f.
peak twitch f.
P terminal f.
shear f.
Starling f.
Venturi f.
forced
f. beat
f. cycle
f. expiratory capacity (FEC)
f. expiratory flow (FEF)
f. expiratory maneuver
f. expiratory spirogram (FES)
f. expiratory technique
f. expiratory time (FET)
f. expiratory volume (FEV)
f. expiratory volume in 1 second (FEV$_1$)
f. expiratory volume in 1 second to forced vital capacity ratio (FEV$_1$/FVC)

f. expiratory volume timed to forced capacity ratio
f. expiratory volume timed to forced vital capacity ratio (FEV/FVC)
f. inspiratory capacity (FIC)
f. inspiratory flow (FIF)
f. inspiratory vital capacity (FIVC)
f. ischemia-reperfusion transition
f. mandatory intermittent ventilation (FMIV)
f. midexpiratory flow (FMF)
f. oscillation (FO)
f. oscillation technique (FOT)
f. respiration
f. vital capacity (FVC)
f. vital capacity analysis (FVCA)
force-frequency relation
force-generating capacity
force-length relation
forceps
Adson f.
Adson arterial f.
Babcock thoracic tissue-holding f.
Barraya f.
Bengolea f.
biopsy f.
bipolar coagulating f.
Bloodwell f.
Boettcher f.
bronchus-grasping f.
Brown-Adson f.
Bycep biopsy f.
Carmalt f.
coagulation f.
Cook flexible biopsy f.
Cooley f.
Cooley-Baumgarten aortic f.
Craafoord pulmonary f.
Craafoord-Sellor hemostatic f.
Crile-Duval lung-grasping f.
Cushing f.
DeBakey arterial f.
DeBakey Atraugrip f.
DeBakey-Colovira-Rumel thoracic f.
DeBakey-Derra anastomosis f.
DeBakey-Diethrich coronary artery f.
DeBakey-Mixter thoracic f.
DeBakey-Péan cardiovascular f.
DeBakey tissue f.
Duracep biopsy f.

NOTES

F

forceps *(continued)*
　　Duval-Crile lung f.
　　Duval lung-grasping f.
　　Englert f.
　　Finochietto f.
　　Fitzgerald f.
　　Foerster f.
　　Fogarty f.
　　Foss cardiovascular f.
　　Fraenkel f.
　　Gemini thoracic f.
　　Gerald f.
　　Gerbode f.
　　Harken f.
　　Hopkins f.
　　Iselin f.
　　Julian thoracic f.
　　Kahler bronchial biopsy f.
　　Magill f.
　　mammary-coronary tissue f.
　　McQuigg-Mixter bronchial f.
　　Mount-Mayfield f.
　　National Institutes of Health mitral valve-grasping f.
　　NIH mitral valve-grasping f.
　　Pilling Weck Y-stent f.
　　Potts bronchial f.
　　Price-Thomas bronchial f.
　　renal artery f.
　　Ruel f.
　　Rugelski arterial f.
　　Rumel thoracic f.
　　Sam Roberts bronchial biopsy f.
　　Samuels f.
　　Scheinmann laryngeal f.
　　Scholten biopsy f.
　　Scholten endomyocardial bioptome and biopsy f.
　　Tuttle thoracic f.
　　Varco thoracic f.
force-velocity-length relation
force-velocity relation
force-velocity-volume relation
Ford equation
forearm blood flow
Foregger
　　F. laryngoscope
　　F. rigid esophagoscope
foregut
foreign
　　f. body
　　f. body aspiration
ForeRunner
　　F. automatic external defibrillator device
　　F. coronary sinus guiding catheter
　　F. defibrillator
foreshortening

fork
　　f. stent
　　f. stenting technique
Forlanini treatment
form
　　Cardioscan standardized evaluation f.
　　M pattern on right atrial wave f.
　　myocardial infarction in dumbbell f.
　　pentamidine in aerosol f.
　　wave f.
formaldehyde
format
　　quad screen f.
　　scanning f.
formation
　　aspergilloma f.
　　coagulum f.
　　fibrin f.
　　hyaline membrane f.
　　impulse f.
　　rouleaux f.
forme fruste
formicans
　　pulsus f.
formicant pulse
formononetin
formoterol fumarate
formula, pl. **formulas, formulae**
　　Bayer Select Pain Relief F.
　　Bazett f.
　　Bazett correction f.
　　biplane f.
　　Bohr f.
　　Brozek f.
　　Cannon f.
　　Devereux f.
　　Framingham f.
　　Fridericia f.
　　Friedewald f.
　　Ganz f.
　　geometric cube f.
　　Gorland f.
　　Gorlin f.
　　Gorlin hydraulic f.
　　Hakki f.
　　Hamilton-Stewart f.
　　heart rate correction f.
　　Impact specialized feeding f.
　　Janz f.
　　f. of Mirsky
　　Penn f.
　　Poiseuille resistance f.
　　Sramek f.
　　Teichholz f.
　　Triaminic AM Decongestant F.

Vicks Formula 44 Pediatric F.
Yeager f.
formulation
Sicilian Gambit f.
Forney syndrome
Forrester
F. syndrome
F. Therapeutic Classification grades
I–IV
forskolin
adenylate cyclase stimulator f.
Fortaz
Forte
Aristocort F.
Enduronyl F.
Robinul F.
fortis
pulsus f.
Fortovase
fortuitum
Mycobacterium f.
fortuitum-chelonel
Mycobacterium f.-c.
forward
f. conduction
f. flow of velocity
f. heart failure
f. pressure waveform
f. stroke volume (FSV)
f. triangle method
f. triangle technique
foscarnet
Foscavir injection
Fos **gene**
fosinopril
f. sodium
F. Versus Amlodipine
Cardiovascular Events Randomized
Trial (FACET)
fosinoprilat
fosinoprilic acid
FOSQ
Functional Outcomes of Sleep
Questionnaire
fossa, pl. **fossae**
antecubital f.
canine f.
Claudius f.
Gerdy hyoid f.
f. glandulae lacrimalis
Malgaigne f.

f. ovalis
supraclavicular f.
Foss cardiovascular forceps
FOT
forced oscillation technique
Fothergill disease
founder effect
four-beam laser Doppler probe
four-chamber view
four-day syndrome
four-hour scan
Fourier
F. analysis of electrocardiogram
F. series analysis
F. transform
F. transform analysis
F. two-dimensional imaging
Fourier-acquired steady-state technique
(FAST)
four-legged cage valve
Fourmentin thoracic index
Fournier gangrene
four-phase Lifestick CPR
four-pole Butterworth filtering
fourth-generation cephalosporin
fourth heart sound (S$_4$)
FOV
field of view
fovea
f. articularis inferior atlantis
f. articularis superior atlantis
f. costalis inferior
f. costalis processus transversi
f. costalis superior
f. dentis atlantis
foveated chest
Fowler
F. single-breath test
F. solution
F. thoracoplasty
Fox green dye
FP
fluticasone propionate
FR139317
F. endothelin A receptor antagonist
Fr
French
fractal
fraction
basilar half ejection f.
blunted ejection f.
CPK-MB f.

NOTES

fraction *(continued)*
    ejection f. (EF)
    f. of expired carbon dioxide
      ($FECO_2$)
    filling f.
    first-third filling f.
    global ejection f.
    global left ventricular ejection f.
    f. of inspired carbon dioxide
      ($FICO_2$)
    f. of inspired oxygen (FIO_2)
    intrapulmonary shunt f. (Q_s/Q_t,
      Qs/Qt)
    left ventricular ejection f. (LVEF)
    light pen-determined ejection f.
    MB f.
    oxygen extraction f. (OEF)
    physiologic dead space f.
    physiologic shunt f.
    regurgitant f.
    rest ejection f.
    right ventricular ejection f. (RVEF)
    shortening f.
    Teichholz ejection f.
    ventriculogram-derived ejection f.
    ventriculographic ejection f.

fractional
    f. area change (FAC)
    f. flow reserve (FFR)
    f. inspired oxygen concentration
      (FIO_2)
    f. myocardial shortening
    f. shortening
    f. velocity reserve (FVR)

fractionation
    electrogram f.

fracture
    anterior rib f.
    cough f.
    double-rib f.
    J retention wire f.
    lead f.
    outlet strut f. (OSF)
    pacemaker lead f.
    plaque f.
    posterior rib f.
    rib f.
    sternal f.

Fraenkel
    F. forceps
    F. node
    F. pneumococcus

fragilis
    Bacteroides f.

fragment
    f. antigen-binding
    antimyosin Fab f.

    antimyosin monoclonal antibody
      with Fab f. (AMA-Fab)
    catheter f.
    crosslinked D f.
    Digibind digoxin immune Fab f.'s
    Digidote digoxin immune Fab f.'s
    Fab f.

fragmentation
    f. myocarditis
    f. of myocardium
    sleep f.

Fragmin
    F. dalteparin sodium injection
    F. During Instability in Coronary
      Artery Disease (FRISC)

frame
    B-scan f.
    Elgiloy f.

Framingham
    F. equation
    F. formula
    F. heart failure criteria
    F. Heart Study (FHS)
    F. risk index

Francisella tularensis

Frank
    F. ECG lead placement system
    F. XYZ orthogonal lead
    F. XYZ orthogonal lead system

frank blood

Frankel treatment

Frank-Starling
    F.-S. curve
    F.-S. law
    F.-S. mechanism
    F.-S. reserve

Frank-Straub-Wiggers-Starling principle

Fräntzel murmur

Franzen needle guide

**Franz monophasic action potential
  catheter**

frappage

Fraser Harlake respirometer

Frater
    F. intracardiac retractor
    F. suture

Fraunhofer zone

FRC
    functional reserve capacity
    functional residual capacity

Frederick pneumothorax needle

Fredrickson
    F. classification
    F. dyslipidemia
    F. hyperlipoproteinemia
      classification
    F., Levy and Lees classification

free
- f. fatty acids (FFA)
- f. radical
- f. root
- f. thyrotoxin index
- f. wall

free-beam laser
free-breathing coronary magnetic resonance angiography
freedom
- Accu-Chek II F.
- F. coronary stent
- F. Force coronary stent

FreeDop
- F. cordless Doppler
- F. portable Doppler unit

free-floating
- f.-f. thrombus (FFT)
- f.-f. vena caval thrombus

free-flowing empyema
freeing up of adhesion
free-radical scavenger
Freestyle
- F. aortic root bioprosthesis
- F. bioprosthetic heart valve
- F. stentless aortic heart valve

free-wall accessory pathway
Freeway Lite portable aerosol compressor
Freezor cryocatheter
Freitag stent
frémissement cattaire
fremitus
- auditory f.
- bronchial f.
- friction f.
- hydatid f.
- pectoral f.
- pericardial f.
- pleural f.
- rhonchal f.
- subjective f.
- tactile f.
- tussive f.
- vocal f.

French (F, Fr)
- Angio-Seal 6 F.
- F. double-lumen catheter
- F. JR4 Schneider catheter
- F. paradox
- F. SAL catheter
- F. scale
- F. shaft catheter
- F. sheath
- F. size
- F. sizing of catheter

Frenchay
- F. Activities Index
- F. Aphasia Screening Test (FAST)

frequency
- breathing f. (BF)
- ciliary beat f.
- critical flicker f.
- f. domain imaging
- dynamic f. response
- fundamental f.
- Larmor f.
- natural f.
- pulse repetition f. (PRF)
- resonant f.
- respiratory f. (f)
- f. response
- f. shifter
- f. to tidal volume (f/V_t)
- f. tracer

frequency-domain analysis
frequens
- pulsus f.

frequent spontaneous premature complex
fresh frozen plasma (FFP)
Fresnel zone
Freund
- F. anomaly
- F. operation

freundii
- *Citrobacter f.*

Frey-Sauerbruch rib shears
friability
- eggshell f.

friable wall
friction
- f. fremitus
- f. murmur
- f. rub
- f. sound

Fridericia formula
Friedewald
- F. approximation
- F. equation
- F. formula

Friedländer
- F. bacillus
- F. bacillus pneumonia

F

NOTES

Friedländer *(continued)*
    F. disease
    F. pneumobacillus
    F. pneumonia
Friedman Splint brace
Friedreich
    F. ataxia
    F. disease
    F. sign
Friedrich rib elevator
FRISC
    Fast Revascularization During Instability
    in Coronary Artery Disease
    Fragmin During Instability in Coronary
    Artery Disease
      FRISC clinical trial
      FRISC II clinical trial
frog breathing
froissement
    bruit de f.
frolement
    bruit de f.
frond
    papillary f.
    sea f.
frontal axis
front wall needle
frosted heart
frosting heart
Frostline linear cryoablation system
frothy sputum
frottement
    bruit de f.
Frouin
    quadrangulation of F.
frozen thorax
FRP
    functional refractory period
fructosamine
Frumil
frusemide
fruste
    forme f.
frustrate systole
FS-069 contrast agent
FSV
    forward stroke volume
fsw
    feet of sea water
FTA-ABS
    fluorescence treponemal antibody
     absorption
    fluorescent treponemal antibody
     absorption
      FTA-ABS test
fTCD
    functional transcranial Doppler
     sonography

FTQ
    Fagerstrom tolerance questionnaire
5-FU
    5-fluorouracil
fucose residue
fucosidosis
FUDR
    fluorodeoxyuridine
fugax
    amaurosis partialis f.
Fugl-Meyer Scale for motor test
Fujinon
    F. flexible bronchoscope
    F. variceal injector
Fukunaga-Hayes unbiased jackknife
    classification
fulguration
    electrical f.
full
    f. caloric density
    f. compensatory pause
    f. PSG
Fuller bivalve trach tube
fuller's earth pneumoconiosis
FullFlow catheter
full-thickness linear lesion
fully automatic pacemaker
fulminans
    purpura f.
fulminant myocarditis
fumagillin
fumarate
    bisoprolol f.
    clemastine f.
    ferrous f.
    formoterol f.
    ibutilide f.
Fumasorb
Fumerin
fumes
    cadmium f.
    cadmium oxide f.
    cobalt f.
    metallic oxide f.
    soldering f.
fumigatus
    Aspergillus f.
function
    atrial transport f.
    auto-threshold f.
    battery cell voltage f.
    bellows f.
    cardiac f.
    cardiovascular f.
    contractile f.
    f. curve
    depressed ventricular f.
    diastolic f.

dopaminergic f.
exercise LV f.
global left ventricular f.
hepatic f.
intramyocardial f.
left atrial appendage f.
left ventricular f.
left ventricular systolic/diastolic f.
lung f.
mechanical contractile f.
mitochondrial f.
myocardial f.
neurohormonal f.
parasympathetic f.
perturbed autonomic nervous
  system f.
phagocytic f.
preserved left ventricular systolic f.
probability density f. (PDF)
pulmonary f. (PF)
pump f.
renal f.
respiratory f.
resting systolic f.
right ventricular f.
sigh f.
sinus node f.
stress perfusion and rest f.
systolic f.
valvular f.
ventilatory f.
ventricular f.

functional
  f. aerobic impairment (FAI)
  f. assessment
  f. block
  f. capacity classification
  f. cardiovascular disease
  f. conduction period (FCP)
  f. congestion
  f. dyspnea
  f. failure to capture
  f. image
  f. imaging
  f. independence measure (FIM)
  f. magnetic resonance imaging
  (fMRI)
  f. magnetic stimulation
  f. mitral regurgitation
  f. MRI
  f. murmur

F. Outcomes of Sleep
  Questionnaire (FOSQ)
f. pacing abnormality
f. pain
f. pulmonary atresia
f. recovery
f. refractory period (FRP)
f. reserve capacity (FRC)
f. residual air
f. residual capacity (FRC)
f. status
f. subtraction
f. transcranial Doppler sonography
  (fTCD)
f. undersensing

functionalism
fundamental
  f. frequency
  f. imaging (FI)
fundi (*pl. of* fundus)
fundoplication
  Belsey Mark II, IV f.
  Belsey two-thirds wrap f.
  Collis-Nissen f.
  Nissen f. (NF)
  Nissen 360-degree wrap f.
  Rossetti modification of Nissen f.
funduliformis
  Bacillus f.
  Bacteroides f.
fundus, pl. **fundi**
funduscopic examination
fungal
  f. endocarditis
  f. infection
fungating mass
fungi (*pl. of* fungus)
Fungizone Intravenous
fungoides
  mycosis f.
fungus, pl. **fungi**
  f. ball
funic
  f. pulse
  f. souffle
funnel
  f. chest
  f. dynamics
  mitral f.
  vascular f.
Furadantin
Furalan

F

NOTES

Furan
Furanite
furcosus
    Bacteroides f.
furifosmin
Furman Type II electrogram
furoate
    mometasone f.
furosemide
Furoside
furrier's
    f. lung
    f. lung disease
furrow
    atrioventricular f.
    Schmorl f.
Fusarium
    F. solani
    F. vasinfectum
fused commissure
fused-tip catheter
fusidic acid

fusiform
    f. aortic aneurysm
    f. bronchiectasis
fusion
    f. beat
    commissural f.
    f. complex
    critical flicker f.
    entrainment with concealed f.
    fusion QRS
Fusobacterium
    F. necrophorum
    F. nucleatum
f/V$_t$
    frequency to tidal volume
FVC
    forced vital capacity
FVCA
    forced vital capacity analysis
FVR
    fractional velocity reserve

G
   cathepsin G.
G₂
   prostaglandin G.
3G4
G5
   G5 massage and percussion
      machine
   G5 Neocussor percussor
Ga
   gallium
⁶⁸Ga
   gallium-68
GABA
   gamma-aminobutyric acid
Gabriel Tucker tube
Gad hypothesis
gadodiamide
gadolinium chelate
gadolinium-diethylenetriamine pentaacetic
   acid (gadolinium-DTPA, Gd-DTPA)
gadolinium-DTPA
   gadolinium-diethylenetriamine
      pentaacetic acid
Gaertner (var. of Gärtner)
Gaffky scale
gag
   g. gene
   g. reflex
Gailliard syndrome
gain
   g. control
   time-compensated g.
   time compensation g. (TCG)
   time-varied g. (TVG)
Gairdner disease
Gaisböck syndrome
gait
   ataxic g.
gaiter perforator
galactophlebitis
galactose
galactosidase deficiency
Galanti-Giusti colorimetric method
Galaxy pacemaker
Galen foramen
Galileo intravascular radiotherapy
   system
GALILEO ventilator
Gallagher bipolar mapping probe
gallamine triethiodide
Gallavardin
   G. murmur
   G. phenomenon
gallbladder disease

gallinatum
   pectus g.
gallium (Ga)
   g.-67
   g.-67 imaging
   g.-67 scan
   g.-67 scintigraphy
   g.-68 (⁶⁸Ga)
   g. imaging
   radiolabeled g.
   g. scan
gallop
   atrial g.
   atrial diastolic g.
   diastolic g.
   filling g.
   presystolic g.
   protodiastolic g.
   g. rhythm
   S₃ g.
   S₄ g.
   S₇ g.
   g. sound
   summation g. (S₇)
   systolic g.
gallopamil
galop
   bruit de g.
GALT
   gut-associated lymphoid tissue
galvanometer
   Einthoven string g.
gambiense
   Trypanosoma g.
Gambro
   G. Lundia Minor hemodialyzer
   G. oxygenator
Gamimune N
gamma
   g. globulin
   g. hydroxybutyrate (GHB)
   g. knife
   g. radiation
   g. radiation therapy system
   g. ray
   g. scintillation camera
gamma-aminobutyric acid (GABA)
gamma-1b
   interferon g.
Gammagard S/D
Gammar-P IV
gammopathy
   polyclonal g.
Gamna-Gandy bodies
ganciclovir (GCV)

G

ganglia
  basal g. (BG)
ganglion
  Bock g.
  Ehrenritter g.
  g. inferius nervi
  g. inferius nervi vagi
  left stellate g.
  petrosal g.
  pharyngeal branch of
    pterygopalatine g.
  stellate g.
  g. superius nervi
  Wrisberg g.
ganglionectomy
ganglionic blocker
ganglioside
gangliosidosis
gangrene
  angiosclerotic g.
  cold g.
  diabetic g.
  dry g.
  embolic g.
  emphysematous g.
  Fournier g.
  gas g.
  hot g.
  intracardiac gas g.
  Raynaud g.
gangrenosa
  angina g.
gangrenous
  g. emphysema
  g. pharyngitis
  g. pneumonia
gannister's disease
Gantanol
Gantrisin Oral
gantry
Gantzer accessory bundle
Ganz
  G.-Edwards coronary infusion
    catheter
  G. formula
gap
  anion g.
  auscultatory g.
  g. conduction phenomenon
  excitable g.
  g. junction
  g. phenomenon
  silent g.
Garamycin injection
Garatec
Garcia aorta clamp
Garfield-Holinger laryngoscope
gargoylism

garlic
  Kwai G.
garment
  antishock g.
  Jobst pressure g.
  pneumatic antishock g. (PASG)
garnet
  yttrium-aluminum-g. (YAG)
Garrett dilator
Gärtner, Gaertner
  G. method
  G. tonometer
  G. vein phenomenon
gas, pl. **gases**
  alveolar g.
  arterial blood g. (ABG)
  blood g.
  capillary blood g. (CBG)
  g. chromatography
  g. chromatography-mass
    spectrometry (GC-MS)
  g. clearance
  g. clearance measurement
  g. clearance method
  g. constant (R)
  g. dilution
  g. embolism
  g. endarterectomy
  g. exchange
  expired g.
  g. gangrene
  ideal alveolar g.
  inspired g.
  intrathoracic g.
  mixed expired g.
  partial pressure of carbon
    monoxide g.
  partial pressure of CO g. (PCO)
  serial blood g.
  suffocating g.
  thoracic g.
  g. trapping
gaseous
  g. microemboli
  g. pulse
Gas-Lyte ABG syringe
gasometer
gasometric
gasometry
gasp reflex
gastri
  Mycobacterium g.
gastric
  g. aspiration
  g. lung
gastric-intrapleural pressure (Pg-Ppl)
gastrocardiac syndrome

Gastrocrom
gastroepiploic artery (GEA)
gastroesophageal
    g. reflux (GER)
    g. reflux disease (GERD)
    g. scintigraphy
    g. sphincter
    g. vestibule
gastrointestinal
    g. flora
    g. symptom
    g. tract
gastropneumonic
gastropulmonary
gate
    acquisition g.
    D g.
    F g.
    H g.
    M g.
gated
    g. averaging
    g. blood-pool angiography
    g. blood-pool cardiac wall motion
      study
    g. blood-pool imaging
    g. blood-pool scanning
    g. blood-pool scintigraphy
    g. blood-pool study (GBPS)
    g. cardiac scan
    g. computed tomography
    g. equilibrium ventriculography,
      frame-mode acquisition
    g. equilibrium ventriculography,
      list-mode acquisition
    g. list mode
    g. nuclear angiogram
    g. radionuclide angiography
    g. sweep magnetic resonance
      imaging
    g. system
    g. technique
    g. view
GateWay Y-adapter rotating hemostatic
  valve
gatifloxacin
gating
    cardiac g.
    electrocardiographic g.
    in-memory g.
    g. mechanism
    prospective g.

    respiratory g.
    R wave g.
    g. signal
Gaucher disease
gauge
    Bourdon g.
    EPMSystems piezoelectric strain g.
    mercury-in-Silastic strain g.
    pounds per square inch g. (psig)
    Silastic strain g.
    strain g.
gaussian
Gauthier bicycle ergometer
gauze
    Surgicel g.
    Teletrast g.
    Xeroform g.
Gazelle balloon dilatation catheter
GBPS
    gated blood-pool study
GC-MS
    gas chromatography-mass spectrometry
Gc protein
GCS
    Glasgow Coma Scale
    graduated compression stockings
GCV
    ganciclovir
GCVF
    great cardiac vein flow
Gd-DTPA
    gadolinium-diethylenetriamine
    pentaacetic acid
Gd-DTPA-enhanced MRI
GDP
    guanosine 5'-diphosphate
GE
    G. CT Advantage high-speed CT
      system
    G. 9800 CT scanner
    G. Lightspeed CT scanner
    G. Signa Horizon SR 120 whole-
      body scanner
    G. Signa 1.5-T MRI
GEA
    gastroepiploic artery
    GEA graft
Gee Gee
gel
    agarose g.
    aluminum hydroxide g.
    Ayr saline nasal g.

NOTES

G

gel (continued)
    Cann-Ease moisturizing nasal g.
    Dermaflex G.
    electrode g.
    fibrin g.
    H.P. Acthar G.
    mucous g.
    Nasal Moist G.
    SDS-polyacrylamide g.

gelatin
    absorbable g.
    g. compression body
    g. compression boot
    g. sponge
    g. sponge slurry
    zinc g.

gelatinase
    92-kDa g.

gelatinous
    g. acute pneumonia
    g. infiltration

gel-filtered platelet (GFP)
gelfiltration
Gelfoam
    G. cookie
    G. sponge
    thrombin-soaked G.
    G. Topical

gelofusine
Gelpi retractor
gelsolin
gel-weave prosthesis
Gem
    G. defibrillator
    G. II DR dual-chamber defibrillator
    G. DR implantable defibrillator
    G. Premier Plus blood
      gas/electrolyte analyzer
    G. SensiCath blood gas monitoring
      system
    G. II VR implantable cardioverter-
      defibrillator

gemcitabine
Gemcor
gemfibrozil
gemifloxacin mesylate
Gemini
    G. DDD pacemaker
    G. Imed pump
    G. thoracic forceps

Gemzar
Gen2 pacemaker
Genabid Oral
Genac Tablet
Genahist Oral
Genamin Expectorant
Genatuss DM

genavense
    Mycobacterium g.
GenBank information system
gene
    actin g.
    angiotensinogen g.
    beta-MHC g.
    beta-myosin heavy-chain g.
    cardiac sodium channel g.
    c-Jun g.
    cyclin A g.
    DCMAG-1 g.
    desmin g.
    D1790G mutant g.
    env g.
    epicardin g.
    g. expression
    FBN1 g.
    Fos g.
    gag g.
    HER2/neu g.
    human ether-a-go-go-related g.
      (HERG)
    human preproendothelin-1 g.
    IL-4 g.
    Jumonji g.
    Jun g.
    kallikrein g.
    methylenetetrahydrofolate
      reductase g.
    MTHFR g.
    MTP g.
    MyBP-C g.
    myosin-binding protein-C g.
    g. secretor
    sodium channel g.
    g. therapy
    g. transcription
    g. transfer injection site
    TT form of MTP g.
    tuple-1 g.
    zinc finger g.
gene-activated erythropoietin
general
    G. Electric Advantx system
    G. Electric Pass-C echocardiograph
      machine
    G. Electric Signa 1.5-T MRI
      system
    g. ward (GW)
    G. Well-Being Index
generalized tuberculosis
generation
    neointimal g.
    thrombin g.
generator
    Angeion 2000 ICD g.
    asynchronous pulse g.

atrial synchronous pulse g.
atrial triggered pulse g.
Aurora pulse g.
bipolar g.
Bird neonatal CPAP g.
Chardack-Greatbatch implantable
  cardiac pulse g.
Closure catheter/radiofrequency g.
Coratomic implantable pulse g.
Cordis Stockert g.
Cordis Theta Sequicor DDD
  pulse g.
Cosmos II multiprogrammable dual-
  chamber cardiac pulse g.
Cosmos II pulse g.
CPI-PRx pulse g.
Cyberlith multiprogrammable
  pulse g.
demand pulse g.
Down's Flow G.
fixed-rate pulse g.
implantable pulse g.
Intec AID cardioverter-
  defibrillator g.
Itrel 1 unipolar pulse g.
magnet application over pulse g.
Maxilith pacemaker pulse g.
Medtronic Cardiorhythm Atakr g.
Medtronic pulse g.
Microlith pacemaker pulse g.
Microny SR+ pulse g.
Minilith pacemaker pulse g.
multiprogrammable pulse g.
Pacesetter Trilogy DR+ pulse g.
PCD ICD g.
g. pocket
Programalith III pulse g.
pulse g.
quadripolar Itrel 2 pulse g.
Radionics g.
Radionics radiofrequency g.
rate-responsive pulse g.
Regency SR pulse g.
Regency SR+ pulse g.
Res-Q ICD g.
SensorMedics G.
single-chamber pulse g.
small-particle aerosol g. (SPAG)
standby pulse g.
Stilith implantable cardiac pulse g.
subpectoral implantation of pulse g.
Synchrony II DDDR pulse g.

Synchrony III DDDR pulse g.
tantalum-178 g.
Trilogy DC, DR, SR pulse g.
ventricular inhibited pulse g.
ventricular synchronous pulse g.
ventricular triggered pulse g.
Ventritex V100, v110 ICD g.
Vivalith II pulse g.
VNUS Closure
  catheter/radiofrequency g.
VPAP II ST-A bilevel flow g.
x-ray g.
GenESA
  G. closed-loop delivery system
  G. system
  G. system for radionuclide imaging
    stress test
genetic
  g. disorder
  g. heterogeneity
  g. hypertrophic cardiomyopathy
  g. locus
  g. transmission
Genic coronary stent delivery system
geniculate
genioglossal
  g. advancement
  g. advancement procedure
genioglossus
Genisis pacemaker
genistein
GenJect
Gen-Minoxidil
Gen-Nifedipine
genomic
genotype
  ACE-II g.
  ACE-DD g.
  ACE-ID g.
  ACE I/D g.
  angiotensin-converting enzyme II g.
  angiotensin-converting enzyme
    DD g.
  angiotensin-converting enzyme
    ID g.
  DD g.
  methylenetetrahydrofolate
    reductase g.
  mitochondrial g.
  MTHFR g.
  QQ g.

G

NOTES

genotype *(continued)*
    QR g.
    TT g.
Gen-Pindolol
Genpril
Gensini
    G. cardiac device
    G. coronary arteriography catheter
    G. coronary catheter
    G. device
    G. index
    G. score
    G. Teflon catheter
GenStent biologic
Gentab-LA
Gent-AK
gentamicin sulfate
Gen-Timolol
Gentle-Flo suction catheter
Gentran
Gentrasul
Genus stent
Geocillin
geometric
    g. cube formula
    g. mean diameter (GMD)
geometry
    left ventricular g.
    normal g.
    g. of stenosis
    ventricular g.
Geopen
George-Lewis technique
George Washington strut
geotrichosis
Geotrichum candidum
GER
    gastroesophageal reflux
Gerald forceps
Gerbode
    G. annuloplasty
    G. defect
    G. forceps
    G. sternal retractor
GERD
    gastroesophageal reflux disease
Gerdy
    G. hyoid fossa
    G. intraauricular loop
Gerhardt
    G. change
    G. syndrome
    G. triangle
Geriatric Depression Scale
Gerlach tonsil
germanate
    bismuth g. (BGO)
germanium-68 external source

germanium sesquioxide
germ cell tumor
gerontology
gestational hypertension
Gesterol injection
Gey
    G. fixative solution
    G. solution
GFP
    gel-filtered platelet
GFR
    glomerular filtration rate
GFT
    gradient field transform
GFX
    grepafloxacin
    GFX 2 coronary stent system
    GFX Micro III stent
    GFX over-the-wire coronary stent
    GFX stent
GG
    Slo-Phyllin GG
GGA
    ground-glass attenuation
GG-Cen
GG/DM
    Kolephrin GG/DM
GHB
    gamma hydroxybutyrate
Ghon
    G. complex
    G. focus
    G. primary lesion
    G. tubercle
ghosting
ghost vessel
GIA
    Global Institute for Asthma
giant
    g. aneurysm
    g. bullous disease
    g. cell
    g. cell aortitis
    g. cell arteritis
    g. cell carcinoma
    g. cell interstitial pneumonitis
    (GIP)
    g. cell myocarditis
    g. cell pneumonia
    g. T wave
    g. v wave
    g. a wave
Gianturco
    G. coil
    G. wool-tufted wire coil
    G. Z stent
Gianturco-Roehm bird's nest vena cava filter

Gianturco-Roubin
    G.-R. in Acute Myocardial
      Infarction (GRAMI)
    G.-R. Flex II stent
    NACI G.-R.
    New Applications for Coronary
      Interventions, G.-R. (NACI
      Gianturco-Roubin)
    G.-R. stent
    G.-R. Stent Acute Closure
      Evaluation (GRACE)
Gibbon-Landis test
Gibson
    G. circularity index
    G. murmur
    G. rule
Giemsa stain
Giertz rib guillotine
Giertz-Shoemaker rib shears
GIK
    glucose, insulin, and potassium
Gilchrist disease
Gill I respirator
**Gill-Jonas modification of Norwood
  procedure**
GIP
    giant cell interstitial pneumonitis
girdle-like action
gitalin
GITS
giving-up/given-up response
GKI
    glucose potassium insulin
glabrata
    Candida g.
    Torulopsis g.
gland
    adrenal g.
    arytenoid g.
    bronchial g.
    esophageal g.
    fibrous capsule of thyroid g.
    Knoll g.
    laryngeal g.
    levator muscle of thyroid g.
    Nuhn g.
    pharyngeal g.
    Philip g.
    Rivinus g.
    sublingual g.

    submucosal g.
    tracheal g.
glandula, pl. glandulae
    capsula fibrosa g.
    glandulae esophageae
    glandulae laryngeae
    g. lingualis anterior
    glandulae pharyngeales
    g. sublingualis
    glandulae tracheales
glandular pharyngitis
Glanzmann thrombasthenia
glare
    veiling g.
Glasgow
    G. Coma Scale (GCS)
    G. sign
glass blower's emphysema
Glassman clamp
glassy degeneration
Glattelast compression pantyhose
Glaucon
Glaxo Wellcome Diskhaler inhaler
glebae
    Acanthamoeba g.
Glenn
    G. anastomosis
    G. anastomosis procedure
    G. operation
    G. procedure
    G. shunt
glibenclamide
Glidecath hydrophilic coated catheter
Glidewire
    G. Gold surgical guidewire
    long taper/stiff shaft G.
    Microvasive G.
    Radiofocus G.
glipizide
Glisson capsule
glissonitis
glistening yellow coronary plaque
global
    g. amnesia
    g. aphasia
    g. cardiac disease
    G. Carotid Artery Stent Registry
    g. ejection fraction
    g. hypokinesis
    G. Institute for Asthma (GIA)
    g. left ventricular ejection fraction
    g. left ventricular function

G

NOTES

global (*continued*)
G. Therapeutics V-Flex stent
g. tissue hypoxia
G. Use of Strategies to Open Occluded Coronary Arteries
G. Utilization of Streptokinase and tPA for Occluded Arteries (GUSTO)
G. Utilization of Streptokinase and tPA for Occluded Coronary Arteries (GUSTO)
g. ventricular dysfunction
globe
bleeding g.
globin
accelerator g. (AcG)
globoid heart
globular
g. heart
g. sputum
g. thrombus
globulin
antithymocyte g.
cytomegalovirus immune g. (CMVIG)
gamma g.
intravenous gamma g. (IVGG)
intravenous immune g.
lymphocyte immune g.
Minnesota antilymphocyte g. (MAG)
rabbit antithymocyte g.
respiratory syncytial virus IV immune g.
Rho(D) immune g.
globus
g. hystericus
g. pharyngis
glomangiosis
pulmonary g.
glomeriform
venous segment of g.
glomerular
g. filtration rate (GFR)
g. hyperfiltration
glomerulonephritis
acute g. (AGN)
crescentic g.
mesangial proliferative g.
pauciimmune g.
glomerulosa
zona g.
glomerulosclerosis
glomus
g. pulmonale
g. tumor
glossectomy

glossopharyngeal
g. breathing
g. nerve
g. neuralgia
glossopharyngeo
ramus communicans cum nervo g.
glossopharyngeus, pl. **glossopharyngei**
glottic atresia
glottidis
atrium g.
glottis respiratoria
glove
compression g.'s
ESP radiation reduction examination g.'s
gloved
g. finger sign
g. fist technique
Glover auricular-appendage clamp
glucagon
glucarate
technetium g.
gluceptate
calcium g.
Gluck rib shears
glucocorticoid
g.-induced hypertension
g. resistance
glucocorticosteroid
glucometer
gluconate
calcium g.
ferrous g.
potassium g.
quinidine g.
Glucophage
glucoronate
trimetrexate g.
glucose
g. exchange
g. intolerance
g. metabolism (rMRGlu)
g. potassium insulin (GKI)
sarcolemmal g.
g. uptake
glucose-6-phosphate dehydrogenase (G6PD)
glucose, insulin, and potassium (GIK)
glucose-6-phosphatase
glucose transporter 4
glucosidase deficiency
Glucotrol
GlucoWatch
glucuronate
glue
fibrin g.
glu-plasminogen
glutamate exchange

glutamer-250
  hemoglobin g.
glutamic-oxaloacetic transaminase (GOT)
glutamic oxalotransaminase
glutaraldehyde
glutaraldehyde-tanned
  g.-t. bovine collagen tube
  g.-t. bovine heart valve
  g.-t. porcine heart valve
glutathione (GSH)
  g. disulfide
glutethimide
Glutose
Glyate
glyburide
glyceraldehyde 3-phosphate
glycerin
Glycerol-T
glyceryl
  g. guaiacolate
  g. trinitrate
glyceryl trinitrate
glycinate
  theophylline sodium g.
glycine site
glycocalicin
  plasma g.
glycocalicine index
glycocalix, glycocalyx
glycoconjugate
  respiratory g. (RGC)
Glycofed
glycogen
  g. cardiomegaly
  g. depletion
  g. loading
  g. phosphorylase
  g. storage disease
  g. storage disease type III
  g. synthase
glycogenated PNA
glycogenosis
  cardiac g.
  g. type III
glycol
  recombinant polyethylene g. (r-PEG)
glycolated
glycolipid antibody
glycolysis
glycolytic enzyme
glycometabolic state

glycopeptide teicoplanin
glycoprotein (GP)
  g. IIb/IIIa antagonist
  g. IIb/IIIa inhibitor
  g. IIb/IIIa receptor
  g. IIb/IIIa receptor antagonist
  multikringle g.
  platelet g.
  platelet membrane g.
  platelet receptor g.
glycopyrrolate
glycoside
  cardiac g.
  digitalis g.
glycosis
glycosphingolipid disorder
glycosylated hemoglobin
glycosylation of intracellular proteins
Glycotuss
Glycotuss-dM
glycyl compound
glycyrrhizinic acid
Glydeine
Glynase PresTab
Glyrol
Glytuss
GM-CSF
  granulocyte/macrophage colony-stimulating factor
GMD
  geometric mean diameter
GMP
  guanosine monophosphate
GMS
  Grocott methenamine silver
  GMS stain
G-myticin
GNB
  gram-negative bacillus
goblet
  g. cell
  g. cell degranulation
  g. cell hypertrophy
  g. cell metaplasia
Godart expirograph
Godwin tumor
Goeltec catheter
Goethlin test
Goetz
  G. bipolar electrode
  G. cardiac device
  G. device

G

NOTES

Gohrbrand cardiac dilator
goiter
    diving g.
    plunging g.
    suffocative g.
    wandering g.
Golaski knitted Dacron graft
Golaski-UMI vascular prosthesis
gold (Au)
    g. marker
    g. salt
Goldberg-MPC mediastinoscope
Goldblatt
    G. kidney
    G. phenomenon
    two-kidney G.
gold-coated Inflow coronary stent
Golden
    S sign of G.
Goldenhar syndrome
Goldflam
    G. disease
    G.-Erb disease
Goldman
    G. cardiac risk index score
    G. index of risk
    G. risk-factor index
gold-195m radionuclide
Goldner trichrome stain
Goldscheider percussion
GoldSeal nasal mask
Goldsmith operation
Goldstein hemoptysis
Golgi
    G. complex
    G. tendon organ
Golub ECG lead
Gomco thoracic drainage pump
gomenol
Gomori methenamine silver stain
gonadal
    g. disease
    g. dysgenesis
gondii
    Toxoplasma g.
gonion to pogonion (GO-POG)
gonococcal endocarditis
gonorrhoeae
    Neisseria g.
Goodale-Lubin
    G.-L. cardiac device
    G.-L. catheter
    G.-L. device
GoodKnight 418A, 418G, 418P CPAP
  system
goodness-of-fit test
Goodpasture syndrome
goose-honk murmur

gooseneck
    g. deformity
    g. outflow tract deformity
    g. snare
Goosen vascular punch
GO-POG
    gonion to pogonion
gordonae
    Mycobacterium g.
Gordon elementary body
Gore-Tex
    G.-T. AF fistula
    G.-T. baffle
    G.-T. bifurcated vascular graft
    G.-T. cardiovascular patch
    G.-T. graft
    G.-T. jump graft
    G.-T. shunt
    G.-T. soft tissue patch
    G.-T. surgical membrane
    G.-T. tube
    G.-T. vascular graft
Goris background subtraction technique
Gorland formula
Gorlin
    G. catheter
    G. constant
    G. equation
    G. formula
    G. and Gorlin equation
    G. hydraulic formula
    G. syndrome
gormanii
    Legionella g.
Gormel Cream
goserelin
GOT
    glutamic-oxaloacetic transaminase
Gott
    G. butterfly heart valve
    G.-Daggett heart valve prosthesis
    G. shunt
Gould
    G. electromagnetic flowmeter
    G.-Godart type 18070 ergometer
    G. Instrument Systems spirometer
    G. PentaCath 5-lumen
      thermodilution catheter
    G. Statham pressure transducer
gout
gouty phlebitis
Gowers
    G. contraction
    G. sign
    G. syndrome
GP
    glycoprotein
gp91^{phox} protein

G6PD
glucose-6-phosphate dehydrogenase
G protein
G$_i$ protein
GRII coronary stent
grabbing technique
GRACE
Gianturco-Roubin Stent Acute Closure Evaluation
gracile habitus
gradational step exercise stress test
grade
Sellers g.
thrombolysis in myocardial infarction flow g. 0–3
thrombus g.
g. 1 through 6 murmur
TIMI flow g. 0–3
TIMI myocardial perfusion g.
graded
g. exercise exercise stress test
g. exercise test (GXT)
gradient
alveolar-arterial oxygen tension g.
alveolocapillary partial pressure g.
aortic pressure g.
aortic valve g. (AVG)
arm-leg g.
atrial-to-pulmonary venous g.
atrioventricular g.
coronary perfusion g.
diastolic g.
Doppler g.
Doppler pressure g.
g. echo-cine MRI
g.-echo imaging
electrochemical g.
elevated g.
g. field transform (GFT)
g. gel electrophoresis
hemodynamic g.
intracavitary pressure g.
intraventricular g.
mitral g.
mitral valve g. (MVG)
peak instantaneous g.
peak instantaneous Doppler g.
peak systolic g. (PSG)
peak transaortic valve g.
pressure g.
pulmonary bed g.
pulmonary valve g.

g. recall echo (GRE)
g. recalled acquisition in a steady state (GRASS)
g. reduction
residual g.
g. reversal image
systolic g.
transaortic g.
transaortic valve g.
transmitral g.
transpulmonary g.
transstenotic pressure g.
transvalvular aortic g.
transvalvular pressure g. (TPG)
ventricular g.
grading
Stary g.
graduated compression stockings (GCS)
graft
activated g.
albumin-coated vascular g.
albuminized woven Dacron tube g.
aldehyde-tanned bovine carotid artery g.
aortic tube g.
aortocoronary bypass g. (ACBG)
aortocoronary snake g.
aortofemoral bypass g. (AFBG)
aortoiliac bypass g.
aortomonoiliac g.
araldehyde-tanned bovine carotid artery g.
Aria coronary artery bypass g.
Artegraft natural collagen vascular g.
autogenic g.
autologous fat g.
bifurcated g.
Biograft g.
Bionit vascular g.
BioPolyMeric vascular g.
Björk-Shiley g.
bypass g.
Carbo-Seal cardiovascular composite g.
collagen-impregnated knitted Dacron velour g.
compressed Ivalon patch g.
Cooley woven Dacron g.
coronary artery bypass g.
Corvita endoluminal g.
Corvita endoprosthesis stent g.

G

NOTES

graft (*continued*)

Cragg endoluminal g.
Cragg Endopro System I/Passager
stent g.
Creech aortoiliac g.
CryoLife valve g.
Dacron Sauvage g.
Dacron tube g.
descending thoracic aorta-to-femoral
artery bypass g.
Diastat vascular access g.
DTAFA bypass g.
Edwards-Tapp arterial g.
Edwards woven Teflon aortic
bifurcation g.
endoluminal stent g.
endoscopic coronary artery
bypass g. (E-CABG)
endovascular g.
endovascular aortic g. (EAG)
EPTFE g.
expanded polytetrafluoroethylene
vascular g.
EXS femoropopliteal bypass g.
Favaloro saphenous vein bypass g.
FEP-ringed Gore-Tex vascular g.
GEA g.
Golaski knitted Dacron g.
Gore-Tex g.
Gore-Tex bifurcated vascular g.
Gore-Tex jump g.
Gore-Tex vascular g.
Hancock pericardial valve g.
Hancock vascular g.
Hemobahn endovascular prosthesis
stent-g.
HUV bypass g.
IEA g.
IMA g.
Impra Distaflo bypass g.
inferior epigastric artery g.
Inoue triple-branched stent g.
InterGard vascular g.
internal mammary artery g.
internal thoracic artery g.
Ionescu-Shiley vascular g.
ITA g.
Jostent coronary stent g.
jump g.
Kimura cartilage g.
knitted polyester crimped g.
left internal mammary artery g.
left internal thoracic artery g.
LIMA g.
LITA g.
lower extremity bypass g.
mammary artery g.
mandrel g.

Meadox g.
Medtronic AneuRx stent g.
mesenteric bypass g.
Microknit arterial g.
Microknit patch g.
Microvel double velour g.
minimally invasive direct coronary
artery bypass g. (MIDCABG)
modified human graft umbilical
vein g.
nonvalved g.
pedicle g.
Perma-Flow coronary g.
Perma-Flow coronary bypass g.
polyfluorotetraethylene g.
Poly-Plus Dacron vascular g.
polytetrafluoroethylene stent g.
portacaval H g.
Post Coronary Artery Bypass G.
(POST-CABG)
PTFE g.
PTFE stent g.
radial artery g.
radial artery g.
g. rejection
renal artery bypass g.
reversed saphenous vein g.
right internal mammary artery g.
right internal thoracic artery g.
RIMA g.
RITA g.
saphenous vein g. (SVG)
SCA-EX 7F g.
Shiley Tetraflex vascular g.
skip g.
snake g.
stent g. (SG)
straight tube g.
subclavian artery bypass g.
T g.
Talent g.
Teflon g.
thoracic-stent g.
transluminally placed endovascular
branched stent g.
Vanguard III endovascular aortic g.
Varivas R denatured homologous
vein g.
VascuLink vascular access g.
g. vasculopathy
Vascutek Gelseal vascular g.
Vascutek knitted vascular g.
Vascutek woven vascular g.
vein g.
Velex woven Dacron vascular g.
velour collar g.
vertebral artery bypass g.
Vitagraft vascular g.

Weavenit patch g.
woven Dacron fabric g.
woven Dacron tube g.
Y g.
Y-shaped g.
GraftAssist vein-graft holder
grafting
    endarterectomy and coronary artery bypass g. (E-CABG)
    endovascular stent g.
    minimally invasive coronary bypass g. (MICABG)
    Port-Access coronary artery bypass g.
graft-seeking catheter
graft-versus-host disease (GVHD)
Graham
    G. law
    G. rib contractor
    G. Steell heart murmur
    G. Steell murmur
grain
    g. dust
    g. handler's disease
    refined g.
GRAMI
    Gianturco-Roubin in Acute Myocardial Infarction
    GRAMI clinical trial
gram-negative
    g.-n. bacillus (GNB)
    g.-n. cocci
    g.-n. endocarditis
    g.-n. organism
    g.-n. pericarditis
gram-positive
    g.-p. bacillus
    g.-p. cocci
    g.-p. organism
Gram stain
granarius
    Sitophilus g.
Grancher
    G. sign
    G. triad
granoplasm
Grant abdominal aortic aneurysmal clamp
granular
    g. cell tumor
    g. pharyngitis
    g. respiration

granulation
    Bayle g.
    cell g.
    g. stenosis
    g. tissue
granule
    aleuronoid g.
    azurophil g.
    Birbeck g.'s
    E.E.S. G.'s
    Fauvel g.'s
    Much g.'s
Granulex
granulocyte activation
granulocyte/macrophage colony-stimulating factor (GM-CSF)
granulocytopenia
granulocytopenic host
granuloma
    cocci g.
    eosinophilic g. (EG)
    hyalinizing g.
    interstitial g.
    necrotizing g.
    noncaseating g.
    pulmonary hyalinizing g.
    sarcoid g.
granulomatosis
    allergic g.
    allergic angiitis and g.
    bronchocentric g. (BCG)
    eosinophilic g.
    Langerhans cell g.
    lymphomatoid g. (LYG)
    talc g.
    Wegener g. (WG)
granulomatous
    g. arteritis
    g. disease
    g. hepatitis
    g. inflammation
    g. mediastinitis
    g. pneumonitis
granulosus
    Echinococcus g.
grapes
    Carswell g.
graphite furnace atomic absorption spectroscopy
Graphtec

G

NOTES

GRASS
gradient recalled acquisition in a steady state
GRASS MRI

Grass
G. neurodata system
G. S88 muscle stimulator

gratus
Strophanthus g.

Gräupner method

Graves disease

gravis
myalgia g.
myasthenia g.

gravitation factor

gray (Gy)
g. hepatization
g. induration
g. infiltration
g. scale

grayout spell

gray-scale ultrasound

Gray-Weale
G.-W. classification
G.-W. plaque

GRE
gradient recall echo

great
g. alveolar cell
g. artery
g. cardiac vein flow (GCVF)
G. Ormond Street tracheostomy
g. vessel
g. vessel disruption
g. vessel tear

Green
monoplanar method of G.

green
g. coffee bean
g. dye curve
g. sputum
g. strep endocarditis

Greene sign

Greenfield
G. filter
G. IVC filter
G. vena cava filter

Gregg
G. cannula
G. phenomenon

Gregory baby profunda clamp

grelot
bruit de g.

grepafloxacin (GFX)

greyout spell

Gricco spell

grid
external g.

Griesinger sign

Griess test

Griggs single-forceps dilatation technique

grinder's
g. asthma
g. phthisis

Grinfeld cannula

grip
devil's g.
NEO-fit endotracheal tube g.
G. Technology stent crimping process
g. torque device

gripping heart

griseofulvin

GRI stent

groaning murmur

Grocco sign

Grocott
G. methenamine silver (GMS)
G. stain

groin
g. approach
g. complication

Grollman
G. catheter
G. pulmonary artery-seeking catheter

Grönblad-Strandberg syndrome

Grondahl esophagoplasty

Grondahl-Finney operation

Groningen voice prosthesis

groove
arterial g.
atrioventricular g.
auriculoventricular g.
A-V g.
bulboventricular g.
conoventricular fold and g.
deltopectoral g.
Harrison g.
laryngotracheal g.
nasopharyngeal g.
pharyngotympanic g.
terminal g.
vascular g.
venous g.
Waterston g.

Groshong double-lumen catheter

gross
g. tracheoesophageal atresia
g. tracheoesophageal fistula

Grossman
G. scale
G. sign

Gross-Pomeranz-Watkins retractor

ground-glass
    g.-g. appearance
    g.-g. attenuation (GGA)
    g.-g. opacification
    g.-g. opacity
    g.-g. pattern
group
    diagnostic-related g. (DRG)
    Digitalis Investigation G. (DIG, DIG study)
    digoxin investigators g. (DIG)
Grover clamp
growth
    dysanaptic g.
    g. factor
    g. hormone
gruberi
    Naegleria g.
gruel
    atheromatous g.
grumous debris
grunt
    diastolic g.
    expiratory g.
Grüntzig
    G. balloon catheter
    G. balloon catheter angioplasty
    G. catheter
    G. femoral stiffening cannula
    G. technique
Grüntzig-Dilaca catheter
GSH
    glutathione
GS Modular pulmonary testing system
GSNO
    S-nitrosoglutathione
G-strophanthin
G-suit
GTP
    guanosine triphosphate
    guanosine 5'-triphosphate
guaiacolate
    glyceryl g.
Guaifed
guaifenesin
    g. and codeine
    g. and dextromethorphan
    hydrocodone and g.
    hydrocodone, pseudoephedrine, and g.
    g. and phenylpropanolamine

    g., phenylpropanolamine, and dextromethorphan
    g., phenylpropanolamine, and phenylephrine
    g. and pseudoephedrine
    g., pseudoephedrine, and codeine
    g., pseudoephedrine, and dextromethorphan
    theophylline and g.
Guaifenex
    G. LA
    G. PSE
GuaiMax-D
Guaipax
Guaitab
Guaituss AC
Guai-Vent/PSE
guanabenz acetate
guanadrel sulfate
guanethidine
    g. monosulfate
    g. sulfate
guanfacine
    g. acetate
    g. hydrochloride
Guangzhou GD-1 prosthetic valve
guanine nucleotide modulatable binding
guanosine
    g. 5'-diphosphate (GDP)
    g. monophosphate (GMP)
    g. triphosphate (GTP)
    g. 5'-triphosphate (GTP)
guanylate cyclase
guanylyl cyclase
Guardian
    G. AICD
    G. ATP 4210 implantable cardioverter-defibrillator
    G. catheter
    G. ICD
    G. pacemaker
Guardwire
    G. angioplasty system
    G. emboli containment system
GuardWire
    PercuSurge G.
guar gum
Gubner-Ungerleider
    G.-U. voltage
    G.-U. voltage criteria
Guedel airway
Guéneau de Mussy point

NOTES

G

Guglielmi detachable coil
GuiaCough Expectorant
Guiaraudon corridor operation for
  atrial fibrillation
Guiatex
Guiatuss
  G. CF
  G. DAC
  G.-DM
Guiatussin
  G. DAC
  G. with Codeine
guidance
  echo g.
  fluoroscopic g.
  G. by Ultrasound Imaging for
    Decision Endpoints (GUIDE)
  G. by Ultrasound Imaging for
    Decision Endpoints II (GUIDE II)
Guidant
  G.-CPI device
  G. CRM pacemaker
  G. defibrillator
  G. Heart Rhythm Technologies
    Linear Ablation system
  G. Multi-Link Tetra coronary stent
    system
  G. stent
  G. TRIAD three-electrode energy
    defibrillation system
GUIDE
  Guidance by Ultrasound Imaging for
    Decision Endpoints
  GUIDE clinical trial
guide
  ACS LIMA g.
  Advanced Cardiovascular Systems
    left internal mammary artery g.
  Amplatz tube g.
  Cor-Flex wire g.
  FL4 g.
  Flexguide intubation g.
  Franzen needle g.
  movable core straight safety
    wire g.
  Müller catheter g.
  Pilotip catheter g.
  Slick stylette endotracheal tube g.
  Slidewire extension g.
  tapered movable core curved
    wire g.
  Tefcor movable core straight
    wire g.
  TEGwire g.
  TrueTorque wire g.
  wire g.

GUIDE II
  Guidance by Ultrasound Imaging for
    Decision Endpoints II
  GUIDE II clinical trial
guidelines
  ACC/AHA pacemaker
    implantation g.
  American College of
    Cardiology/American Heart
    Association Task Force on
    Practice g.
  American Heart Association g.
  clinical practice g. (CPG)
  implantation g.
  McGoon g.
  National Cholesterol Education
    Panel g.
  NCEP g.
  NCEP-II g.
guider
  NL3 g.
guidewire, guide wire
  ACS Amplatz g.
  ACS exchange g.
  ACS extra-support g.
  ACS Hi-Torque Balance g.
  ACS Hi-Torque Balance
    middleweight g.
  ACS LIMA g.
  Advanced Cardiovascular Systems
    exchange g.
  Amplatz Super Stiff g.
  Amplex g.
  atherolytic reperfusion g.
  Athlete g.
  Athlete coronary g.
  Bard Commander PTCA g.
  Becton-Dickinson g.
  Bentson exchange straight g.
  Bentson floppy-tip g.
  Cardiometrics Flowire g.
  catheter g.
  ControlWire g.
  Coons Super Stiff long tip g.
  Cor-Flex g.
  Critikon g.
  Crosswire nitinol hydrophilic g.
  Doppler Flowire g.
  Doppler-tipped angioplasty g.
  Elastorc catheter g.
  EnTre g.
  exchange g.
  Extra Sport coronary g.
  extra-support g.
  FasTrac g.
  FasTrac hydrophilic-coated g.
  flexible g.
  Flex Tip g.

FloMap g.
floppy g.
floppy-tipped g.
FloWire g.
FloWire Doppler g.
fluid-filled pressure monitoring g.
Glidewire Gold surgical g.
heparin-coated g.
Hi-Torque Flex-T g.
Hi-Torque Floppy exchange g.
Hi-Torque Floppy II g.
Hi-Torque Floppy intermediate g.
Hi-Torque Standard g.
hydrophilic coated g.
intravascular Doppler-tipped g.
J g.
J Rosen g.
J-tip g.
Linx exchange g.
Linx extension g.
g. loop
Magic Torque g.
Magnum g.
Micropuncture g.
Microvasive stiff piano wire g.
Monorail g.
Mustang steerable g.
Newton g.
PDT g.
g. perforation
Phantom g.
Phantom cardiac g.
Platinum PLUS g.
Platinum Plus 300-cm g.
Preceder interventional g.
Premo g.
Prima laser g.
Radifocus catheter g.
Redifocus g.
g. reflection
Reflex SuperSoft steerable g.
Roadrunner PC g.
Rotacs g.
safety g.
Schwarten LP g.
Seeker g.
silk g.
Silver Speed hydrophilic g.
SOF-T g.
Sones g.
SOS g.
Spectranetics Prima laser g.

stainless steel g.
steerable angioplastic g.
Superselector Y-K g.
Surpass g.
TAD g.
Taper g.
Tapered Torque g.
g. technique
Teflon-coated g.
Terumo g.
TherOx 0.014 infusion g.
Tomcat PTCA g.
Total Occlusion Trial with
   Angioplasty by Using Laser G.
   (TOTAL)
g. traversal test
Ultra-Select nitinol PTCA g.
USCI Hyperflex g.
Veriflex g.
Wholey Hi-Torque Floppy g.
Wholey Hi-Torque modified J g.
Wholey Hi-Torque standard g.
Wizdom g.
guiding catheter
Guillain-Barré syndrome
guilliermondii
   Candida g.
guillotine
   Giertz rib g.
   rib g.
   Sauerbruch rib g.
Guisez tube
gulae
   plexus g.
Gulf War syndrome
gum
   g. acacia
   g. elastic bougie introducer
   guar g.
   Nicorette G.
   nicotine g.
   polacrilex chewing g.
   Stay Trim Diet G.
gun
   Cobe g.
   skin g.
Gunn- crossing sign
gunshot wound
Günther catheter
gurgling rale
Gurvich biphasic waveform

NOTES

G

GUSTO
Global Utilization of Streptokinase and
tPA for Occluded Arteries
Global Utilization of Streptokinase and
tPA for Occluded Coronary Arteries
Economics and Quality of Life
Substudy of GUSTO (EQOL)
GUSTO IIa, IIb, III, IV
GUSTO protocol
GUSTO study
gut-associated lymphoid tissue (GALT)
Gutgeman auricular appendage clamp
guttural
g. pulse
g. rale
GVHD
graft-versus-host disease
GW
general ward

GW5638
GXT
graded exercise test
Gy
gray
gyri (*pl. of* gyrus)
Gyrocaps
Slo-Phyllin G.
Gyroscan
ACS G.
G. HP Philips 15S whole-body
system
gyrus, pl. **gyri**
angular g. (AG)
inferior frontal g. (IFG)
middle frontal g. (MFG)
superior temporal g. (STG)
supramarginal g. (SMG)

H
    H gate
    H space
    H spike
    H wave
    H zone

h
    h peak
    h plateau
    h wave

H1 receptor
H$_2$
    prostaglandin H.
HA
    Hispanic American
Haake water bath
HAART
    highly active antiretroviral therapy
Haber-Weiss reaction
habit cough
Habitrol Patch
habitual cough
habitus
    gracile h.
HACEK
    Haemophilus aphrophilus, Actinobacillus actinomycetemcomitans, Cardiobacterium hominis, Eikenella corrodens, and *Kingella kingae*
hacking cough
HAD
    Hospital Anxiety and Depression
Hadow balloon
HADS
    Hospital Anxiety and Depression scale
HAEC
    human aortic endothelial cell
H-Ae interval
haematobium
    Schistosoma h.
Haemolite
    H. autologous blood recovery system
    Cell Saver H.
haemolyticus
    Haemophilus h.
Haemonetics
    H. Cell Saver
    H. Cell Saver system
haemophilum
    Mycobacterium h.
Haemophilus
    H. aphrophilus
    H. aphrophilus, Actinobacillus actinomycetemcomitans,

    Cardiobacterium hominis, Eikenella corrodens, and *Kingella kingae* (HACEK)
    H. b conjugate vaccine
    H. endocarditis
    H. haemolyticus
    H. influenzae
    H. parahaemolyticus
    H. parainfluenzae (HPI)
    H. pertussis
Hafnia
HAFOE
    high air flow with oxygen entrainment
Hagar probe
Hageman factor
Hagenbach extension of Poiseuille equation
Haight-Finochietto rib retractor
Haimovici arteriotomy scissors
hair-matrix carcinoma
hairspray thesaurosis
hairy heart
Hakim-Cordis pump
Hakki formula
Hakko Dwellcath catheter
Halbrecht syndrome
Haldane
    H. effect
    H. transformation
Haldane-Priestley
    H.-P. sample
    H.-P. tube
Haldrone
Hales piesimeter
half amplitude pulse duration
half-diluted contrast
half-life
    biological h.-l.
    elimination h.-l.
half-normal saline
half-power distance
Halfprin
half-time
    h.-t. method
    pressure h.-t.
half-value layer
Hall
    H. prosthetic heart valve
    H. sign
    H. valvulotome
Haller plexus
Hallion test
Hall-Kaster prosthetic valve
hallucination
    hypnagogic h.

H

halo
  H. catheter
  h. sheathing
  h. sign
  H. XP electrophysiology catheter
halofantrine
halogenated
  h. hydrocarbon
  h. hydrocarbon propellant
haloperidol
Haloscale respirometer
Halotestin
halothane
Halotussin
  H. AC
  H. DAC
  H. DM
Halsted clamp
Haltran
hamartoma
  myocardial h.
  pulmonary h.
Hamburger test
Hamilton-Stewart formula
Hamilton ventilator
Hamman
  H. click
  H. crunch
  H. disease
  Hamman-Rich syndrome (HRS)
  H. murmur
  H. sign
  H. syndrome
Hammersmith mitral prosthesis
Hamming-Hahn filter
hammocking of posterior mitral leaflet
Hampton hump
Ham test
Hancock
  H. bipolar balloon pacemaker
  H. embolectomy catheter
  H. fiberoptic catheter
  H. hydrogen detection catheter
  H. II porcine bioprosthesis
  H. II tissue valve
  H. luminal electrophysiologic
    recording catheter
  H. mitral valve prosthesis
  H. M.O. bioprosthesis
  H. modified orifice valve
  H. M.O. II bioprosthesis porcine
    valve
  H. M.O. II porcine bioprosthesis
  H. pericardial valve graft
  H. porcine heterograft
  H. porcine valve
  H. temporary cardiac pacing wire
  H. valve

  H. vascular graft
  H. wedge-pressure catheter
hand
  h. agitated solution
  h. injection
hand-crimped stent
Hand-E-Vent
hand-foot-and-mouth disease
handgrip
  h. apexcardiographic test (HAT)
  isometric h.
  h. stress
handheld nebulizer
8500 handheld pulse oximeter series
Handi oxygen sensor
hand-mounted stent
Hand-Schüller-Christian disease
HANE
  hereditary angioneurotic edema
hanging heart
hangout interval
Hank balanced salt solution
Hanley-McNeil method
Hanning window
Hannover classification
hANP
  human atrial natriuretic peptide
Hans
  H. Rudolph nonbreathing valve
  H. Rudolph three-way valve
Hantaan virus
hantavirus pulmonary syndrome
HAPE
  high-altitude pulmonary edema
haploinsuffiency
haplotype
  HLA-DQA1 gene h.
  HLA-DQB1 gene h.
hard
  h. cardiac event
  h. metal disease
  h. metal pneumoconiosis
  h. metal-related lung fibrosis
  h. pulse
hardening
  x-ray beam h.
Hare syndrome
Harken
  H. ball valve
  H. forceps
  H. rib spreader
harmonic
  h. component
  h. content
  h. gray-scale imaging
  h. imaging (HI)
  h. imaging mode
  h. imaging ultrasound technique

h. phase (HARP)
h. phase image
h. power Doppler imaging
Harmonie EEG software
harness
Heart Hugger h.
Heart Hugger sternum support h.
HARP
harmonic phase
Harvard atherosclerosis reversibility
Hospital Admission Risk Profile
HARP image
Harpoon suture anchor
Harrell Y stent
Harrington esophageal diverticulectomy
Harris adapter
Harris-Benedict equation
Harrison groove
harsh
h. murmur
h. respiration
HART
Heparin Aspirin Reperfusion Trial
Hypertension Audit of Risk Factor
Therapy
HART study
Hartmann
H. clamp
H. solution
HARTS
heat-activated recoverable temporary
stent
Hartzler
H. ACX II catheter
H. ACX-II, RX-014 balloon
catheter
H. balloon catheter
H. dilatation catheter
H. Excel catheter
H. LPS dilatation catheter
H. Micro II balloon
H. Micro II catheter
H. Micro-600 catheter
H. Micro XT catheter
H. rib retractor
H. RX-014 balloon catheter
Harvard
H. atherosclerosis reversibility
(HARP)
H. atherosclerosis reversibility
project
H. pump

harvester's lung
Harvey Elite stethoscope
HASHD
hypertensive arteriosclerotic heart disease
Hashimoto thyroiditis
HASMC
human aortic smooth muscle cell
Hassall corpuscle
HAST
high-altitude simulation test
HAT
handgrip apexcardiographic test
hat
bishop's h.
**Hatafuku fundus onlay patch
esophageal repair**
hatchetti
Acanthamoeba h.
Hatle method
hawaiiensis
Drechslera h.
**Hawksley random zero mercury
sphygmomanometer**
Hawthorne effect
Hayek oscillator
Hayfebrol Liquid
hay fever
Haynes 25 material
haze
hilar h.
perihilar h.
hazy
h. appearance
h. infiltrate
h. lesion
Hb
hemoglobin
Hb oximetry
HbCO
carboxyhemoglobin
HbCO$_2$ oximetry
HBDH
hydroxybutyrate dehydrogenase
HBE
His bundle electrogram
HBO
hyperbaric oxygen
HBO therapy
HbO$_2$
oxyhemoglobin
HbO$_2$ oximetry
HbOC vaccine

NOTES

H

315

HBT
> H. Sleuth
> H. Sleuth portable hydrogen monitor

HBW 023

HC
> hypertrophic cardiomyopathy

HCH disk

HCl
> hydrochloride
>> cefepime HCl
>> colesevelam HCl
>> dexmedetomidine HCl
>> levalbuterol HCl
>> losartan potassium HCl
>> moxifloxacin HCl
>> sotalol HCl
>> verapamil HCl

HCM, HCMP
> hypertrophic cardiomyopathy

HCMV
> human cytomegalovirus

HCN
> hydrogen cyanide

HCO₃
> bicarbonate

HCT
> Atacand HCT
> Avapro HCT
> Diovan HCT
> Lotensin HCT

HCTZ
> hydrochlorothiazide

HCVD
> hypertensive cardiovascular disease

HDL
> high-density lipoprotein
>> isolated low HDL
>> nascent HDL
>> pre-beta 1 HDL

HDM
> house dust mite
> HDM allergen

HDU
> high-dependency unit

H&E
> hematoxylin and eosin
> H&E stain

head
> h., neck, or shaft (HNS)
> h., neck, or shaft lesion

headache
> migraine h.
> syncopal migraine h.

head-down tilt test

headgear
> Velstretch/Velcro h.

headhunter angiography catheter

head-out water immersion

Head paradoxical reflex

headpiece
> e-Net h.

head-tilt method

head-up
> h.-u. tilt (HUT)
> h.-u. tilt-induced syncope
> h.-u. tilt-table test (HUTTT)
> h.-u. tilt test

Heaf test

healed tuberculosis

healing
> per primam h.
> per secundum h.

health
> H. level seven (HL7)
> H. Locus of Control Scale
> National Institutes of H. (NIH)

healthcare
> Delay in Accessing Stroke H. (DASH)

health-related quality of life (HRQL, HRQOL)

HealthScan OptiChamber valved holding chamber

HEAP
> Heparin in Early Patency
> HEAP study

heart
> abdominal h.
> acute margin of h.
> H. Aid 80 defibrillator
> air-driven artificial h.
> Akutsu III total artificial h.
> ALVAD artificial h.
> anterior surface of h.
> armor h.
> armored h.
> h. arrest
> artificial h. (AH)
> athlete's h.
> athletic h.
> atrium of h.
> h. attack
> baggy h.
> balloon-shaped h.
> H. Bar snack
> Baylor total artificial h.
> h. beat
> beer h.
> beriberi h.
> Berlin total artificial h.
> h. block
> 3:1 h. block
> 3:2 h. block
> boat-shaped h.
> bony h.

booster h.
boot-shaped h.
bovine h.
CardioWest total artificial h.
cervical h.
h. chamber remodeling
chambers of the h.
chaotic h.
compensatory hypertrophy of the h.
compliance of h.
contour of h.
contracted h.
corticosteroid-treated h.
crisscross h.
crux of h.
decortication of h.
dextroposition of h.
dextroversion of h.
diaphragmatic surface of h.
dilation of h.
h. disease
disordered action of h. (DAH)
donor h.
drop h.
dynamite h.
egg-shaped h.
electrical alternation of h.
electromechanical artificial h.
encased h.
H. and Estrogen-Progestin
  Replacement Study (HERS)
explanted h.
extracorporeal h.
h. failure (HF)
h. failure cell
fatty h.
fatty degeneration of h.
fibroid h.
figure-of-eight h.
flask-shaped h.
focal myocytosis of h.
foramen of veins of h.
frosted h.
frosting h.
globoid h.
globular h.
gripping h.
hairy h.
h. and hand syndrome
hanging h.
Hershey total artificial h.
holiday h.

Holmes h.
horizontal h.
H. hugger harness
hyperthyroid h.
hypoplastic h.
hypoplastic left h.
icing h.
intermediate h.
intracorporeal h.
irritable h.
Jarvik 7, 8 artificial h.
Jarvik 7-70 artificial h.
Jarvik 2000 artificial h.
Kolff-Jarvik artificial h.
H. Laser
h. laser revascularization
H. Laser for TMR
law of the h.
left h.
left auricle of h.
left margin of h.
Liotta total artificial h.
h. loop
luxus h.
h. massage
mechanical h.
mechanical alternation of h.
movable h.
moyamoya of h.
h. murmur
myocytolysis of h.
myxedema h.
h. nebulizer
obtuse margin of h.
one-ventricle h.
orthotopic biventricular artificial h.
orthotopic univentricular artificial h.
H. Outcomes Prevention Evaluation
  (HOPE)
ox h.
paracorporeal h.
parchment h.
pear-shaped h.
pectoral h.
pendulous h.
Penn State total artificial h.
Phoenix total artificial h.
h. position
postischemic h.
pulmonary h.
h. pump
Quain fatty h.

NOTES

H

heart *(continued)*
    h. rate (HR)
    h. rate correction formula
    H. Rate 1-2-3 monitor
    h. rate-pressure product
    h. rate reserve (HRR)
    h. rate variability (HRV)
    h. rate variability test
    recipient h.
    h. reflex
    rheumatism of h.
    right h.
    right auricle of h.
    right margin of h.
    round h.
    RTV total artificial h.
    sabot h.
    semihorizontal h.
    semivertical h.
    senescent h.
    septation of h.
    h. shock protein antigen
    skeleton of h.
    skin h.
    snowman h.
    soldier's h.
    h. sounds S_1, S_2, S_3, S_4
    H. sternum support harness
    stiff h.
    stone h.
    h. stroke
    superoinferior h.
    suspended h.
    swinging h.
    Symbion/CardioWest 100 mL total
      artificial h.
    Symbion Jarvik-7 artificial h.
    Symbion J-7 70-mL ventricle total
      artificial h.
    systemic h.
    tabby cat h.
    h. tamponade
    Taussig-Bing h.
    teardrop h.
    H. Technology Rotablator
    three-chambered h.
    thrush breast h.
    tiger h.
    tiger lily h.
    tobacco h.
    h. tones
    total artificial h. (TAH)
    h. transplant
    h. transplantation
    transverse section of h.
    Traube h.
    triatrial h.
    trilocular h.

    univentricular h.
    University of Akron artificial h.
    upstairs-downstairs h.
    Utah total artificial h.
    h. valve
    h. valve prosthesis
    venous h.
    vertical h.
    Vienna total artificial h.
    waist of h.
    wandering h.
    water-bottle h.
    wooden-shoe h.

HeartBar
heartbeat
HeartCard
    H. cardiac-event recorder
    H. event recorder
    H. monitor
    H. 3X cardiac-event recorder
Heartflo automated anastomosis system
heart-hand syndrome
HeartLine service
heart-lung
    h.-l. bloc
    h.-l. bypass
    h.-l. machine
    h.-l. resuscitation
    h.-l. transplant (HLT)
HeartMate
    H. implantable pneumatic left
      ventricular assist system
    H. implantable ventricular assist
      device
    H. left ventricular assist system
    H. LVAD
    H. pump
    H. vented electric left ventricular
      assist system
Heartport
    H. catheter system
    H. Endoaortic Clamp
    H. Endocoronary Sinus catheter
    H. Endopulmonary Vent
    H. endovascular catheter
    H. Endovenous Drainage cannula
    H. Port-Access system
    H. technique
HEARTrac I Cardiac Monitoring
    system
HeartSaver VAD
Heartscan heart attack prediction test
Heartstream ForeRunner automatic
    external defibrillator
HeartWatch
    H. cardiac-event recorder
    H. III cardiac-event recorder

HearTwave
    H. EP
    H. system
Heartwire lead
heat
    h. load
    h. shock protein (HSP, Hsp, hsp)
    h. stroke
heat-activated recoverable temporary stent (HARTS)
heat-expandable stent
Heath-Edwards
    H.-E. classification
    H.-E. criteria
heating
    ohmic h.
    resistive h.
    volume h.
heat/moisture exchanger (HME)
heat shock protein 47 (HSP47)
heat-treated
    Profilnine H.-T.
heave
    parasternal h.
    precordial h.
    right ventricular h.
heavy metal
Heberden
    H. angina
    H. asthma
    H. node
Hecht pneumonia
HED
    hydroxyephedrine
heel strike
Hegglin syndrome
height
    AR jet h.
    Z score weight-Z score h.
Heim-Kreysig sign
Heimlich
    H. chest drainage valve
    H. heart valve
    H. maneuver
    H. sign
Heinecke method
Heiner syndrome
Heinz body
Heister diverticulum
Heitzman classification
HeLa cell

helical
    h. coil stent
    h. CT
    h. CT scanning
    h. CT venography
helical-tip Halo catheter
helices (*pl. of* helix)
Heliobacter pylori
Helionetics/Acculase excimer laser transmyocardial
heliox
    helium-oxygen mixture
Helistat
helium
    h.-cadmium diagnostic laser
    h. dilution
    h. dilution method
    h.-filled balloon catheter
    h.-oxygen mixture (heliox)
    h. washout
Helix
    H. balloon
    H. PTCA dilatation catheter
helix, pl. **helices**
    amphipathic h.
Heller
    H.-Belsey operation
    H.-Döhle disease
    H. esophagomyotomy
    H.-Nissen operation
Hellige electrocardiographic recorder
HELLP
    hemolysis, elevated liver enzymes, and low platelets
    HELLP syndrome
Helmholtz head coil
helminth
helminthic myocarditis
Helminthosporium
HELP
    heparin-induced extracorporeal low-density lipoprotein precipitation
Hemacor HPH 700 high-performance hemoconcentrator
hemadostenosis
Hemaflex
    H. PTCA sheath with obturator
    H. sheath
hemagglutinin
hemangioendothelioma
    epithelioid h.

NOTES

H

hemangioma
    cavernous h.
    sclerosing h.
hemangioma-thrombocytopenia syndrome
hemangiomatosis
hemangiosarcoma
Hemaquet
    H. introducer
    H. PTCA sheath with obturator
    H. sheath
hemarthrosis
Hemashield
hemathorax
hematin
hematocrit
hematogenous
    h. bacterial dissemination
    h. embolism
    h. metastasis
    h. nodule
    h. tuberculosis
hematologic disease
hematology rocker
hematoma
    aneurysmal h.
    aortic intramural h. (AIH)
    apical h.
    dissecting h.
    intramural h. (IH)
    intraparenchymal h.
    irregular h.
    lobular h.
    parenchymal h. (PH)
    periaortic h.
    pouch h.
    pulmonary h.
    retroperitoneal h.
    round h.
    subdural h. (SDH)
hematopoiesis
hematopoietic
    h. chimerism
    h. system
hematoporphyrin derivative (HPD)
hematosis
hematoxylin
    h. and eosin (H&E)
hematoxylin-eosin stain
hematoxylin-phloxine-safran stain
hematuria
hemautogram
Hemex prosthetic valve
hemianopia
hemiaxial view
hemiazygos vein
hemiblock
    left anterior h. (LAH)
    left anterior superior h. (LASH)

    left middle h.
    left posterior h.
    left posterior inferior h. (LPIH)
    left septal h.
hemic
    h. hypoxia
    h. murmur
    h. systole
hemicardia
hemidesmosome
hemidiaphragm
    h. paralysis
    tenting of h.
hemi-Fontan
    h.-F. operation
    h.-F. procedure
hemifundoplication
    Toupet h.
hemin
hemineglect
    motor-exploratory h.
hemiosteoporosis
hemiparesis
    atactic h.
    ataxic h. (AH)
    pure motor h. (PMH)
hemiplegia
    dense h.
hemisystole
hemithorax
hemitruncus
hemizygosity
hemizygous
Hemobahn endovascular prosthesis stent-graft
hemochromatosis
Hemochron high-dose thrombin time assay
hemoclastic reaction
hemoclip
    Samuels h.
hemoconcentrator
    Biofilter h.
    Biofilter cardiovascular h.
    Hemacor HPH 700 high-performance h.
    Hemocor HPH high-performance h.
HemoCue photometer
hemocyanin
    keyhole-limpet h.
Hemocyte
hemocytometer
hemodialysis
hemodialyzer
    Gambro Lundia Minor h.
hemodilution
    isovolemic h.
    normovolemic h.

hemodynamic
h. abnormality
h. analysis
h. assessment
h. collapse
h. endpoint
h. gradient
h. instability
intraoperative h.'s
h. maneuver
h. measurement
h. mental stress response
h. monitoring
h. principle
h. profile
pulmonary h.'s
h. stability
systemic h.'s
h. tolerance
transvalvular h.'s
h. vise
hemodynamically significant stenosis
hemodynamically-weighted MRI (HW)
hemodynamic-angiographic study
Hemofil M
hemofiltration
continuous arteriovenous h. (CAVH)
continuous venovenous h. (CVVH)
hemoglobin (Hb)
carbon monoxide h.
deoxygenated h.
diaspirin cross-linked h. (DCLHb)
h. glutamer-250
glycosylated h.
oxygenated h.
pyridoxilated stroma-free h. (SFHb)
hemoglobin-based therapeutic system
hemoglobinemia
hemoglobin-oxygen dissociation curve
hemoglobinuria
paroxysmal nocturnal h. (PNH)
Hemolink
H. investigational hemoglobin product or blood substitute
hemolysis
h., elevated liver enzymes, and low platelets (HELLP)
h., elevated liver function tests and low platelets syndrome
hemolytic anemia
HemoMatic blood collection monitor

hemoperfusion
pump-assisted coronary h.
hemopericardium
traumatic h.
hemophagocytic histiocyte
hemopneumopericardium
hemopneumothorax
hemopoietic
hemoptysis
cardiac h.
catamenial h.
coital h.
essential h.
Goldstein h.
oriental h.
hemopump
H. cardiac assist system
Johnson & Johnson h.
Medtronic H.
Nimbus h.
Hemopure oxygen-based therapeutic system
hemorheology
hemorrhage
anticoagulant-related h.
aortic intramural h. (AIH)
CAA-related h.
catastrophic h.
caudate h.
diffuse alveolar h. (DAH)
flame-shaped h.'s
intracavitary h.
intracerebral h. (ICH)
intracranial h. (ICH)
intramural h. (IMH)
intraparenchymal h.
intrapericardial h.
intraventricular h. (IVH)
multiple lobar h. (MLH)
parenchymal h. (PH)
peribronchovascular h.
perimesencephalic pattern of h.
petechial h.
postoperative h. (POH)
primary intracerebral h. (PICH)
pulmonary h.
pulmonary alveolar h.
recurrent lobar h. (RLH)
reperfusion-induced h.
splinter h.
spontaneous intracerebral h. (SICH)
subarachnoid h. (SAH)

NOTES

H

hemorrhage *(continued)*
    supratentorial intracerebral h.
    Surgical Treatment for
      Intracerebral H. (STICH)
    symptomatic h. (SHT)
    thrombolysis-related intracranial h.
      (TICH)
    traumatic h.
hemorrhagic
    h. bronchitis
    h. bronchopneumonia
    h. coagulopathy
    h. cyst
    h. effusion
    h. fever
    h. hereditary telangiectasia
    h. hypotension
    h. infarction (HI)
    h. pericarditis
    h. pleurisy
    h. sputum
    h. stroke
    h. telangiectasia
    h. transformation (HT)
hemosiderin
hemosiderin-laden macrophage
hemosiderosis
    cardiac h.
    essential pulmonary h.
    idiopathic pulmonary h. (IPH)
    pulmonary h.
    transfusional h.
hemostasis valve
hemostat
    Adson h.
    Kelly h.
    Mayo h.
    microfibrillar collagen h.
    mosquito h.
    straight h.
hemostatic
    h. deficiency
    h. occlusive leverage device
      (HOLD)
    h. puncture closure device (HPCD)
    h. sheath
hemoSTATUS assay
HemoTec activated clotting time
  monitor
Hemotene
hemothorax, pl. **hemothoraces (HTX)**
    catamenial h.
    clotted h.
Hemovac
    Arbrook H.
hen-cluck stertor
Henderson-Haggard inhaler
Henderson-Hasselbalch equation

Henke space
Henle
    ascending loop of H.
    H.-Coenen test
    H. elastic membrane
    H. fenestrated membrane
    H. loop
Henoch-Schönlein
    H.-S. purpura
    H.-S. syndrome
    H.-S. vasculitis
Henry-Gauer response
Henry law
HEPA
    high-efficiency particulate air
Hepalean-LCO
Hepalean-LOK
Hepamed-coated Wiktor stent
heparin
    h. arterial filter
    H. Aspirin Reperfusion Trial
      (HART)
    beef-lung h.
    h. block
    calcium h. (CH)
    depolymerized porcine mucosal h.
    h. drip
    H. in Early Patency (HEAP)
    h. flush
    immobilized h.
    h. infusion
    H. Infusion Prior to Stenting
      (HIPS)
    h. injection
    h. lock
    low molecular weight h. (LMWH)
    Preliminary Investigation of Local
      Therapy Using Porous PTCA
      Balloons and Low-Molecular-
      Weight H. (PILOT)
    unfractionated h.
heparin-binding epidermal growth factor
heparin-coated guidewire
heparin-dihydroergotamine
heparin-induced
    h.-i. extracorporeal low-density
      lipoprotein precipitation (HELP)
    h.-i. thrombocytopenia (HIT)
heparinization
heparinized saline
HEPAtech Air Purification system
hepatic
    h. artery
    h. dearterialization
    h. disease
    h. failure
    h. function
    h. hydatid cyst

h. hydrothorax
h. lipase
h. lipoprotein lipase
h. sphincter
h. vein
h. vein catheterization
hepaticopulmonary
hepatis
porta h.
hepatitis
h. A, B, C, D, E
granulomatous h.
viral h.
hepatization
gray h.
red h.
yellow h.
hepatoesophageum
ligamentum h.
hepatofugal flow
hepatojugular
h. reflex
h. reflux (HJR)
h. reflux test
hepatoma
hepatomegaly
hepatopetal flow
hepatopneumonic
hepatopulmonary syndrome (HPS)
hepatosplenomegaly
hepatotoxicity
Hep-Lock injection
heptahelical protein G
heptahydrate
magnesium sulfate h.
heptanal
heptapeptide
Heptest clotting assay
HER2/neu gene
Herceptin
hereditary
h. angioneurotic edema (HANE)
h. ataxia
h. hemorrhagic telangiectasia (HHT)
h. methemoglobinemic cyanosis
heredopathia atactica polyneuritiformis
HERG
human ether-a-go-go-related gene
D-Sotalol block of HERG
HERG potassium channel

Hering
nerve of H.
H. phenomenon
Hering-Breuer reflex
Hermansky-Pudlak syndrome
Herner syndrome
hernia
Béclard h.
Bochdalek h.
congenital diaphragmatic h. (CDH)
diaphragmatic h.
hiatal h.
Larrey h.
Morgagni h.
paraesophageal h.
rolling h.
Serafini h.
sliding hiatal h.
Velpeau h.
herniation
cardiac h.
HERO
Hirulog Early Reperfusion/Occlusion
HERO clinical trial
heroics
heroic snoring
heroin
herpangina pharyngitis
herpes
h. pneumonia
h. simplex
h. simplex pneumonia
h. simplex pneumonitis
h. simplex virus (HSV)
h. zoster
Herpesviridae
herpetic
HERS
Heart and Estrogen-Progestin
Replacement Study
Hershey total artificial heart
herzstoss
Herzyme
Hespan plasma volume expander
Hess capillary test
hetastarch plasma expander
20-HETE
20-hydroxyeicosatetraenoic acid
heterochronicus
pulsus h.
heterogeneity
genetic h.

NOTES

H

323

heterogeneous
 h. attenuation
 h. parenchymal attenuation
 h. plaque
heterogenous emphysema
heterograft
 bovine h.
 Hancock porcine h.
 porcine h.
heterologous
 h. cardiac transplant
 h. surfactant
heterometric autoregulation
heterophony
 phase h.
heterophyiasis
heteroscedastic
heterotaxia
 cardiac h.
heterotaxy
 h. syndrome
 visceral h.
heterotopic
 h. cardiac transplant
 h. heart transplant (HHT)
 h. stimulus
heterotrimeric protein G
heterotypic adhesion
heterozygosity
heterozygote
heterozygous familial
 hypercholesterolemia (hFH)
Hetzel forward triangle method
Heubner
 H. recurrent artery
 H. specific endarteritis
Hewlett-Packard
 H.-P. 77020 A phased-array sector
 scanner
 H.-P. 78720 A SDN monitor
 H.-P. biplane 5-MHz probe
 H.-P. defibrillator
 H.-P. ear oximeter
 H.-P. 500 Echo-Doppler machine
 H.-P. 1000 Echo-Doppler machine
 H.-P. 5 MHz phased-array TEE
 system
 H.-P. omniplane 5-MHz probe
 H.-P. scanner
 H.-P. 2500 SONOS ultrasound
 H.-P. SONOS 1000, 1500, 2500
 ultrasound system
 H.-P. ultrasound
Hexabrix contrast material
Hexadrol Phosphate
hexafluoride
 sulfur h. (SF$_6$)

Hexalen
hexamethonium
hexamethylmelamine
hexapolar catheter
Hexastat
hexaxial reference system
Hexlixate
hexokinase reaction
Hexonate
hexosaminidase deficiency
HF
 heart failure
 high flow
 HF infrared laser
HFA
 Proventil HFA
HFCC
 high-frequency chest wall compression
HFCWO
 high-frequency chest wall oscillation
 HFCWO ventricular resynchronizer
HFEE
 high-frequency epicardial
 echocardiography
HFH
 homozygous familial
 hypercholesterolemia
hFH
 heterozygous familial
 hypercholesterolemia
HFJV
 high-frequency jet ventilation
HFL
 human fetal lung fibroblast
HFO
 high-frequency oscillation
HFOC
 high-flow oxygen conserver
HFPPV
 high-frequency positive pressure
 ventilation
HFV
 high-frequency ventilation
Hg
 mercury
^{195m}Hg
 mercury-195m
H$_1$-H$_2$ interval
HHT
 hereditary hemorrhagic telangiectasia
 heterotopic heart transplant
 hypertensive hypervolemic therapy
HI
 harmonic imaging
 hemorrhagic infarction
HIA
 hyperventilation-induced asthma

hiatal
    h. esophagism
    h. hernia
hiatus
    aortic h.
    h. aorticus
    esophageal h.
    h. esophageus
    h. of facial canal
HIB
    hyperpnea-induced bronchoconstriction
hibernating myocardium
hibernation
    myocardial h.
HibTITER
Hib-VAX
Hi-Care
    H.-C. closed suction and
      pulmonary hygiene system
    H.-C. closed suction system
hiccough, hiccup
Hickman catheter
HICOR system
Hideaway oxygen conserver
Hieshima balloon occluder
Hi-Flex lead
high
    h. air flow with oxygen
      entrainment (HAFOE)
    h. arched palate
    h. blood pressure
    h. density echo
    h. flow (HF)
    h. lung volume
    h. molecular weight dextran
    h. output failure
    H. Oxygen PRM resuscitator
    h. regional wall motion velocity
      (Vhigh)
    h. right atrium
    h. spatial resolution
    h. speed directional coronary
      atherectomy
    h. vacuum (HV)
    h. voltage can (HVC)
high-altitude
    h.-a. pulmonary edema (HAPE)
    h.-a. simulation test (HAST)
high-ceiling diuretic
high-density
    h.-d. electroanatomical and
      entrainment mapping

    h.-d. lipoprotein (HDL)
    h.-d. sector basket catheter
high-dependency unit (HDU)
high-dose
    h.-d. epinephrine
    h.-d. steroid
high-efficiency particulate air (HEPA)
high-energy
    h.-e. laser
    h.-e. transthoracic shock
high-esophageal pH probe
high-fiber diet
high-flow
    h.-f. catheter
    h.-f. oxygen conserver (HFOC)
high-frequency
    3100B h.-f. oscillatory ventilator
    h.-f. burst pacing
    h.-f. chest wall compression
      (HFCC)
    h.-f. chest wall oscillation
      (HFCWO)
    h.-f. chest wall oscillation
      ventricular resynchronizer
    h.-f. epicardial echocardiography
      (HFEE)
    h.-f. jet ventilation (HFJV)
    h.-f. jet ventilator
    h.-f. murmur
    h.-f. oscillation (HFO)
    h.-f. oscillation ventilator
    h.-f. oscillatory ventilation
    h.-f. percussive ventilation
    h.-f. positive pressure ventilation
      (HFPPV)
    h.-f. ventilation (HFV)
high-grade stenosis
high-impedance, low-threshold lead
high-intensity transient signal (HITS)
highly active antiretroviral therapy
    (HAART)
high-output
    h.-o. extended aerosol respiratory
      therapy
    h.-o. heart failure
high-performance liquid chromatography
    (HPLC)
high-pitched murmur
high-pressure
    h.-p. adjunctive percutaneous
      transluminal coronary angioplasty
    h.-p. balloon stenting

NOTES

H

high-pressure *(continued)*
  h.-p. cardiogenic pulmonary edema
  h.-p. edema
  h.-p. inflation technique
  h.-p. liquid chromatography (HPLC)
  h.-p. neurologic syndrome (HPNS)
  h.-p. stent deployment
high-ramp protocol
high-resolution
  h.-r. B-mode ultrasonography
  h.-r. computed tomography (HRCT)
  h.-r. CT (HRCT)
  h.-r. deep penetration 2D
    intracardiac ultrasound
  h.-r. thin section computed
    tomographic
  h.-r. ultrasound
high-risk
  h.-r. angioplasty
  h.-r. phenotype
  h.-r. repolarization abnormality
high-speed
  h.-s. rotational atherectomy (HSRA)
  h.-s. rotation dynamic angioplasty
    catheter
  h.-s. volumetric imaging
Hilal modified headhunter catheter
hilar
  h. adenopathy
  h. clouding
  h. dance
  h. haze
  h. lymphadenopathy
  h. lymph node
Hill
  H. coefficient
  H. phenomenon
  H. sign
Hillis-Müller maneuver
hills-and-valley morphology
Hi-Lo
  H.-L. Evac endotracheal tube
  H.-L. Jet tracheal tube
Hilton sac
hilum
  h. convergence sign
  h. of lung
  h. of lymph node
  h. nodi lymphatici
  h. overlay sign
  pulmonary h.
  h. pulmonis
hilus tuberculosis
Hines-Brown test
hinge
  annulocuspid h.
  h. point
Hinkle-Thaler classification

hip
  h. classification
  h. flexion
Hi-Per
  H.-P. cardiac device
  H.-P. device
  H.-P. Flex exchange wire
hippocratic
  h. angina
  h. sound
  h. succussion
HIPS
  Heparin Infusion Prior to Stenting
  HIPS clinical trial
hirsutum
  cor h.
Hirtz rale
hirudin
  H. for the Improvement of
    Thrombolysis (HIT)
  recombinant h. (r-hirudin)
  H. in Thrombolysis
Hirudo medicinalis
**Hirulog Early Reperfusion/Occlusion
  (HERO)**
His
  bundle of H.
  H. bundle
  H. bundle ablation
  H. bundle catheter
  H. bundle deflection
  H. bundle depolarization
  H. bundle electrocardiogram
  H. bundle electrogram (HBE)
  H. bundle heart block
  H. bundle potential
  H. canal
  H. catheter
  H. deflection
  H. perivascular space
  H. spindle
His-Hass procedure
Hismanal
Hispanic American (HA)
His-Purkinje
  H.-P. conduction
  H.-P. fiber
  H.-P. system
  H.-P. tissue
Histalet
  H. Syrup
  H. X
histaminase
histamine
  h. acid phosphate
  h. challenge
  h. diphosphate
  h. provocation

h. release inhibitory factor (HRIF)
h.-releasing factor (HRF)
His-Tawara node
Histerone Injection
histidine decarboxylase
histiocyte
hemophagocytic h.
palisading h.
histiocytoma
malignant fibrous h. (MFH)
histiocytosis
Langerhans cell h.
primary pulmonary h. X
histiolymphocytic reaction
histocompatibility agent B27
Histocryl Blue tissue adhesive
histogram
DNA h.
h. mode
histologic
histolytica
Entamoeba h.
Torula h.
histolyticus
Cryptococcus h.
histomorphometry
histopathology
Histoplasma
H. capsulatum
H. myocarditis
histoplasmic pericarditis
histoplasmosis
African h.
progressive disseminated h. (PDH)
history
natural h.
pack-year smoking h.
smoking h.
histotoxic hypoxia
Histussin D Liquid
His-ventricular interval
HIT
heparin-induced thrombocytopenia
Hirudin for the Improvement of
Thrombolysis
HIT clinical trial
Hitachi
H. PCT-3600W PET system
H. U-2000 spectrophotometer
Hi-Torque
H.-T. Flex-T guidewire
H.-T. Floppy exchange guidewire

H.-T. Floppy II guidewire
H.-T. Floppy intermediate guidewire
H.-T. Floppy with Pro/Pel
H.-T. Standard guidewire
HITS
high-intensity transient signal
Hitzenberg test
HIV
human immunodeficiency virus
HIV cardiomyopathy
HIV-1 riboprobe
HIVAGEN test
Hivid
Hixson-Vernier protocol
HJR
hepatojugular reflux
HL7
health level seven
HLA
human leukocyte antigen
HLA-6
HLA-129
HLA-A11
HLA-DQA1 gene haplotype
HLA-DQB1 gene haplotype
HLA-DQ gene complex
HLA-DR gene complex
HLHS
hypoplastic left heart syndrome
HLT
heart-lung transplant
HMCAS
hyperdense middle cerebral artery sign
HME
heat/moisture exchanger
Tracheolife HME
HMG-CoA
hydroxymethylglutaryl coenzyme A
3-hydroxy-3-methylglutaryl coenzyme A
HMG CoA-reductase inhibitor
HNS
head, neck, or shaft
HNS lesion
hoarseness
hockey-stick
h.-s. catheter
h.-s. deformity
h.-s. tricuspid valve
HOCM
hypertrophic obstructive cardiomyopathy
Hodgkin
H. disease

NOTES

H

327

Hodgkin *(continued)*
    Hodgkin-Key murmur
    H.-Huxley constant
    H.-Huxley model
Hodgson disease
Hoffman reflex
Hoffrel transesophageal probe
Hohn vessel dilator
hoist
    Temco h.
HOLD
    hemostatic occlusive leverage device
hold
    Children's H.
    H. DM
holder
    Ayers cardiovascular needle h.
    Berry sternal needle h.
    Björk-Shiley heart valve h.
    blade control wire h.
    Castroviejo needle h.
    catheter guide h.
    Comfit endotracheal tube h.
    Cooley Vital microvascular
      needle h.
    Dale tracheostomy tube h.
    DeBakey Vital needle h.
    GraftAssist vein-graft h.
    Lewy chest h.
    LifePort endotracheal tube h.
    needle h.
    NEO-fit neonatal endotracheal
      tube h.
    Thomas LT endotracheal tube h.
    Thomas Quick Block endotracheal
      tube h.
    Vital-Cooley microvascular
      needle h.
    Vital-Ryder microvascular needle h.
    Watson heart valve h.
    wire h.
hole
    bur h.
Holen-Hatle equation
holiday
    dobutamine h.
    h. heart
    h. heart syndrome
Holinger
    H. anterior commissure
      laryngoscope
    H. dissector
holism
Hollenberg treadmill score
Hollenhorst plaque
hollow viscus
Holmes heart
Holmes-Rahe scale

Holmgren-Golgi canal
holmium laser
holmium:yttrium-aluminum-garnet
  (Ho:YAG)
holodiastolic
    h. flow
    h. flow reversal
    h. murmur
holography
    ultrasound h.
holosystolic murmur
Holter
    H. diary
    H.-guided antiarrhythmic drug
      therapy
    Marquette three-channel laser H.
    H. monitor
    H. tube
Holt-Oram syndrome
Holzknecht space
Homans sign
homatropine
    hydrocodone and h.
Hombach
    H. lead placement system
    H. placement of lead
homeometric autoregulation
homeostasis
HomeTrak Plus cardiac event recorder
hominis
    Actinobacillus h.
    Cardiobacterium h.
    Mycoplasma h.
    Pentatrichomonas h.
HomMed Monitoring system
Homochron monitor
homocollateral reconstitution
homocysteine
    plasma h.
    total h. (tHcy)
homocystine
homocystinuria syndrome
homodimer
    alpha-alpha h.
    beta-beta h.
homogeneity
    Breslow-Day test for h.
    tracer h.
homogeneous plaque
homogentisic acid oxidase deficiency
homograft
    aortic h.
    denatured h.
    homovital h.
    h. insertion for pulmonary
      regurgitation
    mitral h.

mitral valve h.
pulmonary artery h.
homologous cardiac transplant
homoscedastic
homotypic adhesion
homovital homograft
homozygosity
homozygote
homozygous
    h. beta-thalassemia
    h. familial hypercholesterolemia
    (HFH)
honeycomb
    h. cyst
    h. lesion
    h. lung
    h. pattern
honeycombing
    h. cyst
    h. of lung
    subpleural h.
Hong Kong influenza
honk
    precordial h.
    systolic h.
honking murmur
hood
    h. O_2
    H. stoma stent
Hood-Westaby T-Y stent
hook
    Adson h.
    barbed h.
    Bryant mitral h.
    Doyen rib h.
hook-and-loop fastener strap
Hooke law
Hoover sign
HOPE
    Heart Outcomes Prevention Evaluation
    Hospital Outcomes Reversibility for the
    Elderly
    HOPE study
hope
    H. bag
    H. Continuous & HELIOX
    nebulizer
    H. resuscitator
    H. sign
Hopkins
    H. aortic clamp

H. forceps
H. Symptom Checklist
Horder spots
horehound lozenge
Horizon
    H. AutoAdjust CPAP system
    H. CPAP device
    H. LT CPAP system
    H. nasal CPAP system
    H. PFT spirometer
    H. surgical ligating and marking
    clip
horizontal
    h. anteroposterior deceleration
    h. deceleration
    h. depression
    h. fissure
    h. heart
    h. long axis
    h. long-axis tomogram
    h. long-axis view
    h. ST segment
    h. ST segment depression
    h. VAS
hormone
    adrenocorticotropic h. (ACTH)
    antidiuretic h. (ADH)
    female h.
    growth h.
    mineralocorticoid h.
    natriuretic h.
    parathyroid h.
    syndrome of inappropriate
    antidiuretic h. (SIADH)
    thyroid-stimulating h. (TSH)
Horner
    H. sign
    H. syndrome
horripilation
horse asthma
horse-race effect
horseshoe
    h. configuration
    h. lung
Horton
    H. arteritis
    H. disease
hose
    Juzo h.
Hosmer-Lemeshow Goodness-of-Fit test
hospital
    H. Admission Risk Profile (HARP)

NOTES

H

hospital *(continued)*
    H. Anxiety and Depression (HAD)
    H. Anxiety and Depression scale
        (HADS)
    Los Angeles Veterans
        Administration H. (LAVA)
    H. Outcomes Reversibility for the
        Elderly (HOPE)
    Veterans Affairs Non-Q-Wave
        Infarction Strategies in H.
        (VANQWISH)
hospital-acquired infection
host
    granulocytopenic h.
    humoral h.
    immunocompetent h.
    nonimmunocompromised h.
host-generated neutrophils recruitment
HOT
    Hypertension Optimal Treatment
    HOT study
hot
    h. gangrene
    h. nose sign
    h. potato voice
    h. spot
    h. wire anemometer
Hotelling T2 test
hot-tip laser probe
hot-wire pneumotachometer
Hounsfield unit (HU)
Hour
    Claritin-D 24 H.
24-hour
    24-h. ambulatory
        electrocardiographic recorder
    24-h. cortisol
12-hour antiplatelet therapy
hourglass
    h. murmur
    h. pattern
    h. stenosis
house
    h. dust mite (HDM)
    h. dust mite allergen
**Housecall transtelephonic monitoring
system**
Howard method
Howel-Evans syndrome
Howell test
Ho:YAG
    holmium:yttrium-aluminum-garnet
    Ho:YAG laser
    Ho:YAG laser angioplasty
Hoyer anastomosis
HP
    hypersensitivity pneumonitis

HP SONOS 30-MHz imaging
    catheter
HP SONOS 2500 transducer
HPA
    hypothalamic-pituitary-adrenal
HPAA
    hypothalamic-pituitary-adrenal axis
H.P. Acthar Gel
HPCD
    hemostatic puncture closure device
HPD
    hematoporphyrin derivative
5-HPETE acid
HPI
    Haemophilus parainfluenzae
H'P interval
HPLC
    high-performance liquid chromatography
    high-pressure liquid chromatography
HPNS
    high-pressure neurologic syndrome
H-proline
HPS
    hepatopulmonary syndrome
HPV
    human papillomavirus
    hypoxic pulmonary vasoconstriction
H-Q interval
H-QRS interval
HR
    heart rate
        HR conduction time
H-R conduction time
HRCT
    high-resolution computed tomography
    high-resolution CT
        diagnostic HRCT
        HRCT scan
HRF
    histamine-releasing factor
        HRF deficiency
HRIF
    histamine release inhibitory factor
HRQL, HRQOL
    health-related quality of life
HRR
    heart rate reserve
HRS
    Hamman-Rich syndrome
HRT
    hyperfractionated radiation
HRV
    heart rate variability
        power spectrum of HRV
        HRV test
H.S.
    Estratest H.S.

HSP, Hsp, hsp
   heat shock protein
      HSP antigen
HSP47
   heat shock protein 47
HSRA
   high-speed rotational atherectomy
      HSRA device
HSS
   hypertrophic subaortic stenosis
HSV
   herpes simplex virus
      HSV meningitis
      HSV pneumonia
HT
   hemorrhagic transformation
      cerebral HT
5HT
   5-hydroxytryptamine
HTLV
   human T-cell lymphotropic virus
      HTLV-I, II
HTN
   hypertension
HTX
   hemothorax
H-type tracheoesophageal fistula
HU
   Hounsfield unit
hub
   catheter h.
   QuickLoad h.
   h. and spoke referral system
Huchard
   H. disease
   H. sign
Hudson
   H. Lifesaver resuscitator
   H. Multi-Vent
Huff coughing
Hufnagel
   H. ascending aortic clamp
   H. prosthetic valve
Hugenholtz method
Hugger
   Bair H.
Hughes-Stovin syndrome
Hull triad
hum
   cervical venous h.
   venous h.

human
   antihemophilic factor (h.)
   h. aortic endothelial cell (HAEC)
   h. aortic smooth muscle cell
      (HASMC)
   h. atrial natriuretic peptide (hANP)
   h. babesiosis
   h. cloned DNA (cDNA)
   h. cosmid library
   h. cytomegalovirus (HCMV)
   cytomegalovirus immune globulin
      intravenous, h.
   h. ether-a-go-go-related gene
      (HERG)
   h. fetal lung fibroblast (HFL)
   h. gene C4B
   h. immunodeficiency virus (HIV)
   h. leukocyte antigen (HLA)
   h. lymphocyte antigen typing
   h. menopausal gonadotropin
      coenzyme A reductase inhibitor
   h. papillomavirus (HPV)
   h. pooled AAT
   h. preproendothelin-1 gene
   h. recombinant deoxyribonuclease
   h. T-cell lymphotropic virus
      (HTLV)
   h. umbilical vein (HUV)
   Velosulin H.
Humate-P
Humatin
humeroperoneal neuromuscular disease
Humibid
   H. DM
   H. L.A.
   H. Sprinkle
humid asthma
humidification
humidified oxygen
humidifier
   Bard-Parker U-Mid/Lo h.
   Bennett Cascade II Servo
      Controlled Heated H.
   bubble h.
   cold-mist h.
   Fischer & Paykel HC100 heated h.
   jet h.
   h. lung
   Mistogen passover h.
   MRT Tidal H.
   OEM 503 h.
   Ohio Bubble h.

NOTES

H

humidifier *(continued)*
    passover h.
    Respironics Oasis h.
    Sullivan HumidAire heated h.
    ThermoFlo h.
    ThermoFloNeo h.
    Whisper Mist h.
humidity
    absolute h.
    relative h.
humming murmur
humming-top murmur
humoral
    h. host
    h. immune defect
hump
    Hampton h.
Humulin L, N, R, U insulin
huN901-DM1 antibody
hunger
    air h.
Hunt
    H. angiographic trocar
    H. and Hess grades I through V
    aneurysm grading system
Hunter
    H. balloon
    H. canal
    H. detachable balloon occluder
    H. operation
    H. syndrome
Hunter-Hurler syndrome
Hunter-Satinsky clamp
Hunter-Sessions balloon
hunting reaction
Huntington chorea
Hurler-Scheie compound
Hurler syndrome
Hurricaine spray
Hürthle
    H. cell tumor
    H. manometer
Hurwitz thoracic trocar
Hustead needle
HUT
    head-up tilt
Hutinel disease
HUTTT
    head-up tilt-table test
HUV
    human umbilical vein
    HUV bypass graft
Huygens principle
H-V
    H.-V. conduction time
    H.-V. interval
HV
    high vacuum

hypervolemic
    HV conduction time
    HV interval
HVC
    high voltage can
HW
    hemodynamically-weighted MRI
hyaline
    h. arterionecrosis
    h. arteriosclerosis
    h. fatty change
    h. membrane disease
    h. membrane formation
    h. thrombus
hyalinizing granuloma
hyalinosis
    arteriolar h.
hyaloserositis
    progressive multiple h.
hyaluronan
hyaluronic
    h. acid
    h. acid polymer
hyaluronidase
Hyate:C
Hybolin
    H. decanoate
    H. Improved Injection
Hybond ECL nitrocellulose membrane
hybrid
    h. revascularization
    h. unit
hybridization
    fluorescence in situ h. (FISH)
    fluorescent in situ h. (FISH)
    in situ h.
Hybritech immunoradiometric assay
Hycamtin
HycoClear Tuss
Hycodan
Hycomine
    H. Compound
    H. Pediatric
Hycotuss
    H. Expectorant Liquid
HYD
    hydrocortisone
hydantoin
hydatid
    h. cyst
    h. fremitus
Hydeltrasol injection
Hydeltra-T.B.A. injection
hydralazine
    h. hydrochloride
    h. and hydrochlorothiazide
    h., hydrochlorothiazide, and
    reserpine

Hydramyn Syrup
Hydrap-ES
hydrate
    chloral h.
    terpin h.
hydration
    systemic h.
hydraulic
    h. resistance
    h. vein stripper
hydrazine
    dimethyl h.
Hydrea
Hydrenox
hydride
    lithium h.
hydrobromic acid
hydrobromide
    hydroxyamphetamine h.
hydrocarbon
    h. aspiration
    halogenated h.
    polycyclic aromatic h. (PAH)
    h. toxicity
HydroCath catheter
Hydrocet
hydrochloric acid
hydrochloride (HCl)
    acebutolol h.
    acecainide h.
    alfentanil h.
    amantadine h.
    amiloride h.
    amiodarone h.
    amprolium h.
    bacampicillin h.
    benazepril h.
    bepridil h.
    betaxolol h.
    bromhexine h.
    carbuterol h.
    carteolol h.
    chlorpromazine h.
    ciprofloxacin h.
    clonidine h.
    clorprenaline h.
    colestipol h.
    cyclopentamine h.
    cyproheptadine h.
    cytarabine h.
    demeclocycline h.
    desipramine h.

diltiazem h.
diphenhydramine h.
dobutamine h.
dopamine h.
doxapram h.
doxepin h.
doxorubicin h.
encainide h.
esmolol h.
esprolol h.
ethambutol h.
ethaverine h.
ethylnorepinephrine h.
fenfluramine h.
fexofenadine h.
fluoxetine h.
guanfacine h.
hydralazine h.
idarubicin h.
isoprenaline h.
isoprophenamine h.
isopropylarterenol h.
isoproterenol h.
isoxsuprine h.
labetalol h.
levamisole h.
lidocaine h.
lincomycin h.
lomefloxacin h.
mecamylamine h.
mechlorethamine h.
mefloquine h.
meperidine h.
mepivacaine h.
methamphetamine h.
methoxamine h.
methoxyphenamine h.
metoclopramide h.
mexiletine h.
minocycline h.
mitoxantrone h.
moexipril h.
Mustargen H.
nalmefene h.
naloxone h.
nicardipine h.
nortriptyline h.
oxytetracycline h.
papaverine h.
phenoxybenzamine h.
phentolamine h.
phenylephrine h.

NOTES

H

hydrochloride *(continued)*
    phenylpropanolamine h.
    prazosin h.
    prenalterol h.
    procainamide h.
    procaine h.
    promethazine h.
    propafenone h.
    propranolol h.
    protokylol h.
    protriptyline h.
    pyridoxine h.
    quinapril h.
    remacemide h.
    rimantadine h.
    sematilide h.
    sertraline h.
    sotalol h.
    spirapril h.
    terazosin h.
    tetracaine h.
    thioridazine h.
    ticlopidine h.
    tiprenolol h.
    tizanidine h.
    tocainide h.
    tolazoline h.
    trazodone h.
    vancomycin h.
    verapamil h.
    yohimbine h.
hydrochlorothiazide (HCTZ)
    amiloride and h.
    benazepril and h.
    bisoprolol and h.
    candesartan, cilexetil and h.
    captopril and h.
    enalapril and h.
    hydralazine and h.
    irbesartan and h.
    lisinopril and h.
    losartan and h.
    losartan potassium h.
    methyldopa and h.
    moexipril and h.
    propranolol and h.
    quinapril and h.
    h. and reserpine
    h. and spironolactone
    h. and triamterene
    valsartan and h.
Hydrocoat hydrophilic coating
hydrocodone
    h. and acetaminophen
    h. bitartrate
    h. and chlorpheniramine
    h. and guaifenesin
    h. and homatropine

    H. PA Syrup
    h., phenylephrine, pyrilamine,
      phenindamine, chlorpheniramine
    h. and phenylpropanolamine
    h. and pseudoephedrine
    h., pseudoephedrine, and
      guaifenesin
Hydrocort
hydrocortisone (HYD)
    h. cyclopentylpropionate
    h. cypionate
    h. hydrogen succinate
    h. sodium phosphate
    h. sodium succinate
    systemic h.
Hydrocortone
    H. Acetate
    H. Acetate Injection
    H. Oral
    H. Phosphate
    H. Phosphate Injection
hydrocyanic acid
HydroDIURIL
HydroDot system
hydroflumethiazide and reserpine
hydrofluoric acid
hydrofluoroalkane
Hydro-Fluserpine
Hydrogel-coated PTCA balloon catheter
hydrogen
    h. appearance time
    h. bromide
    h. chloride
    h. cyanide (HCN)
    h. density
    h. electrodes
    h. fluoride
    h. inhalation technique
    h. ion concentration (pH)
    h. peroxide
    h. sulfide
hydrogen-3 mazindol
Hydrogesic
hydrolase
    lysosomal h.
Hydrolyser
    H. catheter
    H. hydrodynamic thrombectomy
      catheter
    H. thrombectomy catheter
hydrolysis
    ATP h.
    h. of surfactant
Hydromet
hydromorphone
Hydromox
hydronephrosis
Hydropane

Hydro Par
hydropericarditis
hydropericardium
Hydrophed
Hydrophen
hydrophilic
    h. agent
    h. coated guidewire
hydrophobic
    h. drug
hydropneumatosis
hydropneumopericardium
hydropneumothorax
Hydropres
hydrops
    h. fetalis
    h. pericardii
hydroquinidine
Hydro-Serp
Hydroserpine
hydrosoluble asthmogen
hydrosphere
hydrosphygmograph
Hydro-Splint II
hydrostatic
    h. edema
    h. suction
Hydro-T
hydrothorax
    chylous h.
    hepatic h.
Hydrotropine
hydroxide
    potassium h. (KOH)
hydroxocobalamin
hydroxyamphetamine hydrobromide
hydroxyapatite
hydroxybutyrate
    h. dehydrogenase (HBDH)
    gamma h. (GHB)
hydroxychloroquine sulfate
18-hydroxycorticosterone
20-hydroxyeicosatetraenoic acid (20-
    HETE)
hydroxyephedrine (HED)
    carbon-11 h.
hydroxyethyl starch
17-hydroxylase deficiency
hydroxylase deficiency
hydroxyl radical

hydroxymethylglutaryl
    h. coenzyme A (HMG-CoA)
    h. coenzyme A reductase inhibitor
3-hydroxy-3-methylglutaryl
    3-h.-3-m. coenzyme A (HMG-CoA)
    3-h.-3-m. coenzyme A reductase
    3-h.-3-m. coenzyme A reductase
        inhibitor
hydroxyprogesterone caproate
hydroxyproline analysis
5-hydroxypropafenone
11-beta-hydroxysteroid dehydrogenase
hydroxytoluene
    butylated h. (BHT)
5-hydroxytryptamine (5HT)
hydroxyurea
hydroxyzine
    theophylline, ephedrine, and h.
        (TEH)
Hy-Gestrone injection
Hygrobac-Dar heat-moisture exchanger
Hygroton
Hylorel
Hylutin injection
Hynes pharyngoplasty
hyoid
    mandibular plane to h. (MP-H)
    h. myotomy
    h. suspension
hyopharyngeus
Hy-Pam Oral
Hypaque
hyparterial bronchi
hyperabduction syndrome
hyperacute
    h. rejection
    h. T wave
hyperadrenergic activity
hyperaldosteronism
hyperalgesia
hyperalimentation
    intravenous h. (IVH)
hyperalphalipoproteinemia
hyperammonemia
hyperapobetalipoproteinemia
hyperapolipoprotein B syndrome
hyperbaric
    h. chamber
    h. exposure
    h. oxygen (HBO)
    h. oxygenation

NOTES

H

hyperbaric (*continued*)
    h. oxygen therapy
    h. pressure
hypercalcemia
    familial hypocalciuric h.
    h. syndrome
hypercalciuria
hypercapnia
    oxygen-induced h.
    permissive h. (PHC)
hypercapnic
    h. acidosis
    h. challenge
    h. respiratory failure
    h. stimulus
hypercarbia
    oxygen-induced h.
hypercardia
hyperchloremic acidosis
hypercholesterolemia
    false h.
    familial h. (FH)
    heterozygous familial h. (hFH)
    homozygous familial h. (HFH)
    polygenic h.
    h. (types IIa and IIb)
hypercholesterolemic
hyperchylomicronemia
    familial h.
hypercirculation
hypercoagulability
hypercoagulable state
hypercontractile
hypercontractility
hypercortisolemia
hypercortisolism
hypercyanotic
    h. angina
    h. spell
hyperdense middle cerebral artery sign (HMCAS)
hyperdiastole
hyperdicrotic
hyperdicrotism
hyperdynamic
    h. septic shock
    h. state
hyperemia
    active h.
    adenosine-induced h.
    arterial h.
    collateral h.
    fluxionary h.
    passive h.
    peristatic h.
    postocclusal h.
    reactive h.
    venous h.

hyperemic velocity
hypereosinophilia syndrome
hypereosinophilic
    h. heart disease
    h. syndrome
hyperergopathic dilated cardiomyopathy
hyperesthesia
    cutaneous h.
hyperestrogenemia
hyperfibrinogenemia
hyperfiltration
    glomerular h.
Hyperflex tracheostomy tube
hyperfractionated radiation (HRT)
hypergammaglobulinemia
hyperglobulinemia
hyperglycemia
hyperhomocystinemia
hyperinfection
hyperinflated
hyperinflation
    dynamic h.
hyperinsulinemia
hyperinsulinemic euglycemic clamp metabolic state
hyperinsulinism
hyperintense heterogeneous signal
hyperintensity
    deep white matter h. (DWMHI)
    patchy h.
    periventricular h. (PVH, PVHI)
    pontine h. (PHI)
    punctate h.
    white matter h. (WMHI)
hyperirritability
hyperkalemia
hyperkalemic cardioplegia
hyperkinemia
hyperkinesia
hyperkinesis
hyperkinetic
    h. heart syndrome
    h. pulse
    h. state
hyperleukocytic reaction
hyperleukocytosis
hyperlipidemia
    false combined h.
    familial combined h. (FCHL)
    multiple lipoprotein-type h.
    polygenic h.
hyperlipoproteinemia
hyperlucency
hyperlucent
    h. lung
    h. lung syndrome
hypermagnesemia
hypermetabolism

hypernatremia
hypernephroma
hypernitrosopnea
hyperoxaluria
hyperoxia
hyperparathyroidism
hyperperfusion syndrome
hyperphosphatemia
hyperpiesis, hyperpiesia
hyperpietic
hyperpigmentation
hyperplasia
    adrenal h.
    atypical alveolar h.
    bilateral adrenal h.
    congenital adrenal h.
    elastic tissue h.
    intimal h. (IH)
    lymphoid h.
    mucous gland h.
    multifocal micronodular
      pneumocyte h.
    neointimal h.
    nodular lymphoid h.
    synovial sarcoma reactive
      mesothelial h.
    type II cell h.
hyperplastic
    h. mucus-secreting goblet cell
    h. osteoarthritis
hyperplastica
    arteritis h.
hyperpnea
    exercise h.
    h.-induced bronchoconstriction (HIB)
    isocapnic h.
hyperpolarization
    afterspike h. (AHP)
hyperreactivity
    airway h. (AHR)
    bronchial h. (BHR)
    nonspecific bronchial h.
    work-related bronchial h.
hyperreflexia
    autonomic h.
hyperreninemia
hyperresonance
hyperresonant
hyperresponsive airway
hyperresponsiveness
    airway h. (AHR)
    bronchial h. (BHR)

hypersecretion
    airway h.
    mucus h.
hypersecretory
hypersensitive carotid sinus syndrome
hypersensitivity
    aminosalicylic acid h.
    cardioinhibitory carotid sinus h.
    carotid sinus h.
    h. myocarditis
    h. pneumonia
    h. pneumonitis (HP)
    h. vasculitis
hyperserotonemia
    vasculocardiac syndrome of h.
hypersignal
hypersomnia
    idiopathic h.
hypersomnolence
hypersonority
    tympanic h.
hypersphyxia
Hyperstat IV
hypersystole
hypersystolic
hypertelorism
hypertension (HTN)
    accelerated h.
    adrenal h.
    alveolar h.
    arterial h.
    H. Audit of Risk Factor Therapy
      (HART)
    benign h.
    benign intracranial h.
    borderline h. (BHT)
    ceiling effect in h.
    chronic thromboembolic
      pulmonary h. (CTEPH)
    cuffed h.
    H. Detection and Follow-Up
      Program
    diastolic h.
    Dietary Approach to Prevent H.
      (DASH)
    episodic h.
    essential h.
    exercise h.
    familial dyslipidemic h.
    gestational h.
    glucocorticoid-induced h.
    hypoxic pulmonary h.

NOTES

H

hypertension *(continued)*
    idiopathic h.
    induced h.
    intracranial h. (ICH)
    intrathoracic h.
    isolated systolic h.
    labile h.
    left atrial h.
    malignant h.
    masked h.
    mineralocorticoid-induced h.
    neuromuscular h.
    obesity h.
    office h.
    H. Optimal Treatment (HOT)
    oral contraceptive-induced h.
    orthostatic h.
    Page episodic h.
    pale h.
    paroxysmal h.
    pediatric h.
    portal h. (PHT)
    portopulmonary h.
    postcapillary h.
    postpartum h.
    precapillary pulmonary h.
    pregnancy-induced h. (PIH)
    primary h.
    primary pulmonary h. (PPH)
    pulmonary h. (PH, PHT)
    pulmonary artery h. (PAH)
    Quality of Life Trial H. (QoLITY)
    recalcitrant h.
    red h.
    renal h.
    renoprival h.
    renovascular h.
    resistant h.
    resting h.
    retrograde h.
    salt-and-water dependent h.
    secondary h.
    secondary pulmonary h.
    splenoportal h.
    h. standard
    stress-related h.
    systemic h.
    systemic vascular h.
    systemic venous h.
    systolic h.
    thromboembolic pulmonary h.
    venous h.
    white-coat h.
hypertensive
    h. agent
    h. arteriopathy
    h. arteriosclerosis

    h. arteriosclerotic heart disease (HASHD)
    h. cardiovascular disease (HCVD)
    h. crisis
    h. emergency
    h. encephalopathy
    h. heart disease
    h. hypertrophic cardiomyopathy
    h. hypervolemic therapy (HHT)
    h. nephropathy
    h. pulmonary polyarteritis
    h. pulmonary vascular disease
    h. retinopathy
    spontaneously h. (SH)
    h. urgency
    h. vasculopathy
hyperthermia
    cerebral h.
    whole-body h.
hyperthyroid heart
hyperthyroidism
    amiodarone-induced h.
    apathetic h.
hypertonic
    h. saline
    h. saline inhalation
hypertonica
    polycythemia h.
hypertriglyceridemia
hypertriglyceridemic waist
hypertrophic
    h. adenoid
    h. cardiomyopathy (HC, HCM, HCMP)
    h. catarrh
    h. emphysema
    h. obstructive cardiomyopathy (HOCM)
    h. pulmonary osteoarthropathy
    h. smooth muscle layer
    h. subaortic stenosis (HSS)
hypertrophied
    h. apex
    h. myocardium
hypertrophy
    adenotonsillar h.
    apical h.
    asymmetric septal h. (ASH)
    basal-septal h.
    cardiac h.
    compensatory h.
    concentric left ventricular h.
    eccentric h.
    goblet cell h.
    isolated septal h. (ISH)
    left ventricular h. (LVH)
    lipomatous h.
    mucous gland h.

myocardial h.
myocardial cell h.
myocyte h.
pressure-overload h.
right ventricular h. (RVH)
secondary septal h.
septal h.
stretch-induced cardiomyocyte h.
submucosal gland h.
trabecular h.
transcoronary ablation of septal h. (TASH)
ventricular h.
volume load h.
hyperuricemia
hyperuricemic nephropathy
hyperventilation
alveolar h.
eucapneic voluntary h.
h.-induced asthma (HIA)
h. maneuver
h. syndrome
hyperviscosity syndrome
hypervitaminosis
hypervolemia
hypervolemic (HV)
hypha, pl. **hyphae**
hyphemia
Hy-Phen
hypnagogic hallucination
hypnagogue
hypnalgia
hypnesthesia
hypnic
hypnology
Hypnomidate
hypnopompic
hypnosis
hypnotic drug
hypoadrenalism
hypoaeration
hypoalbuminemia
hypoaldosteronism
hyporeninemic h.
hypoalphalipoproteinemia
hypobaric
h. exposure
h. hypoxia
hypobetalipoproteinemia
familial h. (FHBL)
hypocalcemia
hypocapnia

hypocapnic
hypocarbia
hypochloremia
hypochloremic metabolic alkalosis
hypochlorite
hypocholesterolemia
hypochondrial reflex
hypochondriasis
hypodynamia cordis
hypoechoic
hypofunction
hypogammaglobulinemia
hypoglossal nerve
hypoglycemia
hypoglycemic
h. agent
h. syncope
hypokalemia-induced arrhythmia
hypokalemic periodic paralysis
hypokinemia
hypokinesis, hypokinesia
anteromesial h.
cardiac wall h.
global h.
hypokinetic pulse
hypomagnesemia
hyponatremia
hyponatremic-hypertensive syndrome
hypoparathyroidism
hypoperfused myocardium
hypoperfusion
myocardial h.
hypopharyngeal obstruction
hypophosphatemia
hypophyseal-pituitary adrenal axis
hypophyseos
pars pharyngea h.
hypopiesis
orthostatic h.
hypoplasia
isthmic h.
mitral valve h.
h. of right ventricle
right ventricular h.
hypoplastic
h. emphysema
h. heart
h. left heart
h. left heart syndrome (HLHS)
hypopnea
central h.
obstructive h.

NOTES

H

hypopneic
hyporeninemia
hyporeninemic hypoaldosteronism
hyporesonant
hyposphygmia
hyposphyxia
hypostasis
    pulmonary h.
hypostatic
    h. bronchopneumonia
    h. congestion
    h. pneumonia
hyposystole
hypotension
    acute severe h.
    arterial h.
    chronic idiopathic orthostatic h.
    exertional h.
    hemorrhagic h.
    idiopathic orthostatic h.
    intractable h.
    orthostatic h.
    postprandial h.
    postural h.
    vasodilatory h.
    vasovagal h.
hypotensive agent
hypothalamic-pituitary-adrenal (HPA)
    h.-p.-a. axis (HPAA)
hypothermia
    h. blanket
    extracorporeal exchange h.
    h. mattress
    moderate h.
    topical h.
hypothermic fibrillating arrest
hypothesis, pl. **hypotheses**
    fetal origins h.
    Gad h.
    leading circle h.
    lipid h.
    Lyon h.
    Moe h.
    Moe multiple wavelet h.
    monoclonal h.
    null h.
    premature ventricular complex-trigger h.
    response-to-injury h.
    sulfhydryl depletion h.
    Wu-Hoak h.
hypothetical
hypothrombogenic
hypothyroidism
    subclinical h.
hypotonia
hypotonicity
hypotonus, hypotony

Hypovase
hypoventilation
    alveolar h.
    congenital central alveolar h.
    nocturnal h.
hypoviscous
hypovolemia
hypovolemic shock
hypoxanthine
hypoxemia
    arterial h.
    circulatory h.
    intraoperative h.
    refractory h.
    REM sleep-related h.
    rest h.
    h. test
hypoxia
    altitude h.
    alveolar h.
    anemic h.
    circulatory h.
    demand h.
    diffusion h.
    global tissue h.
    hemic h.
    histotoxic h.
    hypobaric h.
    hypoxic h.
    ischemic h.
    myocyte h.
    sleep h.
    stagnant h.
    h. warning system
hypoxic
    h. hypoxia
    h. lap swimming
    h. pulmonary hypertension
    h. pulmonary vasoconstriction (HPV)
    h. response study
    h. spell
    h. syncope
    h. vasoconstriction
hypoxidosis
HypRho-D Mini-Dose
Hyprogest 250
hysteresis
    airway h.
    pacemaker h.
    pacing h.
    rate h.
hysterical
    h. fainting
    h. syncope
hysteric angina
hystericus
    globus h.

hysterosystole
Hy-Tape waterproof adhesive tape
Hytinic
Hytrin
Hytuss
Hytuss-2X

Hyzaar
   H. 50/12.5
   H. 100/25
Hy-Zide
Hyzine-50 Injection

NOTES

I-123
iodine-123
I-123 BMIPP
I-123 BMIPP imaging
I-123 metaiodobenzylguanidine
I-123 MIBG
I-123 MIBG uptake
I-125
I. metaiodobenzylguanidine
I. MIBG
I-309
CC chemokine I.
I_{Ca}
calcium current
I_{Cl}
chloride current
I_F
pacemaker current
I_{Na}
sodium current
2000i
Vapotherm 2000i
IA
intraarterial
IAA
interrupted aortic arch
IAB
intraaortic balloon
IAB catheter
IABC
intraaortic balloon counterpulsation
IABP
intraaortic balloon pulsation
intraaortic balloon pump
intraaortic balloon pumping
IAC
interposed abdominal compression
IAD
implantable atrial defibrillator
intracranial atherosclerotic disease
Metrix IAD
IADL
impairment of activities of daily living
instrumental activities of daily living
Lawton IADL
IAF
idiopathic alveolar fibrosis
IAIA
immune adherence immunosorbent assay
IAQ
indoor air quality
IART
intraatrial reentry tachycardia
iatrogenic
i. atrial septal defect

i. disease
i. disorder
i. pneumothorax
I band
Iberet-Folic-500
iberiotoxin
IBI
internal borderzone infarct
ibopamine
Ibuprin
ibuprofen
Arthritis Foundation I.
pseudoephedrine and i.
Ibuprohm
Ibu-Tab
ibutilide fumarate
IC
inspiratory capacity
ICA
internal carotid artery
ICAM
intercellular adhesion molecule
ICAM-1
intercellular adhesion molecule-1
ICAO
International Civil Aviation Organization
ICAO standard atmosphere
ICAT
intracoronary aspiration thrombectomy
icatibant pretreatment
ICD
implantable cardioverter-defibrillator
Angstrom II ICD
Angstrom MD ICD
Cadence biphasic ICD
Contour High Voltage Can ICD
Contour II ICD
Contour LT V-135D ICD
Contour V-145D ICD
dual-chamber ICD
Guardian ICD
ICD lead
Res-Q Micron ICD
Telectronics Guardian ATP II ICD
transthoracically implanted ICD
Ventritex Cadence ICD
Vitatron Diamond ICD
ICD-9
International Classification of Diseases,
Ninth Revision
ICD-ATP
implantable cardioverter-
defibrillator/atrial tachycardia pacing
ICD-ATP device

ICE
  intracardiac echocardiography
ice
  i. mapping
  i. slush
  slushed i.
iced
  i. saline
  i. saline lavage
ice-pick view
ICEUS
  intracaval endovascular ultrasonography
ICH
  intracerebral hemorrhage
  intracranial hemorrhage
  intracranial hypertension
    infratentorial ICH
    supratentorial ICH
ICHD pacemaker code
ichorous pleurisy
icing heart
ICO
  intracellular organism
ICOPER
  International Cooperative Pulmonary
  Embolism Registry
Icorel
ICP
  intracranial pressure
ICRT
  intracoronary radiation therapy
ICS
  intracellular-like, calcium-bearing
  crystalloid solution
    ICS cardioplegic solution
ICSD
  International Classification of Sleep
  Disorders
ICSS
  International Carotid Stenting Study
icteric sputum
ictometer
ICTP
  type I collagen telopeptide
ictus
  i. cordis
  i. sanguinis
ICUS
  intracoronary ultrasound
ICV
  internal cerebral vein
ICV-10 ventilator
ICXA
  intermediate circumflex artery
ID
  immunodiffusion
Idamycin PFS

idarubicin
  i. hydrochloride
IDC
  idiopathic dilated cardiomyopathy
IDCS
  diffuse cutaneous scleroderma
  antitopoisomerase IDCS
IDDM
  insulin-dependent diabetes mellitus
ideal
  i. alveolar gas
  I. cardiac device
  I. device
ideational apraxia
ideomotor apraxia
idiojunctional rhythm
idiomotor apraxia
idionodal rhythm
idiopathic
  i. acute eosinophilic pneumonia
  i. alveolar fibrosis (IAF)
  i. arteritis of Takayasu
  i. bradycardia
  i. brown induration
  i. cardiomegaly
  i. cardiomyopathy
  i. central sleep apnea
  i. cyclic edema
  i. dilated cardiomyopathy (IDC)
  i. dilation
  i. hypereosinophilic syndrome
  (IHES)
  i. hypersomnia
  i. hypertension
  i. hypertrophic subaortic stenosis
  (IHSS)
  i. interstitial fibrosis
  i. interstitial pneumonia
  i. long Q-T interval syndrome
  i. myocarditis
  i. orthostatic hypotension
  i. pericarditis
  i. pulmonary fibrosis (IPF)
  i. pulmonary hemosiderosis (IPH)
  i. restrictive cardiomyopathy
  i. right atrial dilation
  i. thrombocytopenia
  i. thrombocytopenic purpura (ITP)
  i. unilobar emphysema
  i. venoocclusive disease
  i. ventricular fibrillation
  i. ventricular tachycardia (IVT)
idiopathica cystica
idiosyncratic asthma
idioventricular
  i. bradycardia
  i. kick

i. rhythm
i. tachycardia
IDIS
intraoperative digital subtraction
IDIS angiography system
IDIS system
IDL
intermediate-density lipoprotein
idoxuridine
IDV
intermittent demand ventilation
IE
infective endocarditis
I:E
inspiratory to expiratory ratio
I:E ratio
IE-2 riboprobe
IEA
inferior epigastric artery
IEA graft
IEL
internal elastic lamina
IEM
internal elastic membrane
IEM rupture
Ifex
IFG
inferior frontal gyrus
IFL
inferior frontal lobe
IFN
interferon
ifosfamide
Ig
immunoglobulin
Igaki-Tamai stent
IgE
serum I.
IgE-sensitized cell
IGF
insulin-like growth factor
IGF-1 overexpression
IgG
immunoglobulin-G
ACLA IgG
IgG avidity test
IgG1–4
IgM
ACLA I.
IGT
impaired glucose tolerance

IH
intimal hyperplasia
intramural hematoma
IHD
ischemic heart disease
IHES
idiopathic hypereosinophilic syndrome
IHSS
idiopathic hypertrophic subaortic stenosis
Ikorel
IL
interleukin
IL 1640 blood gas/electrolyte
system
IL GEMPCL testing system
IL GEM Premier Plus testing
system
IL GEMSensiCath ABG system
IL IMPACT testing system
IL Synthesis analyzer
IL Synthesis testing system
IL-10
I. production
recombinant human I. (rhuIL-10)
IL-4 gene
ILD
interstitial lung disease
ileal artery
ileocolic artery
Iletin
beef Lente I. II
Lente I.
ileus
meconium i.
ILHDL
isolated low high-density lipoprotein
iliac
i. artery
i. artery occlusion
i. steal
i. vein
i. vein thrombosis
iliofemoral venous system
iliopopliteal bypass
Illinois Test of Psycholinguistic Abilities (ITPA)
illness
catabolic i.
decompression i.
Illumen-8 guiding catheter
illusion
oculostenotic i.

NOTES

Iloprost
Ilosone
    I. Oral
    I. Pulvules
Ilotycin
ILUS
    intraluminal ultrasound
    ILUS catheter
IM
    Rocephin IM
IMA
    inferior mesenteric artery
    internal mammary artery
    IMA graft
    IMA retractor
IMAB
    internal mammary artery bypass
image
    i. aliasing
    amplitude i.
    i. analysis
    i. bundle
    CK i.
    color kinesis i.
    3D SPGR i.
    ejection-fraction i.
    ejection shell i.
    equilibrium i.
    FLAIR i.
    fluid-attenuated inversion
      recovery i.
    functional i.
    gradient reversal i.
    harmonic phase i.
    HARP i.
    i. intensifier
    paradox i.
    parametric i.
    phase i.
    phase-encoded velocity i.
    respiratory-gated 2 D segmented-
      FLASH MRCA i.
    SE i.
    short-axis i.
    stress washout myocardial
      perfusion i.
    supine rest gated equilibrium i.
    three-dimensional spoiled gradient-
      recalled acquisition i.
    T1-weighted i.
    T2-weighted i.
    VMap dynamic flow-based i.
Imagecath
    Baxter I.
    I. rapid exchange angioscope
Image-Measure morphometry software
Imagent contrast agent

imager
    SONOS 2000 ultrasound i.
    SONOS 5500 ultrasound i.
    I. Torque selective catheter
Image-View system
ImageVue software
imaging
    acoustic i.
    ADC i.
    adenosine nuclear perfusion i.
    adenosine radionuclide perfusion i.
    A-FAIR i.
    i. agent
    Aloka color Doppler system for
      blood flow i.
    antifibrin antibody i.
    antimyosin antibody i.
    apparent diffusion coefficient i.
    arrhythmia-insensitive flow-sensitive
      alternating inversion recovery i.
    biplane i.
    black-blood magnetic resonance i.
    blood-pool i.
    breathhold, turbo-flash tagged i.
    cardiac blood-pool i.
    i. chain
    chemical shift i. (CSI)
    color kinesis i.
    color tissue Doppler i.
    continuous-wave Doppler i.
    diffusion tensor i. (DTI)
    diffusion-weighted i. (DWI)
    digital subtraction i.
    digital vascular i.
    dipyridamole-thallium i.
    direct Fourier transformation i.
    Doppler tissue i. (DTI)
    Doppler transesophageal color
      flow i.
    double-oblique i.
    3D tagged magnetic resonance i.
    duplex i.
    echocardiographic strain rate i.
    echo planar i. (EPI)
    electrocardiographic gated SPECT
      myocardial perfusion i.
    exercise i.
    exercise tomographic TI-201 i.
    Fourier two-dimensional i.
    frequency domain i.
    functional i.
    functional magnetic resonance i.
      (fMRI)
    fundamental i. (FI)
    gallium i.
    gallium-67 i.
    gated blood-pool i.
    gated sweep magnetic resonance i.

gradient-echo i.
harmonic i. (HI)
harmonic gray-scale i.
harmonic power Doppler i.
high-speed volumetric i.
I-123 BMIPP i.
I. Including MCID high-resolution image processing
indium-111-labeled lymphocyte i.
infarct-avid i.
Integris cardiovascular i.
krypton-81m ventilation i.
long-echo-train-length fast-spin-echo i., long-ETL FSE i.
magnetic resonance i. (MRI)
magnetic source i. (MSI)
mask-mode cardiac i.
MCD i.
myocardial perfusion i.
native tissue harmonic i.
nuclear magnetic resonance i. (NMRI)
nuclear perfusion i.
parametric i.
perfusion-weighted i.
pharmacologic stress i.
pharmacologic stress perfusion i.
phase i.
planar myocardial i.
planar thallium i.
platelet i.
power motion i.
pulsed Doppler tissue i.
pulse inversion harmonic i.
PYP i.
pyrophosphate i.
radionuclide i.
radiopharmaceutical i.
real-time perfusion i.
redistribution i.
rest-redistribution thallium-201 i.
rubidium-82 i.
second harmonic i. (SHI)
sestamibi i.
sestamibi perfusion i.
single-photon emission computed tomographic i.
single-photon emission tomography i.
SPECT i.
SPET i.
spin-echo i.

stress-redistribution-reinjection thallium-201 i.
stress SPECT perfusion i.
stress thallium-201 myocardial perfusion i.
i. study
tagged magnetic resonance i.
^{99m}Tc-sestamibi i.
^{99m}Tc-tetrofosmin i.
teboroxime i.
technetium-99m i.
technetium-99m MIBI i.
technetium (Tc)-99m sestamibi tomographic i.
thallium perfusion i.
thallium SPECT i.
three-dimensional tagged magnetic resonance i.
tissue Doppler i. (TDI)
tomographic radionuclide i.
transient response i. (TRI)
ultrasonic integrated backscatter i.
velocity-encoded cine-magnetic resonance i. (VE-cMRI)
ventilation/perfusion i.
video i.
i. window
xenon lung ventilation i.
imaging-angioplasty balloon catheter
Imatron
    I. C-150 scanner
    I. C-100 system
    I. C-100 tomographic scanner
    I. Ultrafast CT scanner
imazodan
imbalance
    acid-base i.
    electrolyte i.
    protease-antiprotease i.
    sympathovagal i.
imciromab pentetate
Imdur
IMED
    I. infusion device
    I. infusion pump
I-Methasone
imglucerase
IMGU
    insulin-mediated glucose uptake
IMH
    intramural hemorrhage

NOTES

I-123-MIBG
iodine-123 metaiodobenzylguanidine
123I-MIBG-SPECT
imidazoline
i. receptor (I-receptor)
i. receptor agonist
imipenem and cilastatin
imipramine
immediate silhouette
immersion
head-out water i.
immitis
Coccidioides i.
Dirofilaria i.
immobilized heparin
immotile cilia syndrome
ImmuCyst
immune
i. adherence immunosorbent assay
(IAIA)
i. thrombocytopenia
immune-mediated
i.-m. disease
i.-m. membranous nephritis
immunity
cell-mediated i.
Immuno
Feiba VH I.
immunoassay
AfeCTA i.
enzyme i. (EIA)
nifedipine enzyme i.
Thrombus Precursor Protein i.
immunoblot
antiphosphotyrosine i.
immunoblotting
immunochemical abnormality
immunocompetent host
immunocompromised
immunodeficiency
immunodetected
immunodiffusion (ID)
immunofluorescence
cytometric indirect i.
immunofluorescent technique
immunoglobulin (Ig)
i.-G (IgG)
respiratory syncytial virus i. (RSV-
IG)
varicella-zoster i. (VZIG)
immunological theory
immunometric sandwich method
immunonephelometer
BNA-100-Behring Diagnostics i.
immunonephelometry
rate i.
immunoperoxidase stain
immunoprecipitation

immunoprecipitin analysis
immunoprophylaxis
immunoradiometric assay (IRMA)
immunoreactivity
endothelin-1 i.
immunoregulator
IMREG-1 i.
immunoseparation
immunosorbent
immunostaining technique
immunosuppressant
immunosuppression
postinjury i.
i. therapy
immunosuppressive
immunotherapy
immunoturbidimetric assay
Imovax vaccine
IMPACT
integrilin to Manage Platelet Aggregation
to Prevent Coronary Thrombosis
Integrilin to Manage Platelet Aggregation
to Prevent Coronary Thrombosis
IMPACT Clinical Trial
impaction
mucoid i.
Impact specialized feeding formula
IMPACT-Stent
integrilin to Minimize Platelet
Aggregation and Coronary Thrombosis
in Stenting
Integrilin to Minimize Platelet
Aggregation and Coronary Thrombosis
in Stenting
IMPACT-Stent clinical trial
impaired
i. glucose tolerance (IGT)
i. relaxation mitral flow pattern
impairment
i. of activities of daily living
(IADL)
ciliary i.
conduction i.
functional aerobic i. (FAI)
restrictive functional i.
ventricular systolic i.
IMP-Capello arm support
impedance
acoustic i.
i. aggregometry
aortic i.
arterial i.
atrial lead i.
battery cell i.
i. catheter
lead i.
i. modulus
pacemaker i.

pacing lead i.
i. plethysmography (IPG)
thoracic i.
i. threshold valve (ITV)
transthoracic i.
i. variables
vascular i.
ventricular i.
impeller pump
impending respiratory failure
imperfecta
osteogenesis i.
implant
adrenal medullary i.
annuloplasty band i.
Biocell RTV i.
Biomatrix ocular i.
bioresorbable i.
Core-Vent i.
defibrillator i.
SynerGraft i.
Zoladex I.
implantable
i. atrial defibrillator (IAD)
i. cardioverter-defibrillator (ICD)
i. cardioverter-defibrillator/atrial
tachycardia pacing (ICD-ATP)
i. cardioverter-defibrillator lead
i. cardioverter electrode
i. left ventricular assist system
(IPLVAS)
i. loop recorder
i. pulse generator
**Implantaid Di-Lock cardiac lead
introducer**
implantation
i. guidelines
i. metastasis
Optimal Stent I. (OSTI)
prophylactic implantable
cardioverter-defibrillator i.
rescue stent i.
i. response
stent i.
transcatheter valve i.
implosion effect
Import vascular access port
impotence
vasculogenic i.
Impra Distaflo bypass graft
impressio cardiaca pulmonis

improvement
deterioration following i. (DFI)
ImPulse
I. electronic oxygen conserving
device
I. Oxygen Conserving Device
impulse
afferent i.
apex i.
apical i. (AI)
cardiac i.
i. conduction
ectopic i.
escape i.
i. formation
overlapping biphasic i. (OLBI)
paradoxic rocking i.
point of maximal i.
point of maximum i. (PMI)
i. propagation
right parasternal i.
i. summation
systolic apical i.
impure flutter
IMREG-1 immunoregulator
IMT
intimal-medial thickness
Imulyse tPA ELISA kit
IMV
intermittent mandatory ventilation
intermittent mechanical ventilation
^{111}In
indium-111
in
i. situ hybridization
i. situ thrombosis
i. vitro
i. vitro allergy test
i. vitro pharmacology
i. vivo
i. vivo gene transfer
inactivated poliovirus vaccine
inactivation
recovery from i.
tumor suppressor gene i.
inactive tuberculosis
inactivity
physical i.
inaequalis
pulsus i.
inamrinone

NOTES

INCA
infant nasal cannula assembly
INCA system
Incardia valve system
Incenti-neb nebulizer
incentive
i. spirometer
i. spirometry
incessant
i. atrial tachycardia
i. tachycardia
i. ventricular tachycardia
inch
pounds per square i. (psi)
incidence
peak i.
incident
i. pressure waveform
vascular i.
incidental murmur
incision
clamshell i.
collar i.
fish-mouth i.
ladder i.
longitudinal midline i.
median sternotomy i.
pleuropericardial i.
racquet i.
stab i.
sternal-splitting i.
stocking-seam i.
thoracotomy i.
transverse i.
incisura
i. apicis cordis
cardiac i.
i. cardiaca pulmonis sinistri
i. pulse
incisure
thoracic i.
incline
treadmill i.
inclusion
Rocha-Lima i.
i. technique of Bentall
incognitus
Mycoplasma i.
incompetence, incompetency
aortic i.
cardiac i.
cardiac valvular i.
chronotropic i.
mitral i.
muscular i.
pulmonary i.
pulmonic i.
pyloric i.

relative i.
tricuspid i.
valvular i.
incomplete
i. atrioventricular block
i. atrioventricular dissociation
i. A-V dissociation
i. thrombosis
incongruens
pulsus i.
incontinentia pigmenti syndrome
increased
i. afterload
i. contractility
increased-permeability pulmonary edema
increment
work rate i.
incremental
i. atrial pacing
i. threshold loading
i. ventricular pacing
incrementation
couch i.
incrementing response
IND
investigational new drug
IND status
Indacrinone
indanyl carbenicillin
indapamide
indecainide
Indec Systems TapeMeasure
computerized planimetry
Indeflator
ACS I.
I. Plus 20
Inderal LA
Inderide
indeterminate single ventricle
index, pl. **indices, indexes**
airway reactivity i. (ARI)
ankle-arm i.
ankle-brachial i. (ABI)
apnea i. (AI)
apnea-hypopnea i. (AHI)
arm-ankle indices
arousal i.
asynchrony i.
atherectomy i.
atherogenicity i.
atrial stasis i.
Barthel i.
Baseline Dyspnea I. (BDI)
body mass i. (BMI)
brachial-ankle i.
breath-holding i. (BHI)
Breuer-Hering deflation i.
Broders i.

Calgary Sleep Apnea Quality of Life I.
cardiac i. (CI)
cardiac output i.
cardiac risk i.
cardiac work i. (CWI)
carotid augmentation i.
Chapman i.
Charlson comorbidity i.
chemotherapeutic i.
chest i.
Cholesterol-Saturated Fat I. (CSFI)
compliance, rate, oxygenation, and pressure i.
contractile work i.
coronary prognostic i.
cortical arousal i. (CAI)
Crown-Crisp i.
Detsky modified risk i.
diastolic amplitude time i. (DATI)
diastolic pressure-time i. (DPTI)
Doppler-derived i.
Dubois i.
Duke Activity Status I. (DASI)
Eagle risk score i.
eccentricity i.
ejection phase i.
end-diastolic volume i. (EDVI)
end-systolic force-velocity i.
end-systolic volume i. (ESVI)
exercise i.
Fischl i.
Fourmentin thoracic i.
Framingham risk i.
free thyrotoxin i.
Frenchay Activities I.
General Well-Being I.
Gensini i.
Gibson circularity i.
glycocalicine i.
Goldman i. of risk
Goldman risk-factor i.
isovolumetric phase i.
isovolumic i.
ITPA i.
late potential parameter i.
laterality i. (LI)
left atrial emptying i.
left ventricular diastolic phase i.
left ventricular mass i.
left ventricular stroke volume i. (LVSVI)

left ventricular stroke work i. (LVSWI)
i. lesion
Lewis i.
lipid-laden macrophage i.
MB i.
Miller index
mitral valve closure i.
movement arousal i. (MAI)
myocardial band i.
myocardial jeopardy i.
oxygen consumption i.
oxyhemodynamic i.
penile-brachial pressure i.
performance i. (PI)
Pneumonia Severity I. (PSI)
polysomnographic i.
ponderal i.
Positive Symptom Distress I. (PSDI)
Pourcelot i.
pulmonary vascular resistance i. (PVRI)
QTI:QT i.
Quality of Well-Being I.
Quetelet i.
Rapid Shallow Breathing I. (RSBI)
regional wall motion i.
Reid i.
relaxation time i.
respiratory disturbance i. (RDI)
right ankle i.
right ventricular end-diastolic volume i. (RVEDVI)
right ventricular end-systolic volume i. (RVESVI)
risk i.
Ritchie Articular I.
Robinson i.
Rohrer i. (RI)
saturation i.
Schneider i.
segmental pressure i.
semiquantitative i.
shock i.
Sleep Apnea Quality of Life I. (SAQLI)
smoothness i.
Sokolow electrocardiographic i.
sphericity i.
stiffness i.
stroke i.

NOTES

index *(continued)*
 stroke volume i. (SVI)
 stroke work i. (SWI)
 i. of suspicion
 systemic vascular resistance i.
  (SVRI)
 systolic pressure time i. (SPTI)
 tension-time i.
 TIMI frame count i.
 total apexcardiographic relaxation
  time i. (TARTI)
 total peripheral resistance i. (TPRI)
 i. value
 vascular resistance i.
 ventricular stroke work i.
 viability i.
 volume thickness i. (VTI)
 wall motion i. (WMI)
 wall motion score i. (WMSI)
 weaning i. (WI)
 Wood units i.
 Youden i.
indicator
 i. dilution method
 i. dilution technique
 elective replacement i. (ERI)
 electric replacement i. (ERI)
 SPI-Lite sleep position i.
 xylol pulse i.
indifferent electrode
indinavir
indirect
 i. diuretic
 i. lead
 i. murmur
InDirect primary stenting concept
indium-111 (^{111}In)
 i.-labeled lymphocyte imaging
 i. scintigraphy
Indocin
 I. I.V. injection
 I. Oral
indocyanine
 i. dilution curve
 i. green
 i. green angiography
 i. green dye
 i. green indicator dilution technique
 i. green method
indomethacin
indoor air quality (IAQ)
indoramin
induced
 i. hypertension
 i. pneumothorax
inducibility
inducible
 i. arrhythmia

 i. nitric oxide synthase (iNOS)
 i. nitric oxide synthetase (iNOS)
 i. polymorphic ventricular
  fibrillation
 i. polymorphic ventricular
  tachycardia
induction
 rapid sequence i. (RSI)
 sputum i.
induration
 gray i.
 idiopathic brown i.
 red i.
indurative
 i. myocarditis
 i. pleurisy
 i. pneumonia
industrial anthrax
indux
 rale i.
indwelling
 i. central venous catheter
 i. line
inelastic load
inert gas narcosis
inertia
inertial effect
In-Exsufflator respiratory device
infant
 I. Airflow and effort sensor
 i. Ambu resuscitator
 continuous noninvasive monitoring
  of ventilated i.'s
 I. Flow Nasal CPAP system
 I. Flow noninvasive nasal CPAP
  system
 i. nasal cannula assembly (INCA)
 i. respiratory distress syndrome
  (IRDS)
 I. Resuscitation system
 I. Star 100 ventilator
 I. Star 200 ventilator
 I. Star Ventilator 500/950
infantile
 i. arteritis
 i. beriberi
 i. lobar emphysema
infarct *(See also* infarction*)*
 acute multiple brain i.'s (AMBI)
 i. artery
 i. artery patency
 brain i. (BI)
 i. bulging
 caudate i.
 cerebral i.
 embolic i.
 i. expansion
 i. extension

insular i.
internal borderzone i. (IBI)
internal capsule i.'s
lacunar i. (LACI)
partial anterior circulation i.
  (PACI)
perforating artery i. (PAI)
pontine i. (PI)
posterior circulation i. (POCI)
pulmonary i.
red i.
i. scar
silent cerebral i. (SCI)
subcortical junctional i.
i. thinning
total anterior circulation i. (TACI)
watershed i.
i. zone wall motion

infarct-avid
  i.-a. hot-spot scintigraphy
  i.-a. imaging
  i.-a. myocardial scintigraphy

infarction (*See also* infarct)
  acute diaphragmatic myocardial i.
  age-undetermined myocardial i.
  anterior myocardial i. (AMI)
  anterior wall myocardial i.
  anteroinferior myocardial i.
  anterolateral myocardial i.
  anteroseptal myocardial i. (ASMI)
  apical i.
  atherothrombotic brain i. (ABI)
  atrial i.
  atrial myocardial i.
  Canadian Assessment of
    Myocardial I. (CAMI)
  cardiac i.
  cerebral i.
  cerebrovascular i. (CVI)
  cocaine-induced myocardial i.
  Cohort of Rescue Angioplasty in
    Myocardial I. (CORAMI)
  coitus-induced myocardial i.
  completed myocardial i.
  complicated myocardial i.
  diaphragmatic myocardial i.
  evolving myocardial i.
  family history of myocardial i.
  Gianturco-Roubin in Acute
    Myocardial I. (GRAMI)
  hemorrhagic i. (HI)
  H-form myocardial i.

inferior myocardial i.
inferior wall myocardial i. (IWMI)
inferolateral myocardial i.
Integrilin and Tenecteplase in
  Acute Myocardial I. (INTEGRITI)
Intravenous Streptokinase in Acute
  Myocardial I. (ISAM)
ischemic cerebral i.
juvenile myocardial i.
lacunar i. (LI)
large-vessel i. (LVI)
lateral medullary i. (LMI)
lateral myocardial i.
malignant middle cerebral artery i.
  (mMCAI)
Maximal Individual Therapy in
  Acute Myocardial I. (MITRA)
medial medullary i. (MMI)
myocardial i. (MI)
National Registry of Myocardial I.
  (NRMI)
non-Q-wave myocardial i. (non-Q
  MI, NQWMI)
nontransmural myocardial i. (NTMI)
posterior myocardial i.
postmyocardial i.
Primary Angioplasty in
  Myocardial I. (PAMI)
pulmonary i.
Q wave myocardial i.
recurrent myocardial i.
right ventricular i.
Roesler-Bressler i.
ruled out for myocardial i.
  (romied)
rule out myocardial i. (ROMI)
silent brain i. (SBI)
silent cerebral i. (SCI)
silent myocardial i. (SMI)
small-vessel i. (SVI)
Stenting for Acute Myocardial I.
  (STAMI)
Stenting in Acute Myocardial I.
  (STENTIM)
Stenting with Elective Wiktor Stent
  in Acute Myocardial I.
  (STENTIM-2)
Stent Primary Angioplasty for
  Myocardial I. (STENT PAMI)
striatocapsular i.
stuttering myocardial i.
subacute myocardial i.

NOTES

infarction *(continued)*
    subendocardial myocardial i.
    Thrombin Inhibition in
      Myocardial I. (TIMI)
    Thrombolysis in Myocardial I.
      (TIMI)
    Thrombolysis and Thrombin
      Inhibition in Myocardial I.
    Thrombolytic Trial of Eminase in
      Acute Myocardial I. (TEAM)
    thrombotic brain i. (TBI)
    through-and-through myocardial i.
    transmural myocardial i.
    unstable angina/non-Q-wave
      myocardial i. (UA/NQMI)
    watershed i.
    i. with shock
infarctlet
infarct-related
    i.-r. artery (IRA)
    i.-r. vessel
Infasurf
InfCM
    inflammatory cardiomyopathy
infected
    i. aneurysm
    i. myxoma
    i. secretion
infection
    acute lower respiratory tract i.
      (ALRI)
    adenoviral type 40/41 i.
    bacterial i.
    bacterial respiratory tract i.
    community-acquired i.
    coronavirus i.
    endemic fungal i.
    endobronchial i.
    fungal i.
    hospital-acquired i.
    laryngeal i.
    laryngotracheal i.
    MAC i.
    MAI i.
    miliary i.
    Mycobacterium avium complex i.
    Mycobacterium avium-
      intracellulare i.
    mycotic i.
    nosocomial i.
    opportunistic i.
    pleuropulmonary i.
    primary i.
    pyogenic i.
    recurrent respiratory i. (RRI)
    respiratory i.
    respiratory tract i.
    rhinocerebral i.

    secondary i.
    spirochetal i.
    staphylococcal i.
    streptococcal i.
    systemic i.
    upper respiratory i. (URI)
    varicella-zoster i.
    viral respiratory i.
infectious
    i. asthmatic bronchitis
    i. bronchiolitis
    i. endocarditis
    i. esophagitis
    i. mononucleosis
infective
    i. asthma
    i. embolism
    i. endocarditis (IE)
    i. exacerbation
    i. pericarditis
    i. thrombosis
    i. thrombus
InFed injection
inferior
    i. accessory fissure
    arteria glutealis i.
    i. articular facet of atlas
    i. border of lung
    i. constrictor muscle of pharynx
    i. costal facet
    i. costal pit
    i. epigastric artery (IEA)
    i. epigastric artery graft
    i. esophageal sphincter
    fovea costalis i.
    i. frontal gyrus (IFG)
    i. frontal lobe (IFL)
    i. ganglion of glossopharyngeal
      nerve
    i. laryngeal artery
    i. laryngeal cavity
    i. laryngeal vein
    i. lingular bronchopulmonary
      segment [S V]
    i. lobe of left/right lung
    macular arteriole i.
    i. mesenteric artery (IMA)
    i. mesenteric artery retractor
    i. mesenteric vascular occlusion
    i. myocardial infarction
    i. parietal/superior temporal lobe
      (IPSTL)
    i. phrenic lymph node
    i. thyroid artery
    i. thyroid vein
    i. tracheobronchial lymph node
    i. triangle sign
    i. vena cava (IVC)

i. vena cava occlusion
vena laryngea i.
i. wall myocardial infarction
(IWMI)
inferior-axis flutter
inferiores
nodi lymphoidei phrenici i.
nodi lymphoidei
tracheobronchiales i.
inferioris
rami esophageales arteriae
thyroideae i.
inferius
tuberculum thyroideum i.
inferoapical
inferobasal wall
inferobasilar
inferolateral
i. myocardial infarction
i. segment
inferoseptal segment
infestans
Triatoma i.
infestation
parasitic i.
infiltrate
alveolar i.
Assmann tuberculous i.
bronchiolar inflammatory i.
bronchopneumonic i.
diffuse interstitial i.
fibrous i.
fleeting i.
fluffy alveolar i.
hazy i.
inflammatory i.
inflammatory cellular i.
infraclavicular i.
interstitial i.
linear i.
lobar i.
migratory pulmonary i.
nodular i.
patchy i.
peribronchiolar inflammatory i.
perivascular eosinophilic i.'s
perivascular lymphocytic i.
reticulonodular i.
strandy i.
streaky i.
Wasserman-positive pulmonary i.
infiltrating lobular carcinoma

infiltration
cardiac i.
epituberculous i.
gelatinous i.
gray i.
patchy i.
subepicardial fatty i.
infiltrative cardiomyopathy
Infiltrator local drug delivery device
Infiniti
I. catheter
I. catheter introducer system
inflammation
adhesive i.
cap i.
granulomatous i.
lymphoplasmacytic i.
neutrophil-induced pulmonary i.
peribronchiolar granulomatous i.
inflammatoria
dysphagia i.
inflammatory
i. adhesion
i. airway disease
i. cardiomyopathy (InfCM)
i. cellular infiltrate
i. cytokine
i. infiltrate
i. myofibroblastic tumor
i. pericarditis
i. pseudotumor (IPT)
i. reaction
inflation
balloon i.
oscillating balloon i.
i. pressure
i. reflex
inflow
I. Dynamics Antares coronary stent
i. tract
turbulent diastolic mitral i.
InFlow Flex stent
influenza, pl. **influenzae**
i. A, B, C
Asian i.
i. bacillus
endemic i.
Hong Kong i.
i. pneumonia
Port Charles i.
Russian i.
Texas i.

NOTES

influenza *(continued)*
    i. tracheobronchitis
    Victoria i.
    i. virus pneumonia
    i. virus vaccine
influenzae
    Haemophilus i.
    nontypeable *Haemophilus i.* (NTHI)
influenzal pneumonia
Influenzavirus
infraclavicular
    i. infiltrate
    i. triangle
infracristal
infracubital bypass
infradiaphragmatic
    i. portion
    i. venous flow
infrahisian
    i. block
    i. conduction system
infranodal extrasystole
infrared
    i. thermography
    i. thermometer
infrared-pulsed laser
infrarenal abdominal aortic aneurysm
infrasegmental vein
Infrasonics ventilator
infrasonic ventilator
Infrasurf
infratentorial ICH
infrequens
    pulsus i.
infundibula (*pl. of* infundibulum)
infundibular
    i. atresia
    i. obstruction
    i. septal defect
    i. stenosis
    i. wedge resection
infundibulectomy
    Brock i.
infundibulum, gen. **infundibuli,**
    pl. **infundibula**
    i. of lung
    tendo infundibuli
Infusaid infusion pump
InfusaSleeve
    I. II catheter
    Kaplan-Simpson I.
    LocalMed I.
Infuse-A-Port pump
infuser
    Critikon pressure i.
infusion
    Adenoscan i.
    adrenomedullin i.

    brain-heart i.
    bretylium i.
    cardioplegia i.
    ergonovine i.
    heparin i.
    intracoronary acetylcholine i.
    isoproterenol i.
    nitroprusside i.
    volume i.
ingravescent apoplexy
INH
    isoniazid
inhalant
    antifoaming i.
    i. antigen
inhalation
    i. agent
    Atrovent Aerosol I.
    i. bronchography
    i. challenge test
    hypertonic saline i.
    isoproterenol sulfate i.
    NebuPent I.
    oxygen i.
    i. pneumonia
    i. therapy
    tobramycin solution for i.
    toxic fume i.
    i. tuberculosis
inhalational
    i. anesthesia
    i. anesthetic
inhaled
    i. antibiotic
    i. bronchodilator
    i. radioaerosol technique
Inhale deep lung delivery system
inhaler
    AeroBid Oral Aerosol I.
    AeroDose i.
    albuterol i.
    AREx i.
    Azmacort Oral I.
    Beclovent Oral I.
    Beconase AQ Nasal I.
    breath-actuated i. (BAI)
    Combivent i.
    Diskus i.
    dry powder i. (DPI)
    Glaxo Wellcome Diskhaler i.
    Henderson-Haggard i.
    Intal Oral I.
    ipratropium i.
    Junker i.
    Leiras metered-dose powder i.
    metered-dose i. (MDI)
    metered solution i. (MSI)
    nicotine i.

Nicotrol I.
pressurized metered-dose i. (pMDI)
Spiral Mark V portable ultrasonic
   drug i.
Spiros i.
Tape Based i.
Tilade i.
Vancenase AQ I.
Vanceril Oral I.
Inhibace
inhibited
   atrial demand-i. (AAI)
   i. pacing
inhibition
   leukotriene i.
   magnet i.
   neutral endopeptidase i. (NEP-I,
      NEPi)
   phosphodiesterase III i. (PDE3I)
   IIb/IIa platelet i.
   potassium i.
   Prevention of Events with ACE I.
      (PEACE)
   Ramipril Angiotensin Converting
      Enzyme I. (RACE)
inhibitor
   ACE i.
   acyl-CoA:cholesterol
      acyltransferase i.
   alpha-2-plasmin i.
   alpha-1 proteinase i.
   angiotensin-converting enzyme i.
      (ACEI, ACEi)
   atriopeptidase i.
   beta-lactamase i.
   bronchial mucus i.
   carbonic anhydrase i.
   caspase i.
   cholinesterase i.
   complement i.
   converting enzyme i.
   cyclooxygenase i.
   direct thrombin i.
   endopeptidase i.
   glycoprotein IIb/IIIa i.
   HMG CoA-reductase i.
   human menopausal gonadotropin
      coenzyme A reductase i.
   hydroxymethylglutaryl coenzyme A
      reductase i.
   3-hydroxy-3-methylglutaryl coenzyme
      A reductase i.

IIb/IIIa i.
Kuntiz-type i.
leukotriene i.
lipoprotein-associated coagulation i.
   (LACI)
MAO i.
mast cell i.
metalloproteinase i.
monoamine oxidase i. (MAOI)
mucus i.
Na$^+$/H$^+$ exchange i. (NHEI)
neutral endopeptidase i.
oxysterol i.
PDE isoenzyme i.
phosphodiesterase i. (PDE, PDE-I)
phosphodiesterase isoenzyme i.
plasminogen activator i. (PAI)
platelet aggregation i.
platelet glycoprotein IIb/IIIa i.
protease i. (PI)
proton pump i.
reductase i.
renin i.
secretory leukocyte protease i.
   (SLPI)
secretory leukoprotease i. (SLPI)
secretory leukoproteinase i. (SLPI)
thromboxane synthetase i.
tissue factor pathway i. (TFPI)
vasopeptidase i. (VPI)
inhibitor-1
   plasminogen activator i. (PAI-1)
inhomogeneity
initial apnea
initiative
   NIH *Xenopus* I.
   Women's Health I. (WHI)
Injectable
   Cardizem I.
injection
   Abbokinase i.
   Activase i.
   Adenocard i.
   Adlone i.
   Adrucil i.
   A-hydroCort i.
   Amcort i.
   A-methaPred i.
   Amikin i.
   Andro-L.A. i.
   Andropository i.
   Apresoline i.

NOTES

injection *(continued)*
AquaMEPHYTON i.
Arfonad i.
Aristocort Forte i.
Aristocort Intralesional i.
Aristospan Intra-articular i.
Aristospan Intralesional i.
Articulose-50 i.
Baci-IM i.
Bactocill i.
Bena-D i.
Benadryl i.
Benahist i.
Ben-Allergin-50 i.
Benoject i.
Bicillin L-A i.
blood patch i.
bolus i.
bolus intravenous i.
Brethine i.
Brevibloc i.
Bricanyl i.
Bronkephrine i.
Cafcit i.
i. catheter
Caverject i.
Celestone Phosphate i.
CellCept intravenous for i.
Cel-U-Jec i.
Ceredase i.
Chlor-Pro i.
Chlor-Trimeton i.
Cipro i.
Cleocin Phosphate i.
Compazine i.
Cortone Acetate i.
Cortrosyn i.
Corvert i.
Crysticillin A.S. i.
Cyklokapron i.
Cytoxan i.
dalteparin sodium i.
daptomycin for i.
DDAVP i.
Decadron i.
Delatest i.
Delatestryl i.
Demadex i.
depAndro i.
depMedalone i.
Depoject i.
Depo-Medrol i.
Depopred i.
Depo-Provera i.
D.H.E. 45 i.
Diflucan i.
Dihyrex i.
Dilocaine i.

Diprivan i.
D-Med i.
Dobutrex i.
Dopram i.
Doxychel i.
Duo-Trach i.
Duraclon i.
Duralone i.
Duralutin i.
Duratest i.
Durathate i.
dye i.
Edecrin Sodium i.
Enlon i.
epoprostenol sodium for i.
ergonovine i.
Ethamolin i.
Everone i.
Flolan i.
Floxin i.
Foscavir i.
Fragmin dalteparin sodium i.
Garamycin i.
Gesterol i.
hand i.
heparin i.
Hep-Lock i.
Histerone i.
Hybolin Improved i.
Hydeltrasol i.
Hydeltra-T.B.A. i.
Hydrocortone Acetate i.
Hydrocortone Phosphate i.
Hy-Gestrone i.
Hylutin i.
Hyzine-50 i.
Indocin I.V. i.
InFed i.
Intropin i.
iopromide i.
isosorbide dinitrate i.
Jenamicin i.
Keflin i.
Kefurox i.
Kenaject i.
Kenalog i.
Key-Pred i.
Key-Pred-SP i.
Konakion i.
Lasix i.
lepirudin rDNA i.
Levophed i.
Lincocin i.
Lincorex i.
Liquaemin i.
Lovenox i.
Lyphocin i.
Medralone i.

I

meropenem for i.
Metro I.V. i.
Minocin I.V. i.
M-Prednisol i.
mycophenolate mofetil intravenous for i.
Nafcil i.
Nallpen i.
Narcan i.
Nebcin i.
negative-contrast i.
Neosar i.
Nervocaine i.
Netromycin i.
Neucalm-50 i.
Neutrexin i.
Nitro-Bid I.V. i.
Normodyne i.
Nydrazid i.
Oncovin i.
Osmitrol i.
Pentacarinat i.
Pentam-300 i.
Permapen i.
Pfizerpen-AS i.
Phenazine i.
Phenergan i.
Pitressin i.
Predaject i.
Predalone i.
Predcor i.
Predicort-50 i.
Prednisol TBA i.
Priscoline i.
Pro-Depo i.
Prodrox i.
Prometh i.
Prorex i.
Prostaphlin i.
Prostin VR Pediatric i.
Prothazine i.
Quiess i.
Refludan i.
Retrovir i.
Reversol i.
Rifadin i.
root i.
Solu-Cortef i.
Solu-Medrol i.
Sotradecol i.
Sublimaze i.
Tac-3 i.

Tac-40 i.
Tensilon i.
Terramycin I.M. i.
Tesamone i.
tinzaparin sodium i.
Toposar i.
Trandate i.
Triam-A i.
Triam Forte i.
Triamonide i.
Tridil i.
Tri-Kort i.
Trilog i.
Trilone i.
Triostat i.
Trisoject i.
Ultravist i.
Unipen i.
Ureaphil i.
Vancocin i.
Vancoled i.
VePesid i.
V-Gan i.
Vibramycin i.
Vistacon-50 i.
Vistaquel i.
Vistaril i.
Vistazine i.
Vumon i.
Wycillin i.
Zinacef i.

injector
flow i.
Fujinon variceal i.
Medrad Mark IV angiographic i.
Mill-Rose esophageal i.
modified Mark IV R-wave-triggered power i.
power i.
pressure i.
Viamonte-Hobbs dye i.

injury
acute chemical i.
acute lung i. (ALI)
aortic i.
aspiration lung i.
blowout i.
blunt i.
blunt chest i.
blunt pulmonary i.
blunt torso i.
brachial plexus i.

NOTES

injury *(continued)*
    chest wall i.
    chronic recurrent chemical i.
    contrecoup i.
    diastolic current of i.
    diffuse lung i.
    early lung i.
    early pulmonary i.
    electrical i.
    femoral vascular i.
    intrathoracic i.
    ischemic-reperfusion i.
    late lung i.
    late pulmonary i.
    lipid-induced lung i.
    lung i.
    median nerve i.
    mesangial immune i.
    myocardial i.
    penetrating i.
    penetrating chest i.
    phrenic nerve crush i.
    pulmonary i.
    pulmonary parenchymal i.
    radionecrosis i.
    reperfusion i.
    systolic current of i.
    thermal i.
    thoracic i.
    thoracic crush i.
    vascular i.
    ventilator-associated lung i. (VALI)
    ventilator-induced lung i. (VILI)
Injury Severity Score (ISS)
inlet
    thoracic i.
    ventricular i.
in-memory gating
inner city asthma
InnerVasc sheath
Innervase
    I. dilatable percutaneous vascular
    access device
innervation
    autonomic sensory i.
innocent
    i. heart murmur
    i. murmur
    i. murmur of elderly
Innohep
innominate
    i. aneurysm
    i. artery
    i. vein
Innovace
Innovar
Innovator Holter system
Inocor

inoculation
inogatran
Inokucki vascular stapler
INOmax
inorganic
    i. acid
    i. acid vapor
    i. dust
    i. dust disease
    i. murmur
iNOS
    inducible nitric oxide synthase
    inducible nitric oxide synthetase
inosine
inositol triphosphate
inotrope
    negative i.
inotropic
    i. agent
    i. arrhythmia
    i. effect
    i. support
inotropy
Inoue
    I. balloon
    I. balloon catheter
    I. balloon mitral valvotomy
    I. balloon technique
    I. endovascular stent-graft
    I. self-guiding balloon
    I. single-balloon technique
    I. technique
    I. triple-branched stent graft
INOvent delivery system
INR
    international normalized ratio
    target INR
insert
    EverGrip clamp i.
    Koala vascular i.
insertion
    percutaneous catheter i.
    retrograde catheter i.
    route of i.
    wire i.
InSight system
insipidus
    nephrogenic diabetes i.
insipiratory limb
insomnia
insomniac
insonation
    angle of i.
insonified
inspiration
    crowing i.
    duration of i. (T_I)
    sustained maximal i. (SMI)

inspirator
inspiratory
- i. airflow
- i. capacity (IC)
- i. center
- i. dyspnea
- i. to expiratory ratio (I:E)
- i. flow rate
- i. loading
- i. murmur
- i. muscle fatigue
- i. occlusion pressure
- i. positive airway pressure (IPAP)
- i. rale
- i. reserve capacity (IRC)
- i. reserve volume (IRV)
- i. resistance and positive expiratory pressure (IR-PEP)
- i. stridor
- i. threshold load (ITL)
- i. time (T_I)
- i. view
- i. vital capacity (IVC)

InspirEase device
inspired gas
inspirometer
Inspiron
- I. AccurOx Mask
- I. device
- I. Instromedix computer

Inspirx incentive spirometer
inspissated
instability
- catheter i.
- circulatory i.
- hemodynamic i.
- microsatellite i.

instantaneous
- i. electrical axis
- i. spectral peak velocity
- i. vector

Insta-Pulse heart rate monitor
InStent
- I. CarotidCoil stent
- I. VascuCoil stent

in-stent
- i.-s. neointimal proliferation
- i.-s. restenosis (ISR)
- i.-s. thrombosis

instillation
- intracavitary i.
- lavage i.

institute
- National Heart, Lung, Blood I. (NHLBI)

instrument
- arterial oscillator endarterectomy i.
- blood sampling i.
- Cooley neonatal i.'s
- Diamond-Lite titanium i.'s
- EndoWrist i.
- KinetiX i.'s
- K x-ray fluorescence i.
- Matsuda titanium surgical i.'s
- Medicon i.
- Multi-Dop X/TCD transcranial Doppler i.
- NeoKnife electrosurgical i.
- Neuro-Trace i.
- Pneumo-Needle reusable i.
- Stratus i.
- Wolvek sternal approximation fixation i.

instrumental activities of daily living (IADL)
instrumentation
- angiographic i.
- EEG and PSG i.
- MIDA CoroNet i.

insudate
insufficiency
- aortic i.
- aortic valvular i.
- arterial i.
- atrioventricular valve i.
- cardiac i.
- cerebrovascular i.
- coronary i.
- deep venous i. (DVI)
- distal vascular i.
- mitral i.
- multivalve i.
- myocardial i.
- periprosthetic valve aortic i.
- pulmonary i.
- pulmonic i.
- renal i.
- respiratory i.
- rheumatic mitral i.
- Sternberg myocardial i.
- tricuspid i.
- valvular i.
- velopharyngeal i.

NOTES

insufficiency (continued)
    venous i.
    venous valvular i.
insufflation
    thoracoscopic talc i.
    tracheal gas i. (TGI)
insufflator
    Venturi i.
Insuflon device
insula
insular infarct
insulation
    i. failure
    lead i.
insulin
    beef i.
    glucose potassium i. (GKI)
    Lente i.
    Lente Iletin I, II, L i.
    NPH Iletin i.
    pork i.
    i. preparation
    regular purified pork i.
    i. resistance
    I. Resistance Atherosclerosis Study (IRAS)
    i. resistance syndrome
    I. Riabead II radioimmunoassay
    i. shock
insulin-dependent diabetes mellitus (IDDM)
insulin-like growth factor (IGF)
insulin-mediated glucose uptake (IMGU)
insult
    cardiac i.
    vascular i.
InSync
    I. cardiac resynchronization device
    I. multisite cardiac stimulator
    I. stimulator
intact valve
Intal
    I. Nebulizer Solution
    I. Oral Inhaler
Intec
    I. AID cardioverter-defibrillator generator
    I. implantable defibrillator
Integra
    I. catheter
    I. II balloon
integral
    paced depolarization i.
    velocity time i.
integrated
    i. bipolar sensing
    i. lead system

integration
    digital color Doppler velocity profile i.
    vertical i.
integrator
    Medical Graphics pneumotachograph with volume i.
integrilin
    I. to Manage Platelet Aggregation to Prevent Coronary Thrombosis (IMPACT)
    I. to Minimize Platelet Aggregation and Coronary Thrombosis in Stenting (IMPACT-Stent)
    I. and Tenecteplase in Acute Myocardial Infarction (INTEGRITI)
integrin
    i. blocker
    i. signaling
integrin-dependent pathway
Integris
    I. cardiac imaging system
    I. cardiovascular imaging
    I. 3D RA
    I. H5000 digital x-ray imaging system
INTEGRITI
    Integrilin and Tenecteplase in Acute Myocardial Infarction
    INTEGRITI Clinical Trial
Integrity
    I. AFx AutoCapture pacing system
    I. AFx pacemaker
intellectual dysfunction
Intellicath pulmonary artery catheter
intelligent CPAP
intensifier
    image i.
intensity
    echo i.
    intravascular signal i.
    reduced signal i.
    spatial i.
    waxing and waning in i.
intensivist
intentionem
    per primam i.
    per secundum i.
intention-to-treat (ITT)
interaction
    adhesin-receptor i.
    leukocyte-endothelial cell i.
    lung-liver i.
interalveolar
    i. communication
    i. septa

interarterial
  i. communication
  i. shunt
interarytenoid notch
interatrial
  i. block
  i. conduction time
  i. septum
interbronchiolar communication of Martin
intercadence
intercadent
intercalary
intercellular
  i. adhesion molecule (ICAM)
  i. adhesion molecule-1 (ICAM-1)
  i. coupling
intercept angle
intercidens
  pulsus i.
intercostal
  i. catheter
  external i.
  internal i.
  i. mammary vessel
  i. nerve block
  i. retraction
  i. space
intercurrens
  pulsus i.
interdependence
  ventricular i.
interdigitating coil stent
interectopic interval
interelectrode
  i. distance
  i. space
interest
  region of i. (ROI)
interface
  I. arterial blood filter
  electrode-skin i.
  lung-wall i.
  Monarch Mini Mask nasal i.
  sputum-epithelium i.
  Ultimate Seal gel i.
interfascicular fibrous tissue
interference
  i. beat
  dissociation by i.
  i. dissociation

electromagnetic
  interference/radiofrequency i.
  (EMI/RFI)
interferon (IFN)
  i. alfa-2a
  i. alfa-2b
  i. alfa-2b and ribavirin combination
  pack
  i. alpha
  alpha-i.
  i. gamma-1b
InterGard vascular graft
interlaced scanning
interlead
  i. QT dispersion
  i. QT variability
interleukin (IL)
  IL-2
  IL-3
  IL-4
  IL-5
  IL-6
  IL-7
  IL-8
  IL-9
  IL-10
  IL-11
  circulating IL-6
  PEG IL-2
interlobar
  i. effusion
  i. empyema
  i. pleurisy
  i. surface of lung
interlobular
  i. emphysema
  i. pleurisy
  i. septa
  i. septum
interlobularis
  pneumonia i.
intermediary vesicle
intermediate
  i. bronchus
  i. circumflex artery (ICXA)
  i. coronary syndrome
  i. heart
  i. laryngeal cavity
  i. probability
intermediate-density lipoprotein (IDL)
Intermedics
  I. atrial antitachycardia pacemaker

NOTES

Intermedics *(continued)*
 I. lead
 I. Marathon dual-chamber rate-responsive pacemaker
 I. Marathon VVI single-chamber pacemaker
 I. RES-Q implantable cardioverter-defibrillator
 I. Stride pacemaker
intermedius
 bronchus i.
 ramus i.
intermesenteric arterial anastomosis
intermittence, intermittency
intermittens
 dyskinesia i.
 pulsus i.
 pulsus respiratione i.
intermittent
 i. claudication
 i. coronary sinus occlusion
 i. demand ventilation (IDV)
 i. mandatory ventilation (IMV)
 i. mechanical ventilation (IMV)
 i. percussive ventilation (IPV)
 i. pneumatic compression (IPC)
 i. positive pressure (IPP)
 i. positive pressure breathing (IPPB)
 i. positive pressure ventilation (IPPV)
 i. pulse
 i. sinus arrest
interna
 lamina elastica i.
internal
 i. adhesive pericarditis
 i. borderzone infarct (IBI)
 i. branch of superior laryngeal nerve
 i. capsule
 i. capsule infarcts
 i. cardioversion
 i. carotid artery (ICA)
 i. cerebral vein (ICV)
 i. diameter
 i. elastic lamina (IEL)
 i. elastic membrane (IEM)
 i. elastic membrane rupture
 i. intercostal
 i. jugular vein
 i. mammary artery (IMA)
 i. mammary artery bypass (IMAB)
 i. mammary artery catheter
 i. mammary artery graft
 i. mammary artery graft angiography
 i. mammary vessel

 i. pneumatic stabilization
 i. pudendal vein
 i. reed switch
 i. respiration
 i. thoracic artery (ITA)
 i. thoracic artery graft
 i. thoracic vein
international
 I. Carotid Stenting Study (ICSS)
 I. Classification of Diseases, Ninth Revision (ICD-9)
 I. Classification of Sleep Disorders (ICSD)
 I. Cooperative Pulmonary Embolism Registry (ICOPER)
 I. Joint Efficacy Comparison of Thrombolytics
 i. normalized ratio (INR)
 I. Society for Heart and Lung Transplant
 I. Society for Heart Transplantation (ISHT)
 I. Staging System for Lung Cancer (ISSLC)
 I. Standards Organization (ISO)
 I. Stroke Trial (IST)
 I. Study of Infarct Survival (ISIS)
International Civil Aviation Organization (ICAO)
internodal
 i. conduction
 i. pathway
 i. tract of Bachmann
internum
 pericardium i.
interpleural space
interpolated
 i. beat
 i. extrasystole
 i. premature complex
interposed abdominal compression (IAC)
interposition of Dacron tube
Interpret ultrasound catheter
interpulmonary septum
interquartile range
interrogation
 deep Doppler velocity i.
 i. device
 Doppler i.
 stereoscopic i.
interrupted
 i. aortic arch (IAA)
 i. pledgeted suture
 i. respiration
interruption
 aortic arch i.
 azygoportal i.

intersegmental
  i. artery
  i. part of pulmonary vein
intersegmentales
  partes i.
Intersept cardiotomy reservoir
Interspec XL ultrasound
interstitial
  i. disease
  i. distribution
  i. edema
  i. emphysema
  i. fibrosis
  i. fluid
  i. granuloma
  i. infiltrate
  i. lung disease (ILD)
  i. marking
  i. nodule
  i. pattern
  i. and perivascular collagen
    network
  i. plasma cell pneumonia
  i. pneumonia
  i. pneumonitis
  i. pulmonary edema
  i. pulmonary fibrosis (IPF)
  i. space
interstitium
  axial i.
  cardiac i.
  lung i.
  peripheral i.
intersystole
intersystolic period
Intertach II pacemaker
Intertech
  I. anesthesia breathing circuit
  I. Mapleson D nonrebreathing
    circuit
  I. nonrebreathing modified Jackson-
    Rees circuit
  I. Perkin-Elmer gas sampling line
Intertherapy intravascular ultrasound
interval
  A-A i.
  A_1-A_2 i.
  A-C i.
  Ae-H i.
  AH i.
  A_2 incisural i.
  A-N i.

AN i.
A_2 to opening snap i.
atrial escape i.
atriocarotid i.
atrioventricular i.
auriculoventricular i.
automatic capacitor formation i.
A-V i.
A-V delay i.
Bazett corrected QT i.
B-H i.
c-a i.
cardioarterial i.
confidence i. (CI)
coupling i.
critical coupling i.
electromechanical i.
escape i.
fetal PR i.
f-f i.
filtered atrial rate i. (FARI)
flutter R i.
H-Ae i.
hangout i.
H_1-H_2 i.
His-ventricular i.
H'P i.
H-Q i.
H-QRS i.
H-V i.
HV i.
interectopic i.
isoelectric i.
isometric i.
isovolumic i.
JT i.
long PP i.
magnet pacing i.
P-A i.
PA i.
pacemaker escape i.
passive i.
P-H i.
P-J i.
postsphygmic i.
P-P i.
P-Q i.
PR i.
P-R i.
presphygmic i.
prolongation of P-R i.
Q-H i.

NOTES

interval *(continued)*
    Q-M i.
    QR i.
    QRB i.
    QRS i.
    QRS-T i.
    Q-S$_2$ i.
    QS$_2$ i.
    QT i.
    QTc i.
    Q-U i.
    right ventricular systolic time i.
    R-P i.
    RR i.
    R-R′ i.
    RS-T i.
    short coupling i.
    sphygmic i.
    S-QRS i.
    S$_1$-S$_2$ i.
    ST i.
    stimulus-T i.
    symptom-free i.
    systolic time i. (STI)
    TP i.
    V-A i.
    VA i.
    V-H i.
interval-dependent potentiation
interval-strength relation
intervalvular fibrosa
intervention
    Myocardial Infarction Triage and I. (MITI)
    New Applications for Coronary I.'s (NACI)
    New Approaches to Coronary I. (NACI)
    percutaneous coronary i. (PCI)
    Postmenopausal Estrogen/Progestin I. (PEPI)
    vagomimetic i.
interventional
    i. cardiac catheterization
    i. cardiologist
    i. echocardiography
    i. radiology
    i. study
interventricular
    i. foramen
    i. septal motion
    i. septal rupture
    i. septal thickness (IVS)
    i. septum
    i. septum aneurysm
    i. sulcus
    i. vein
intervertebral disk

interview
    Alexithymia Provoked Response I.
intestinal
    i. ischemia
    i. lipodystrophy
intima
    aortic tunica i.
intimal
    i. atheroma
    i. defect
    i. erosion
    i. flap
    i. hyperplasia (IH)
    i. proliferation
    i. tear
    i. thickening
intimal-medial
    i.-m. thickening
    i.-m. thickness (IMT)
Intimax vascular catheter
INTIME
    Intravenous tPA for Treatment of Infarcting Myocardium Early
    INTIME clinical trial
intolerance
    carbohydrate i.
    exercise i.
    glucose i.
intoxication
    alcohol i.
    digitalis i.
intraalveolar
    i. deposit
    i. pressure
intraaortic
    i. balloon (IAB)
    i. balloon catheter
    i. balloon counterpulsation (IABC)
    i. balloon device
    i. balloon pulsation (IABP)
    i. balloon pump (IABP)
    i. balloon pumping (IABP)
intraarterial (IA)
    i. counterpulsation
    i. gene transfer
    i. thrombosis
intraatrial
    i. activation sequence
    i. baffle
    i. block
    i. conduction
    i. conduction time
    i. reentrant tachycardia
    i. reentry tachycardia (IART)
    i. shunting
intrabronchial
intracardiac
    i. accelerometer

i. amobarbital sodium procedure
i. atrial activation sequence
i. catheter
i. ECG
i. echocardiography (ICE)
i. electrocardiography
i. electrogram
i. electrophysiologic study
i. electrophysiology
i. event
i. gas gangrene
i. lead
i. mapping
i. mass
i. navigation
i. pacing
i. pressure
i. pressure curve
i. shunt
i. sucker
i. thrombus
i. tumor
intracaval
i. device
i. endovascular ultrasonography (ICEUS)
intracavitary
i. air meniscus
i. electrocardiography
i. hemorrhage
i. instillation
i. pressure-electrogram dissociation
i. pressure gradient
intracavity mass
intracellular
i. calcium concentration
i. caveolae
i. lipid
i. magnesium
i. organism (ICO)
i. tyrosine protein kinase
intracellulare
Mycobacterium i.
intracellular-like, calcium-bearing crystalloid solution (ICS)
intracerebral hemorrhage (ICH)
IntraCoil self expanding nitinol stent
intracoronary
i. acetylcholine infusion
i. angioscopy
i. artery radiation
i. aspiration thrombectomy (ICAT)

i. beta-radiation
i. Doppler flow wire
i. radiation
i. radiation therapy (ICRT, IRT)
i. sonicated meglumine
i. stenting
I. Stenting and Antithrombotic regimen (ISAR)
i. stenting of de novo narrowing
i. stent placement
i. thrombolysis balloon valvuloplasty
i. ultrasonography
i. ultrasound (ICUS)
i. vascular ultrasound (IVUS)
intracorporeal heart
intracranial
i. aneurysm
i. atherosclerotic disease (IAD)
i. fusiform aneurysm
i. hemorrhage (ICH)
i. hypertension (ICH)
i. microembolic signal
i. pressure (ICP)
intractable
i. aspiration
i. hypotension
IntraDop
intragraft thrombus
intrahisian block
intralesion restenosis
Intralipid
intralobar
intralobular line
intraluminal
i. dissection
i. flap
i. plaque
i. thrombus
i. ultrasound (ILUS)
IntraLuminal Safe-Steer guidewire system
intramucosal pH (pH$_{im}$)
intramural
i. coronary arteries
i. hematoma (IH)
i. hemorrhage (IMH)
i. thrombosis
i. thrombus
intramyocardial
i. conduction delay
i. function

NOTES

intramyocardial *(continued)*
- i. prearteriolar vessel
- i. pressure
- i. sinusoid

Intra-Op autotransfusion system
intraoperative
- i. cell salvage
- i. digital subtraction (IDIS)
- i. digital subtraction angiography
- i. echocardiography (IOE)
- i. hemodynamics
- i. hypoxemia
- i. mapping
- i. vascular angiography (IVA)

intraparenchymal
- i. hematoma
- i. hemorrhage

intraparietal sulcus (IPS)
intrapericardial
- i. hemorrhage
- i. pressure
- i. sign

intraperitoneal rupture
intraplaque LDL oxidation
intrapleural
- i. catheter
- i. catheter analgesia
- i. oncotic pressure
- i. rupture
- i. sealed drainage unit
- i. space

intrapulmonary
- i. percussive ventilation (IPV)
- i. rheumatoid nodule
- i. shunt
- i. shunt fraction (Q_s/Q_t, Qs/Qt)
- i. shunting
- i. vascular dilation

intrapulmonic
intrarectal
intrastent
- i. minimal lumen cross-sectional area (ISMLCSA)
- i. recurrent disease
- i. restenosis (IR)

intrathoracic
- i. gas
- i. gas compression
- i. hypertension
- i. injury
- i. pressure
- i. PTLPD
- i. thyroid

intratracheal tube
intrauterine
- i. pneumonia
- i. respiration

intravariability

intravascular
- i. aggregate
- i. bronchoalveolar tumor
- i. catheter electrode
- i. Doppler
- i. Doppler-tipped guidewire
- i. elastogram
- i. fetal air sign
- i. foreign body retrieval
- i. gene transfer
- i. MRI
- i. oxygenator (IVOX)
- i. perfluorochemical emulsion
- i. pressure
- i. procoagulant factor
- i. red light therapy (IRLT)
- i. signal intensity
- i. stent
- i. thrombus
- i. ultrasound (IVUS)
- i. ultrasound catheter
- i. volume

intravenous (IV)
- i. analgesia
- CellCept i.
- i. digital subtraction angiography (IVDSA)
- Fungizone I.
- i. gamma globulin (IVGG)
- i. glucose tolerance test (IVGTT)
- i. hyperalimentation (IVH)
- i. immune globulin
- i. immunoglobulin therapy
- Saventrine I.
- I. Streptokinase in Acute Myocardial Infarction (ISAM)
- I. tPA for Treatment of Infarcting Myocardium Early (INTIME)

intraventricular
- i. aberration
- i. block (IVB)
- i. catheter (IVC)
- i. conduction
- i. conduction delay
- i. conduction pattern
- i. gradient
- i. hemorrhage (IVH)

intravital
- i. capillary video microscopy
- i. microscopy

Intrepid
- I. balloon catheter
- I. PTCA catheter

intrinsic
- i. activity
- i. asthma
- i. deflection
- i. depolarization

i. disease
i. positive end-expiratory pressure (PEEPi)
i. sympathomimetic activity
intrinsicoid deflection
introduced
percutaneous i.
introducer
Angestat hemostasis i.
Angetear tearaway i.
aortic assist balloon i.
Avanti i.
Cardak percutaneous catheter i.
Check-Flo i.
Ciaglia percutaneous tracheostomy i.
Davol pacemaker i.
Desilets i.
Desilets-Hoffman catheter i.
Encapsulon sheath i.
Fast-Cath Duo i.
FasTrac i.
gum elastic bougie i.
Hemaquet i.
I. II sheath
Implantaid Di-Lock cardiac lead i.
Littleford/Spector i.
LPS Peel-Away i.
Micropuncture Peel-Away i.
Mullins catheter i.
Nottingham i.
Razi cannula i.
i. sheath
888 i. sheath
split-sheath i.
Tuohy-Borst i.
UMI transseptal Cath-Seal catheter i.
USCI i.
introducer/endoscope
Czaja-McCaffrey rigid stent i.
intron
i. 16
i. A
Intropin
I. injection
intubated patient
intubation
catheter-guided endoscopic i. (CAGEIN)
endotracheal i.

mainstem i.
nasotracheal i.
O'Dwyer i.
orotracheal i.
RSI orotracheal i.
i. time
tracheal i.
intussusception
Invacare
I. ConnectO2 Telemetry System home oxygen system
I. nasal prongs
I. Venture HomeFill complete home oxygen system
I. Venture HomeFill oxygen system
invasive
i. assessment
i. monitoring
i. pressure measurement
i. pulmonary aspergillosis (IPA)
Inventory
Beck Depression I.
Cloninger Temperament and Character I.
Edinburgh Handedness I. (EHI)
State-Trait Anger Expression I. (STAXI)
State-Trait Anxiety I.
inversa
angina i.
inverse-ratio ventilation (IRV)
Inversine
inversion
shallow T-wave i.
T wave i.
U wave i.
ventricular i.
inversus
dextrocardia with situs i.
levocardia with situs i.
situs i.
inverted
i. buttoned device
i. T wave
i. V technique
investigation
bypass angioplasty revascularization i. (BARI)
Coronary Angioplasty versus Bypass Revascularization i. (CABRI)

NOTES

investigation *(continued)*
  Coronary Artery Bypass
  Revascularization Investigation
  (CABRI)
investigational
  i. new drug (IND)
  i. new drug status
investigator
  atrial fibrillation i.
Invirase
INVM
  isolated noncompaction of the ventricular
  myocardium
inward-going rectification
INX stent
Iobid DM
iodide
  metocurine i.
  potassium i.
  saturated solution of potassium i.
  (SSKI)
iodine
  lithium i. (LiI)
  radiolabeled i.
iodine-123 (I-123)
  i. heptadecanoic acid radioactive
  tracer
  i. metaiodobenzylguanidine (I-123-
  MIBG)
  i. metaiodobenzylguanidine uptake
iodine-125 isotope
iodine-131 MIBG scintigraphy
iodophenylpentadecanoic acid
iodoquinol
IOE
  intraoperative echocardiography
iohexol
Iohexol contrast
Iomeron
ion
  calcium i.
  i. channel
  chloride i.
  potassium i.
  i. pump
  sodium i.
Ionescu
  I. method
  I. trileaflet valve
Ionescu-Shiley
  I.-S. pericardial patch
  I.-S. pericardial valve
  I.-S. pericardial xenograft
  I.-S. valve
  I.-S. valve prosthesis
  I.-S. vascular graft
ionic mechanism
ionizing radiation (IR)

ionophore
  calcium i. A23187
ion-selective electrode (ISE)
Ionyx lead
iopamidol
Iopamiro
iopromide injection
I-orthoiodohippurate
iothalamate meglumine contrast medium
ioversol
ioxaglate
  i. meglumine
  i. meglumine contrast medium
  i. sodium
  sodium meglumine i.
IPA
  invasive pulmonary aspergillosis
IPAP
  inspiratory positive airway pressure
IPC
  intermittent pneumatic compression
  ischemic preconditioning
  IPC boots
IPCO-Partridge defibrillator
IPF
  idiopathic pulmonary fibrosis
  interstitial pulmonary fibrosis
IPG
  impedance plethysmography
IPH
  idiopathic pulmonary hemosiderosis
IPLVAS
  implantable left ventricular assist system
IPP
  intermittent positive pressure
IPPB
  intermittent positive pressure breathing
IPPV
  intermittent positive pressure ventilation
Iprafen
ipratropium
  i. and albuterol
  i. bromide
  i. inhaler
IPS
  intraparietal sulcus
ipsilateral stroke
IPSTL
  inferior parietal/superior temporal lobe
IPT
  inflammatory pseudotumor
IPV
  intermittent percussive ventilation
  intrapulmonary percussive ventilation
IQ nasal mask
IR
  intrastent restenosis
  ionizing radiation

IRA
infarct-related artery
IRAS
Insulin Resistance Atherosclerosis Study
irbesartan and hydrochlorothiazide
IRC
inspiratory reserve capacity
IRDS
infant respiratory distress syndrome
I-receptor
imidazoline receptor
Irex Exemplar ultrasound
iridium strand
iridodonesis
irinotecan
Iris
I. coronary stent
I. II stent
IRLT
intravascular red light therapy
IRMA
immunoradiometric assay
IRMA blood gas analysis system
IRMA SL blood glucose strip
tester
IRMA system
iron
i. chelator
colloidal i. (CI)
i. dextran complex
i. lung
serum i.
i. storage disease
irox Si-Carbide
IR-PEP
inspiratory resistance and positive
expiratory pressure
irradiation
endovascular i. (EI)
prophylactic brain i. (PCI)
total axial node i. (TANI)
total body i. (TBI)
total lymphoid i. (TLI)
irregular
i. discrete lesion
i. hematoma
i. rhythm
irregularis
pulsus i.
irregularly
i. irregular cardiac rhythm

i. irregular pulse
i. irregular rhythm
irrespirable
irreversible
i. airway obstruction
i. shock
Irri-Cath suction system
irrigated
i. catheter ablation
i. coiled catheter
irritable heart
irritant
i. receptor
respiratory i.
i. rhinitis
i. sinusitis
**irritant-associated vocal cord
dysfunction**
irritant-induced asthma
IRT
intracoronary radiation therapy
IRV
inspiratory reserve volume
inverse-ratio ventilation
**Irvine viable organ-tissue transport
system (IVOTTS)**
Isaacs-Ludwig arteriole
ISAM
Intravenous Streptokinase in Acute
Myocardial Infarction
ISAM clinical trial
Isambert disease
ISAR
Intracoronary Stenting and
Antithrombotic regimen
ISAR clinical trial
ischemia
asymptomatic cardiac i. (ACI)
brachiocephalic i.
cardiac i.
cerebral i.
clandestine myocardial i.
colonic i.
delayed cerebral i. (DCI)
dobutamine-induced i.
exercise-induced i.
exercise-induced silent myocardial i.
extremity i.
intestinal i.
Laser Angioplasty for Critical I.
(LACI)
limb i.

NOTES

ischemia (*continued*)
>   low-flow i.
>   manifest i.
>   mental stress-induced i.
>   mesenteric i.
>   mucosal i.
>   myocardial i. (MI)
>   nonocclusive mesenteric i.
>   recurrent mesenteric i.
>   regional i.
>   silent i.
>   silent myocardial i.
>   subendocardial i.
>   Thrombin Inhibition in
>   Myocardial I. (TIMI-7, TRIM)
>   transient i.
>   transient mesenteric i.
>   vertebrobasilar territory i. (VBI)

ischemia-driven revascularization
ischemia-guided medical therapy
ischemia-induced
>   i.-i. intracellular acidosis
>   i.-i. intramyocardial conduction
>   delay

ischemia/reperfusion-induced apoptosis
ischemic
>   i. burden
>   i. cardiomyopathy
>   i. cascade
>   i. cerebral infarction
>   i. contracture of left ventricle
>   i. core
>   i. ECG change
>   i. event
>   i. heart disease (IHD)
>   i. hypoxia
>   i. leukoaraiosis
>   i. mitral regurgitation
>   i. myocardium
>   i. necrosis
>   i. paralysis
>   i. penumbra
>   i. pericarditis
>   i. preconditioning (IPC)
>   i. rest angina
>   i. stroke
>   i. sudden death
>   i. threshold
>   i. zone

ischemic-reperfusion injury
ischemic-type preconditioning stimulus
ISDN
>   isosorbide dinitrate

ISE
>   ion-selective electrode

Iselin forceps
isethionate
>   aerosolized pentamidine i.

>   pentamidine i.
>   piritrexim i.

ISH
>   isolated septal hypertrophy

ISHT
>   International Society for Heart
>   Transplantation
>   ISHT Registry

ISIS
>   International Study of Infarct Survival

Ismelin
ISMLCSA
>   intrastent minimal lumen cross-sectional
>   area

IS-5-MN
>   isosorbide-5-mononitrate

Ismo
ISO
>   International Standards Organization

isoactin switch
isobutyl 2-cyanoacrylate
isocapnia
isocapnic, isocapneic
>   i. condition
>   i. hyperpnea

isocenter system
isochoric
Isoclor Expectorant
isocratic elution
isocyanate
>   methyl i.

isocyanate-induced asthma
isodiametric bipolar screw-in lead
isodiphasic complex
isoechoic
isoelectric
>   i. interval
>   i. line
>   i. period
>   i. point
>   i. ST segment

isoenzyme
>   CPK i.
>   myocardial muscle creatine
>   kinase i. (CK-MB)

isoetharine
>   Arm-a-Med I.
>   Dey-Lute I.
>   I. Inhalation Solution USP 1%

isoflavone
isoflurane
isoform
>   Apo E3 i.
>   CYP1A2 i.
>   CYP3A i.
>   CYP2C9 i.
>   CYP2C19 i.
>   CYP2D6 i.

isoglycemia
isointense heterogeneous signal
isolated
    i. cerebral thromboangiitis obliterans disease
    i. CTAO
    i. dextrocardia
    i. dysarthria
    i. ectopic beat
    i. heat perfusion
    i. low HDL
    i. low high-density lipoprotein (ILHDL)
    i. noncompaction of the ventricular myocardium (INVM)
    i. parietal endocarditis
    i. septal hypertrophy (ISH)
    i. systolic hypertension
    i. T wave
isomer
    dextro i.
isomerism
isometric
    i. contraction
    i. contraction period
    i. exercise
    i. handgrip
    i. handgrip test
    i. interval
    i. period of cardiac cycle
    i. relaxation period
    i. sports
isometrically contracting myocardial preparation
isomyosin switch
isoniazid (INH)
    rifampin and i.
isonitrile
    carbomethoxyisopropyl i.
    methoxyisobutyl i. (MIBI)
    technetium-99m hexakis 2-methyoxyisobutyl i.
    technetium-99m methoxyisobutyl i.
Isopaque
8-iso-PGF$_{2alpha}$
    8-iso-prostaglandin F$_{2alpha}$
isoprenaline
    i. hydrochloride
    i. sulfate
isoprophenamine hydrochloride

isopropylarterenol hydrochloride
8-iso-prostaglandin F$_{2alpha}$ (8-iso-PGF$_{2alpha}$)
isoproterenol
    Arm-a-Med i.
    Dey-Dose i.
    Dispos-a-Med i.
    i. hydrochloride
    i.-induced vasovagal syncope
    i. infusion
    i. and phenylephrine
    i. stress test
    i. sulfate
    i. sulfate inhalation
    i. tilt-table test
    i. tilt test
Isoptin SR
Isopto Atropine
Isordil
isorhythmic dissociation
isosorbide
    i. dinitrate (ISDN)
    i. dinitrate injection
    i. mononitrate
isosorbide-5-mononitrate (IS-5-MN)
Isospora belli
IsoStent
    I. BX
    I. stent
isotonic
    i. contraction
    i. exercise
isotope
    iodine-125 i.
isotypic
Isovex
isovolemic hemodilution
isovolume
    i. flow
    i. pressure-flow curve
    i. shifting
isovolumetric
    i. contractility
    i. phase index
    i. relaxation
    i. relaxation period (IVRP)
isovolumic
    i. index
    i. interval
    i. period
    i. pressure decay
    i. relaxation

NOTES

isovolumic *(continued)*
    i. relaxation period
    i. relaxation time (IVRT)
    i. systole
Isovue contrast medium
isoxsuprine hydrochloride
ISR
    in-stent restenosis
isradipine
Israel Benzedrine vaporizer
israelii
    Actinomyces i.
    Nocardia i.
ISS
    Injury Severity Score
ISSLC
    International Staging System for Lung
      Cancer
IST
    International Stroke Trial
I-STATE bedside blood testing device
i-STAT handheld analyzer
isthmectomy
isthmic hypoplasia
isthmus, pl. **isthmi**
    aortic i.
    cavotricuspid i.
    Krönig i.
    i. line
    posterior i.
    septal i.
    subeustachian i.
    thyroid i.
    tricuspid-inferior vena cava i.
isthmus-dependent atrial flutter
Isuprel Mistometer
ITA
    internal thoracic artery
    ITA graft
ITC balloon catheter
iterative presyncope
ITL
    inspiratory threshold load
ITP
    idiopathic thrombocytopenic purpura
ITPA
    Illinois Test of Psycholinguistic Abilities
    ITPA index
itraconazole
Itrel
    I. 3 spinal cord stimulation system
    I. 1 unipolar pulse generator
I-Tropine
ITT
    intention-to-treat

ITV
    impedance threshold valve
IV
    intravenous
      Gammar-P IV
      Hyperstat IV
      Merrem IV
      IV Persantine
      Vasotec IV
IVA
    intraoperative vascular angiography
IVAC
    I. electronic thermometer
    I. ventilator
    I. volumetric infusion pump
Ivalon
    I. plug
    I. sponge
IVA-S2000
IVB
    intraventricular block
IVC
    inferior vena cava
    inspiratory vital capacity
    intraventricular catheter
      IVC thrombosis
IVDSA
    intravenous digital subtraction
      angiography
Ivemark syndrome
ivermectin
IVGG
    intravenous gamma globulin
IVGTT
    intravenous glucose tolerance test
IVH
    intravenous hyperalimentation
    intraventricular hemorrhage
IV-Heart nebulizer
IVOTTS
    Irvine viable organ-tissue transport
      system
IVOX
    intravascular oxygenator
IVRP
    isovolumetric relaxation period
IVRT
    isovolumic relaxation time
IVS
    interventricular septal thickness
IVT
    idiopathic ventricular tachycardia
      IVT percutaneous catheter
      introducer sheath

I

IVUS
    intracoronary vascular ultrasound
    intravascular ultrasound
      IVUS catheter
      coronary IVUS

    3D IVUS
      IVUS-guided balloon angioplasty
Ivy bleeding time
IWMI
    inferior wall myocardial infarction

NOTES

J
joule
J curve
J exchange wire
J guidewire
J junction
J-loop technique
J orthogonal electrode
J point
J point electrical axis
J retention wire
J retention wire fracture
J Rosen guidewire
J wave
J wire
J5 lipopolysaccharidase
JA
juxtaarticular
JA lesion
Jaa Amp
Jaa-Prednisone
Jabaley-Stille Super Cut Scissors
Jaccoud
J. dissociated fever
J. sign
jacket
Bonchek-Shiley cardiac j.
cardiac cooling j.
cuirass j.
Medtronic cardiac cooling j.
Willock respiratory j.
jacket-type chest dressing
Jackman
J. coronary sinus electrode catheter
J. orthogonal catheter
Jackson
J. bistoury
J. cane-shaped tracheal tube
J. safety triangle
J. sign
J. syndrome
Jackson-Trousseau dilator
Jacobaeus
J. procedure
J. thoracoscope
Jacobaeus-Unverricht thoracoscope
Jacobson
J. microbulldog clamp
J. modified vessel clamp
Jacobson-Potts clamp
Jacquet apparatus
Jaeger
J. body plethysmography system
J. ER 900 electromagnetically
braked cycle ergometer

J. Flowscreen spirometer
J. LE3000 treadmill
J. MasterLab Pro pneumotachograph
spirometer
Jaffe method
Jahnke anastomosis clamp
Jahnke-Barron heart support net
jail
stent j.
jailed side branch
Jak
Janus kinase
Jako laryngoscope
Jak/Stat
Janus kinase/signal transducer and
activator of transcription
Jak/Stat pathway
Jamar
J. hand dynamometer
J. model 0030J4 dynamometer
James
J. accessory tracts
J. bundle
J. exercise protocol
J. fiber
Jamshidi needle
Janeway
J. lesion
J. sphygmomanometer
Janus
J. kinase (Jak)
J. kinase/signal transducer and
activator of transcription (Jak/Stat)
J. syndrome
Janz formula
japonicum
Schistosoma j.
Jarvik
J. 7, 8 artificial heart
J. 7-70 artificial heart
J. 2000 artificial heart
Jatene
J. arterial switch procedure
J.-Macchi prosthetic valve
J. technique
Javid
J. carotid artery bypass clamp
J. shunt
jaw
j. reflex (JR)
j. thrust maneuver
jaw-thrust/head-tilt maneuver
Jebsen Hand Function Test
jeikeium
Corynebacterium j.

J

jejunal artery
jejunostomy
    percutaneous endoscopic j. (PEJ)
jelly
    cardiac j.
    electrode j.
Jenamicin injection
Jenkins Activity Survey
Jenner emphysema
jeopardized myocardium
jeopardy
    myocardial j.
    j. score
jerk
    dormescent j.
jerkin plethysmograph
jerky
    j. pulse
    j. respiration
Jervell and Lange-Nielsen syndrome
Jesberg esophagoscope
JET
    junctional ectopic tachycardia
jet
    anteriorly directed j.
    aortic stenosis j.
    Doppler color j.
    eccentric stenotic j.
    j. effect
    j. humidifier
    j. lesion
    mitral regurgitant j.
    mosaic j.
    j. nebulizer
    patent ductus arteriosus flow j.
    regurgitant j.
    residual j.
    saline j.
    signal-void j.
    stenotic j.
    tricuspid regurgitant j.
    turbulent j.
    j. velocity
    j. ventilation
Jeune syndrome
Jewel
    J. AF implantable arrhythmia
    management device
    J. AF implantable defibrillator
    J. atrial fibrillation dual chamber
    device
    J. pacer-cardioverter-defibrillator
    J. PCD
Jinotti closed suctioning system
J & J stent
JL4
    Judkins left 4
    JL4 catheter

JL5
    Judkins left 5
    JL5 catheter
JNK
    c-Jun N-terminal kinase
Jobst
    J. extremity pump
    J. pressure garment
    J.-Stride support stockings
    J.-Stridette support stockings
    J. VPGS stockings
Job syndrome
Johnson
    J. & Johnson biliary stent
    J. & Johnson coronary stent
    J. & Johnson hemopump
    J. & Johnson Interventional
    Systems
    J. and Johnson Interventional
    Systems stent
joint
    j. deformity
    tuberculosis of bones and j.'s
Joklik medium
Jomed stent
Jonas modification of Norwood
  procedure
Jones criteria
Jonnson maneuver
Jopamiro 370
jordanis
    Legionella j.
Jorgenson thoracic scissors
josamycin
Josephson
    J. catheter
    J. quadpolar mapping electrode
    J. quadripolar catheter
Jostent
    J. Bifurcation stent
    J. coronary stent
    J. coronary stent graft
    J. Flex stent
    J. Plus stent
    J. Sidebranch stent
    J. stent
Jostra
    J. arterial blood filter
    J. cardiotomy reservoir
    J. catheter
joule (J)
JP lead
JR
    jaw reflex
    Aerolate JR
JR4
    Judkins right 4
    JR4 catheter

JR5
 Judkins right 5
  JR5 catheter
J-shaped
  J.-s. pacemaker electrode
  J.-s. tube
JT
 junctional tachycardia
  JT interval
JTc value
J-tip guidewire
JTV519 1,4-benzothiazepine derivative
Judkins
  J. coronary catheter
  J. curve LAD catheter
  J. curve LCX catheter
  J. curve STD catheter
  J. 4 diagnostic catheter
  6-French J. catheter
  J. guiding catheter
  J. left 4 (JL4)
  J. left 5 (JL5)
  J. pigtail left ventriculography
   catheter
  J. right 4 (JR4)
  J. right 5 (JR5)
  J. selective coronary arteriography
  J. technique
  J. torque control catheter
Judkins-Sones technique
jugular
  j. bulb catheter placement
   assessment
  j. embryocardia
  j. pulse
  j. vein
  j. venous arch
  j. venous catechol spillover
  j. venous distention (JVD)
  j. venous pressure (JVP)
  j. venous pulse
  j. venous pulse tracing
jugulodigastric lymph node
juice
  purple grape j.
Julian thoracic forceps
Jumonji gene
jump graft
jumping thrombosis
junction
  adherens j.
  atrioventricular j. (AVJ)

  A-V j.
  cardioesophageal j.
  costochondral j.
  esophagogastric j.
  gap j.
  J j.
  loose j.
  QRS-ST j.
  saphenofemoral j.
  sinotubular j.
  ST j.
  sternochondral j.
  tight j.
  tracheoesophageal j.
  triadic j.
junctional
  atrioventricular j.
  j. axis
  j. bigeminy
  j. bradycardia
  j. complex
  j. depression
  j. ectopic tachycardia (JET)
  j. escape
  j. escape beat
  j. escape rhythm
  j. extrasystole
  j. parasystole
  j. reciprocating tachycardia
  j. rhythm
  j. tachycardia (JT)
Jun **gene**
Junker inhaler
Junod procedure
Juquitiba virus
Jürgensen sign
jute worker's lung
Juvenelle clamp
juvenile
  j. arrhythmia
  j. myocardial infarction
  j. pattern
  j. rheumatoid arthritis
juvenum
  cor j.
juxtaarticular (JA)
  j. lesion
juxtacapillary receptor
juxtacardiac pleural pressure
juxtaductal coarctation
juxtaesophageal lymph node

NOTES

J

Juzo
  J. hose
  J. shrinker
  J. stockings
J-Vac
JVD
  jugular venous distention

JVP
  jugular venous pressure
J-wire
  J-w. lead

K
    potassium
       K current
       K 54 lead
       K stylet
       K x-ray fluorescence instrument
K-37 pediatric arterial blood filter
KAAT II Plus intraaortic balloon pump
Kabikinase
KabiVitrum
Kahler bronchial biopsy forceps
Kairos pacemaker
Kalcinate
Kales scoring method
kaliuresis
kallidinogenase inactivator unit
kallikrein
       k. 1 (KLK1)
       k. gene
       k. inactivating unit (KIU)
kallikrein-bradykinin system
kallikrein-kinin (KK)
Kallmann syndrome
Kalos pacemaker
Kaltostat
       K. wound packing dressing
       K. wound packing material
Kamen-Wilkenson endotracheal tube
Kampmeier foci
Kampo medicine
kanamycin
kangaroo
       k. care
       K. pump
kansasii
       Mycobacterium k.
Kantor-Berci video laryngoscope
Kantrowitz
       K. pacemaker
       K. thoracic clamp
kaolinosis
kaolin pneumoconiosis
Kaon
Kaopectate
Kaplan-Meier
       K.-M. event-free survival curve
       K.-M. life table
       K.-M. method
Kaplan-Simpson InfusaSleeve
kapok asthma
Kaposi sarcoma (KS)
Kappa 400 Series pacemaker
karaya asthma
Kardegic

Karell diet
Karhunen-Loeve procedure
Karmen units
Karmody venous scissors
Karnofsky rating scale
Karolinska quality of life questionnaire
Karplus sign
Kartagener
       K. syndrome
       K. triad
Kasabach-Merritt syndrome
Kasser-Kennedy method
Kaster mitral valve prosthesis
Katayama fever
Kattus
       K. exercise stress test
       K. treadmill protocol
Katz activities of daily living score
Katzen
       K. infusion wire
       K. long balloon dilatation catheter
Katz-Wachtel phenomenon
Kaufman pneumonia
Kawai bioptome
Kawasaki
       K. disease
       K. syndrome
Kawashima intraventricular tunnel
Kay
       K. annuloplasty
       K. balloon
Kayexalate enema
Kay-Shiley caged-disk valve
K^+ channels
KCl
    potassium chloride
kDa, kd
    kilodalton
Kearns-Sayre syndrome
keel
    McNaught k.
keeled chest
Keflex
Keflin injection
Keftab
Kefurox injection
Kefzol
Keith
       K. bundle
       K. node
Keith-Flack node
Keith-Wagener-Barker (KWB)
Kellner questionnaire
Kellock sign

Kelly
> K. clamp
> K. hemostat
> K.-Wick vascular tunneler

keloidal
Kelvin Sensor pacemaker
Kempner diet
Kenacort
> K. Oral
> K. Syrup
> K. Tablet

Kenaject Injection
Kenalog injection
Kendall
> K. compression stockings
> K. Sequential Compression device

Kendal nasal prongs
Kennedy area-length method
Kenonel
Kensey
> K. atherectomy catheter
> K. rotation atherectomy extrusion

Kent
> K. bundle
> K. bundle ablation
> bundle of Stanley K.
> K. fiber
> K.-His bundle
> K. pathway
> K. potential

Keofeed feeding tube
keratin pearls
Kerley A, B, C lines
Kerlone Oral
Kernan-Jackson bronchoscope
Kern technique
kerosene pneumonitis
Keshan disease
ketamine
ketanserin
Ketek
ketoacidosis
ketoconazole
ketone
> D-Phe-L-Pro-L-Arg-chloromethyl k.
> (PPACK)

ketoprofen
ketorolac
ketotifen
Kety-Schmidt method
keV
> kiloelectron volt

key
> ResCue K.
> Walking with Angina-Learning
> is K. (WALK)

keyhole-limpet hemocyanin
keyhole surgery

Key-Pred Injection
Key-Pred-SP injection
Keystone PF analyzer
kg/m^2
> kilogram per meter squared

KI antigen
kick
> atrial k.
> idioventricular k.

kidney
> Ask-Upmark k.
> flea-bitten k.
> Goldblatt k.
> polycystic k.

Kiel classification of lymphoma
Kienbock phenomenon
**Kiethly-DAS series 500 data-acquisition
system**
Kifa catheter material
Kikuchi disease
killer
> natural k. (NK)

Killian bundle
Killian-Lynch laryngoscope
Killip
> K. heart disease classification
> K.-Kimball heart failure
> classification
> K. wire

kilodalton (kDa, kd)
45-kilodalton protein
kiloelectron volt (keV)
kilogram
> milligrams per k. (mg/kg)
> milliliter per k. (mL/kg)
> k. per meter squared (kg/m^2)

kilohm
kilopascal (kPa)
kilopond (KP)
> k. meter (KPM)

kilovolt (kV)
Kimmelstiel-Wilson syndrome
Kim-Ray
> K.-R. Greenfield antiembolus filter
> K.-R. Greenfield caval filter
> K.-R. thermodilution

Kimura cartilage graft
kinase
> adrenergic receptor k. (ARK)
> adrenergic receptor k. 1 (ARK-1)
> beta-adrenergic receptor k.
> c-Jun N-terminal k. (JNK)
> creatine k. (CK)
> extracellularly responsive k. (ERK)
> extracellular-regulated k. (ERK)
> extracellular signal-regulated k.
> focal adhesion k. (FAK)
> intracellular tyrosine protein k.

Janus k. (Jak)
mitogen-activated protein k.
(MAPK)
mitogen-activated protein kinase k.
phosphorylase k.
protein k.
protein k. A
protein k. C (PKC)
Ras mitogen-activated protein k.
serine k.
serum creatine k.
Src k.
threonine protein k.

Kindt carotid artery clamp
kinesiological electromyogram
kinesis
color k. (CK)
kinetics
first-order k.
zero-order k.
kinetic therapy
KinetiX
K. instrument
K. ventilation monitor
kinetocardiogram
kinetocardiograph
King
K. ASD umbrella closure
K. biopsy method
K. bioptome
K. cardiac device
K. double umbrella closure system
K. guiding catheter
K. of Hearts event recorder
K. of Hearts Express cardiac-event
recorder
K. of Hearts Express 3X cardiac-
event recorder
K. of Hearts Holter monitor
K. interlocking device
K. multipurpose catheter
kingae
Haemophilus aphrophilus,
Actinobacillus
actinomycetemcomitans,
Cardiobacterium hominis,
Eikenella corrodens, and
Kingella k. (HACEK)
Kingella k.
kinin
endogenous k.
kininogen

kinked aorta
kinky-hair disease
Kinsey
K. atherectomy
K. atherectomy catheter
K. rotation atherectomy extrusion
angioplasty
Kinyoun stain
Kirklin fence
Kirkorian-Touboul method
Kirstein method
Kisch reflex
kissing
k. balloon angioplasty
k. balloon technique
k. stent
k. stenting
k. tonsil
Kistner tracheal button
kit
AeroGear asthma action k.
Alatest Latex-specific IgE allergen
test k.
Arrow pneumothorax k.
AsthmaPACK personal asthma
care k.
BioSource Cytoscreen SAA k.
BiPort hemostasis introducer
sheath k.
Cordis lead conversion k.
cyanide antidote k.
Daiichi Radioisotope Labs. Techne
MAA k.
Denver Pleurx pleural catheter/home
drainage k.
Enzygnost F1+2 ELISA k.
Enzygnost TAT complex k.
Euro-Collins multiorgan
perfusion k.
Fergus percutaneous introducer k.
Imulyse tPA ELISA k.
MDI k.
neonatal internal jugular
puncture k.
No Pour Pak suction catheter k.
Oncor ApopTaq k.
percutaneous access k. (PAK)
percutaneous catheter introducer k.
Per-fit percutaneous tracheostomy k.
Pleurx drainage and catheter k.
Pleurx pleural catheter/home
drainage k.

K

NOTES

383

kit *(continued)*
    Portex Per-Fit tracheostomy k.
    Pro-Vent ABG k.
    Pro-Vent arterial blood gas k.
    Pro-Vent arterial blood sampling k.
    Pulsator dry heparin arterial blood
        gas k.
    RNeasy MINI k.
    Sub-4 Platinum Plus wire k.
    thermodilution catheter introducer k.
    TintElize PAI-1 ELISA k.
    TriPort hemostasis introducer
        sheath k.
    UniPort hemostasis introducer
        sheath k.
    Virgo anticardiolipin screening
        ELISA test k.
    Yamasa assay k.
KIU
    kallikrein inactivating unit
KK
    kallikrein-kinin
    KK system
KL-6
    serum KL-6
Klebsiella
    K. oxytoca
    K. pneumonia
    K. pneumoniae
    K. pneumoniae subsp. *ozaenae*
    K. rhinoscleromatis
Klebs-Loeffler bacillus
Kleihauer-Betke test
Kleihauer test
Klein transseptal introducer sheath
Klein-Waardenburg syndrome
Klerist-D Tablet
Klinefelter syndrome
Klippel-Feil syndrome
Klippel-Trenaunay-Weber syndrome
KLK1
    kallikrein 1
knee
    k. extension
    medial inferior artery of k.
    medial superior artery of k.
knife, pl. **knives**
    A-K diamond k.
    A-OK ShortCut k.
    Bailey-Glover-O'Neill
        commissurotomy k.
    Beaver k.
    k. blade
    Bosher commissurotomy k.
    Derra k.
    Derra commissurotomy k.
    gamma k.
    Lebsche sternal k.

    Neoflex bendable k.
    roentgen k.
    UltraCision ultrasonic k.
    valvotomy k.
    k. wound
**KnightStar 335 respiratory-support
    system**
knitted
    k. polyester crimped graft
    k. sewing ring
    k. vascular prosthesis
knives *(pl. of* knife*)*
knob
    aortic k.
knock
    pericardial k.
Knoll gland
knuckle
    aortic k.
    B k.
    cervical aortic k.
    k. sign
Ko-Airan bleeding control procedure
Koala
    K. vascular clamp
    K. vascular insert
Koate-HP
Koch
    K. bacillus
    K. node
    K. old tuberculin
    K. phenomenon
    triangle of K.
    K. triangle
    K. tuberculin
    K.-Weeks bacillus
Kocher-Cushing reflex
Koelner Vitaport accelerometer
Koffex DM
Koffex-DM Children
Koga treatment
KoGENate
KOH
    potassium hydroxide
Kohlrausch vein
Kohn pore
KoKo
    K. Moe PF/spirometry filter
    K. research-grade spirometer
    K. rhythm ECG
    K. Rhythm ECG recorder
    K. rhythm PC-based ECG
    K. Trek research-grade spirometer
Kolephrin GG/DM
Kolff-Jarvik artificial heart
Kolmogorov-Smirnov procedure
Konakion injection

Kondoleon-Sistrunk elephantiasis procedure
Konica KFDR-S laser film scanner
Konigsberg catheter
Konno
    K. biopsy method
    K. bioptome
    K. operation
    K. procedure
Konton catheter
Kontron
    K. balloon
    K. balloon catheter
    K. intraaortic balloon pump
Konyne 80
Koplik spot
Kopp asthma
Korányi
    K. auscultation
    K. sign
Korean hemorrhagic fever
Korotkoff
    K. phase I–V
    K. sound
Kostmann syndrome
Kotonkan virus
KP
    kilopond
kPa
    kilopascal
KPM
    kilopond meter
^{81m}Kr
    krypton-81m
Krebs
    K. buffer
    K. cycle
    K.-Henseleit buffer
    K.-Henseleit solution
    K. solution
Kredex
Kreiselman unit
Kreysig sign
Krichenko criteria
kringle
Krishaber disease
KRM-1648/Isoniazid
Krogh
    K. apparatus spirometer
    K. spirometer
Kronecker center
Krönig
    K. area

    K. isthmus
    K. step
Krovetz-Gessner equation
Krukenberg vein
krypton-81m (^{81m}Kr)
    k. ventilation imaging
KS
    Kaposi sarcoma
k-space segmentation
K-Sponge
Kugel
    K. anastomosis
    K. anastomotic artery
Kugelberg-Welander
    K.-W. disease
    K.-W. syndrome
Kuhn
    K. mask
    K. tube
Kuhnt postcentral vein
Kulchitsky cell
Kuntiz-type inhibitor
Kuntz
    nerve of K.
Kurten vein stripper
Kussmaul
    K. breathing
    K. disease
    K.-Kien respiration
    K.-Maier disease
    K. paradoxical pulse
    K. respiration
    K. sign
    K. symptom
    K. syndrome
kV
    kilovolt
    kV fluoroscopy
Kveim
    K. antigen skin test
    K. reaction
    K.-Siltzbach test
    K. test
Kwai Garlic
KWB
    Keith-Wagener-Barker
    KWB classification
Kwelcof
kymogram
kymograph
kymography
kymoscope
kyphoscoliosis

K

NOTES

L
    L. 67 lead
    L. loop
    L. stylet
LA
  left atrium
    Dexone LA
    Guaifenex LA
    Inderal LA
L.A.
    Dexasone L.A.
    Humibid L.A.
    Solurex L.A.
    Theoclear L.A.
LAA
  left atrial appendage
    LAA contraction
    LAA filling
    LAA thrombi
La:A
  left atrial to aortic
    La:A ratio
LAARS
  LDL Apheresis Atherosclerosis
  Regression Study
LABA
  laser-assisted balloon angioplasty
labeled FFA scintigraphy
labeling
    TdT-mediated dUTP nick-end l.
    (TUNEL)
labetalol hydrochloride
labile
    l. blood pressure
    l. hypertension
    l. pulse
laboratory
    Core Exercise Testing L.
    Venereal Disease Research L.
    (VDRL)
Laborde method
labored respiration
Labrador lung
Labtron stethoscope
laceration
    parenchymal l.
LACI
  lacunar infarct
  Laser Angioplasty for Critical Ischemia
  lipoprotein-associated coagulation
    inhibitor
    LACI Study
lacidipine
Lacipil

lacrimalis
    fossa glandulae l.
lacrymans
    Serpula l.
LACS
  lacunar syndrome
lactamase
    beta l.
lactate
    amrinone l.
    l. dehydrogenase
    l. extraction
    milrinone l.
    Ringer l.
    sodium l.
    l. threshold
lactea
    macula l.
lactic
    l. acid
    l. acid concentration
    l. acid dehydrogenase
    l. acidosis
    l. acid transport
    l. dehydrogenase (LDH)
LactiCare-HC
Lactobacillus
lacuna, pl. **lacunae**
lacunar
    l. angina
    l. infarct (LACI)
    l. infarction (LI)
    l. stroke
    l. syndrome (LACS)
LAD
  left anterior descending
  left atrial dimension
  left axis deviation
    LAD artery
LADA
  left anterior descending artery
ladder
    l. diagram
    l. incision
    L. of Life score
Laënnec
    L. catarrh
    L. cirrhosis
    L. pearl
    L. sign
Laerdal
    L. infant resuscitator
    L. Resusci Folding Bag II
    L. resuscitator
    L. silicon resuscitator

L

laevis
  Xenopus l.
Laevovist
LAF
  left atrial enlargement
LAFS
  long-axis fractional shortening
Laguna Negra virus
LAH
  left anterior hemiblock
laid-back
  l.-b. balloon occlusion aortography
  l.-b. view
laidlawii
  Acholeplasma l.
LAIS laser
laiteuse
  tache l.
lakes
  venous l.
LAM
  lymphangioleiomyomatosis
LAMA
  laser-assisted microanastomosis
LAMB
  lentigines, atrial myxoma, mucocutaneous
  myxomas, and blue nevi
  LAMB syndrome
Lambert
  L. aortic clamp
  L.-Beer law
  canal of L.
  L.-Eaton myasthenic syndrome
  L.-Kay aortic clamp
  L.-Kay clamp
lambertosis
Lambl excrescence
lamella
  elastic l.
lamifiban
lamina
  elastic l.
  l. elastica interna
  external elastic l. (EEL)
  internal elastic l. (IEL)
laminar blood flow
laminated
  l. clot
  l. connective tissue
  l. thrombus
laminin
  l. antibody
laminography
lamivudine
  zidovudine and l.
lamp
  Wood l.
Lamprene

Lam procedure
lamreotide
LAN
  local area network
Lanacaps
  Ferralyn L.
Lanaphilic topical
lanata
  Digitalis l.
lanatoside C
Lancisi sign
Landolfi sign
Landouzy-Dejerine
  L.-D. dystrophy
  facioscapulohumeral dystrophy
  of L.-D.
  L.-D. syndrome
Landry-Guillain-Barre syndrome
Landry Vein Light Venoscope
lanetoplase
Lange calipers
Langendorff
  L. apparatus
  L. heart preparation
Langer axillary arch
Langerhans
  L. cell granulomatosis
  L. cell histiocytosis
  L. giant cell
Langevin updating procedure
Langhans
  L. cell
  L.-type giant cell
Laniazid Oral
Lannelongue foramen
Lanophyllin-GG
lanoteplase
Lanoxicaps
Lanoxin
lansingensis
  Legionella l.
lanuginosum
  Stemphylium l.
Lanz low-pressure cuff endotracheal
  tube
LAO
  left anterior oblique
  LAO position
LAP
  laser-assisted palatoplasty
laparotomy sponge
Laplace
  L. law
  L. mechanism
  L. principle
  L. relationship
Laplacian mapping
lapping murmur

Lap Sac
LAR
    Sandostatin L.
Largactil
large
    l. cell carcinoma
    l. cell carcinoma with rhabdoid
      phenotype
    l. cell undifferentiated carcinoma
large-bore
    l.-b. angiocatheter
    l.-b. catheter
    l.-b. chest tube
    l.-b. slotted aspirating needle
    l.-b. trocar
large-caliber chest tube
large-tip electrode
large-vessel
    l.-v. disease
    l.-v. infarction (LVI)
large-volume aspiration
L-arginine
Lariam
Larmor frequency
Laron syndrome (LS)
Larrey
    L. hernia
    L. space
LARS
    Laser Angioplasty in Restenosed Stents
    LARS Clinical Trial
    LARS Retrospective USA Registry
Larus high-pressure rapid exchange
  balloon catheter
larva migrans
laryngalgia
laryngea
    angina l.
    arteria l.
    prominentia l.
    protuberantia l.
laryngeae
    glandulae l.
laryngeal
    l. aperture
    l. atresia
    l. bursa
    l. cleft
    l. cough reflex test (LCR)
    l. crisis
    l. gland
    l. infection

    l. mask airway (LMA)
    l. nerve
    l. part of pharynx
    l. pharynx
    l. pouch
    l. prominence
    l. rale
    l. reflex
    l. stridor
    l. syncope
    l. tonsil
    l. vein
    l. ventricle
    l. vertigo
    l. web
laryngectomee
laryngeus
    Syngamus l.
laryngis
    cartilago l.
    cartilago sesamoidea l.
    cavitas l.
    cavum l.
    corniculum l.
    phlebectasia l.
    sacculus l.
    tunica mucosa l.
    ventriculus l.
    vestibulum l.
laryngismus
    l. paralyticus
    l. stridulus
laryngitis
    atrophic l.
    catarrhal l.
    chronic catarrhal l.
    croupous l.
    diphtheritic l.
    membranous l.
    phlegmonous l.
    l. sicca
    l. stridulosa
    subglottic l.
    syphilitic l.
    tuberculous l.
    vestibular l.
Laryngoflex reinforced endotracheal
  tube
laryngomalacia
laryngopharynx
laryngoscope
    Benjamin binocular slimline l.

L

NOTES

laryngoscope *(continued)*
    Benjamin pediatric l.
    Bizzari-Guiffrida l.
    Broyles anterior commissure l.
    Bullard intubating l.
    Dedo-Pilling l.
    Foregger l.
    Garfield-Holinger l.
    Holinger anterior commissure l.
    Jako l.
    Kantor-Berci video l.
    Killian-Lynch l.
    Lindholm operating l.
    Machida fiberoptic l.
    MacIntosh l.
    Magill l.
    Ossoff-Karlan l.
    Sanders intubation l.
    shadow-free l.
    Shapshay-Healy l.
    Storz-Hopkins l.

laryngoscopy
    direct l.
    mirror-image l.
    suspension l.

laryngospasm

laryngotracheal
    l. diverticulum
    l. groove
    l. infection

laryngotracheitis

laryngotracheobronchitis

larynx
    artificial l.
    cartilages of l.
    cavity of l.
    Cooper-Rand intraoral artificial l.
    Nu-Vois artificial l.
    saccule of l.
    tuberculosis of l.
    ventricular band of l.
    vestibule of l.

LASAR
    Local Alcohol and Stent Against
    Restenosis
        LASAR Clinical Trial

LASEC
    left atrial spontaneous echo contrast

laser
    l. ablation
    alexandrite l.
    l. angioplasty
    L. Angioplasty for Critical
        Ischemia (LACI)
    L. Angioplasty in Restenosed
        Stents (LARS)
    ArF excimer l.
    argon ion l.

argon pumped tuneable dye l.
balloon-centered argon l.
l. bronchoscopy
cool-tip l.
coumarin pulsed dye l.
CVX-300 XeCl excimer l.
l. delivery catheter
l. Doppler flowmeter
dye l.
Eclipse holmium l.
Eclipse TMR l.
ELCA l.
erbium:YAG l.
excimer cool l.
excimer gas l.
l. fiber
l. firing
flashlamp-pulsed Nd:YAG l.
fluorescence-guided smart l.
free-beam l.
Heart L.
helium-cadmium diagnostic l.
HF infrared l.
high-energy l.
holmium l.
Ho:YAG l.
infrared-pulsed l.
LAIS l.
low-energy l.
Lumonics YAG l.
l. maze operation
MCM smart l.
microsecond pulsed flashlamp
    pumped dye l.
mid-infrared pulsed l.
Nd:YAG l.
neodymium:yttrium-aluminum-
    garnet l.
PhotoGenica V-Star l.
pulsed dye l.
Q-switched Nd:YAG l.
l. revascularization
rotational ablation l.
ruby l.
Spectranetics l.
spectroscopy-directed l.
Surgica K6 l.
Surgilase 150 l.
THC:YAG l.
l. thermal angioplasty
thulium-holmium-chromium:yttrium-
    aluminum-garnet l.
thulium-holmium:YAG l.
l. transmyocardial revascularization
    (TMR)
l. tube
tunable dye l.
tunable pulsed dye l.

ultraviolet l.
XeCl excimer l.
xenon chloride excimer l.
YAG l.
laser-assisted
l.-a. balloon angioplasty (LABA)
l.-a. microanastomosis (LAMA)
l.-a. palatoplasty (LAP)
l.-a. uvulopalatopharyngoplasty
l.-a. uvulopalatoplasty (LAUP)
laser-balloon angioplasty
Laserdish
L. electrode
L. pacing lead
laser-Doppler flowmetry
laser-induced
l.-i. arterial fluorescence (LIAF)
l.-i. thrombosis
Laserpor pacing lead
Laserprobe
L. catheter
L.-PLR Flex catheter
laserscope YAG/1064
LASH
left anterior superior hemiblock
Lasix
L. injection
L. Oral
L. Special
Lassa
L. fever
L. virus
LATE
Late Assessment of Thrombolytic
Efficacy
LATE Study
late
l. afterdepolarization
l. angioplasty complication
l. apical systolic murmur
l. apnea
l. arterial switch
L. Assessment of Thrombolytic
Efficacy (LATE)
l. cyanosis
l. death
l. deceleration
l. diastole
l. diastolic murmur
l. diastolic potential (LDP)
l. lung injury
l.-peaking systolic murmur

l. potential parameter
l. potential parameter index
l. proarrhythmic effect
l. progressing stroke (LPS)
l. pulmonary injury
l. reperfusion
l. silhouette
l. sudden death
l. systole
l. systolic murmur
latent
l. empyema
l. pleurisy
lateral
l. basal bronchopulmonary segment
[S IX]
l. basal segmental artery of right
lung
l. cephalometry
l. flail chest
l. frontal bone window (LFBW)
l. jugular lymph node
l. medullary infarction (LMI)
l. mesocardium
l. myocardial infarction
l. pharyngeal space
l. sac
l. thrombus
l. view
l. wall (LW)
lateralis
arteria genus superior l.
ramus anterior l.
laterality index (LI)
lateropharyngeum
spatium l.
laterosporus
Bacillus l.
latex balloon
lathyrogen
Lathyrus odoratus
latis dual-lumen graft-cleaning catheter
latissimus
l. dorsi
l. dorsi muscle
l. dorsi procedure
Latrodectus
Latson multipurpose catheter
Laubry-Soulle syndrome
laudanosine
LAUP
laser-assisted uvulopalatoplasty

L

NOTES

Laurell
    L. method
    rocket immunoelectrophoretic
      method of L.
Laurence-Moon-Bardet-Biedl syndrome
Laurence-Moon-Biedl syndrome
laurentii
    Cryptococcus l.
LAVA
    Los Angeles Veterans Administration
    Hospital
    LAVA Diet Trial
lavage
    bronchial l.
    bronchoalveolar l. (BAL)
    continuous pericardial l.
    diagnostic peritoneal l. (DPL)
    iced saline l.
    l. instillation
    pericardial l.
    pleural l.
    tracheobronchial l.
law
    all or none l.
    Beer L.
    Bowditch l.
    Boyle l.
    Boyle Gay-Lusac l.
    Charles l.
    Dalton l.
    Dalton-Henry l.
    Du Bois-Reymond l.
    Einthoven l.
    Frank-Starling l.
    Graham l.
    l. of the heart
    Henry l.
    Hooke l.
    Lambert-Beer L.
    Laplace l.
    Louis l.
    Marey l.
    Ohm l.
    Poiseuille l.
    Starling l.
    Sutton l.
    Torricelli l.
Lawton
    L. IADL
    L. Instrumental Activities of Daily
      Living scale
LAX
  long axis
laxa
    cutis l.
layer
    adventitial l.
    fascial l.

    half-value l.
    hypertrophic smooth muscle l.
    M cell l.
    mucous l.
    peribronchiolar l.
    subendocardial l.
lazaraoid
LBBB
    left bundle-branch block
LBD
    left brain damage
LBNP
    lower body negative pressure
LBT
    loaded breathing test
LC
    lymphangitic carcinomatosis
LC+
    Advantx LC+
LCA
    left coronary artery
LCAT
    lecithin-cholesterol acyltransferase
LCCA
    left common carotid artery
LCCE
    length contraction compensation element
LCD
    liquid crystal display
LCF
    left circumflex
    lymphocyte chemoattractant factor
    LCF coronary artery
LCL
    Levinthal-Coles-Lillie
    LCL bodies
LCR
    laryngeal cough reflex test
    ligase chain reaction
LCVA
    left hemisphere stroke
LCX
    left circumflex artery
    left circumflex coronary artery
LDD
    lead locking device
LDH
    lactic dehydrogenase
    LDH flip
LDL
    low-density lipoprotein
    LDL Apheresis Atherosclerosis
      Regression Study (LAARS)
    LDL direct blood test
    LDL direct test
    native LDL (n-LDL)
    oxidative modification of LDL
      (oxLDL, ox-LDL)

oxidized LDL
LDL pattern B
LDP
late diastolic potential
LE
lupus erythematosus
LEAD
lower extremity arterial disease
lead
3.3 l.
A 67 l.
ABC l.
Accufix II DEC pacing l.
Accufix pacemaker l.
active fixation l.
active fixation pacemaker l.
Aescula left ventricular l.
Aescula left ventricular IV l.
American Pacemaker Corporation l.
aVF l.
aVL l.
aVR l.
barbed epicardial pacing l.
barb-tip l.
bifurcated J-shaped tined atrial
  pacing and defibrillation l.
Biocontrol Technology/Coratomic l.
Biopore TM l.
Biotronik l.
bipolar l.
bipolar limb l.'s
Brilliant l.
Cadence TVL nonthoracotomy l.
capped l.
CapSure cardiac pacing l.
CapSure Fix l.
CapSure SP l.
CapSure VDD l.
Cardiac Control Systems l.
CB l.
CCS endocardial pacing l.
CF l.
chest l.
CL l.
Cordis Ancar pacing l.
coronary sinus l.
CPI endocardial defibrillation/rate-
  sensing/pacing l.
CPI Endotak SQ electrode l.
CPI/Guidant l.
CPI porous tined-tip bipolar
  pacing l.

CPI Sentra endocardial l.
CPI Sweet Tip l.
CR l.
Daig Corporation l.
Daig/Medcor l.
dedicated bipolar l.
direct l.
l. dislodgment
dual-coil transvenous l.
EASYTRAK coronary venous l.
Einthoven l.
Ela ventricular pacing l.
electrocardiographic l.'s
Elema l.'s
ELWRITE l.
ELWRITE pediatric l.
Encor l.
endocardial l.
endocardial balloon l.
endocardial bipolar l.
EndoLoc l.
Endotak C transvenous l.
Endotak C tripolar
  pacing/sensing/defibrillation l.
Endotak C tripolar transvenous l.
Endotak DSP l.
Endotak Picotip defibrillation l.
epicardial l.
esophageal l.
Fast-Pass endocardial l.
finned pacemaker l.
fishhook l.
floating l.
l. fracture
Frank XYZ orthogonal l.
Golub ECG l.
Heartwire l.
Hi-Flex l.
high-impedance, low-threshold l.
Hombach placement of l.'s
ICD l.
l. impedance
implantable cardioverter-
  defibrillator l.
indirect l.
l. insulation
Intermedics l.
intracardiac l.
Ionyx l.
isodiametric bipolar screw-in l.
JP l.
J-wire l.

L

NOTES

lead *(continued)*
    K 54 l.
    L 67 l.
    Laserdish pacing l.
    Laserpor pacing l.
    left ventricular transvenous l.
    Lewis l.
    Lifeline l.
    limb l.
    l. locking device (LDD)
    Low-Flex l.
    Mason-Likar placement of ECG l.
    Medtronic l.'s
    Medtronic Spring l.
    Microtip l.
    monitor l.'s
    MR l.
    myocardial l.
    Myopore l.
    Nehb D l.
    Nine-Turn l.
    nonintegrated transvenous
      defibrillation l.
    nonintegrated tripolar l.
    Oscor atrial l.
    Oscor pacing l.
    Osypka atrial l.
    over-the-wire pacing l.
    pacemaker l.'s
    Pacesetter l.
    Pacesetter AutoCapture l.
    Pacesetter/St. Jude l.
    Pacesetter Tendril DX steroid-
      eluting active-fixation pacing l.
    pediatric l.
    permanent cardiac pacing l.
    Permathane l.
    Pisces l.
    l. placement
    l. poisoning
    Polyflex l.
    Polyrox fractal active fixation l.
    PolySafe A-track l.
    Precept l.
    precordial l.
    l. reversal
    reversed arm l.'s
    scalar l.'s
    screw-in l.
    screw-on l.
    segmented ring tripolar l.
    semidirect l.
    silicone l.
    single-pass l.
    Sorin l.
    Spectraflex l.
    Sprint Model 6942
      tachyarrhythmia l.

    Sprint Model 6943
      tachyarrhythmia l.
    SRT l.
    standard limb l.
    Stela electrode l.
    steroid-eluting pacemaker l.
    Stop at Ring l.
    Stop at Tip l.
    SVC l.
    Sweet Tip l.
    Sweet Tip bipolar l.
    Synox fractal pacemaker l.
    l. system
    Target Tip l.
    Telectronics Accufix pacing l.
    temporary pervenous l.
    Tenax l.
    Tendril l.
    Tendril DX implantable pacing l.
    Tendril DX pacing l.
    Tendril DX steroid-eluting active-
      fixation pacing l.
    Tendril SDX pacing l.
    ThinLine l.
    ThinLine EZ bipolar cardiac
      pacing l.
    ThinLine EZ bipolar pacemaker l.
    ThinLine EZ pacing l.
    three-turn epicardial l.
    l. threshold
    TIJ l.
    transcutaneous l.
    Transvene-RV l.
    transvenous l.
    transvenous defibrillator l.
    tripolar l.
    two-turn epicardial l.
    Unipass endocardial pacing l.
    unipolar l.
    unipolar J-tined passive-fixation l.
    unipolar limb l.'s
    unipolar precordial l.
    Uni-Silicone l.
    V l.
    ventricular l.
    Vitatron l.
    V-Pace transluminal pacing l.
    V1/V6 l.'s
    Wilson l.

12-lead
    12-l. echocardiogram
    12-l. electrocardiogram
    12-l. electrocardiography
    12-l. voltage-duration product
      criteria
15-lead echocardiogram
3-lead electrocardiogram
6-lead electrocardiogram

16-lead electrocardiogram
leading
 l. circle concept
 l. circle hypothesis
 l. edge
 l. edge enhancement
lead-letter marker
lead/zirconium/titanium (LZT)
leaflet
 adherent l.
 anterior l.
 anterior mitral l. (AML)
 aortic valve l.
 bowing of mitral valve l.
 calcified mitral l.
 cleft anterior l.
 cleft of aortic l.
 C valvular l.
 doming of l.
 dysplastic mitral valvar l.
 flail l.
 hammocking of posterior mitral l.
 mitral l.
 mitral valve l.
 l. motion
 posterior l.
 prolapsed middle scallop of
  posterior l.
 prolapsing mitral valvar l.
 tethered l.
 l. thickening
 tricuspid valvular l.
 valvular l.
 l. vegetation
leak
 alveolar l.
 baffle l.
 paraprosthetic l.
 perivalvular l.
 shunt l.
 silent trace l.
leakage
 spectral l.
**Leaman classification of coronary
disease**
LEAP low-energy all-purpose collimator
Lebsche sternal knife
lecithin
**lecithin-cholesterol acyltransferase
(LCAT)**
lecithin/sphingomyelin (L/S)
Lecompte maneuver

LED
 light-emitting diode
LEDC
 low energy direct current
Ledercillin VK Oral
ledge
 eccentric l.
 limbic l.
Lee-White method
left
 l. anterior descending (LAD)
 l. anterior descending artery
  (LADA)
 l. anterior hemiblock (LAH)
 l. anterior oblique (LAO)
 l. anterior oblique position
 l. anterior oblique projection
 l. anterior superior hemiblock
  (LASH)
 l. aortic angiography
 l. apical cap
 apicoposterior branch of l.
 l. atrial abnormality
 l. atrial angiography
 l. atrial to aortic (La:A)
 l. atrial appendage (LAA)
 l. atrial appendage area
 l. atrial appendage flow velocity
 l. atrial appendage function
 l. atrial appendage stunning
 l. atrial diameter
 l. atrial dimension (LAD)
 l. atrial emptying index
 l. atrial enlargement (LAF)
 l. atrial hypertension
 l. atrial isolation procedure
 l. atrial myxoma
 l. atrial partitioning
 l. atrial pressure
 l. atrial spontaneous echo contrast
  (LASEC)
 l. atrium (LA)
 l. auricle of heart
 l. axis deviation (LAD)
 l. brain damage (LBD)
 l. bundle-branch block (LBBB)
 l. circumflex (LCF)
 l. circumflex artery (LCX)
 l. circumflex coronary artery
  (LCX)
 l. common carotid artery (LCCA)
 l. coronary artery (LCA)

NOTES

L

left (*continued*)

l. coronary artery of stomach
l. coronary catheter
l. crus of diaphragm
l. dominant coronary circulation
l. heart
l. heart bypass
l. heart catheter
l. heart catheterization
l. hemisphere damage (LHD)
l. hemisphere stroke (LCVA)
l. inferior pulmonary vein
l. internal jugular vein
l. internal mammary artery (LIMA)
l. internal mammary artery graft
l. internal thoracic artery (LITA)
l. internal thoracic artery graft
l. Judkins catheter
l. lateral projection
l. lower lobe
l. main bronchus
l. main coronary artery (LMCA)
l. main coronary artery disease
l. main coronary disease (LMC)
l. main coronary stenosis
l. main disease (LMD)
l. main equivalency
l. main stem coronary artery disease (LMS-CAD)
l. margin of heart
l. median vein
l. middle hemiblock
l. posterior hemiblock
l. posterior inferior hemiblock (LPIH)
l. pulmonary artery (LPA)
l. recurrent laryngeal nerve
l. septal hemiblock
l. stellate ganglion
l. stellate ganglionic blockade (LSGB)
l. subclavian artery (LSCA)
l. superior pulmonary vein
l. upper lobe (LUL)
l. ventricle (LV)
l. ventricular aneurysm
l. ventricular angiography
l. ventricular apex
l. ventricular assist device (LVAD)
l. ventricular assist system (LVAS)
l. ventricular assist system implantable pump
l. ventricular bypass pump
l. ventricular cavity dilation
l. ventricular cavity obstruction ring
l. ventricular chamber compliance
l. ventricular contractility

l. ventricular diastolic phase index
l. ventricular diastolic pressure
l. ventricular diastolic relaxation
l. ventricular dysfunction (LVD)
l. ventricular dyskinesis
l. ventricular ejection fraction (LVEF)
l. ventricular ejection time (LVET)
l. ventricular end-diastolic dimension (LVEDD)
l. ventricular end-diastolic pressure (LVEDP)
l. ventricular end-diastolic volume (LVEDV)
l. ventricular end-systolic dimension (LVESD)
l. ventricular end-systolic stress
l. ventricular epicardium
l. ventricular failure
l. ventricular filling pressure
l. ventricular force
l. ventricular function
l. ventricular geometry
l. ventricular hypertrophy (LVH)
l. ventricular inflow tract obstruction
l. ventricular internal diastolic diameter (LVIDD)
l. ventricular internal diastolic dimension (LVIDD)
l. ventricular-left atrial crossover dynamics
l. ventricular mass
l. ventricular mass index
l. ventricular muscle compliance
l. ventricular myxoma
l. ventricular outflow tract (LVOT)
l. ventricular outflow tract obstruction (LVOTO)
l. ventricular outflow tract velocity
l. ventricular output
l. ventricular power
l. ventricular pressure-volume curve
l. ventricular puncture
l. ventricular reduction (LVR)
l. ventricular relaxation
l. ventricular-right atrial communication murmur
l. ventricular stroke volume
l. ventricular stroke volume index (LVSVI)
l. ventricular stroke work index (LVSWI)
l. ventricular sump catheter
l. ventricular systolic/diastolic function
l. ventricular systolic dimension (LVSD)

l. ventricular systolic dysfunction
l. ventricular systolic performance
l. ventricular systolic pressure
l. ventricular tension
l. ventricular transvenous lead
l. ventricular unloading
l. ventricular wall
l. ventricular wall motion abnormality
l. ventricular wall stress
l. ventriculography
left-heart contour
left-sided
l.-s. heart failure
l.-s. innominate trunk
left-to-right shunt
leftward ventricular septal bowing (LVSB)
Legend pacemaker
Legionella
L. anisa
L. birminghamensis
L. bozemanii
L. cincinnatiensis
L. dumoffii
L. feeleii
L. gormanii
L. jordanis
L. lansingensis
L. longbeachae
L. micdadei
L. oakridgensis
L. pneumonia
L. pneumoniae
L. pneumophila
L. wadsworthii
legionellosis
Legionnaire
L. disease
L. pneumonia
Legroux remission
Lehman
L. cardiac device
L. device
L. ventriculography catheter
leiomyoma, pl. **leiomyomata**
leiomyosarcoma
Leiras metered-dose powder inhaler
Leishmania
leishmaniasis
Leitner syndrome
Lell esophagoscope

lemakalim
Lemierre
L. disease
L. syndrome
Lemmon sternal elevator
LemonPrep electrode lotion
lemon squeezer
Lenègre
L. disease
L. syndrome
length
antegrade block cycle l.
atrial fibrillation cycle l. (AFCL)
atrial-paced cycle l.
basic cycle l. (BCL)
basic drive cycle l.
block cycle l.
chordal l.
l. contraction compensation element (LCCE)
cycle l. (CL)
drive cycle l.
flutter cycle l.
lesion l. (LL)
paced cycle l.
pacing cycle l.
sinus cycle l.
l. of stay (LOS)
tachycardia cycle l.
ventricular tachycardia cycle l. (VTCL)
Wenckebach cycle l.
length-active tension curve
length-dependent activation
length-resting tension relation
length-tension
l.-t. curve (LT)
l.-t. relation
LENI
lower extremity noninvasive
Lennarson tube
Lennert lymphoma
lensed fiber-tip laser delivery catheter
lenta
endocarditis l.
Lente
L. Iletin
L. Iletin I, II, L insulin
L. insulin
lenticulostriate artery
lentiginosis
lentigo, pl. **lentigines**

L

NOTES

lentigo *(continued)*
 lentigines, atrial myxoma,
  mucocutaneous myxomas, and
  blue nevi (LAMB)
 lentigines, electrocardiographic
  abnormalities, ocular hypertelorism,
  pulmonary stenosis, abnormalities
  of genitalia, retardation of
  growth, and deafness (LEOPARD)
lentis
 ectopia l.
Lenz syndrome
Leocor hemoperfusion system
LEOPARD
 lentigines, electrocardiographic
  abnormalities, ocular hypertelorism,
  pulmonary stenosis, abnormalities of
  genitalia, retardation of growth, and
  deafness
  LEOPARD syndrome
lepirudin
 l. rDNA
 l. rDNA injection
Lepley-Ernst tracheal tube
leprae
 Mycobacterium l.
lepromin test
leptin
leptospiral pneumonia
leptospirosis
Leptotrichia buccalis
lercapidipine
Leredde syndrome
Leriche syndrome
Lerman-Means scratch
Lescol XL
lesion
 aorto-ostial l.
 bifurcation l. (BL)
 bifurcational coronary l.
 bird's nest l.
 Blumenthal l.
 Bracht-Wächter l.
 braid-like l.
 branch l.
 calcified l.
 cavitary l.
 coin l.
 complex l.
 connective tissue l.
 continuous full-thickness linear l.
 coronary artery l.
 cryoablation l.
 culprit l.
 cystic l.
 deep white matter l. (DWML)
 dendritic l.
 de novo coronary l.

dilatable l.
discrete coronary l.
dottering of l.
eccentric l.
enhancing l.
epicardial radiofrequency atrial l.
fibrocalcific l.
fibromusculoelastic l.
fibrous cap l.
full-thickness linear l.
Ghon primary l.
hazy l.
head, neck, or shaft l.
HNS l.
honeycomb l.
index l.
irregular discrete l.
JA l.
Janeway l.
jet l.
juxtaarticular l.
l. length (LL)
Libman-Sacks l.
linear l.
Lohlein-Baehr l.
long l.
macrovascular coronary l.
monotypic l.
mucocutaneous l.
multifocal l.
nonbacterial thrombotic
 endocardial l.
onion scale l.
ostial l.
parenchymal l.
plexiform l.
polypoidal l.
pulmonary coin l.
punctate mucosal l.
restenosis l.
satellite l.
smooth l.
space-occupying l.
spot l.
stenotic l.
synchronous airway l.'s
tandem l.
target l.
type Va l.
type Vb l.
type Vc l.
ulcerated l.
vegetative l.
wear-and-tear l.
wire-loop l.
lesser
 l. circulation
 l. resection

lethal arrhythmia
letrozole
Letterer-Siwe disease
leucine
leucovorin
Leudet
    bruit de L.
leukemia
    acute lymphocytic l. (ALL)
    acute myelocytic l. (AML)
leukemic cell lysis pneumopathy
Leukeran
leukoaraiosis
    ischemic l.
leukocidin
leukocyte
    l. elastase
    polymorphonuclear l. (PMN)
leukocyte-endothelial
    l.-e. cell adhesion cascade
    l.-e. cell adhesion molecule
    l.-e. cell interaction
leukocytoblastic vasculitis
leukocytoclastic angiitis
leukocytosis
    transient l.
leukoencephalopathy
    cerebral autosomal dominant
      arteriopathy with subcortical
      infarct and l. (CADASIL)
    l. disease
    progressive multifocal l. (PML)
LeukoNet Filter
Leukos pacemaker
leukostasis
    pulmonary l.
Leukotrap red cell storage system
leukotriene
    l. A_4
    l. antagonist
    l. B4 (LTB4)
    l. biosynthesis
    l. C
    l. C_4
    cysteinyl l. (cys-LT)
    l. D_4
    l. E
    l. E_4
    l. inhibition
    l. inhibitor
    l. modifier
leumedin

leuprolide acetate
Leutrol
Lev
    L. classification
    L. disease
    L. syndrome
levalbuterol
    l. HCl
    l. HCl inhalation solution
levamisole hydrochloride
Levaquin
Levatol
levator muscle of thyroid gland
LeVeen
    L. peritoneovenous shunt
    L. plaque-cracker
level
    air-fluid l.
    beta-thromboglobulin l.
    blood oxygen l.
    dig l.
    digoxin l.
    ELF l.'s
    malondialdehyde l.
    multiple shunt l.'s
    myofibrillar calcium l.
    peak and trough l.'s
    plasma nicotine l.
    predose l.
    reflecting l.
    renin l.
    sarcolemmal l.
    serum renin l.
    total homocysteine l. (tHcy)
    triglyceride l.
    trough l.
    trough and peak l.'s
level-dependent
    blood oxygenation l.-d. (BOLD)
Levenberg-Marquardt algorithm
Levin catheter
Levine
    L. grade 1–6 cardiac murmur
    L.-Harvey classification
    L. sign
Levinson-Durbin recursion
Levinthal-Coles-Lillie (LCL)
levoatriocardinal vein
levocardia
    l. malposition
    mixed l.
    l. with situs inversus

L

NOTES

levocardiogram
levodopa
Levo-Dromoran
levofloxacin
levogram
levoisomer
levoisomerism
Levophed injection
levorphanol
levosimendan
Levo-T
Levothroid
levothyroxine
levotransposed position
levotransposition
levoversion
Levovist contrast
Levoxyl
Levy Chimeric Faces Test
Lewis
    L. index
    L. lead
    L. lines
    L.-Pickering test
    P substance of L.
    L.-Tanner procedure
    L. thoracotomy
    L. upper limb cardiovascular
      disease
Lewy chest holder
Lewy-Rubin needle
Lexxel 5-2.5
Leycom volume conductance catheter
Leyden crystal
LFB
    low-flow cardiopulmonary bypass
LFBW
    lateral frontal bone window
LFCT
    lung-to-finger circulation time
LFT
    liver function test
LGV
    lymphogranuloma venereum
LHD
    left hemisphere damage
LHMT
    low-range heparin management test
LI
    lacunar infarction
    laterality index
LIAF
    laser-induced arterial fluorescence
Libman-Sacks
    L.-S. disease
    L.-S. endocarditis
    L.-S. lesion
    L.-S. syndrome

library
    Cochrane L.
    human cosmid l.
licheniformis
    Bacillus l.
lichenoides
    tuberculosis l.
licorice
    Chinese l.
Liddle
    L. aorta clamp
    L. syndrome
lidocaine hydrochloride
Lidodan
lidoflazine
LidoPen I.M. Injection Auto-Injector
Liebermann-Burchard test
Liebermeister
    L. rule
    L. sign
Liebow
    L. classification
    usual interstitial pneumonia of L.
lienis
    porta l.
lifarizine
LIFE
    lung imaging fluorescence endoscope
life
    L. Care Pump
    l. change unit
    l. force
    health-related quality of l. (HRQL,
      HRQOL)
    quality of l.
    stroke-specific quality of l. (SS-
      QOL)
    Study of Economics and Quality
      of L. (SEQOL)
    L. Suit
Lifecare ventilator
lifeguard lung
Lifeline
    L. electrode
    L. lead
Life-Pack 5 cardiac monitor
Lifepak
    L. defibrillator
    L. 5 monitor/defibrillator
    L. 7 monitor/defibrillator
Lifepath AAA endovascular graft
system
LifePort endotracheal tube holder
Lifesaver disposable resuscitator bag
Lifescan
LifeShirt monitor
LifeStick
    L. cardiopulmonary resuscitation

L. CPR device
L. resuscitation device

Lifestream coronary dilation catheter
lifestyle
sedentary l.
life-support
life-years
quality-adjusted l.-y. (QALY)
lift
parasternal systolic l.
tongue-jaw l.
ligament
Cooper l.
costoclavicular l.
Marshall l.
pericardiosternal l.
pulmonary l.
Teutleben l.
ventricular l.
vestibular l.
ligamentum, pl. **ligamenta**
ligamenta anularia trachealia
l. arteriosum
l. hepatoesophageum
l. latum pulmonis
l. phrenicocolicum
l. pulmonale
l. teres cardiopexy
ligand
l. binding
Fas l. (FasL)
macromolecular l.
l. plus 1, 2, 3
ligase chain reaction (LCR)
ligation
Bardenheurer l.
l. clip
Linton radical vein l.
thoracic duct l.
variceal l.
varicose vein stripping and l.
ligature
Stannius l.
light
L. chain
L. criteria
L.-emitting diode (LED)
L. microscopy
L. pen
L. pen-determined ejection fraction
Questran L.

L. stroke
L. Talker device
Lightweight and portable Sullivan nasal CPAP
lightwire
lignan
Lignieres test
lignocaine
M l.
LiI
lithium iodine
LiI battery
Likert
L. 5-point scale
L. scale (LS)
Lilienthal-Sauerbruch
L.-S. retractor
L.-S. rib spreader
Lillehei-Kaster
L.-K. cardiac valve prosthesis
L.-K. mitral valve prosthesis
L.-K. pivoting-disk prosthetic valve
Lillehei pacemaker
Lilliput oxygenator
LIMA
left internal mammary artery
LIMA graft
LIMA-Lift
L.-L. tool
LIMA-Loop
L.-L. tool
limb
anacrotic l.
l. blood flow
claudicant l.
insipiratory l.
l. ischemia
l. lead
l. salvage
thoracic l.
limb-girdle
l.-g. dystrophy of Erb
l.-g. muscular dystrophy
limbic ledge
limb-kinetic apraxia
lime
bruit de l.
limit
Nyquist l.
limitation
airflow l.

L

NOTES

limitation *(continued)*
    chronic airflow l. (CAL)
    flow l. (FL)
limited
    l. Doppler examination
    l. ventricular reserve
LIMITS
    Liquaemin in Myocardial Infarction
    during Thrombolysis with Saruplase
    LIMITS Clinical Trial
limonite pneumoconiosis
Lincocin
    L. injection
    L. Oral
lincomycin hydrochloride
Lincorex injection
lincosamide
Linctus
    L. Codeine Blac
    L. With Codeine phosphate
Lindbergh pump
Lindesmith operation
Linde Walker Oxygen Program
Lindholm
    L. operating laryngoscope
    L. tracheal tube
line
    anterior axillary l. (AAL)
    anterior junction l.
    arterial l. (A-line)
    arterial mean l.
    Beau l.'s
    Cantlie l.
    central venous l.
    Commander PTCA wire l.
    Conradi l.
    Correra l.
    costophrenic septal l.
    CVP l.
    Fleischner l.
    indwelling l.
    Intertech Perkin-Elmer gas
      sampling l.
    intralobular l.
    isoelectric l.
    isthmus l.
    Kerley A, B, C l.'s
    Lewis l.'s
    Linton l.
    M l.'s
    midaxillary l.
    midclavicular l. (MCL)
    paraspinal l.
    pleural l.
    pleuroesophageal l.
    posterior junction l.
    l. sepsis
    septal l.

    tram l.
    Z l.
    Zahn l.'s
    zero velocity l.
linear
    l. ablation
    l. echo
    l. echodensity
    l. infiltrate
    L. KGT tonometer
    l. lesion
    l. local shortening map
    l. phonocardiograph
    l. stenosis
linearity
    amplitude l.
    count-rate l.
**linear-phased radiofrequency catheter
ablation**
linezolid
lingoscope
**Lingraphica system treatment
technology**
linguae
    corpus l.
    dorsum l.
    radix l.
    raphe l.
    septum l.
    tunica mucosa l.
    venae dorsales l.
    vena profunda l.
    vinculum l.
lingual
    l. bone
    l. branch
    l. branch of facial nerve
    l. plexus
    l. quinsy
    l. thyroid
    l. tonsil
    l. vein
lingualis
    arteria l.
    plexus periarterialis arteriae l.
    rami isthmi faucium nervi l.
    tonsilla l.
lingula
    l. of left lung
    l. pulmonis sinistri
lingulaplasty
lingular
    l. bronchus
    l. pneumonia
lingularis
    vena l.
linoleic acid
linsidomine

Linton
L. elastic stockings
L. flap
L. line
L. radical vein ligation
L. vein stripper

Linx
L. exchange guidewire
L. extension guidewire
L. extension wire
L.-EZ cardiac device
L. guidewire extension
L. guidewire extension cardiac device

liothyronine
liotrix
Liotta
L.-BioImplant low profile bioprosthesis prosthetic valve
L. total artificial heart

LIP
lymphocytic interstitial pneumonitis
lymphoid interstitial pneumonitis

lipase
diacylglycerol l.
hepatic l.
hepatic lipoprotein l.
lipoprotein l. (LPL)

lipedema
lipemia
postprandial l. (PPL)

LIPID
Long-Term Intervention with Pravastatin in Ischemic Disease
lipid-A
LIPID Study

lipid
l. accumulation
l. core
l. core density
endogenous l.
exogenous l.
extracellular l.
l. hypothesis
intracellular l.
l. panel
l. peroxidation product
l. peroxide
l. pneumonia
renomedullary l.
l. risk factor
sarcolemma l.

l. solubility
l. triad

Lipidil
lipid-induced lung injury
lipid-laden
l.-l. macrophage
l.-l. macrophage index
l.-l. macrophage semiquantitation

lipid-lowering
l.-l. agent
l.-l. therapy

lipidosis, pl. **lipidoses**
lipid-rich plaque
Lipitor
lipoarabinomannan
lipocardiac
lipodystrophy
intestinal l.

lipofuscinosis
neuronal ceroid l.

lipogenic theory of atherosclerosis
lipohyalinosis
lipoides
arcus l.

lipoid pneumonia
lipolysis
lipoma, pl. **lipomata**
lipomatous hypertrophy
lipoparticle
lipoperoxide
lipophilic drug
lipophilicity
properties of l.

lipopolysaccharidase
J5 l.

lipopolysaccharide
l.-induced thrombocytopenia
l. vaccine

lipoprotein
alpha l.
beta l.
high-density l. (HDL)
intermediate-density l. (IDL)
isolated low high-density l. (ILHDL)
l. lipase (LPL)
low-density l. (LDL)
malondialdehyde modified low-density l. (MDA-LDL)
pre-beta l.
remnant l. (RLP)
remnant-like particle l.

NOTES

L

lipoprotein *(continued)*
 RLP l.
 small low-density l.
 triglyceride-rich l. (TRL)
 very-low-density l. (VLDL)
lipoprotein(a) (Lp(a))
lipoprotein-associated coagulation inhibitor (LACI)
lipoproteinemia
liposarcoma
liposomal
 amphotericin B (liposomal)
Liposorber LA-15 system
Liposyn
lipothymia
Lipovnik virus
lipoxygenase
 5-l.
 l. pathway
LIP/PLH complex
lip pursing
Liprostin
Liquaemin
 L. injection
 L. in Myocardial Infarction during
 Thrombolysis with Saruplase
 (LIMITS)
liquefaciens
 Serratia l.
liquefaction necrosis
Liquibid
Liqui-Caps
 Vicks 44 Non-Drowsy Cold &
 Cough L.-C.
liquid
 Anaplex l.
 Brontex L.
 Chlorafed l.
 Contac Cough Formula L.
 l. crystal display (LCD)
 Detussin l.
 Entuss-D l.
 Hayfebrol l.
 Histussin D l.
 Hycotuss Expectorant L.
 Naldecon DX Adult l.
 oxygen-carrying perfluorochemical l.
 L. Pred
 L. Pred Oral
 Rhinosyn l.
 Rhinosyn-PD l.
 Rhinosyn-X l.
 Ryna l.
 Ryna-C l.
 l. scintillation spectrophotometer
 Tyrodone l.
 ULR L.
liquifying expectorant

Liqui-Gels
 Alka-Seltzer Plus Flu & Body
 Aches Non-Drowsy L.-G.
 Robitussin Severe Congestion L.-G.
LiquiVent
LIS
 lung injury score
lisinopril and hydrochlorothiazide
Lissajou loop
Listeria monocytogenes
list mode
LITA
 left internal thoracic artery
 LITA graft
Lite Blade
Liteguard minidefibrillator
liter
 millimoles per l. (mmol/L)
 l. per minute (Lpm)
 l.'s per minute per meter squared
 (Lpm/m^2)
lithium
 l. battery
 l. hydride
 l. iodine (LiI)
 l. iodine battery
 l. pacemaker
 l. powered pacemaker
lithomyxoma
 cardiac l.
Litten
 L. diaphragm sign
 L. phenomenon
Little disease
Littleford/Spector introducer
Littman
 L. class II pediatric stethoscope
 L. defibrillation pad
Litwak left atrial-aortic bypass
livedo
 l. reticularis
 l. vasculitis
livedoid dermatitis
liver
 cardiac l.
 cirrhosis of l.
 l. flap
 l. function test (LFT)
 l. palm
 right triangular ligament of l.
Livewire TC ablation catheter
livida
 asphyxia l.
Livierato
 L. reflex
 L. sign
 L. test

living
    activities of daily l. (ADL)
    impairment of activities of daily l. (IADL)
    instrumental activities of daily l. (IADL)
    l. related transplant (LRT)
    L. with Heart Failure
LIZ-88 ablation unit
LL
    lesion length
L-looping of the ventricle
LMA
    laryngeal mask airway
LMA-Unique
LMC
    left main coronary disease
LMCA
    left main coronary artery
LMD
    left main disease
    low molecular weight dextran
LMI
    lateral medullary infarction
LMS-CAD
    left main stem coronary artery disease
LMWH
    low molecular weight heparin
L-NAME
    N^G-nitro-L-arginine methyl ester
L-NMMA
    N^G-monomethyl-L-arginine
load
    chronic volume l.
    elastic l.
    electronic pacemaker l.
    exercise l.
    heat l.
    inelastic l.
    inspiratory threshold l. (ITL)
    L. model WLP-450 electromagnetically braked cycle ergometer
    whole-body amyloid l.
loaded breathing test (LBT)
loading
    bretylium l.
    discontinuous incremental threshold l.
    glycogen l.
    incremental threshold l.
    inspiratory l.

    methionine l.
    relaxation l.
    saline l.
    volume l.
lobar
    l. atelectasis
    l. bronchus
    l. collapse
    l. emphysema
    l. infiltrate
    l. pneumonia
lobares
    bronchi l.
lobe
    inferior frontal l. (IFL)
    inferior parietal/superior temporal l. (IPSTL)
    left lower l.
    left upper l. (LUL)
    right lower l. (RLL)
    right middle l. (RML)
    right upper l. (RUL)
    side l.
lobectomize
lobectomy
    sleeve l.
    video-assisted thoracic surgical non-rib-spreading l. (VNSSL)
lobeline sulfate
lobular
    l. consolidation
    l. hematoma
    l. pneumonia
lobule
    pulmonary l.
    secondary pulmonary l.
    superior parietal l. (SPL)
lobus
    l. azygos pulmonis dextri
    l. dexter
    l. medius pulmonis dextri
LOC
    LOC guidewire extension
local
    L. Alcohol and Stent Against Restenosis (LASAR)
    l. area network (LAN)
    l. asphyxia
    l. organ procurement area
    l. reaction
    l. syncope
LocaLisa technique

L

NOTES

localization
  anatomic l.
localized
  l. obstructive emphysema
  l. pericarditis
  l. sacculation
LocalMed
  L. catheter infusion sleeve
  L. InfusaSleeve
Lochol
LoCholest
loci (*pl. of* locus)
lock
  L. Clamshell device
  heparin l.
locking
  l. device
  l. stylet
LOCM
  low osmolality contrast material
  low osmolality contrast media
locular cyst
loculated
  l. cyst
  l. effusion
  l. emphysema
  l. empyema
loculation
locus, pl. **loci**
  l. ceruleus
  chymase gene l.
  genetic l.
  quantitative trait l. (QTL)
lodaxamide
Lode BV Excalibur braked cycle
  ergometer
Loeffler bacillus
Loesche classification
lofexidine
Löffler
  L. disease
  L. endocardial fibrosis
  L. endocarditis
  L. parietal fibroplastic endocarditis
  L. pneumonia
  L. syndrome
Löfgren syndrome
Lo-Fold balloon
logarithmic
  l. dynamic range
  l. phonocardiograph
Lohlein-Baehr lesion
Lombardi sign
lomefloxacin hydrochloride
lomustine
London
  L. School of Hygiene
  Cardiovascular Rose Questionnaire

  L. School of Hygiene and Tropical
  medicine sphygmomanometer
lone atrial fibrillation
long
  l. ACE fixed-wire balloon catheter
  l. axial oblique view
  l. axis (LAX)
  L. Bare Stent Registry
  L. Brite Tip guiding catheter
  l. dissection
  l. iliac artery occlusion
  l. lesion
  L. over-the-wire balloon catheter
  l. PP interval
  l. pulse
  l. QT syndrome (LQTS)
  l. Q-TU syndrome
  L. surpass 30 PTCA perfusion
  catheter
  l. taper/stiff shaft Glidewire
Long-Acting
  Sinex L.-A.
long-acting nitrate
long-axis
  l.-a. fractional shortening (LAFS)
  l.-a. parasternal view
  echocardiogram
  l.-a. shortening velocity
  l.-a. view
longbeachae
  Legionella l.
Longdwel Teflon catheter
long-echo-train-length fast-spin-echo
  imaging, long-ETL FSE imaging
longitudinal
  l. analysis
  l. arteriography
  l. dissociation
  l. midline incision
  l. narrowing
  l. relaxation time
long-leg venography technique
Longmire valvotomy
long-term
  l.-t. care (LTC)
  l.-t. care facility
  L.-t. Intervention with Pravastatin
  in Ischemic Disease (LIPID)
  l.-t. oxygen therapy (LTOT)
long-time recording
LONG WRIST
  Washington Radiation for In-Stent
  Restenosis Trial for Long Lesions
Loniten Oral
loop
  atrial vector l.
  bulboventricular l.
  Cannon endarterectomy l.

cine l.
clockwise l.
cortico-pallido-nigra-thalamo
  cortical l.
corticostriatocerebellar l.
D l.
l. diuresis
l. diuretic
elliptical l.
exercise tidal flow-volume l.
  (ETFVL)
flow volume l.
Gerdy intraauricular l.
guidewire l.
heart l.
Henle l.
L l.
Lissajou l.
maximum flow-volume l. (MFVL)
maxi-vessel l.'s
memory l.
l. monitor
P l.
peratriotomy l.
peritricuspid l.
pressure-volume l.
QRS l.
reentrant l.
rigid monopolar l.
sewing ring l.
T l.
tidal l.
tidal flow-volume l. (TFVL)
U l.
Uresil radiopaque silicone band
  vessel l.'s
U-shaped catheter l.
vector l.
ventricular pressure-volume l.
video l.
loose junction
Lopid
Lopressor
Lo-Profile II catheter
Lo-Pro tracheal tube
Lorabid
loracarbef
loratadine
lorazepam
lorcainide
Lorcet Plus
Lore-Lawrence trachea tube

Lorelco
Lortat-Jacob approach
LOS
  length of stay
**Los Angeles Veterans Administration
  Hospital (LAVA)**
losartan
  l. and hydrochlorothiazide
  Optimal Therapy in Myocardial
    Infarction with the Angiotensin II
    Antagonist L. (OPTIMAAL)
  Optimal Trial in Myocardial
    Infarction with the Angiotensin II
    Antagonist L. (OPTIMAAL)
  l. potassium
  l. potassium HCl
  l. potassium hydrochlorothiazide
loss
  l. of capture
  l. of consciousness
  signal l.
  volume l.
lossy
Lotensin HCT
lotion
  LemonPrep electrode l.
lotrafiban
Lotrel
Louis
  L. angle
  L. law
Louisiana pneumonia
loupe magnification
lovastatin
  Expanded Clinical Evaluation of L.
    (EXCEL)
Lovenox injection
Loven reflex
loversol
low
  l. cardiac output syndrome
  l. energy direct current (LEDC)
  l. flow rate
  l. molecular weight dextran (LMD)
  l. molecular weight heparin
    (LMWH)
  l. osmolality contrast material
    (LOCM)
  l. osmolality contrast media
    (LOCM)
  l.-output failure
  l.-output heart failure

NOTES

low *(continued)*
    L. Profile Port vascular access
    l. septal atrium
low-chloride St. Thomas solution
low-density lipoprotein (LDL)
low-dose
    l.-d. bile-acid sequestrant
    l.-d. dobutamine cine MRI
Lowell pleural needle
Löwenberg cuff sign
low-energy
    l.-e. intracardiac cardioversion
    l.-e. laser
    l.-e. synchronized cardioversion
lower
    l. airway
    l. body negative pressure (LBNP)
    l. extremity arterial disease (LEAD)
    l. extremity bypass graft
    l. extremity noninvasive (LENI)
    l. lobe bronchus
    l. lobe of lung
    l. nodal extrasystole
    l. nodal rhythm
    l. respiratory tract
    l. respiratory tract smear
    l. ribs
    L. rings
    L.-Shumway cardiac transplant
lowering
    antihypertensive and lipid l. (ALL)
low-esophageal pH probe
low-fat diet
Low-Flex lead
low-flow
    l.-f. cardiopulmonary bypass (LFB)
    l.-f. ischemia
low-frequency murmur
low-methionine diet
low-molecular-weight
Lown
    L. arrhythmia
    L. class 4a or 4b ventricular ectopic beat
    L. classification
    L.-Edmark waveform
    L.-Gagong-Levine syndrome
    L. grading system
    L. technique
    L. and Woolf method
low-pass filter
low-pitched murmur
low-plaque coarctation
low-pressure tamponade
low-prime circuitry

low-profile
    l.-p. balloon-positioning catheter
    l.-p., semi-compliant balloon
low-ramp protocol
low-range heparin management test (LHMT)
low-reflow phenomenon
low-salt
    l.-s. diet
    l.-s. syndrome
low-sodium
    l.-s. diet
    l.-s. syndrome
low-speed rotation angioplasty catheter
low-viscosity mucus
lozenge
    horehound l.
Lozide
Lozol
LP
    lung perfusion
    LP stent
LPA
    left pulmonary artery
Lp(a)
    lipoprotein(a)
L-phenylalinine mustard
LPIH
    left posterior inferior hemiblock
LPL
    lipoprotein lipase
Lpm
    liter per minute
Lpm/m^2
    liters per minute per meter squared
LPS
    late progressing stroke
    LPS Peel-Away introducer
LQTS
    long QT syndrome
    LQTS Study
LRT
    living related transplant
LS
    Laron syndrome
    Likert scale
L/S
    lecithin/sphingomyelin
    L/S ratio
LSCA
    left subclavian artery
L-selectin
LSGB
    left stellate ganglionic blockade
LT
    length-tension curve
    lung transplant

LT V-105 implantable cardioverter-defibrillator

LTB4
  leukotriene B4
LTC
  long-term care
    LTC facility
LTOT
  long-term oxygen therapy
LTx
  lung transplant
LTX PTCA catheter
L-type calcium blocker
lubeluzole
lubricity
Lucas-Championnière disease
Lucchese mitral valve dilator
lucency
lucent defect
Luciani-Wenckebach atrioventricular block
luciferase reporter phages
lucigenin
Ludiomil
Ludwig
  L. angina
  L. angle
Luer-Lok
  L.-L. connector
  L.-L. needle
  L.-L. needle tip
  L.-L. port
Luer tracheal tube
lues
luetic
  l. aneurysm
  l. aortitis
  l. disease
Lufyllin
Lugol solution
Lukens thymus retractor
Luke procedure
LUL
  left upper lobe
Lumaguide catheter
lumbar
  l. part of diaphragm
  l. sympathectomy
lumbricoides
  Ascaris l.
Lumelec pacing catheter
lumen, pl. **lumina**

airway l.
aortic l.
l. of artery
bronchial l.
conduit l.
double l. (DL)
esophageal l.
false l.
l. finder
plaque l.
single l.
vessel l.
Luminal
luminal
  l. diameter
  l. encroachment
  l. narrowing
  l. recoil
  l. widening
luminescence
luminogram
luminology
  coronary l.
Lumonics YAG laser
lunata
  Curvularia l.
lung
  l. abscess
  l. acinus
  aerated l.
  AIDS-related lymphoma of the l. (ARLL)
  air-conditioner l.
  aluminum l.
  anterior border of l.
  anterior descending segmental artery of right l.
  apex of l.
  l. architecture
  artificial l.
  atrium of l.
  azygos lobe of right l.
  base of l.
  Bible printer's l.
  l. biopsy
  bird-breeder's l.
  bird-fancier's l.
  black l.
  blast l.
  brown induration of l.
  l. bud
  l. capacity

L

NOTES

lung *(continued)*
l. carcinoma
cardiac l.
cardiac impression on l.
cardiac notch of left l.
cheese worker's l.
coal miner's l.
coin lesion of l.
collapsed l.
collier's l.
l. compliance
consolidation of l.
l. contusion
costal surface of l.
cystic disease of l.
decortication of l.
detergent worker's l.
l. diffusion
drowned l.
dynamic compliance of l.
l. dysfunction
edema of l.
l. edema
l. elasticity
l. elastic recoil
l. elastic recoil pressure (Pel)
end-stage l.
l. entrapment
eosinophilic l.
esophageal l.
essential brown induration of l.
farmer's l.
l. fever
fibrocystic l.
fibroid l.
l. fibrosis
fish meal l.
fissure of l.
flock-worker's l.
l. fluke
l. function
furrier's l.
gastric l.
harvester's l.
hilum of l.
honeycomb l.
honeycombing of l.
horseshoe l.
humidifier l.
hyperlucent l.
l. imaging fluorescence endoscope (LIFE)
inferior border of l.
inferior lobe of left/right l.
infundibulum of l.
l. injury
l. injury score (LIS)
interlobar surface of l.

l. interstitium
iron l.
jute worker's l.
Labrador l.
lateral basal segmental artery of right l.
lifeguard l.
lingula of left l.
lower lobe of l.
malt worker's l.
l. marking
mason's l.
l. mass
l. mechanics
medial surface of l.
mediastinal part of l.
mesentery of l.
middle lobe of right l.
miller's l.
miner's l.
mold worker's l.
l. morphometry
mushroom worker's l.
l. nodule
non-reexpanding l.
oblique fissure of l.
l. perfusion (LP)
pigeon-breeder's l.
pigeon-fancier's l.
pigment induration of the l.
pizza l.
polycystic l.
posterior basal segmental artery of right l.
postperfusion l.
pump l.
l. reexpansion
respirator l.
l. retractor
rheumatoid l.
root of l.
l. scan
l. scanning
scleroderma l.
shock l.
silo-filler's l.
silver polisher's l.
l. sliding
stiff l.
l. stone
superior lobe of right/left l.
thresher's l.
l. tissue destruction
l. transfer capacity
l. transplant (LT, LTx)
transverse fissure of the right l.
trapped l.
trench l.

tuberculosis of l.'s
unilateral hyperlucency of the l.
unilateral hyperlucent l.
unilateral nonfunctioning l.
l. unit
upper lobe of l.
l. uptake
uremic l.
vanishing l.
vernal edema of l.
vertebral part of the costal surface
of the l.
l. volume
l. volume reduction surgery
(LVRS)
l. washings
welder's l.
wet l.
white l.
wood pulp worker's l.
lunger
chronic l.
lung-liver interaction
Lungmotor
lungs
lung-to-finger circulation time (LFCT)
lung-wall interface
lungworm
lunula, pl. **lunulae**
lupoid
Lupron
L. Depot
L. Depot-3 Month
L. Depot-4 Month
L. Depot-Ped
lupus
l. anticoagulant
l. anticoagulant disorder
cerebral l.
l. erythematosus (LE)
l. pernio
l. pleuritis
lupus-associated valve disease
Luria conflicting tasks
Lurselle
Luschka
L. cartilage
foramen of L.
L. tonsil
lusitaniae
Candida l.
lusitropic abnormality

lusitropy
lusoria
dysphagia l.
Lutembacher
L. complex
L. syndrome
lutetium
motexafin l.
l. texaphyrin
Lutrin
Lutz-Splendore-Almeida disease
Luxtec fiberoptic system
luxury perfusion
luxus
l. heart
l. perfusion
LV
left ventricle
LV end-diastolic diameter
LVAD
left ventricular assist device
HeartMate LVAD
Novacor LVAD
vented-electric HeartMate LVAD
LVAS
left ventricular assist system
LVAS implantable pump
LVD
left ventricular dysfunction
LVEDD
left ventricular end-diastolic dimension
LVEDP
left ventricular end-diastolic pressure
LVEDV
left ventricular end-diastolic volume
LVEF
left ventricular ejection fraction
LVESD
left ventricular end-systolic dimension
LVET
left ventricular ejection time
LVH
left ventricular hypertrophy
LVI
large-vessel infarction
LVIDD
left ventricular internal diastolic diameter
left ventricular internal diastolic
dimension
LVOT
left ventricular outflow tract

NOTES

LVOTO
 left ventricular outflow tract obstruction
LVR
 left ventricular reduction
LVRS
 lung volume reduction surgery
LVSB
 leftward ventricular septal bowing
LVSD
 left ventricular systolic dimension
LVSVI
 left ventricular stroke volume index
LVSWI
 left ventricular stroke work index
LW
 lateral wall
lwoffi
 Acinetobacter l.
lycopene
Lycoperdon
lycoperdonosis
Lycopodium
lycopodium asthma
LYG
 lymphomatoid granulomatosis
Lyme
 L. borreliosis
 L. disease
 L. titer
lymphadenitis
 tuberculous l.
lymphadenopathy
 hilar l.
lymphangiectasis
 chronic pulmonary cystic l.
lymphangioendothelioma
lymphangioleiomyomatosis (LAM)
lymphangioma
lymphangiomatosis
 diffuse pulmonary l.
lymphangiomyomatosis
 pulmonary l.
lymphangitic
 l. carcinoma
 l. carcinomatosis (LC)
 l. spread
lymphangitis carcinomatosa
Lymphapress compression therapy
lymphatic
 l. channel
 l. dilation
 l. edema
 obtuse marginal l.
 subclavian l.
lymphatici
 hilum nodi l.
lymphedema praecox

lymph node
lymphocyte
 l. chemoattractant factor (LCF)
 l. concentration
 l. immune globulin
 T l.
 l. transformation test
lymphocytic
 l. infiltrative disorder
 l. interstitial pneumonitis (LIP)
lymphoepithelioma-like carcinoma
lymphogranuloma venereum (LGV)
lymphohematogenous drainage system
lymphoid
 l. alveolitis
 l. hyperplasia
 l. interstitial pneumonia
 l. interstitial pneumonitis (LIP)
lymphokine
lymphoma
 African Burkitt l.
 AIDS-related l. (ARL)
 B cell l.
 Burkitt l.
 Kiel classification of l.
 Lennert l.
 nodular sclerosing Hodgkin l.
 noncleaved cell l.
 non-Hodgkin l.
 primary effusion l.
 primary pulmonary non-Hodgkin l.
  (PPL)
 pulmonary l.
 pyothorax-associated l.
lymphomatoid granulomatosis (LYG)
lymphoplasma
lymphoplasmacytic inflammation
lymphoreticular granulomatous vasculitis
lymphosarcoma
lymphotoxin
Lyo-Ject
 Cardizem L.-J.
 L.-J. syringe
Lyon-Horgan procedure
Lyon hypothesis
lyophilize
lyophilized powder
Lyphocin injection
Lyra
 L. 2020 implantable cardioverter
 L. 2020 implantable cardioverter-
  defibrillator
 L. laser system
lysate
Lysatec rtPA
lyse
lysed artery

lysine
　　l. acetylsalicylate
　　l.-binding site
lysis
　　clot l.
　　myofibrillar l.
　　spontaneous l.
　　l. time
Lysodren
lysophosphatidic acid
lysophosphatidylcholine scavenger
lysophospholipase
lysosomal
　　l. enzyme

　　l. hydrolase
　　l. thiolprotease
lysosome
lysozyme
lys-plasminogen
　　recombinant l.-p.
Lyssavirus
lysylbradykinin
LZT
　　lead/zirconium/titanium
　　LZT crystal

NOTES

L

M

M cell layer
M gate
M lignocaine
M lines
M pattern on right atrial wave
form
M protein

99m

sodium pertechnetate Tc 99m

M$_1$

mitral first sound

M$_2$

mitral second sound

M6/C cylinder carrying case
M6 oxygen cylinder
m7E3 Fab
MA

mixed apnea

mA

milliampere

MAA

macroaggregated albumin
mandibular advancement appliance
MAA perfusion lung scintigraphy

MAAS

Multicenter Antiatherosclerotic Study

MABP

mean arterial blood pressure

MAC

malignancy-associated change
membrane attack complex
minimal alveolar concentration
mitral annular calcium
mitral annulus calcification
multiaccess catheter
Mycobacterium avium complex
MAC infection

MAC-1

beta-2-integrin MAC-1

MacCallum patch
MACE

major adverse cardiac event
Mayo Asymptomatic Carotid
Endarterectomy
MACE clinical trial

Macewen sign
Mach

M. band
M. effect

Machado-Guerreiro test
Machida fiberoptic laryngoscope
machine

Aloka echocardiograph m.

Apogee CX 100 Interspec
ultrasound m.
Bird m.
Burdick ECG m.
bypass m.
Century heart-lung m.
Cobe-Stockert heart-lung m.
Corometrics-Aloka
echocardiograph m.
Crafoord-Senning heart-lung m.
General Electric Pass-C
echocardiograph m.
G5 massage and percussion m.
heart-lung m.
Hewlett-Packard 500 Echo-
Doppler m.
Hewlett-Packard 1000 Echo-
Doppler m.
May-Gibbon heart-lung m.
Respironics CPAP m.
Respitrace m.
Sullivan V Elite Real Time Clock
CPAP m.
Toshiba electrocardiography m.

machinery murmur
MacIntosh

M. blade anesthesia
M. laryngoscope

Mackenzie polygraph
Mackler tube
Macleod syndrome
MacNamara protocol
macroaggregated

m. albumin (MAA)
m. albumin perfusion lung
scintigraphy
m. albumin scintigraphy

macroangiopathy

coronary m.

Macrobid
macrocardia
Macrodantin
Macrodex
macroembolus
macroglobulin

alpha-2 m.

macroglobulinemia

Waldenström m.

macroglossia
macrolide

m. antibiotic
m. antimicrobial
m. antimicrobial agent

macromolecular ligand
macromolecule

M

macrophage
alveolar m.
foamy m.
hemosiderin-laden m.
m. inflammatory protein (MPI)
m. inflammatory protein-1 (MIP-1)
lipid-laden m.
tissue-infiltrating m. (TIM)
macroreentrant
m. atrial tachycardia
m. circuit
macrosteatosis
macrovascular
m. artery disease
m. coronary lesion
Mac stent
macula, pl. **maculae**
m. albida
m. lactea
m. tendinea
macular arteriole inferior
maculopapular rash
MAC-VU electrocardiograph
MAD
mandibular advancement device
MadCAM-1
mucosal addresin cell adhesion molecule-1
MADRS
Montgomery-Asberg Depression Rating Scale
Maestro implantable cardiac pacemaker
MAG
Minnesota antilymphocyte globulin
Magan
Magellan monitor
Magic
M. Torque guidewire
M. Wallstent
M. Wallstent stent
Magill
M. forceps
M. laryngoscope
M. Safety Clear Plus endotracheal tube
magna
arteria anastomotica auricularis m.
auricularis m.
Magnascanner
Picker M.
magnesium
m. carbonate ($MgCO_3$)
m. deficiency
intracellular m.
m. oxide
m. salicylate
serum m.
m. sulfate

m. sulfate heptahydrate
m. supplementation
magnet
m. application over pulse generator
bronchoscopic m.
m. check
Equen m.
m. inhibition
m. pacing interval
m. rate
m. resonance angiography
m. wire
magnetic
m. moment
m. relaxation time
m. resonance angiography (MRA)
m. resonance coronary angiography (MRCA)
m. resonance flowmetry (MRF)
m. resonance imaging (MRI)
m. resonance signal
m. resonance spectography
m. resonance spectroscopy (MRS)
m. resonance venography (MRV)
m. source imaging (MSI)
m. valve resistor
magnetite pneumoconiosis
magnetization
spatial modulation of m. (SPAMM)
magnetocardiogram (MCG)
magnetocardiograph
magnetocardiography
Magnevist
magnification
loupe m.
magnitude
average pulse m.
peak m.
Magnolia biondii
Magnum
M. guidewire
M.-Meier system
magnus
pulsus m.
Magovern-Cromie ball-cage prosthetic valve
Mag-Ox 400
Magsal
Mahaim
M. bundle
M. fiber
M.-type tachycardia
Mahalanobis distance
Mahler
M. Baseline Dyspnea Index questionnaire
M. sign
mahogany flush

MAI
>movement arousal index
>*Mycobacterium avium-intracellulare*
>>MAI complex
>>MAI infection

Maigret-50

main
>m. bundle
>m. pulmonary artery (MPA)
>m. renal vein
>m. stem bronchus
>unprotected left m. (ULM)

mainstem
>m. coronary artery
>m. intubation

maintained
>adequate hemostasis m.

major
>m. adverse cardiac event (MACE)
>*Babesia m.*
>ductus sublingualis m.
>m. fissure
>pectoralis m.

Makin murmur

malabsorption

maladie de Roger

malaise

malar flush

malaria

malariae
>*Plasmodium m.*

malarial pneumonitis

malayi
>*Brugia m.*

maleate
>azatadine m.
>chlorpheniramine m.
>dexchlorpheniramine m.
>enalapril m.
>ergonovine m.
>methysergide m.
>nomifensine m.
>timolol m.
>trimipramine m.

malformation
>angiographically occult intracranial vascular m. (AOIVM)
>arteriovenous m. (AVM)
>atrioventricular m. (AVM)
>congenital m.
>congenital cystic adenomatoid m.
>cystic adenomatoid m.

>Ebstein m.
>Mondini pulmonary arteriovenous m.
>neural crest m.
>pulmonary arteriovenous m. (PAVM)
>Taussig-Bing m.
>Uhl m.

malfunction
>pacemaker m.

Malgaigne fossa

malignancy
>cutaneous m.
>de novo m.
>mesenchymal m.
>posttransplantation m.
>primary cardiac m.

malignancy-associated
>m.-a. change (MAC)
>m.-a. phlebitis

malignant
>m. arrhythmia
>m. beat
>m. carcinoid syndrome
>m. endocarditis
>m. fibrous histiocytoma (MFH)
>m. hypertension
>m. mesothelioma
>m. middle cerebral artery infarction (mMCAI)
>m. pleural effusion
>m. pleural mesothelioma (MPM)
>m. superior vena caval syndrome
>m. SVC syndrome
>m. thrombocytopenia
>m. vasovagal syndrome
>m. ventricular arrhythmia (MVA)
>m. ventricular tachyarrhythmia
>m. ventricular tachycardia

malinger

Mallampati score

mall asthma

malleable retractor

Mallergan-VC with Codeine

Mallinckrodt
>M. angiographic catheter
>M. cuffed endotracheal tube
>M. Hi-Care Pulmonary Hygiene system
>M. radioimmunoassay
>M. vertebral catheter

M

NOTES

417

Mallory
>M. RM-1 cell pacemaker
>M. stain

Mallory-Weiss
>M.-W. syndrome
>M.-W. tear

malmoense
>*Mycobacterium m.*

malnutrition
>alcoholic m.
>kwashiorkor-like m.
>myocardial m.
>protein-calorie m.

malondialdehyde (MDA)
>m. level
>m. modified low-density lipoprotein
> (MDA-LDL)

**Maloney mercury-filled esophageal
dilator**

malonylcoenzyme A, malonyl-CoA

malperfused segment

malperfusion phenomenon

malpighian vesicle

malposition
>crisscross heart m.
>double-outlet left ventricle m.
>double-outlet right ventricle m.
>m. of great arteries (MGA)
>levocardia m.
>mesocardia m.
>single ventricle m.

maltase deficiency

Malteno valve

maltophilia
>*Pseudallescheria m.*
>*Pseudomonas m.*
>*Stenotrophomonas m.*
>*Xanthomonas m.*

malt worker's lung

malum cordis

mammary
>m. artery
>m. artery graft
>m. souffle
>m. souffle murmur
>m. souffle sound

mammary-coronary tissue forceps

man
>radiation equivalent in m. (rem)

management
>atrial fibrillation followup
> investigation of rhythm m.
> (AFFIRM)
>data base m.
>Platelet Receptor Inhibition for
> Ischemic Syndrome M. (PRISM)
>postprocedural m.
>real-time position m. (RPM)

>SenDx Relay data m.
>Total Atherosclerosis M. (TAM)
>Trial of Antihypertensive
> Interventions and M. (TAIM)
>ventilator m.

mandatory
>m. minute volume (MMV)
>synchronized intermittent m.

mandibular
>m. advancement appliance (MAA)
>m. advancement device (MAD)
>m. plane to hyoid (MP-H)

mandibulopharyngeal

Mandol

mandrel, mandril
>m. graft

mandrin

maneuver
>Addison m.
>Adson m.
>breathhold m.
>cold pressor testing m.
>costoclavicular m.
>Ejrup m.
>forced expiratory m.
>Heimlich m.
>hemodynamic m.
>Hillis-Müller m.
>hyperventilation m.
>jaw thrust m.
>jaw-thrust/head-tilt m.
>Jonnson m.
>Lecompte m.
>Mattox m.
>Miller m.
>modified Miller m. (MM)
>Mueller m.
>Müller m.
>nonpanting m.
>panting m.
>peak expiratory m.
>Sellick m.
>submaximal m.
>Valsalva m. (VS)

maneuverability

**manganese superoxide dismutase (Mn-
SOD)**

manidipine

manifest
>m. ischemia
>Morse m.
>m. vector

manifold
>Morse m.

manipulation
>catheter m.

manmade vitreous fiber (MMVF)

mannequin

manner
>Creech m.
>m. of Creech
>DeBakey-Creech m.
>m. of DeBakey-Creech

Mannkopf sign
manofluorography (MFG)
manometer
>aneroid m.
>Dinamap ultrasound blood
>pressure m.
>Hürthle m.
>Mercury Medical Airway
>Pressure M.
>Posey Cufflator tracheal cuff
>inflator and m.
>single-patient use m.

manometer-tipped catheter
manometry
>esophageal m.

Manoplax
Mansfield
>M. Atri-Pace 1 catheter
>M. balloon
>M. bioptome
>M. orthogonal electrode catheter
>M. Polaris electrode
>M. Scientific dilatation balloon
>catheter
>M. Valvuloplasty Registry
>M.-Webster catheter

mansoni
>*Schistosoma m.*

Mantoux test
manual
>M. edge detection
>PACE Physician M.
>M. resuscitation baffle
>M. resuscitation bag
>M. ventilation

manubrium
MAO
>monoamine oxidase
>MAO inhibitor

MAOI
>monoamine oxidase inhibitor

MAP
>mean airway pressure
>mean arterial pressure
>mitogen-activated protein
>monophasic action potential

map
>electroanatomical m.
>linear local shortening m.
>maximum voltage m.
>polar coordinate m.

MAPD
>monophasic action potential duration

MAPK
>mitogen-activated protein kinase
>MAPK pathway

maple bark disease
Mapper hemostasis EP mapping sheath
mapping
>activation sequence m.
>advanced cardiac m.
>atrial activation m.
>Biosense left ventricular m.
>body surface Laplacian m. (BSLM)
>bull's-eye polar coordinate m.
>cardiac m.
>catheter m.
>m. catheter
>cavotricuspid isthmus m.
>color-coded flow m.
>color flow m.
>digital phase m. (DPM)
>Doppler color flow m. (DCFM)
>Doppler flow m.
>electromagnetic m.
>electromechanical m.
>electromechanical left ventricular m.
>electrophysiologic m.
>endocardial m.
>endocardial m. of ventricular
>tachycardia
>entrainment m.
>EP m.
>flow m.
>high-density electroanatomical and
>entrainment m.
>ice m.
>intracardiac m.
>intraoperative m.
>Laplacian m.
>MRI velocity m.
>multisite m.
>noncontact m.
>noncontact endocardial m.
>pace-m.
>pulsed-wave Doppler m.
>retrograde atrial activation m.
>Revelation microcatheter for EP m.

M

NOTES

mapping *(continued)*
    simultaneous catheter m.
    spectral temporal m.
    spectral turbulence m.
    tachycardia pathway m.
    ventricular m.
mapping/ablation catheter
maprotiline
MAPS
    Multivessel Angioplasty Prognosis Study
MAR
    mean atrial rate
    MAR algorithm
marantic
    m. endocarditis
    m. thrombosis
    m. thrombus
marasmic
    m. thrombosis
    m. thrombus
marasmus
Marathon guiding catheter
Marax bronchodilator
Marbach-Weil technique
Marburg virus
MARCATOR
    Multicenter American Research Trial
    with Cilazapril after Angioplasty to
    Prevent Transluminal Coronary
    Obstruction and Restenosis
marcescens
    Serratia m.
Marcillin
Marek disease
Marey law
Marfan syndrome
margarine
    Benecol m.
    sitostanol ester m.
Margesic H
margin
    costal m.
    rib m.
marginal
    m. artery of colon
    m. artery of Drummond
    m. branch #1
    m. circumflex artery
    obtuse m. (OM)
    m. rale
marginatum
    erythema m.
margo
    m. anterior pulmonis
    m. inferior pulmonis
Marie-Bamberger syndrome
Marie syndrome
marine oil

Marinol
marinum
    Mycobacterium m.
Marion-Clatworthy side-to-end vena caval shunt
MARISA
    Monotherapy Assessment of Ranolazine
    in Stable Angina
    MARISA clinical trial
mark
    alignment m.
    M. IV respiratory pacemaker
    M. VI cooling vest
marker
    m. annotation
    breath m.
    m. catheter
    CD63 platelet activation m.
    CD62p (p-selectin) platelet
     activation m.
    m. channel
    CYFRA 21-1 tumor m.
    dual m.
    gold m.
    lead-letter m.
    plaque m.
    predictive survival m.
    radiopaque end m.
    serum m.
    tumor m.
    vein graft ring m.
marking
    bronchial m.
    bronchovesicular m.
    interstitial m.
    lung m.
    perihilar m.
    pulmonary m.
    pulmonary vascular m.
    vascular m.
Markov process
Marlex
Marmine Oral
marmorata
    cutis m.
marneffei
    Penicillium m.
Maroteaux-Lamy syndrome
Marpres
Marquest Respirgard II nebulizer
Marquette
    M. Case-12 electrocardiographic
     system
    M. Case-12 exercise system
    M. electrocardiograph
    M. 8000 Holter monitor
    M. Holter recorder

M. Responder 1500 multifunctional defibrillator
M. Series 8000 Holter analyzer
M. three-channel laser Holter
M. treadmill

Marriott method

MARS

Monitored Atherosclerosis Regression Study

Marshall

M. bundle
M. fold
M. ligament
M. oblique vein

marsupialization

Marthritic

Martin

interbronchiolar communication of M.

Martorell syndrome

Mary Allen Engle ventricle

MAS

meconium aspiration syndrome
Motor Assessment Scale

Masimo Set

mask

AccurOx m.
ACE detachable m.
AeroChamber m.
AirSep CPAP bilevel nasal m.
AirSep Nasal CPAP m.
AirSep Ultimate Nasal m.
Bili m.
BLB m.
BLB oxygen m.
Boothby-Lovelace-Bulbulian oxygen m.
ComfortSeal m.
EasiVEnt valved holding chamber m.
ecchymotic m.
Finney m.
GoldSeal nasal m.
Inspiron AccurOx M.
IQ nasal m.
Kuhn m.
meter m.
Mirage nasal m.
Nic the Asthmatic Dragon aerosol m.
nonrebreathing m.
oxygen m.

partial rebreathing m.
PEP m.
Phantom nasal m.
RBS face m.
rebreathing m.
Rendell-Baker face m.
reservoir face m.
Res Medication Bubble Mask nasal m.
Rudolph Full Face m.
SCRAM face m.
SealEasy resuscitation m.
Series 7900 face m.
Series 7900 mouth breathing face m.
Series 8900 nasal and mouth breathing face m.
Sullivan Mirage nasal m.
thermoplastic head m.
Ultimate nasal m.
Venti m.
ventilation m.
Venturi m.
Vickers Ventimask Mark 2 m.

masked hypertension

mask-mode

m.-m. cardiac imaging
m.-m. subtraction

Mason-Likar

M.-L. 12-lead ECG system
M.-L. limb lead modification
M.-L. placement of ECG lead

mason's lung

MASS

Medicine, Angioplasty, or Surgery Study

mass

achromatic m.
cardiac m.
echodense m.
echogenic m.
m. effect
false m.
fat-free m. (FFM)
fibrotic m.
fungating m.
intracardiac m.
intracavity m.
left ventricular m.
lung m.
m. median aerodynamic diameter (MMAD)
myocardial m.

M

NOTES

mass *(continued)*
    pleural m.
    ventricular m.
massage
    cardiac m.
    carotid sinus m.
    closed chest m.
    closed chest cardiac m.
    direct cardiac m.
    external cardiac m.
    heart m.
    open chest m.
    open chest cardiac m.
    vapor m.
mass-flow anemometer
Massier solution
massive
    m. aspiration
    m. collapse
    m. pneumonia
    m. thrombus
Masson
    M. body
    M. trichrome stain
MAST
    military antishock trousers
    Multicenter Acute Stroke Trial
    MAST suit
mast
    m. cell
    m. cell inhibitor
    m. cell protease
Mastadenovirus
Master
    M. exercise stress test
    M. Flow Pumpette pump
    M. test
    M. two-step exercise test
master
    change description m. (CDM)
    SpaceLabs Event M.
MasterScreen Body plethysmograph
mastocytosis syndrome
Masy angioscope
MAT
    multifocal atrial tachycardia
Matas
    M. aneurysmectomy
    M. test
match defect
matching
    afterload m.
    ventilation/perfusion m.
MATE
    Medicine versus Angioplasty for
      Thrombolytic Exclusions
    MATE Clinical Trial

material
    Biobrane/HF graft m.
    Biograft bovine heterograft m.
    Carbo-Seal graft m.
    Cellolite m.
    contrast m.
    embolized foreign m.
    fibrinohematic m.
    Haynes 25 m.
    Hexabrix contrast m.
    Kaltostat wound packing m.
    Kifa catheter m.
    low osmolality contrast m.
      (LOCM)
    MycroMesh graft m.
    Myoview contrast m.
    nonionic contrast m.
    PermaMesh m.
    Soludrast contrast m.
    Stellite ring m.
    Zenotech graft m.
maternally inherited cardiomyopathy
matrix
    extracellular m. (ECM)
    m. metalloproteinase (MMP)
    m. mode
    myocardial collagen m.
    subendothelial m.
    m. synthesis
    vascular m.
matrix-degrading
    m.-d. neutral metalloproteinase
    m.-d. neutral MMP
Matson-Alexander rib stripper
Matson rib elevator
Matsuda titanium surgical instrument
matter
    temporoparietal white m. (TPWM)
    white m. (WM)
Mattox
    M. aorta clamp
    M. maneuver
mattress
    apnea alarm m.
    Bedge antireflux m.
    eggcrate m.
    hypothermia m.
    Roho m.
    m. suture
    TheraKair m.
maturation
    affinity m.
Maugeri syndrome
Mavik
max
    VO_2 m.
      maximum oxygen consumption

Maxair
    M. Autohaler
    M. Inhalation Aerosol
Maxaquin Oral
MAXBlend oxygen/air blender
Maxepa
MaxForce balloon dilatation catheter
Maxilith pacemaker pulse generator
maxillomandibular
    m. advancement (MMA)
    m. advancement procedure
    m. osteotomy (MMO)
maximal
    m. breathing capacity
    m. exercise systolic pressure (MESP)
    m. expiratory flow rate (MEFR)
    m. expiratory flow volume (MEFV)
    m. expiratory mouth pressure (P_{Emax})
    m. expiratory pressure (MEP)
    m. flow-volume envelope (MFVL)
    m. forced expiratory flow (FEFmax)
    M. Individual Therapy in Acute Myocardial Infarction (MITRA)
    m. inspiratory flow rate (MIFR)
    m. inspiratory mouth pressure (P_{Imax})
    m. inspiratory pressure (MIP)
    m. midexpiratory flow (MMEF, MMF)
    m. midexpiratory flow rate (MMEFR)
    m. sniff-induced esophageal pressure (Pessniff)
    m. sniff-induced gastric pressure (Pgasniff)
    m. sniff-induced transdiaphragmatic pressure (Pdisniff)
    m. sustainable ventilatory capacity (MSVC)
    m. velocity (V_{MAX})
    m. ventilation (MV)
    m. ventilation rate (MVR)
    m. vital capacity (MVC)
Maxima Plus plasma resistant fiber oxygenator
maximum
    m. breathing capacity (MBC)

    m. expiratory airflow-static lung elastic recoil pressure (MFSR)
    m. expiratory flow at 50% vital capacity (MEF_{50})
    m. expiratory pressure (MEP)
    m. flow rate
    m. flow-volume loop (MFVL)
    m. inspiratory pressure (MIP)
    m. medical therapy
    m. midexpiratory flow rate (MMEF, MMF)
    m. negative potential
    m. oxygen consumption (VO_2 max)
    m. oxygen uptake
    m. predicted heart rate (MPHR)
    m. sensory rate
    m. tolerated dose (MTD)
    m. ventricular elastance (Emax)
    m. voltage map
    m. voluntary contraction (MVC)
    m. voluntary ventilation (MVV)
    m. walking time
Maxi-Myst vaporizer
Maxipime
Maxivent
maxi-vessel loops
Maxzide
Mayaro virus
Mayer wave
May-Gibbon heart-lung machine
May-Grünwald-Giemsa stain
Mayo
    M. Asymptomatic Carotid Endarterectomy (MACE)
    M. classification
    M. exercise treadmill protocol
    M. hemostat
maze
    m. ablation
    m. III surgery
    m. procedure
Mazicon
mazindol
    hydrogen-3 m.
MB
    microbubble
    myocardial band
    myocardial bridging
    MB band
    MB enzymes of CPK
    MB fraction
    MB index

M

NOTES

MBC
maximum breathing capacity
MBF
myocardial blood flow
MBIP
model-based image processing
MBP
mean arterial blood pressure
MBq
megabecquerel
MBTS
modified Blalock-Taussig shunt
MBV
mitral balloon valvotomy
MCA
middle cerebral artery
MCAF
monocyte chemotactic and activating
factor
MCAO
middle cerebral artery occlusion
McArdle
M. disease
M. syndrome
MCAS modular clip application
MCC
mucociliary clearance
McCort sign
MCD
molecular coincidence detection
MCD imaging
McDowall reflex
MCE
myocardial contrast echocardiography
MCFSR
mean circumferential fiber-shortening
rate
MCG
magnetocardiogram
McGill
M.-Melzack Pain Questionnaire
M. Pain Questionnaire
McGinn-White sign
McGoon
M. guidelines
M. technique
McHenry protocol
mCi
millicurie
MCL
midclavicular line
MCM smart laser
McNaught keel
MCP
monocyte chemoattractant protein
MCP-1
monocyte chemoattractant protein-1
monocyte chemotactic protein-1

McPheeters treatment
McQuigg-Mixter bronchial forceps
MC4-R
melanocortin-4 receptor
MCT
monocarboxylate/proton cotransporter
monocarboxylate transporter
MCT Oil
MCV
mean corpuscular volume
MDA
malondialdehyde
MDA-LDL
malondialdehyde modified low-density
lipoprotein
MDBP
mean resting diastolic blood pressure
MDC
Metoprolol in Dilated Cardiomyopathy
Multicenter Dilated Cardiomyopathy
MDC Clinical Trial
MDCM
mildly dilated congestive cardiomyopathy
M/D 4 defibrillator system
MDF
myocardial depressant factor
MDI
metered-dose inhaler
methylene diphenyl diisocyanate
MDI kit
MDILog
M. microelectronic monitor
M. therapy monitoring device
MDP
methylene diphosphonate
MDR
multidrug-resistant
MDRSP
multidrug-resistant *Streptococcus
pneumoniae*
MDR-TB
multidrug-resistant tuberculosis
MDS
minimum data set
myocardial depressant substance
MDS system
MDV
myocardial Doppler velocity
Meadows syndrome
Meadox
M.-Cooley woven low-porosity
prosthesis
M. graft
M. graft sizer
M. Teflon felt pledget
M. woven velour prosthesis
mean
m. airway pressure (MAP)

arterial m.
m. arterial blood pressure (MABP, MBP)
m. arterial pressure (MAP)
m. atrial rate (MAR)
m. atrial rate algorithm
m. circumferential fiber-shortening rate (MCFSR)
m. contrast enhancement
m. corpuscular volume (MCV)
m. diastolic left ventricular pressure
m. electrical axis
m. forced midexpiratory flow
m. inspiratory flow (MIF)
m. manifest vector
m. midexpiratory flow rate ($FEF_{25-75\%}$)
m. normalized systolic ejection rate
m. pulmonary artery pressure (MPAP, PAPm)
m. pulmonary artery wedge pressure (MPAWP)
m. QRS axis
m. reference diameter (MRD)
m. resting diastolic blood pressure (MDBP)
m. right atrial pressure
m. systolic left ventricular pressure
m. vector

Means-Lernan mediastinal crunch
measles pneumonia
measure
adjunctive m.
ancillary m.
CD4+ m.
functional independence m. (FIM)
measured
m. data
m. output
measurement
automated cardiac flow m. (ACM)
automated cardiac output m. (ACOM)
blood flow m.
cardiac output m.
coronary blood flow m.
Doppler m.
gas clearance m.
hemodynamic m.
invasive pressure m.
M-mode m.

morphometric m.
physiologic m.
PR-AC m.
pressure m.
quantitative coronary angiography caliper m.
Reid index m.
spectral Doppler velocity m.
splenic perfusion m.
thermodilution m.
transstenotic pressure gradient m.
venous flow m.

Measurin
meat, eggs, dairy, invisible fat, condiments, snacks (MEDICS)
meat-wrapper's asthma
mebendazole
mecalil provocation
mecamylamine hydrochloride
mechanical
m. alternation
m. alternation of heart
m. cardiopulmonary resuscitation
m. contractile function
m. cough
m. debulking
m. dyssynchrony
m. heart
m. obstruction
m. pleurodesis
m. prosthesis
m. thrombectomy
m. trauma
m. valve
m. VAS
m. ventilation (MV)
m. ventilatory support
m. visual analogue scale

mechanics
fluid m.
lung m.
mechanic's bronchitis
mechanism
m. of action
compensatory m.
coronary steal m.
deglutition m.
fixation m.
Frank-Starling m.
gating m.
ionic m.
Laplace m.

M

NOTES

mechanism *(continued)*
    peeling-back m.
    pinchcock m.
    postsynaptic cholinergic m.
    reentrant m.
    sinus m.
    Starling m.
    steal m.
    triggering m.
    vertical deceleration m.
    wave-speed m.
mechanocardiography
mechanoelectrical feedback
mechanoreceptor
mechanoreflex
mechanosensor
mechanotransduction
mechlorethamine hydrochloride
meclofenamate sodium
Meclomen Oral
meconium
    m. aspiration
    m. aspiration syndrome (MAS)
    m. ileus
Medasonics NeuroGuard CDS
ultrasound
MEDDARS cardiac catheterization
analysis system
Medex
    M. coronary C1 stent
    M. transducer
MedGraphics
    M. 1085 body plethysmograph
    series
    M. Breeze PF software
    M. Cardio O2 system
    M. CPE 2000 electronically braked
    bicycle
    M. CPX/D metabolic cart
    M. model 1085 body
    plethysmograph
media
    aortic tunica m.
    arterial m.
    low osmolality contrast m.
    (LOCM)
    m. thickness
medial
    m. basal branch of pulmonary
    artery
    m. inferior artery of knee
    m. medullary infarction (MMI)
    m. necrosis
    m. superior artery of knee
    m. surface of lung
    m. tear
medialis
    arteria genus superior m.

median
    m. nerve injury
    m. sternotomy
    m. sternotomy incision
    m. survival time (MST)
medianus
    ramus m.
mediastinal
    m. adenopathy
    m. amyloidosis
    m. crunch
    m. emphysema
    m. fibrosis
    m. flutter
    m. lymph node
    m. lymph node biopsy
    m. node biopsy
    m. part of lung
    m. pleura
    m. pleurisy
    m. shadow
    m. shift
    m. space
    m. sump filter
    m. thickening
    m. wedge
    m. widened
    m. widening
mediastinale
    septum m.
mediastinalis
    pleura m.
mediastinitis
    acute m.
    descending necrotizing m. (DNM)
    fibrosing m.
    fibrous m.
    granulomatous m.
mediastinoscope
    Goldberg-MPC m.
mediastinoscopy
    Chamberlain m.
mediastinotomy
mediastinum
    superior vascular m.
mediator
    pyrogenic m.
    m. receptor antagonist
    vasoactive m.
MedicAIR
    M. PLUS spirometer
    M. PLUS spirometry station
medical
    M. Graphics Cardiopulmonary
    Exercise System 2001
    M. Graphics pneumotachograph
    with volume integrator

m. intensive care unit (MICU)
M. Research Council questionnaire

medicamentosa
rhinitis m.

medication
bolus of m.
m. monitoring event system
(MEMS)
mucoactive m.
presyncopal m.
M. Use Studies (MUST)

medication-use evaluation (MUE)

medicinalis
Hirudo m.

medicine
American College of Sports M.
(ACSM)
Angioplasty Compared to M.
(ACME)
M., Angioplasty, or Surgery Study
(MASS)
digital imaging and communications
in m. (DICOM)
evidence-based m. (EBM)
Kampo m.
M. versus Angioplasty for
Thrombolytic Exclusions (MATE)

Medicon
M. instrument
M. rib spreader

Medicopaste

MEDICS
meat, eggs, dairy, invisible fat,
condiments, snacks

Medi-Facts system

Mediflex-Bookler device

Medi-graft vascular prosthesis

Medigraphics 2000 analyzer

Medihaler
M.-Epi
M. Ergotamine
M.-Iso

MEDILOG 4000 ambulatory ECG recorder

Medimet

Medinol
M. NIRside slotted stent
M. NIR stent

mediomalacia vasculativa aortae

medionecrosis
m. of aorta

m. aortae
m. aortae idiopathica cystica

MediPort

Medipren

Medi-Quet tourniquet

MEDIS off-line quantitative coronary angiography

Medi-Strumpf stockings

Meditape

Medi-Tech
M.-T. balloon catheter
M.-T. catheter system
M.-T. multipurpose basket
M.-T. steerable catheter
M.-T. wire

Mediterranean
M. anemia
M. fever

Medi-Tuss AC

medium
Adenoscan contrast m.
Amipaque contrast m.
Angio-Conray contrast m.
m. chain triglycerides
Conray contrast m.
contrast m.
Eagle m.
fibrinolytic m.
iothalamate meglumine contrast m.
ioxaglate meglumine contrast m.
Isovue contrast m.
Joklik m.
metrizamide contrast m.
nonionic contrast m.
Optiray contrast m.
polygelin colloid contrast m.
QW3600 contrast m.
SHU-454 contrast m.
Urografin-76 contrast m.

Medi vascular stockings

Medivent
M. self-expanding coronary stent
M. vascular stent

Medlar body

Med-Neb respirator

Medos mechanical circulatory support system

Medrad Mark IV angiographic injector

Medralone injection

Medrol
M. Dosepak

M

NOTES

427

Medrol *(continued)*
    M. Oral
    M. Veriderm Cream
medroxyprogesterone
    m. acetate (MPA)
    estrogen, m.
Medtel pacemaker
Medtronic
    M. Activitrax rate-responsive
      unipolar ventricular pacemaker
    M. AneuRx stent graft
    M. AVE S660 coronary stent
    M. beStent stent
    M. bipolar pacemaker
    M. cardiac cooling jacket
    M. Cardiorhythm Atakr generator
    M. connector
    M. defibrillator implant support
      device
    M. Elite DDDR pacemaker
    M. Elite II pacemaker
    M. Evergreen balloon
    M. external cardioverter-defibrillator
    M. external tachyarrhythmia control
      device
    M. Gem automatic implantable
      defibrillator
    M. Hancock II tissue valve
    M. Hancock II valve
    M. Hemopump
    M. Hemopump cardiac assist
      device
    M. Hemopump system
    M. Inspire implantable device
    M. Intact bioprosthetic valve
    M. INTACT porcine bioprosthesis
    M. Interactive Tachycardia
      Terminating system
    M. interventional vascular stent
    M. Jewel AF arrhythmia
      management device
    M. Jewel AF 7250 dual-chamber
      implantable cardioverter-defibrillator
    M. Jewel AF implantable
      arrhythmia management device
    M. Jewel 7219D and C device
    M. Kappa 400 pacemaker
    M. lead
    M. Micro Jewel II defibrillator
    M. Micro Jewel II implantable
      defibrillator
    M. Mosaic bioprosthetic valve
    M. Octopus tissue stabilizing
      device
    M. Octopus tissue stabilizing
      system
    M. Octopus 2+ tissue stabilizing
      system

    M. PCD implantable cardioverter-
      defibrillator
    M. pulse generator
    M. Pulsor Intrasound pain reliever
    M. radiofrequency receiver
    M. RF 5998 pacemaker
    M. SPO pacemaker
    M. SP 502 pacemaker
    M. Spring lead
    M. Sympios pacemaker
    M. SynchroMed pump
    M. temporary pacemaker
    M. Thera DR pacemaker
    M. Thera I-series cardiac
      pacemaker
    M. tip
    M. Transvene electrode
    M. Transvene 6937 electrode
      catheter
    M. Transvene endocardial lead
      system
    M. Transvene lead system
    M. tremor control therapy device
    M. Zuma guiding catheter
Medtronic-Alcated pacemaker
Medtronic-Byrel-SX pacemaker
Medtronic-Hall
    M.-H. device
    M.-H. heart valve prosthesis
    M.-H. monocuspid tilting-disk valve
    M.-H. prosthetic heart valve
    M.-H. tilting-disk valve prosthesis
Medtronic-Hancock device
medulla
    adrenal m.
    m. oblongata
    rostral ventrolateral m. (RVLM)
    ventrolateral m. (VLM)
medullary collecting duct
Med-Xcor
Med-X stent
MEF_{50}
    maximum expiratory flow at 50% vital
      capacity
mefenamic acid
mefloquine hydrochloride
Mefoxin
MEFR
    maximal expiratory flow rate
MEFV
    maximal expiratory flow volume
megabecquerel (MBq)
megacardia
Megacart electrocardiograph
Megace
Megacillin Susp
megaelectron volt (MeV)

megaesophagus
megahertz (MHz)
megaloblastic anemia
megalocardia
MegaSonics PTCA catheter
megaterium
    Bacillus m.
megaunit (MU)
megestrol acetate
meglumine
    m. diatrizoate enema study
    intracoronary sonicated m.
    ioxaglate m.
Meier-Magnum system
Meigs syndrome
meiosis
meizothrombin
melaninogenica
    Prevotella m.
melaninogenicus
    Bacteroides m.
melanocortin-4 receptor (MC4-R)
melanoderma cachecticorum
melanoma
    Clark classification of malignant m.
melanotic carcinoma
melena
melenic stool
melioidosis
melitensis
    Brucella m.
Mellaril
mellitus
    diabetes m. (DM)
    insulin-dependent diabetes m.
    (IDDM)
    noninsulin-dependent diabetes m.
    (NIDDM)
melphalan
Melrose solution
Meltzer
    M. method
    M. sign
Melzack-Wall gate theory
membranacea
    angina m.
    pars m.
membranaceous
membrane
    adventitious m.
    alveolar-capillary m.
    alveolar hyaline m.

    alveolocapillary m.
    antibasement m.
    m. attack complex (MAC)
    basement m.
    bronchial mucous m.
    cell m.
    m. channel
    cricothyroid m.
    cuprophane m.
    m. current
    DeBove m.
    m. diffusing capacity (Dm)
    external elastic m. (EEM)
    Gore-Tex surgical m.
    Henle elastic m.
    Henle fenestrated m.
    Hybond ECL nitrocellulose m.
    internal elastic m. (IEM)
    polyacrylonitrile m.
    m. potential
    Preclude pericardial m.
    m. rupture
    sarcolemmal m.
    schneiderian respiratory m.
    serous m.
    suprapleural m.
    syncytiovascular m. (SVM)
membrane-bound membrane-type
metalloproteinase (MT-MMP)
membrane-stabilizing activity
membranous
    m. bronchitis
    m. croup
    m. laryngitis
    m. pharyngitis
    m. pulmonary atresia
    m. septum
    m. wall of trachea
memory
    cardiac m.
    m. catheter
    m. loop
MemoryTrace
    M. AT
    M. AT ambulatory cardiac monitor
Memotherm stent
MEMS
    medication monitoring event system
Menadol
mendelian disorder
Mendelson syndrome
Menghini needle

M

NOTES

Ménière syndrome
meningeal coccidioidomycosis
meningitic respiration
meningitidis
    Neisseria m.
meningitis, pl. meningitides
    HSV m.
    Mollaret m.
meningococcal
    m. pericarditis
    m. vaccine
meningococcemia
meningococcus
meningoencephalitis
meniscus
    intracavitary air m.
mental
    m. clouding
    m. status
    m. stress
    m. stress-induced ischemia
Menzel-Glaser SuperFrost/Plus
  electrically charged microscope slides
MEP
    maximal expiratory pressure
    maximum expiratory pressure
    motor provoked potential
meperidine hydrochloride
mephentermine
Mephyton Oral
mepivacaine hydrochloride
Mepron
mEq
    milliequivalent
meralluride
mercaptomerin sodium
6-mercaptopurine
Mercator atrial high-density array
  catheter
Mercuhydrin
mercury (Hg)
    M. Medical Airway Pressure
    Manometer
    millimeters of m. (mmHg)
    m. poisoning
    m. vapor
mercury-in-rubber strain gauge
  plethysmograph
mercury-in-Silastic strain gauge
mercury-195m (^{195m}Hg)
Merendino technique
Meridia
meridian
    m. echocardiogram
    m. echocardiography
Meridian pacemaker
meridional
    m. end-systolic stress (mESS)

    m. ESS (mESS)
    m. wall stress
MERIT-HF
    Metoprolol CR/XL Controlled Release
    Randomized Intervention Trial in Heart
    Failure
merodiastolic
meromyosin
meropenem for injection
merosystolic
Merrem IV
Mersilene
    M. braided nonabsorbable suture
    M. suture
MES
    microembolic signal
mesangial
    m. cell
    m. immune injury
    m. proliferative glomerulonephritis
mesangium
mesaortitis
mesarteritis
mesenchymal
    m. cell
    m. intimal cell
    m. malignancy
mesenchymal-derived tumor
mesenchyme
mesenteric
    m. angiography
    m. arteritis
    m. artery
    m. artery occlusion
    m. bypass graft
    m. ischemia
    m. vascular occlusion
mesentery of lung
mesh stent
mesna
mesocardia malposition
mesocardium
    arterial m.
    dorsal m.
    lateral m.
mesocaval shunt
mesoderm
    precardiac m.
mesodermal tumor
mesodiastolic
mesophlebitis
mesopneumonium
mesopulmonum
mesosystolic
mesothelial
    m. cell
    m. tumor

mesothelioma
    benign fibrous m.
    biphasic m.
    desmoplastic m.
    diffuse malignant pleural m.
     (DMPM)
    epithelioid m.
    malignant m.
    malignant pleural m. (MPM)
    pleural m.
    sarcomatoid m.
MESP
    maximal exercise systolic pressure
mESS
    meridional end-systolic stress
    meridional ESS
messenger
    m. ribonucleic acid (mRNA)
    second m.
Messerklinger endoscope
Mester test
Mestinon
mesylate
    bitolterol m.
    deferoxamine m.
    Desferal M.
    dihydroergotamine m.
    doxazosin m.
    gemifloxacin m.
    phentolamine m.
    saquinavir m.
    tirilazad m.
MET
    metabolic equivalent of task
    estimated MET
Meta
    M. DDDR pacemaker
    M. II pacemaker
    M. MV pacemaker
    M. rate-responsive pacemaker
metaanalysis
metabolator
    Sanborn m.
metabolic
    m. acidosis
    m. alkalosis
    m. cart
    m. encephalopathy
    m. equivalent
    m. equivalent of task (MET)
    m. parameter determination
    m. rate meter

    m. syndrome
    m. vasodilatory capacity
metabolism
    aerobic m.
    anaerobic m.
    arachidonate m.
    cerebral rate of glucose m.
     ($CMRGI_c$)
    cerebral rate of oxygen m.
     ($CMRO_2$)
    extracelluar matrix m.
    glucose m. (rMRGlu)
    myocardial m.
    oxidative m.
    respiratory m.
    substrate m.
metabolite
    arachidonic acid m.
    m. correction
    prostacyclin m.
metaboreceptor
metaboreflex
    muscle m.
    m. response
metacholin
metachronous lung cancer
Metahydrin
metaiodobenzylguanidine (MIBG)
    I-123 m.
    I-125 m.
metal
    m. fume fever (MFF)
    heavy m.
    m. sewing ring
    trace m.
metallic
    m. breath sounds
    m. click
    m. echo
    m. oxide fumes
    m. rale
    m. tinkle
metalloproteinase, metalloprotease
    m. inhibitor
    matrix m. (MMP)
    matrix-degrading neutral m.
    membrane-bound membrane-type m.
     (MT-MMP)
    tissue inhibitor of m. (TIMP)
    tissue inhibitor of m.-3 (TIMP-3)
metamorphosing respiration
metam sodium

M

NOTES

metamyelocyte
MetaPhor agarose
metaplasia
    cellular m.
    goblet cell m.
    peribronchiolar m.
metaplastic mucus-secreting cell
Metaplus arterial pump with disposable
metapneumonic
    m. empyema
    m. pleurisy
Metaprel
metaproterenol
    Arm-a-Med M.
    Dey-Dose M.
    m. sulfate
metaraminol bitartrate
metarteriole
metastasectomy
    pulmonary m.
metastasis, pl. **metastases**
    cannonball metastases
    cardiac m.
    contact m.
    hematogenous m.
    implantation m.
    tumor, nodes, m. (TNM)
metastatic
    m. calcification
    m. carcinoid syndrome
    m. carcinoma
    m. disease
    m. nodule
    m. phenotype
    m. pneumonia
    m. sarcoma
metazoal myocarditis
Metenix
metenkephalin
meter (*See also* flowmeter)
    ExacTech blood glucose m.
    kilopond m. (KPM)
    m. mask
    metabolic rate m.
    MicroRint portable airway
      resistance m.
    OxySAT oxygen saturation m.
    m. per second (m/sec)
    m.'s per second squared
    pH M.
    ventilation m.
metered-dose
    m.-d. inhaler (MDI)
    m.-d. spray
metered solution inhaler (MSI)
metformin
methacholine
    m. bronchoprovocation challenge

    m. challenge test
    m. chloride
    m. reaction
    m. reactivity
    m. response
    reversal speed of
      bronchoconstriction in response
      to m. (r-Sm)
    speed of bronchoconstriction in
      response to m. (Sm)
    m. test
methamphetamine hydrochloride
methanesulfonanilide derivative
methanesulfonate
    phentolamine m.
methemoglobin
methemoglobinemia
methicillin-sensitive right-sided
    endocarditis
methicillin sodium
methimazole
methionine loading
method
    Alfieri m.
    Allain m.
    Anderson-Keys m.
    Antyllus m.
    area-length m.
    Arvidsson dimension-length m.
    atrial extrastimulus m.
    biplane area-length m.
    Bland-Altman m.
    body box m.
    Bohr isopleth m.
    Bonferroni m.
    Brasdor m.
    Brisbane m.
    Brown-Dodge m.
    Burow quantitative m.
    Carrel m.
    catheter introduction m.
    Cavalieri m.
    Celermajer m.
    chromogenic m.
    Clauss m.
    closed circuit m.
    conductance catheter m.
    constant-flow m.
    Cribier m.
    CryoLife Single Step dilution m.
    Cutler-Ederer m.
    cyanmethemoglobin m.
    cyanogen bromide m.
    Danielson m.
    Defares rebreathing m.
    Devereux-Reichek m.
    digital color Doppler velocity
      integration m.

digitized caliper m.
Dodge area-length m.
Douglas bag collection m.
Dow m.
downstream sampling m.
dye-dilution m.
dynamic m.
edge-detection m.
Eggleston m.
Eicken m.
estimated Fick m.
Eve m.
Fick m.
Fick oxygen m.
flow convergence m.
forward triangle m.
Galanti-Giusti colorimetric m.
Gärtner m.
gas clearance m.
Gräupner m.
half-time m.
Hanley-McNeil m.
Hatle m.
head-tilt m.
Heinecke m.
helium dilution m.
Hetzel forward triangle m.
Howard m.
Hugenholtz m.
immunometric sandwich m.
indicator dilution m.
indocyanine green m.
Ionescu m.
Jaffe m.
Kales scoring m.
Kaplan-Meier m.
Kasser-Kennedy m.
Kennedy area-length m.
Kety-Schmidt m.
King biopsy m.
Kirkorian-Touboul m.
Kirstein m.
Konno biopsy m.
Laborde m.
Laurell m.
Lee-White m.
Lown and Woolf m.
Marriott m.
Meltzer m.
Monte Carlo multiway sensitivity
  analysis m.
Murphy m.

Narula m.
Ogata m.
Oliver-Rosalki m.
open circuit m.
Orsi-Grocco m.
oxygen step-up m.
Pachon m.
Penaz volume-clamp m.
Penn m.
phenylephrine ramp m.
planimetry m.
polarographic m.
prick-test m.
prism m.
proximal flow convergence m.
pulse m.
Purmann m.
pyramid m.
m. of Quinones
Rackley m.
m. of Rackley
Raff-Glantz derivative m.
rebreathing m.
Rechtschaffen scoring m.
Roche-Microwell plate
  hybridization m.
root inclusion m.
Sandler-Dodge area-length m.
Satterthwaite m.
Scarpa m.
Schiller m.
Schüller m.
Shimazaki area-length m.
Sigma m.
Silvester m.
sliding scale m.
Stanford biopsy m.
steady-state m.
Stegemann-Stalder m.
Strauss m.
Theden m.
thermodilution m.
Thom flap laryngeal
  reconstruction m.
Thompson-Hatina m.
Thrombo-Wellcotest m.
Tomita m.
triphenyl tetrazolium staining m.
TUNEL m.
Van Slyke m.
von Claus chronometric m.
V-slope m.

M

NOTES

method *(continued)*
    Wardrop m.
    Weir m.
    Weiss logarithmic m.
    Welcker m.
    Westergren m.
    Willett-Stampfer m.
    Wilson-White m.
methohexital
methotrexate
methoxamine
    m. hydrochloride
methoxsalen
methoxyisobutyl
    m. isonitrile (MIBI)
    m. isonitrile single-photon emission computed tomography (MIBI-SPECT)
2-methoxyisobutyl isonitrile
    technetium hexakis 2-m. i.
methoxyphenamine hydrochloride
8-methoxypsoralen
methyclothiazide
    m. and cryptenamine tannates
    m. and deserpidine
    m. and pargyline
methyl
    M. bromide
    M. isocyanate
    Oreton M.
    M. prednisolone
methyldichloroarsine
methyldopa
    chlorothiazide and m.
    m. and hydrochlorothiazide
methylene
    m. blue
    m. diphenyl diisocyanate (MDI)
    m. diphenyl diisocyanate asthma
    m. diphosphonate (MDP)
methylenetetrahydrofolate
    m. reductase (MTHFR)
    m. reductase gene
    m. reductase genotype
methylisocyanate
methylphenidate
methylprednisolone (MTP)
    m. acetate
    sodium m.
    m. succinate
methyltestosterone
    estrogen, m.
    Premarin With M.
methylxanthine
methysergide maleate
Meticorten Oral
metoclopramide hydrochloride
metocurine iodide

metolazone
metoprolol
    m. CR
    M. CR/XL Controlled Release Randomized Intervention Trial in Heart Failure (MERIT-HF)
    M. in Dilated Cardiomyopathy (MDC)
    m. OROS tablet
    m. succinate
    m. tartrate
    M. and Xamoterol Infarction Study (MEXIS)
Metras catheter
Metrix
    M. atrial defibrillation system
    M. Atrioverter
    M. IAD
    M. implantable atrial defibrillator
metrizamide contrast medium
metrocyte
Metro I.V. injection
metronidazole
Metroxamine
metyrosine
Metzenbaum scissors
MeV
    megaelectron volt
Mevacor lovastatin tablet
mevalonate acid
mevinolin
Mewi-5 sidehole infusion catheter
Mewissen infusion catheter
Mexican bean weevil asthma
mexiletine hydrochloride
MEXIS
    Metoprolol and Xamoterol Infarction Study
Mexitil
Meyer cartilage
Meyerding retractor
Mezlin
mezlocillin sodium
MFAT
    multifocal atrial tachycardia
MFF
    metal fume fever
MFG
    manofluorography
    middle frontal gyrus
MFH
    malignant fibrous histiocytoma
MFSR
    maximum expiratory airflow-static lung elastic recoil pressure
MFVL
    maximal flow-volume envelope
    maximum flow-volume loop

mg
> fluvastatin sodium 80 mg

MGA
> malposition of great arteries

Mgb
> myoglobulin

MGC Cardi-O2 cycle ergometer

MgCO₃
> magnesium carbonate

mg/kg
> milligrams per kilogram
>> mg/kg per day

MHA-TP
> microhemagglutination *Treponema pallidum*
>> MHA-TP test

M-HEART
> Multi-Hospital Eastern Atlantic Restenosis Trial

MHHP
> Minnesota Heart Health Program

MHz
> megahertz

MI
> myocardial infarction
> myocardial ischemia
>> elevation MI
>> Enoxaparin and TNK-tPA with/without GP IIb/IIIa Inhibitor as Reperfusion Strategy in ST Elevation MI (ENTIRE)
>> non-Q MI
>>> non-Q-wave myocardial infarction

mibefradil

MIBG
> metaiodobenzylguanidine
>> I-123 MIBG
>> I-125 MIBG

MIBI
> methoxyisobutyl isonitrile
>> MIBI SPECT
>> MIBI stress test
>> technetium-99m MIBI

MIBI-SPECT
> methoxyisobutyl isonitrile single-photon emission computed tomography
>> Tc-99 MIBI-SPECT

MIC
> minimum inhibitory concentration

MICABG
> minimally invasive coronary bypass grafting

mica pneumoconiosis

Micardis

micdadei
> *Legionella m.*
> *Tatlockia m.*

Michelson bronchoscope

miconazole

Micor catheter

MICRhoGAM

Micrins microsurgical suture

Micro
> M. Delta/Max Delta system
> M. II stent
> M. Minix pacemaker
> M. Mist nebulizer
> M. Plus spirometer
> M. stent
> M. Stent II
> 6 M. Stent PL

microaerosol

MicroAir
> M. handheld nebulizer
> M. Model NE U03

microalbuminuria

microanastomosis
> laser-assisted m. (LAMA)

microaneurysm
> Charcot-Bouchard m.

microangiopathic anemia

microangiopathy
> cerebral m. (CMA)
> coronary m.
> thrombotic m.

microarousal scoring

microarray analysis

microaspiration

microatelectasis

microatheroma

microatheromatosis

microballoon
> Rand m.

microbiologic brushing

microbrushing

microbubble (MB)
> m. persistence

microbulldog clip

Micro-Bumintest
> Bayer Corp. M.-B.

microcalcification

Microcap handheld capnograph

microcardia

M

NOTES

microcatheter
    Cardima Pathfinder m.
    end-hole Tracker m.
    Excelsior 1018 m.
    Pathfinder m.
    Pathfinder mini m.
    Revelation endocardial m.
    Terumo SP hydrophilic-polymer-coated m.
    Tracker m.
microcavitation
microcentrum
MicroChamber
microcirculation
microcirculatory
    m. adaptation
    m. vasoconstriction
MicroCO carbon monoxide monitor
Micrococcus
microcontaminant
microcrystal
microdensitophotometric quantification
microdialysis
MicroDigitrapper-HR
MicroDigitrapper-S apnea screening device
microelectrode
    tungsten m.
microemboli
    gaseous m.
microembolic signal (MES)
microembolism
microembolization
microfibril
microfibrillar collagen hemostat
microfilaria
microflora
    bronchial m.
MicroGard
MicroGas 7650 transcutaneous monitoring system
micrognathia
Micro-Guide catheter
MicroHartzler ACS balloon catheter system
microhemagglutination *Treponema pallidum* **(MHA-TP)**
microinfarct
microinvasive
Microjet Quark portable pump
microjoule
Micro-K 10
Microknit
    M. arterial graft
    M. patch graft
    M. vascular graft prosthesis
MicroLab ML3300

microlaryngoscope
    Dedo-Jako m.
microlaryngoscopy
    Thornell m.
Microlith
    M. pacemaker pulse generator
    M. P pacemaker
microlithiasis
    pulmonary alveolar m.
Microloop
MicroLoop
    M. II
    M. II handheld spirometer
    M. ML3535
micromanometer
    m. catheter
    m. catheter system
    catheter-tip m. system
micromanometry
MicroMewi multiple sidehole infusion catheter
Micromonospora
micromultiplane transesophageal echocardiographic probe
Micronase
micronebulizer
    Bird m.
microNefrin
microneurography
microneutralization test
micronized progesterone
micron needle
micronodular dissemination
Micronor
Micron Res-Q implantable cardioverter-defibrillator
micronutrient balance
Microny SR+ pulse generator
microorganism
microparticle
microphage
    fat-laden m.
Micropolyspora faeni
micropuncture
    M. guidewire
    M. introducer needle
    m. introducer set
    M. Peel-Away introducer
microreentry
MicroRint portable airway resistance meter
Microsampler device
microsatellite instability
microscope
    acoustic m.
    electron m.
    epi illuminated m.
    scanning electron m. (SEM)

microscopic polyangiitis
microscopy
    darkfield m.
    electron m.
    intravital m.
    intravital capillary video m.
    light m.
microsecond pulsed flashlamp pumped dye laser
Microsoftrac catheter
microsomal triglyceride transfer protein (MTP)
MicroSpacer
microsphere
    m. perfusion scintigraphy
    polystyrene latex m.
    radiolabeled m.
    Ultrasound Contrast M.
microsphygmy
microsphyxia
Micross
    M. dilatation catheter
    M. SL balloon
microsteatosis
Microstent stent
Microstream carbon dioxide measuring technology
Microsulfon
MicroTach
    M. pneumotach
    M. pneumotachometer
Microthin P2 pacemaker
microthromboembolism
    pulmonary m.
microthrombosis
microthrombus
microti
    Babesia m.
    Mycobacterium m.
Microtip lead
microtome
    Cryo-Cut m.
    Stadie-Riggs m.
Micro-Tracer portable ECG
microvascular
    m. angina
    m. angiopathy (MVA)
    m. artery disease
    m. clamp
    m. decompression (MVD)
    m. dysfunction
    m. flow distribution

    m. free flap
    m. permeability
Microvasive
    M. Glidewire
    M. Rigiflex TTS balloon
    M. stiff piano wire guidewire
Microvel double velour graft
Microvena
    M. Amplatz Goose Neck snare
    M. Das Angel Wings occluder
MicroVent ventilator
microvessel
MicroView sheath-based IVUS catheter
microvolt T-wave alternans
microwave cardiac ablation system
Microzide
Mictrin
micturition syncope
MICU
    medical intensive care unit
MIDA
    M. CoroNet instrumentation
    M. 1000 monitoring system
Midamor
MIDAS
    Multicenter Isradipine/Diuretic Atherosclerosis Study
    Myocardial Infarction Data Acquisition System Study
midaxillary line
midazolam
MIDCAB
    Patency, Outcomes and Economics of M. (POEM)
    M. procedure
    M. system
MidCab
MIDCABG
    minimally invasive direct coronary artery bypass graft
midclavicular line (MCL)
midcoronary artery bypass
middiastolic
    m. murmur
    m. rumble
middle
    m. capsular artery
    m. cerebral artery (MCA)
    m. cerebral artery occlusion (MCAO)
    m. constrictor muscle of pharynx
    m. frontal gyrus (MFG)

M

NOTES

middle *(continued)*
    m. lobe bronchus
    m. lobe of right lung
    m. lobe syndrome
    m. ribs
midepigastric bruit
midexpiratory phase
mid-infrared pulsed laser
midinspiratory
midline shift
midlung zone
midnodal
    m. extrasystole
    m. rhythm
midodrine
midriff
midsagittal plane
midsystolic
    m. buckling
    m. buckling of mitral valve
    m. click syndrome
    m. closure of aortic valve
    m. dip
    m. murmur
    m. notching
midventricle
midventricular (MV)
midwall shortening
MIF
    mean inspiratory flow
mifarmonab
MIFR
    maximal inspiratory flow rate
migraine
    m. headache
    syncopal m.
    m. syncope
migrans
    erythema m.
    larva m.
    ocular larva m.
    thrombophlebitis m.
    visceral larva m.
migrated tumor
migrating
    m. pacemaker
    m. phlebitis
migration
    neural crest m.
    stent m.
migratory
    m. pneumonia
    m. pulmonary infiltrate
    m. thrombus
Mijnhard
    M. electrical cycloergometer
    M. Valugraph
Mikity-Wilson disease

Mikros pacemaker
Mikro-Tip
    M.-T. angiocatheter
    M.-T. micromanometer-tipped
    catheter
    M.-T. transducer
Milano
mild-intensity exercise
**mildly dilated congestive
cardiomyopathy (MDCM)**
Miles vena cava clip
miliary
    m. coccidioidomycosis
    m. embolism
    m. infection
    m. pattern
    m. tuberculosis
milieu
military
    m. antishock trousers (MAST)
    m. pattern
milk
    m. scan
    m. scintigraphy
milk-alkali syndrome
mill
    m. house murmur
    m. wheel, millwheel
    m. wheel murmur
Millar
    M. asthma
    M. Doppler catheter
    2F M. Instrument catheter
    M. Mikro-Tip catheter pressure
    transducer
    M. MPC-500 catheter
    M. TCB-500 transducer
mille-feuilles effect
Millenia
    M. balloon catheter
    M. portable vital sign monitor
    M. PTCA catheter
Miller
    M. elastic stain
    M. Fisher variant
    M. index
    M. maneuver
    M. septostomy catheter
milleri
    Streptococcus m.
miller's
    m. asthma
    m. lung
milliamperage
milliampere (mA)
millicurie (mCi)
milliequivalent (mEq)

milligrams
    m. per kilogram (mg/kg)
    m. per kilograms per day
millijoule (mJ)
Milliknit
    M. Dacron prosthesis
    M. vascular graft prosthesis
milliliter (mL)
    nanograms per m.
    m. per kilogram (mL/kg)
millimeters of mercury (mmHg)
millimole (mmol)
    m. per liter (mmol/L)
million
    m. international unit (MIU)
    parts per m. (ppm)
milliosmole (mOsm)
Millipore filter
millisecond (ms, msec)
milliunit (mU)
Millivent vascular graft prosthesis
millivolt (mV)
Mill-Rose
    M.-R. esophageal injector
    M.-R. Protected Specimen
      microbiology brush
millwheel (*var. of* mill wheel)
milrinone lactate
Miltex rib spreader
Miltner constraint compliance device
Milton edema
Mima-Herellea
mimetic
mineralocorticoid hormone
mineralocorticoid-induced hypertension
miner's
    m. asthma
    m. lung
    m. phthisis
Mingograf
    M. 62 6-channel electrocardiograph
    M. 82 recorder
Mingograph
mini
    m. arousal
    21 M. device
    M. Mental State Examination
      (MMSE)
    m. stroke
    M. Thin Asthma Relief
miniballoon
Minibird II

Miniclinic
    A-V M.
minicoil
MINI Crown stent
minidefibrillator
    Liteguard m.
Mini-Dose
    HypRho-D M.-D.
Mini-Gamulin Rh
MiniHEART low-flow nebulizer
26 Mini II device
Minilith pacemaker pulse generator
minimal
    m. alveolar concentration (MAC)
    m. leak technique
    m. luminal diameter (MLD)
minimally
    m. invasive coronary bypass
      grafting (MICABG)
    m. invasive direct coronary artery
      bypass
    m. invasive direct coronary artery
      bypass graft (MIDCABG)
    m. invasive direct coronary artery
      bypass procedure
    m. invasive procedure (MIP)
    m. invasive valve repair (MIVR)
    m. invasive valve replacement
      (MIVR)
Mini-Motionlogger Actigraph
minimum
    m. bactericidal concentration
    m. data set (MDS)
    m. data set system
    m. inhibitory concentration (MIC)
    m. lumen diameter (MLD)
Mini-Neb nebulizer
MiniOX
    M. IA oxygen analyzer
    M. oxygen analyzer
    M. 1000 oxygen analyzer
    M. 3000 Oxygen Monitor
Minipress
Mini-Profile
    M.-P. catheter
    M.-P. dilatation catheter
Miniscope MS-3
ministernotomy
Mini-Torr Plus NIPB monitor
Minitran Patch
Minix pacemaker
Minizide

M

NOTES

Minnesota
    M. antilymphocyte globulin (MAG)
    M. classification of ECG
    M. code
    M. criteria for high R wave
    M. ECG classification
    M. Heart Health Program (MHHP)
    M. Impedance Cardiograph
    M. Leisure Time Physical Activity
      Questionnaire
    M. Living with Heart Failure
      questionnaire
    M. Q-QS code
Minocin
    M. I.V. injection
    M. Oral
minocycline hydrochloride
Minodyl
minor
    m. fissure
    pectoralis m.
minores
    ductus sublinguales m.
minoxidil
Minoxigaine
Mintezol
Minuet DDD pacemaker
minute
    alveolar ventilation per m. (V_A)
    beats per m. (bpm)
    liter per m. (Lpm)
    m. output
    oxygen consumption per m. (VO_2)
    physiological dead space ventilation
      per m. (V_D)
    m. ventilation (V_E)
    m. volume
6-minute
    6-m. corridor walk test
    6-m. walking test (6-MWT)
minute-gun cough
Miochol
Miochol-E
miosphygmia
MIP
    maximal inspiratory pressure
    maximum inspiratory pressure
    minimally invasive procedure
MIP-1
    macrophage inflammatory protein-1
MIPm
Mipron digital computer-assisted
  calipers
mirabilis
    Proteus m.
Mirage
    M. nasal mask
    M. over-the-wire balloon catheter

mirror
    m. image dextrocardia
    m. movement
    van Helmont m.
mirror-image
    m.-i. brachiocephalic branching
    m.-i. laryngoscopy
    m.-i. lung syndrome
Mirsky
    formula of M.
    M. thick wall model
misery perfusion
mismatch
    ventilation/perfusion m.
    $\dot{V}/\dot{Q}$ m.
mismatching
    afterload m.
missed
    m. beat
    m. ostium sequence (MOS)
missense mutation
miss rate
mist
    AsthmaHaler M.
    Ayr saline nasal m.
    Bronitin M.
    Bronkaid M.
    cool m.
    Primatene M.
    m. tent
Mistogen
    M. nebulizer
    M. passover humidifier
Mistometer
    Isuprel M.
mite
    house dust m. (HDM)
Mithracin
MITI
    Myocardial Infarction Triage and
    Intervention
    MITI Project
mitis
    Streptococcus m.
mitochondrial
    m. biogenesis
    m. calcium deposition
    m. cardiomyopathy
    m. enzyme
    m. function
    m. genotype
    m. oxidative phosphorylation
    m. respiration
mitochondrion, pl. mitochondria
mitogen
mitogen-activated
    m.-a. kinase pathway
    m.-a. protein (MAP)

m.-a. protein kinase (MAPK)
m.-a. protein kinase kinase
mitogenic radiation
mitomycin
mitomycin, vinblastine, cisplatin (MVP)
mitotane
mitoxantrone hydrochloride
MITRA
Maximal Individual Therapy in Acute
Myocardial Infarction
MITRA clinical trial
mitral
m. annular area
m. annular calcification
m. annular calcium (MAC)
m. annulus calcification (MAC)
m. area
m. atresia
m. balloon commissurotomy
m. balloon valvotomy (MBV)
m. buttonhole
m. click
m. commissurotomy
m. E to F slope
m. E velocity curve
m. E-wave transmission
m. facies
m. first sound (M_1)
m. funnel
m. gradient
m. homograft
m. incompetence
m. insufficiency
m. leaflet
m. leaflet tip
m. murmur
m. opening snap (MOS)
m. orifice (MO)
m. prolapse murmur
m. prosthesis
m. regurgitant jet
m. regurgitation (MR)
m. regurgitation artifact
m. regurgitation murmur
m. restenosis
m. second sound (M_2)
m. stenosis (MS)
m. stenosis murmur
m. tap
m. valve (MV)
m. valve aneurysm
m. valve anulus

m. valve area (MVA)
m. valve billowing
m. valve closure index
m. valve commissurotomy
m. valve dilator
m. valve echocardiography
m. valve endocarditis
m. valve gradient (MVG)
m. valve homograft
m. valve hypoplasia
m. valve leaflet
m. valve prolapse (MVP)
m. valve prolapse syndrome
m. valve regurgitation
m. valve replacement (MVR)
m. valve valvotomy
m. valvotomy
m. valvulitis
m. valvuloplasty
mitrale
P m.
mitralis
facies m.
mitralism
mitralization
mitral-septal apposition
Mitroflow Synergy PC stented pericardial valve
mitrotricuspid facies
MIU
million international unit
mivacurium
mivazerol
MIVR
minimally invasive valve repair
minimally invasive valve replacement
mix
oncology m.
mixed
m. alveolar-interstitial pneumonitis
m. aneurysm
m. angina
m. apnea (MA)
m. asthma
m. beat
m. expired gas
m. flora
m. hematopoietic chimerism
m. levocardia
m. neurally mediated syncope
m. thrombus
m. venous blood

NOTES

M

mixed (*continued*)
    m. venous oxygen saturation
        (SvO$_2$)
mixed-dust pneumoconiosis
mixing
    convective gas m.
MixOMask
    OEM Venturi M.
mixture
    helium-oxygen m. (heliox)
mizoribine
mJ
    millijoule
MK-383
MK-499
MKIII
ML3300
    MicroLab M.
ML3535
    MicroLoop M.
mL
    milliliter
MLD
    minimal luminal diameter
    minimum lumen diameter
MLH
    multiple lobar hemorrhage
M-line protein
mL/kg
    milliliter per kilogram
MLR
    myocardial laser revascularization
        MLR procedure
MM
    modified Miller maneuver
MMA
    maxillomandibular advancement
MMAD
    mass median aerodynamic diameter
mMCAI
    malignant middle cerebral artery
    infarction
MMEF, MMF
    maximal midexpiratory flow
    maximum midexpiratory flow rate
MMEFR
    maximal midexpiratory flow rate
mmHg
    millimeters of mercury
MMI
    medial medullary infarction
MMO
    maxillomandibular osteotomy
M-mode
    motion mode
        M-mode echocardiogram
        M-mode echocardiography
        M-mode measurement

        omnidirectional M-mode
        M-mode recording
        M-mode stripchart recording
        M-mode transducer
mmol
    millimole
mmol/L
    millimoles per liter
MMP
    matrix metalloproteinase
        MMP-2
        MMP-9
        matrix-degrading neutral MMP
MMSE
    Mini Mental State Examination
MMTT
    Multicenter Myocarditis Treatment Trial
MMV
    mandatory minute volume
MMVF
    manmade vitreous fiber
Mn-SOD
    manganese superoxide dismutase
MO
    mitral orifice
Mobidin
mobile
    carina sharp and m.
    cor m.
    m. coronary care unit
    m. myxoma
    m. vegetation
mobilization
    secretion m.
Mobin-Uddin
    M.-U. filter system
    M.-U. sieve
    M.-U. vena cava filter
Mobitz
    M. II A-V heart block
    M. block
    M. second-degree block
    M. type A-V block
    M. type I A-V block
    M. type I, II atrioventricular block
    M. type II SA block
    M. types of atrioventricular block
MOCHA
    Multicenter Oral Carvedilol in Heart-
    Failure Assessment
        MOCHA Study
modafinil
modality
    pacing m.
    therapeutic m.
mode
    A-m.
    AAI m.

AAI rate-responsive m.
AAT m.
auto decremental m.
demand m.
fixed-rate m.
gated list m.
harmonic imaging m.
histogram m.
list m.
matrix m.
motion m. (M-mode)
noise-reversion m.
OOO m.
overdrive m.
pacing m.
passive m.
patient activator m.
rate-drop response m.
RDR m.
M. Selection Trial in Sinus Node
  Dysfunction (MOST)
m. switching
VDD m.
VDI m.
VVT m.

model
M. 6260 aspirator
M. 500 ECG/pulse oximeter
Hodgkin-Huxley m.
Mirsky thick wall m.
M. O2T oxygen analyzer
M. 326 portable aspirator
M. 40-400 Pruitt-Inahara shunt
Torricelli m.
Tracheostomy T.O.M.
  anatomical m.
windkessel m.

model-based image processing (MBIP)
moderate hypothermia
moderate-ramp protocol
moderator band
modification
A-V nodal m.
Mason-Likar limb lead m.
Mullins m.

modified
m. Blalock-Taussig shunt (MBTS)
m. brachial technique
m. Bruce protocol
m. Ellestad protocol
m. Fontan procedure

m. human graft umbilical vein
  graft
m. Mark IV R-wave-triggered
  power injector
m. Miller maneuver (MM)
m. multifactorial index of cardiac
  risk
m. Rashkind PDA occluder
m. Seldinger technique
m. shuttle test

modifier
leukotriene m.

MODS
multiple organ dysfunction syndrome

modulation
autonomic m.
brightness m.
rate m.

module
Capnostat Mainstream carbon
  dioxide m.
Co-Oximeter m.
Research Pneumotach System
  instrumentation m.

modulus
impedance m.
Peterson elastic m.
Young m.

Moduretic
Moe
M. hypothesis
M. multiple wavelet hypothesis
M. multiple wavelet hypothesis of
  atrial defibrillation

Moersch bronchoscope
moexipril
m. hydrochloride
m. and hydrochlorothiazide

mofetil
mycophenolate m.

**Mogul 3F steerable decapolar
  electrophysiology diagnostic**
moiety-conserved cycle
moist
Nasal M.
m. rale

moisturizer
Cann-Ease nasal m.
RoEzIt skin m.

mol
mole

M

NOTES

mold worker's lung
mole (mol)
molecular
    m. chemotherapy
    m. coincidence detection (MCD)
molecular-weight dextran
molecule
    cell adhesion m. (CAM)
    circulating adhesion m. (CAM)
    endothelium-leukocyte adhesion m.
     (E-LAM)
    E-selectin cell adhesion m.
    intercellular adhesion m. (ICAM)
    leukocyte-endothelial cell
     adhesion m.
    proatherothrombogenic m.
    P-selectin cell adhesion m.
    soluble adhesion m.
    soluble intracellular adhesion m.
     (sICAM)
molecule-1
    intercellular adhesion m. (ICAM-1)
    mucosal addresin cell adhesion m.
     (MadCAM-1)
    vascular cell adhesion m. (VCAM-
     1)
Molina needle catheter
Mol-Iron
Mollaret meningitis
mollis
    pulsus m.
molluscum contagiosum
Molnar disk
Moloney murine leukemia virus
molsidomine
molybdenum
moment
    magnetic m.
Momentum DR pacemaker
mometasone furoate
Monafed DM
Monaghan
    M. respirator
    M. 300 ventilator
Monaldi drainage system
Monarch Mini Mask nasal interface
Monark bicycle ergometer
Mönckeberg
    M. arrhythmia
    M. arteriosclerosis
    M. degeneration
    M. sclerosis
Monday
    M. dyspnea
    M. fever
Mondini pulmonary arteriovenous
  malformation

Mondor
    M. disease
    M. syndrome
Monge disease
Monilia albicans
monilial esophagitis
moniliasis
    chronic mucocutaneous m.
moniliformis
    Streptobacillus m.
Monit
Monitan
monitor
    Accucap CO_2/O_2 m.
    Accucom cardiac output m.
    Accutracker II ambulatory blood
     pressure m.
    Acuson V5M m.
    Acuson V5M transesophageal
     echocardiographic m.
    aerosol inhalation m. (AIM)
    AID-Check m.
    AM1 asthma m.
    ambulatory Holter m.
    AMI infant apnea m.
    APM-2000 vital signs m.
    apnea m.
    Arrhythmia Net arrhythmia m.
    automatic oscillometric blood
     pressure m.
    AvoSure PT m.
    Bedfont carbon monoxide m.
    Bedfont EC60 Gastrolyzer
     hydrogen m.
    bedside m.
    bioimpedance m.
    Biotrack coagulation m.
    BioZ.com cardiac output m.
    blood perfusion m. (BPM)
    CA m.
     cardiac-apnea monitor
    Caire Messenger Reporter m.
    Capintec nuclear VEST m.
    Capnocheck Plus NIPB m.
    cardiac m.
    cardiac apnea m.
    cardiac-apnea m. (CA monitor)
    CardioBeeper CB 12L cardiac m.
    Cardiocap/5 m.
    CardioDiary heart m.
    Cardioguard 4000
     electrocardiographic m.
    Cardiovit AT-10 m.
    Carity transportable m.
    Chronicle implantable
     hemodynamic m.
    Colin ambulatory BP m.
    Commucor A+V Patient m.

Corometrics m.
CO Sleuth carbon monoxide m.
CO_2SMO Plus m.
CO_2SMO Plus continuous
noninvasive respiratory profile m.
Cricket pulse oximetry m.
Criticare $ETCO_2/SpO_2$ m.
Datascope Accutor bedside m.
DeltaTrac II metabolic m.
Digitrapper MkIII sleep m.
Dinamap m.
Dinamap Accutorr A1, 3 blood
pressure m.
Dinamap blood pressure m.
Doplette m.
Doppler-Cavin m.
Doppler fetal heart m.
DynaPulse 5000A blood
pressure m.
EcoCheck oxygen m.
EC50 TOXCO breath carbon
monoxide m.
electrocardiographic
transtelephonic m.
electronic fetal m.
endotracheal cardiac output m.
(ECOM)
event m.
event recorder m.
Finapres blood pressure m.
HBT Sleuth portable hydrogen m.
HeartCard m.
Heart Rate 1-2-3 m.
HemoMatic blood collection m.
HemoTec activated clotting
time m.
Hewlett-Packard 78720 A SDN m.
Holter m.
Homochron m.
Insta-Pulse heart rate m.
KinetiX ventilation m.
King of Hearts Holter m.
m. leads
Life-Pack 5 cardiac m.
LifeShirt m.
loop m.
Magellan m.
Marquette 8000 Holter m.
MDILog microelectronic m.
MemoryTrace AT ambulatory
cardiac m.
MicroCO carbon monoxide m.

Millenia portable vital sign m.
MiniOX 3000 Oxygen M.
Mini-Torr Plus NIPB m.
MRM-2 oxygen consumption m.
Nellcor Nl000 $ETCO_2/SpO_2$ m.
Nellcor Symphony blood
pressure m.
Nellcor Symphony N-3100
noninvasive blood pressure m.
Neotrend multiparameter blood
gas m.
$NICO_2$ noninvasive cardiac
output m.
noninvasive m.
Novametrix NICO cardiac
output m.
NoxBOX m.
Ohio Vortex respiration m.
Ohmeda 6200, 6300 CO_2 m.
Omega 5600 noninvasive blood
pressure m.
One Touch blood glucose m.
OSD m.
O2SMO Plus respiratory profile m.
OxyData Plus oxygen m.
PAM2, PAM3 m.'s
Paramed Cardivon 9200
noninvasive blood pressure m.
Paratrend 7 continuous blood
gas m.
Paratrend 7+ multiparameter blood
gas m.
patient M.
PeakLog m.
Physios CTM 01 cardiac
transplant m.
Pick and Go m.
Polar Vantage XL heart rate m.
Porta-Resp m.
Pressurometer blood pressure m.
PrinterNOx nitric oxide/nitrogen
dioxide m.
Propaq Encore vital signs m.
Pulse Pro heart rate m.
Puritan Bennett 7250 metabolic m.
Q-TRAK IAQ m.
RIP portable sleep m.
Rossmax automatic wristwatch
blood pressure m.
SpaceLabs Holter m.
TCM30 transcutaneous oxygen m.
three-channel Holter m.

M

NOTES

445

monitor *(continued)*
TINA m.
transcutaneous oxygen m. (TCOM)
Trans-Scan 2100 noninvasive physiological m.
transtelephonic exercise m. (TEM)
Tri-Met apnea m.
VentCheck m.
VentCheck handheld respiratory m.
VenTrak respiratory mechanics m.
vest ambulatory ventricular function m.
video m.
V.I.P. Bird volume m.
VitalCare 506DX m.
Vitalograph BreathCO M.
Vitalograph pulmonary m.
WinABP ambulatory blood pressure m.
7200 with 7250 metabolic m.
monitor/defibrillator
Lifepak 5 m.
Lifepak 7 m.
Monitored Atherosclerosis Regression Study (MARS)
monitoring
ambulatory m.
ambulatory blood pressure m. (ABPM)
ambulatory electrocardiographic m. (AEM)
ambulatory Holter m. (AHM)
ambulatory oximetry m. (AOM)
beat-by-beat hemodynamic m.
Doptone m.
endotracheal cardiac output m. (ECOM)
hemodynamic m.
invasive m.
physiologic m.
physiological m.
pleural space m.
pulse oximetry m. (POM)
transtelephonic ambulatory m. (TAM)
transtelephonic arrhythmia m. (TTM)
transtelephonic cardiac event m.
Moniz carotid siphon
Monneret pulse
monoamine
m. oxidase (MAO)
m. oxidase inhibitor (MAOI)
monobactam
monoballoon
monocarboxylate/proton cotransporter (MCT)
monocarboxylate transporter (MCT)

monocardiogram
Mono-Cedocard
Monocid
Monoclate-P
monoclonal
m. antibody 3G4
m. antimyosin antibody
m. hypothesis
m. theory of atherogenesis
MonoClone immunoenzymetric assay
monocrotaline
monocrotic pulse
monocrotism
monocrotus
pulsus m.
monocyte
m. chemoattractant protein (MCP)
m. chemoattractant protein-1 (MCP-1)
m. chemotactic and activating factor (MCAF)
m. chemotactic protein-1 (MCP-1)
surface adherent m. (SAM)
transcardiac m.
monocytic leukemoid reaction
monocytogenes
Listeria m.
monodisperse
Monodox Oral
monofilament
m. absorbable suture
m. polypropylene suture
Semmes-Weinstein m.
monofoil catheter
monoform tachycardia
Mono-Gesic
monohydrate
cefadroxil m.
cephalexin m.
Monojector
Monoket
Monolyth oxygenator
monomer
actin m.
fibrin m. (FM)
monometer-tipped catheter
N^G**-monomethyl-L-arginine (L-NMMA)**
monomorphic ventricular tachycardia (MVT)
mononeuritis multiplex
Mononine
mononitrate
isosorbide m.
mononuclear cell
mononucleosis
infectious m.
monophasic
m. action potential (MAP)

m. action potential duration (MAPD)
m. complex
m. contour of QRS complex
m. pulse
m. shock therapy
m. waveform
monophonic wheeze
monophosphate
adenosine m. (AMP)
cyclic adenosine m. (cAMP)
cyclic guanosine m. (cGMP)
cyclic nucleotide adenosine m.
guanosine m. (GMP)
monoplace chamber
monoplanar method of Green
monopolar temporary electrode
Monopril
Monorail
M. angioplasty catheter
M. guidewire
M. imaging catheter
M. Speedy balloon
monoresistance
monosaturated fat
Monostrut cardiac valve prosthesis
monosulfate
guanethidine m.
monotest
R-lactate enzyme m.
monotherapy
M. Assessment of Ranolazine in Stable Angina (MARISA)
monotypic lesion
Mono-Vacc
Monovial
Cardizem M.
monoxide
carbon m. (CO)
diffusing capacity of lung for carbon m. (DLCO)
monoxide-oximetry
monoxime
butanedione m.
Monro
foramen of M.
Monte Carlo multiway sensitivity analysis method
montelukast sodium
Montgomery
M. Safe-T-Tube

M. speaking valve
M. tracheostomy
Montgomery-Asberg Depression Rating Scale (MADRS)
month
Lupron Depot-3 M.
Lupron Depot-4 M.
Moody friction factor
moon face
Moore
M. procedure
M. tracheostomy button
mopamidol
Moraxella
M. catarrhalis
M. nonliquefaciens
morbidity
morbid obesity
Morbillivirus
morcellation
Morch respirator
Morestin syndrome
Moretz clip
Morgagni
M. disease
foramen of M.
M. hernia
M. nodule
Morgagni-Adams-Stokes
M.-A.-S. syncope
M.-A.-S. syndrome
Morganella morganii
morganii
Morganella m.
moribund
moricizine
moriens
ultimum m.
morphine
morphologic
morphology
hills-and-valley m.
QRS m.
valvular m.
windsock m.
morphometric measurement
morphometry
aerosol-derived airway m. (ADAM)
airway m.
lung m.
Morquio-Brailsford disease
Morquio syndrome

M

NOTES

morrhuate sodium
Morrow procedure
Morse
>M. manifest
>M. manifold

mortality rate (MR)
Mortara Instruments ELI-100XR 12-lead ECG
mortis
>myocardial rigor m.

Morton cough
MOS
>missed ostium sequence
>mitral opening snap

mosaic
>M. cardiac bioprosthesis
>m. jet
>m. jet signals
>m. pattern
>m. perfusion
>M. porcine bioprosthetic heart valve

Moschcowitz
>M. disease
>M. sign
>M. test

Moses sign
Mosher life-saving tracheal tube
mOsm
>milliosmole

mosquito
>m. clamp
>m. hemostat

moss-agate sputum
Mosso sphygmomanometer
MOST
>Mode Selection Trial in Sinus Node Dysfunction

motexafin lutetium
motility
>esophageal m.
>receptor for hyaluronan-mediated m. (RHAMM)

motion
>atrioventricular junction m.
>chest wall m.
>cusp m.
>diastolic m.
>m. display echo
>endocardial m.
>fetal atrial wall m.
>fetal ventricular wall m.
>infarct zone wall m.
>interventricular septal m.
>leaflet m.
>m. mode (M-mode)
>paradoxic wall m.
>plaque m.

>precordial m.
>regional wall m.
>right ventricular wall m.
>segmental wall m.
>septal wall m.
>systolic anterior m. (SAM)
>tricuspid annular m. (TAM)
>ventricular wall m.
>wall m.
>whorl m.

motoneuron
motor
>M. Assessment Scale (MAS)
>M. Club Assessment test of motor activity
>m.-exploratory hemineglect
>m. neglect
>m. provoked potential (MEP)

motoricity
motorized transducer pullback device
Motrin IB Sinus
MOTT
>mycobacteria other than tuberculosis

mottling
>m. of extremities
>quantum m.

Moulaert
>muscle of M.

moulin
>bruit de la roue de m.

Mounier-Kuhn syndrome
mountain sickness
Mount-Mayfield forceps
Moure esophagoscope
mouse
>pleural m.

mousetail pulse
Mousseau-Barbin esophageal tube
mouth of aneurysm
mouthpiece
>pneumotach disposable m.
>SafeTway m.
>SafeTway pediatric m.

mouth-to-mouth
>m.-t.-m. respiration
>m.-t.-m. resuscitation
>m.-t.-m. ventilation

movable
>m. core straight safety wire guide
>m. heart
>m. pulse

Movat
>M. pentachrome
>M. stain

movement
>air m.
>ameboid m.
>anomalous m.

m. arousal index (MAI)
ciliary m.
circus m.
m. disorder
mirror m.
nonrapid eye m. (NREM)
periodic leg m. (PLM)
precordial m.
quality of m. (QOM)
rapid eye m. (REM)
m.-related cortical potential (MRCP)
M. Science physiotherapy
vessel wall m.
moxalactam
Moxam
moxibustion
moxifloxacin HCl
moxonidine
moyamoya
m. disease
m. of heart
Moynahan syndrome
Moynihan respirator
MPA
main pulmonary artery
medroxyprogesterone acetate
MPAP
mean pulmonary artery pressure
MPAWP
mean pulmonary artery wedge pressure
MP-H
mandibular plane to hyoid
MPHR
maximum predicted heart rate
MPI
macrophage inflammatory protein
MPM
malignant pleural mesothelioma
MPO
myeloperoxidase
M-Prednisol injection
M-protein serotype
MPS
myocardial protection system
MPT
multiple-parameter telemetry
MR
mitral regurgitation
mortality rate
MR 290 humidification chamber
MR lead

MRA
magnetic resonance angiography
3D TOF MRA
TOF MRA
MRCA
magnetic resonance coronary
angiography
respiratory gated MRCA
MRCP
movement-related cortical potential
MRD
mean reference diameter
MRF
magnetic resonance flowmetry
MRFIT
Multiple Risk Factor Intervention Trial
MRI
magnetic resonance imaging
CASL-PI MRI
cine gradient-echo MRI
continuous arterial spin-labeled
perfusion MRI (CASL-PI MRI)
diffusion MRI
diffusion-weighted MRI
DSC MRI
dynamic susceptibility contrast-
enhanced MRI
FLASH MRI
functional MRI
Gd-DTPA-enhanced MRI
GE Signa 1.5-T MRI
gradient echo-cine MRI
GRASS MRI
hemodynamically-weighted MRI
(HW)
intravascular MRI
low-dose dobutamine cine MRI
perfusion imaging MRI
perfusion-weighted MRI (PWI)
Philips ACS NT 1.5 Gyroscan
MRI
Siemens Magnetom 1.5-T MRI
spin-echo MRI
MRI stroke
ThromboScan MRI
Toshiba MRT 200 MRI
T2-weighted MRI
MRI velocity mapping
MRI-identified stroke
MRM-2 oxygen consumption monitor
mRNA
messenger ribonucleic acid

M

NOTES

mRNA *(continued)*
    osteopontin mRNA
    skeletal alpha-actin mRNA
MRS
    magnetic resonance spectroscopy
MRT Tidal Humidifier
MRV
    magnetic resonance venography
MRX-113 contrast agent
MRX-408 contrast agent
MS
    mitral stenosis
        MS Classique balloon dilatation
        catheter
        MS Classique catheter
MS-3
    Miniscope MS-3
MS-857
ms
    millisecond
MS-325 contrast agent
MS-CIS SV stent
MSD Enteric Coated ASA
m/sec
    meter per second
msec
    millisecond
MSI
    magnetic source imaging
    metered solution inhaler
        MSI pulmonary drug delivery
MSLT
    Multiple Sleep Latency Test
MSM-BMS stent
MSM-CIS system
MSM-Stent
    M.-S. stent
    M.-S. SV stent
MSNA
    muscle sympathetic nerve activity
MSOF
    multisystem organ failure
MSPECT
    three-dimensional M.
MST
    median survival time
    MST cryoprobe
MSVC
    maximal sustainable ventilatory capacity
MT-100 ECG Holt system
MTB
    Mycobacterium tuberculosis
MTC catheter
MTD
    maximum tolerated dose
    MTD test
MTHFR
    methylenetetrahydrofolate reductase

MTHFR gene
MTHFR genotype
MT-MMP
    membrane-bound membrane-type
    metalloproteinase
MTP
    methylprednisolone
    microsomal triglyceride transfer protein
    MTP gene
M-type alpha 1-antitrypsin
MU
    megaunit
mU
    milliunit
Much
    M. bacillus
    M. granules
mucicarmine stain
mucin
    epithelial m.
mucinous
    m. adenocarcinoma
    m. carcinoma
mucoactive
    m. medication
    m. therapy
mucociliary
    m. clearance (MCC)
    m. efficiency
    m. escalator
    m. system
    m. transport
mucocutaneous
    m. lesion
    m. lymph node syndrome
mucoepidermoid carcinoma
mucoepithelial dysplasia
Muco-Fen-DM
Muco-Fen-LA
mucogenicum
    Mycobacterium m.
mucoid
    m. exopolysaccharide
    m. impaction
    m. medial degeneration
mucokinetic
mucolipidosis, pl. **mucolipidoses**
    m. III
mucolytic
    classic m.
    peptide m.
mucomembranous
Mucomyst
mucopolysaccharide
    acid m. (AMP)
mucopolysaccharidosis,
    pl. **mucopolysaccharidoses**
mucopurulent sputum

mucopus
Mucor
Mucor-Absidia
Mucoraceae
mucoregulatory agent
mucoretention cyst
mucormycosis
    pulmonary m.
mucosa
    airway m.
    m. of bronchus
    esophageal m.
    region of respiratory m.
    respiratory m.
    tracheal m.
mucosal
    m. addresin cell adhesion
      molecule-1 (MadCAM-1)
    m. edema
    m. ischemia
mucoserous
Mucosil
mucous
    m. cell
    m. desiccation
    m. gel
    m. gland hyperplasia
    m. gland hypertrophy
    m. layer
    m. plugging
    m. rale
    m. sheets
    m. thread
mucoviscidosis
mucus
    m. hypersecretion
    m. inhibitor
    low-viscosity m.
    oyster mass of m.
    m. plug
    m. production
    m. retention
    m. secretion
    tenacious m.
    thick and sticky m.
    m. transport
    viscid m.
    m. viscosity
MUE
    medication-use evaluation

Mueller
    M. maneuver
    M. sign
Muerto Canyon virus
muffled heart sounds
MUGA
    multiple gated acquisition
    MUGA cardiac blood pool scan
    MUGA exercise stress test
    MUGA scan
    MUGA scanning
**Mui Scientific 6-channel esophageal
pressure probe**
Muller
    M. banding
    M. test
Müller
    M. catheter guide
    M. experiment
    M. maneuver
    M. sign
    M. vena caval clamp
Mullins
    M. blade and balloon septostomy
    M. blade technique
    M. cardiac device
    M. catheter introducer
    M. dilator
    M. modification
    M. modification of transseptal
      catheterization
    M. sheath
    M. sheath/dilator
    M. sheath system
    M. transseptal catheter
    M. transseptal catheterization sheath
    M. transseptal sheath
multiaccess catheter (MAC)
multiaxis accelerometer
multibreath nitrogen washout technique
multicanalicular rupture
multicellular stent
multicenter
    M. Acute Stroke Trial (MAST)
    M. American Research Trial with
      Cilazapril after Angioplasty to
      Prevent Transluminal Coronary
      Obstruction and Restenosis
      (MARCATOR)
    M. Antiatherosclerotic Study
      (MAAS)
    M. Dilated Cardiomyopathy (MDC)

M

NOTES

multicenter *(continued)*
  M. Investigation for the Limitation of Infarct Size
  M. Isradipine/Diuretic Atherosclerosis Study (MIDAS)
  M. Myocarditis Treatment Trial (MMTT)
  M. Oral Carvedilol in Heart-Failure Assessment (MOCHA)
  M. Stents Ticlopidine (MUST)
  M. Stent Study (MUST)
  M. Ultrasound Stent in Coronary Artery Disease (MUSIC)
  M. Unsustained Tachycardia Trial (MUSTT)
Multicor II cardiac pacemaker
multicrystal gamma camera
multidisciplinary pulmonary rehabilitation program
Multi-Dop X/TCD transcranial Doppler instrument
multidrug-resistance
multidrug-resistant (MDR)
  m.-r. *Streptococcus pneumoniae* (MDRSP)
  m.-r. tuberculosis (MDR-TB)
multielectrode
  m. basket catheter
  m. impedance catheter
  m. probe
multielement linear array
multifactorial cough
Multifit system risk management of heart attack patient
multiflanged Portnoy catheter
Multiflex catheter
Multi-Flex stent
multifocal
  m. atrial tachycardia (MAT, MFAT)
  m. lesion
  m. micronodular pneumocyte hyperplasia
  m. supraventricular tachyarrhythmia
multiform
  m. premature ventricular complex
  m. tachycardia
multiforme
  erythema m.
multigated angiography
Multigon 500M non-contrast-enhanced TCD
multihead detector
Multi-Hospital Eastern Atlantic Restenosis Trial (M-HEART)
multiinfarct dementia
multikringle glycoprotein
multilamellar body

multilayer design catheter
Multileaf collimator device
multilesion angioplasty
Multi-Link
  M.-L. Ascent stent
  M.-L. coronary stent system
  M.-L. Duet stent
  M.-L. Solo stent
  M.-L. Tetra coronary stent system
  M.-L. Tristar balloon
Multilith pacemaker
multilobar disease
multilocular cyst
multilocularis
  Echinococcus m.
multimer assay
multinucleated giant cell
Multipax
multiplace chambers
multiplanar reconstruction technique
multiplane
  m. echocardiography
  m. transesophageal echocardiography
multiple
  m. CVIs
  m. embolism
  m. gated acquisition (MUGA)
  m. gated acquisition cardiac blood pool scan
  m. gated acquisition scan
  m. lentigines syndrome
  m. lipoprotein-type hyperlipidemia
  m. lobar hemorrhage (MLH)
  m. meningotheloid nodule
  m. organ dysfunction syndrome (MODS)
  m. point electrode
  M. Risk Factor Intervention Trial (MRFIT)
  m. sclerosis
  m. shunt levels
  M. Sleep Latency Test (MSLT)
  m. system atrophy
multiple-balloon valvuloplasty
multiple-organ
  m.-o. dysfunction
  m.-o. failure
multiple-parameter telemetry (MPT)
multiple-trauma patient
multiplex
  m. catheter
  mononeuritis m.
  m. neuropathy
multipolar
  m. catheter
  m. catheter electrode
  m. electrode catheter
multiprogrammable pulse generator

Multipurpose-SM catheter
multisensor catheter
multisite
    m. biventricular pacing
    m. mapping
    m. pacing
MultiSPIRO
    M. Clear Advantage pulmonary
      function filter
    M. computerized spirometry
    M. DX-Portable spirometry
    M. The Peak peak flowmeter
Multistage Maximal Effort exercise
  stress test
multisystem organ failure (MSOF)
multitargeted antifolate
Multitest cell-mediated immunity system
multivalve insufficiency
multivalvular
    m. disease
    m. disease murmur
Multi-Vent
    Hudson M.-V.
multivessel
    M. Angioplasty Prognosis Study
      (MAPS)
    m. coronary artery disease
    m. coronary artery obstruction
    m. disease (MVD)
multiwire gamma camera
multocida
    Pasteurella m.
mupirocin
muqueux
    rales m.
mural
    m. aneurysm
    m. endocarditis
    m. endocardium
    m. thrombi
    m. thrombosis
    m. thrombus
Murat sign
Murgo pressure contour
mu rhythm
murmur
    accidental m.
    amphoric m.
    anemic m.
    aneurysmal m.
    aortic m.
    aortic-left ventricular tunnel m.

aortic-mitral combined disease m.
aortic regurgitation m.
aortic stenosis m.
apex m.
apical mid-diastolic heart m.
apical systolic heart m.
arterial m.
atriosystolic m.
atrioventricular flow rumbling m.
attrition m.
Austin Flint m.
basal diastolic m.'s
bellows m.
blood m.
blowing m.
blubbery diastolic m.
brain m.
Bright m.
bronchial collateral artery m.
Cabot-Locke m.
carcinoid m.
cardiac m.
cardiopulmonary m.
cardiorespiratory m.
Carey Coombs m.
Carey Coombs short mid-
  diastolic m.
carotid artery m.
click m.
coarse m.
Cole-Cecil m.
congenital m.
continuous m.
continuous heart m.
cooing m.
Coombs m.
crescendo m.
crescendo-decrescendo m.
Cruveilhier-Baumgarten m.
decrescendo m.
deglutition m.
diamond ejection m.
diamond-shaped m.
diastolic m.
diastolic decrescendo m.
direct m.
Docke m.
dove coo musical m.
Duroziez m.
dynamic m.
early diastolic m.
early-peaking systolic m.

M

NOTES

murmur *(continued)*
ejection m.
end-diastolic m.
endocardial m.
end-systolic m.
Eustace Smith m.
exit block m.
exocardial m.
expiratory m.
extracardiac m.
Fisher m.
Flint m.
Fräntzel m.
friction m.
functional m.
Gallavardin m.
Gibson m.
goose-honk m.
grade 1 through 6 m.
Graham Steell m.
Graham Steell heart m.
groaning m.
Hamman m.
harsh m.
heart m.
hemic m.
high-frequency m.
high-pitched m.
Hodgkin-Key m.
holodiastolic m.
holosystolic m.
honking m.
hourglass m.
humming m.
humming-top m.
incidental m.
indirect m.
innocent m.
innocent m. of elderly
innocent heart m.
inorganic m.
inspiratory m.
lapping m.
late apical systolic m.
late diastolic m.
late-peaking systolic m.
late systolic m.
left ventricular-right atrial
  communication m.
Levine grade 1–6 cardiac m.
low-frequency m.
low-pitched m.
machinery m.
Makin m.
mammary souffle m.
middiastolic m.
midsystolic m.
mill house m.

mill wheel m.
mitral m.
mitral prolapse m.
mitral regurgitation m.
mitral stenosis m.
multivalvular disease m.
muscular m.
musical m.
noninvasive m.
nun's m.
nun's venous hum m.
obstructive m.
organic m.
outflow m.
pansystolic m.
Parrot m.
patent ductus arteriosus m.
pathologic m.
pericardial m.
physiologic m.
pleuropericardial m.
prediastolic m.
presystolic m.
primary pulmonary hypertension m.
protodiastolic m.
pulmonary m., pulmonic m.
rasping m.
reduplication m.
regurgitant m.
respiratory m.
Roger m.
rumbling diastolic m.
Rytand m.
scratchy m.
seagull m.
seesaw m.
Steell m.
stenosal m.
Still m.
subclavian m.
subclavicular m.
systolic m.
systolic apical m.
systolic ejection m. (SEM)
systolic regurgitant m.
to-and-fro m.
transmitted m.
Traube m.
tricuspid m.
vascular m.
venous m.
ventricular septal defect m.
vesicular m.
water wheel m.
whooping m.

Murphy
M. method
M. percussion

Murray score
muscarinic
    m. agonist
    m. receptor
    m. stimulation
muscle
    accessory m.
    accessory inspiratory m.
    airway smooth m. (ASM)
    anterior papillary m. (APM)
    m. artifact
    m. bridge
    bronchial smooth m.
    bronchoesophageal m.
    cardiac m.
    Chassaignac axillary m.
    m. ergoreceptor
    m. fraction enzyme of CPK (CPK-MM, CPK-3)
    m. immunocytochemical study
    latissimus dorsi m.
    m. metaboreflex
    m. of Moulaert
    Oehl m.
    papillary m.
    pectinate m.
    pleuroesophageal m.
    posterior cricoarytenoid m.
    posterior papillary m. (PPM)
    rectus abdominis m.
    Reisseisen m.
    m. relaxant
    ribbon m.'s
    serratus anterior m.
    skeletal m.
    m. stiffness
    strap m.
    m. sympathetic nerve activity (MSNA)
    m. of thorax
    m. trabeculation
    trachealis m.
    transversus nuchae m.
    venous smooth m.
muscles
muscular
    m. bridging
    m. coat of bronchus
    m. coat of esophagus
    m. coat of trachea
    m. contraction
    m. dystrophy

    m. incompetence
    m. murmur
    m. subaortic stenosis
    m. venous pump
    m. ventricular septal defect (MVSD)
musculoskeletal pain
musculus
    m. bronchoesophageus
    m. diaphragma
    m. levator glandulae thyroideae
    m. pleuroesophageus
mush clamp
mushroom
    m. dust
    m. worker's disease
    m. worker's lung
MUSIC
    Multicenter Ultrasound Stent in Coronary Artery Disease
    MUSIC clinical trial
musical
    m. bruit
    m. murmur
    m. rale
Musset sign
MUST
    Medication Use Studies
    Multicenter Stents Ticlopidine
    Multicenter Stent Study
    MUST clinical trial
Mustang steerable guidewire
Mustard
    M. atrial baffle
    M. operation
    M. procedure
    M. repair
mustard
    L-phenylalinine m.
    nitrogen m.
Mustard/Senning procedure
Mustargen Hydrochloride
MUSTT
    Multicenter Unsustained Tachycardia Trial
Mutamycin
mutant allele
mutation
    factor V Leiden m.
    missense m.
    SCN5A m.
    thrombophilic factor V Leiden m.

M

NOTES

mute
  m. reflex
  m. toe sign
muzolimine
MV
  maximal ventilation
  mechanical ventilation
  midventricular
  mitral valve
mV
  millivolt
MVA
  malignant ventricular arrhythmia
  microvascular angiopathy
  mitral valve area
MVC
  maximal vital capacity
  maximum voluntary contraction
MVD
  microvascular decompression
  multivessel disease
  myocardial vasodilation
MVE-50 implantable myocardial electrode
MVG
  mitral valve gradient
MVO$_2$
  myocardial oxygen consumption
MVP
  mitomycin, vinblastine, cisplatin
  mitral valve prolapse
    MVP catheter
MVR
  maximal ventilation rate
  mitral valve replacement
MVSD
  muscular ventricular septal defect
MVT
  monomorphic ventricular tachycardia
MVV
  maximum voluntary ventilation
    MVV ventilator
6-MWT
  6-minute walking test
myalgia gravis
Myambutol
myasthenia
  m. cordis
  m. gravis
  m. gravis pseudoparalytica
myasthenic crisis
MyBP-C
  myosin-binding protein-C
    MyBP-C gene
mycetoma
MycoAKT latex bead agglutination test

mycobacteria
  nontuberculous m. (NTM)
  m. other than tuberculosis (MOTT)
mycobacterial
  m. disease
Mycobacterium
  M. abscessus
  M. africanum
  M. aquae
  M. avium
  M. avium complex (MAC)
  M. avium complex infection
  M. avium-intracellulare (MAI)
  M. avium-intracellulare complex
  M. avium-intracellulare infection
  M. bovis
  M. chelonae
  M. fortuitum
  M. fortuitum-chelonel
  M. gastri
  M. genavense
  M. gordonae
  M. haemophilum
  M. intracellulare
  M. intracellulare, Battey bacillus
  M. kansasii
  M. leprae
  M. malmoense
  M. marinum
  M. microti
  M. mucogenicum
  M. peregrinum
  M. phlei
  M. scrofulaceum
  M. simiae
  M. smegmatis
  M. szulgai
  M. terrae
  M. thermoresistable
  M. tuberculosis (MTB)
  M. ulcerans
  M. vaccae
  M. xenopi
Mycobutin Oral
mycology
mycophenolate
  m. mofetil
  m. mofetil capsule
  m. mofetil intravenous for injection
  m. mofetil oral suspension
  m. mofetil tablet
Mycoplasma
  M. faucium
  M. hominis
  M. incognitus
  M. pneumoniae
  M. xenopi
mycoplasmal pneumonia

mycoplasmosis
Mycoscint
mycosis
    m. fungoides
    Posadas m.
    pulmonary m.
Mycostatin Topical
mycotic
    m. aortic aneurysm
    m. aortography
    m. endocarditis
    m. infection
MycroMesh graft material
mycroPhylax implantable cardioverter-
    defibrillator
mydriatic
myectomy
    septal m.
myeloma
myelonecrosis
myeloperoxidase (MPO)
myelosuppression
Myers Solution
Mykrox
Mylar catheter
Myleran
Myminic Expectorant
myocardial
    m. abscess
    m. adrenergic signaling
    m. angiogenesis
    m. anoxia
    m. band (MB)
    m. band enzymes of CPK (CPK-MB, CPK-2)
    m. band index
    m. bed
    m. blood flow (MBF)
    m. blush
    m. bridge
    m. bridging (MB)
    m. cell hypertrophy
    m. clamp
    m. cold-spot perfusion scintigraphy
    m. collagen matrix
    m. concussion
    m. contractility
    m. contrast echocardiography (MCE)
    m. contrast echo study
    m. contusion
    m. creatine phosphate

m. depolarization
m. depressant factor (MDF)
m. depressant substance (MDS)
m. depression
m. disarray
m. disease
m. Doppler velocity (MDV)
m. edema
m. electrode
m. endothelin
m. energy
m. failure
m. fiber shortening
m. fibrosis
m. fibrous scar
m. fractional flow reserve (FFR_{myo})
m. function
m. hamartoma
H-form m. infarction
m. hibernation
m. hypertrophy
m. hypoperfusion
m. indirect calorimetry
m. infarction (MI)
M. Infarction Data Acquisition System
M. Infarction Data Acquisition System Study (MIDAS)
m. infarction in dumbbell form
M. Infarction Triage and Intervention (MITI)
m. infiltrative process
m. infundibular stenosis
m. injury
m. insufficiency
m. ischemia (MI)
m. ischemic syndrome
m. jeopardy
m. jeopardy index
m. lactate extraction
m. laser revascularization (MLR)
m. laser revascularization procedure
m. lead
m. long-chain fatty acid uptake defect
m. malnutrition
m. mass
m. metabolism
m. muscle creatine kinase isoenzyme (CK-MB)
m. necrosis
m. oxygen consumption (MVO_2)

M

NOTES

myocardial (*continued*)
>   m. oxygen demand
>   m. oxygen supply
>   m. oxygen uptake
>   m. perforation
>   m. perfusion
>   m. perfusion imaging
>   m. perfusion scintigraphy
>   m. perfusion study
>   m. protection
>   m. protection system (MPS)
>   m. remodeling
>   m. repolarization
>   m. reserve
>   m. revascularization
>   m. rigor mortis
>   m. rupture
>   m. salvage
>   m. scar tissue
>   m. scintigraphy
>   m. sinusoid
>   m. sparing
>   m. stiffness
>   m. stunning
>   m. tension
>   m. tissue
>   m. vasodilation (MVD)
>   m. viability
>   m. viability scintigraphy

myocardiograph

myocardiopathy
>   alcoholic m.
>   chagasic m.

myocardiorrhaphy

myocardiotomy

myocarditic

myocarditis
>   acute isolated m.
>   asymptomatic m.
>   atrial m.
>   bacterial m.
>   burned out viral m.
>   cardiac sarcoidosis m.
>   chronic m.
>   clostridial m.
>   coxsackievirus m.
>   cryptococcal m.
>   diphtheritic m.
>   echovirus m.
>   Fiedler m.
>   fragmentation m.
>   fulminant m.
>   giant cell m.
>   helminthic m.
>   *Histoplasma* m.
>   hypersensitivity m.
>   idiopathic m.
>   indurative m.

>   metazoal m.
>   parenchymatous m.
>   peripartum m.
>   protozoal m.
>   rheumatic m.
>   rickettsial m.
>   spirochetal m.
>   syphilitic m.
>   toxic m.
>   tuberculoid m.
>   viral m.

myocardium
>   dysfunctional m.
>   dyssynergic m.
>   fragmentation of m.
>   hibernating m.
>   hypertrophied m.
>   hypoperfused m.
>   ischemic m.
>   isolated noncompaction of the ventricular m. (INVM)
>   jeopardized m.
>   postischemic m.
>   reperfused m.
>   senescent m.
>   spongy m.
>   stunned m.
>   underperfused m.
>   viable m.
>   vulnerable m.

myocardosis
>   Reisman m.

myocyte
>   amplifying m.
>   Anichkov m.
>   cardiac m.
>   m. deenergization
>   m. hypertrophy
>   m. hypoxia
>   m. magnesium stores
>   m. metabolic activity
>   m. necrosis

myocytolysis
>   coagulative m.
>   m. of heart

myoendocarditis

myofascial

myofibril

myofibrillar
>   m. ATPase
>   m. calcium level
>   m. disarray
>   m. lysis

myofibroblast

myofibrosis cordis

myofilament
>   m. calcium responsiveness
>   m. contractile activation

myogenic theory
myoglobin assay
myoglobinuria
myoglobulin (Mgb)
    m. cardiac diagnostic test
myoglobulinuria
myointimal plaque
myolysis
    cardiotoxic m.
myomalacia cordis
myopathia cordis
myopathy
    centronuclear m.
    myotubular m.
    nemaline m.
    tachycardia-induced m.
myopericarditis
myopexy
myoplasmic calcium
myoplasty
myopleuropericarditis
Myopore lead
Myoscint
myosin
    cardiac m.
    m. heavy chain
    m. light chain
myosin-binding
    m.-b. protein-C (MyBP-C)
    m.-b. protein-C gene
myosin-specific antibody
myositis
MYOtherm XP cardioplegia delivery
  system
myotomy
    hyoid m.
    septal m.
myotomy-myectomy-septal resection
myotonia congenita
myotonic muscular dystrophy

myotubular myopathy
Myoview contrast material
MyoVive
Myowire II cardiac electrode
Myphetane DC
myrtillus
    Vaccinium m.
Mystic balloon catheter
Mytussin
    M. AC
    M. DAC
    M. DM
myurous
myurus
    pulsus m.
myxedema
    m. heart
    pretibial m.
myxedematous
myxoma, pl. myxomata
    atrial m.
    cardiac m.
    familial atrial m.
    infected m.
    left atrial m.
    left ventricular m.
    mobile m.
    petrified cardiac m.
    right atrial m.
    right ventricular m.
    stone-like m.
    m. tumor
    ventricular m.
myxomatous
    m. change
    m. degeneration
    m. proliferation
    m. pulmonary embolism
    m. valve disease

M

NOTES

N

N cell
N High Sensitivity CRP assay
N region

N=1 trial

Number Equal to One; Single Patient
Trial

N₂

nitrogen
N_2 oximetry

N/2 artifact
n-3 fatty acid
n-6 fatty acid
N-13

nitrogen-13
N-13 ammonia
N-13 ammonia uptake

***N*-acetylneuraminic acid**
***N*-acetyl procainamide (NAPA)**
Nachlas tube
NACI

New Applications for Coronary
Interventions
New Approaches to Coronary
Intervention
NACI clinical trial
NACI Gianturco-Roubin
New Applications for Coronary
Interventions, Gianturco-Roubin
NACI Palmaz-Schatz
NACI registry

NACI DCA

New Approaches to Coronary
Intervention Registry Directional
Coronary Atherectomy
NACI DCA study

NACPTAR

North American Cerebral Transluminal
Angioplasty Registration

nacre dust asthma
NAD

nicotinamide adenine dinucleotide

nadir of QRS complex
nadolol
Nadopen-V
nadroparin calcium
Naegleria gruberi
NAEP

National Asthma Education Program

NAEPP

National Asthma Education and
Prevention Program

nafamostat
nafate

cefamandole n.

nafazatrom
Nafcil injection
nafcillin sodium
naftidrofuryl
Nagle exercise stress test
Na⁺/H⁺

N. exchange inhibitor (NHEI)
N. exchanger (NHE)

nail

n. bed
cyanosis of n. beds
n.-fold skin
n.-patella disease
n. pulse
n.-to-nail bed angle

NaK-ATPase
Nakayama

N. anastomosis
N. anastomosis apparatus

nalbuphine hydrochloride
Naldecon

N. DX Adult Liquid
N. Senior EX

Nalfon
nalidixic acid
Nallpen injection
nalmefene hydrochloride
naloxone hydrochloride
naltrexone
NAME

nevi, atrial myxoma, myxoid
neurofibromas, and epheledes
NAME syndrome

Namic

N. angiographic syringe
N. catheter

NAMIS

Nifedipine Angina Myocardial Infarction
Study

**N-13 ammonia positron emission
tomography**
nandrolone decanoate
NANIPER

nonallergic noninfectious perennial
rhinitis

nanograms per milliliter
nanomole (nmol)
Nanos 01 pacemaker
NAPA

N-acetyl procainamide

nape

transverse muscle of n.

napkin-ring

n.-r. calcification

napkin-ring *(continued)*
    n.-r. defect
    n.-r. stenosis
Naprosyn
naproxen
Naqua
Narcan injection
Narco
    N. Biosystems recorder
    N. Physiograph-6B recorder
narcolepsy
Narcomatic flowmeter
narcosis
    inert gas n.
    nitrogen n.
narcotic
NARES
    nonallergic rhinitis with eosinophilia
narrow communication
narrow-complex tachycardia
narrowed pulse pressure
NarrowFlex intraaortic balloon catheter
narrowing
    atherosclerotic n.
    eccentric n.
    intracoronary stenting of de
      novo n.
    longitudinal n.
    luminal n.
    ostial n.
    restenotic n.
Narula method
Nasabid
Nasacort AQ
nasal
    n. airway
    n. asthma
    n. cannula
    Concentraid N.
    n. continuous positive airway
      pressure (NCPAP, nCPAP)
    n. CPAP
    n. CPAP system
    DDAVP N.
    Drixoral N.
    n. flaring
    N. Moist
    N. Moist Gel
    n. nicotine spray (NNS)
    n. nocturnal ventilation (NNV)
    n. part of pharynx
    n. pharynx
    n. polyposis
    n. pool technique
    n. positive pressure ventilation
      (NPPV)
    n. prongs
    n. steroid (NS)

    triamcinolone inhalation, n.
    n. vibrissa
Nasalcrom Nasal Solution
Nasalide Nasal Aerosol
Nasarel
nascent HDL
NASCET
    North American Symptomatic Carotid
    Endarterectomy Trial
nasi
    ala n.
    regio respiratoria tunicae
      mucosae n.
nasobronchial reflex
nasogastric
    n. tube
    n. tube feeding (NTF)
nasopharyngeal (NP)
    n. carcinoma
    n. groove
    n. reflux
    n. secretion
    n. wash
nasopharyngitis
nasopharyngoscopy
nasopharynx
nasosinus-bronchial reflex
nasotracheal
    n. intubation
    n. suction
    n. tube
Nathan test
national
    N. Asthma Education and
      Prevention Program (NAEPP)
    N. Asthma Education Program
      (NAEP)
    N. Cholesterol Education Program
      (NCEP)
    N. Cholesterol Education Program
      guidelines
    N. Emphysema Treatment Trial
      (NETT)
    N. Health and Nutrition
      Examination Survey
    N. Health and Nutrition
      Examination Survey I
    N. Health Service (NHS)
    N. Heart, Lung, Blood Institute
      (NHLBI)
    N. Heart, Lung, Blood
      Institute/National Asthma
      Education Prevention Program
      (NHLBI/NAEPP)
    N. High Blood Pressure Education
      Program (NHBPEP)
    N. Home Oxygen Patients
      Association

N. Institutes of Health (NIH)
N. Institutes of Health left ventriculography catheter
N. Institutes of Health marking catheter
N. Institutes of Health mitral valve-grasping forceps
N. Institutes of Health Stroke Scale (NIHSS)
N. Institutes of Neurological Disorders and Stroke (NINDS)
N. Institutes of Neurological Disorders and Stroke-Tissue Plasminogen Activator Stroke Trial (NINDS-TPAST)
N. Lung Health Education Program (NLHEP)
N. Nosocomial Infection Surveillance
N. Registry of Myocardial Infarction (NRMI)

native
n. coarctation
n. coronary anatomy
n. coronary artery
n. LDL (n-LDL)
n. tissue harmonic imaging
n. valve
n. valve endocarditis (NVE)
n. valve fibroplastic endocarditis
n. vessel

Natrecor
Natrilix
natriuresis
natriuretic
n. hormone
n. peptide

natural
n. frequency
n. history
n. killer (NK)
n. resistance macrophage-associated protein (Nramp)

Naturetin
Naughton
N. cardiac exercise treadmill test
N. graded exercise stress test
N. protocol
N. treadmill protocol

Nauheim
N. bath
N. treatment

NavAblator catheter
Navelbine
Navidrex
Navier-Stokes equation
navigation
intracardiac n.
navigator echo signal
Naviport deflectable tip guiding catheter
Navistar catheter
Navius stent
n-BCA
n-butyl cyanoacrylate
NBIH cardiac device
NBTE
nonbacterial thrombotic endocarditis
n-butyl cyanoacrylate (n-BCA)
NC
N. balloon
N. Bandit ball
N. Bandit catheter
N. Cobra balloon
NCA
normal coronary arteries
NCEP
National Cholesterol Education Program
NCEP guidelines
NCEP-II guidelines
NCEP Step-One Diet
N95-Companion
NCPAP, nCPAP
nasal continuous positive airway pressure
Aladdin^{II} NCPAP
NCPAP therapy
NCV
nerve conduction velocity
NDA
new device angioplasty
Nd:YAG
neodymium:yttrium-aluminum-garnet
Nd:YAG laser
NE
norepinephrine
near
n. field
n. patient test (NPT)
near-fainting
near-field visualization
near-gain
near-infrared
n.-i. cerebral oximetry
n.-i. spectroscopy (NIRS, NIS)

N

NOTES

near-syncope
nebacumab
Nebcin injection
nebivolol
NebuChamber
Nebuhaler
Nebules
    Ventolin N.
nebulization
    aqueous solution for n.
    continuous albuterol n. (CAN)
    wet n.
nebulized
    n. bronchodilator
    n. Ig therapy
    n. tobramycin
nebulizer
    Acorn II n.
    AeroEclipse breath actuated n.
    aerosol n.
    AeroSonic personal ultrasonic n.
    AeroTech II n.
    air-powered n.
    Babbington-type n.
    baffled jet n.
    BESTNEB n.
    Centimist n.
    N. Chronolog
    compressor-generated n. (CGN)
    Compu-Neb ultrasonic n.
    DeVilbiss n.
    handheld n.
    Heart n.
    Hope Continuous & HELIOX n.
    Incenti-neb n.
    IV-Heart n.
    jet n.
    Marquest Respirgard II n.
    MicroAir handheld n.
    Micro Mist n.
    MiniHEART low-flow n.
    Mini-Neb n.
    Mistogen n.
    PermaNeb reusable n.
    Pulmo-Aide n.
    Respirgard II n.
    Schuco n.
    Sidestream n.
    small-volume n. (SNV, SVN)
    Sonix 2000 ultrasonic n.
    Tote-A-Neb n.
    Twin Jet n.
    ultrasonic n.
    UniHEART IV universal n.
    UniHEART universal n.
    Updraft handheld n.
    VixOne small-volume n.
NebuPent Inhalation

Necator americanus
necessitatis
    empyema n.
neck
    transverse artery of n.
necrobacillosis
necrobiosis lipoidica diabeticorum
necrobiotic nodule
necroformis
    Bacillus n.
necrolysis
    toxic epidermal n.
necrophorum
    Fusobacterium n.
necrophorus
    Sphaerophorus n.
necropsy
necrosis, pl. necroses
    avascular n.
    coagulation n.
    contraction band n.
    cystic medial n.
    digital n.
    dirty n.
    embolic n.
    Erdheim cystic medial n.
    n. factor
    fibrinoid n.
    ischemic n.
    liquefaction n.
    medial n.
    myocardial n.
    myocyte n.
    pressure n.
    renal cortical n.
    tissue n.
    tubular n.
necrotic cyst
necrotisans
    phlebitis nodularis n.
necrotizing
    n. angiitis
    n. arterial disease
    n. arteriolitis
    n. bronchopneumonia
    n. granuloma
    n. granulomatous vasculitis
    n. pneumonia
    n. vasculitis
nedocromil sodium
needle
    Abrams n.
    Adson aneurysm n.
    Aldrete n.
    argon n.
    Arrow-Fischell EVAN n.
    arterial n.
    n. aspirate

aspirating n.
Atraloc n.
atraumatic n.
Becton-Dickinson Teflon-sheathed n.
Bengash n.
beveled thin-walled n.
Brockenbrough n.
Brockenbrough curved n.
Brughleman n.
butterfly n.
Cardiopoint n.
Chiba n.
Cooley aortic vent n.
Cope pleural biopsy n.
Cope thoracentesis n.
Cournand n.
Cournand-Grino angiography n.
Cournand-Potts n.
Crown n.
Curry n.
DLP cardioplegic n.
Dos Santos n.
ergonomic vascular access n.
  (EVAN)
Ethalloy n.
eyeless n.
Fergie n.
Ferguson n.
Fischer pneumothoracic n.
Flynt n.
Frederick pneumothorax n.
front wall n.
27G n.
n. holder
Hustead n.
Jamshidi n.
large-bore slotted aspirating n.
Lewy-Rubin n.
Lowell pleural n.
Luer-Lok n.
Menghini n.
micron n.
Micropuncture introducer n.
Nordenstrom Rotex II biopsy n.
O'Brien airway n.
olive-tipped n.
PercuCut biopsy n.
percutaneous cutting n.
pilot n.
polytef-sheathed n.
Potts n.

Potts-Cournand n.
Quincke-point spinal n.
Ranfac n.
Rashkind septostomy n.
Retter n.
Riley n.
Rochester n.
root n.
Ross n.
Rotex n.
Rotex II biopsy n.
Safe Step blood-collection n.
scalp vein n.
Seldinger n.
slotted n.
standard n.
steel-winged butterfly n.
Stifcore aspiration n.
Stifcore biopsy injection n.
THI n.
thin-walled n.
thoracentesis n.
n. thoracostomy
Tru-Cut biopsy n.
UMI n.
Venflon n.
Vim-Silverman n.
Wang transbronchial n.
Wasserman n.
Zavala lung biopsy n.
needlepoint electrocautery
Needle-Pro needle protection device
NEEP
  negative end-expiratory pressure
NEFA
  nonesterified fatty acid
  NEFA scintigraphy
nefazodone
Neff percutaneous access set
negative
  n. chronotropism
  n. contrast
  n. end-expiratory pressure (NEEP)
  n. expiratory pressure (NEP)
  n. inotrope
  n. intrapleural pressure
  n. predictive value (NPV)
  n. pressure
  n. pressure ventilation (NPV)
  n. remodeling
  n. treppe

NOTES

negative *(continued)*
    n. T wave
    n. U wave
negative-contrast
    n.-c. injection
    n.-c. intravascular ultrasound
NegGram
neglect
    motor n.
    perceptual-sensory n.
    unilateral spatial n. (USN)
    visuospatial n.
Negri body
Negus bronchoscope
Negus-Broyles bronchoscope
Nehb D lead
Neisseria
    N. catarrhalis
    N. gonorrhoeae
    N. meningitidis
neisserial
nelfinavir
Nellcor
    N. N2500 ETCO$_2$ multigas
      analyzer
    N. N1000 ETCO$_2$/SpO$_2$ monitor
    N. N200 pulse oximeter
    N. Puritan Bennett (NPB)
    N. Puritan Bennett Sandman 2.4
      polysomnogram
    N. Symphony blood pressure
      monitor
    N. Symphony N-3100 noninvasive
      blood pressure monitor
    N. Symphony N-3000 pulse
      oximeter
nemaline myopathy
Nembutal
NENAR
    noneosinophilic nonallergic rhinitis
neoadjuvant chemotherapy
neoangiogenesis
neocapilarization
Neo-Codema
Neo-Durabolic
neodymium:yttrium-aluminum-garnet
  (Nd:YAG)
    n.-a.-g. laser
neoendothelium
Neofed
NEO-fit
    N.-f. endotracheal tube grip
    N.-f. neonatal endotracheal tube
      holder
Neoflex bendable knife
neoformans
    Cryptococcus n.
neoglottis

neointima
neointimal
    n. generation
    n. hyperplasia
    n. hyperplastic response
    n. proliferation
    n. ridge
    n. tear
    n. thickening
    n. tissue
NeoKnife electrosurgical instrument
neolumen
neomycin sulfate
neonatal
    Exosurf N.
    N. internal jugular puncture kit
    N. Y TrachCare
neonate respiratory distress syndrome
  (NRDS)
neonatorum
    apnea n.
    asphyxia n.
neoplasia
neoplasm
    extrathoracic n.
neoplastic
    n. cavity
    n. cell
    n. disease
    n. pericarditis
neopterin
    serum n.
Neoral cyclosporine capsule
Neosar injection
Neo-Sert umbilical vessel catheter
  insertion set
Neos M pacemaker
Neo-Synephrine
    N.-S. 12 Hour Nasal Solution
NeoTect
Neo-Therm neonatal skin temperature
  probe
Neothylline
Neotrend
    N. multiparameter blood gas
      monitor
    N. system
neovascularization
NeoVO-2-R volume control resuscitator
NEP
    negative expiratory pressure
    neutral endopeptidase
Nephril
nephritis, pl. **nephritides**
    familial n.
    immune-mediated membranous n.
    tuberculous n.
Nephro-Fer

nephrogenesis
nephrogenic diabetes insipidus
nephrogram
nephron
nephropathic cardiomyopathy
nephropathy
    analgesic n.
    diabetic n.
    hypertensive n.
    hyperuricemic n.
nephrosclerosis
nephrostolithotomy
    percutaneous n. (PCNL)
nephrotic syndrome
nephrotoxicity
NEP-I, NEPi
    neutral endopeptidase inhibition
neprilysin
Neptune high-pressure PTCA balloon
  catheter
Nernst equation
nerve
    accelerator n.
    accompanying artery of ischiadic n.
    accompanying artery of median n.
    n. action potential
    aortic n.
    axillary n.
    brachial n.
    cardiac sensory n.
    cardiopulmonary splanchnic n.'s
    carotid sinus n.
    n. conduction velocity (NCV)
    cranial n.'s I–XII
    esophageal branches of the
      vagus n.
    external branch of superior
      laryngeal n.
    faucial branches of lingual n.
    glossopharyngeal n.
    n. of Hering
    hypoglossal n.
    inferior ganglion of
      glossopharyngeal n.
    internal branch of superior
      laryngeal n.
    n. of Kuntz
    laryngeal n.
    left recurrent laryngeal n.
    lingual branch of facial n.
    pharyngeal branch of
      glossopharyngeal n.

    pharyngeal branch of vagus n.
    phrenic n.
    right recurrent laryngeal n.
    sensory n.
    sympathetic n.
    thoracic n.
    trigeminal n.
    ulnar n.
    vagus n.
nervi
    ganglion inferius n.
    ganglion superius n.
Nervocaine Injection
nervorum
    vasa n.
nervosa
    anorexia n.
    dysphagia n.
nervous
    n. asthma
    n. respiration
    n. system
    n. tachypnea
nesiritide
Nestor guiding catheter
Nestrex
nest of veins
net
    n. absorption
    Arrhythmia N.
    Jahnke-Barron heart support n.
netilmicin sulfate
Netromycin injection
NETT
    National Emphysema Treatment Trial
network
    Chiari n.
    fibrillar collagen n.
    interstitial and perivascular
      collagen n.
    local area n. (LAN)
    Organ Procurement and
      Transplantation N. (OPTN)
    Platelet IIb/IIIa Antagonist for the
      Reduction of Acute Coronary
      Syndrome Events in a Global
      Organization N. (PARAGON)
    Purkinje n.
Neubauer artery
Neucalm-50 Injection
neuf
    bruit de cuir n.

NOTES

N

Neupogen
neural
    n. crest malformation
    n. crest migration
neuralgia
    glossopharyngeal n.
neurally
    n. mediated syncopal syndrome
    n. mediated syncope (NMS)
    n. mediated vasovagal syncope
    (NMVS)
neurapraxia
neurenteric cyst
neurilemoma
neuritis
    optic n.
neuroblastoma
neurocardiac
neurocardial syncope
neurocardiogenic syncope
neurocirculatory asthenia
neurodegenerative disease
neurodiagnostics
neuroendocrine
    n. theory
    n. tumor
neuroepithelial body
neurofibrillary tangle
neurofibroma
neurofibromatosis
neurogenic
    n. abnormality
    n. pulmonary edema
    n. theory
    n. tumor
neurohormonal
    n. arterial constriction
    n. function
neurohormone
neurohumoral
    n. factors
    n. stimulus
neurokinin A (NKA)
neuroleptic
neurologic
    n. DCS
    n. deficit
    n. examination
    n. status
neurological disorder
neuromediated syncope
neuromuscular
    n. blockade
    n. blocking agent (NMBA)
    n. disease
    n. disorder
    n. hypertension
neuromyopathic disorder

neuromyopathy
    carcinomatous n.
neuronal ceroid lipofuscinosis
neuron-specific enolase (NSE)
neuropathy
    angiopathic n.
    diabetic n.
    diabetic autonomic n. (DAN)
    multiplex n.
    peripheral n.
    vasculitic n.
neuropeptide
neuropeptide Y
Neuroperfusion pump
neuroprotection
neuroprotective
    n. agent
    n. drug
neurosis, pl. neuroses
    anxiety n.
    cardiac n.
neurosyphilis
neuroticism
neurotoxic effect
Neuro-Trace instrument
Neurotrac II EEG
neurotransmission
    sympathetic n.
neurotransmitter substance
neurovascular bundle
NeuroVasx
    N. catheter
    N. submicroinfusion catheter
neuroxanthoendothelioma
neutral
    n. endopeptidase (NEP)
    n. endopeptidase inhibition (NEP-I,
    NEPi)
    n. endopeptidase inhibitor
Neutrexin injection
neutriceutical
neutron activation analysis
neutropenia
neutropenic angina
neutrophil
    n. elastase
    polymorphonuclear n. (PMN)
    segmented n.'s
neutrophilia
    pleural fluid n.
neutrophil-induced pulmonary
  inflammation
NEV
    noninvasive extrathoracic ventilator
nevi (pl. of nevus)
Neville
    N. stent
    N. tracheal prosthesis

nevirapine
nevobilol
nevus, pl. **nevi**
    n. araneus
    nevi, atrial myxoma, myxoid
    neurofibromas, and ephelides
    (NAME)
    lentigines, atrial myxoma,
    mucocutaneous myxomas, and
    blue nevi (LAMB)
new
    N. Applications for Coronary
    Interventions (NACI)
    N. Applications for Coronary
    Interventions, Gianturco-Roubin
    (NACI Gianturco-Roubin)
    N. Applications for Coronary
    Interventions, Palmaz-Schatz
    N. Approaches to Coronary
    Intervention (NACI)
    N. Approaches to Coronary
    Intervention Registry Directional
    Coronary Atherectomy (NACI
    DCA)
    N. Approaches to Coronary
    Interventions registry
    N. device angioplasty (NDA)
    N. Glucorder analyzer
    N. Orleans endarterectomy stripper
    N. Weavenit Dacron prosthesis
    N. York Heart Association
    (NYHA)
    N. York Heart Association
    functional classification (I–IV)
newborn
    persistent pulmonary hypertension
    of n. (PPHN)
    respiratory distress syndrome of
    the n.
    transient tachypnea of n. (TTNB)
NewLife
    N. Elite concentrator
    N. oxygen concentrator
Newport
    N. E100M ventilator
    N. ventilator
    N. Wave VM200
Newton
    N. catheter
    N. guidewire
    N. law of motion and variables
NexStent carotid stent

Nexus
    N. coronary stent
    N. 2 linear ablation catheter
NF
    Nissen fundoplication
NF-ATc protein
NF-kappa-B
    nuclear factor-κB
N-geneous HDL cholesterol test
NH
    N. region
    N. region of A-V node
NHBPEP
    National High Blood Pressure Education
    Program
NHE
    Na^+/H^+ exchanger
NHEI
    Na^+/H^+ exchange inhibitor
NHLBI
    National Heart, Lung, Blood Institute
NHLBI/NAEPP
    National Heart, Lung, Blood
    Institute/National Asthma Education
    Prevention Program
NHS
    National Health Service
Niacels
niacin
niacinamide
niacin/lovastatin
    extended-release n.
Niaspan
NiCad
    nickel-cadmium
nicardipine hydrochloride
Nic the Asthmatic Dragon aerosol
mask
nickel
    salt of n.
nickel-cadmium (NiCad)
    n.-c. battery
Nickerson-Kveim test
nicking
    arteriovenous n.
Nicks procedure
niclofolan
Nicobid
Nicoderm Patch
nicofuranose
Nicoladoni-Branham sign
Nicoladoni sign

N

NOTES

Nicolar
Nicolet
 N. Biomedical UltraSom
  computerized sleep analysis
 N./EME Muller and Moll probe
  fixation device
NICO$_2$ noninvasive cardiac output
 monitor
nicorandil
Nicorette
 N. Gum
 N. Plus
Nicostatin
nicotinamide adenine dinucleotide (NAD)
2-nicotinamidoethyl nitrate
nicotine
 crystalline n.
 n. gum
 n. inhaler
 n. nasal spray
 n. transdermal patch
Nicotinex
nicotinic acid
Nicotrol
 N. Inhaler
 N. NS nasal spray
 N. Patch
nicoumalone
NIDDM
 noninsulin-dependent diabetes mellitus
nidulans
 Aspergillus n.
nidus
Niemann-Pick disease
nifedipine
 N. Angina Myocardial Infarction
  Study (NAMIS)
 n. enzyme immunoassay
Niferex
niger
 Aspergillus n.
night
 N. Owl pocket polygraph
 n. terrors
NightBird nasal CPAP
nightsweats
Niglycon
nigra
 cardiopathia n.
nigrum
 Epicoccum n.
NIH
 National Institutes of Health
  NIH cardiomarker catheter
  NIH left ventriculography catheter
  NIH marking catheter
  NIH mitral valve-grasping forceps
  NIH Xenopus Initiative

Nihon Kohden
 N. K. CFV-3000
 N. K. model 4412P
  polysomnogram
 N. K. Polygraph system
NIHSS
 National Institutes of Health Stroke Scale
Nikaidoh-Bex technique
Nikaidoh translocation
nikethamide
Niko-Fix
Nilandron
Nilstat Topical
nilutamide
Nimbex
Nimbus hemopump
nimesulide
nimodipine
Nimotop
NINDS
 National Institutes of Neurological
  Disorders and Stroke
NINDS-TPAST
 National Institutes of Neurological
  Disorders and Stroke-Tissue
  Plasminogen Activator Stroke Trial
Nine-Turn lead
NI-NR
 no infection-no rejection
NIP
 nonspecific chronic interstitial
  pneumonitis
NIPB
 noninvasive blood pressure
nipple
 aortic n.
NIPPV
 noninvasive positive pressure ventilation
Nipride
NIPS
 noninvasive programmed stimulation
NIR
 N. Adante monorail catheter shaft
 N. 5 Cell stent
 N. 7 Cell stent
 N. 9 Cell stent
 N. ON Ranger
 N. Primo Monorail stent
 N. Royal stent
 N. stent
 N. with SOX coronary stent
  system
 N. with SOX over-the-wire
  coronary stent system
NIROYAL
 N. Advance stent
 N. Elite stent

NIRS, NIS
  near-infrared spectroscopy
Nisocor
nisoldipine
Nissen
  N. 360-degree wrap fundoplication
  N. fundoplication (NF)
niter paper
NiteView polysomnography system
nitinol
  n. filter
  n. mesh stent
  n. petal
  n. polymeric compound
  n. self-expandable stent
  n. self-expanding coil stent
  n. snare
  n. thermal memory stent
nitrate
  long-acting n.
  2-nicotinamidoethyl n.
  peroxyacetyl n.
  n. resistance
nitrendipine
nitric
  n. oxide (NO)
  n. oxide synthase (NOS, NOS1)
  n. oxide synthase gene therapy
  n. oxide system
nitrite
  amyl n.
  sodium n.
Nitro-Bid
  N.-B. I.V. injection
  N.-B. Ointment
  N.-B. Oral
nitroblue tetrazolium
Nitrocap
Nitrocels
Nitrocine Oral
Nitro-Dial
Nitrodisc Patch
Nitro-Dur Patch
Nitrodyl
nitrofurantoin
Nitrogard Buccal
nitrogen (N_2)
  n.-13 (N-13)
  n.-13 ammonia
  blood urea n. (BUN)
  n. curve
  n. dioxide (NO_2)

  n. mustard
  n. narcosis
  n. oxide
  n. washout technique
nitroglycerin-induced dilation
nitroglycerin transdermal patch
nitroglycerol
Nitroglyn Oral
nitroimidazole
Nitrolin
Nitrolingual Translingual Spray
Nitrol Ointment
Nitromed
Nitronet
Nitrong
  N. Oral Tablet
  N. SR
Nitropress
nitroprusside
  n. infusion
  sodium n.
  n. sodium
NitroQuick sublingual tablets
nitrosopnea
nitrosothiol
Nitrospan
Nitrostat Sublingual
Nitro TD
Nitrotym
nitrotyrosine
nitrous oxide
Nitrovas
nitrovasodilator
NIV
  noninvasive ventilation
NIVS
  noninvasive ventilatory support
Nizoral Oral
NK
  natural killer
  NK cell
NKA
  neurokinin A
NKK Hema Tracer 1 aggregometer
NK-104 stain
NL3 guider
n-LDL
  native LDL
NLHEP
  National Lung Health Education Program
N-link Flexi Segment

N

NOTES

NMBA
neuromuscular blocking agent
NMDA
N-methyl-D-aspartate
NMDA receptor
N-methyl-D-aspartate (NMDA)
nmol
nanomole
NMR
nuclear magnetic resonance
NMR diffusometry
NMR relaxometry
NMR spectroscopy
NMR topography
NMRI
nuclear magnetic resonance imaging
NMS
neurally mediated syncope
NMVS
neurally mediated vasovagal syncope
N^G**-nitro-L-arginine methyl ester (L-NAME)**
NNS
nasal nicotine spray
NNT
number needed to treat
NNV
nasal nocturnal ventilation
NO
nitric oxide
NO₂

nitrogen dioxide
no
n. atrial pacing
n. infection-no rejection (NI-NR)
N. Surgery on Site (NoSOS)
NOA model 280 nitric oxide analyzer
Nobis aortic occluder
Nocardia
N. asteroides
N. brasiliensis
N. caviae
N. israelii
N. transvalensis
nocardiosis
nociceptive threshold
nocturia
nocturnal
n. angina
n. asthma
n. cardiovascular blunting
n. dyspnea
n. hypoventilation
n. oximetry
n. oximetry screening
n. oxygenation
n. polysomnogram (NPSG)
n. polysomnography
n. ventilation
n. walking
nod
bishop's n.
nodal
n. arrhythmia
n. artery
n. beat
n. bigeminy
n. bradycardia
n. escape
n. escape rhythm
n. extrasystole
n. paroxysmal tachycardia
n. premature contraction
n. reentrant tachycardia
n. rhythm
n. tachycardia
n. tissue
node
Aschoff-Tawara n.
atrioventricular n. (AVN)
A-V n.
axillary lymph n.'s
azygos n.
bifurcation lymph n.
bronchopulmonary lymph n.
carinal lymph n.
compact A-V n.
Cruveilhier n.'s
Delphian n.
dual atrioventricular n.
Flack n.
Fraenkel n.
Heberden n.
hilar lymph n.
hilum of lymph n.
His-Tawara n.
inferior phrenic lymph n.
inferior tracheobronchial lymph n.
jugulodigastric lymph n.
juxtaesophageal lymph n.
Keith n.
Keith-Flack n.
Koch n.
lateral jugular lymph n.
lymph n.
mediastinal lymph n.'s
NH region of A-V n.
Osler n.
paratracheal lymph n.
perihilar lymph n.'s
prelaryngeal lymph n.
pretracheal lymph n.
pulmonary lymph n.
n. of Ranvier
retropharyngeal lymph n.
S-A n.

sentinel n.
shotty n.'s
singer's n.
sinuatrial n. (SAN, SN)
sinus n. (SN)
subaortic lymph n.
subcarinal n.
superior phrenic lymph n.
superior tracheobronchial lymph n.
supraclavicular lymph n.
Tawara atrioventricular n.
teacher's n.
tracheal lymph n.

nodi (*pl. of* nodus)
nodofascicular
nodohisian bypass tract
nodosa

arteritis n.
periarteritis n.
polyarteritis n.

nodose arteriosclerosis
nodosum

erythema n.

nodoventricular

n. fiber
n. tract

nodular

n. arteriosclerosis
n. infiltrate
n. interlobular septal thickening
n. lymphoid hyperplasia
n. opacity
n. pulmonary amyloidosis
n. sarcoidosis
n. sclerosing Hodgkin lymphoma
n. sclerosis
n. vasculitis

nodularity
nodule

acinar n.
Albini n.
Arantius n.
Aschoff n.
Bianchi n.'s
calcified n.
Caplan n.
centrilobular n.
cold n.
hematogenous n.
interstitial n.
intrapulmonary rheumatoid n.
lung n.

metastatic n.
Morgagni n.
multiple meningotheloid n.
necrobiotic n.
peribronchiolar n.
perilymphatic n.
random n.
rheumatoid n.
round pneumonia n.
solitary pulmonary n. (SPN)
subcutaneous n.
warm n.
Wegener n.

nodus, pl. **nodi**

n. atrioventricularis
nodi lymphoidei bronchopulmonales
nodi lymphoidei juxtaesophageales
  pulmonales
nodi lymphoidei paratracheales
nodi lymphoidei phrenici inferiores
nodi lymphoidei phrenici superiores
nodi lymphoidei prelaryngeales
nodi lymphoidei pretracheales
nodi lymphoidei pulmonales
nodi lymphoidei retropharyngeales
nodi lymphoidei tracheobronchiales
  inferiores
nodi lymphoidei tracheobronchiales
  superiores
n. sinuatrialis
n. sinuatrialis echo

noise

n. reversion
n.-reversion mode

noisy chest
nolbufine
no-leak technique
Nolex LA
Nolvadex tablet
nomatopic stimulus
nomifensine maleate
nomogram

Radford n.

non

conditio sine qua n.

nonacute total occlusion
nonagenarian
nonallergic

n. noninfectious perennial rhinitis
  (NANIPER)
n. rhinitis with eosinophilia
  (NARES)

N

NOTES

nonarticulated stent
nonasthmatic eosinophilic bronchitis
nonatheromatous intimal thickening
nonatopic asthma
nonbacteremic
nonbacterial
>   n. thrombotic endocardial lesion
>   n. thrombotic endocarditis (NBTE)
>   n. verrucous endocarditis

nonballoon therapy
noncalcified valve
noncardiac
>   n. angiography
>   n. surgery
>   n. syncope

noncardiogenic pulmonary edema
noncaseating granuloma
noncavitary
noncleaved cell lymphoma
noncollagenous pneumoconiosis
noncommitted biphasic shock therapy
noncommunicating air space
noncompensatory pause
noncompliant
>   n. balloon
>   n. ventricle

nonconotruncal anomaly
noncontact
>   n. endocardial mapping
>   n. mapping

noncoronary
>   n. cusp
>   n. sinus

noncrushing vascular clamp
nondecremental retrograde
    ventriculoatrial conduction
nondepolarizing drug
nondisjunction
nondominant vessel
Non-Drowsy
>   Comtrex Maximum Strength N.-D.
>   Drixoral N.-D.

nonejection systolic click
noneosinophilic nonallergic rhinitis
    (NENAR)
nonessential
nonesterified fatty acid (NEFA)
nonexcitatory
>   n. contractility-modulation electric
>   signal
>   n. signal

nonexertional angina
nonexpansional dyspnea
nonfatal cardiac event
nonfenestrated endothelium
nonflotation catheter
nonflow-directed catheter
nonfluent aphasia

nongenomic
nonglycoside inotropic agent
nonhemodynamic effect
non-Hodgkin lymphoma
nonhomogeneous pulmonary time-
    constant distribution
nonhypercapnic respiratory failure
nonimmunocompromised host
noninducible
noninfectious complication
noninfective valve endocarditis
noninhalation
Nonin Onyx pulse oximeter
noninsulin-dependent diabetes mellitus
    (NIDDM)
nonintegrated
>   n. transvenous defibrillation lead
>   n. tripolar lead

nonintubated patient
noninvasive
>   n. assessment
>   n. blood pressure (NIPB)
>   n. evaluation
>   n. extrathoracic ventilator (NEV)
>   n. face mask ventilation
>   lower extremity n. (LENI)
>   n. mechanical ventilation
>   n. monitor
>   n. murmur
>   n. positive pressure ventilation
>   (NIPPV, NPPV)
>   n. positive pressure ventilatory
>   support
>   n. programmed stimulation (NIPS)
>   n. temporary pacemaker
>   n. test
>   n. ventilation (NIV)
>   n. ventilation with positive pressure
>   n. ventilatory support (NIVS)

nonionic
>   n. contrast material
>   n. contrast medium

nonischemic dilated cardiomyopathy
nonliquefaciens
>   *Moraxella n.*

nonnecrotizing angiitis
nonobstructive valve thrombosis
nonocclusive mesenteric ischemia
nonoperative closure
nonostial plaque
nonpanting maneuver
nonparametric data
nonparoxysmal atrioventricular
    junctional tachycardia
nonpenetrating rupture
nonpharmacologic measure of treatment
nonphasic sinus arrhythmia
nonpitting edema

nonpressor dose
nonprimary ventricular fibrillation
nonpyramidal hemimotor syndrome
non-Q MI
nonquinolone antibiotic
non-Q-wave myocardial infarction (non-Q MI, NQWMI)
nonrapid eye movement (NREM)
nonrebreathing
    n. mask
    n. valve
non-reexpanding lung
nonreset nodus sinuatrialis
nonreversibility
nonrheumatic
    n. AF
    n. valvular aortic stenosis
nonsegmental
    n. disease
    n. perfusion defect
nonselective coronary angiography
non-sensing
    atrial n.-s.
nonsinusoidal waveform
non-small
    n.-s. cell carcinoma
    n.-s. cell lung cancer (NSCLC)
    n.-s. cell lung carcinoma (NSCLC)
    n.-s. cell tumor
nonspecific
    n. bronchial hyperreactivity
    n. challenge test
    n. chronic interstitial pneumonitis (NIP)
    n. climatic change
    n. idiopathic pulmonary fibrosis
    n. interstitial pneumonia (NSIP)
    n. interstitial pneumonitis (NSIP)
    n. intraventricular block
    n. lung fibrosis
    n. pneumonitis
    n. T-wave aberration
    n. T-wave abnormality
nonsteroidal
    n. antiinflammatory agent
    n. antiinflammatory drug (NSAID)

nonsuppressible
    n. arrhythmia
    n. ventricular tachycardia
nonsurgical septal reduction therapy (NSRT)
nonsustained ventricular tachycardia (NSVT)
nonthoracotomy
    n. defibrillation lead system
    n. lead implantable cardioverter-defibrillator
    n. system antitachycardia device (NTS-AICD)
nonthrombogenic
nontransmural myocardial infarction (NTMI)
nontransplanted
nontraumatizing catheter
nontuberculous mycobacteria (NTM)
nontypeable *Haemophilus influenzae* (NTHI)
nonuniform
    n. direct cardiac compression
    n. rotational defect (NURD)
nonvalved graft
nonvalvular atrial fibrillation (NVAF)
nonvenereal syphilis
nonventilated patient
Noonan syndrome
Noon A-V fistula clamp
no-phase wrap
No Pour Pak suction catheter kit
NoProfile
    N. balloon
    N. balloon catheter
noradrenaline
Norcet
Norcuron
Nordach treatment
Nordenstrom Rotex II biopsy needle
Nordryl Oral
no-reflow
    n.-r. phenomenon
    n.-r. syndrome
Norelco allergen reducer
norepinephrine (NE)
    n. bitartrate
    fasting plasma n.
    n. uptake-1
norethindrone
norfloxacin
Norisodrine

N

NOTES

Norlutate
Norlutin
normal
- n. coronary arteries (NCA)
- n. electrical axis
- n. geometry
- n. intravascular pressure
- n. saline
- n. sinus rhythm (NSR)
- n. vital capacity (NVC)

normalization of inverted T wave
Normiflo
normobaric environment
Normocap capnometer
normocapnia
normocholesterolemic
Normodyne
- N. injection
- N. Oral

normokinesia
normolipidemic
normomagnesemia
normonatremic
normoperfused
Normotensin
normotension
normotensive pneumothorax
normothermic cardioplegia
normovolemia
normovolemic (NV)
- n. hemodilution

normoxia
Normozide
Noroxin Oral
Norpace CR
Norpramin
NOR-Q.D.
Norris
- N. score
- N. test

Nor-tet Oral
north
- N. American blastomycosis
- N. American Cerebral Transluminal Angioplasty Registration (NACPTAR)
- N. American Inoue Balloon registry
- N. American Symptomatic Carotid Endarterectomy Trial (NASCET)

Northern
- N. blot
- N. hybridization analysis

Norton flow-directed Swan-Ganz thermodilution catheter
nortriptyline hydrochloride
Norvasc

norvegicus
- *Rattus n.*

norverapamil
Norvir
Norwalk agent
Norwood
- N. operation
- N. operation for hypoplastic left-sided heart
- N. repair
- N. univentricular heart procedure

NOS
- nitric oxide synthase

NOS1
- nitric oxide synthase

nose
- n. clip
- respiratory region of tunica mucosa of n.

Nosema connori
no-sigh period
nosocomial
- n. aspiration
- n. disease
- n. endocarditis
- n. infection
- n. pathogen
- n. pneumonia (NP)

nosocomii
- angina n.

nosology
- Berlin n.

NoSOS
- No Surgery on Site

Nostrilla
notch
- anacrotic n.
- aortic n.
- atrial n.
- cardiac n.
- dicrotic n.
- interarytenoid n.
- Sibson n.
- sternal n.
- suprasternal n.
- thyroid n.

notching
- midsystolic n.
- rib n.

notha
- angina n.
- peripneumonia n.
- pneumonia n.

Nottingham
- N. Extended Activities of Daily Living scale
- N. Health profile

N. introducer
N. Sensory Assessment test
Nova
N. II pacemaker
N. Microsonics Image Vue system
N. MR pacemaker
N. Rectal
Novacode Q-wave score
Novacor
N. DIASYS cardiac device
N. left ventricular assist device
N. left ventricular assist system
N. LVAD
N. mechanical circulatory support
system
Novafed
Novametrix
N. ETCO$_2$ multigas analyzer
N. NICO cardiac output monitor
N. pulse oximeter
N. Tidal Wave handheld
capnograph
Novamoxin
Novantrone
Novasen
Novastan
Novastent stent
Novo
N.-Atenol
N.-AZT
N.-Captopril
N.-Chlorpromazine
N.-Clonidine
N.-Cloxin
N.-Cromolyn
N.-Digoxin
N.-Diltazem
N.-Dipiradol
N.-Hydrazide
N.-Hydroxyzine
N.-Hylazin
N.-Lexin
N.-Medopa
N.-Metoprolol
N.-Nifedin
N.-Pen-VK
N.-Pindol
N.-Prazin
N.-Prednisolone
N.-Prednisone
N.-Reserpine
N.-Rythro Encap

N.-Salmol
N.-Semide
N.-Spiroton
N.-Tamoxifen
N.-Thalidone
N.-Timol
N.-Triamzide
N.-Trimel
N.-Veramil
novo
de n.
saphenous vein graft de n.
(SAVED)
Novolin 70/30
NovoSeven
Novoste catheter
NoxBOX monitor
Nozovent nasal-valve dilator
NP
nasopharyngeal
nosocomial pneumonia
NPB
Nellcor Puritan Bennett
NPB-40 handheld pulse oximeter
NPB-75
NPB-75 handheld capnograph
NPB-75 handheld capnograph/pulse
oximeter
NPB-190 pulse oximeter
NPB-195 pulse oximeter
NPB-290 pulse oximeter
NPB-295 pulse oximeter
NPB VentNet
NPH Iletin insulin
NPPV
nasal positive pressure ventilation
noninvasive positive pressure ventilation
N-propanol
NPSG
nocturnal polysomnogram
NPT
near patient test
NPV
negative predictive value
negative pressure ventilation
NQWMI
non-Q-wave myocardial infarction
NR
Organidin NR
Tussi-Organidin NR
Tussi-Organidin DM NR

N

NOTES

Nramp

natural resistance macrophage-associated protein

NRDS

neonate respiratory distress syndrome

NREM

nonrapid eye movement

NREM sleep

NRMI

National Registry of Myocardial Infarction

NS

nasal steroid

NS echo

NSAID

nonsteroidal antiinflammatory drug

NSCLC

non-small cell lung cancer

non-small cell lung carcinoma

NSE

neuron-specific enolase

NSIP

nonspecific interstitial pneumonia

nonspecific interstitial pneumonitis

NSR

normal sinus rhythm

NSRT

nonsurgical septal reduction therapy

NSVT

nonsustained ventricular tachycardia

N-terminal

N-t. proANF

N-t. proatrial natriuretic factor

NTF

nasogastric tube feeding

NTHI

nontypeable *Haemophilus influenzae*

NTM

nontuberculous mycobacteria

NTMI

nontransmural myocardial infarction

NTS-AICD

nonthoracotomy system antitachycardia device

NTZ Long Acting Nasal Solution

Nu

N.-Amoxi

N.-Ampi

N.-Atenol

N.-Capto

N.-Cephalex

N.-Clonidine

N.-Cloxi

N.-Cotrimox

N.-Diltiaz

N.-Hydral

N.-Iron

N.-Medopa

N.-Metop

N.-Nifedin

N.-Pen-VK

N.-Pindol

N.-Prazo

N.-Propranolol

N.-Timolol

N.-Trake Weiss emergency airway system

N.-Triazide

N.-Trim dietary fat substitute

N.-Verap

N.-Vois artificial larynx

nuchal rigidity

nuclear

n. factor-κB (NF-kappa-B)

n. magnetic resonance (NMR)

n. magnetic resonance imaging (NMRI)

n. pacemaker

n. perfusion imaging

n. probe

n. stent

n. ventricular function study (NVFS)

nucleatum

Fusobacterium n.

nuclei (*pl. of* nucleus)

nucleic acid direct amplification test

nucleotide

total adenine n. (TAN)

nucleus, pl. **nuclei**

caudate n.

suprachiasmatic n.

n. tractus solitarius

vein of caudate n.

Nucofed Pediatric Expectorant

Nucotuss

Nuhn gland

null

n. hypothesis

n. point

number

N. Equal to One; Single Patient Trial (N=1 trial)

n. needed to treat (NNT)

representative CT (Hounsfield) n.

Reynolds n.

Strouhal n.

Wasserman n.

Numed

N. intracoronary Doppler catheter

NuMED single balloon

nummiform

nummular

n. aortitis

n. sputum

nummulation

nun's
    n. murmur
    n. venous hum murmur
Nuprin
NURD
    nonuniform rotational defect
Nurolon suture
nutcracker esophagus
nutraceutical (*var. of* nutriceutical)
Nutracort
Nutraplus topical
nutriceutical, nutraceutical
nutrient cardioplegia
nutrition
    enteral n.
    parenteral n.
Nuvance
Nuvolase 660 laser system
NV
    normovolemic
NVAF
    nonvalvular atrial fibrillation
NVC
    normal vital capacity

NVE
    native valve endocarditis
NVFS
    nuclear ventricular function study
Nyboer esophageal electrode
Nycore
    N. cardiac device
    N. device
    N. pigtail catheter
Nydrazid injection
NYHA
    New York Heart Association
    NYHA functional classification
       I–IV
nylon
    Xcelon n.
Nyomin
Nyquist limit
nystatin
Nystat-Rx
Nystex Topical

NOTES

N

Ω (*var. of* ohm)
O

    O antigen
    O point of cardiac apex pulse

O$_2$

    oxygen
    ambulatory O$_2$
    AVD O$_2$
        arteriovenous oxygen difference
    hood O$_2$
    O$_2$ radical
    O$_2$ via nasal cannula

O2 Advantage conserving device
O2SMO Plus respiratory profile monitor
OA

    occipital artery
    occupational asthma
    oral appliance

OAD

    obstructive airway disease

oakridgensis

    Legionella o.

OARS

    Optimal Atherectomy Restenosis Study

OASIS

    Organization to Assess Strategies for Ischemic Syndromes
    OASIS-2 clinical trial
    OASIS clinical trial

Oasis thrombectomy system
oat

    o. cell
    o. cell carcinoma

OB

    obliterative bronchiolitis

obesity

    exogenous o.
    o. hypertension
    morbid o.
    Roux-en-Y o.
    waist/hip ratio for upper body o.

obesity-hypoventilation syndrome
oblique

    o. fissure
    o. fissure of lung
    left anterior o. (LAO)
    right anterior o. (RAO)
    o. sinus

obliterans

    arteriosclerosis o.
    arteritis o.
    bronchiolitis o. (BO)
    bronchiolitis fibrosa o.
    bronchitis o.

    cerebral thromboangiitis o. (CTAO)
    endarteritis o.
    pericarditis o.
    phlebitis o.
    thromboangiitis o.

obliterating

    o. pericarditis
    o. phlebitis

obliteration

    coil o.

obliterative

    o. bronchiolitis (OB)
    o. bronchitis
    o. cardiomyopathy
    o. pericarditis
    o. pleuritis
    o. vascular disease

oblongata

    medulla o.

O'Brien airway needle
obscuration

    aortic o.

Observer's Assessment of Alertness/Sedation Scale
obstruction

    airflow o.
    airway o. (AO)
    aortic o.
    aortic arch vessel o.
    baffle o.
    chronic airflow o. (CAO)
    chronic upper respiratory o.
    coronary artery o.
    dynamic intracavitary o.
    embolic o.
    endobronchial o.
    extracranial carotid o.
    extrathoracic airway o.
    fixed airflow o.
    hypopharyngeal o.
    infundibular o.
    irreversible airway o.
    left ventricular inflow tract o.
    left ventricular outflow tract o. (LVOTO)
    mechanical o.
    multivessel coronary artery o.
    outflow tract o.
    pulmonary vascular o. (PVO)
    retropalatal o.
    reversible airway o.
    right ventricular inflow o.
    right ventricular outflow o.
    stop-valve airway o.
    subaortic o.

O

obstruction (*continued*)
    subpulmonary o.
    subvalvular o.
    upper airway o. (UAO)
    vena cava o.
    vena caval o.
    ventricular inflow tract o.
    ventricular outflow tract o.

obstructive
    o. airway disease (OAD)
    o. atelectasis
    o. edema
    o. emphysema
    o. hypertrophic cardiomyopathy
    o. hypopnea
    o. lung disease (OLD)
    o. murmur
    o. pneumonia
    o. shock
    o. sleep apnea (OSA)
    o. sleep apnea-induced
      cardiovascular change
    o. sleep apnea syndrome (OSAS)
    o. thrombus
    o. valve thrombosis
    o. ventilatory defect
    o. ventilatory dysfunction

obturating embolism
obturator
    Fitch o.
    Hemaflex PTCA sheath with o.
    Hemaquet PTCA sheath with o.

obtuse
    o. marginal (OM)
    o. marginal artery (OMA)
    o. marginal branch (OMB)
    o. marginal coronary artery
    o. marginal lymphatic
    o. margin of heart

OCBAS
    Optimal Coronary Balloon Angioplasty
    versus Stent
    OCBAS clinical trial

occipital artery (OA)
occipitalis
    basilaris ossis o.

occluder
    air clamp inflatable vessel o.
    Amplatzer o.
    Amplatzer septal o.
    ASDOS umbrella o.
    o. balloon wash-out technique
    Bard Clamshell septal o.
    Brockenbrough curved-tip o.
    CardioSeal o.
    CardioSeal septal o.
    catheter-tip o.
    clamshell septal o.

    Crile tip o.
    double-disk o.
    Flo-Rester vascular o.
    Hieshima balloon o.
    Hunter detachable balloon o.
    Microvena Das Angel Wings o.
    modified Rashkind PDA o.
    Nobis aortic o.
    Pediatric Cardiology Devices
      Sideris Buttoned device o.
    PFO-Star o.
    square-shaped o.
    STARFLex o.
    tilting-disk o.
    tip o.

occludin
occluding thrombus
occlusion
    angioplasty-related vessel o.
    arterial o.
    balloon o.
    Balloon Angioplasty Versus Rotacs
      for Total Chronic Coronary O.
      (BAROCCO)
    balloon coronary o. (BCO)
    balloon test o. (BTO)
    basilar artery o. (BAO)
    branch retinal artery o. (BRAO)
    branch retinal vein o. (BRVO)
    branch vessel o.
    central retinal artery o. (CRAO)
    chronic coronary O.'s
    chronic total o. (CTO)
    coronary o.
    coronary artery o.
    coronary branch o.
    Excimer Laser Angioplasty in
      Coronary Total O. (EXACTO)
    femoral artery o.
    femoral vein o.
    iliac artery o.
    inferior mesenteric vascular o.
    inferior vena cava o.
    intermittent coronary sinus o.
    long iliac artery o.
    mesenteric artery o.
    mesenteric vascular o.
    middle cerebral artery o. (MCAO)
    nonacute total o.
    recurrent mesenteric vascular o.
    side branch o.
    Stenting in Chronic Coronary O.
      (SICCO)
    superior mesenteric vascular o.
    temporary unilateral pulmonary
      artery o.
    transcatheter o.

transcatheter coil o.
venous mesenteric vascular o.
occlusive
    o. disease
    o. thromboaortopathy
    o. thrombus
occult
    o. cardiogenic shock
    o. pericardial constriction
    o. pericarditis
occupational
    o. asthma (OA)
    o. asthmogen
    o. health and safety (OHS)
    o. lung disease
Ochrobacterium anthropi
ochrometer
ochronosis
Ochsner-Mahorner
    O.-M. echocardiogram
    O.-M. test
OCT
    optical coherence tomography
octafluoropropane
octapolar catheter
Octocaine
Octomyces etiennei
Octopus 3 tissue stabilization system
octreotide
Ocugram
ocular larva migrans
oculocardiac reflex
oculocraniosomatic disease
oculomucocutaneous syndrome
oculopharyngeal reflex
oculoplethysmography (OPG)
oculoplethysmography-Gee
oculopneumoplethysmography
oculostenotic illusion
oculovagal reflex
OD
    outer diameter
Odam defibrillator
odds ratio (OR)
ODN
    oligodeoxynucleotide
odorans
    Alcaligenes o.
odoratus
    Lathyrus o.
odor-triggered panic attack

ODTS
    organic dust toxic syndrome
O'Dwyer intubation
odynophagia
OEF
    oxygen extraction fraction
Oehler symptoms
Oehl muscle
OEM
    O. 503 humidifier
    O. Venturi MixOMask
O$_2$ER
    oxygen extraction ratio
Oertel treatment
off-axis
office
    o. angina
    o. hypertension
off-pump
    o.-p. coronary artery bypass (OPCAB)
    o.-p. vascular surgery
ofloxacin
Ogata method
OGTT
    oral glucose tolerance test
OHD
    organic heart disease
Ohio
    O. Bubble humidifier
    O. critical care ventilator
    O. Hope resuscitator
    O. Vortex respiration monitor
ohm, Ω
    O. law
Ohmeda
    O. 6200, 6300 CO$_2$ monitor
    O. ETCO$_2$ multigas analyzer
    O. handheld oximeter
    O. pulse oximeter
    O. 3800 pulse oximeter
    O. 3770 spot-check handheld pulse oximeter
    O. thoracic suction regulator
ohmic heating
ohmmeter
Ohnell
    X wave of O.
OHS
    occupational health and safety
OHT
    orthotopic heart transplant

O

NOTES

OIA
    osmotically induced asthma
oil
    o.-aspiration pneumonia
    canola o.
    o. embolism
    emu o.
    fish o.
    marine o.'s
    MCT O.
    o. mist asthma
    progesterone O.
    rapeseed o.
    O. Red O stain
    trypsin, balsam peru, and castor o.
ointment
    Nitro-Bid O.
    Nitrol O.
    Whitfield o.
    Xylocaine Topical O.
OKT3
    O. antibody
    Orthoclone O.
OKT4A
OLB
    open lung biopsy
Olbert
    O. balloon
    O. balloon catheter
OLBI
    overlapping biphasic impulse
OLD
    obstructive lung disease
Olean
oleate
    ethanolamine o.
oleogomenol
olestra
Oligella
oligemia
oligemic shock
oligodeoxynucleotide (ODN)
    antisense o.
oligonucleotide
oliguria
Oliver-Rosalki method
Oliver sign
olive-tipped
    o.-t. Magnum wire
    o.-t. needle
olivopontocerebellar atrophy
olprinone
Olympix II PTCA dilatation catheter
Olympus
    O. bioptome
    O. GIF-EUM2 echoendoscope
    O. One-Step Button tube

OM
    obtuse marginal
    OM coronary artery
OM-1
    first obtuse marginal artery
OM-2
    second obtuse marginal artery
OMA
    obtuse marginal artery
omapatrilat
    O. in Persons with Enhanced Risk
    of Atherosclerotic Events
    (OPERA)
OMB
    obtuse marginal branch
omega
    O. 5600 noninvasive blood
    pressure monitor
    O. stent
omega-3 unsaturated fatty acids
Omega-NV balloon
omental wrap
omentopexy
omeprazole
omni
    O. analyzer
    O. SST balloon
    O. tract retractor system
Omni-Atricor pacemaker
Omnicarbon
    O. heart valve prosthesis
    O. prosthetic heart valve
OmniCath atherectomy catheter
Omnicef
Omnicor
    O. pacemaker
    O. Programmer
omnidirectional M-mode
Omniflex
    O. balloon
    O. balloon catheter
OmniHIB
Omni-Orthocor pacemaker
Omnipaque
Omnipen
Omnipen-N
OmniPlane TEE
Omniscience
    O. single leaflet cardiac valve
    prosthesis
    O. tilting-disk valve
    O. tilting-disk valve prosthesis
    O. valve device
    O. valve prosthesis
Omni-Stanicor pacemaker
OmniStent
omnivore

omotracheale
 trigonum o.
omphalitis
omphalocele
omphalomesenteric
 o. duct
 o. vein
 o. vessel
Omsk hemorrhagic fever
Oncaspar
Oncet
Onchocerca volvulus
oncology mix
Onconase
Oncor ApopTaq kit
oncostatin M
oncotic pressure
Oncovin injection
Ondine's curse breathing
one-block claudication
one-flight exertional dyspnea
one-hole
 o.-h. angiographic catheter
 o.-h. angioplastic catheter
One Touch blood glucose monitor
one-ventricle heart
one-vessel angioplasty
onion-bulb dilation
onion scale lesion
onset
 sudden rate o.
Ontak
On-X
 O.-X mechanical bi-leaflet
  prosthetic heart valve
 O.-X prosthetic valve
onychograph
Onyvul
Onyx
oocyte
 Xenopus o.
OOH-SCD
 out-of-hospital sudden cardiac death
OOO mode
opacification
 alveolar o.
 amorphous parenchymal o.
 faint o.
 ground-glass o.
 selective graft o.
opacify

opacity
 ground-glass o.
 nodular o.
 vitreous o.
OPC-18790
OPCAB
 off-pump coronary artery bypass
open
 o. atrial disk
 o. bronchus sign
 o. chest cardiac massage
 o. chest cardiac resuscitation
 o. chest massage
 o. circuit method
 o. heart surgery
 o. lung approach
 o. lung biopsy (OLB)
 O. Pivot heart valve
 o. pneumothorax
 o. surgery (OS)
 o. tuberculosis
Open-Cath
 Abbokinase O.-C.
opening
 esophageal o.
 fistulous o.
 o. pressure
 o. snap
open-label ACE-inhibitor therapy
OpenSail
 O. balloon catheter
 O. coronary dilatation catheter
OPERA
 Omapatrilat in Persons with Enhanced
 Risk of Atherosclerotic Events
 OPERA clinical trial
operation
 Abbe o.
 Anel o.
 arterial switch o.
 atrial baffle o.
 Babcock o.
 Barnard o.
 Beck I, II o.
 Bentall o.
 Berger o.
 bidirectional Glenn o.
 Blalock-Hanlon o.
 Blalock-Taussig o.
 Brock o.
 cautery-assisted palatal stiffening o.
 (CAPSO)

O

NOTES

operation *(continued)*
 Cox maze o.
 Damus-Kaye-Stansel o.
 DKS o.
 electrode catheter ablation o.
 encircling endocardial
  ventriculotomy o.
 endocardial to epicardial
  resection o.
 Estlander o.
 fenestrated Fontan o.
 Fontan o.
 Freund o.
 Glenn o.
 Goldsmith o.
 Grondahl-Finney o.
 Heller-Belsey o.
 Heller-Nissen o.
 hemi-Fontan o.
 Hunter o.
 Konno o.
 laser maze o.
 Lindesmith o.
 Mustard o.
 Norwood o.
 Norwood o. for hypoplastic left-
  sided heart
 Palma o.
 Potts o.
 Ransohoff o.
 Rastan o.
 Rastelli o.
 Sawyer o.
 second-look o.
 Senning o.
 switch o.
 talc o.
 Tanner o.
 transcatheter closure of atrial septal
  defect o.
 Trendelenburg o.
 triangular resection of leaflet o.
 valve-conserving o.
 Waterston o.
operculum
OPG
 oculoplethysmography
OPG-Gee test
ophthalmic
ophthalmoplegia
ophthalmotonometry
opiate
opioid
Opisthorchis
Opitz syndrome
OPO
 organ procurement organization

opportunistic
 o. infection
 o. pneumonia
opsoclonia
opsonin
opsonization
opsonophagocytic receptor
Opta 5 catheter
OPTI
 O. 1 pH/blood gas analyzer
 O. 1 portable blood analyzer
optic
 o. atrophy
 o. disk
 o. neuritis
optical
 o. coherence tomography (OCT)
 o. fiber catheter
 O. Sensors stand-alone arterial
  blood gas monitoring system
Opticath oximeter catheter
OptiChamber valved holding chamber
Optichin disk test
Opti-Flex
Opti-Flow
 O.-F. catheter
 Vas-Cath O.-F.
Optihaler
OptiHaler drug delivery system
Optima
 O. MP pacemaker
 O. MPT Series III pacemaker
 O. SPT pacemaker
OPTIMAAL
 Optimal Therapy in Myocardial
  Infarction with the Angiotensin II
  Antagonist Losartan
 Optimal Trial in Myocardial Infarction
  with the Angiotensin II Antagonist
  Losartan
optimal
 O. Atherectomy Restenosis Study
  (OARS)
 O. Coronary Balloon Angioplasty
  versus Stent (OCBAS)
 O. Stent Implantation (OSTI)
 O. Stent Implantation Trial-I
 O. Stent Implantation Trial-IIA
 O. Stent Implantation Trial-IIB
 O. Therapy in Myocardial
  Infarction with the Angiotensin II
  Antagonist Losartan (OPTIMAAL)
 O. Trial in Myocardial Infarction
  with the Angiotensin II
  Antagonist Losartan (OPTIMAAL)

OPTIME-CHF
  Outcomes of a Prospective Trial of
  Intravenous Milrinone for
  Exacerbations of Chronic Heart Failure
Optimine
**Opti-Qvue Mixed Venous
  Saturation/CCO pulmonary artery
  catheter system**
Optiray
  O. 320
  O. contrast
  O. contrast medium
Optiscope catheter
Optison
  O. contrast
  O. contrast agent
  O. injectable suspension
OPTN
  Organ Procurement and Transplantation
  Network
Optrin
OPUS
  Orbofiban in Patients with Unstable
  Coronary Syndromes
    OPUS Clinical Trial
Opus
  O. cardiac troponin I assay
  O. pacemaker
OR
  odds ratio
Oracle
  O. Focus catheter
  O. Focus imaging catheter
  O. Focus PTCA catheter
  O. Micro catheter
  O. Micro intravascular ultrasound
    catheter
  O. Micro Plus
  O. Micro Plus catheter
  O. Micro Plus PTCA catheter
oral
  Achromycin V O.
  o. airflow in liters per second
    (V_O)
  Alazine O.
  Aller-Chlor O.
  AllerMax O.
  Altace O.
  Amen O.
  o. anticoagulant therapy
  Anxanil O.
  o. appliance (OA)

Apresoline O.
Aristocort O.
Atarax O.
Atolone O.
Atozine O.
Bactocill O.
Banophen O.
Beepen-VK O.
Belix O.
Benadryl O.
Betapace O.
Betapen-VK O.
Bio-Tab O.
Blocadren O.
Brethine O.
Bricanyl O.
Calm-X O.
o. candidiasis
Cardioquin O.
Cartrol O.
Catapres O.
CeeNU O.
Ceftin O.
Celestone O.
Cerespan O.
Chlo-Amine O.
Chlorate O.
Chlor-Trimeton O.
Cipro O.
Cleocin HCl O.
Cleocin Pediatric O.
Compazine O.
o. contraceptive-induced
  hypertension
Cortef O.
Cortone Acetate O.
Curretab O.
Cycrin O.
Cyklokapron O.
Cytomel O.
Cytoxan O.
Decadron O.
Delta-Cortef O.
Deltasone O.
Demadex O.
Diflucan O.
Dimetabs O.
Dormarex 2 O.
Dormin O.
Doryx O.
Doxy O.
Doxychel O.

NOTES

O

oral *(continued)*

Dramamine O.
Durrax O.
Dynacin O.
Edecrin O.
E.E.S. O.
E-Mycin O.
Eryc O.
EryPed O.
Ery-Tab O.
Erythrocin O.
Eryzole O.
Flagyl O.
o. flecainide therapy
o. flora
Floxin O.
Flumadine O.
Gantrisin O.
Genabid O.
Genahist O.
o. glucose tolerance test (OGTT)
O. Glycoprotein IIb/IIIa Receptor Blockade to Inhibit Thrombosis (ORBIT)
Hydrocortone O.
Hy-Pam O.
Ilosone O.
Indocin O.
Kenacort O.
Kerlone O.
Laniazid O.
o. L-Arginine system
Lasix O.
Ledercillin VK O.
Lincocin O.
Liquid Pred O.
Loniten O.
Marmine O.
Maxaquin O.
Meclomen O.
Medrol O.
Mephyton O.
Meticorten O.
Minocin O.
Monodox O.
Mycobutin O.
Nitro-Bid O.
Nitrocine O.
Nitroglyn O.
Nizoral O.
Nordryl O.
Normodyne O.
Noroxin O.
Nor-tet O.
Orasone O.
Orinase O.
Oxsoralen-Ultra O.
Panmycin O.

o. part of pharynx
Pavabid O.
Pavased O.
Pavatine O.
Paverolan O.
PCE O.
PediaCare O.
Pediapred O.
Pediazole O.
Penetrex O.
Pen.Vee K O.
o. pharynx
Phenameth O.
Phendry O.
Phenergan O.
Phenetron O.
poliovirus vaccine, live, trivalent, o.
Prednicen-M O.
Prelone O.
Proglycem O.
Prostaphlin O.
Prothazine O.
Protostat O.
Provera O.
Quinalan O.
Quinora O.
Retrovir O.
Rifadin O.
Rimactane O.
Robicillin VK O.
Robitet O.
Sporanox O.
Sterapred O.
Sumycin O.
Tega-Vert O.
Telachlor O.
Teldrin o.
Teline O.
Terramycin O.
Tetracap O.
Tetralan O.
Tetram O.
Trandate O.
o. triamcinolone inhalation
o. tuberculosis
Unipen O.
Uri-Tet O.
Vamate O.
Vancocin O.
Vasotec O.
V-Cillin K O.
Veetids O.
VePesid O.
Vibramycin O.
Videx O.
Vistaril O.
Xylocaine O.

Oralet
    Fentanyl O.
oral-inhalation dexamethasone
oralis
    Bacteroides o.
Orasone Oral
Orbenin
ORBIT
    Oral Glycoprotein IIb/IIIa Receptor
      Blockade to Inhibit Thrombosis
    ORBIT clinical trial
orbofiban
    O. in Patients with Unstable
      Coronary Syndromes (OPUS)
orciprenaline sulfate
Ordrine AT Extended Release Capsule
Oregon tunneler
Oreopoulos-Zellerman catheter
Oretic
Oreticyl
Oreton Methyl
organ
    Golgi tendon o.
    o. procurement organization (OPO)
    O. Procurement and Transplantation
      Network (OPTN)
    o. transplantation system
organic
    o. dust
    o. dust pneumoconiosis
    o. dust toxic syndrome (ODTS)
    o. heart disease (OHD)
    o. murmur
    o. phosphorus
Organidin NR
organism
    Cox o.
    encapsulated o.
    gram-negative o.
    gram-positive o.
    intracellular o. (ICO)
    pleuropneumonia-like o. (PPLO)
organization
    O. to Assess Strategies for
      Ischemic Syndromes (OASIS)
    Extracorporeal Life Support O.
      (ELSO)
    International Standards O. (ISO)
    organ procurement o. (OPO)
    World Health O. (WHO)
organized thrombus

organizing
    o. empyema
    o. pneumonia
organoid pattern
organophosphate
Orgaran
oriental hemoptysis
orifice
    aortic o.
    atrioventricular o.
    cardiac o.
    effective regurgitant o. (ERO)
    esophagogastric o.
    flow across o.
    mitral o. (MO)
    pulmonary o.
    o. of pulmonary trunk
    regurgitant o.
    stent-jail o.
    o. of superior vena cava
    tricuspid o.
    valvular o.
orificial
    o. stenosis
    o. tuberculosis
origin
    anomalous o.
original
    Doan's O.
    O. Pink Tape waterproof adhesive
      tape
Orimune
Orinase Oral
Orion balloon
orlistat
Orlowski stent
Ormazine
Ornish
    O. diet
    O. theory
ornithosis
oroendotracheal tube
orofiban
oropharyngeal tularemia
oropharynx
    crowded o.
orotracheal
    o. intubation
    o. tube
orphan
    enteric cytopathogenic human o.
      (ECHO)

O

NOTES

orphan (*continued*)
  enterocytopathogenic human o. (ECHO)
  respiratory and enteric o. (REO)
Orsi-Grocco method
ORT
  orthodromic reciprocating tachycardia
orthoarteriotony
orthocardiac reflex
Orthoclone OKT3
Ortho Cytofluorograf 50-H flow cytometer
orthodeoxia
orthodox sleep
orthodromic
  o. atrioventricular reciprocating tachycardia
  o. A-V reentrant tachycardia
  o. circus movement tachycardia
  o. reciprocating tachycardia (ORT)
orthogonal
  o. electrocardiogram
  o. lead system
  o. plane
  o. view
orthograde conduction
Orthomyxoviridae virus
orthomyxovirus
orthopercussion
orthopnea
  three-pillow o.
  two-pillow o.
orthopneic
orthosis
  ankle-foot o. (AFO)
orthostasis autoregulation
orthostatic
  o. dyspnea
  o. hypertension
  o. hypopiesis
  o. hypotension
  o. syncope
  o. tachycardia
orthostatism
  vasovagal o.
orthotopic
  o. biventricular artificial heart
  o. cardiac transplant
  o. heart transplant (OHT)
  o. univentricular artificial heart
Orudis
Oruvail
oryzae
  Aspergillus o.
  Rhizopus o.
OS
  open surgery

OSA
  obstructive sleep apnea
OSAS
  obstructive sleep apnea syndrome
Osborne wave
Osciflator balloon inflation syringe
oscillating
  o. balloon inflation
  o. dilation
  o. paraboloid
  o. saw
oscillation
  external chest wall o.
  forced o. (FO)
  high-frequency o. (HFO)
  high-frequency chest wall o. (HFCWO)
  o. technique
oscillator
  Hayek o.
oscillatory afterpotential
oscillometer
oscillometric signal
oscilloscope
Oscor
  O. atrial lead
  O. pacing lead
OSD
  OSD monitor
  Profilate OSD
oseltamivir phosphate
OSF
  outlet strut fracture
Osler
  O. node
  O. sign
  O. triad
Osler-Weber-Rendu
  O.-W.-R. disease
  O.-W.-R. syndrome
OSM2 in vitro oximeter
Osmitrol
  O. injection
osmolality
osmolarity
osmometer
osmoregulation
osmoregulatory
osmotaxis
osmotic
  o. challenge
  o. diuretic
  o. pressure
osmotically induced asthma (OIA)
ossification
  pulmonary o.
ossifying pneumonitis
Ossoff-Karlan laryngoscope

osteitis
 caseous o.
 o. deformans
 o. tuberculosa multiplex cystica
osteoarthritis
 hyperplastic o.
osteoarthropathy
 hypertrophic pulmonary o.
 pneumogenic o.
 pulmonary o.
 pulmonary hypertrophic o.
osteochondroma
osteogenesis imperfecta
osteonecrosis
 dysbaric o.
osteoplastica
 tracheopathia o.
osteopontin
 o. messenger ribonucleic acid
 o. mRNA
osteoradionecrosis
osteosarcoma
osteosynthesis
 exit surgical o.
 plastic surgical o.
 surgical o.
osteotomy
 anterior inferior mandibular o.
 (AIMO)
 bilateral sagittal split ramus o.'s
 (BSSRO)
 maxillomandibular o. (MMO)
OSTI
 Optimal Stent Implantation
 OSTI-I clinical trial
 OSTI-IIA clinical trial
 OSTI-IIB clinical trial
ostia (*pl. of* ostium)
ostial
 o. lesion
 o. narrowing
 o. stenosis
Ostia stent
ostium, pl. **ostia**
 coronary o.
 o. primum
 o. primum defect
 o. secundum
 o. secundum defect
 solitary coronary o.
 o. trunci pulmonalis
 ostia venarum pulmonalium

Ostwald viscometer
Osypka
 O. atrial lead
 O. Cereblate electrode
 O. rotational angioplasty
otopharyngeal tube
Ototemp 3000
ototoxicity
OTW
 over-the-wire
 over the wire
  OTW perfusion catheter
  OTW thrombolytic brush
ouabain
Outcomes of a Prospective Trial of Intravenous Milrinone for Exacerbations of Chronic Heart Failure (OPTIME-CHF)
outer diameter (OD)
outflow
 o. cardiac patch
 o. murmur
 o. tract
 o. tract obstruction
outlet strut fracture (OSF)
out-of-hospital sudden cardiac death (OOH-SCD)
output
 cardiac o. (CO)
 o. circuit
 continuous cardiac o. (CCO)
 Fick cardiac o.
 left ventricular o.
 measured o.
 minute o.
 pacemaker o.
 postoperative low cardiac o.
 (PLCO)
 stroke o.
 thermodilution cardiac o.
outside-in signaling
ovale
 foramen o.
 patent foramen o. (PFO)
 Plasmodium o.
oval foramen
ovalis
 anulus o.
 fossa o.
overdilation
overdistention
 alveolar o.

O

NOTES

overdrive
    o. mode
    o. pacing
    o. suppression
overexpression
    beta-2 AR o.
    cardiac-specific o.
    IGF-1 o.
    TIMP-3 o.
    tissue inhibitor of metalloproteinase-3 o.
overflow wave
Overholt-Jackson bronchoscope
Overholt procedure
overhydration
overinflation
    congenital lobar o.
overlap
    o. syndrome
    o. vasculitis
overlapping biphasic impulse (OLBI)
overlay
    psychogenic o.
overload
    circulatory o.
    diastolic o.
    pressure o.
    volume o.
overreactivity
    physiological o.
override
    aortic o.
overriding aorta
oversampling
oversedation
oversensing
    afterpotential o.
    o. pacemaker
oversewing
overshoot phenomenon
over-the-wire, over the wire (OTW)
    o.-t.-w. balloon dilatation system
    o.-t.-w. pacing lead
    o.-t.-w. probe
    o.-t.-w. PTCA balloon catheter
overventilation
Owens
    O. balloon
    O. balloon catheter
    O. Lo-Profile dilatation catheter
Owren
    O. disease
    O. factor V deficiency
oxacillin sodium
oxalate
    calcium o.
oxalosis

oxalotransaminase
    glutamic o.
oxamniquine
oxandralone
oxazepam
oxazolidinone
Oxford
    O. Handicap Scale
    O. Medilog frequency-modulated recorder
    O. technique
ox heart
Oxicom-2000 analyser
oxidase
    cytochrome c o.
    monoamine o. (MAO)
    xanthine o.
oxidation
    intraplaque LDL o.
oxidative
    o. metabolism
    o. modification of LDL (oxLDL, ox-LDL)
    o. phosphorylation
    o. stress
oxide
    cadmium o.
    endothelial nitric o. (ecNOS)
    endothelium-derived nitric o. (EDNO)
    exhaled nitric o. (eNO, ENO)
    expired nitric o. (eNO, ENO)
    magnesium o.
    nitric o. (NO)
    nitrogen o.
    nitrous o.
    stannic o.
    tin o.
oxidized
    o. cellulose
    o. LDL
OxiFlow
Oxilan
OxiLink oximeter probe cover
oximeter
    American Optical o.
    Armstrong handheld pulse o.
    AutoCorr portable pulse o.
    BI-OX III ear o.
    CO_2SMO capnograph/pulse o.
    Cricket pulse o.
    Cricket recording pulse o.
    Criticare pulse o.
    Datascope pulse o.
    Datex-Ohmeda pulse o.
    Dinamap pulse o.
    ear o.
    FingerPrint handheld pulse o.

Hewlett-Packard ear o.
Model 500 ECG/pulse o.
Nellcor N200 pulse o.
Nellcor Symphony N-3000 pulse o.
Nonin Onyx pulse o.
Novametrix pulse o.
NPB-40 handheld pulse o.
NPB-75 handheld
  capnograph/pulse o.
NPB-190 pulse o.
NPB-195 pulse o.
NPB-290 pulse o.
NPB-295 pulse o.
Ohmeda handheld o.
Ohmeda pulse o.
Ohmeda 3800 pulse o.
Ohmeda 3770 spot-check handheld
  pulse o.
OSM2 in vitro o.
Oximetrix 3 o.
Oxypleth pulse o.
OxyTemp handheld pulse o.
Oxytrak pulse o.
Palco Laboratories Model 400
  pulse o.
Palco Model 300 pulse o.
pulse o.
3800 pulse o.
Respironics 920P handheld pulse o.
Respironics 930 pulse o.
SensorMedics SAT-TRAK pulse o.
SpaceLabs pulse o.
SpotCheck+ handheld pulse o.
Tidal Wave Sp capnometer/pulse o.
oximetric catheter
Oximetrix
O. 3 oximeter
O. 3 System
oximetry
carbon monoxide o. (CO-oximetry)
central venous o.
cerebral o.
CO o.
CO_2 o.
finger o.
Hb o.
$HbCO_2$ o.
HbO_2 o.
N_2 o.
near-infrared cerebral o.
nocturnal o.
OxiScan overnight pulse o.

oxygen saturation as measured
  using pulse o. (SpO_2)
PCO_2 o.
PO_2 o.
reflectance o.
spectrophotometric o.
OxiScan
O. overnight pulse oximetry
O. oximetry program
O. oximetry recording and
  reporting system
Oxisensor II adult sensor
**Oxismart Advanced Signal Processing
  and Alarm Technology**
oxitropium bromide
oxLDL, ox-LDL
oxidative modification of LDL
oxolamine
oxothiazolidine
oxotremorine
oxprenolol
Oxsoralen Topical
Oxsoralen-Ultra Oral
oxtriphylline
Oxycel
Oxycure topical oxygen system
OxyData
O. oxygen fuel cells
O. Plus oxygen monitor
Oxyfill oxygen refilling system
oxygen (O_2)
o.-15
aqueous o.
blood o.
blow-by o.
o. capacity
o. consumption (VO_2)
o. consumption index
o. consumption per minute (VO_2)
o. content
o. cost
O. Cost Diagram questionnaire
cytotoxic singlet o.
o. debt
o. delivery (Do_2)
o. dissociation curve
o. entrainment
o. exchange
o. extraction
o. extraction fraction (OEF)
o. extraction ratio (O_2ER)
fraction of inspired o. (FIO_2)

NOTES

O

oxygen *(continued)*
    humidified o.
    hyperbaric o. (HBO)
    o. inhalation
    o. mask
    o. paradox
    partial pressure of o. (PO_2)
    partial pressure of inspiratory o. (P_{IO_2})
    o. poisoning
    o. radical
    o. radical scavenger
    o. saturation (So_2)
    o. saturation as measured using pulse oximetry (SpO_2)
    o. saturation of the hemoglobin of arterial blood
    o. step-up method
    supplemental o.
    o. tension
    o. tent
    o. therapy
    o. toxicity
    T-piece o.
    o. transport
    o. uptake

oxygenated hemoglobin

oxygenation
    apneic o.
    bubble o.
    disk o.
    extracorporeal membrane o. (ECMO)
    film o.
    hyperbaric o.
    nocturnal o.
    pump o.
    rotating disk o.
    screen o.

oxygenator
    Affinity o.
    Bentley o.
    Biocor 200 high performance o.
    bubble o.
    Capiox-E bypass system o.
    Cobe Optima hollow-fiber membrane o.
    DeBakey heart pump o.
    disk o.
    extracorporeal membrane o.
    extracorporeal pump o.
    Gambro o.
    intravascular o. (IVOX)
    Lilliput o.
    Maxima Plus plasma resistant fiber o.
    Monolyth o.
    plasma-resistant fiber o. (PRF)
    pump o.
    Sarns membrane o. (SMO)

oxygen-binding capacity

oxygen-carrying
    o.-c. capacity
    o.-c. perfluorochemical liquid

oxygen-diffusing capacity

oxygen-induced
    o.-i. hypercapnia
    o.-i. hypercarbia

oxyhemodynamic index

oxyhemoglobin (HbO_2)
    o. dissociation curve
    o. saturation

Oxy-Hood pressurizer

Oxylator-EM 100 automatic resuscitation and inhalation system

OxyLead interconnect cable

Oxylite ambulatory oxygen system

Oxymatic
    O. conserver
    O. electronic oxygen conserver
    O. oxygen conserver

Oxymax

oxymetazoline

Oxymizer device

Oxypleth pulse oximeter

oxypurinol

OxySAT oxygen saturation meter

oxysterol inhibitor

OxyTemp handheld pulse oximeter

oxytetracycline hydrochloride

OxyTip sensor

oxytoca
    Klebsiella o.

Oxytrak pulse oximeter

Oxy-Ultra-Lite ambulatory oxygen system

oyster mass of mucus

ozaenae
    Klebsiella pneumoniae subsp. *o.*

ozone

P

pressure
P cell
P congenitale
P duration
P loop
P mitrale
P pulmonale
P pulmonale syndrome
P substance of Lewis
P synchronous pacing
P terminal force
P vector
P wave
P wave amplitude
P wave axis
P wave triggered ventricular
pacemaker

P_{Emax}
maximal expiratory mouth pressure
P_{Imax}
maximal inspiratory mouth pressure
P_{IO_2}
partial pressure of inspiratory oxygen
P_T
total pressure
P2
pulmonic second heart sound
p22^{phox} protein
p24
p. antigen
p. antigen test
P-32 BXI-15 BetaStent
p47^{phox} protein
p67^{phox} protein
P-A
P-A conduction time
P-A interval
PA
pressure augmentation
pulmonary angiography
pulmonary artery
pulmonary autograft
Adalat PA
PA banding
PA conduction time
PA filling pressure
PA interval
PA 120 Osypka radiofrequency
probe
PA Watch position-monitoring
catheter
PA-1648
P&A
percussion and auscultation

Pa
pascal
pAAT
plasma alpha 1-antitrypsin
PAC
premature atrial contraction
pulmonary artery catheterization
**Paceart complete pacemaker patient
testing system**
Pace bipolar pacing catheter
paced
p. cycle length
p. depolarization integral
p. rhythm
p. ventricular evoked response
Pacefinder
Pacejector
pacemaker
AAI p.
AAT p.
Accufix p.
Acculith p.
Activitrax p.
Activitrax II p.
Activitrax single-chamber
responsive p.
Activitrax variable rate p.
activity-guided p.
activity-sensing p.
Actros p.
p. adaptive rate
adaptive-rate p.
Addvent atrioventricular p.
AEC p.
Aequitron p.
Affinity p.
AFP p.
AFP II p.
p. afterpotential
AICD-B p.
AICD-BR p.
Alcatel p.
American Optical Cardiocare p.
American Optical R-inhibited p.
p. amplifier refractory period
Amtech-Killeen p.
antitachycardia p. (ATP)
AOO p.
Arco atomic p.
Arco lithium p.
p. artifact
artificial p.
Arzco p.
Astra T4, T6 p.
atrial asynchronous p.

pacemaker (*continued*)
  atrial-based p.
  atrial demand-inhibited p.
  atrial demand-triggered p.
  atrial synchronous
    noncompetitive p.
  atrial synchronous ventricular
    inhibited p.
  atrial tracking p.
  atrial triggered noncompetitive p.
  atrial triggered ventricular-
    inhibited p.
  atrial VOO p.
  Atricor Cordis p.
  atrioventricular sequential p.
  p. augmentor
  Aurora dual-chamber p.
  Autima II dual-chamber p.
  automatic p.
  p. automaticity
  Avius sequential p.
  A-V sequential p.
  A-V synchronous p.
  Axios 04 p.
  Basix p.
  Betacel-Biotronik p.
  bifocal demand DVI p.
  Biorate p.
  Biotronik p.
  bipolar p.
  breathing p.
  p. burst pacing
  Byrel SX p.
  Byrel SX/Versatrax p.
  p. can
  p. capture
  cardiac p.
  Cardio-Pace Medical Durapulse p.
  p. catheter
  Chardack-Greatbatch p.
  Chardack Medtronic p.
  Chorus DDD p.
  Chorus RM rate-responsive dual-
    chamber p.
  Chronocor IV external p.
  Chronos 04 p.
  Circadia dual-chamber rate-
    adaptive p.
  circadian p.
  Classix p.
  p. code system
  Command PS p.
  committed mode p.
  Cook p.
  Coratomic R wave inhibited p.
  Cordis Atricor p.
  Cordis Chronocor IV p.
  Cordis Ectocor p.

Cordis fixed-rate p.
Cordis Gemini cardiac p.
Cordis Multicor p.
Cordis Omni Stanicor Theta
  transvenous p.
Cordis Sequicor cardiac p.
Cordis Stanicor unipolar
  ventricular p.
Cordis Synchrocor p.
Cordis Ventricor p.
Cosmos 283 DDD p.
Cosmos II p.
Cosmos II DDD p.
Cosmos pulse-generator p.
CPI p.
CPI Astra p.
CPI DDD p.
CPI Maxilith p.
CPI Microthin DI, DII lithium-
  powered programmable p.
CPI Minilith p.
CPI Ultra II p.
CPI Vista-T p.
crosstalk p.
p. current (I_F)
Cyberlith p.
Cybertach automatic-burst atrial p.
Cybertach 60 bipolar p.
Daig ESI-II or DSI-III screw-in
  lead p.
Dart p.
Dash p.
Dash single-chamber rate-adaptic p.
DDD p.
DDI mode p.
Delta p.
Delta TRS p.
demand p.
Devices, Ltd. p.
Dialog p.
Diplos M 05 p.
Discovery DDDR p.
Dromos p.
DSI-III screw-in lead p.
dual-chamber p.
dual-chamber Medtronic Kappa
  400 p.
dual-demand p.
Durapulse p.
DVI p.
ECT p.
Ectocor p.
ectopic p.
ectopic atrial p.
Ela Chorus DDD p.
Elecath p.
electric cardiac p.
p. electrode

Electrodyne p.
electronic p.
Elema p.
Elema-Schonander p.
Elevath p.
Elite p.
Elite dual-chamber rate-
responsive p.
Encor p.
p. endocarditis
end-of-life p.
Endotak p.
Enertrax 7l00 p.
Entity p.
Ergos O_2 dual-chamber rate-
responsive p.
escape p.
p. escape interval
external p.
p. failure
fixed-rate p.
fully automatic p.
Galaxy p.
Gemini DDD p.
Gen2 p.
Genisis p.
Guardian p.
Guidant CRM p.
Hancock bipolar balloon p.
p. hysteresis
p. impedance
Integrity AFx p.
Intermedics atrial antitachycardia p.
Intermedics Marathon dual-chamber
rate-responsive p.
Intermedics Marathon VVI single-
chamber p.
Intermedics Stride p.
Intertach II p.
Kairos p.
Kalos p.
Kantrowitz p.
Kappa 400 Series p.
Kelvin Sensor p.
p. lead
p. lead fracture
Legend p.
Leukos p.
Lillehei p.
lithium p.
lithium powered p.
Maestro implantable cardiac p.

p. malfunction
Mallory RM-1 cell p.
Mark IV respiratory p.
Medtel p.
Medtronic Activitrax rate-responsive
unipolar ventricular p.
Medtronic-Alcated p.
Medtronic bipolar p.
Medtronic-Byrel-SX p.
Medtronic Elite DDDR p.
Medtronic Elite II p.
Medtronic Kappa 400 p.
Medtronic RF 5998 p.
Medtronic SP 502 p.
Medtronic SPO p.
Medtronic Sympios p.
Medtronic temporary p.
Medtronic Thera DR p.
Medtronic Thera I-series cardiac p.
Meridian p.
Meta DDDR p.
Meta II p.
Meta MV p.
Meta rate-responsive p.
Microlith P p.
Micro Minix p.
Microthin P2 p.
migrating p.
Mikros p.
Minix p.
Minuet DDD p.
Momentum DR p.
Multicor II cardiac p.
Multilith p.
Nanos 01 p.
Neos M p.
noninvasive temporary p.
Nova II p.
Nova MR p.
nuclear p.
Omni-Atricor p.
Omnicor p.
Omni-Orthocor p.
Omni-Stanicor p.
Optima MP p.
Optima MPT Series III p.
Optima SPT p.
Opus p.
p. output
p. output reprogramming
p. output voltage
oversensing p.

NOTES

P

pacemaker *(continued)*

Pacesetter p.
Pacesetter Addvent 2060 LR p.
Pacesetter Affinity p.
Pacesetter 2060 LR p.
Pacesetter Regency SC+ p.
Pacesetter Synchrony p.
Paragon II p.
Pasar tachycardia reversion p.
PDx pacing and diagnostic p.
pervenous p.
phantom p.
Phoenix 2 p.
Phymos 3D p.
physiologic p.
piezoelectric crystal-based p.
Pinnacle p.
p. pocket
Polyflex p.
p. potential
Precept DR p.
Prima p.
primary p.
Prism-CL p.
Programalith p.
Programalith A-V p.
Programalith II p.
Programalith III p.
programmable p.
programmer p.
Prolog p.
Pulsar p.
Pulsar DDD p.
Pulsar NI implantable p.
P wave triggered ventricular p.
QT interval sensing p.
Quantum p.
rate-modulated p.
rate-responsive p.
reedswitch of p.
p. reedswitch
Reflex 8220 p.
reflex p.
refractory period of electronic p.
Relay cardiac p.
SAVVI p.
Seecor p.
P. Selection in the Elderly (PASE)
p. sensitivity
Sensolog II, III p.
Sensor p.
Sequicor III p.
shifting p.
Siemens-Elema p.
smart p.
SmartTracking on the Marathon p.
Solus p.
Sorin p.

p. sound
Spectrax SX, SX-HT, SXT, VL, VM, VS p.
p. spike
standby p.
Stanicor p.
p. stimulus artifact
Stride cardiac p.
subsidiary atrial p.
Swing DR1 DDDR p.
Symbios 7006 p.
Synchrony I, II p.
p. syndrome
Synergyst DDD p.
Synergyst II p.
Tachylog p.
Telectronics p.
p. telemetry
temperature-sensing p.
Thermos p.
p. threshold
tined lead p.
transmural antitachycardia p.
transthoracic p.
Trios M p.
Triumph VR p.
Ultra p.
p. undersensing
Unilith p.
unipolar p.
unipolar atrial p.
unipolar sequential p.
Unity-C p.
Unity-C cardiac p.
Unity VDDR p.
universal p.
VAT p.
VDD p.
Ventak AICD p.
Ventak PRx p.
ventricular asynchronous p.
ventricular demand-inhibited p.
ventricular demand-triggered p.
Versatrax II 7000A p.
Vigor p.
Vigor DDDR p.
Vigor DR p.
Vista 4, T, TRS p.
Vitatron Diamond p.
Vitatron Diamond II p.
VOO p.
VVD mode p.
VVI p.
VVIR p.
wandering p.
wandering atrial p. (WAP)
Zoll NTP noninvasive p.

Zyrel p.
Zytron p.
pacemaker-mediated tachycardia (PMT)
PACE Physician Manual
Paceport catheter
Pacerone 200 mg tablet
Pacer-Tracer
Pacesetter

P. Addvent 2060 LR pacemaker
P. Affinity pacemaker
P. APS II 3004 programmer
P. APS pacemaker programmer
P. AutoCapture lead
P. lead
P. 2060 LR pacemaker
P. pacemaker
P. Regency SC+ pacemaker
P. Synchrony pacemaker
P. Tendril DX steroid-eluting
  active-fixation pacing lead
P. Trilogy DR+ pulse generator

Pacesetter/St. Jude lead
pace-terminable
pace-terminate
Pacewedge dual-pressure bipolar pacing
  catheter
Pachon

P. method
P. test

pachypleuritis
PACI

partial anterior circulation infarct

pacing

AAI p.
AAI-RR p.
AAT p.
acceleration-guided activity p.
activity-guided p.
antitachycardia p. (ATP)
AOO p.
asynchronous p.
atrial incremental p.
atrial overdrive p.
atrial septum septal p.
atrial train p.
atrioventricular synchronous p.
autodecremental p.
biatrial p.
biventricular p.
burst p.
burst atrial p.
cardiac p.

P. in Cardiomyopathy Study
  (PICS)
p. catheter
closed-loop p.
p. code
p. counter
p. cycle length
DDD p.
DDDR p.
DDI p.
DDIR p.
decremental atrial p.
demand p.
diaphragmatic p.
direct His bundle p. (DHBP)
dual-chamber p.
dual-site right atrial p.
p. duration
DVI p.
endocardial p.
epicardial p.
external high-output ramp p.
high-frequency burst p.
p. hysteresis
implantable cardioverter-
  defibrillator/atrial tachycardia p.
  (ICD-ATP)
incremental atrial p.
incremental ventricular p.
inhibited p.
intracardiac p.
p. lead impedance
p. modality
p. mode
multisite p.
multisite biventricular p.
no atrial p.
overdrive p.
pacemaker burst p.
permanent p.
P synchronous p.
RAMP p.
rapid p.
rapid atrial p.
rapid-burst p.
Rate Modulated P. (RAMP)
rate-responsive p.
rate-responsive ventricular p.
right atrial p.
right ventricular outflow tract p.
right ventricular septal p.
RVOT p.

NOTES

P

pacing *(continued)*
    sequential p.
    shock p.
    p. spike
    p. stimulus
    subthreshold p.
    suprathreshold p.
    p. system analyzer
    temporary p.
    threshold p.
    p. threshold
    trains of ventricular p.
    transatrial p.
    transesophageal atrial p. (TAP, TEAP)
    transesophageal echocardiography with p. (TEEP)
    trichambered p.
    triggered p.
    underdrive p.
    univentricular p.
    VAT p.
    VDD p.
    ventricular p.
    ventricular safety p.
    VOO p.
    VVI p.
    VVIR p.
    VVI-RR p.
    VVI/VVIR p.
    VVT p.
pacing-induced
    p.-i. angina
    p.-i. heart failure
Pacis
pack
    AeroGear fanny p.
    interferon alfa-2b and ribavirin combination p.
    RIK fluid-filled head p.
package
    SX/DX computerized spirometry p.
pack-year smoking history
paclitaxel
PaCO$_2$
    arterial partial pressure of CO$_2$
PACS
    partial anterior circulation syndrome
PACT
    Philadelphia Association of Clinical Trials
    Plasminogen Activator Angioplasty Compatibility Trial
    Prehospital Application of Coronary Thrombolysis
    Prescription Analyses and Cost
    Prourokinase in Acute Coronary Thrombosis

    PACT clinical trial
    PACT study
PACU
    postanesthesia care unit
PAD
    peripheral arterial disease
    public access defibrillation
    public access defibrillator
    pulsatile assist device
pad
    digitizing p.
    electrode p.
    Littman defibrillation p.
    pericardial fat p.
    pharyngoesophageal p.'s
    p. sign
    Signa P.
    SomaSensor p.
PADCAB
    perfusion-assisted direct coronary artery bypass
paddles
    anteroposterior p.
    cardioversion p.
    defibrillation p.
    defibrillator p.
    electrode p.
PADP
    pulmonary artery diastolic pressure
PAE
    postantibiotic effect
Paecilomyces variotii
PAF
    paroxysmal atrial fibrillation
    platelet activating factor
PAG
    pulmonary angiography
PAGE
    perfluorocarbon-associated gas exchange
Page episodic hypertension
Paget disease of bone
Paget-von Schrötter
    Paget-von Schrötter syndrome
    P.-v. S. venous thrombosis
PAH
    polycyclic aromatic hydrocarbon
    pulmonary artery hypertension
PAI
    perforating artery infarct
    plasminogen activator inhibitor
PAI-1
    plasminogen activator inhibitor-1
pain
    anginal p.
    atypical chest p.
    burning p.
    calf p.
    chest p.

crushing chest p.
dream p.
dull p.
Emergency Room Assessment of
Sestamibi for Evaluation of
Chest P. (ERASE)
p.-free walking time (PFWT)
functional p.
musculoskeletal p.
p., pallor, paraesthesia,
pulselessness, paralysis, prostration
(PPPPPP)
phantom p.
pleuritic chest p.
psychogenic p.
pulmonary p.
rest p.
staccato p.
Study of Nitroglycerin and
Chest P. (SNAP)
waxing and waning chest p.

paired
p. beats
p. electrical stimulation
p. stimulus

PAK
percutaneous access kit
Denver PAK

palatal surgery
palate
high arched p.

palatina
tonsilla p.

palatine tonsil
palatini
tensor p.

palatopharyngeal sphincter
palatoplasty
laser-assisted p. (LAP)

palatovaginal canal
Palco
P. Laboratories Model 400 pulse
oximeter
P. Model 300 pulse oximeter

pale
p. hypertension
p. thrombus

paleopneumoniae
Peptostreptococcus p.

palestinensis
Acanthamoeba p.

palisading histiocyte

palivizumab
palliation
palliative surgery
pallida
asphyxia p.

pallidum
microhemagglutination *Treponema p.*
(MHA-TP)
Treponema p.

pallor
palm
liver p.
tripe p.

Palma operation
palmar
p. arch
carpal arch p.
p. click
p. erythema
p. xanthoma

palmare
xanthoma striatum p.

Palmaz
P. balloon-expandable iliac stent
P. stent
P. vascular stent

Palmaz-Schatz (PS)
P.-S. balloon-expandable stent
P.-S. coronary stent
P.-S. Crown stent
NACI P.-S.
New Applications for Coronary
Interventions, P.-S.
P.-S. PS-204 stent
P.-S. stent (PSS)

palmi (*pl. of* palmus)
palmic
palmitate
C-11 p.
clofazimine p.
colfosceril p.

palmitic acid
palmitoylcarnitine
palmodic
palmoscopy
palmus, pl. **palmi**
palpation
bimanual precordial p.

palpatio cordis
palpitation
paroxysmal p.
premonitory p.

NOTES

P

PALS
pediatric life support
palsy
pseudobulbar p.
suprabulbar p.
Palv
alveolar pressure
2-PAM
2-pralidoxime
PAM2, PAM3 monitors
Pamax
Pamelor
PAMI
Primary Angioplasty in Myocardial
Infarction
PAMI clinical trial
PAMI II clincal trial
p-**aminosalicylic acid**
pamoate
pyrantel p.
Panacet 5/500
panacinar emphysema
panbronchiolitis
diffuse p. (DPB)
pancarditis
panchamber enlargement
Pancoast
P. syndrome
P. tumor
panconduction defect
pancreas
pancreatic
p. dornase
p. enzyme
p. extract
p. polypeptide (PP)
pancreaticopleural fistula
pancreatin asthma
pancreatitis
pancreatopleural fistula
pancuronium bromide
pandiastolic
panel
Cholestech LDX system with TC
and Glucose P.
lipid p.
p. of reactive antibodies (PRA)
South Florida RAST p.
thyroid p.
panel-reactive antibody (PRA)
pang
breast p.
Panhematin
panhyperemia
panhypogammaglobulinemia
panic disorder
paninspiratory
Panje voice button

panlobular emphysema
Panlukast
Panmycin Oral
panniculitis
panning
panophthalmitis
pansystolic
p. flow
p. murmur
pantaloon
p. embolism
p. patch
Panther balloon
panting maneuver
pantoprazole sodium
pantothenate synthetase
pantyhose
Glattelast compression p.
Panwarfin
panzerherz
PAO$_2$
alveolar oxygen partial pressure
PaO$_2$
arterial oxygen partial pressure
PAOD
peripheral arterial occlusive disease
PAOP
pulmonary artery occlusion pressure
PAP
positive airway pressure
pulmonary artery pressure
papain
Papanicolaou solution
papaverine hydrochloride
paper
asthma p.
niter p.
Papercuff
papilla
Bergmeister p.
papillary
p. adenocarcinoma
p. carcinoma
p. fibroelastoma (PES)
p. frond
p. muscle
p. muscle abscess
p. muscle of conus arteriosus
p. muscle dysfunction
p. muscle rupture (PMR)
p. muscle syndrome
p. muscle tip
p. muscle traction
p. tumor
papilledema
papillitis
papillomatosis
recurrent respiratory p.

papillomavirus
　　human p. (HPV)
papillotome
　　Wilson-Cook p.
PAPm
　　mean pulmonary artery pressure
Pappenheim stain
papulonecrotic tuberculosis
papulosis
　　atrophic p.
PAPV
　　partial anomalous pulmonary veins
　　peak hyperemic average velocity
　　positive airway pressure ventilation
PAPVC
　　partial anomalous pulmonary venous
　　　connection
PAPVD
　　partial anomalous pulmonary venous
　　　drainage
PAPVR
　　partial anomalous pulmonary venous
　　　return
PAR
　　pulse amplitude ratio
paraaminobenzoic acid
paraaminosalicylate sodium
paraaminosalicylic acid (PAS, PASA)
paraaortic bodies
paraboloid
　　oscillating p.
paracentesis
　　p. pericardii
　　p. thoracis
paracetamol sensitivity
parachute
　　p. deformity
　　p. mitral valve
paracicatricial emphysema
Paracoccidioides brasiliensis
paracoccidioidin skin test
paracoccidioidomycosis
paracorporeal heart
paracrine
　　p. factor
　　p. signaling
paradigm
paradox
　　calcium p.
　　French p.
　　p. image

　　oxygen p.
　　thoracoabdominal p.
paradoxic
　　p. embolism
　　p. embolus
　　p. pulse
　　p. rocking impulse
　　p. split of S_2
　　p. wall motion
paradoxical
　　p. aberrancy
　　p. bronchospasm
　　p. cerebral embolism
　　p. embolism
　　p. embolization
　　p. embolus
　　p. respiration
　　p. vasoconstriction
paradoxically split S_2 sound
paradoxus
　　p. parvus et tardus
　　pulsus p.
paraesophageal hernia
paraffin block
paraffinoma
paraganglioma tumor
PARAGON
　　Platelet IIb/IIIa Antagonist for the
　　Reduction of Acute Coronary
　　Syndrome Events in a Global
　　Organization Network
　　PARAGON clinical trial
Paragon
　　P. coronary stent
　　P. II pacemaker
　　P. nitinol stent
　　P. PAS stent
paragonimiasis
Paragonimus westermani
parahaemolyticus
　　Haemophilus p.
　　Vibrio p.
parahilar
　　p. fibrosis
　　p. region
parahisian accessory pathway
parainfluenzae
　　Haemophilus p. (HPI)
parainfluenza virus
parallel shunt
paralysis
　　diaphragmatic p.

NOTES

P

paralysis *(continued)*
    diphtheric p.
    diphtheritic p.
    hemidiaphragm p.
    hypokalemic periodic p.
    ischemic p.
    periodic p.
    phrenic nerve p.
    respiratory p.
    sleep p.
    tick p.
    vasomotor p.
    Volkmann ischemic p.
paralytica
    dysphagia p.
paralytic chest
paralyticus
    laryngismus p.
    thorax p.
paramagnetic substance
Paramed Cardivon 9200 noninvasive blood pressure monitor
paramedian frontal bone window (PMFBW)
paramedic
parameter
    late potential p.
    portable monitor of respiratory p.'s (PMRP)
    systemic hemodynamic p.'s
paramethasone acetate
parametric
    p. image
    p. imaging
Paramyxoviridae virus
Paramyxovirus
paraneoplastic
    p. pemphigus
    p. syndrome
paraoxonase polymorphism
paraplane echocardiography
Paraplatin
parapneumonic effusion
paraprosthetic leak
parapsilosis
    Candida p.
paraquat
pararrhythmia
parasagittal plane
paraseptal
    p. emphysema
    p. pathway
parasitic
    p. cardiomyopathy
    p. infestation
paraspinal line
parasternal
    p. examination

    p. heave
    p. long axis
    p. long-axis view
    p. long-axis view echocardiogram
    p. short axis
    p. short-axis view
    p. short-axis view echocardiogram
    p. systolic lift
    p. systolic thrill
    p. view
    p. window
parasympathetic
    p. function
    p. nerve fibers
    p. nervous system
parasympathomimetic
parasynapsis
parasyndesis
parasystole
    atrial p.
    junctional p.
    pure p.
    ventricular p.
parasystolic
    p. beat
    p. ventricular tachycardia
parathyroid hormone
paratracheal
    p. chain
    p. lymph node
    p. region
paratracheales
    nodi lymphoidei p.
Paratrend
    P. 7 continuous blood gas monitor
    P. 7+ multiparameter blood gas monitor
paravalvular
parchemin
    bruit de p.
parchment
    p. heart
    p. right ventricle
parenchyma
    pulmonary p.
parenchymal
    p. amyloidosis
    p. asbestosis
    p. aspergillosis
    p. disease
    p. fibrosis
    p. hematoma (PH)
    p. hemorrhage (PH)
    p. laceration
    p. lesion
    p. sarcoidosis

parenchymatous
    p. myocarditis
    p. pneumonia
parenteral
    Coly-Mycin M P.
    P. nutrition
paresis
    faciobrachiocrural p.
pargyline
    methyclothiazide and p.
Parham band
paries membranaceus tracheae
parietal
    p. ball
    p. band
    p. endocarditis
    p. pericardiectomy
    p. pericardium
    p. pleura
    p. pleural damage
    p. thrombus
parietalis
    pleura p.
parietooccipital artery
PARIS
    Peripheral Artery Radiation
    Investigational Study
    Persantine and Aspirin Reinfarction
    Study
    Port Access Recovery Improvement
    Study
Park
    P. aneurysm
    P. blade septostomy
    P. blade septostomy catheter
Parks 800 bidirectional Doppler
flowmeter
Parlodel
parnaparin
paromomycin sulfate
paroxetine
paroxysmal
    p. atrial fibrillation (PAF)
    p. atrial tachycardia (PAT)
    p. atrial tachycardia with aberrancy
    p. burst
    p. cough
    p. hypertension
    p. junctional tachycardia
    p. nocturnal dyspnea (PND)
    p. nocturnal hemoglobinuria (PNH)
    p. nodal tachycardia

    p. palpitation
    p. pulmonary edema
    p. reentrant supraventricular
    tachycardia
    p. sinus tachycardia
    p. sleep
    p. supraventricular arrhythmia
    p. supraventricular tachycardia
    (PSVT)
    p. tachycardia
    p. ventricular tachycardia
paroxysm of coughing
parrot
    p. fever
    P. murmur
pars, pl. **partes**
    p. abdominalis esophagi
    p. basalis arteriae pulmonalis
    p. cervicalis esophagi
    p. costalis diaphragmatis
    partes intersegmentales
    p. intralobaris intersegmentalis
    venae posterioris lobi superioris
    pulmonis dextri
    p. lumbalis diaphragmatis
    p. mediastinalis pulmonis
    p. membranacea
    p. nasalis pharyngis
    p. oralis pharyngis
    p. pharyngea hypophyseos
    p. thoracica esophagi
Parsonnet
    P. coronary probe
    P. dilator
    P. epicardial retractor
    P. pulse generator pouch
PART
    Prevention of Atherosclerosis with
    Ramipril Therapy
    PART Clinical Trial
part
    certified distinct P. (CDP)
partes (*pl. of* pars)
partial
    p. anomalous pulmonary veins
    (PAPV)
    p. anomalous pulmonary venous
    connection (PAPVC)
    p. anomalous pulmonary venous
    drainage (PAPVD)
    p. anomalous pulmonary venous
    return (PAPVR)

NOTES

P

partial (*continued*)
  p. anterior circulation infarct (PACI)
  p. anterior circulation syndrome (PACS)
  p. atrioventricular canal
  p. autobullectomy
  p. A-V canal defect
  p. chordal-sparing mitral valve replacement
  p. confluens sinuum thrombosis
  p. encircling endocardial ventriculotomy
  p. heart block
  p. intermixed fibrosis
  p. liquid ventilation (PLV)
  p. occlusion inferior vena cava clip
  p. pressure of carbon dioxide (PCO_2)
  p. pressure of carbon monoxide gas
  p. pressure of CO gas (PCO)
  p. pressure of end-tidal CO_2 ($PETCO_2$)
  p. pressure of inspiratory oxygen (P_{IO_2})
  p. pressure of oxygen (PO_2)
  p. rebreathing mask
  p. thromboplastin time (PTT)
partially coagulated effusion
particle
  Amberlite p.'s
  Dane p.
  remnant-like lipoprotein p. (RLP)
particulate respirator
partition
  atrial p.
partitioning
  left atrial p.
parts per million (ppm)
Partuss LA
Parvolex
parvus
  p. alternans
  pulsus p.
Parzen window
PAS
  paraaminosalicylic acid
  peripheral access system
  posterior airway space
  PAS port
  venarum pulmonum PAS
P.A.S.
  P. Port
  P. Port catheter
  P. Port Fluoro-Free

PASA
  paraaminosalicylic acid
Pasar tachycardia reversion pacemaker
pascal (Pa)
  P. principle
PASE
  Pacemaker Selection in the Elderly
  Physical Activity Scale for the Elderly Evaluation
  PASE Quality-of-Life Study
PASG
  pneumatic antishock garment
PASP
  pulmonary artery systolic pressure
PASS
  Piracetam in Acute Stroke Study
  Postural Assessment Scale for Stroke Patient
  Practical Applicability of Saruplase Study
  Prehospital Applicability of Saruplase Study
passage
  adiabatic fast p.
  P. exchange balloon
Passager
  P. device
  P. endoprosthesis
  P. stent
passive
  p. clot
  p. congestion
  p. edema
  p. hyperemia
  p. interval
  p. mode
  p. smoking
  p. tilting
passover humidifier
Passy-Muir
  P.-M. O2 Adapter
  P.-M. tracheostomy speaking valve
paste
  electrode p.
Pasteurella
  P. aerogenes
  P. multocida
pasteurellosis
PASYS
  P. cardiac pacing system
  P. ST cardiac pacing system
PAT
  paroxysmal atrial tachycardia
patch
  AcuSeal cardiovascular p.
  Adcon-C Resorbable liquid p.
  p. angioplasty
  atrial septal defect p.
  autologous blood p.

autologous pericardial p.
BioGlue surgical p.
buspirone transdermal p.
cardiac p.
CardioFix pericardium p.
Carrel p.
chest wall p.
p. closure
Dacron intracardiac p.
defibrillation p.
Deponit P.
electrodispersive skin p.
epicardial p.
epicardial defibrillator p.
extrapericardial p.
Fluoropassiv thin-wall carotid p.
Gore-Tex cardiovascular p.
Gore-Tex soft tissue p.
p. graft reconstruction
Habitrol P.
Ionescu-Shiley pericardial p.
MacCallum p.
Minitran P.
Nicoderm P.
nicotine transdermal p.
Nicotrol P.
Nitrodisc P.
Nitro-Dur P.
nitroglycerin transdermal p.
outflow cardiac p.
pantaloon p.
pericardial p.
Peyer p.
polypropylene intracardiac p.
ProStep P.
p. repair
retropectoral p.
sandwich p.
Silastic p.
SJM pericardial p.
soldier's p.'s
Stat-padz defibrillator p.
subcutaneous p.
Teflon felt p.
Teflon intracardiac p.
transannular p.
Transdermal-NTG P.
Transderm-Nitro P.
patch-coil system
patch-graft
   p.-g. angioplasty
   Dacron onlay p.-g.

patchplasty
patchy
   p. atelectasis
   p. consolidation
   p. hyperintensity
   p. infiltrate
   p. infiltration
patency
   catheter p.
   coronary bypass graft p.
   epicardial artery p.
   epicardial vessel p.
   Heparin in Early P. (HEAP)
   infarct artery p.
   P., Outcomes and Economics of
     MIDCAB (POEM)
   probe p.
   stent p.
   TIMI p.
   vein graft p.
   venous coronary graft p.
PATENT
   Prourokinase and tPA Enhancement of
     Thrombolysis Trial
patent
   p. bronchus sign
   p. ductus arteriosus (PDA)
   p. ductus arteriosus flow jet
   p. ductus arteriosus murmur
   p. ductus arteriosus umbrella
   p. foramen ovale (PFO)
   P. Foramen Ovale in Cryptogenic
     Stroke Study (PICSS)
Pathfinder
   P. catheter
   P. microcatheter
   P. microcatheter system
   P. mini microcatheter
Pathocil
pathogen
   nosocomial p.
pathogenesis
pathogenicity
pathologic murmur
pathology
   coexistent p.
pathophysiology
pathostimulation
pathway
   accessory p. (AP)
   antegrade internodal p.
   anterior internodal p.

NOTES

P

pathway (*continued*)
    atrio-His p.
    atrioventricular node p.
    Bachmann p.
    concealed accessory p.
    conduction p.
    diacylglycerate p.
    Fas-Fas ligand p.
    FasL p.
    fast p.
    final common p.
    free-wall accessory p.
    integrin-dependent p.
    internodal p.
    Jak/Stat p.
    Kent p.
    lipoxygenase p.
    MAPK p.
    mitogen-activated kinase p.
    parahisian accessory p.
    paraseptal p.
    reentrant p.
    retinohypothalamic p.
    retrograde fast p.
    scavenger cell p.
    selective past p.
    septal p.
    shunt p.
    slow p.
    slow A-V node p.
    slow and fast A-V nodal p.
    surgical ablation of p.
    Thorel p.
patient
    p. activator mode
    p. circuit wye
    p. compliance
    intubated p.
    p. monitor
    Multifit system risk management of
      heart attack p.'s
    multiple-trauma p.
    nonintubated p.
    nonventilated p.
    P. Outcomes Research Team Study
      (PORT, PORTS)
    Postural Assessment Scale for
      Stroke P. (PASS)
patient-controlled
    p.-c. analgesia (PCA)
    p.-c. analgesic (PCA)
patient-triggered recording
Patil stereotactic system
pattern
    abdominal paradox breathing p.
    airspace-filling p.
    airway p.
    alveolar p.

    alveolar-filling p.
    ballerina-foot p.
    butterfly p.
    candle flame p.
    cephalization of pulmonary flow p.
    circadian p.
    circadian blood pressure p.
    concave p.
    contraction p.
    crochetage p.
    deer-antler vascular p.
    diastolic filling p.
    dip-and-plateau p.
    disturbed circadian blood
      pressure p.
    eggshell p.
    embryonic phenotype p.
    fishnet p.
    ground-glass p.
    honeycomb p.
    hourglass p.
    impaired relaxation mitral flow p.
    interstitial p.
    intraventricular conduction p.
    juvenile p.
    miliary p.
    military p.
    mosaic p.
    organoid p.
    Poincar plot p.
    QR p.
    QS p.
    respiratory p.
    respiratory alternans breathing p.
    restrictive physiology mitral
      flow p.
    reticular p.
    reticulonodular p.
    salt and pepper p.
    sawtooth p.
    scintillating speckle p.
    scooped p.
    sine wave p.
    sinusoidal strut p.
    S_1Q_3 p.
    $S_1Q_3T_3$ p.
    torpedo-shaped p.
    upstroke p.
    uptake-mismatch p.
    vascular p.
    ventricular contraction p.
    W p.
    watershed p.
patty
    cottonoid p.
PAU
    penetrating aortic ulcer
    penetrating atherosclerotic ulcer

pauciimmune glomerulonephritis
Paulin venography technique
pause
- compensatory p.
- full compensatory p.
- noncompensatory p.
- postectopic p.
- postextrasystolic p.
- preautomatic p.
- sinus p.
- sinus exit p.
- ventricular p.

pause-dependent arrhythmia
PAV
- proportional assist ventilation

Pavabid Oral
Pavased Oral
Pavatine Oral
pavementing
Pavenik monodisk device
Paveral Stanley Syrup With Codeine Phosphate
Paverolan Oral
Pavlov reflex
PAVM
- pulmonary arteriovenous malformation

PAVSD
- pulmonary atresia with ventricular septal defect

Pavulon
PAW
- pulmonary artery wedge

PAWP
- pulmonary artery wedge pressure

Pax3 deficiency
Paxene
Paykel scale
PBC
- perfusion balloon catheter

PBMC
PBP
- percutaneous balloon pericardiotomy

PBS
- phosphate-buffered saline

PBV
- percutaneous balloon valvuloplasty
- pulmonary balloon valvuloplasty
- pulmonary blood volume

PBZ
- Pyribenzamine

PC
- posterior circulation

- posterior circumflex artery
- pressure control

PCA
- patient-controlled analgesia
- patient-controlled analgesic
- posterior cerebral artery
  - fetal-type PCA
  - PCA system

PCB
- protected catheter brushing

PCBS
- percutaneous cardiopulmonary bypass support

PCD
- primary ciliary dyskinesia
- programmable cardioverter-defibrillator
  - PCD ICD generator
  - Jewel PCD
  - PCD Transvene implantable cardioverter-defibrillator
  - PCD Transvene implantable cardioverter-defibrillator system

PCE Oral
PCF
- peak cough flow

PCI
- percutaneous coronary intervention
- prophylactic brain irradiation

PCIRV
- pressure-controlled inverse ratio ventilation

PCIS
- postcardiac injury syndrome

PCNA
- proliferating cell nuclear antigen

PCNL
- percutaneous nephrostolithotomy

PCO
- partial pressure of CO gas

PCO$_2$
- partial pressure of carbon dioxide
  - PCO$_2$ oximetry

PCoA
- posterior communicating artery

P-congenitale
PCP
- *Pneumocystis carinii* pneumonia

PCPB
- percutaneous cardiopulmonary bypass

PCPS
- percutaneous cardiopulmonary support

NOTES

P

PCR

polymerase chain reaction
PCR assay
PCR test

PCr

phosphocreatine

PCRA

percutaneous coronary rotational
atherectomy

PCS

proximal coronary sinus

PCV

pressure-controlled ventilation

PCW

pulmonary capillary wedge

PCWP

pulmonary capillary wedge pressure

PD

postural drainage
pure dysarthria
PD 123319 AT receptor agonist
PD 2000 defibrillator

PDA

patent ductus arteriosus
posterior descending artery
snare-assisted coil occlusion of
PDA
PDA umbrella

PDB

preperitoneal distention balloon
PDB preperitoneal distention
balloon system

PDE

phosphodiesterase inhibitor
PDE isoenzyme inhibitor

PDE-I

phosphodiesterase inhibitor

PDE3I

phosphodiesterase III inhibition

P-dextrocardiale

PDF

probability density function

PDGF

platelet-derived growth factor

PDH

progressive disseminated histoplasmosis
pyruvate dehydrogenase

PDHRF

platelet-derived histamine-releasing factor

Pdisniff

maximal sniff-induced
transdiaphragmatic pressure

PD&P

postural drainage and percussion

PDPV

postural drainage, percussion and
vibration

PDT

percutaneous dilatational tracheostomy
percutaneous dilational tracheostomy
PDT guidewire

PDUFA

Prescription Drug User Fee Act

PDx pacing and diagnostic pacemaker

PE

cisplatin, etoposide
pulmonary embolism
pulmonary emphysema
PE balloon
PE Plus II peripheral balloon
catheter

**PE-85-I-2 implantable pronged unipolar
electrode**

PEA

pulseless electrical activity

PEACE

Prevention of Events with ACE
Inhibition
PEACE study

peak

p. airway pressure (Ppeak)
p. A velocity
p. cough flow (PCF)
p. diastolic filling rate
p. ejection velocity (V_{pe})
p. emptying rate
p. E velocity
p. exercise
p. exercise oxygen consumption
(VO_2)
p. exercise ventilation (V_E)
p. expiratory flow (PEF)
p. expiratory flow rate (PEFR)
p. expiratory maneuver
p. filling rate (PFR)
p. flowmeter (PFM)
p. flow rate
h p.
p. hyperemic average velocity
(PAPV)
p. incidence
p. inspiratory flow (PIF)
p. inspiratory flow rate (PIFR)
p. instantaneous Doppler gradient
p. instantaneous gradient
p. jet flow rate
p. lengthening rate
p. magnitude
p. oxygen uptake
p. respiratory ratio (RER)
p. shortening rate
p. systolic aortic pressure (PSAP)
p. systolic gradient (PSG)
p. systolic gradient pressure
p. systolic velocity

p. tidal expiratory flow (PTEF)
p. tidal inspiratory flow (PTIF)
p. transaortic flow velocity
p. transaortic valve gradient
p. and trough
p. and trough levels
p. twitch force
p. VO_2
p. workload
p. work rate (Wmax)

peaked P wave
PeakLog monitor
The PEAK peak flowmeter
PEAP

positive end-airway pressure

pearl

p.-and-string sign
keratin p.
Laënnec p.
p. sign
string of p.'s

pear-shaped heart
peau d'orange
Pecor intraaortic balloon catheter
pecorum

Chlamydia p.

pectinate muscle
pectoral

ectopia cordis p.
p. emulation
p. fascia
p. fremitus
p. heart
p. tea

pectoralgia
pectoralis

p. fascia
p. major
p. minor

pectoriloquous bronchophony
pectoriloquy

aphonic p.
whispered p.
whispering p.

pectoris

angina p.
angor p.
stable angina p. (SAP)
unstable angina p. (UAP)
variant angina p. (VAR)

pectorophony

pectus

p. carinatum
p. deformity
p. excavatum
p. gallinatum
p. recurvatum

pedal

p. edema
p. pulse

pedal-mode ergometer
PediaCare Oral
Pediacof
Pediapred Oral
pediatric

Benylin P.
P. Cardiology Devices Sideris
    Buttoned device occluder
p. cardiomyopathy
Cleocin P.
Codamine P.
Cycofed P.
Exosurf P.
Fedahist Expectorant P.
P. Finger Clip Sensor
Hycomine P.
p. hypertension
p. lead
p. life support (PALS)
p. pigtail catheter
Robitussin P.
P. universal bite block B117
p. vascular clamp

Pediazole Oral
pedicle graft
Pedi-Dri
Pedituss
Pedoff continuous wave transducer
pedunculated thrombus
PedvaxHIB
peel

pericardial p.
pleural p.
visceral p.

Peel-Away

P.-A. banana catheter
P.-A. catheter
P.-A. introducer set

peel-away sheath
peeling-back mechanism
PEEP

positive end-expiratory pressure
PEEP valve

NOTES

P

PEEPi
    intrinsic positive end-expiratory pressure
Peep-Keep II adapter
PEF
    peak expiratory flow
%PEF
    percent predicted peak expiratory flow
2110 PEF/FEV₁ DiaryCard
pefloxacin
PEFR
    peak expiratory flow rate
PEG
    P. interleukin-2
    P. tube
PEG-ADA
    pegademase bovine
pegademase bovine (PEG-ADA)
pegaspargase
PEG-LES
    polyethylene glycol electrolyte lavage
    solution
PE-60-I-2 implantable pronged unipolar electrode
PEJ
    percutaneous endoscopic jejunostomy
    PEJ tube
PE-60-K-10 implantable unipolar endocardial electrode
PE-85-K-10 implantable unipolar endocardial electrode
PE-60-KB implantable unipolar endocardial electrode
PE-85-KB implantable unipolar endocardial electrode
PE-85-KS-10 implantable unipolar endocardial electrode
Pel
    lung elastic recoil pressure
PELA
    peripheral excimer laser angioplasty
PELCA
    Percutaneous Excimer Laser Coronary
    Angioplasty
    PELCA Registry
Pelger-Huet cell
pellagra
pellet
    Testopel P.
pellucidum
    pineal p.
    septum p.
Pelorus stereotactic system
Pel-V
    elastic pressure-volume
Pemco prosthetic valve
pemphigus
    paraneoplastic p.
PE-MT balloon dilatation catheter

pen
    light p.
Penaz volume-clamp method
penbutolol sulfate
PenChant stent delivery system
penciclovir
pencil percussion
pendelluft phenomenon
Penderluft syndrome
pendulous heart
pendulum
    cor p.
    p. rhythm
    p. test
penetrance
penetrating
    p. aortic ulcer (PAU)
    p. atherosclerotic ulcer (PAU)
    p. chest injury
    p. injury
    p. rupture
    p. thoracic trauma
penetration
penetrator artery
Penetrex Oral
penicillin
    benzathine benzyl p.
    p. G
    p. G benzathine
    p. G benzathine and procaine
    combined
    p. G, parenteral, aqueous
    p. G procaine
    p.-nonsusceptible *Streptococcus
    pneumoniae* (PNSP)
    p. phenoxymethyl
    p.-resistant
    p.-resistant *Streptococcus
    pneumoniae* (PRSP)
    semisynthetic p.
    p. VK
    p. V potassium
penicilliosis
Penicillium marneffei
penile-brachial pressure index
penis
    cavernous vein of p.
Penlon infant resuscitator
Penn
    P. Convention criteria
    P. formula
    P. method
    P. State TAH
    P. State total artificial heart
    P. State ventricular assist device
pentaacetate
    diethylenetriamine p.-a. (DTPA)
Pentacarinat injection

PentaCath catheter
Pentacef
pentachloride
    antimony p.
pentachrome
    Movat p.
pentaerythritol tetranitrate
pentagastrin
pentalogy
    Cantrell p.
    p. of Fallot
    Fallot p.
Pentalumen catheter
pentamidine
    p. in aerosol form
    aerosolized p.
    p. isethionate
Pentam-300 injection
pentane
PentaPace QRS catheter
pentasaccharide
Pentatrichomonas hominis
Pentax bronchoscope
pentazocine
pentetate
    imciromab p.
pentobarbital
Pentothal Sodium
pentoxifylline
pentraxin
penumbra
    ischemic p.
Pen-Vee
Pen.Vee K
    P. K. Oral
PEP
    positive expiratory pressure
    preejection period
    PEP mask
PEPI
    Postmenopausal Estrogen/Progestin
    Intervention
    PEPI Clinical Trial
Pepper
    P. Medical Antidisconnect Device
    strap
    P. Medical tube neck band
peppermint test
Peptavlon
peptic
    p. aspiration pneumonitis

    p. esophagitis
    p. ulcer
peptide
    adrenomedullin p.
    atrial natriuretic p. (ANP)
    brain natriuretic p. (BNP)
    B-type natriuretic p. (BNP)
    calcitonin gene-related p. (CGRP)
    C-type natriuretic p. (CNP)
    dendroaspis natriuretic p. (DNP)
    human atrial natriuretic p. (hANP)
    p. mucolytic
    natriuretic p.
    procollagen type III
      aminoterminal p. (PIIIP)
    TFF-domain p.
    tick anticoagulant p.
    trefoil factor family domain p.
    vasoactive intestinal p. (VIP)
    vasoconstrictor p.
    vasorelaxant p.
peptidoglycan
peptidomimetic
Peptococcus constellatus
Peptostreptococcus
    P. anaerobius
    P. asaccharolyticus
    P. evolutus
    P. paleopneumoniae
    P. prevotii
    P. productus
per
    p. primam healing
    p. primam intentionem
    p. secundum healing
    p. secundum intentionem
peratriotomy loop
Per-C-Cath
perceived exertion
percent
    p. of maximum predicted heart
    rate
    p. predicted peak expiratory flow
    (%PEF)
perceptual-sensory neglect
perchloric acid
percholesterolemia
Perclose
    P./Prostar device
    P. vascular closure device
    P. vascular surgical closure system

NOTES

Percor
> P. DL-II intraaortic ball
> P. DL-II intraaortic balloon catheter
> P. dual-lumen-II intraaortic ball

Percor-Stat-DL catheter
PercuCut biopsy needle
PercuGuide
percussion
> p. and auscultation (P&A)
> chest p.
> coin p.
> p. dullness
> fist p.
> Goldscheider p.
> Murphy p.
> pencil p.
> piano p.
> Plesch p.
> p. and postural drainage (P&PD)
> postural drainage and p. (PD&P)
> slapping p.
> p. sound
> strip p.
> tangential p.
> threshold p.
> p. wave

percussor
> G5 Neocussor p.
> Vibracare p.

PercuSurge GuardWire
percutaneous
> p. access kit (PAK)
> p. aortic balloon valvuloplasty
> p. approach
> p. balloon angioplasty
> p. balloon aortic valvuloplasty
> p. balloon mitral valvuloplasty
> p. balloon pericardiotomy (PBP)
> p. balloon pulmonic valvuloplasty
> p. balloon valvuloplasty (PBV)
> p. brachial sheath
> p. cannulated screw
> p. cardiopulmonary bypass (PCPB)
> p. cardiopulmonary bypass support (PCBS)
> p. cardiopulmonary support (PCPS)
> p. catheter insertion
> p. catheter introducer kit
> p. coronary intervention (PCI)
> p. coronary rotational atherectomy (PCRA)
> p. cutting needle
> p. dilatational tracheostomy (PDT)
> p. dilational tracheostomy (PDT)
> p. endoscopic gastrostomy tube
> p. endoscopic jejunostomy (PEJ)
> p. endoscopic jejunostomy tube

> P. Excimer Laser Coronary Angioplasty (PELCA)
> p. extrapleural analgesia
> p. femoral
> p. intraaortic balloon counterpulsation
> p. intraaortic balloon counterpulsation catheter
> p. intracoronary angioscopy
> p. intrapericardial fibrin-glue infusion therapy
> p. introduced
> p. laser angioplasty
> p. left heart bypass (PLHB)
> p. mechanical mitral commissurotomy
> p. mechanical thrombectomy (PMT)
> p. mechanical thrombectomy system
> p. mitral balloon commissurotomy (PMBC)
> p. mitral balloon valvotomy (PMBV)
> p. mitral balloon valvuloplasty (PMBV)
> p. mitral commissurotomy (PMC)
> p. mitral valvuloplasty (PMV)
> p. myocardial laser revascularization
> p. myocardial revascularization (PMR)
> p. myocardial revascularization procedure
> p. needle aspiration biopsy
> p. needle biopsy
> p. nephrostolithotomy (PCNL)
> p. occlusion of ductus
> p. patent ductus arteriosus closure
> p. pericardiocentesis
> p. radiofrequency catheter
> p. radiofrequency catheter ablation
> p. revascularization
> p. rotational thrombectomy (PRT)
> p. rotational thrombectomy catheter
> p. technique
> p. thrombolytic device (PTD)
> p. tracheotomy
> p. transatrial mitral commissurotomy
> p. transhepatic cardiac catheterization
> p. transluminal
> p. transluminal angioplasty (PTA)
> p. transluminal angioscopy (PTAS)
> p. transluminal balloon valvuloplasty
> p. transluminal coronary
> p. transluminal coronary angioplasty (PTCA)

p. transluminal coronary
revascularization (PTCR)
p. transluminal myocardial
revascularization (PTMR)
p. transluminal renal angioplasty
(PTRA)
p. transluminal rotational
atherectomy (PTRA)
p. transluminal septal myocardial
ablation (PTSMA)
p. transmyocardial laser
revascularization (PMR)
p. transmyocardial revascularization
(PTMR)
p. transthoracic needle biopsy
(PTNB)
p. transtracheal bronchography
p. transtracheal jet ventilation
(PTJV)
p. transvenous mitral
commissurotomy (PTMC)
p. tunnel
PerDUCER
P. percutaneous pericardial device
P. pericardial access device
peregrinum
Mycobacterium p.
perennial allergic rhinitis
Perez sign
Per-fit percutaneous tracheostomy kit
perflenapent
p. emulsion
p. injectable emulsion
perflubron
perfluorocarbon (PFC)
**perfluorocarbon-associated gas exchange
(PAGE)**
**perfluorocarbon-exposed sonicated
dextrose albumin (PESDA)**
perflutren
Definity p.
perforating
p. artery
p. artery infarct (PAI)
perforation
cardiac p.
esophageal p.
guidewire p.
myocardial p.
septal p.
ventricular p.

perforator
gaiter p.
septal p.
· **performance**
cardiac p.
p. index (PI)
left ventricular systolic p.
ventricular p.
perfringens
Clostridium p.
PerfTrak
P. display
P. perfusion waveform display
perfuse
perfusion
p. balloon catheter (PBC)
p. balloon PTCA
p. bed
blood p.
bradykinin p.
cardiac p.
p. catheter
cerebral p.
cool head-warm body p.
p. defect
p. imaging MRI
isolated heat p.
lung p. (LP)
luxury p.
luxus p.
misery p.
mosaic p.
myocardial p.
p. pressure
regional p.
remote access p. (RAP)
root p.
p. scan
p. scintigraphy
splanchnic bed p.
stuttering of p.
p. via collateral
**perfusion-assisted direct coronary artery
bypass (PADCAB)**
perfusion/ventilation
perfusion-weighted
p.-w. imaging
p.-w. MRI (PWI)
periaccretio pericardii
Periactin

NOTES

P

periaortic
   p. abscess
   p. hematoma
periapical
periarteriolar fibrosis
periarteritis nodosa
peribronchial
   p. cuffing
   p. desquamation
   p. fibrosis
   p. pneumonia
   p. sheath
peribronchiolar
   p. airspace consolidation
   p. consolidation
   p. granulomatous inflammation
   p. inflammatory infiltrate
   p. layer
   p. metaplasia
   p. nodule
peribronchiolitis
peribronchitis
peribronchovascular
   p. disease
   p. distortion
   p. hemorrhage
   p. thickening
pericarbon
   p. bioprosthesis
   p. pericardial prosthesis
pericardectomy
pericardia (*pl. of* pericardium)
pericardiaca
   pleura p.
pericardiacophrenica
   arteria p.
pericardiac tumor
pericardial
   p. baffle
   p. basket
   p. biopsy
   p. calcification
   p. constraint
   p. cyst
   p. disease
   p. echo
   p. effusion
   p. fat pad
   p. flap
   p. fluid
   p. fremitus
   p. friction rub
   p. friction sound
   p. knock
   p. lavage
   p. murmur
   p. patch
   p. peel

   p. poudrage
   p. pressure
   p. reflex
   p. rub
   p. sac
   p. sling
   p. symphysis
   p. tamponade
   p. tap
   p. teratoma
   p. well
   p. window
pericardicentesis
pericardiectomy
   parietal p.
   visceral p.
pericardii
   accretio p.
   concretio p.
   hydrops p.
   paracentesis p.
   periaccretio p.
   synechia p.
pericardiocentesis
   echo-guided p.
   percutaneous p.
pericardiology
pericardiophrenic artery
pericardioplasty
pericardiorrhaphy
pericardioscopy
pericardiosternal ligament
pericardiostomy
pericardiotomy
   percutaneous balloon p. (PBP)
   p. scissors
   subxiphoid limited p.
pericarditic
pericarditis
   acute fibrinous p.
   adhesive p.
   amebic p.
   bacterial p.
   calcific p.
   p. calculosa
   p. callosa
   carcinomatous p.
   cholesterol p.
   chronic constrictive p.
   constrictive p.
   drug-associated p.
   drug-induced p.
   dry p.
   effusive-constrictive p.
   epistenocardiac p.
   p. epistenocardica
   fibrinous p.
   fibrous p.

gram-negative p.
hemorrhagic p.
histoplasmic p.
idiopathic p.
infective p.
inflammatory p.
internal adhesive p.
ischemic p.
localized p.
meningococcal p.
neoplastic p.
p. obliterans
obliterating p.
obliterative p.
occult p.
postinfarction p.
postoperative p.
purulent p.
radiation-induced p.
rheumatic p.
serofibrinous p.
serous p.
p. sicca
Sternberg p.
subacute p.
suppurative p.
transient p.
traumatic p.
tuberculous p.
uremic p.
p. villosa
viral p.
p. with effusion
pericarditis-myocarditis syndrome
pericardium, pl. **pericardia**
absent p.
adherent p.
bread-and-butter p.
calcified p.
CardioFix p.
congenitally absent p.
diaphragmatic p.
dropsy of p.
empyema of p.
p. externum
p. fibrosum
fibrous p.
p. internum
parietal p.
p. serosum
shaggy p.

thickened p.
visceral p.
pericardosis
pericardotomy
pericentriolar
periciliary fluid
perielectrode fibrosis
periesophageal
Periflow
P. peripheral balloon angioplasty-
infusion catheter
P. peripheral balloon catheter
Periflux PF 1 D blood-flowmeter
perigraft
p. flow
p. thrombosis
perihilar
p. adenopathy
p. haze
p. lymph node
p. marking
periinfarction conduction defect (PICD)
periinfarction
p. block
p. zone
perilymphatic
p. distribution
p. nodule
perimembranous ventricular septal defect
perimesencephalic pattern of hemorrhage
Perimount RSR pericardial bioprosthesis
perimuscular plexus
perimyocarditis
perimyocytic fibrosis
perimyoendocarditis
perimysial
p. fibrosis
p. plexus
perimysium
perindoprilat
perindopril erbumine
perineal artery
perinodal tissue
perinodular emphysema
perinuclear cisterna
period
absolute refractory p. (ARP)
accessory pathway effective
refractory p. (APERP)
p. of accommodation

NOTES

P

period *(continued)*
  alveolar p.
  antegrade refractory p.
  atrial effective refractory p.
  atrial refractory p.
  atrioventricular refractory p.
  blanking p.
  canalicular p.
  diastolic filling p.
  effective conduction p. (ECP)
  effective refractory p. (ERP)
  ejection p.
  functional conduction p. (FCP)
  functional refractory p. (FRP)
  intersystolic p.
  isoelectric p.
  isometric p. of cardiac cycle
  isometric contraction p.
  isometric relaxation p.
  isovolumetric relaxation p. (IVRP)
  isovolumic p.
  isovolumic relaxation p.
  no-sigh p.
  pacemaker amplifier refractory p.
  postinfarction p.
  postsphygmic p.
  postventricular atrial refractory p.
    (PVARP)
  preejection p. (PEP)
  preisovolumic contraction p.
  presphygmic p.
  pulse p.
  refractory p.
  relative refractory p. (RRP)
  right ventricular refractory p.
    (RVERP)
  saccular p.
  sigh p.
  systolic ejection p. (SEP)
  TAB p.
  total atrial blanking p.
  total atrial refractory p. (TARP)
  ventricular effective refractory p.
    (VERP)
  p. of ventricular filling
  ventriculoatrial effective
    refractory p.
  vulnerable p.
  Wenckebach p.
periodic
  p. breathing
  p. edema
  p. leg movement (PLM)
  p. limb movement disorder
    (PLMD)
  p. paralysis
  p. polyserositis
  p. respiration

periodicity
  A-V node Wenckebach p.
  circadian p.
  Wenckebach p.
perioperative antibiotic
periorbital edema
periosteotome
  Alexander-Farabeuf p.
periosteum
peripartal heart disease
peripartum
  p. cardiomyopathy
  p. myocarditis
peripharyngeal space
peripharyngeum
  spatium p.
peripheral
  p. access system (PAS)
  p. airspace
  P. AngioJet system
  p. arterial disease (PAD)
  p. arterial occlusive disease
    (PAOD)
  p. arteriosclerosis
  p. artery
  p. artery bypass
  P. Artery Radiation Investigational
    Study (PARIS)
  p. artery tonometry
  p. atherectomy system
  p. atherosclerotic disease
  p. blood eosinophilia
  p. blood smear
  p. chemoreceptor
  p. circulation
  p. cyanosis
  p. disease
  p. edema
  p. excimer laser angioplasty
    (PELA)
  p. interstitial disease
  p. interstitium
  p. laser angioplasty (PLA)
  p. muscle strength (PMS)
  p. neuropathy
  p. paracicatricial emphysema
  p. pulmonic stenosis
  p. resistance
  p. resistance unit (PRU)
  p. stigmata
  p. vascular disease (PVD)
  p. vascular resistance
  p. vasoconstriction
  p. vasodilation
  p. vasodilator effect
  p. zone radioaerosol clearance
peripherally inserted catheter (PIC)
peripneumonia notha

periprosthetic
> p. mitral regurgitation
> p. valve abscess
> p. valve aortic insufficiency

peripylephlebitis
peristaltic wave
peristasis
peristatic hyperemia
Peri-Strips
perisystole
perisystolic
perithelium
> Eberth p.

peritoneal
> continuous cyclic p.
> p. dialysis

peritracheal
Peritrate SA
peritricuspid loop
peritubular capillary (PTC)
perivalvular leak
perivascular
> p. canal
> p. edema
> p. eosinophilic infiltrates
> p. fibrosis
> p. lymphocytic infiltrate
> p. rupture
> p. sheath
> p. spaces

periventricular hyperintensity (PVH, PVHI)
Perles
> Tessalon P.

Perma-Flow
> P.-F. coronary bypass graft
> P.-F. coronary graft

PermaMesh material
PermaNeb reusable nebulizer
permanent
> p. atrial tachycardia
> p. cardiac pacing lead
> p. junctional reciprocating tachycardia (PJRT)
> p. pacemaker placement
> p. pacing

Permapen injection
Permathane lead
permeability
> airway p.
> alveolar p. (AP)

> endothelial p.
> microvascular p.

permissive hypercapnia (PHC)
pernio
> lupus p.

peroneal
> p. artery
> p. muscular atrophy

peroxidase
> airway p. (APO)
> avidin-biotin p.

peroxide
> hydrogen p.
> lipid p.

peroxisome
> p. proliferator-activated receptor (PPAR)
> p. proliferator-activated receptor gamma (PPAR-gamma)
> p. proliferator response element (PPRE)

peroxyacetyl nitrate
peroxyl radical-trapping potential
peroxynitrite
perpetual arrhythmia
perpetuus
> pulsus irregularis p.

Per-Q-Cath percutaneously inserted central venous catheter
Persantine
> P. and Aspirin Reinfarction Study (PARIS)
> P.-isonitrile stress test
> IV P.
> P. thallium stress test

persidomine
persistence
> microbubble p.

persistent
> p. atrioventricular canal
> p. common atrioventricular canal
> p. ductus arteriosus
> p. fetal circulation
> p. ostium primum
> p. pulmonary hypertension of newborn (PPHN)
> p. shunt
> p. truncus arteriosus

personal
> P. Best peak flowmeter
> p. heart device (PHD)

NOTES

P

Perspex
    P. block
    P. button
persulfate salt
pertechnetate sodium
Perthes
    P. syndrome
    P. test
Pertofrane
pertubation
perturbed
    p. autonomic nervous system
      function
    p. carotid baroreceptor
Pertussin
    P. CS
    P. ES
pertussis
    Bordetella p.
    Haemophilus p.
    p. toxin
peruana
    verruga p.
pervenous
    p. catheter
    p. pacemaker
PES
    papillary fibroelastoma
    programmed electrical stimulation
PESDA
    perfluorocarbon-exposed sonicated
      dextrose albumin
Pesend
    end-expiratory esophageal pressure
PESP
    postextrasystolic potentiation
Pessniff
    maximal sniff-induced esophageal
      pressure
pestis
    Yersinia p.
PET
    polyethylene terephthalate
    positron emission tomography
    PET balloon
    PET balloon atherectomy device
    Rb-82 PET
    PET scan
    PET scanning
    PET with C-11 acetate
petal
    nitinol p.
petal-fugal flow
PETCO$_2$
    partial pressure of end-tidal CO_2
petechia, pl. petechiae
petechial hemorrhage
Peterson elastic modulus

pethidine
petiolous epiglottiditis
Petit sinus
Petriellidium boydii
petrified cardiac myxoma
Petrillium
petrosal ganglion
Peyer patch
Peyrot thorax
PF
    pulmonary function
PFC
    perfluorocarbon
PFF
    polymer fume fever
Pfizerpen-AS injection
PFM
    peak flowmeter
      TruZone PFM
PFO
    patent foramen ovale
PFO-Star occluder
PFR
    peak filling rate
PFS
    Adriamycin PFS
    Folex PFS
    Idamycin PFS
    Tarabine PFS
    Vincasar PFS
PFSDQ
    Pulmonary Functional Status and
      Dyspnea Questionnaire
PFT
    pulmonary function test
PFTKit disposable set
Pfuhl-Jaffé sign
PFWT
    pain-free walking time
Pgasniff
    maximal sniff-induced gastric pressure
PGCMS
    Philadelphia Geriatric Center Morale
      Scale
PGF
    primary graft failure
PGI$_2$
    prostacyclin
P-glycoprotein
Pg-Ppl
    gastric-intrapleural pressure
PGVS
    postganglionic vagal stimulation
PH
    parenchymal hematoma
    parenchymal hemorrhage
    pulmonary hypertension
      PH conduction time

P-H
    P.-H. conduction time
    P.-H. interval
pH
   hydrogen ion concentration
   intramucosal pH (pH$_{im}$)
   pH Meter
   scalp pH
pH$_{im}$
   intramucosal pH
phacoma
phage
   luciferase reporter p.
phagocyte
phagocytic
   p. function
   p. pneumonocyte
phagocytose
phagocytosis
phalangis
   corpus p.
phalanx
   body of p.
Phalen stress test
Phanatuss Cough Syrup
phantom
   p. aneurysm
   P. cardiac guidewire
   P. guidewire
   P. nasal mask
   P. nasal mask CPAP
   p. pacemaker
   p. pain
   p. sponge
   p. tumor
   P. V Plus catheter
pharmacodynamics
pharmacoeconomics
pharmacokinetics
pharmacologic
   p. environment
   p. stress
   p. stress echocardiography
   p. stress imaging
   p. stress perfusion imaging
pharmacological cardioversion
pharmacology
   in vitro p.
pharmacomechanic thrombolysis
Pharmacopeia
   United States P. (USP)
pharmacotherapy

pharyngalgia
pharyngea, pl. **pharyngeae**
   arteria p.
   venae pharyngeae
pharyngeal
   p. arch
   p. artery
   p. branch
   p. branch of descending palatine artery
   p. branch of glossopharyngeal nerve
   p. branch of inferior thyroid artery
   p. branch of pterygopalatine ganglion
   p. branch of vagus nerve
   p. canal
   p. collapsibility
   p. crisis
   p. gland
   p. lymphatic ring
   p. nervous plexus
   p. pouch
   p. pouch syndrome
   p. raphe
   p. reflex
   p. ridge
   p. space
   p. tonsil
   p. tubercle of basilar part of occipital bone
   p. vein
pharyngeales
   glandulae p.
pharyngealis
   tonsilla p.
pharyngeus
   plexus nervosus p.
   recessus p.
pharyngis, pl. **pharynges**
   cavitas p.
   cavum p.
   globus p.
   pars nasalis p.
   pars oralis p.
   raphe p.
   tunica mucosa p.
   tunica muscularis p.
pharyngitis
   acute p.
   arcanobacterial p.
   atrophic p.

NOTES

pharyngitis *(continued)*
    catarrhal p.
    chronic p.
    croupous p.
    diphtheric p.
    diphtheritic p.
    follicular p.
    gangrenous p.
    glandular p.
    granular p.
    herpangina p.
    membranous p.
    phlegmonous p.
    plague p.
    p. sicca
    p. ulcerosa
pharyngobranchial duct
pharyngoconjunctival fever
pharyngoepiglottic
pharyngoesophageal
    p. cushions
    p. pads
    p. sphincter
pharyngoglossal
pharyngoglossus
pharyngolaryngeal
pharyngomaxillary space
pharyngometer
    Eccovision acoustic p.
pharyngonasal cavity
pharyngooral
pharyngopalatine
pharyngopalatinus
pharyngoparalysis
pharyngoplasty
    Hynes p.
pharyngoscopy
pharyngospasm
pharyngostaphylinus
pharyngotracheal lumen airway (PTL, PTLA)
pharyngotympanic groove
pharynx
    constrictor muscle of p.
    inferior constrictor muscle of p.
    laryngeal p.
    laryngeal part of p.
    middle constrictor muscle of p.
    nasal p.
    nasal part of p.
    oral p.
    oral part of p.
    raphe of p.
phase
    p. angle
    convalescent p.
    ejection p.
    fibrinopurulent p.

    harmonic p. (HARP)
    p. heterophony
    p. image
    p. image analysis
    p. imaging
    Korotkoff p. I–V
    midexpiratory p.
    plateau p.
    supernormal recovery p.
    terminal p.
    venous p.
    vulnerable p.
    washout p.
phased
    p. array receiver coil
    p. array sector scanner
    p. array sector transducer
    p. array study
    p. array system
    p. array technology
    p. array ultrasonographic device
phase-encoded velocity image
phasic
    p. excursion
    p. intragraft flow velocity
    p. sinus arrhythmia
PHC
    permissive hypercapnia
PHD
    personal heart device
Phemister elevator
Phenadex Senior
Phenameth
    P. DM
    P. Oral
Phenazine injection
phenazopyridine
    sulfisoxazole and p.
Phendry Oral
Phenergan
    P. injection
    P. Oral
    P. VC With Codeine
    P. With Codeine
Phenetron Oral
phen-fen
    phentermine and fenfluramine
Phenhist Expectorant
phenindamine tartrate
phenindione sensitivity
phenobarbital
    theophylline, ephedrine, and p.
phenolformaldehyde
phenomenon
    AFORMED p.
    Anrep p.
    Aschner p.
    Ashley p.

Ashman p.
Austin Flint p.
blush p.
Bowditch p.
cascade p.
coronary steal p.
diaphragm p.
diaphragmatic p.
dip p.
Duckworth p.
Ehret p.
embolic p.
Gallavardin p.
gap p.
gap conduction p.
Gärtner vein p.
Goldblatt p.
Gregg p.
Hering p.
Hill p.
Katz-Wachtel p.
Kienbock p.
Koch p.
Litten p.
low-reflow p.
malperfusion p.
no-reflow p.
overshoot p.
pendelluft p.
preconditioning p.
Raynaud p.
recoil p.
reentry p.
R-on-T p.
Schellong-Strisower p.
Splendore-Hoeppli p.
staircase p.
steal p.
treppe p.
Venturi p.
warm-up p.
washout p.
Wenckebach p.
Williams p.
Woodworth p.
zone 1 p.
phenothiazine
phenotype
high-risk p.
large cell carcinoma with
rhabdoid p.
metastatic p.

Pi MM p.
Pi MZ p.
Pi SS p.
Pi SZ p.
Pi ZZ p.
phenoxybenzamine hydrochloride
phenoxymethyl
penicillin p.
phenprocoumon
phentermine and fenfluramine (phen-fen)
phentolamine
p. hydrochloride
p. mesylate
p. methanesulfonate
phenyl
p. aminosalicylate
p. salicylate
phenylalkylamine
phenylbutazone sensitivity
phenylephrine
guaifenesin, phenylpropanolamine,
and p.
p. hydrochloride
isoproterenol and p.
p. ramp method
Phenylfenesin L.A.
phenylpropanolamine
caramiphen and p.
guaifenesin and p.
p. hydrochloride
hydrocodone and p.
p. toxicity
phenytoin
pheochromocytoma
Phe-Pro-boro-Arg
Pherazine
P. VC w/ Codeine
P. w/DM
P. with Codeine
PHI
pontine hyperintensity
Phialophora verrucosa
Philadelphia
P. Association of Clinical Trials
(PACT)
P. Geriatric Center Morale Scale
(PGCMS)
Philip gland
Philips
P. ACS NT 1.5 Gyroscan MRI

NOTES

P

Philips *(continued)*
  P. Integris 3000 biplane digital subtraction angiography
  P. Integris HP 3000
  P. Medical Systems Tomoscan AVE1 CT spiral scanner
  P. Medical Systems Tomoscan SR 7000 CT spiral scanner
  P. Somoscan 310 CT scanner
phlebarteriectasia
phlebectasia laryngis
phlebemphraxis
phlebitis
  adhesive p.
  blue p.
  chlorotic p.
  descending p.
  gouty p.
  malignancy-associated p.
  migrating p.
  p. nodularis necrotisans
  p. obliterans
  obliterating p.
  plastic p.
  puerperal p.
  sclerosing p.
  superficial p.
phlebodynamics
phlebogenous
phlebogram
phlebograph
phlebography
phlebolithiasis
phlebomanometer
phleborrheogram
  Cranley-Grass p.
phlebostasis
phlebotomize
phlebotomy
  bloodless p.
phlegm
phlegmasia
  p. alba dolens
  p. cerulea dolens
phlegmonosa
  angina p.
phlegmonous
  p. laryngitis
  p. pharyngitis
phlei
  Mycobacterium p.
Phoenix
  P. 2 pacemaker
  P. total artificial heart
phonarteriogram
phonarteriography
Phonate

phonoangiography
  carotid p.
phonocardiogram
phonocardiograph
  linear p.
  logarithmic p.
  spectral p.
  stethoscopic p.
phonocardiographic transducer
phonocardiography
phonocatheter
phonoechocardiogram
phonoscope
phonoscopy
phosducin
phosgene
phosphatase
  acid p.
  alkaline p. (AP)
phosphate
  Aralen P.
  azapetine p.
  p.-buffered saline (PBS)
  chloroquine p.
  Cleocin P.
  codeine p.
  Decadron P.
  dexamethasone sodium p. (DSP)
  disopyramide p.
  etoposide p.
  Hexadrol P.
  histamine acid p.
  hydrocortisone sodium p.
  Hydrocortone P.
  Linctus With Codeine p.
  myocardial creatine p.
  oseltamivir p.
  Paveral Stanley Syrup With Codeine P.
  polyribosylribitol p. (PRP)
  primaquine p.
  sodium p.
  triciribine p. (TCN-P)
phosphatidylcholine (PtdCho)
  dipalmitoyl p. (DPPC)
phosphatidylinositol
phosphatidylserine
phosphine
phosphinic acid
phosphocreatine (PCr)
phosphodiesterase
  p. enzyme
  p. III inhibition (PDE3I)
  p. inhibitor (PDE, PDE-I)
  p. isoenzyme inhibitor
  sphingomyelin p.
phosphofructokinase
phosphoinositide

phosphoinositol
phosphokinase
    creatine p. (CPK)
phospholamban
phospholipase A$_2$, B, C
phospholipid
    surfactant p.
phospholipidosis
    alveolar p.
phosphomonoesterase
phosphorus
    organic p.
    p. tribomide
phosphorus-31 magnetic resonance spectroscopy (^{31}P-MRS)
phosphorycholine
phosphorylase
    glycogen p.
    p. kinase
    thymidine p.
phosphorylation
    mitochondrial oxidative p.
    oxidative p.
Phospho-Soda
    Fleet P.-S.
photoablation
photoaffinity
photoangioplasty
photobiological response
photochemical air pollution
photocoagulation
PhotoDerm VL device
photodiode
photodisruption
photodynamic therapy (PTD)
PhotoFix alpha pericardial bioprosthesis
Photofrin
PhotoGenica V-Star laser
photohemotachometer
Photo-Mask-and Etch-on-a-Tube (PMEOAT)
photometer
    HemoCue p.
photometry
    emission flame p.
photomicrography
photomultiplier
photon
    annihilation p.
photopeak
photoplethysmography (PPG)
photoprotection

photoreactivation
photoresection
photosensitizing reaction
photostethoscope
phren
phrenic
    p. artery
    p. nerve
    p. nerve crush injury
    p. nerve paralysis
    p. pleura
phrenica
    pleura p.
phrenicocolic
phrenicocolicum
    ligamentum p.
phrenicocostal sinus
phrenicogastric
phrenicoglottic
phrenicohepatic
phrenicosplenic
phrenocardia
phrenocolic
phrenogastric
phrenohepatic
PHRT
    procarbazine, hydroxyurea, radiotherapy
    PHRT protocol
PHT
    portal hypertension
    pulmonary hypertension
phthalic anhydride irrigatant-induced asthma
phthinoid
    p. bronchitis
    p. chest
phthisis
    aneurysmal p.
    bacillary p.
    black p.
    collier's p.
    diabetic p.
    fibroid p.
    grinder's p.
    miner's p.
    potter's p.
    pulmonary p.
    stone-cutter's p.
phycomycosis
Phylax
    P. A-V dual-chamber implantable cardioverter-defibrillator

NOTES

P

Phylax *(continued)*
    P. 06 implantable cardioverter-defibrillator
phylaxis
Phyllocontin Tablet
phyllosilicate
Phymos 3D pacemaker
physical
    P. Activity Scale for the Elderly Evaluation (PASE)
    p. inactivity
    p. stimulus
    P. Work Capacity exercise stress test
physical therapy *(var. of* physiotherapy*)*
physiochemical
Physio-Control Lifestat sphygmomanometer
physiodensitometry
physiologic
    p. congestion
    p. dead space
    p. dead space fraction
    p. dead space ventilation (V_D/V_T)
    p. measurement
    p. monitoring
    p. murmur
    p. pacemaker
    p. pattern release (PPR)
    p. shunt fraction
    p. third heart sound
physiological
    p. dead space ventilation per minute (V_D)
    p. monitoring
    p. overreactivity
    p. split of S_2
    p. stress
physiologically split S_2 sound
physiology
    constrictive p.
    Damus-Kaye-Stansel procedure for single ventricle p.
    Eisenmenger p.
Physios
    P. CTM 01 cardiac transplant monitor
    P. CTM 01 noninvasive cardiac transplant monitoring system
physiotherapy, physical therapy
    chest p.
    Movement Science p.
phytanic acid accumulation
Phytis stent
phytoestrogen
    soy p.
phytohemagglutinin
phytonadione

phytopneumoconiosis
PI
    performance index
    pontine infarct
    protease inhibitor
    alpha-1 PI
    PI MRI technique
Pi
    P. MM phenotype
    P. MZ phenotype
    P. SS phenotype
    P. SZ phenotype
    P. ZZ phenotype
pial collateralization
piano percussion
piaulement
    bruit de p.
PIC
    peripherally inserted catheter
PICA
    posterior inferior cerebellar artery
    posterior inferior communicating artery
Piccolino
    P. balloon
    P. Monorail catheter
PICD
    periinfarction conduction defect
pi cell
PICH
    primary intracerebral hemorrhage
Pick
    P. and Go monitor
    P. syndrome
Picker
    P. CS scanner
    P. Dyna Mo collimator
    P. Edge 1.5-T scanner
    P. Magnascanner
    P. PQ 2000 CT scanner
    P. Vista HPQ MRI scanner
    P. VISTAR image analysis system
    P. VOXEL image analysis system
pickwickian syndrome
Picornaviridae virus
Pico-ST II low-profile balloon catheter
picrosirius red stain
PICS
    Pacing in Cardiomyopathy Study
PICSS
    Patent Foramen Ovale in Cryptogenic Stroke Study
PICTURE
    Post Intracoronary Treatment Ultrasound Result Evaluation
    PICTURE study
PIE
    pulmonary infiltrate with eosinophilia
    pulmonary infiltration with eosinophilia

pulmonary interstitial emphysema
PIE syndrome

Pie
P. Medical CAAS II analysis system

piechaudii
Alcaligenes p.

Pielograf
Pierce-Donachy Thoratec ventricular assist device
Pierre Robin syndrome
piesimeter
Hales p.

piesis
Piezo
P. Electric Snore Sensor
P. PLM sensor

piezoelectric
p. crystal
p. crystal-based pacemaker
p. ultrasound transducer

PIF
peak inspiratory flow

PIFR
peak inspiratory flow rate

pigeon-breast deformity
pigeon-breeder's
p.-b. disease
p.-b. lung

pigeon chest
pigeon-fancier's lung
piggyback
pigment induration of the lung
pigskin
pigtail
p. catheter
p. rotation catheter

PIH
pregnancy-induced hypertension

PIIIP
procollagen type III aminoterminal peptide

PI3-kinase
pillar
tonsillar p.

Pilling
P. bronchoscope
P. microanastomosis clamp
P. Weck Y-stent forceps

pillow-shaped balloon
pilocarpine iontophoresis test

PILOT
Preliminary Investigation of Local Therapy Using Porous PTCA Balloons and Low-Molecular-Weight Heparin
PILOT clinical trial

pilot
Asymptomatic Cardiac Ischemia P. (ACIP)
p. needle

Pilotip
P. catheter
P. catheter guide

pilsicainide
Pima
pimobendan
PIMS
programmable implantable medication system

pinacidil
pinchcock mechanism
pincushion distortion
Pindac
pindolol
pineal pellucidum
pine resin
pinhole
p. balloon rupture
p. VSD

pink
p. puffer
p. sputum
p. tetralogy of Fallot

pinked up
Pinkerton .018 balloon catheter
Pinnacle
P. introducer sheath
P. pacemaker

pinocytosis
pinocytotic
pinosome
Pins
P. sign
P. syndrome

pioglitazone
PIOPED
Prospective Investigation of Pulmonary Embolism Diagnosis
PIOPED study

PIP
plasma cell interstitial pneumonitis
positive inspiratory pressure

pipecuronium bromide

NOTES

P

piperacillin and tazobactam sodium
piperanometozine
piperazine citrate
pipobroman
Pipracil
Piracetam in Acute Stroke Study (PASS)
pirbuterol
    p. acetate
    p. acetate inhalation aerosol
pirenzepine
piretanide
pirfenidone
piriform, pyriform
piriform sinus
piriform thorax
piritrexim isethionate
pirmenol
pirodavir
Pirogoff angle
pirolazamide
piroximone
Pirquet reaction
PISA
    proximal isovelocity surface area
Pisces lead
pistol
    pistol shot
    pistol shot femoral sound
    p. shot sound
    p. shot of Traube
piston pulse
pit
    inferior costal p.
Pitressin injection
pitting edema
Pittman IMA retractor
Pittsburgh
    P. pneumonia
    P. pneumonia agent
Pitt talking tracheostomy tube
pivampicillin
pivot
    P. balloon
    p. point
pixel
pizza lung
Pizzolatto stain
PJC
    premature junctional contraction
P-J interval
PJRT
    permanent junctional reciprocating tachycardia
PKC
    protein kinase C
PL
    6 Micro Stent P.

PLA
    peripheral laser angioplasty
PLAC
    Pravastatin Limitation of Atherosclerosis in Coronary Arteries
    PLAC study
PLAC-2
    Pravastatin, Lipids, and Atherosclerosis in the Carotid Arteries
    PLAC-2 study
placebo
placement
    Angiography Versus Intravascular Ultrasound-Directed Coronary Stent P. (AVID)
    carotid angioplasty and stent p.
    catheter-directed thrombolysis and endovascular stent p.
    intracoronary stent p.
    lead p.
    permanent pacemaker p.
    prophylactic filter p.
    stent p.
    temporary pacemaker p.
    Thoracoport p.
placental
    p. barrier
    p. circulation
    p. respiration
plague
    bubonic p.
    p. pharyngitis
    p. pneumonia
    pneumonic p.
PLA-I platelet antigen
planar
    p. myocardial imaging
    p. myocardial scintigraphy
    p. thallium imaging
    p. thallium scintigraphy
    p. thallium test
    p. xanthoma
plane
    Addison p.
    axial p.
    circular p.
    coronal p.
    cove p.
    midsagittal p.
    orthogonal p.
    parasagittal p.
    sagittal p.
    short-axis p.
    sternal p.
    sternoxiphoid p.
    transaxial p.
planigraphy
planimeter

planimetry
    Indec Systems TapeMeasure
      computerized p.
    p. method
    p. volume
planithorax
plantar ischemia test
plant toxicity
plaque
    p. area
    atheromatous p.
    atherosclerotic p.
    p. burden
    calcified p.
    carcinoid p.
    carotid p.
    complex p.
    disrupted p.
    p. disruption
    echogenic p.
    echolucent p.
    p. embolization
    equistenotic p.
    fibrofatty p.
    fibrolipoid p.
    fibrous p.
    p. fissure
    p. fissuring
    p. fracture
    glistening yellow coronary p.
    Gray-Weale p.
    heterogeneous p.
    Hollenhorst p.
    homogeneous p.
    intraluminal p.
    lipid-rich p.
    p. lumen
    p. marker
    p. motion
    myointimal p.
    nonostial p.
    pleural p.
    p. prolapse
    protuberant p.
    p. rupture
    senile p.
    shelf of p.
    p. shift
    p. stabilization
    p. strutting
    submucosal p.
    ulcerated p.
    unstable p.
    p. volume
    white p.
    yellow p.
plaque-cracker
    LeVeen p.-c.
Plaquenil
plaquing
plasma
    p. alpha 1-antitrypsin (pAAT)
    p. beta-thromboglobulin
    p. catecholamine
    p. cell interstitial pneumonitis (PIP)
    p. cell pneumonia
    p. coagulation system
    p. colloid osmotic pressure
    p. endothelin
    p. endothelin concentration
    p. erythropoietin
    p. exchange column
    p. extravasation
    p. exudation
    p. fibrinogen
    fresh frozen p. (FFP)
    p. glycocalicin
    p. homocysteine
    p. homocysteine concentration
    p. nicotine level
    p. oncotic pressure
    platelet-poor p. (PPP)
    platelet-rich p. (PRP)
    p. protein exudation
    p. renin
    p. renin activity (PRA)
    p. retinol
    p. skimming
    p. thromboplastin antecedent
    p. thromboplastin component
    p. volume
    p. volume expander
    zoster immune p. (ZIP)
plasmagel
plasmahaut
plasmakinin
plasmalemma
Plasma-Lyte A
Plasmanate
plasmapheresis
Plasma-Plex bottle
plasma-resistant fiber oxygenator (PRF)
Plasmatein
plasmatic vascular destruction

NOTES

P

plasmin
plasminemia
plasminogen
    p. activator
    P. Activator Angioplasty
      Compatibility Trial (PACT)
    p. activator inhibitor (PAI)
    p. activator inhibitor-1 (PAI-1)
plasminogen-streptokinase complex
Plasmodium
    P. embolism
    P. *falciparum*
    P. *malariae*
    P. *ovale*
    P. *vivax*
plastic
    p. bronchitis
    p. endocarditis
    p. phlebitis
    p. pleurisy
    p. polymer
    p. sewing ring
    p. surgical osteosynthesis
plasticity
    cortical p.
    skeletal muscle p.
plasty
    endoventricular circular patch p.
    sliding p.
plate
    polar p.
    pole p.
    Strasburger cell p.
    p. thrombosis
    p. thrombus
    trach p.
    tracheostomy p.
plateau
    h p.
    p. phase
    p. pulse
    p. response
    ventricular p.
platelet
    p. activating factor (PAF)
    p. activation
    p. activity
    p.-aggregating factor
    p. aggregation
    p. aggregation inhibitor
    p. antibody
    p. consumption
    p. factor 4
    gel-filtered p. (GFP)
    p. glycoprotein
    p. glycoprotein IIb/IIIa blockade
    p. glycoprotein IIb/IIIa blocker
    p. glycoprotein IIb/IIIa inhibitor

    P. Glycoprotein IIb/IIIa in Unstable
      Angina; Receptor Suppression
      Using Integrilin Therapy
      (PURSUIT)
    hemolysis, elevated liver enzymes,
      and low p.'s (HELLP)
    P. IIb/IIIa Antagonist for the
      Reduction of Acute Coronary
      Syndrome Events in a Global
      Organization Network
      (PARAGON)
    P. IIb/IIIa Underpinning the
      Receptor for Suppression of
      Unstable Ischemia Trial
      (PURSUIT)
    p. imaging
    IIb/IIa p. inhibition
    p. membrane glycoprotein
    p. receptor glycoprotein
    P. Receptor Inhibition for Ischemic
      Syndrome Management (PRISM)
    P. Receptor Inhibition for Ischemic
      Syndrome Management in Patients
      Limited to Very Unstable Signs
      and Symptoms (PRISM-PLUS)
    p. thrombosis
    p. thrombus
platelet-derived
    p.-d. growth factor (PDGF)
    p.-d. histamine-releasing factor
      (PDHRF)
plateletpheresis
platelet-poor plasma (PPP)
platelet-rich plasma (PRP)
platelike atelectasis
platform
    Complete stent delivery p.
    TomTec echo p.
Platinol
    P.-AQ
platinum
    p. coil
    p.-iridium electrode
    P. Plus 300-cm guidewire
    p. PLUS guidewire
    salt of p.
    p. wire
platypnea
    p.-orthodeoxia syndrome
platysma
Plavix
PLCO
    postoperative low cardiac output
plecaronil
pledget
    Dacron p.
    Meadox Teflon felt p.
    polypropylene p.

p.-supported
Teflon p.
pledgeted mattress suture
PlegiaGuard
pleiotropic cytokine
Plendil
plenus
pulsus p.
pleomorphic
p. premature ventricular complex
p. tachycardia
Plesch
P. percussion
P. test
Pletal
plethora
plethoric
plethysmograph
body p.
BPXG body p.
jerkin p.
MasterScreen Body p.
MedGraphics model 1085 body p.
mercury-in-rubber strain gauge p.
pressure p.
pressure-compensated flow p.
respiratory inductance p. (RIP)
Respitrace p.
Respitrace inductive p.
volume-displacement p.
plethysmography
cuff p.
impedance p. (IPG)
respiratory inductance p. (RIP)
serial impedance p.
servocontrolled p.
strain-gauge p.
thermistor p.
pleura, pl. **pleurae**
adipose folds of the p.
black p.
cavum pleurae
cervical p.
costal p.
p. costalis
costodiaphragmatic recess of p.
costomediastinal recess of p.
cupula of p.
cupula pleurae
diaphragmatic p.
p. diaphragmatica
discission of p.

fibrin bodies of p.
mediastinal p.
p. mediastinalis
parietal p.
p. parietalis
p. pericardiaca
phrenic p.
p. phrenica
plicae adiposae pleurae
p. pulmonalis
pulmonary p.
visceral p.
p. visceralis
pleuracentesis (*var. of* pleurocentesis)
pleuracotomy
pleural
p. abrasion
p. adhesion
p. amyloidosis
p. aspergillosis
p. biopsy
p. bleb
p. calculus
p. cap
p. cavity
p. crackle
p. cupula
p. disease
p. effusion
p. empyema
p. fibrin ball
p. fluid
p. fluid neutrophilia
p. fremitus
p. friction rub
p. lavage
p. line
p. mass
p. meniscus sign
p. mesothelioma
p. mouse
p. peel
p. plaque
p. poudrage
p. pressure (Ppl)
p. rale
p. reaction
p. recess
p. rings
p. sac
p. scarring
p. sclerosant

NOTES

P

pleural *(continued)*
  p. shock
  p. sinus
  p. sliding
  p. space
  p. space evacuation
  p. space monitoring
  p. suction
  p. surface
  p. tag
  p. tap
  p. tent
  p. thickening
  p. toilet
  p. tube
  p. villi
pleurales
  recessus p.
  villi p.
pleuralgia
pleuralis
  cavitas p.
pleurectomy
  thorascopic apical p.
Pleur-evac
  P.-e. autotransfusion system
  P.-e. device
  P.-e. suction
pleurisy
  acute p.
  adhesive p.
  blocked p.
  cholesterol p.
  chronic p.
  chyliform p.
  chylous p.
  circumscribed p.
  costal p.
  diaphragmatic p.
  diffuse p.
  double p.
  dry p.
  encysted p.
  exudative p.
  fibrinous p.
  hemorrhagic p.
  ichorous p.
  indurative p.
  interlobar p.
  interlobular p.
  latent p.
  mediastinal p.
  metapneumonic p.
  plastic p.
  primary p.
  productive p.
  proliferating p.
  pulmonary p.

  pulsating p.
  purulent p.
  sacculated p.
  secondary p.
  serofibrinous p.
  serous p.
  single p.
  suppurative p.
  tuberculous p.
  typhoid p.
  visceral p.
  wet p.
  p. with effusion
pleuritic
  p. chest pain
  p. pneumonia
  p. rub
pleuritis
  fibrinous acute p.
  lupus p.
  obliterative p.
  rheumatoid p.
  tuberculous p.
pleuritogenous
pleurocentesis, pleuracentesis
pleurodesis
  chemical p.
  doxycycline p.
  mechanical p.
  talc p.
  thorascopic talc p.
pleurodural fistula
pleurodynia
pleuroesophageal
  p. fistula
  p. line
  p. muscle
pleuroesophageus
  musculus p.
pleurogenic pneumonia
pleurogenous
pleurography
pleurolith
pleuroparenchymal abnormality
pleuroparietopexy
pleuropericardial
  p. cyst
  p. incision
  p. murmur
  p. rub
  p. window
pleuropericarditis
pleuroperitoneal
  p. canal
  p. cavity
  p. fold
  p. shunt
  p. shunting

pleuropneumonectomy
pleuropneumonia-like organism (PPLO)
pleuropulmonary
    p. blastoma
    p. infection
pleuroscopy
pleurovisceral
Pleurx
    P. drainage and catheter kit
    P. pleural catheter
    P. pleural catheter/home drainage
      kit
plexectomy
plexiform lesion
PlexiPulse
    P. compression device
    P. device
plexogenic
    p. pulmonary
    p. pulmonary arteriopathy
plexopathy
    brachial p.
plexus
    ascending pharyngeal p.
    Batson p.
    brachial p.
    esophageal nervous p.
    p. gulae
    Haller p.
    lingual p.
    p. nervosus esophageus
    p. nervosus pharyngeus
    p. periarterialis arteriae lingualis
    p. periarterialis arteriae pharyngeae
      ascendentis
    perimuscular p.
    perimysial p.
    pharyngeal nervous p.
    p. pulmonalis
    pulmonary nervous p.
PLHB
    percutaneous left heart bypass
pliability
PLIC
    posterior limb of the internal capsule
plica, pl. **plicae**
    plicae adiposae pleurae
plicamycin
plication
PLLA
    poly-L-lactic acid

PLM
    periodic leg movement
PLMD
    periodic limb movement disorder
plombage
plop
    cardiac tumor p.
    tumor p.
plot
    box p.
    box-and-whisker p.
    bull's-eye p.
    whisker p.
plug
    Alcock catheter p.
    collagen p.
    Dittrich p.
    Ivalon p.
    mucus p.
    Shiley decannulation p.
    Teflon Bardic p.
    Traube p.
plugged telescoping catheter
plugging
    mucous p.
PlugStation earplug station
plumb-line sign
Plummer
    P. disease
    P.-Vinson syndrome
    P. water-filled pneumatic
      esophageal dilator
plunging goiter
plurilocular
plus
    CO_2SMO P.
    Duramist P.
    2010 P. Holter system
    ligand p. 1, 2, 3
    Lorcet P.
    Nicorette P.
    Oracle Micro P.
    Tri-Tannate P.
Plussq1 software
PLV
    partial liquid ventilation
PMBC
    percutaneous mitral balloon
      commissurotomy
PMBV
    percutaneous mitral balloon valvotomy
    percutaneous mitral balloon valvuloplasty

NOTES

P

PMC
    percutaneous mitral commissurotomy
    premotor cortex
pMDI
    pressurized metered-dose inhaler
PM-DM
    polymyositis-dermatomyositis
PMEOAT
    Photo-Mask-and Etch-on-a-Tube
PMF
    progressive massive fibrosis
PMFBW
    paramedian frontal bone window
PMH
    pure motor hemiparesis
PMI
    point of maximum impulse
P-mitrale
PML
    progressive multifocal
        leukoencephalopathy
PMN
    polymorphonuclear leukocyte
    polymorphonuclear neutrophil
PMR
    papillary muscle rupture
    percutaneous myocardial
        revascularization
    percutaneous transmyocardial laser
        revascularization
PMRP
    portable monitor of respiratory
        parameters
³¹P-MRS
    phosphorus-31 magnetic resonance
        spectroscopy
PMS
        P.-Amantadine
        P.-Erythromycin
        P.-Hydroxyzine
        P.-Isoniazid
        P.-Levothyroxine Sodium
        P.-Methylphenidate
        P.-Progesterone
        P.-Pyrazinamide
        P.-Sodium Cromoglycate
PMS
    peripheral muscle strength
        PMS Integris angiogram
PMT
    pacemaker-mediated tachycardia
    percutaneous mechanical thrombectomy
        PMT AccuSpan tissue expander
        Thrombex PMT
PMV
    percutaneous mitral valvuloplasty
        PMV 2000 clear tracheostomy &
            ventilator speaking valve

PMV 2001 purple tracheostomy &
    ventilator speaking valve
PMV 2000 series speaking valve
PMV 005 tracheostomy valve
PMV 007 tracheostomy &
    ventilator speaking valve
PNA
    glycogenated P.
PND
    paroxysmal nocturnal dyspnea
    postnasal drip
PND-Rh
    postnasal drip due to rhinitis
PNDS
    postnasal drainage syndrome
    postnasal drip syndrome
PND-Si
    postnasal drip due to sinusitis
pneocardiac reflex
pneopneic reflex
PNET
    primitive neuroectodermal tumor
pneumatic
        p. antishock garment (PASG)
        p. compression stockings
        p. cuff
        p. hammer disease
        p. tourniquet
        p. trousers
pneumatics
pneumatocardia
pneumatocele
pneumatohemia
pneumatonometer
        Digibind p.
pneumatosis coli
pneumectomy
pneumobacillus
        Friedländer p.
pneumobulbar
pneumocardial
pneumocentesis
pneumococcal
        p. empyema
        p. pneumonia
        p. vaccine
pneumococcosis
pneumococcus, pl. **pneumococci**
        Fraenkel p.
pneumoconiosis
        antimony p.
        arc welder's p.
        asbestos p.
        bauxite p.
        coal worker's p. (CWP)
        collagenous p.
        fuller's earth p.
        hard metal p.

kaolin p.
limonite p.
magnetite p.
mica p.
mixed-dust p.
noncollagenous p.
organic dust p.
rheumatoid p.
shale p.
p. siderotica
silicotic p.
talc p.
tungsten carbide p.
pneumocystic
Pneumocystis
    P. carinii
    P. carinii pneumonia (PCP)
    P. choroidopathy
    P. pneumonia
    P. pneumonitis
pneumocystosis
pneumocyte
    type II p.
PNEUMO disposable pneumotachometer
pneumodynamics
pneumogastric
pneumogenic osteoarthropathy
pneumogram
pneumograph
pneumohemia
pneumohemothorax
pneumohydropericardium
pneumohydrothorax
pneumomediastinography
pneumomediastinum
Pneumomist
pneumomycosis
pneumonectomy
    extrapleural p. (EPP)
    simultaneously stapled p. (SSP)
Pneumo-Needle reusable instrument
pneumonia
    abortive p.
    acute interstitial p. (AIP)
    adenoviral p.
    p. alba
    alcoholic p.
    amebic p.
    anthrax p.
    apex p.
    apical p.
    p. aposthematosa

aspiration p.
atypical p.
bacillary p.
bacterial p.
bacterial pneumococcal p.
bilious p.
bronchial p.
bronchiolitis obliterans with
  organizing p. (BOOP)
Buhl desquamative p.
Candida p.
Carrington p.
caseous p.
catarrhal p.
central p.
cerebral p.
cheesy p.
Chlamydia p.
chronic eosinophilic p. (CEP)
chronic fibrous p.
cold agglutinin p.
community-acquired p. (CAP)
congenital aspiration p.
contusion p.
core p.
Corrigan p.
croupous p.
cryptogenic organizing p. (COP)
deglutition p.
Desnos p.
desquamative interstitial p. (DIP)
p. dissecans
double p.
Eaton agent p.
embolic p.
Enterobacter p.
eosinophilic p.
ephemeral p.
ether p.
exogenous lipid p.
fibrinous acute lobar p.
fibrous p.
Friedländer p.
Friedländer bacillus p.
gangrenous p.
gelatinous acute p.
giant cell p.
Hecht p.
herpes p.
herpes simplex p.
HSV p.
hypersensitivity p.

NOTES

P

pneumonia *(continued)*
    hypostatic p.
    idiopathic acute eosinophilic p.
    idiopathic interstitial p.
    indurative p.
    influenza p.
    influenzal p.
    influenza virus p.
    inhalation p.
    p. interlobularis
    p. interlobularis purulenta
    interstitial p.
    interstitial plasma cell p.
    intrauterine p.
    Kaufman p.
    Klebsiella p.
    Legionella p.
    Legionnaire p.
    leptospiral p.
    lingular p.
    lipid p.
    lipoid p.
    lobar p.
    lobular p.
    Löffler p.
    Louisiana p.
    lymphoid interstitial p.
    massive p.
    measles p.
    metastatic p.
    migratory p.
    mycoplasmal p.
    necrotizing p.
    nonspecific interstitial p. (NSIP)
    nosocomial p. (NP)
    p. notha
    obstructive p.
    oil-aspiration p.
    opportunistic p.
    organizing p.
    parenchymatous p.
    peribronchial p.
    Pittsburgh p.
    plague p.
    plasma cell p.
    pleuritic p.
    pleurogenic p.
    pneumococcal p.
    Pneumocystis p.
    Pneumocystis carinii p. (PCP)
    polymicrobial p.
    postobstructive p.
    primary atypical p.
    primary eosinophilic p.
    primary influenza p.
    progressive p.
    Proteus p.
    purulent p.

    Reisman p.
    rheumatic p.
    rickettsial p.
    Scopulariopsis sp. p.
    secondary p.
    segmental p.
    septic p.
    Serratia p.
    staphylococcal p.
    Stoll p.
    streptococcal p.
    superficial p.
    suppurative p.
    terminal p.
    toxemic p.
    transplant p.
    traumatic p.
    Trichosporon beigelii p.
    tuberculous p.
    tularemic p.
    TWAR p.
    typhoid p.
    unilateral p.
    unresolved p.
    uremic p.
    usual interstitial p. (UIP)
    vagus p.
    varicella p.
    ventilator-associated p. (VAP)
    viral p.
    walking p.
    wandering p.
    white p.
    woolsorter's p.
pneumoniae
    Bacillus p.
    Chlamydia p.
    Diplococcus p.
    Klebsiella p.
    Legionella p.
    multidrug-resistant *Streptococcus* p.
      (MDRSP)
    Mycoplasma p.
    penicillin-resistant *Streptococcus* p.
      (PRSP)
    Streptococcus p.
Pneumonia Severity Index (PSI)
pneumonic
    p. fever
    p. plague
pneumonitis
    acute interstitial p. (AIP)
    acute lupus p. (ALP)
    acute radiation p.
    aspiration p.
    bronchiolitis with interstitial p.
      (BIP)
    chemical p.

cholesterol p.
CMV p.
cryptogenic organizing p. (COP)
cytomegalovirus p.
desquamative interstitial p. (DIP)
eosinophilic p.
giant cell interstitial p. (GIP)
granulomatous p.
herpes simplex p.
hypersensitivity p. (HP)
interstitial p.
kerosene p.
lymphocytic interstitial p. (LIP)
lymphoid interstitial p. (LIP)
malarial p.
mixed alveolar-interstitial p.
nonspecific p.
nonspecific chronic interstitial p.
  (NIP)
nonspecific interstitial p. (NSIP)
ossifying p.
peptic aspiration p.
plasma cell interstitial p. (PIP)
Pneumocystis p.
radiation p.
uremic p.
usual interstitial p. (UIP)
varicella p.

pneumonoconiosis
bauxite p.
rheumatoid p.

pneumonocyte
phagocytic p.

pneumonopathy
eosinophilic p.

pneumonoresection
pneumonotherapy
pneumoparotid
pneumopathy
leukemic cell lysis p.
seropositive nonsyphilitic p.

Pneumopent
pneumopericardium
tension p.
ventilator-induced p.

pneumoperitoneum
pneumopexy
pneumophila
Legionella p.
pneumoplethysmography
pneumopleuritis
pneumopleuroparietopexy

pneumoresection
pneumoscope
pneumoscrotum
pneumosilicosis
pneumosintes
Bacteroides p.
Pneumo Sleeve
pneumotach
p. disposable mouthpiece
MicroTach p.
pneumotachogram
pneumotachograph
Fleisch p.
flow-sensing p.
Silverman-Lilly p.
pneumotachometer
hot-wire p.
MicroTach p.
PNEUMO disposable p.
pneumotaxic center
pneumotherapy
pneumothorax, pl. **pneumothoraces**
artificial p.
catamenial p.
clicking p.
closed chest p.
extrapleural p.
iatrogenic p.
induced p.
normotensive p.
open p.
pressure p.
primary spontaneous p. (PSP)
pure p.
secondary p.
simultaneous bilateral
  spontaneous p. (SBSP)
spontaneous p. (SP)
tension p.
therapeutic p.
traumatic p.
unilateral p.
valvular p.
ventilator-induced p.
pneumotomy
Pneumotron ventilator
Pneumovax 23
pneumovirus
pneuPAC
p. resuscitator
p. ventilator

NOTES

P

PneuView
    P. single lung simulator
    P. ventilator system
    P. ventilator testing and training system
PNH
    paroxysmal nocturnal hemoglobinuria
PNPB
    positive-negative pressure breathing
PNS
    posterior nasal spine
    PNS Unna boot
PNSP
    penicillin-nonsusceptible *Streptococcus pneumoniae*
^{31}P nuclear magnetic resonance spectroscopy
Pnu-Imune 23
PO$_2$
    partial pressure of oxygen
    PO$_2$ oximetry
POC
    point-of-care
    polyolefin copolymer
    POC balloon
    POC Bandit catheter
    POC blood gas test
    POC test
POCI
    posterior circulation infarct
pocket
    abdominal p.
    generator p.
    pacemaker p.
    regurgitant p.
    retropectoral p.
    P. SPO$_2$T
    p. of Zahn
Pocket-Dop II
Pockethaler
    Vancenase P.
PocketPeak peak flowmeter
POCS
    posterior circulation syndrome
POCT
    point-of-care testing
    POCT device
pod
    rigid p.
podagra
POEM
    Patency, Outcomes and Economics of MIDCAB
    POEM study

POEMS
    polyneuropathy, organomegaly, endocrinopathothy, monoclonal gammopathy and skin changes
    POEMS syndrome
POET
    pulse oximeter/end tidal CO$_2$
pogonion
    gonion to p. (GO-POG)
POH
    postoperative hemorrhage
poikilocytosis
Poincar plot pattern
point
    A p.
    p. of Arrhigi
    Boyd p.
    p. of care test
    Castellani p.
    p. of critical stenosis
    cut p.
    D p.
    de Mussy p.
    E p.
    equal-pressure p. (EPP)
    Erb p.
    exit p.
    Guéneau de Mussy p.
    hinge p.
    isoelectric p.
    J p.
    p. of maximal impulse
    p. of maximum impulse (PMI)
    null p.
    pivot p.
    p. tenderness
    Z p.
pointes
    quinidine-induced torsade de p.
    torsade de p. (TDP, TdP)
point-of-care (POC)
    p.-o.-c. analysis
    p.-o.-c. testing (POCT)
    p.-o.-c. testing device
Poiseuille
    P. equation
    P. law
    P. resistance formula
poisoning
    arsenic p.
    arsine gas p.
    fluorocarbon p.
    lead p.
    mercury p.
    oxygen p.
Poisson regression
pokkuri
polacrilex chewing gum

Poladex
polar
  p. coordinate map
  P. Electro sport tester
  p. plate
  P. Vantage XL heart rate monitor
Polaramine
polarcardiography
Polaris
  P. CPAP system
  P. electrode
  P. Mansfield/Webster deflectable tip
  P. steerable diagnostic catheter
polarity
  reverse p.
polarization
  electrochemical p.
  fluorescence p.
polarographic method
pole plate
Polhemus-Schafer-Ivemark syndrome
polichinelle
  voix de p.
poliomyelitis
poliovirus
  p. vaccine, live, trivalent, oral
Polisar-Lyons tracheal tube
polixus
  Rhodnius p.
pollen asthma
pollution
  air p.
  photochemical air p.
poloxamer 188
polyacrylamide gel electrophoresis
polyacrylonitrile membrane
polyamidamine
polyamide
polyaminocarbonates polymer
polyangiitis
  microscopic p.
polyanion precipitation procedure
polyarteritis
  disseminated p.
  hypertensive pulmonary p.
  p. nodosa
polyarthritis
polyblennia
polycarbonate urethane
polycardia
polychondritis
  relapsing p.

Polycillin
Polycitra-K
polyclonal gammopathy
polycrotic
polycrotism
polycyclic aromatic hydrocarbon (PAH)
polycystic
  p. kidney
  p. kidney disease
  p. lung
  p. tumor
polycythemia
  compensatory p.
  p. hypertonica
  p. vera
polydactyly
polyene
polyestradiol
polyether alcohol asthma
polyethylene
  p. glycol electrolyte lavage solution
    (PEG-LES)
  p. terephthalate (PET)
  p. terephthalate balloon
Polyflex
  P. lead
  P. pacemaker
polyfluorotetraethylene graft
Polygam S/D
polygelin colloid contrast medium
polygenic
  p. hypercholesterolemia
  p. hyperlipidemia
**polyglandular autoimmune syndrome
  type II**
polyglycolic acid
polygonal arcade
polygraph
  Mackenzie p.
  Night Owl pocket p.
polyhedral surface reconstruction
PolyHeme
Poly-Histine CS
polyhydroxybutyrate polymer
polylactic
  p. acid
  p. acid stent coating
poly-L-lactic, poly-l-lactic
  p.-L.-l. acid (PLLA)
  p.-L.-l. acid stent
polymer
  p. fume fever (PFF)

NOTES

P

polymer *(continued)*
    hyaluronic acid p.
    plastic p.
    polyaminocarbonates p.
    polyhydroxybutyrate p.
    polyphosphate esters p.
polymerase
    p. chain reaction (PCR)
    Taq DNA p.
polymeric endoluminal paving stent
POLY-MESAM recording unit
polymetabolic syndrome
polymicrobial pneumonia
polymorphic
    p. premature ventricular complex
    p. slow wave
    p. ventricular tachycardia
polymorphism
    ACE deletion/insertion p.
    adducin p.
    angiotensin-converting enzyme
      deletion/insertion p.
    paraoxonase p.
    restriction fragment length p.
      (RFLP)
polymorphonuclear
    p. leukocyte (PMN)
    p. neutrophil (PMN)
polymorphous ventricular tachycardia
Polymox
polymyalgia rheumatica syndrome
polymyositis
polymyositis-dermatomyositis (PM-DM)
polymyxa
    Bacillus p.
polymyxin
polynet
polyneuritiformis
    heredopathia atactica p.
polyneuropathy
    ascending p.
    Roussy-Lévy p.
polyneuropathy, organomegaly, endocrinopathothy, monoclonal gammopathy and skin changes (POEMS)
polyolefin
    p. copolymer (POC)
    p. copolymer balloon
polyorganophosphazene-coated stent
polyostotic fibrous dysplasia
polyp
    bronchial p.
    bronchial inflammatory p.
    cardiac p.
polypeptide
    atrial natriuretic p. (ANP)
    pancreatic p. (PP)

polyphaga
    Acanthamoeba p.
polyphenol
    red wine p.
polyphosphate esters polymer
polyphosphoinositide
polyploidy
Poly-Plus Dacron vascular graft
polypoidal lesion
polypoid bronchitis
polyposis
    nasal p.
polypous endocarditis
polypropylene
    p. intracardiac patch
    p. pledget
    p. stent
polyribosylribitol phosphate (PRP)
polyribosylribitol phosphate-diphtheria toxoid conjugate (PRP-D)
Polyrox fractal active fixation lead
polysaccharide-iron complex
polysaccharide storage disease
PolySafe A-track lead
polyserositis
    familial paroxysmal p.
    periodic p.
polysomatic
polysomaty
polysome
polysomnogram (PSG)
    Nellcor Puritan Bennett Sandman 2.4 p.
    Nihon Kohden model 4412P p.
    nocturnal p. (NPSG)
    SensorMedics model 4100
    Somnostar p.
polysomnographic
    p. index
    p. study
polysomnography (PSG)
    nocturnal p.
polysplenia
Polystan
    P. cardiotomy reservoir
    P. perfusion cannula
    P. venous return catheter
polystyrene latex microsphere
polytef
polytef-sheathed needle
polytetraflouroethylene-covered stent
polytetrafluoroethylene (PTFE)
    expanded p. (EPTFE)
    predilated p.
    p. prosthesis
    p. stent graft
polythiazide
    prazosin and p.

polyunsaturated fat
polyurethane
    p. foam
    p. foam embolus
polyuria
polyvinyl
    p. chloride (PVC)
    p. chloride balloon
    p. chloride tube
    p. prosthesis
POM
    pulse oximetry monitoring
Pompe disease
POMS 20/50 oxygen conservation device
ponderal index
ponderance
    ventricular p.
Pondimin
Pondocillin
ponopalmosis
Ponstel
Pontiac fever
pontine
    p. hyperintensity (PHI)
    p. infarct (PI)
    p. ischemic rarefaction
Pontocaine
pool
    blood p.
poor
    p. expiratory effort
    p. R wave progression
poorly
    p. differentiated carcinoma
    p. reversible asthma
popliteal
    p. aneurysm
    p. artery
    p. pulse
poppet
    ball p.
    barium-impregnated p.
    prosthetic p.
    Silastic p.
popping sensation
porcelain aorta
porcine
    p. bioprosthesis
    p. heterograft
    p. prosthesis
    p. prosthetic valve

    p. valve
    p. xenograft
pore
    Kohn p.
porfimer
pork
    p. insulin
    P. NPH Iletin II
    P. Regular Iletin II
porphyria
    acute intermittent p. (AIP)
porphyrin
Porstmann technique
PORT
    Patient Outcomes Research Team Study
    postoperative radiotherapy
    PORT electrode
port
    P. Access Recovery Improvement
      Study (PARIS)
    p. access technique
    chest p.
    Import vascular access p.
    Luer-Lok p.
    PAS p.
    Q P.
    SEA p.
    side p.
    side arm pressure p.
porta, pl. **portae**
    p. hepatis
    p. lienis
    p. pulmonaris
    p. pulmonis
portable
    p. aerosol delivery device
    AutoSet P. II
    p. chest radiograph
    p. monitoring device
    p. monitor of respiratory
      parameters (PMRP)
    Pulsair .5 liquid oxygen p.
    p. volume ventilator
Port-A-Cath
    P.-A.-C. device
    P.-A.-C. implantable catheter system
portacaval
    p. anastomosis
    p. H graft
    p. shunt
    p. transposition

NOTES

P

Port-Access
P.-A. coronary artery bypass grafting
P.-A. minimally invasive cardiac surgery
St. Jude Medical P.-A.
portae (*pl. of* porta)
Portagen diet
portal
p. circulation
p. hypertension (PHT)
p. pyemia
p. vein
p. vein thrombosis
Porta Pulse 3 defibrillator
Porta-Resp monitor
Port Charles influenza
Porter sign
Portex
P. Neo-Vac meconium suction device
P. Per-Fit tracheostomy kit
P. Per-Fit tracheostomy tube
P. Soft-Seal cuff system
P. ThermoVent heat and moisture exchanger
portion
infradiaphragmatic p.
portogram
portography
computed tomography angiographic p. (CTAP)
splenic p.
portoportal anastomosis
portopulmonary
p. hypertension
p. shunt
portosystemic anastomosis
portovenography
PORTS
Patient Outcomes Research Team Study
Posadas
P. mycosis
P.-Wernicke disease
Posey Cufflator tracheal cuff inflator and manometer
Posicor
position
Andral decubitus p.
body p.
electrical heart p.
heart p.
LAO p.
left anterior oblique p.
levotransposed p.
RAO p.
right anterior oblique p.
scalloped subcoronary p.

semilateral supine p.
shock p.
Trendelenburg p.
tricuspid p.
positional obstructive sleep apnea syndrome
positioner
CAS-8000V general angiography p.
Thornton anterior p. (TAP)
positioning
prone p.
positive
p. afterpotential
p. airway pressure (PAP)
p. airway pressure ventilation (PAPV)
p. chronotropism
p. end-airway pressure (PEAP)
p. end-expiratory pressure (PEEP)
p. expiratory pressure (PEP)
p. inspiratory pressure (PIP)
p. pressure
p. pressure mechanical ventilation
p. pressure ventilation
p. support ventilator (PSV)
P. Symptom Distress Index (PSDI)
p. symptom total (PST)
p. treppe
positive-negative pressure breathing (PNPB)
Positrol
P. cardiac device
P. II catheter
positron emission tomography (PET)
Possis Medical AngioJet thrombectomy catheter
POST
Posterior Stroke Trial
Potassium-Channel Opening Stroke Trial
post
p. balloon angioplasty restenosis
p. bypass spasm
P. Coronary Artery Bypass Graft (POST-CABG)
P. Intracoronary Treatment Ultrasound Result Evaluation (PICTURE)
postabsorptive state
postanesthesia
p. care unit (PACU)
p. pulmonary edema
postangioplasty
postantibiotic effect (PAE)
postbronchodilator
postbypass
POST-CABG
Post Coronary Artery Bypass Graft
POST-CABG clinical trial

postcapillary hypertension
postcardiac injury syndrome (PCIS)
postcardiotomy
    p. psychosis syndrome
    p. syndrome
postcardioversion pulmonary edema
postcatheterization
postcoital asthma
postcommissurotomy syndrome
postcontrast echocardiogram
postdiastolic
postdicrotic
postdiphtheritic stenosis
postdiuresis scan
postdrive depression
postductal
postectopic pause
posterior
    p. airway space (PAS)
    p. approach
    p. basal segmental artery of right lung
    p. branch of right superior
    p. cerebral artery (PCA)
    p. circulation (PC)
    p. circulation infarct (POCI)
    p. circulation syndrome (POCS)
    p. circumflex artery (PC)
    p. communicating artery (PCoA)
    p. cricoarytenoid muscle
    p. descending artery (PDA)
    p. inferior cerebellar artery (PICA)
    p. inferior communicating artery (PICA)
    p. isthmus
    p. junction line
    p. leaflet
    p. left ventricular wall motion on echocardiogram
    p. limb of the internal capsule (PLIC)
    p. lung zone
    p. myocardial infarction
    p. nasal spine (PNS)
    p. papillary muscle (PPM)
    p. Q wave
    p. rib fracture
    P. Stroke Trial (POST)
    p. tibial pulse
    p. upper lung zone
    p. wall (PW)
    p. wall thickness

posteroinferior dyskinesis
posterolateral thoracotomy
posteroseptal wall
postesophageal
postexercise
    p. echocardiogram
    p. scan
postextrasystolic
    p. aberrancy
    p. beat
    p. pause
    p. potentiation (PESP)
    p. T wave
postganglionic vagal stimulation (PGVS)
posthemothorax
posthyperventilation apnea
postictal state
postimiotic
postinfarct, post infarct
    p. ventricular remodeling
postinfarction
    p. angina
    p. pericarditis
    p. period
    p. syndrome
postinfectious bradycardia
postinfective bradycardia
postinflammatory
postinjury
    p. empyema
    p. immunosuppression
postintervention
postischemic
    p. dysfunction
    p. heart
    p. myocardium
postmenopausal
    P. Estrogen/Progestin Intervention (PEPI)
    p. estrogen/progestin interventions study
postmicturition syncope
postmitotic
postmortem
    p. clot
    p. thrombus
postmyocardial
    p. infarction
    p. infarction syndrome
postnasal
    p. catarrh
    p. drainage syndrome (PNDS)

NOTES

postnasal *(continued)*
    p. drip (PND)
    p. drip due to rhinitis (PND-Rh)
    p. drip due to sinusitis (PND-Si)
    p. drip syndrome (PNDS)
postobstructive
    p. atelectasis
    p. pneumonia
postocclusal hyperemia
Post-Op
    Emerson P.-O.
postoperative
    p. chest radiograph
    p. endocarditis
    p. hemorrhage (POH)
    p. low cardiac output (PLCO)
    p. pericarditis
    p. radiotherapy (PORT)
postpartum
    p. cardiomyopathy
    p. hypertension
postperfusion
    p. arrhythmia
    p. lung
    p. psychosis
    p. syndrome
postpericardiotomy syndrome (PPS)
postpharyngeal space
postphlebitic syndrome
postpneumonectomy tuberculous empyema
postpneumonic
postprandial
    p. angina
    p. blood sugar
    p. hypotension
    p. lipemia (PPL)
postprimary tuberculosis
postprocedural management
postpump syndrome
postrandomization
postrema
postrenal azotemia
postresuscitative death
postrheumatic cusp retraction
postsphygmic
    p. interval
    p. period
poststenotic dilation
poststreptococcal inflammatory process
poststroke pruritus
postsynaptic cholinergic mechanism
posttest
    Tukey-Kramer p.
postthrombolytic therapy
posttransfusion syndrome

posttransplantation
    p. lymphoproliferative disorder (PTLPD, PTLD)
    p. malignancy
posttraumatic
    p. ARDS
    p. pulmonary pseudocyst
posttussive
    p. emesis
    p. syncope
postural
    P. Assessment Scale for Stroke Patient (PASS)
    p. drainage (PD)
    p. drainage of infected secretion
    p. drainage and percussion (PD&P)
    p. drainage, percussion and vibration (PDPV)
    p. hypotension
    p. orthostatic tachycardia syndrome (POTS)
    p. syncope
posture
    Stern p.
    p. technique
posturing
    decerebrate p.
    posturing decerebrate p.
postventricular
    p. atrial blanking (PVAB)
    p. atrial refractory period (PVARP)
Potain sign
potassium (K)
    p. aminosalicylate
    amoxicillin and clavulanate p.
    canrenoate p.
    p. chloride (KCl)
    p. chloride cardioplegia
    p. citrate and citric acid
    p. gluconate
    glucose, insulin, and p. (GIK)
    p. hydroxide (KOH)
    p. inhibition
    p. iodide
    P. Iodide Enseals
    p. ion
    losartan p.
    penicillin V p.
    ticarcillin and clavulanate p.
    p. wasting
Potassium-Channel Opening Stroke Trial (POST)
potassium-sparing diuretic
potassium-wasting diuretic
potential
    action p.
    bioelectric p.
    cardiac action p.

compound motor action p. (CMAP)
electrical p.
fibrillation p.
His bundle p.
Kent p.
late diastolic p. (LDP)
maximum negative p.
membrane p.
monophasic action p. (MAP)
motor provoked p. (MEP)
movement-related cortical p.
  (MRCP)
nerve action p.
pacemaker p.
peroxyl radical-trapping p.
putative slow pathway p.
resting membrane p.
sensory nerve action p. (SNAP)
somatosensory evoked p. (SSEP)
total peroxyl radical-trapping
  antioxidant p. (TRAP)
transmembrane p.
ventricular late p. (VLP)

potentiation
interval-dependent p.
postextrasystolic p. (PESP)
twitch p.

potentiator
potroom asthma
POTS
postural orthostatic tachycardia syndrome
Pott aneurysm
Pottenger sign
potter's
p. asthma
p. phthisis
Potts
P. anastomosis
P. bronchial forceps
P.-Cournand needle
P. needle
P. operation
P. procedure
P. shunt
P.-Smith anastomosis
pouch
Cardio-Cool myocardial
  protection p.
p. hematoma
laryngeal p.
Parsonnet pulse generator p.
pharyngeal p.

poudrage
Beck epicardial p.
pericardial p.
pleural p.
talc p.
pounds
p. per square inch (psi)
p. per square inch gauge (psig)
Pourcelot index
povidone-iodine
powder
budesonide inhalation p.
fluticasone propionate inhalation p.
fluticasone propionate and
  salmeterol inhalation p.
lyophilized p.
powdered tantalum
power
p. Doppler ultrasound
p. failure
P. Grip Over the Wire Stent
  Delivery system
P. Grip stent
p. injector
left ventricular p.
p. motion imaging
resolving p.
spectral p.
p. spectral analysis
p. spectral density (PSD)
p. spectrum of HRV
ventricular p.
Powerheart
P. AECD
P. automatic external cardioverter-
  defibrillator
Powerlink endoluminal graft system
PP
pancreatic polypeptide
pulse pressure
PPACK
D-Phe-L-Pro-L-Arg-chloromethyl ketone
PPAR
peroxisome proliferator-activated receptor
PPAR-gamma
peroxisome proliferator-activated receptor
  gamma
PPD
purified protein derivative
PPD skin test
PPD test
Tine Test PPD

NOTES

P

545

P&PD
> percussion and postural drainage

Ppeak
> peak airway pressure

PPG
> photoplethysmography

PPH
> primary pulmonary hypertension

PPHN
> persistent pulmonary hypertension of newborn

P-P interval

PPL
> postprandial lipemia
> primary pulmonary non-Hodgkin lymphoma
> > PPL skin test

Ppl
> pleural pressure

PPLO
> pleuropneumonia-like organism

PPM
> posterior papillary muscle

ppm
> parts per million

PPP
> platelet-poor plasma

PPPPPP
> pain, pallor, paraesthesia, pulselessness, paralysis, prostration

PPR
> physiologic pattern release
> > PPR verapamil

PPRE
> peroxisome proliferator response element

PPS
> postpericardiotomy syndrome

pPTCA
> primary percutaneous transluminal coronary angioplasty

P-pulmonale

P-Q, PQ
> > P-Q interval
> > P-Q segment depression

P:QRS ratio

P-R
> > P-R interval
> > P-R segment

PR
> pulmonary regurgitation
> > PR interval
> > PR segment

PRA
> panel of reactive antibodies
> panel-reactive antibody
> plasma renin activity

PR-AC measurement

Practical Applicability of Saruplase Study (PASS)

practitioner
> respiratory care p. (RCP)

practolol

^{32}P radioactive stent

praecox
> ascites p.
> lymphedema p.

PRAISE
> Prospective Randomized Amlodipine Survival Evaluation

2-pralidoxime (2-PAM)

pranlukast

Pravachol

Pravastatin
> P. Limitation of Atherosclerosis in Coronary Arteries (PLAC)

pravastatin
> P., Lipids, and Atherosclerosis in the Carotid Arteries (PLAC-2)
> p. sodium

prawn asthma

praxis

praziquantel

prazosin
> p. hydrochloride
> p. and polythiazide

PRCCT
> Prospective Randomized Controlled Clinical Trials

preamplifier
> Arzco p.

prearteriole

preatheroma

preautomatic pause

pre-beta
> p.-b. 1 HDL
> p.-b. lipoprotein

precapillary
> p. anastomosis
> p. arteriole
> p. pulmonary hypertension
> p. sphincter

precardiac mesoderm

precatheterization

Preceder interventional guidewire

Precedex

Precept
> P. DR pacemaker
> P. lead

precipitation
> heparin-induced extracorporeal low-density lipoprotein p. (HELP)

precipitin

precipitous drop in blood pressure

PRECISE
Prospective Randomized Evaluation of
Carvedilol in Symptoms and Exercise
PRECISE study
Preclude pericardial membrane
preconditioning
ischemic p. (IPC)
p. phenomenon
p. signal
precordial
p. A wave
p. bulge
p. catch syndrome
p. electrocardiography
p. heave
p. honk
p. lead
p. motion
p. movement
p. pulse
p. ST depression
p. ST segment
p. thrill
p. thump
precordialgia
precordium
quiet p.
precoronary angioplasty
Precose
Pred
Liquid P.
Predaject injection
Predalone injection
Predator balloon catheter
Predcor injection
predeposit autologous donation
prediastole
prediastolic murmur
Predicort-50 injection
predicrotic
PREDICT
Prospective Randomized Evaluation of
Diltiazem CD Trial
PREDICT score
predictive
p. survival marker
p. value
predictor
APACHE CV Risk P.
Corazonix P.
univariate p.
predilated polytetrafluoroethylene

predischarge test
Prednicen-M
P.-M. Oral
prednisolone
methyl p.
p. systemic
Prednisol TBA injection
prednisone
predominant emphysema
predose level
preductal
preeclampsia
preejectional left ventricular wall
preejection period (PEP)
preexcitation
p. syndrome
ventricular p.
preexisting condition
pregnancy
anaphylactoid syndrome of p.
pregnancy-induced hypertension (PIH)
prehospital
P. Applicability of Saruplase Study
(PASS)
P. Application of Coronary
Thrombolysis (PACT)
preinfarction
p. angina
p. syndrome
preisovolumic contraction period
prekallikrein
prelaryngeales
nodi lymphoidei p.
prelaryngeal lymph node
**Preliminary Investigation of Local
Therapy Using Porous PTCA
Balloons and Low-Molecular-Weight
Heparin (PILOT)**
preload
cardiac p.
p. reduction
p. reserve
ventricular p.
Prelone Oral
Premarin With Methyltestosterone
premature
p. atherosclerosis
p. atrial beat
p. atrial complex
p. atrial contraction (PAC)
p. atrial extrastimulus

NOTES

P

premature *(continued)*
    p. atrioventricular junctional complex
    p. beat
    p. contraction
    p. diastolic distention
    p. excitation
    p. junctional beat
    p. junctional contraction (PJC)
    p. stimulus
    p. systole
    p. valve closure
    p. ventricular beat (PVB)
    p. ventricular complex
    p. ventricular complex-trigger hypothesis
    p. ventricular contraction (PVC)
prematurity
    chronic pulmonary insufficiency of p.
    retinopathy of p. (ROP)
premedication
premeiotic
Premilene suture
premitotic
premonitory
    p. palpitation
    p. syndrome
premotor cortex (PMC)
premounted stent
prenalterol hydrochloride
prenylamine
preoperative antibiotic
preparation
    insulin p.
    isometrically contracting myocardial p.
    Langendorff heart p.
preperitoneal
    p. distention balloon (PDB)
    p. fat
preprandial
prerenal azotemia
presacral edema
Presaril
presaturation pulse
presbycardia
presbyesophagus
presbylaryngia
prescription
    P. Analyses and Cost (PACT)
    P. Drug User Fee Act (PDUFA)
    exercise p.
presentation
    roentgenographic p.
preservation
    tissue p.

preserved left ventricular systolic function
preshaped catheter
presphygmic
    p. interval
    p. period
Press-mate SAT
pressor
    p. drug
    p. effect
pressoreceptive
pressoreceptor
    p. reflex
pressosensitive
pressosensitivity
    reflexogenic p.
pressure (P)
    abr maximal inspiratory mouth p.
    absolute p.
    airway-esophageal balloon p.
    alveolar p. (Palv)
    alveolar capillary intravascular p.
    alveolar carbon dioxide p.
    alveolar oxygen partial p. (PAO$_2$)
    ambient p.
    aortic blood p. (AoBP)
    aortic dicrotic notch p.
    aortic pullback p.
    arterial p.
    arterial blood p. (ABP)
    arterial carbon dioxide p.
    arterial dicrotic notch p.
    arterial oxygen partial p. (PaO$_2$)
    ascending aortic p.
    ascending aortic blood p.
    atmospheres of p.
    atmospheric p.
    atrial p.
    atrial filling p.
    p. augmentation (PA)
    average mean p. (AMP)
    back p.
    barometric p.
    beat-to-beat finger arterial p.
    bilevel positive airway p. (BiPAP)
    blood p. (BP)
    capillary wedge p.
    carbon dioxide p.
    cardiovascular p.
    central venous p. (CVP)
    cerebral perfusion p. (CPP)
    chest wall elastic recoil p. (Pth)
    coaxial p.
    colloid oncotic p. (COP)
    colloid osmotic p.
    compliance, rate, oxygenation, and p.
    continuous positive air p.

continuous positive airway p.
(CPAP)
p. control (PC)
p. controller
p. conversion
coronary perfusion p.
coronary venous p.
cricoid p.
p. cycled ventilation
p. cycled ventilator
p. decay
diastolic p.
diastolic blood p. (DBP)
diastolic filling p. (DFP)
differential blood p.
distal coronary perfusion p.
Donders p.
Doppler p.
downstream venous p.
dynamic p.
elastic recoil p.
end-diastolic p. (EDP)
end-diastolic left ventricular p.
end-expiratory esophageal p.
(Pesend)
endocardial p.
end-systolic left ventricular p.
expiratory positive airway p.
(EPAP)
femoral artery p.
filling p.
gastric-intrapleural p. (Pg-Ppl)
p. gradient
P. Guide pressure wire
p. half-time
p. half-time technique
high blood p.
hyperbaric p.
inflation p.
p. injector
inspiratory occlusion p.
inspiratory positive airway p.
(IPAP)
inspiratory resistance and positive
expiratory p. (IR-PEP)
intermittent positive p. (IPP)
intraalveolar p.
intracardiac p.
intracranial p. (ICP)
intramyocardial p.
intrapericardial p.
intrapleural oncotic p.

intrathoracic p.
intravascular p.
intrinsic positive end-expiratory p.
(PEEPi)
jugular venous p. (JVP)
juxtacardiac pleural p.
labile blood p.
left atrial p.
left ventricular diastolic p.
left ventricular end-diastolic p.
(LVEDP)
left ventricular filling p.
left ventricular systolic p.
lower body negative p. (LBNP)
lung elastic recoil p. (Pel)
maximal exercise systolic p.
(MESP)
maximal expiratory p. (MEP)
maximal expiratory mouth p.
(P_{Emax})
maximal inspiratory p. (MIP)
maximal inspiratory mouth p.
(P_{Imax})
maximal sniff-induced esophageal p.
(Pessniff)
maximal sniff-induced gastric p.
(Pgasniff)
maximal sniff-induced
transdiaphragmatic p. (Pdisniff)
maximum expiratory p. (MEP)
maximum expiratory airflow-static
lung elastic recoil p. (MFSR)
maximum inspiratory p. (MIP)
mean airway p. (MAP)
mean arterial p. (MAP)
mean arterial blood p. (MABP,
MBP)
mean diastolic left ventricular p.
mean pulmonary artery p. (MPAP,
PAPm)
mean pulmonary artery wedge p.
(MPAWP)
mean resting diastolic blood p.
(MDBP)
mean right atrial p.
mean systolic left ventricular p.
p. measurement
narrowed pulse p.
nasal continuous positive airway p.
(NCPAP, nCPAP)
p. necrosis
negative p.

NOTES

P

pressure *(continued)*
negative end-expiratory p. (NEEP)
negative expiratory p. (NEP)
negative intrapleural p.
noninvasive blood p. (NIPB)
noninvasive ventilation with
  positive p.
normal intravascular p.
oncotic p.
opening p.
osmotic p.
p. overload
p. overload-induced aortic valve
  calcific thickening
PA filling p.
peak airway p. (Ppeak)
peak systolic aortic p. (PSAP)
peak systolic gradient p.
perfusion p.
pericardial p.
plasma colloid osmotic p.
plasma oncotic p.
p. plethysmograph
pleural p. (Ppl)
p. pneumothorax
positive p.
positive airway p. (PAP)
positive end-airway p. (PEAP)
positive end-expiratory p. (PEEP)
positive expiratory p. (PEP)
positive inspiratory p. (PIP)
precipitous drop in blood p.
PSG p.
pullback p.
pulmonary p.
pulmonary arterial p.
pulmonary arterial end-diastolic p.
pulmonary arterial wave p.
pulmonary artery p. (PAP)
pulmonary artery diastolic p.
  (PADP)
pulmonary artery occlusion p.
  (PAOP)
pulmonary artery occlusive
  wedge p.
pulmonary artery systolic p.
  (PASP)
pulmonary artery wedge p.
  (PAWP)
pulmonary capillary wedge p.
  (PCWP)
pulmonary hypertension p.
pulmonary vascular p.
pulmonary wedge p. (PWP)
p. pulse
pulse p. (PP)
p. pulse differentiation
radial artery systolic p. (RASP)

p. recovery
resting p.
right atrial p. (RAP)
right ventricular diastolic p.
right ventricular end-diastolic p.
  (RVEDP)
right ventricular peak systolic p.
right ventricular systolic p. (RVSP)
self-adjusting nasal continuous
  positive airway p. (APAP)
p. sling
sniff nasal inspiratory p.
p. stasis
stump p.
supersystemic pulmonary artery p.
p. support ventilation (PSV)
systemic arterial p. (SAP)
systemic mean arterial p. (SMAP)
systolic p.
systolic blood p. (SBP)
systolic left ventricular p.
p. time product (PTP)
torr p.
total p. (P_T)
p. tracing
transdiaphragmatic p.
p. transducer
p. transducer airflow sensor
transesophageal p.
transmural p.
transmyocardial perfusion p.
transpulmonary p.
transthoracic p.
twitch gastric p.
upper airway closing p. (UACP)
upper airway opening p. (UAOP)
p. urticaria
variable positive airway p. (VPAP)
venous p.
p. ventilator
ventricular diastolic p.
ventricular filling p.
p. wave
p. waveform
wedge p.
widening of pulse p.
zero end-expiratory p. (ZEEP)
zero end-inspiratory p.
zero-flow p. (Pzf, ZFP)
pressure-compensated
p.-c. flow
p.-c. flow plethysmograph
pressure-controlled
p.-c. inverse ratio ventilation
  (PCIRV)
p.-c. respirator
p.-c. ventilation (PCV)
p.-c. ventilation technique

pressure-flow relationship
pressure-like
    p.-l. sensation
    p.-l. sensation in chest
pressure-natriuresis curve
pressure-overload hypertrophy
pressure-regulated
    p.-r. volume control (PRVC)
    p.-r. volume control ventilation
pressure-volume
    p.-v. analysis
    p.-v. curve
    p.-v. data
    p.-v. diagram
    elastic p.-v. (Pel-V)
    p.-v. loop
    p.-v. relation
pressurized metered-dose inhaler (pMDI)
pressurizer
    Oxy-Hood p.
Pressurometer blood pressure monitor
PresTab
    Glynase P.
Presto
    P. cardiac device
    P.-Flash spirometry system
    P. spirometry system
presyncopal
    p. episode
    p. medication
    p. spell
presyncope
    iterative p.
presystole
presystolic
    p. gallop
    p. murmur
    p. pressure and volume
    p. pulsation
    p. thrill
pretibial
    p. edema
    p. myxedema
pretracheal
    p. lymph node
pretracheales
    nodi lymphoidei p.
pretreatment
    icatibant p.
Pretz-D
prevalence

Prevel sign
PREVENT
    Prevention of Recurrent Venous Thromboembolism
    Program in Ex Vivo Vein Graft Engineering via Transfection
    Proliferation Reduction with Vascular Energy Trial
    Prospective Randomized Evaluation of the Vascular Effects of Norvasc Trial
    PREVENT clinical trial
prevention
    P. of Atherosclerosis with Ramipril Therapy (PART)
    Centers for Disease Control and P. (CDC)
    P. of Events with ACE Inhibition (PEACE)
    P. of Recurrent Venous Thromboembolism (PREVENT)
    secondary p.
    Trials of Hypertension P. (TOHP)
    Vitamin Intervention for Stroke P. (VISP)
preventricular stenosis
Preveon
prevertebral space
Prevotella melaninogenica
prevotii
        Peptostreptococcus p.
Prevue system
PRF
    plasma-resistant fiber oxygenator
    pulse repetition frequency
Price-Thomas bronchial forceps
prickle cell carcinoma
prick-test method
Priftin
Prima
    P. laser guidewire
    P. pacemaker
    P. Total Occlusion Device
    P. Total Occlusion system
Primacor
primaquine
    p. phosphate
    p. phosphate antimalarial
primary
    P. Angioplasty in Myocardial Infarction (PAMI)
    p. atelectasis
    p. atypical pneumonia

NOTES

P

primary *(continued)*
   p. bronchus
   p. cardiac arrhythmia
   p. cardiac malignancy
   p. cardiomyopathy
   p. ciliary dyskinesia (PCD)
   p. closure
   p. coccidioidomycosis
   p. complex
   p. effusion lymphoma
   p. electrical disease
   p. endocardial fibroelastosis
   p. eosinophilic pneumonia
   p. fibroproliferative pulmonary
     vasculopathy
   p. graft failure (PGF)
   p. hypertension
   p. infection
   p. influenza pneumonia
   p. intracerebral hemorrhage (PICH)
   p. isolated chylopericardium
   p. lung carcinoma
   p. pacemaker
   p. percutaneous transluminal
     coronary angioplasty (pPTCA)
   p. pleural aspergillosis
   p. pleurisy
   p. pleuropulmonary disease
   p. pulmonary histiocytosis X
   p. pulmonary hypertension (PPH)
   p. pulmonary hypertension murmur
   p. pulmonary non-Hodgkin
     lymphoma (PPL)
   p. pulmonary parenchymal disease
   p. restrictive cardiomyopathy
   p. sensorimotor cortex (SM1)
   p. spontaneous pneumothorax (PSP)
   p. systemic amyloidosis
   p. thrombus
   p. tuberculosis
   p. ventricular fibrillation
   p. ventricular tachycardia (PVT)
Primatene Mist
Primaxin
prime
   P. balloon
   crystalloid p.
   P. ECG mapping system
   RR p.
   RSR p. (rSR′)
primed lymphocyte test
priming
   p. dose
   retrograde autologous p.
primitive
   p. aorta
   p. neuroectodermal tumor (PNET)
primordial catheter tube

primum
   p. atrial septal defect
   ostium p.
   persistent ostium p.
   septum p.
Principen
principle
   Beer-Lambert p.
   Castaneda p.
   Fick p.
   Frank-Straub-Wiggers-Starling p.
   hemodynamic p.
   Huygens p.
   Laplace p.
   Pascal p.
Prinivil
Prinizide
PrinterNOx
   P. nitric oxide/nitrogen dioxide
     monitor
   P. nitric oxide with MKII analyzer
Prinzide
Prinzmetal
   P. angina
   P. effect
   P. variant angina
Priscoline injection
PRISM
   Platelet Receptor Inhibition for Ischemic
     Syndrome Management
   PRISM study
Prism-CL pacemaker
prism method
PRISM-PLUS
   Platelet Receptor Inhibition for Ischemic
     Syndrome Management in Patients
     Limited to Very Unstable Signs and
     Symptoms
   PRISM-PLUS Study
privet cough
proaccelerin
proadrenomedullin
Pro-Air
ProAmatine
Pro-Amox
Pro-Ampi
proANF
   proatrial natriuretic factor
   N-terminal proANF
proarrhythmia
proarrhythmic effect
proatherosclerotic factor
proatherothrombogenic molecule
proatrial natriuretic factor (proANF)
probability
   Cooperman event p.
   p. density function (PDF)
   intermediate p.

**Pro-Bal Protected balloon-tipped
 catheter**
proband
probe
  acoustic impedance p.
  acradinium-ester-labeled nucleic
   acid p.
  ambulatory ventricular function p.
  AngeLase combined mapping-
   laser p.
  p. balloon catheter
  P. balloon-on-wire dilatation system
  P. balloon-on-wire dilation system
  Bard p.
  bipolar circumactive p. (BICAP)
  blood-flow p.
  cardiac p.
  P. cardiac device
  Chandler V-pacing p.
  coronary artery p.
  Delalande Spectradop 2 4-MHz p.
  digoxigenin-labeled DNA p.
  DNA p.
  Doppler flow p.
  Doppler velocity p.
  Dymer excimer delivery p.
  echo p.
  esophageal temperature p.
  four-beam laser Doppler p.
  Gallagher bipolar mapping p.
  Hagar p.
  Hewlett-Packard biplane 5-MHz p.
  Hewlett-Packard omniplane 5-
   MHz p.
  high-esophageal pH p.
  Hoffrel transesophageal p.
  hot-tip laser p.
  low-esophageal pH p.
  micromultiplane transesophageal
   echocardiographic p.
  Mui Scientific 6-channel esophageal
   pressure p.
  multielectrode p.
  Neo-Therm neonatal skin
   temperature p.
  nuclear p.
  over-the-wire p.
  PA 120 Osypka radiofrequency p.
  Parsonnet coronary p.
  p. patency
  Radiometer p.
  Robicsek vascular p.

  scintillation p.
  p. shield
  Siemens-Elema AB pulse
   transducer p.
  Silverstein stimulator p.
  Spectraprobe-Max p.
  transcranial Doppler p.
  transesophageal p.
  transesophageal echo p.
  Typ Vasocope III Doppler p.
  Vasoscope 3 Doppler p.
Probeta
probing sheath exchange catheter
probucol
procainamide
  N-acetyl p. (NAPA)
  p. hydrochloride
procaine
  p. hydrochloride
  penicillin G p.
Procanbid
Procan SR
procarbazine
  cyclophosphamide, doxorubicin,
   methotrexate, p. (CAMP)
  p., hydroxyurea, radiotherapy
   (PHRT)
  p., hydroxyurea, radiotherapy
   protocol
Procardia XL
procaterol
Procath electrophysiology catheter
procedure
  Alliston p.
  Anderson p.
  arterial switch p.
  atrial maze p.
  Batista p.
  Batista left ventriculectomy p.
  Bentall p.
  Bernstein p.
  bidirectional Glenn p. (BDG)
  Bing-Taussig heart p.
  Björk method of Fontan p.
  Blalock-Taussig p.
  Brock p.
  cardiac hybrid revascularization p.
  Chamberlain p.
  Charles p.
  cherry-picking p.
  Clagett p.
  Cockett p.

NOTES

P

procedure *(continued)*
    compartment p.
    corridor p.
    Damian graft p.
    Damus-Kaye-Stansel p.
    Damus-Stansel-Kaye p.
    deairing p.
    debubbling p.
    debulking p.
    domino p.
    double switch p.
    Effler-Groves mode of Allison p.
    esophageal sling p.
    fenestrated Fontan p.
    Fontan p.
    Fontan-Baudet p.
    Fontan-Kreutzer p.
    Fontan modification of Norwood p.
    genioglossal advancement p.
    Gill-Jonas modification of
      Norwood p.
    Glenn p.
    Glenn anastomosis p.
    hemi-Fontan p.
    His-Hass p.
    intracardiac amobarbital sodium p.
    Jacobaeus p.
    Jatene arterial switch p.
    Jonas modification of Norwood p.
    Junod p.
    Karhunen-Loeve p.
    Ko-Airan bleeding control p.
    Kolmogorov-Smirnov p.
    Kondoleon-Sistrunk elephantiasis p.
    Konno p.
    Lam p.
    Langevin updating p.
    latissimus dorsi p.
    left atrial isolation p.
    Lewis-Tanner p.
    Luke p.
    Lyon-Horgan p.
    maxillomandibular advancement p.
    maze p.
    MIDCAB p.
    minimally invasive p. (MIP)
    minimally invasive direct coronary
      artery bypass p.
    MLR p.
    modified Fontan p.
    Moore p.
    Morrow p.
    Mustard p.
    Mustard/Senning p.
    myocardial laser revascularization p.
    Nicks p.
    Norwood univentricular heart p.
    Overholt p.
    percutaneous myocardial
      revascularization p.
    polyanion precipitation p.
    Potts p.
    Quaegebeur p.
    Rashkind p.
    Rastan-Konno p.
    Rastelli p.
    Ross p.
    Ross aortic valve replacement p.
    Sade modification of Norwood p.
    salting-out p.
    Schenk-Eichelter vena cava plastic
      filter p.
    Schonander p.
    Senning-Rastelli p.
    Senning transposition p.
    septation p.
    Simplate p.
    Somnoplasty p.
    Sondergaard p.
    Stansel p.
    Sugiura p.
    switch p.
    Thal p.
    tonsillar somnoplasty p.
    transjugular balloon valvuloplasty p.
    Vineberg cardiac
      revascularization p.
    Waterston-Cooley p.
    Womack p.

process
    consolidative p.
    costal pit of transverse p.
    Grip Technology stent crimping p.
    Markov p.
    myocardial infiltrative p.
    poststreptococcal inflammatory p.
    vocal p.
    xiphisternal p.
    xiphoid p.

processing
    film p.
    Imaging Including MCID high-
      resolution image p.
    model-based image p. (MBIP)
    signal p.

processor
    Cobe 2991 cell P.

prochlorperazine
procoagulant
procollagen
    type I p.
    type III p.
    p. type III aminoterminal peptide
      (PIIIP)
proconvertin
    p. blood coagulation factor

p. prothrombin conversion
accelerator
Procort
Procrit
ProCross
P. Rely balloon
P. Rely over-the-wire balloon
catheter
proctacyclin
Procytox
Pro-Depo injection
prodromal symptom
prodrome
Prodrox injection
prodrug
combretastatin A4 p. (CA4P)
product
Autoplex Factor VIII inhibitor
bypass p.
BioBypass gene-based drug
delivery p.
calcium p.
CFC-free p.
double p.
fibrin degradation p.
fibrinogen degradation p.
fibrinogen-fibrin degradation p.
fibrin split p.
heart rate-pressure p.
lipid peroxidation p.
pressure time p. (PTP)
rate pressure p.
Respironics Great Performers P.'s
production
carbon dioxide p.
energy p.
IL-10 p.
mucus p.
sputum p.
venous carbon dioxide p. (VCO_2)
ventilation/carbon dioxide p.
(VE/VCO_2)
productive
p. bronchitis
p. cough
p. pleurisy
p. sputum
p. tuberculosis
productus
Peptostreptococcus p.
proepileptic action

Profen
P. II DM
P. LA
profibrinolytic
Profilate OSD
profile
aortic valve velocity p.
Astra p.
Burke Stroke Time-Oriented p.
(BUSTOP)
coronary risk p.
deflated p.
flow p.
hemodynamic p.
Hospital Admission Risk P.
(HARP)
Nottingham Health p.
P. Plus balloon dilatation catheter
risk factor p.
serum lipid p.
Sickness Impact p. (SIP)
sound intensity p.
ultra low p. (ULP)
profilin
Profilnine heat-treated
Proflex 5 catheter
Pro-Flo XT catheter
profound systemic vasodilation
profunda
p. femoris artery
p. femoris vein
reconstitution via p.
vena circumflexa iliaca p.
profundaplasty
profusion
progeria
Progestasert
progestational agent
progesterone
continuous p.
cyclic p.
micronized p.
p. oil
progestin
Proglycem Oral
prognosis
Prograf
Prograft bifurcated endograft
program
Air Wise p.
APT p.

NOTES

P

program *(continued)*
    azimilide supraventricular arrhythmia p.
    Cholesterol Reduction in Seniors P. (CRISP)
    Cholesterol Reduction in Seniors P., United States (CRISP-US)
    expedited recovery p.
    P. in Ex Vivo Vein Graft Engineering via Transfection (PREVENT)
    Hypertension Detection and Follow-Up P.
    Linde Walker Oxygen P.
    Minnesota Heart Health P. (MHHP)
    multidisciplinary pulmonary rehabilitation p.
    National Asthma Education P. (NAEP)
    National Asthma Education and Prevention P. (NAEPP)
    National Cholesterol Education P. (NCEP)
    National Heart, Lung, Blood Institute/National Asthma Education Prevention P. (NHLBI/NAEPP)
    National High Blood Pressure Education P. (NHBPEP)
    National Lung Health Education P. (NLHEP)
    OxiScan oximetry p.
    SENTRY Antimicrobial Surveillance P.
    SleepGen polysomnography data entry p.
    SMILE p.
    SomnoStar LabManager multifunction p.
    Spofford-Christopher oxygen optimizing p. (SCOOP)
    Stroke Education P. (SEP)
    Systolic Hypertension in the Elderly P. (SHEP)
    University Group Diabetes P. (UGDP)
    WALK p.
Programalith
    P. II pacemaker
    P. III pacemaker
    P. A-V pacemaker
    P. pacemaker
    P. III pulse generator
programmability
programmable
    p. cardioverter-defibrillator (PCD)

    p. implantable medication system (PIMS)
    p. pacemaker
programmed
    p. cut-off rate
    p. electrical stimulation (PES)
    p. ventricular stimulation (PVS)
programmer
    Omnicor P.
    Pacesetter APS II 3004 p.
    Pacesetter APS pacemaker p.
programmer pacemaker
progression
    poor R wave p.
    R wave p.
progressive
    p. disseminated histoplasmosis (PDH)
    p. dyspnea
    p. interstitial pulmonary fibrosis
    p. massive fibrosis (PMF)
    p. multifocal leukoencephalopathy (PML)
    p. multiple hyaloserositis
    p. parenchymal restriction
    p. pneumonia
    p. pump failure
    p. scanning
    p. systemic sclerosis (PSS)
    p. thrombus
ProHIBiT
proinflammatory
    p. cytokine
    p. substance
proiosystole, proiosystolia
proischemic
project
    bronchoscopy quality improvement p.
    Cooperative Cardiovascular P.
    Harvard atherosclerosis reversibility p.
    MITI P.
    Stanford Coronary Risk Intervention P. (SCRIP)
    Stanford Coronary Risk Intervention Reversibilty P.
    Surveillance of Work-related Occupational Respiratory Disease p.
    SWORD p.
    Technology Assessment Methods P. (TAM)
projection
    anterior p.
    anterior oblique p.
    anteroposterior p.
    left anterior oblique p.

left lateral p.
right anterior oblique p.
spider p.
steep left anterior oblique p.
projector
Tagarno 3SD cineangiography p.
prolactin-producing decidual cell
prolapse
aortic valve p.
bileaflet p.
p. coil
mitral valve p. (MVP)
plaque p.
tricuspid valve p.
unileaflet p.
valvular p.
prolapsed
p. middle scallop of posterior
leaflet
p. mitral valve syndrome
prolapsing mitral valvar leaflet
Prolastin
prolate ellipse
Proleukin
proliferans
endarteritis p.
proliferating
p. cell nuclear antigen (PCNA)
p. pleurisy
proliferation
in-stent neointimal p.
intimal p.
myxomatous p.
neointimal p.
P. Reduction with Vascular Energy
Trial (PREVENT)
proliferative bronchiolitis
Prolog pacemaker
prolongation
p. of expiration
p. of P-R interval
prolonged
p. pulmonary eosinophilia
p. Q-T interval syndrome
Proloprim
Prometa
Prometh
P. injection
P. VC With Codeine
promethazine
p. and codeine
p. and dextromethorphan

p. hydrochloride
p., phenylephrine, and codeine
Promethist With Codeine
Promine
prominence
laryngeal p.
subcutaneous bursa of the
laryngeal p.
prominentia laryngea
prominent pulmonary vein
Promit
promyelocyte
prone positioning
Pronestyl
P.-SR
prongs
Allegiance nasal p.
Invacare nasal p.
Kendal nasal p.
nasal p.
Pro-Tech nasal p.
Sims nasal p.
Taema nasal p.
Uno nasal p.
Pronova suture
propafenone
p. hydrochloride
propagated thrombus
propagating thrombosis
propagation
impulse p.
p. of R wave
p. of thrombus
propantheline
Propaq Encore vital signs monitor
Pro/Pel
P. coating
P. coating cardiac device
Hi-Torque Floppy with P.
propellant
halogenated hydrocarbon p.
propensity
systemic thrombotic p.
propeptide
aminoterminal p.
property
p.'s of lipophilicity
vagolytic p.
prophylactic
p. antibiotic
p. aspirin regimen
p. brain irradiation (PCI)

NOTES

P

557

prophylactic (*continued*)
   p. filter placement
   p. implantable cardioverter-defibrillator implantation
   p. therapy
   p. thoracostomy
prophylaxis
   PulStar compression device for DVT p.
   SBE p.
propidium iodide stain
propionate
   fluticasone p. (FP)
   salmeterol and fluticasone p.
Propionibacterium acnes
propionyl-L-carnitine
Proplex T
propofol
proportional assist ventilation (PAV)
propranolol
   p. hydrochloride
   p. and hydrochlorothiazide
proprius
   sacculus p.
Propulsid
propylthiouracil (PTU)
prorenin
Prorex injection
ProSom
prospective
   p. gating
   P. Investigation of Pulmonary Embolism Diagnosis (PIOPED)
   P. Randomized Amlodipine Survival Evaluation (PRAISE)
   P. Randomized Controlled Clinical Trials (PRCCT)
   P. Randomized Evaluation of Carvedilol in Symptoms and Exercise (PRECISE)
   P. Randomized Evaluation of Diltiazem CD Trial (PREDICT)
   P. Randomized Evaluation of the Vascular Effects of Norvasc Trial (PREVENT)
prostacyclin (PGI$_2$)
   p. metabolite
prostaglandin
   p. D2
   p. E, E1
   p. G$_2$
   p. H$_2$
Prostaphlin
   P. injection
   P. Oral
Prostar
   P. 9F percutaneous vascular surgery system

P. 11F percutaneous vascular surgery system
P. XL hemostatic puncture closure device
P. XL 8 suture mediated closure system
P. XL 10 suture mediated closure system
ProStep Patch
prosthesis, pl. **prostheses**
   Alvarez p.
   Angelchik antireflux p.
   antireflux p.
   aortic p.
   ball-and-cage p.
   ball valve p.
   Barnard mitral valve p.
   Baxter mechanical valve p.
   Beall disk valve p.
   Beall mitral valve p.
   Bentall cardiovascular p.
   bifurcated aortofemoral p.
   bifurcation p.
   bileaflet p.
   Bionit vascular p.
   Bivona-Colorado voice p.
   Björk-Shiley aortic valve p.
   Björk-Shiley convexoconcave 60-degree valve p.
   Björk-Shiley floating disk p.
   Blom-Singer indwelling low-pressure voice p.
   Braunwald-Cutter ball valve p.
   caged ball valve p.
   Capetown aortic valve p.
   Carbomedics cardiac valve p.
   Carbo-Seal ascending aortic p.
   cardiac valve p.
   Carpentier annuloplasty ring p.
   Carpentier-Edwards aortic valve p.
   Carpentier-Edwards glutaraldehyde-preserved porcine xenograft p.
   Carpentier-Rhone-Poulenc mitral ring p.
   Cartwright heart p.
   Cartwright valve p.
   collar p.
   Cooley-Bloodwell mitral valve p.
   Cooley Dacron p.
   Cross-Jones disk valve p.
   Cutter aortic valve p.
   Cutter-Smeloff aortic valve p.
   Dacron-covered Delerin frame of valve p.
   DeBakey ball valve p.
   DeBakey Vasculour-II vascular p.
   Delrin frame of valve p.
   De Vega p.

duckbill voice p.
Duromedics valve p.
Edwards Teflon intracardiac patch p.
EndoPro p.
esophageal p.
gel-weave p.
Golaski-UMI vascular p.
Gott-Daggett heart valve p.
Groningen voice p.
Hammersmith mitral p.
Hancock mitral valve p.
heart valve p.
Ionescu-Shiley valve p.
Kaster mitral valve p.
knitted vascular p.
Lillehei-Kaster cardiac valve p.
Lillehei-Kaster mitral valve p.
Meadox-Cooley woven low-porosity p.
Meadox woven velour p.
mechanical p.
Medi-graft vascular p.
Medtronic-Hall heart valve p.
Medtronic-Hall tilting-disk valve p.
Microknit vascular graft p.
Milliknit Dacron p.
Milliknit vascular graft p.
Millivent vascular graft p.
mitral p.
Monostrut cardiac valve p.
Neville tracheal p.
New Weavenit Dacron p.
Omnicarbon heart valve p.
Omniscience single leaflet cardiac valve p.
Omniscience tilting-disk valve p.
Omniscience valve p.
pericarbon pericardial p.
polytetrafluoroethylene p.
polyvinyl p.
porcine p.
Rashkind double-disk occluder p.
Sauvage filamentous p.
Sorin bicarbon bileaflet p.
Sorin mitral valve p.
Starr-Edwards aortic valve p.
Starr-Edwards ball valve p.
Starr-Edwards cardiac valve p.
Starr-Edwards disk valve p.
Starr-Edwards heart valve p.
Starr-Edwards mitral p.

stentless p.
stentless porcine aortic valve p.
St. Jude heart valve p.
St. Jude valve p.
supraannular p.
Teflon trileaflet p.
Teflon woven p.
tilting-disk aortic valve p.
Ultra Low resistance voice p.
USCI Sauvage EXS side-limb p.
vascular graft p.
Wada hingeless heart valve p.
Weavenit p.
Wesolowski vascular p.
woven Teflon p.
woven-tube vascular graft p.

prosthetic
p. aortic valve
p. ball valve
p. cardiac valve
p. poppet
p. ring annuloplasty
St. Jude composite p.
p. valve endocarditis (PVE)
p. valve regurgitation (PVR)
p. valve sewing ring
p. valve sound
p. valve stenosis (PVS)
p. valve thrombosis
p. valve vegetation

Prostin VR Pediatric injection
prostration
pain, pallor, paraesthesia, pulselessness, paralysis, p. (PPPPPP)

protamine sulfate
Protara
protease
p. inhibitor (PI)
mast cell p.

protease-antiprotease imbalance
Pro-Tech nasal prongs
protected
p. brush
p. catheter brushing (PCB)
p. specimen brush (PSB)
p. specimen brushing (PSB)

protection
airway p.
automated boundary p. (ABP)
myocardial p.

NOTES

P

protection *(continued)*
    Short Transitional Edge P.
    (S.T.E.P.)
protective
    p. block
    p. ventilation
    p. zone
protector
    pulse-ox p.
Protégé 31 Low Loss stationary liquid oxygen system
Protegra
protein
    activator p. (AP)
    alpha-B-crystallin p.
    amyloid A p.
    amyloid precursor p. (APP)
    bone morphogenetic p. type 2 (BMP-2)
    BvgS p.
    p. C
    cardiac gap junction p.
    CD45 cell surface p.
    p. C deficiency
    cholesteryl ester transfer p. (CETP)
    Clara cell secretory p.
    coagulation p.
    contractile p.
    C-reactive p. (CRP)
    CTLA4Ig p.
    cytosolic p.
    p. electrophoresis
    enhanced green fluorescent p. (*eGFP*)
    eosinophil cationic p. (ECP)
    ESAT-6 p.
    G p.
    G_i p.
    Gc p.
    glycosylation of intracellular p.'s
    $gp91^{phox}$ p.
    heat shock p. (HSP, Hsp, hsp)
    45-kilodalton p.
    p. kinase
    p. kinase A
    p. kinase C (PKC)
    M p.
    macrophage inflammatory p. (MPI)
    microsomal triglyceride transfer p. (MTP)
    mitogen-activated p. (MAP)
    M-line p.
    monocyte chemoattractant p. (MCP)
    myosin-binding p.-C (MyBP-C)
    natural resistance macrophage-associated p. (Nramp)
    NF-ATc p.
    $p22^{phox}$ p.

    $p47^{phox}$ p.
    $p67^{phox}$ p.
    rat urine p.
    recognition p.
    rhoGDI p.
    p. S
    p. S-100B
    p. S deficiency
    secretory leukoprotease inhibitor p.
    STAT4 p.
    STAT6 p.
    surfactant p. (SP)
    Tamm-Horsfall p.
    thrombus precursor p. (TpT)
    ToxR p.
    tyrosine phosphorylated p.
protein-1
    macrophage inflammatory p. (MIP-1)
    monocyte chemoattractant p. (MCP-1)
    monocyte chemotactic p. (MCP-1)
protein-A
proteinase
protein-B
protein-C
    myosin-binding p.-C. (MyBP-C)
protein-calorie
    p.-c. deficiency
    p.-c. malnutrition
proteinosis
    alveolar p.
    pulmonary alveolar p.
proteinuria
proteoglycan
proteolysis
    quantum p.
proteolytic enzyme
Proteus
    P. mirabilis
    P. pneumonia
    P. syndrome
    P. vulgaris
Protex swivel adapter
Prothazine
    P.-DC
    P. injection
    P. Oral
prothrombin
    p. G20210A mutated allele
    p. time (PT)
    p. time/partial thromboplastin time (PT/PTT)
prothrombinase complex
prothrombosis
    systemic p.
prothrombotic state

protocol
    ABC p.
    Astrand-Rhyming p.
    Balke p.
    Balke treadmill p.
    Balke-Ware treadmill p.
    BARI p.
    Bruce p.
    Bruce treadmill p.
    cardiac rehabilitation p.
    chronotropic exercise assessment p. (CAEP)
    continuous ramp p.
    Cornell p.
    Cornell exercise p.
    Cornell modification of the Bruce p.
    Ellestad p.
    exsanguination p.
    GUSTO p.
    high-ramp p.
    Hixson-Vernier p.
    James exercise p.
    Kattus treadmill p.
    low-ramp p.
    MacNamara p.
    Mayo exercise treadmill p.
    McHenry p.
    moderate-ramp p.
    modified Bruce p.
    modified Ellestad p.
    Naughton p.
    Naughton treadmill p.
    PHRT p.
    procarbazine, hydroxyurea, radiotherapy p.
    RAMP antitachycardia p.
    RAMP-based p.
    RAMP treadmill p.
    Reeves treadmill p.
    reinjection p.
    resident assessment p. (RAP)
    rest metabolism/stress perfusion p.
    Sheffield modification of Bruce treadmill p.
    Sheffield treadmill p.
    standard Bruce p.
    Stanford treadmill exercise p.
    step treadmill p.
    TAMI p.
    therapist-driven p. (TDP)
    USAFSAM treadmill exercise p.
    weaning p.
    Weber-Janicki cardiopulmonary exercise p.
    Westminster drug-free p.

protodiastolic
    p. gallop
    p. murmur
    p. rumble

protofibril

protokylol hydrochloride

proton
    p.-beam radiotherapy
    p. density
    p. pump inhibitor
    p. spectroscopy

Protonix

protooncogene

protooncogenic effect

protoplasmic block

protoporphyrin

protoporphyrin IX

Protostat Oral

protoveratrine A and B

protozoal myocarditis

protozoan

Pro-Trin

protriptyline hydrochloride

protruding atheroma

protuberantia laryngea

protuberant plaque

prourokinase
    P. in Acute Coronary Thrombosis (PACT)
    recombinant p.
    P. and tPA Enhancement of Thrombolysis Trial (PATENT)

Pro-Vent
    P.-V. ABG kit
    P.-V. arterial blood gas kit
    P.-V. arterial blood sampling kit

Proventil HFA

Provera Oral

Providencia

Provigil

provocation
    bronchial p.
    histamine p.
    mecalil p.
    p. test

Provocholine

Provox speaking valve

NOTES

P

prowazekii
  Rickettsia p.
ProWrap expansion
proxetil
  cefpodoxime p.
proximal
  p. convoluted tubule
  p. coronary sinus (PCS)
  p. and distal portion of vessel
  p. flow convergence method
  p. isovelocity surface area (PISA)
  p. segment
  p. stenosis
PRP
  platelet-rich plasma
  polyribosylribitol phosphate
PRP-D
  polyribosylribitol phosphate-diphtheria
  toxoid conjugate
  PRP-D vaccine
PRP-OMPC vaccine
PRR
  pulmonary reimplantation response
PR/RP ratio
PRSP
  penicillin-resistant *Streptococcus*
    pneumoniae
PRT
  percutaneous rotational thrombectomy
PRU
  peripheral resistance unit
prudent diet
Pruitt-Inahara
  P.-I. balloon-tipped perfusion
    catheter
  P.-I. carotid shunt
Pruitt vascular shunt
prune
  p. juice expectoration
  p. juice sputum
pruning
  branch vessel p.
pruritus
  poststroke p.
Prussian helmet sign
PRVC
  pressure-regulated volume control
  PRVC ventilation
PRx Endotak-Sub-Q array
PS
  Palmaz-Schatz
  pulmonary sequestration
  pulmonic stenosis
  PS 153 stent
psammoma bodies
psammosarcoma
PSAP
  peak systolic aortic pressure

PSA stationary oxygen system
PSB
  protected specimen brush
  protected specimen brushing
PSD
  power spectral density
PSDI
  Positive Symptom Distress Index
P-selectin
  P.-s. cell adhesion molecule
  P.-s. expression
P-Series sleep monitoring system
Pseudallescheria
  P. boydii
  P. maltophilia
  P. stutzeri
pseudallescheriasis
pseudangina, pseudoangina
pseudo
  p. R′ wave
  p. S wave
pseudoalternating current
pseudoaneurysm
  arterial p.
  femoral p.
pseudoangina (*var. of* pseudangina)
pseudoapoplexy
pseudoasthma
pseudo-A-V block
pseudobronchiectasis
pseudobulbar palsy
Pseudo-Car DM
pseudocavitation
pseudocholinesterase deficiency
pseudochylothorax
pseudocirrhosis
pseudocoarctation of aorta
pseudocomplication
pseudocroup
pseudocylindrical bronchiectasis
pseudocyst
  posttraumatic pulmonary p.
  pulmonary p.
pseudodextrocardia
pseudodiastolic
pseudodiphtheriticum
  Bacillus p.
pseudodisappearance criterion
pseudoephedrine
  acetaminophen, dextromethorphan,
    and p.
  acrivastine and p.
  carbinoxamine and p.
  chlorpheniramine and p.
  p. and dextromethorphan
  guaifenesin and p.
  p. HCl
  hydrocodone and p.

p. and ibuprofen
triprolidine and p.
pseudofusion beat
Pseudo-Gest Plus Tablet
pseudohypoparathyroidism
pseudohypotension
pseudoinfarction
pseudointermittent
pseudo-Kaposi sarcoma
pseudolumen
pseudolupus
pseudo-Mahaim fiber
pseudomalfunction
pseudomallei
    Pseudomonas p.
pseudomembranous
    p. angina
    p. *Aspergillus* tracheobronchitis
    p. bronchitis
    p. croup
    p. tracheobronchial aspergillosis
    p. tracheobronchitis
pseudomonad
Pseudomonas
    P. aeruginosa
    P. cepacia
    P. elastase
    P. exotoxin
    P. maltophilia
    P. pseudomallei
    P. stutzeri
pseudomucinous
pseudonormalization
    p. of T wave
    T-wave p.
pseudoparalytica
    myasthenia gravis p.
pseudopericarditis
pseudopneumonia
pseudopodia
pseudo-P pulmonale
pseudothrombocytopenia
pseudotruncus arteriosus
pseudotuberculosis
    Yersinia p.
pseudotumor
    inflammatory p. (IPT)
pseudotumoral mediastinal amyloidosis
pseudoxanthoma
    p. elasticum
    p. elasticum syndrome

PSG
    peak systolic gradient
    polysomnogram
    polysomnography
        full PSG
        PSG pressure
PSI
    Pneumonia Severity Index
psi
    pounds per square inch
psig
    pounds per square inch gauge
P-sinistrocardiale
psittaci
    Chlamydia p.
psittacosis inclusion bodies
psoriasis
PSP
    primary spontaneous pneumothorax
PSS
    Palmaz-Schatz stent
    progressive systemic sclerosis
    pure sensory syndrome
PST
    positive symptom total
PSV
    positive support ventilator
    pressure support ventilation
PSVT
    paroxysmal supraventricular tachycardia
psychic akinesia
psychocardiac reflex
psychogenic
    p. cough
    p. dyspnea
    p. overlay
    p. pain
    p. syncope
psychological
    p. factor
    p. stimulus
psychosis
    postperfusion p.
psychosocial
    P. Adjustment to Illness Scale
    P. factor
psychostimulant
psychotherapy
psychotropic agent
psyllium
PT
    prothrombin time

NOTES

P

PTA
  percutaneous transluminal angioplasty
PTAS
  percutaneous transluminal angioscopy
PTB
  pulmonary tuberculosis
PTC
  peritubular capillary
PTCA
  percutaneous transluminal coronary
    angioplasty
    perfusion balloon PTCA
    Reopro for Acute Myocardial
      Infarction and Primary PTCA
    Stenting of Total Occlusion versus
      PTCA (STOP)
PTCR
  percutaneous transluminal coronary
    revascularization
PTD
  percutaneous thrombolytic device
  photodynamic therapy
    Arrow-Trerotola PTD
PtdCho
  phosphatidylcholine
PTEF
  peak tidal expiratory flow
pteronyssimus
    Dermatophagoides p.
pterygoid chest
PTFE
  polytetrafluoroethylene
    PTFE closure
    PTFE-covered stent
    PTFE graft
    PTFE stent graft
Pth
  chest wall elastic recoil pressure
PTIF
  peak tidal inspiratory flow
PTJV
  percutaneous transtracheal jet ventilation
PTL
  pharyngotracheal lumen airway
PTLA
  pharyngotracheal lumen airway
PTLPD, PTLD
  posttransplantation lymphoproliferative
    disorder
    intrathoracic PTLPD
PTMC
  percutaneous transvenous mitral
    commissurotomy
PTMR
  percutaneous transluminal myocardial
    revascularization
  percutaneous transmyocardial
    revascularization

PTNB
  percutaneous transthoracic needle biopsy
PTP
  pressure time product
PTP-gamma
PT/PTT
  prothrombin time/partial thromboplastin
    time
PTRA
  percutaneous transluminal renal
    angioplasty
  percutaneous transluminal rotational
    atherectomy
PTSMA
  percutaneous transluminal septal
    myocardial ablation
PTT
  partial thromboplastin time
PTU
  propylthiouracil
public
    p. access defibrillation (PAD)
    p. access defibrillator (PAD)
puerile respiration
puerperal
    p. phlebitis
    p. thrombosis
puff
    p. of smoke
    veiled p.
puffball
puffer
    pink p.
puffing sound
Puig
    P. Massana annuloplasty ring
    P. Massana-Shiley annuloplasty ring
    P. Massana-Shiley annuloplasty
      valve
pullback
    aortic p.
    p. pressure
    pullback atherectomy device
pulley
pull-through
    station p.-t.
Pulmanex
Pulmicort
    P. Respules
    P. Turbuhaler
pulmo
    p. dexter
    p. sinister
Pulmo-Aide
    P.-A. aerosol compressor/nebulizer
    P.-A. nebulizer
    P.-A. Traveler
pulmoaortic canal

Pulmocare
Pulmo-Graph
pulmolith
PulmoMate aerosol compressor/nebulizer
Pulmo-Mist compressor
pulmonale
    acute cor p.
    acutely decompensated cor p.
    atrium p.
    chronic cor p.
    cor p.
    glomus p.
    ligamentum p.
    P p.
    pseudo-P p.
pulmonales
    nodi lymphoidei p.
    nodi lymphoidei
     juxtaesophageales p.
    venae p.
pulmonalis
    arteria p.
    ostium trunci p.
    pars basalis arteriae p.
    pleura p.
    plexus p.
    sinus trunci p.
    sulcus p.
    truncus p.
    valva trunci p.
pulmonalium
    ostia venarum p.
pulmonaris
    porta p.
pulmonary
    p. acid aspiration syndrome
    p. acinus
    p. actinomycosis
    p. adenomatosis
    p. agenesis
    p. air embolism
    p. alveolar hemorrhage
    p. alveolar microlithiasis
    p. alveolar proteinosis
    p. alveolus
    p. amebiasis
    p. amyloidosis
    p. angiogram
    p. angiography (PA, PAG)
    p. anthrax
    p. aplasia
    p. arch

p. area
p. arterial end-diastolic pressure
p. arterial pressure
p. arterial system
p. arterial wave pressure
p. arterial web
p. arteriolar resistance
p. arterioplasty
p. arteriovenous fistula
p. arteriovenous malformation
  (PAVM)
p. arteritides
p. artery (PA)
p. artery band
p. artery banding
p. artery catheterization (PAC)
p. artery diastolic pressure (PADP)
p. artery homograft
p. artery hypertension (PAH)
p. artery occlusion pressure
  (PAOP)
p. artery occlusive wedge pressure
p. artery pressure (PAP)
p. artery rupture
p. artery sling
p. artery steal
p. artery stenosis
p. artery systolic pressure (PASP)
p. artery wedge (PAW)
p. artery wedge pressure (PAWP)
p. aspergillosis
p. atresia
p. atresia with ventricular septal
  defect (PAVSD)
p. autograft (PA)
p. autograft valve
p. A-V O_2 difference
p. balloon valvuloplasty (PBV)
p. barotrauma
basal part of left and right
  inferior p.
p. bed
p. bed gradient
p. blastoma
p. blood flow
p. blood volume (PBV)
p. botryomycosis
p. branch of autonomic
p. branch stenosis
p. bulla
p. calcification
p. capillary blood volume (Vc)

NOTES

P

pulmonary *(continued)*
  p. capillary wedge (PCW)
  p. capillary wedge pressure (PCWP)
  p. cavitation
  p. cavity
  p. circulation
  p. coccidioidomycosis
  p. coin lesion
  p. component of second heart sound
  p. cone
  p. congestion
  p. consolidation
  p. contusion
  p. conus
  p. cryptococcosis
  p. cyanosis
  p. DCS
  p. diffusion capacity (D_{CO})
  p. disease anemia syndrome
  p. dysmaturity syndrome
  p. dyspnea
  p. edema
  p. effusion
  p. embolectomy
  p. embolism (PE)
  p. embolization
  p. embolus
  p. emphysema (PE)
  p. epithelium
  p. failure
  p. fever
  p. fibrosis
  p. flotation catheter
  p. function (PF)
  P. Functional Status and Dyspnea Questionnaire (PFSDQ)
  p. function status
  p. function test (PFT)
  p. gas exchange
  p. glomangiosis
  p. hamartoma
  p. heart
  p. hematoma
  p. hemodynamics
  p. hemorrhage
  p. hemosiderosis
  p. hilum
  p. hyalinizing granuloma
  p. hyperinfection syndrome
  p. hypertension (PH, PHT)
  p. hypertension pressure
  p. hypertrophic osteoarthropathy
  p. hypostasis
  p. incompetence
  p. infarct
  p. infarction

p. infarction syndrome
p. infiltrates with eosinophilia syndrome
p. infiltrate with eosinophilia (PIE)
p. infiltration with eosinophilia (PIE)
p. injury
p. insufficiency
p. interstitial edema
p. interstitial emphysema (PIE)
p. leukostasis
p. ligament
p. lobule
p. lymphangiomyomatosis
p. lymph node
p. lymphoma
p. marking
p. meniscus sign
p. metastasectomy
p. microthromboembolism
p. mucormycosis
p. murmur
p. mycosis
p. nervous plexus
p. notch sign
p. orifice
p. ossification
p. osteoarthropathy
p. outflow tract
p. pain
p. parenchyma
p. parenchymal injury
p. parenchymal window
p. phthisis
p. pleura
p. pleurisy
plexogenic p.
p. pressure
p. pseudocyst
p. pulse
p. rale
p. reexpansion
p. regurgitation (PR)
p. reimplantation response (PRR)
p. resistance
p. restriction
p. ridge
p. sarcoidosis
p. scintigraphy
p. sequestration (PS)
p. shunt
p. sinus
p. sling syndrome
p. stenosis
p. sulcus
p. surfactant
p. system
p. systemic blood flow ratio

p. target sign
p. thromboembolism
p. toilet
p. transpiration
p. trunk
p. tuberculosis (PTB)
p. valve anomaly
p. valve area
p. valve disease
p. valve echocardiography
p. valve gradient
p. valve restenosis
p. valve stenosis
p. valve vegetation
p. valvotomy
p. valvular regurgitation
p. valvular stenosis
p. valvuloplasty
p. vascular bed
p. vascular marking
p. vascular obstruction (PVO)
p. vascular obstructive disease
p. vascular pressure
p. vascular reactivity
p. vascular redistribution
p. vascular resistance (PVR)
p. vascular resistance index (PVRI)
p. vasculature
p. vasculitis
p. vasoconstriction
p. vasodilation
p. vein
p. venoocclusive disease (PVOD)
p. venous atrium
p. venous congestion
p. venous connection
p. venous connection anomaly
p. venous drainage
p. venous flow (PVF)
p. venous return
p. venous return anomaly
p. ventilation
p. wedge angiography
p. wedge pressure (PWP)
pulmonary-to-systemic flow ratio
  (Qp/Qs)
pulmonic
aortic end p.
p. area
p. closure sound
p. endocarditis
p. incompetence

p. insufficiency
p. murmur
p. regurgitation
p. second heart sound (P2)
p. stenosis (PS)
p. tricuspid
p. valve
p. valve closure sound
p. valve stenosis
pulmonis
alveoli p.
apex p.
basis p.
facies costalis p.
facies interlobares p.
facies medialis p.
facies mediastinalis p.
fissura obliqua p.
hilum p.
impressio cardiaca p.
ligamentum latum p.
margo anterior p.
margo inferior p.
pars mediastinalis p.
porta p.
pulmonitis
pulmonocoronary reflex
pulmonologist
Pulmopak pump
PulmoSonic
PulmoSphere
PulmoTrack acoustic PF test
pulmowrap
Pulmozyme
Pulsair .5 liquid oxygen portable
Pulsar
P. DDD pacemaker
P. Max sensor
P. NI implantable pacemaker
P. pacemaker
pulsate
pulsatile
p. assist device (PAD)
p. flow
pulsating
p. empyema
p. pleurisy
pulsation
intraaortic balloon p. (IABP)
presystolic p.
suprasternal p.

NOTES

P

Pulsator
    P. dry heparin arterial blood gas kit
    P. syringe
pulse (*See also* pulsus)
    abdominal p.
    abrupt p.
    alternating p.
    amplitude of p.
    p. amplitude
    p. amplitude ratio (PAR)
    anacrotic p.
    anadicrotic p.
    arterial p.
    atrial liver p.
    atrial venous p.
    Bamberger bulbar p.
    bigeminal p.
    bigeminal bisferious p.
    bisferious p.
    bounding p.
    brachial p.
    bulbar p.
    cannonball p.
    capillary p.
    carotid p.
    catacrotic p.
    catadicrotic p.
    catatricrotic p.
    centripetal venous p.
    collapsing p.
    cordy p.
    Corrigan p.
    coupled p.
    C point of cardiac apex p.
    p. curve
    CV wave of jugular venous p.
    p. deficit
    dicrotic p.
    digitalate p.
    dorsalis pedis p.
    p. duration
    elastic p.
    entoptic p.
    filiform p.
    formicant p.
    F point of cardiac apex p.
    funic p.
    f wave of jugular venous p.
    gaseous p.
    p. generator
    guttural p.
    hard p.
    hyperkinetic p.
    hypokinetic p.
    incisura p.
    intermittent p.
    p. inversion harmonic imaging

    irregularly irregular p.
    jerky p.
    jugular p.
    jugular venous p.
    Kussmaul paradoxical p.
    labile p.
    long p.
    p. method
    Monneret p.
    monocrotic p.
    monophasic p.
    mousetail p.
    movable p.
    nail p.
    O point of cardiac apex p.
    p. oximeter
    3800 p. oximeter
    p. oximeter/end tidal CO_2 (POET)
    p. oximetry device
    p. oximetry monitoring (POM)
    paradoxic p.
    pedal p.
    p. period
    piston p.
    plateau p.
    popliteal p.
    posterior tibial p.
    precordial p.
    presaturation p.
    p. pressure (PP)
    pressure p.
    P. Pro heart rate monitor
    pulmonary p.
    quadrigeminal p.
    quick p.
    Quincke p.
    radial p.
    p. rate
    p. repetition
    p. repetition frequency (PRF)
    respiratory p.
    reversed paradoxical p.
    Riegel p.
    SF wave of cardiac apex p.
    soft p.
    spike-and-dome p.
    sustained p.
    tense p.
    thready p.
    tibial p.
    tidal wave p.
    p. tracing
    trigeminal p.
    triphammer p.
    triple-humped pressure p.
    p. trisection
    undulating p.
    unequal p.

vagus p.
venous p.
vermicular p.
water hammer p.
p. wave
p. wave duration
p. wave velocity (PWV)
p. width
wiry p.
x depression of jugular venous p.
x descent of jugular venous p.
y depression of jugular venous p.
y descent of jugular venous p.

pulsed
p. Doppler echocardiography
p. Doppler flowmetry
p. Doppler tissue imaging
p. dye laser
p. laser ablation
p. wave (PW)

PulseDose
P. EX2000D oxygen conserver
P. oxygen conserver
P. oxygen delivery technology
P. portable compressed oxygen system

pulsed-wave
p.-w. Doppler (PWD)
p.-w. Doppler mapping
2-MHz p.-w. Doppler transducer
p.-w. tissue Doppler (PWTD)

pulse-height analyzer
pulseless
p. bradycardia
p. disease
p. electrical activity (PEA)
p. idioventricular rhythm

pulse-ox protector
PulseSpray infusion system
pulsimeter, pulsometer
Pulsox-5
Pulsoxymeter P.

Pulsoxymeter Pulsox-5
PulStar compression device for DVT prophylaxis
pulsus
p. alternans
p. anadicrotus
p. bigeminus
p. bisferiens
p. caprisans
p. catacrotus

p. catadicrotus
p. celer
p. celerrimus
p. cordis
p. debilis
p. differens
p. duplex
p. durus
p. filiformis
p. fluens
p. formicans
p. fortis
p. frequens
p. heterochronicus
p. inaequalis
p. incongruens
p. infrequens
p. intercidens
p. intercurrens
p. irregularis
p. irregularis perpetuus
p. magnus
p. mollis
p. monocrotus
p. myurus
p. paradoxus
p. parvus
p. parvus et tardus
p. plenus
p. pseudointermittens
p. quadrigeminus
p. rarus
p. respiratione intermittens
p. tardus
p. tremulus
p. trigeminus
p. vacuus
p. venosus
p. vibrans

pultaceous debris
Pulvinal
Pulvules
Cinobac P.
Co-Pyronil 2 P.
Ilosone P.
Seromycin P.

Pumactant
pumilus
Bacillus p.

pump
Abbott infusion p.
abdominothoracic p.

NOTES

P

pump (continued)
Acat 1 intraaortic balloon p.
Accupressure infusion p.
Affinity blood p.
angle port p.
aortic balloon p.
AutoCat intraaortic balloon p.
AVCO balloon p.
Axiom double sump p.
balloon p.
Bard cardiopulmonary support p.
Bard TransAct intra-aortic
balloon p.
Barron p.
Baxter Flo-Gard 8200 volumetric
infusion p.
Bio-Medicus p.
blood p.
BVS p.
CADD-Plus intravenous infusion p.
cardiac balloon p.
cardiopulmonary bypass p.
centrifugal p.
Cobe double blood p.
Cordis Hakim p.
Cormed ambulatory infusion p.
p. current
Datascope intraaortic balloon p.
Datascope System 90 balloon p.
Datascope System 90 intraaortic
balloon p.
DeBakey VAD continuous-axial-
flow p.
ECMO p.
Emerson p.
p. failure
p. failure death
Flowtron DVT p.
p. function
Gemini Imed p.
Gomco thoracic drainage p.
Hakim-Cordis p.
Harvard p.
heart p.
HeartMate p.
IMED infusion p.
impeller p.
Infusaid infusion p.
Infuse-A-Port p.
intraaortic balloon p. (IABP)
ion p.
IVAC volumetric infusion p.
Jobst extremity p.
KAAT II Plus intraaortic
balloon p.
Kangaroo p.
Kontron intraaortic balloon p.

left ventricular assist system
implantable p.
left ventricular bypass p.
Life Care P.
Lindbergh p.
p. lung
LVAS implantable p.
Master Flow Pumpette p.
Medtronic SynchroMed p.
Microjet Quark portable p.
muscular venous p.
Neuroperfusion p.
p. oxygenation
p. oxygenator
Pulmopak p.
respiratory p.
roller p.
sump p.
SynchroMed programmable p.
Thoratec p.
Travenol infusion p.
volumetric infusion p.
pump-assisted coronary hemoperfusion
Pumpette
Stat 2 P.
pumping
intraaortic balloon p. (IABP)
pumpkin-seeding
punch
Abrams pleural biopsy p.
p. biopsy
disposable aortic rotating p.
Goosen vascular p.
punctate
p. hyperintensity
p. mucosal lesion
puncture
apical left ventricular p.
direct cardiac p.
left ventricular p.
tracheoesophageal p.
transcricothyroid p.
transseptal p.
venous p.
ventricular p.
pup cell
pupil
Argyll Robertson p.
Pura
P. stent
P.-Vario-AL stent
P.-Vario-AS stent
P.-Vario-A stent
P.-Vario stent
pure
p. dysarthria (PD)
p. flutter
p. motor hemiparesis (PMH)

p. motor stroke
p. parasystole
p. pneumothorax
p. sensorimotor stroke
p. sensory stroke
p. sensory syndrome (PSS)
purified
p. protein derivative (PPD)
p. protein derivative test
p. protein derivative of tuberculin
purifier
Air Supply air p.
Bemis Air P.
purine nucleotides adenosine triphosphate
purinergic action
purinoceptors
endothelial p.
Puritan
P. All Purpose
P. Bennett Aeris 590 concentrator
P. Bennett ETCO$_2$ multigas analyzer
P. Bennett 7250 metabolic monitor
P. Bennett OxiClip PC20 conserver
P. Bennett ventilator
P. Bubble-Jet
Purkinje
P. cell
P. conduction
P. disease
P. fiber
P. image tracker
P. network
P. system
P. tumor
Purmann method
puromucous
purple grape juice
purpose
Puritan All P.
purpura
allergy p.
anaphylactoid p.
p. fulminans
Henoch-Schönlein p.
idiopathic thrombocytopenic p. (ITP)
thrombotic thrombocytopenic p. (TTP)
purpurea
Digitalis p.

purr
purring thrill
pursed-lip breathing
pursestring suture
pursing
lip p.
PURSUIT
Platelet Glycoprotein IIb/IIIa in Unstable Angina; Receptor Suppression Using Integrilin Therapy
Platelet IIb/IIIa Underpinning the Receptor for Suppression of Unstable Ischemia Trial
purulent
p. effusion
p. pericarditis
p. pleurisy
p. pneumonia
p. sputum
purulenta
pneumonia interlobularis p.
pushability
pusher wire
putative slow pathway potential
putrid
p. bronchitis
p. empyema
PVAB
postventricular atrial blanking
PVARP
postventricular atrial refractory period
PVB
premature ventricular beat
PVC
polyvinyl chloride
premature ventricular contraction
PVD
peripheral vascular disease
PVE
prosthetic valve endocarditis
PVF
pulmonary venous flow
PVF K
PVH, PVHI
periventricular hyperintensity
PVO
pulmonary vascular obstruction
PVOD
pulmonary venoocclusive disease
PVR
prosthetic valve regurgitation
pulmonary vascular resistance

NOTES

PVRI
> pulmonary vascular resistance index

PVS
> programmed ventricular stimulation
> prosthetic valve stenosis

PVT
> primary ventricular tachycardia

P-V-Tussin

PW
> posterior wall
> pulsed wave

P-wave duration

PWD
> pulsed-wave Doppler

PWI
> perfusion-weighted MRI

PWP
> pulmonary wedge pressure

PWTD
> pulsed-wave tissue Doppler

PWV
> pulse wave velocity
> PWV Medical SphygmoCor system

pycnogenol

pyemia
> arterial p.
> portal p.

pyemic embolism

pyknosis

pylori
> *Heliobacter p.*

pyloric incompetence

pyocyanine

pyogenes
> *Streptococcus p.*

pyogenic infection

Pyopen

pyopneumopericardium

pyopneumothorax

pyothorax-associated lymphoma

PYP
> pyrophosphate
> PYP imaging
> PYP scan

pyramid method

pyrantel pamoate

pyrazinamide (PZA)
> rifampin, isoniazid, and p.

pyrexia

Pyribenzamine (PBZ)

pyridazinone dinitrile

pyridoxilated
> stroma-free hemoglobin p. (SFHb)
> p. stroma-free hemoglobin (SFHb)

pyridoxine hydrochloride

pyriform (*var. of* piriform)

pyrimethamine
> sulfadoxine and p.

pyrogenic mediator

pyrogen reaction

pyroglycolic acid suture

pyrolytic carbon

pyrophosphate (PYP)
> p. imaging
> p. scan
> p. scintigram
> p. scintigraphy
> technetium p.
> technetium-99m p.

pyruvate dehydrogenase (PDH)

pyruvic acid

PZA
> pyrazinamide

Pzf
> zero-flow pressure

Q

Q fever
Q Port
Q wave
Q wave myocardial infarction
Q wave regression

14q

chromosome 14q

QALY

quality-adjusted life-years

QCA

quantitative coronary angiography
quantitative coronary arteriography

Q-cath

Q.-c. catheter
Q.-c. catheterization recording system

QC 253 CO-oximetry control

QCT

quantitative computed tomography

QCU

qualitative coronary ultrasound

Q-H interval

Q-M interval

QMV

quadricusp mitral valve

QOLHS

Quality of Life Hypertension Study

QoLITY

Quality of Life Trial Hypertension

QOM

quality of movement

Q-Plex Cardio-Pulmonary Exercise system

Qp/Qs

flow ratio
pulmonary-to-systemic flow ratio

Q$_s$/Q$_t$, Qs/Qt

intrapulmonary shunt fraction

QQ genotype

QR, Q-R

QR genotype
QR interval
QR pattern

QRB interval

QRS

QRS alternans
QRS axis
QRS change
QRS complex
QRS complex configuration
QRS complex duration
QRS contour
fusion QRS
QRS interval

QRS loop
QRS morphology
slurring of QRS
QRS synchronous atrial defibrillation shocks
QRS vector

QRS-ST junction

QRS-T

Q.-T angle
Q.-T complex
Q.-T interval
Q.-T value

QS

QS complex
QS deflection
QS pattern
QS wave

Q-S$_2$ interval

QS$_2$ interval

Qs/Qt (*var. of* Q$_s$/Q$_t$)

Q-Stress

Q.-S. treadmill
Q.-S. treadmill stress test

Q-switched Nd:YAG laser

QT, Q-T

QT corrected for heart rate (QTc)
QT dispersion (QTd)
QT interval
QT interval dispersion
QT interval duration
QT interval sensing pacemaker
QT syndrome
QT ventilation

QTc

QT corrected for heart rate
QTc interval

QTd

QT dispersion

QTd-S

QTd-V

QTI:QT index

QTL

quantitative trait locus

QTp/QTe

ratio of QTp/QTe

QT/QTc dispersion

Q-TRAK IAQ monitor

Q-TU interval syndrome

quad

q. coughing
q. screen format

QuadPolar electrode

quadpolar w/Damato curve catheter

quadrangular resection

quadrangulation of Frouin

quadratum
    foramen q.
quadrature
    q. birdcage coil
    q. head coil
quadricusp
    q. mitral valve (QMV)
    q. stentless mitral bioprosthetic
    valve
quadricuspid
quadrigeminal
    q. pulse
    q. rhythm
quadrigeminus
    pulsus q.
quadrigeminy
quadriparesis
quadriplegia
quadripolar
    q. catheter
    q. diagnostic catheter
    q. electrode catheter
    q. Itrel 2 pulse generator
    q. pacing catheter
    q. Quad electrode
    q. steerable electrode catheter
    q. steerable mapping/ablation
    catheter
    q. thermocouple-equipped ablation
    catheter
quadruple rhythm
quadruplet
Quaegebeur procedure
Quain
    Q. fatty degeneration
    Q. fatty heart
qualitative coronary ultrasound (QCU)
Quality
    Q. of Well-Being Index
    Q. of Well-Being Scale
    questionnaire
quality
    q. control
    indoor air q. (IAQ)
    q. of life
    Q. of Life Hypertension Study
    (QOLHS)
    Q. of Life Trial Hypertension
    (QoLITY)
    q. of movement (QOM)
quality-adjusted
    q.-a. life years
    q.-a. life-years (QALY)
Quanticor catheter
quantification
    acoustic q. (AQ)
    digital echo q. (DEQ)

microdensitophotometric q.
    shunt q.
quantify
Quantison contrast agent
quantitative
    q. arteriography
    q. computed tomography (QCT)
    q. coronary angiographic analysis
    q. coronary angiography (QCA)
    q. coronary angiography caliper
    measurement
    q. coronary arteriography (QCA)
    q. Doppler
    q. edge-detection angiography
    q. left ventriculography
    q. trait locus (QTL)
    q. two-dimensional echocardiography
    q. wall motion score (QWMS)
quantum
    q. mottling
    Q. pacemaker
    q. proteolysis
    Q. PSV
    Q. TTC balloon dilator
QuantX color quantification tool
Quartet system
quartile range
quartisternal
quartz transducer
quasisinusoidal biphasic waveform
quaternary ammonium atropine
    derivative
Quattro mitral valve
Queckenstedt sign
Queensland
    Q. fever
    Q. tick typhus
quellung reaction
Queltuss
Quénu-Muret sign
quercetin
Quervain rib spreader
query fever
Quest
    Q. MPS myocardial protection
    system
    Q. MPS system
    Tranquility Q.
questionnaire
    Asthma Quality of Life Q.
    (AQLQ)
    Childhood Asthma Q. (CAQ)
    Chronic Respiratory Q. (CRQ)
    Cognitive Failures Q. (CFQ)
    Coping Strategies q.
    Dyspnea Scale q.
    Fagerstrom tolerance q. (FTQ)

Functional Outcomes of Sleep Q.
(FOSQ)
Karolinska quality of life q.
Kellner q.
London School of Hygiene
Cardiovascular Rose Q.
Mahler Baseline Dyspnea Index q.
McGill-Melzack Pain Q.
McGill Pain Q.
Medical Research Council q.
Minnesota Leisure Time Physical
Activity Q.
Minnesota Living with Heart
Failure q.
Oxygen Cost Diagram q.
Pulmonary Functional Status and
Dyspnea Q. (PFSDQ)
Quality of Well-Being Scale q.
Rose Q.
Seattle Angina Q.
Sickness Impact Profile q.
St. George Respiratory Q. (SGRQ)
Questran Light
Quetelet index
Quibron
Q.-T
Q.-T/SR
quick
q. prothrombin time
q. pulse
QuickCal algorithm
QuickDraw venous cannula
QuickFlash arterial catheter
QuickFlow
Q. DPS
Q. DPS distal perfusion system
QuickFurl
Q. DL
Q. SL balloon
QuickLoad hub
Quick test
Quiess Injection
QUIET
Quinapril Ischemic Event Trial
quiet
q. breath sounds
q. chest
q. heart sounds
q. precordium

Quik-Chek external pacer tester
Quik-Coff electrical cough stimulator
Quik-Prep
quinacrine
Quinaglute Dura-Tabs
Quinalan Oral
quinapril
q. hydrochloride
q. and hydrochlorothiazide
Q. Ischemic Event Trial (QUIET)
quinaprilat
Quinatime
Quincke
Q. disease
Q. edema
Q. pulse
Q. sign
Quincke-point spinal needle
quinestrol
quinethazone
Quinidex Extentabs
quinidine
q. gluconate
q.-induced torsade de pointes
q. sulfate
q. syncope syndrome
quinine sulfate
quinolone
Quinones
method of Q.
Quinora Oral
quinsy
lingual q.
Q-U interval
Quinton
Q. PermCath catheter
Q.-Scribner shunt
Q. Synergy cardiac information
management system
Q. tube
quinupristin
quotient
respiratory q. (RQ)
$\dot{V}/\dot{Q}$ q.
QVAR Inhalation Aerosol
QW3600 contrast medium
QWMS
quantitative wall motion score

NOTES

R
gas constant
roentgen
R axis
R on T ventricular premature
contraction
R unit
R wave
R wave amplitude
R wave gating
R wave progression
R wave upstroke
R1 rapid exchange balloon dilatation catheter
R3
Reopro Readministration Registry
RA
rheumatoid arthritis
right atrium
rotational atherectomy
RA 523 blood gas/CO-oximetry
control
RA cell
Integris 3D RA
RAA
right atrial appendage
RAAS
renin-angiotensin-aldosterone system
rAAT
recombinant alpha-1 antitrypsin
rabbit
r. antithymocyte globulin
r.-ear sign
r. fever
rabies
Rabinov venography technique
RACAT
rapid acquisition computed axial
tomography
RACE
Ramipril Angiotensin Converting
Enzyme Inhibition
RACE study
racemic
r. epinephrine
r. warfarin sodium
racemose aneurysm
Rackley
method of R.
R. method
racquet incision
RAD
reactive airways disease
regional alveolar damage

right axis deviation
RAD Airway laryngeal blade
rad
radiation absorbed dose
radarkymography
Radford nomogram
radial
r. approach
r. artery
r. artery graft
r. artery systolic pressure (RASP)
r. pulse
RADIANCE
Randomized Assessment of Digoxin on
Inhibitors of the Angiotensin
Converting Enzyme
RADIANCE study
radiant heat device (RHD)
radiata
corona r.
radiation
r. absorbed dose (rad)
Biological Effects of Ionizing R.
r. equivalent in man (rem)
extended field r. (EFR)
r. fibrosis
gamma r.
hyperfractionated r. (HRT)
r.-induced atherosclerosis
r.-induced pericarditis
intracoronary r.
intracoronary artery r.
ionizing r. (IR)
r. lung disease
mitogenic r.
r. pneumonitis
r. safety
secondary r.
r. therapy
radical
free r.
hydroxyl r.
O_2 r.
oxygen r.
radicle
radiculitis
cervical r.
Radifocus
R. catheter guidewire
R. wire
Radii-T catheter
RadiMedical fiberoptic pressure-monitoring wire
radioactive
r. iodinated serum albumin (RISA)

radioactive *(continued)*
  r. stent
  r. tantalum
  r. xenon test
radioallergosorbent test (RAST)
radiocardiogram
radiocardiography
radiocontrast dye
radiodense
radiodermatitis
Radiofocus Glidewire
radiofrequency (RF)
  r. ablater
  r. ablation (RFA)
  r.-assisted valvotomy
  r. catheter ablation
  r. current (RFC)
  r. electrophrenic respiration
  r. energy
  r. hot balloon
  r. percutaneous myocardial
    revascularization (RF-PMR)
radiograph
  chest r. (CXR)
  portable chest r.
  postoperative chest r.
radiographic
  r. cephalometry
  r. technique
radiography
  digital r.
  dual-energy digital r.
radioimmunoassay (RIA)
  Coat-a-Count r.
  Insulin Riabead II r.
  Mallinckrodt r.
radioimmunotherapy
  Study of Monoclonal Antibody R.
    (SMART)
radioisotope
radioisotopic study
radiolabeled
  r. fibrinogen
  r. gallium
  r. iodine
  r. microsphere
radioligand binding assay
radiologic scimitar syndrome
radiologist
  thoracic r.
radiology
  interventional r.
radiolucent
Radiometer probe
radiometry
  BACTEC r.
radionecrosis injury

Radionics
  R. generator
  R. radiofrequency generator
  R. RFG-35
radionuclide
  r. angiocardiography
  r. angiography
  r. cineangiocardiography
  gold-195m r.
  r. imaging
  r. perfusion lung scanning
  radionuclide perfusion lung
    scanning
  r. scanning
  r. study
  r. technique
  r. ventriculography (RNV)
radiopacity
radiopaque
  r. calibrated catheter
  r. end marker
  radiopaque ERCP catheter
  r. tantalum stent
radiopharmaceutical imaging
radiotelemetry
radiotherapy (XRT)
  continuous hyperfractionated
    accelerated r. (CHART)
  postoperative r. (PORT)
  procarbazine, hydroxyurea, r.
    (PHRT)
  proton-beam r.
radiotracer
RadiStop radial compression system
radius
  R. self-expanding stent
  thrombocytopenia-absent r. (TAR)
  thrombocytopenia with absence
    of r.
radix
  r. basalis anterior venae
  r. linguae
radon
RADS
  reactive airways disease syndrome
  reactive airways dysfunction syndrome
Raeder-Harbitz syndrome
RAE endotracheal tube
Raff-Glantz derivative method
ragpicker's disease
ragsorter's disease
Rahn-Otis sample
railroad track sign
rake retractor
rale
  amphoric r.
  atelectatic r.
  basilar r.

bibasilar r.
border r.
bronchial r.
bronchiectatic r.
bubbling r.
cavernous r.
cellophane r.
clicking r.
coarse r.
collapse r.
consonating r.
crackling r.
crepitant r.
r. de retour
dry r.
extrathoracic r.
gurgling r.
guttural r.
Hirtz r.
r. indux
inspiratory r.
laryngeal r.
marginal r.
metallic r.
moist r.
mucous r.
r.'s muqueux
musical r.
pleural r.
pulmonary r.
r. redux
r.'s and rhonchi
sibilant r.
Skoda r.
snoring r.
sonorous r.
subcrepitant r.
tracheal r.
Velcro r.
vesicular r.
wet r.
whistling r.

RALES
    Randomized Aldactone Evaluation Study
raloxifene
ramacemide
Raman
    R. spectography
    R. spectroscopy
rami (*pl. of* ramus)

R

ramipril
    R. Angiotensin Converting Enzyme
      Inhibition (RACE)
Ramirez shunt
Ramond sign
RAMP
    Rate Modulated Pacing
    RAMP antitachycardia protocol
    RAMP-based protocol
    RAMP pacing
    RAMP treadmill protocol
ramus, pl. **rami**
    r. anterior descendens
    r. anterior lateralis
    rami bronchiales
    r. communicans cum nervo
      glossopharyngeo
    rami esophageales
    rami esophageales aortae thoracicae
    rami esophageales arteriae gastricae
      sinistrae
    rami esophageales arteriae
      thyroideae inferioris
    rami esophagei
    rami esophagei nervi laryngei
      recurrentis
    rami esophagei nervi vagi
    r. intermedius
    r. intermedius artery
    r. internus nervi laryngei superioris
    rami isthmi faucium nervi lingualis
    r. lobi medii arteriae pulmonalis
      dextrae
    r. medianus
    r. posterior descendens
    r. posterior venae pulmonalis
      dextrae superioris
    rami pulmonales systematis
      autonomici
Rand
    R. appropriateness selection criteria
    R. microballoon
Randall-Baker Soucek (RBS)
Randomized
    R. Intervention Treatment of
      Angina (RITA)
randomized
    R. Aldactone Evaluation Study
      (RALES)
    R. Assessment of Digoxin on
      Inhibitors of the Angiotensin
      Converting Enzyme (RADIANCE)

NOTES

randomized *(continued)*
    r. clinical trial (RCT)
    R. Efficacy Study of Tirofiban for Outcomes and Restenosis (RESTORE)
    R. Evaluation of Salvage Angioplasty with Combined Utilization of Endpoints (RESCUE)
    r. trials
random nodule
random-zero sphygmomanometer
Ranfac needle
range
    dynamic r.
    interquartile r.
    logarithmic dynamic r.
    quartile r.
range-alternating current
range-gated transducer
Ranger
    R. balloon
    NIR ON R.
    R. over-the-wire balloon catheter
ranging
    echo r.
ranine artery
Ranke complex
Rankin Disability Scale
ranolazine
Ransohoff operation
Ranvier
    node of R.
RAO
    right anterior oblique
    RAO angulation
    RAO position
    RAO view
RAP
    remote access perfusion
    resident assessment protocol
    right atrial pressure
    RAP cannula
rapamycin
rape
    bruit de scie ou de r.
rapeseed oil
raphe
    r. linguae
    pharyngeal r.
    r. pharyngis
    r. of pharynx
rapid
    r. acquisition computed axial tomography (RACAT)
    r. antigen-detection test
    r. atrial pacing
    r. depolarization

    r. eye movement (REM)
    r. filling
    r. filling wave
    r. nonsustained ventricular tachycardia
    r. pacing
    r. plasma test
    r. sequence induction (RSI)
    R. Shallow Breathing Index (RSBI)
    r. troponin T
    r. y descent
rapid-burst pacing
Rapidgraft arterial vessel substitute
Rapidlab 800 Critical Care system
Rapidpoint access/Rapidpoint Coag
RapidScore software feature
Rappaport-Sprague stethoscope
rappel
    bruit de r.
RAPPORT
    Reopro in Acute Myocardial Infarction and Primary PTCA Organization and Randomized Trial
rarefaction
    pontine ischemic r.
rarus
    pulsus r.
RAS
    rotational atherectomy system
rash
    erythematous maculopapular r.
    maculopapular r.
Rashkind
    R. balloon atrial septostomy
    R. balloon technique
    R. cardiac device
    R. double-disk occluder prosthesis
    R. double umbrella
    R. double umbrella device
    R. hooked device
    R. procedure
    R. septostomy
    R. septostomy balloon catheter
    R. septostomy needle
    R. umbrella
    R. umbrella device
Ras mitogen-activated protein kinase
Rasmussen
    R. aneurysm
    R. syndrome
Rasor blood pumping system (RBPS)
RASP
    radial artery systolic pressure
raspatory
    Coryllos rib r.
    rib r.
rasping murmur

RAST
  radioallergosorbent test
Rastan-Konno procedure
Rastan operation
Rastelli
  R. conduit
  R. operation
  R. procedure
rate
  atrial tachycardia detection r.
    (ATDR)
  baseline fetal heart r.
  baseline variability of fetal heart r.
  beat-to-beat variability of fetal
    heart r.
  beginning-of-life r.
  complication r.
  count r.
  critical r.
  disintegration r.
  ejection r.
  end-of-life r. (EOL)
  erythrocyte sedimentation r. (ESR)
  expiratory flow r.
  fetal heart r.
  flow r.
  glomerular filtration r. (GFR)
  heart r. (HR)
  r. hysteresis
  r. immunonephelometry
  inspiratory flow r.
  low flow r.
  magnet r.
  maximal expiratory flow r.
    (MEFR)
  maximal inspiratory flow r. (MIFR)
  maximal midexpiratory flow r.
    (MMEFR)
  maximal ventilation r. (MVR)
  maximum flow r.
  maximum midexpiratory flow r.
    (MMEF, MMF)
  maximum predicted heart r.
    (MPHR)
  maximum sensory r.
  mean atrial r. (MAR)
  mean circumferential fiber-
    shortening r. (MCFSR)
  mean midexpiratory flow r. ($FEF_{25-75\%}$)
  mean normalized systolic
    ejection r.

  miss r.
  R. Modulated Pacing (RAMP)
  r. modulation
  mortality r. (MR)
  pacemaker adaptive r.
  peak diastolic filling r.
  peak emptying r.
  peak expiratory flow r. (PEFR)
  peak filling r. (PFR)
  peak flow r.
  peak inspiratory flow r. (PIFR)
  peak jet flow r.
  peak lengthening r.
  peak shortening r.
  peak work r. (Wmax)
  percent of maximum predicted
    heart r.
  r. pressure product
  programmed cut-off r.
  pulse r.
  QT corrected for heart r. (QTc)
  repetition r.
  respiratory r. (RR, R-R)
  resting metabolic r. (RMR)
  sed r.
  sedimentation r. (sed rate)
  slew r. (SR)
  r. smoothing
  stroke ejection r.
  submaximal heart r.
  submaximum heart r.
  Svedberg flotation r.
  systolic ejection r. (SER)
  target heart r. (THR)
  time forced expiratory r.
  time-to-peak filling r.
  transvalvular flow r.
  ventilator r.
  Westergren erythrocyte
    sedimentation r.
  Wintrobe sedimentation r.
  work r.
rate-adaptive device
rate-dependent
  r.-d. angina
  r.-d. bundle branch block
rate-drop
  r.-d. response (RDR)
  r.-d. response mode
  r.-d. sensing
rate-modulated pacemaker

NOTES

R

rate-responsive
> dual-chamber r.-r.
> r.-r. pacemaker
> r.-r. pacing
> r.-r. pulse generator
> single-chamber, r.-r.
> r.-r. ventricular pacing

Rathke pouch tumor
rating
> Borg dyspnea r.
> r. of perceived breathing difficulty (RPBD)
> r. of perceived exertion (RPE)

ratio
> AH:HA r.
> ankle-brachial blood pressure r.
> aorta-left atrium r.
> aortic root r.
> cardiothoracic r. (CT, CTR)
> 0 to 10 category r. (CR-10)
> conduction r.
> contrast r.
> dead-space gas volume to tidal gas volume r. (V_{DS}/V_T)
> dead space:tidal volume r.
> E/A wave r.
> E:I r.
> embolus-to-blood r. (EBR)
> end-systolic volume r.
> r. of expiration time and total time of breathing cycle (tE/tTOT)
> flow r. (Qp/Qs)
> forced expiratory volume timed to forced capacity r.
> forced expiratory volume timed to forced vital capacity r. (FEV/FVC)
> I:E r.
> r. of ingested saturated fat and cholesterol to calories
> r. of inspiration time and total time of breathing cycle (tI/tTOT)
> inspiratory to expiratory r. (I:E)
> r. of inspiratory time to total cycle time (T_I/T_{TOT})
> international normalized r. (INR)
> La:A r.
> L/S r.
> odds r. (OR)
> oxygen extraction r. (O_2ER)
> peak respiratory r. (RER)
> P:QRS r.
> PR/RP r.
> pulmonary systemic blood flow r.
> pulmonary-to-systemic flow r. (Qp/Qs)
> pulse amplitude r. (PAR)
> r. of QTp/QTe

> renal vein renin r.
> residual volume/total lung capacity r.
> resistance r.
> respiratory exchange r. (RER)
> R/Q wave r.
> RV/TLC r.
> sex r.
> shunt r.
> signal-to-noise r.
> subendocardial to epicardial resting perfusion r.
> systolic velocity r.
> r. of tidal expiratory flow at 25% of tidal volume and peak tidal expiratory flow $(TEF_{25}/PTEF)$
> r. of tidal expiratory and inspiratory flow at 50% of tidal volume (TEF_{50}/TIF_{50})
> transmitral Doppler E:A r.
> transmitral E:A r.
> trough-to-peak r.
> V/C r.
> velocity r. (VR)
> ventilation/perfusion r.
> waist-to-hip r. (WHR)

rationalization
rattle of return
Rattus
> *R. norvegicus*
> *R. norvegicus* allergen

rat urine protein
Rauchfuss triangle
Raudilan PB
Raudixin
Raudolfin
Raulerson syringe
Rautaharju ECG criteria
Rauverid
Rauwolfia
> *R.* alkaloid
> *R.* extract
> *R. serpentina*

rauwolscine
RAVES
> Reduced Anticoagulation in Saphenous Vein Graft Stent

Raw
> airway resistance

Raxar
ray
> beta r.
> gamma r.
> r. sum
> x-r.

Rayleigh scattering
Raynaud
> R. disease

R. gangrene
R. phenomenon
R. sign
R. syndrome
RayTec sponge
Razi cannula introducer
RB
respiratory bronchiolitis
Rb
rubidium
RBBB
right bundle-branch block
RBC
Ultra Tag R.
RBD
right brain damage
Rb-82 PET
rubidium-82 positron emission
tomography
RBPS
Rasor blood pumping system
RBS
Randall-Baker Soucek
RBS face mask
RCA
right coronary artery
rotational coronary atherectomy
RCBF
renal cortical blood flow
rCBF
regional cerebral blood flow
RCCA
right common carotid artery
RCFR
relative coronary flow reserve
RCP
respiratory care practitioner
RCT
randomized clinical trial
cutting balloon RCT
RCVA
right cerebrovascular accident
RCVR
renal cortical vascular resistance
RDF
Adriamycin R.
RDI
respiratory disturbance index
rDNA
lepirudin r.

RDR
rate-drop response
RDR mode
RDS
respiratory distress syndrome
**RDX coronary radiation catheter
delivery system**
reabsorbable suture
reaction
allergic r.
anaphylactoid r.
Arthus-type r.
cholera vaccine r.
egg-yellow r.
Eisenmenger r.
Fernandez r.
fibrinolytic r.
fight-or-flight r.
Haber-Weiss r.
hemoclastic r.
hexokinase r.
histiolymphocytic r.
hunting r.
hyperleukocytic r.
inflammatory r.
Kveim r.
ligase chain r. (LCR)
local r.
methacholine r.
monocytic leukemoid r.
photosensitizing r.
Pirquet r.
pleural r.
polymerase chain r. (PCR)
pyrogen r.
quellung r.
reverse transcriptase polymerase
chain r. (RT-PCR)
smallpox vaccine r.
vagal r.
vasovagal r.
Weil-Felix r.
xanthine oxidase r.
reactivation tuberculosis
reactive
r. airways disease (RAD)
r. airways disease syndrome
(RADS)
r. airways dysfunction syndrome
(RADS)
r. dilation
r. hyperemia

R

NOTES

reactive *(continued)*
  r. upper airways dysfunction
    syndrome (RUDS)
reactivity
  cerebrovascular r. (CVR)
  methacholine r.
  pulmonary vascular r.
  vascular r.
reader
  Fisher Micro-capillary Tube R.
Read test
reagin
Rea-Lo
real-time
  r.-t. echocardiography
  r.-t. perfusion imaging
  r.-t. position management (RPM)
  r.-t. position management tracking
    system
  r.-t. position management-tracking
    system/catheter (RPM)
  r.-t. telemetry
  r.-t. three-dimensional
    echocardiography
  r.-t. ultrasound
reassessment
Reaven syndrome
Rebar-18 micro catheter
Rebetron
rebound angina
rebreathing
  r. bag
  r. mask
  r. method
  r. technique
recainam
recalcitrant
  r. hypertension
  r. obstructive airways disease
recall antigen
recalled
  spoiled gradient r. (SPGR)
recanalization
  balloon occlusive intravascular lysis
    enhanced r.
  coronary r.
  excimer vascular r.
  r. versus recannulization
recannulization
  recanalization versus r.
receiver
  Medtronic radiofrequency r.
receptive aphasia
receptor
  A$_{2A}$ adenosine r.
  adrenergic r. (AR)
  A-II r.
  alpha r.

alpha-1-adrenergic r.
IIb/IIIa r. antagonist
beta r.
beta-1 r.
beta-adrenergic r. (βAR, BAR)
cholinergic r.
chylomicron remnant r.
dopamine D2 r. (DD2R)
endothelin A, B r.'s
epithelial 5′-nucleotide r.
Fas r.
Fc r.'s
glycoprotein IIb/IIIa r.
H1 r.
r. for hyaluronan-mediated motility
  (RHAMM)
imidazoline r. (I-receptor)
irritant r.
juxtacapillary r.
melanocortin-4 r. (MC4-R)
muscarinic r.
NMDA r.
opsonophagocytic r.
peroxisome proliferator-activated r.
  (PPAR)
peroxisome proliferator-activated r.
  gamma (PPAR-gamma)
ryanodine r.
stretch r.
tachykinin r.
β$_2$-receptor
receptor-operated calcium channel
recess
  costodiaphragmatic r.
  pleural r.
  Rosenmüller r.
  subphrenic r.
  superior omental r.
  supratonsillar r.
recessed balloon septostomy catheter
recessus
  r. pharyngeus
  r. pleurales
Rechtschaffen scoring method
recipient heart
reciprocal
  r. beat
  r. bigeminy
  r. regulation
  r. rhythm
  r. ST depression
reciprocating
  r. macroreentry orthodromic
    tachycardia
  r. rhythm
reciprocity
reclosure
recoarctation of aorta

recognition protein
recoil
elastic r.
luminal r.
lung elastic r.
r. phenomenon
r. wave
recombinant
r. alpha-1 antitrypsin (rAAT)
r. alteplase
r. desulfatohirudin
r. hirudin (r-hirudin)
r. human antithrombin III
r. human IL-10 (rhuIL-10)
r. human relaxin
r. human vascular endothelial
growth factor (rhVEGF)
r. lys-plasminogen
r. polyethylene glycol (r-PEG)
r. prourokinase
r. reteplase
r. tissue plasminogen activator
(rtPA)
r. tissue-type plasminogen activator
r. urokinase (r-UK)
Recombinate
recompression
reconstitution
homocollateral r.
r. via collateral
r. via profunda
reconstruction
aortic r.
arterial r.
bifurcated vein graft for
vascular r.
Cabral coronary r.
patch graft r.
polyhedral surface r.
right ventricular outflow tract r.
Sheen airway r.
stent r.
record
Algoform patient r.
recorder
circadian event r.
Del Mar Avionics three-channel r.
DM-400 Holter ECG cassette r.
Eigon CardioLoop r.
event r.
HeartCard cardiac-event r.
HeartCard event r.

HeartCard 3X cardiac-event r.
HeartWatch cardiac-event r.
HeartWatch III cardiac-event r.
Hellige electrocardiographic r.
HomeTrak Plus cardiac event r.
24-hour ambulatory
electrocardiographic r.
implantable loop r.
King of Hearts event r.
King of Hearts Express cardiac-
event r.
King of Hearts Express 3X
cardiac-event r.
KoKo Rhythm ECG r.
Marquette Holter r.
MEDILOG 4000 ambulatory
ECG r.
Mingograf 82 r.
Narco Biosystems r.
Narco Physiograph-6B r.
Oxford Medilog frequency-
modulated r.
Reveal insertable loop r.
Reveal Plus insertable loop r.
Scole Alta II 3-channel
precalibrated Holter AM r.
SNAP sleep r.
Vas r.
videotape r.
recording
bipolar esophageal r.
cineloop r.
Doppler r.
long-time r.
M-mode r.
M-mode stripchart r.
patient-triggered r.
2120 R. Spirometer
time-based event r.
transtelephonic r.
X, Y, Z r.'s
recovery
fluid-attenuated inversion r.
(FLAIR)
r. from inactivation
functional r.
pressure r.
recrossability
recrudescence
recruitable collateral vessel
recruitment
alveolar r.

NOTES

recruitment *(continued)*
    capillary r.
    host-generated neutrophils r.
rectal
    Nova R.
rectification
    anomalous r.
    inward-going r.
rectilinear
    r. biphasic shock
    r. biphasic waveform
    r. scan
    r. ST-segment depression
rectivirgula
    Saccharopolyspora r.
rectocardiac reflex
rectus abdominis muscle
recurrence
    early ischemic r. (EIR)
    familial r.
    r. risk
recurrent
    r. infective exacerbation
    r. lobar hemorrhage (RLH)
    r. mesenteric ischemia
    r. mesenteric vascular occlusion
    r. myocardial infarction
    r. respiratory infection (RRI)
    r. respiratory papillomatosis
recurrentis
    rami esophagei nervi laryngei r.
recurring
    R. Figures test for short-time
        memory
    R. Words test for short-time
        memory
recursion
    Levinson-Durbin r.
recurvatum
    pectus r.
red
    r. atrophy
    r. cedar asthma
    r. coronary thrombus
    r. hepatization
    r. hypertension
    r. induration
    r. infarct
    r. light therapy (RLT)
    r. soft coral asthma
    r. system
    r. thrombus
    r. wine polyphenol
Redha cut catheter
Redifocus guidewire
RediFurl TaperSeal IAB catheter
redilation

redistribution
    r. imaging
    pulmonary vascular r.
    vascular r.
reduced
    r. afterload
    R. Anticoagulation in Saphenous
        Vein Graft Stent (RAVES)
    r. signal intensity
reducer
    Norelco allergen r.
reducing
    r. event
    r. valve
reductase
    3-hydroxy-3-methylglutaryl coenzyme
        A r.
    r. inhibitor
    methylenetetrahydrofolate r.
        (MTHFR)
reduction
    absolute risk r. (ARR)
    afterload r.
    gradient r.
    left ventricular r. (LVR)
    preload r.
    relative risk r. (RRR)
    stapled lung r.
redundant cusp syndrome
reduplication murmur
redux
    rale r.
REE
    resting energy expenditure
reedswitch
    pacemaker r.
    r. of pacemaker
reed ventriculorrhaphy
reelevation
    ST r.
    ST-segment r.
Reel syndrome
reendothelialization
reentrant
    r. arrhythmia
    r. atrial tachycardia
    r. circuit
    r. excitation
    r. loop
    r. mechanism
    r. pathway
    r. supraventricular tachycardia
    r. ventricular tachyarrhythmia
reentry
    anatomical r.
    anisotropic r.
    atrial r.
    atrioventricular nodal r.

R

A-V nodal r.
bundle-branch r. (BBR)
dual-loop intraatrial r.
figure-of-eight intraatrial r.
r. phenomenon
Schmitt-Erlanger model of r.
sinus nodal r.
r. theory
ventricular r.
r. waveform
wavelength of r.
Reeves treadmill protocol
reexpansion
lung r.
pulmonary r.
reexploration
surgical r.
refeeding syndrome
reference
r. catheter
r. electrode
r. phantom CT
r. value
r. vessel diameter (RVD)
refill
transcapillary r.
refined
r. flour
r. grain
reflectance oximetry
reflected pressure waveform
reflecting level
reflection
guidewire r.
reflex
abdominocardiac r.
Abrams heart r.
r. angina
aortic r.
Aschner r.
Aschner-Dagnini r.
r. asthma
atriopressor r.
auriculopressor r.
Babinski r.
Bainbridge r.
baroreceptor r.
Bezold-Jarisch r.
bregmocardiac r.
Breuer-Hering inflation r.
r. bronchoconstriction
cardiac depressor r.

carotid sinus r.
chemoreceptor r.
Churchill-Cope r.
coronary r.
r. cough
cough r.
r. cough test
craniocardiac r.
Cushing r.
depressor r.
diving r.
Erben r.
esophagosalivary r.
exercise pressor r.
eyeball compression r.
eyeball-heart r.
gag r.
gasp r.
Head paradoxical r.
heart r.
hepatojugular r.
Hering-Breuer r.
Hoffman r.
hypochondrial r.
inflation r.
jaw r. (JR)
Kisch r.
Kocher-Cushing r.
laryngeal r.
Livierato r.
Loven r.
McDowall r.
mute r.
nasobronchial r.
nasosinus-bronchial r.
oculocardiac r.
oculopharyngeal r.
oculovagal r.
orthocardiac r.
r. pacemaker
R. 8220 pacemaker
Pavlov r.
pericardial r.
pharyngeal r.
pneocardiac r.
pneopneic r.
pressoreceptor r.
psychocardiac r.
r. pulmonary arterial
    vasoconstriction
pulmonocoronary r.
rectocardiac r.

NOTES

587

reflex *(continued)*
    respiratory r.'s
    RIII r.
    sinus r.
    sneeze r.
    r. stimulation
    suck r.
    R. SuperSoft steerable guidewire
    r. sympathetic dystrophy
    r. sympathoexcitation
    r. tachycardia
    vagal r.
    r. vagal bronchoconstriction
    vascular r.
    r. vasoconstriction
    vasoconstrictive r.
    r. vasodilation
    vasopressor r.
    venorespiratory r.
    viscerocardiac r.
ReFlex ENT Wand
Re/Flex filter
reflexogenic pressosensitivity
Reflotron bedside theophylline test
Refludan injection
reflux
    abdominojugular r.
    cardioesophageal r.
    erosive r.
    esophageal r.
    r. esophagitis
    extraesophageal r.
    gastroesophageal r. (GER)
    hepatojugular r. (HJR)
    nasopharyngeal r.
    transvalvular r.
    valvular r.
    venous r.
reform
    capacitor r.
refractoriness
    dispersion of r.
refractory
    r. congestive heart failure
    r. hypoxemia
    r. to medical therapy
    r. period
    r. period of electronic
    r. period of electronic pacemaker
    r. shock
    r. tachycardia
Ref-Star EP catheter
Refsum
    R. disease
    R. syndrome
Regency
    R. SR+ pulse generator
    R. SR pulse generator

regimen
    antithrombotic r.
    dosage r.
    exercise r.
    Intracoronary Stenting and
      Antithrombotic r. (ISAR)
    prophylactic aspirin r.
    stepped-care antihypertensive r.
    titration r.
region
    AN r.
    r. of interest (ROI)
    N r.
    NH r.
    parahilar r.
    paratracheal r.
    r. of respiratory mucosa
    watershed r.
regional
    r. alveolar damage (RAD)
    r. cerebral blood flow (rCBF)
    r. dyssynergy
    r. ischemia
    r. myocardial blood flow (RMBF)
    r. oxygen saturation (rSO$_2$)
    r. perfusion
    r. vasodilation
    r. wall motion
    r. wall motion abnormality
    r. wall motion index
regio respiratoria tunicae mucosae nasi
registration
    flow-time r.
    North American Cerebral
      Transluminal Angioplasty R.
      (NACPTAR)
registry
    balloon valvuloplasty r. (BVR)
    Cardiac Ablation R. (CAR)
    Cardiovascular Information R.
      (CVIR)
    ELCA r.
    ELSO r.
    Global Carotid Artery Stent R.
    International Cooperative Pulmonary
      Embolism R. (ICOPER)
    ISHT R.
    LARS Retrospective USA R.
    Long Bare Stent R.
    Mansfield Valvuloplasty R.
    NACI r.
    New Approaches to Coronary
      Interventions r.
    North American Inoue Balloon r.
    PELCA R.
    Reopro Readministration R. (R3)
Regitine

REGRESS
    Regression Growth Evaluation Statin
    Study
regression
    arteriographic r.
    coronary plaque r.
    r. equation
    R. Growth Evaluation Statin Study
      (REGRESS)
    Poisson r.
    Q wave r.
    xanthoma r.
regular
    R. (Concentrated) Iletin II U-500
    R. Iletin I
    r. purified pork insulin
    r. rate and rhythm (RRR)
    r. sinus rhythm (RSR, rSR′)
regularly irregular rhythm
regulation
    reciprocal r.
regulator
    aluminum oxygen r.
    Boehringer suction R.
    cystic fibrosis transmembrane r.
      (CFTR)
    cystic fibrosis transmembrane
      conductance r.
    Easy/Dial Reg oxygen r.
    Ohmeda thoracic suction r.
regulon
    BvgAS r.
regurgitant
    r. fraction
    r. jet
    r. jet area (RJA)
    r. murmur
    r. orifice
    r. orifice area (ROA)
    r. pocket
    r. volume (RVol)
    r. wave
regurgitation
    aortic r. (AR)
    aortic valve r.
    atrioventricular valve r.
    commissural mitral r.
    faint pulmonary r.
    functional mitral r.
    homograft insertion for
      pulmonary r.
    ischemic mitral r.

    mitral r. (MR)
    mitral valve r.
    periprosthetic mitral r.
    prosthetic valve r. (PVR)
    pulmonary r. (PR)
    pulmonary valvular r.
    pulmonic r.
    Sellers classification of mitral r.
    semilunar valve r.
    tricuspid r. (TR)
    valvular r.
rehabilitation
    American Association of
      Cardiovascular and Pulmonary R.
      (AACVPR)
    cardiac r.
    r. exercise
    vocational r.
    work r.
rehalation
Rehbein rib spreader
Reich-Nechtow clamp
Reid
    R. classification
    R. index
    R. index measurement
Reil
    ball of R.
    band of R.
reinfarction
reinfection tuberculosis
reinfusion
Reinhoff
    R. clamp
    R. rib spreader
    R. swan neck clamp
    R. thoracic scissors
reinjection protocol
Reisman
    R. myocardosis
    R. pneumonia
Reisseisen muscle
Reiter
    R. disease
    R. syndrome
reject control
rejection
    acute r. (AR)
    acute allograft r.
    acute cellular xenograft r.
    acute lung r.
    allograft r.

R

NOTES

rejection *(continued)*
r.-associated pulmonary fibrosis
r. cardiomyopathy
r. cardiomyopathy transplant
delayed xenograft r. (DXR)
graft r.
hyperacute r.
no infection-no r. (NI-NR)
relapsing
r. fever
r. polychondritis
relation
concentration-effect r.
diastolic pressure-volume r.
end-systolic pressure-volume r.
end-systolic stress-dimension r.
force-frequency r.
force-length r.
force-velocity r.
force-velocity-length r.
force-velocity-volume r.
interval-strength r.
length-resting tension r.
length-tension r.
pressure-volume r.
resting length-tension r.
tension-length r.
ventilation/perfusion r.
ventricular end-systolic pressure-
volume r.
relationship
Fick r.
Laplace r.
pressure-flow r.
stress-shortening r.
relative
r. cardiac volume
r. coronary flow reserve (RCFR)
r. humidity
r. incompetence
r. inspiratory effort (RIE)
r. lymphocyte count
r. mitral stenosis
r. refractory period (RRP)
r. risk (RR, R-R)
r. risk reduction (RRR)
r. wall thickness (RWT)
relaxant
muscle r.
smooth muscle r.
relaxation
r. atelectasis
atrial r.
diastolic r.
dynamic r.
endothelium-dependent vascular r.
endothelium-independent vascular r.
endothelium-mediated r.

isovolumetric r.
isovolumic r.
left ventricular r.
left ventricular diastolic r.
r. loading
smooth muscle r.
stress r.
r. technique
r. time
r. time index
ventricular r.
relaxin
recombinant human r.
relaxometry
NMR r.
Relay cardiac pacemaker
release
Acutrim Precision R.
allergen-induced mediator r.
catecholamine r.
physiologic pattern r. (PPR)
sustained r.
Relenza
Relia-Vac drain
relief
Mini Thin Asthma R.
Vicks DayQuil Sinus Pressure &
Congestion R.
reliever
Arthritis Foundation Pain R.
Medtronic Pulsor Intrasound pain r.
REM
rapid eye movement
REM sleep
REM sleep-related hypoxemia
rem
radiation equivalent in man
remacemide hydrochloride
Remac system
remedial psychological stressor
Remedy
R. Sleep Therapy
R. sleep therapy system
Remicade
remifentanil
remission
Legroux r.
remnant
chylomicron r.
r. lipoprotein (RLP)
remnant-like
r.-l. lipoprotein particle (RLP)
r.-l. particle lipoprotein
remodeling
adverse ventricular r.
airway r.
arterial r.
atrial reverse r.

concentric r.
coronary r.
flow-responsive r.
heart chamber r.
myocardial r.
negative r.
postinfarct ventricular r.
reverse r.
vascular r.
ventricular r.
remote
r. access perfusion (RAP)
r. access perfusion cannula
removal
extracorporeal carbon dioxide r.
REMstar Reliance CPAP system
Renaissance spirometry system
renal
r. angiography
r. arteriography
r. artery
r. artery bypass graft
r. artery disease
r. artery forceps
r. artery-reverse saphenous vein
bypass
r. azotemia
r. blood vessel
r. cortical blood flow (RCBF)
r. cortical necrosis
r. cortical vascular resistance
(RCVR)
r. cyst
r. dialysis
r. diet
r. dyspnea
r. failure
r. fistula
r. function
r. hypertension
r. insufficiency
r. juxtaglomerular cell
r. kallikrein-kinin system
r. parenchymal disease
r. plasma flow (RPF)
r. transplant
r. tuberculosis
r. vein
r. vein renin ratio
r. venography
renal-splanchnic steal
Rendell-Baker face mask

Rendu-Osler-Weber
R.-O.-W. disease
R.-O.-W. syndrome
Renese
renin
r. angiotensin
r. inhibitor
r. level
plasma r.
renin-angiotensin-aldosterone
r.-a.-a. cascade
r.-a.-a. system (RAAS)
renin-angiotensin blocker
Renografin-76
sonicated R.
renography
captopril r.
renomedullary lipid
renoprival hypertension
renopulmonary
Renormax
renovascular
r. angiography
r. hypertension
Renovist
Rentamine
Rentrop
R. catheter
R. classification
REO
respiratory and enteric orphan
REO virus
reocclusion
reoperation
Reopro
R. for Acute Myocardial Infarction
and Primary PTCA
R. in Acute Myocardial Infarction
and Primary PTCA Organization
and Randomized Trial
(RAPPORT)
R. Readministration Registry (R3)
Reovirus
repair
Alfieri r.
Allison hiatal hernia r.
Boerema hernia r.
Brom r.
cap r.
DeBakey-Creech aneurysm r.
Effler hiatal hernia r.
endovascular r. (EVR)

R

NOTES

repair *(continued)*
   Fontan r.
   Hatafuku fundus onlay patch
      esophageal r.
   minimally invasive valve r.
      (MIVR)
   Mustard r.
   Norwood r.
   patch r.
   Senning atrial baffle r.
reparative cardiac surgery
repeat
   r. balloon mitral valvotomy
   r. revascularization
**Repel-CV bioresorbable adhesion-barrier
film**
reperfused myocardium
reperfusion
   r. arrhythmia
   Calcium Antagonist in R. (CARE)
   r. catheter
   r. edema
   emergency r.
   r. injury
   late r.
   r. pulmonary edema
   r. therapy
reperfusion-induced hemorrhage
reperfusion/occlusion
   Hirulog Early r/o (HERO)
repetition
   pulse r.
   r. rate
   r. time (TR)
repetitive
   r. monomorphic ventricular
      tachycardia
   r. paroxysmal ventricular
      tachycardia
   r. stunning
rephasing
   even-echo r.
replacement
   aortic valve r. (AVR)
   battery elective r.
   blood r.
   composite valve graft r.
   Cosgrove mitral valve r.
   minimally invasive valve r.
      (MIVR)
   mitral valve r. (MVR)
   partial chordal-sparing mitral
      valve r.
   supraannular mitral valve r.
      (SMVR)
   total chordal-sparing mitral valve r.
   valve r. (VR)
repletion

replication
repolarization
   benign early r. (BER)
   early r. (ER)
   early rapid r.
   final rapid r.
   myocardial r.
representative CT (Hounsfield) number
repression
reprogramming
   pacemaker output r.
reptilase
RER
   peak respiratory ratio
   respiratory exchange ratio
RERA
RES-701-1
Rescaps-D Capsule
Rescriptor
ReSCU
   Respiratory Special Care Unit
RESCUE
   Randomized Evaluation of Salvage
      Angioplasty with Combined Utilization
      of Endpoints
   RESCUE study
rescue
   r. angioplasty
   citrovorum r.
   r. shock
   r. stent implantation
ResCue Key
research
   Agency for Health Care Policy
      and R. (AHCPR)
   R. Medical straight multiple-holed
      aortic cannula
   R. on Instability in Coronary
      Artery Disease (RISC)
   R. Pneumotach System
      instrumentation module
resection
   activation map-guided surgical r.
   atrial septal r.
   bronchial sleeve r.
   r. clamp
   endocardial r.
   endocardial-to-endocardial r.
   infundibular wedge r.
   lesser r.
   myotomy-myectomy-septal r.
   quadrangular r.
   segmental lung r.
   septal r.
   Torek r. of thoracic esophagus
Resectisol Irrigation Solution
reserpine
   chlorothiazide and r.

hydralazine, hydrochlorothiazide, and r.
hydrochlorothiazide and r.
hydroflumethiazide and r.

reserve
r. air
blood flow r.
breathing r. (BR)
cardiac r.
cardiopulmonary r.
r. cell carcinoma
contractile r.
coronary r.
coronary arterial r.
coronary flow r. (CFR)
coronary flow velocity r. (CFVR, CVR)
coronary vascular r.
coronary vasodilator r.
diastolic r.
Doppler Endpoints Stenting International Investigation: Coronary Flow R. (DESTINI-CFR)
extraction r.
flow r.
fractional flow r. (FFR)
fractional velocity r. (FVR)
Frank-Starling r.
heart rate r. (HRR)
limited ventricular r.
myocardial r.
myocardial fractional flow r. (FFR$_{myo}$)
preload r.
relative coronary flow r. (RCFR)
respiratory r.
stenotic flow r. (SFR)
systolic r.
vasodilator r.
ventricular r.

reservoir
Biocor softshell venous r.
Cardiometrics cardiotomy r.
cardiotomy r.
Cobe cardiotomy r.
double bubble flushing r.
r. face mask
Intersept cardiotomy r.
Jostra cardiotomy r.
Polystan cardiotomy r.

Scimed extracorporeal silicone rubber r.
Shiley cardiotomy r.
William Harvey cardiotomy r.

reset
r. nodus sinuatrialis
sinus node r.

resident assessment protocol (RAP)

residual
r. air
r. capacity
r. deep vein thrombosis
r. DVT
r. gradient
r. jet
r. lung capacity
r. shunt
r. stenosis
r. volume (RV)
r. volume/total lung capacity (RV/TLC)
r. volume/total lung capacity ratio

residue
fucose r.

resin
anion exchange r.
bile acid binding r.
cholestyramine r.
epoxy r.
pine r.
thermosetting r.

resistance
afterload r.
airway r. (Raw)
aortic valve r.
cerebrovascular r. (CVR)
coronary vascular r.
elastic r.
expiratory r.
glucocorticoid r.
hydraulic r.
insulin r.
r. to movement of lung tissue (Rti)
nitrate r.
peripheral r.
peripheral vascular r.
pulmonary r.
pulmonary arteriolar r.
pulmonary vascular r. (PVR)
r. ratio
renal cortical vascular r. (RCVR)

NOTES

resistance *(continued)*
    respiratory r. (Rrs)
    stenosis r.
    systemic vascular r. (SVR)
    total airway r. (Rtot)
    total peripheral r. (TPR)
    total pulmonary r. (TPR)
    r. training (RT)
    valve r.
    vascular r.
    vascular peripheral r.
    r. vessel
resistant hypertension
Resistex
    R. expiratory resistance exerciser
    R. PEP therapy device
resistive heating
resistor
    fixed orifice r.
    magnetic valve r.
    spring-loaded r.
    threshold r.
    underwater seal r.
    water column r.
    weighted ball r.
Res Medication Bubble Mask nasal mask
resolution
    energy r.
    Fibrinolytic and Aggrastat ST Elevation R. (FASTER)
    high spatial r.
    spatial r.
    ST r.
    ST segment r.
    temporal r.
resolving power
resonance
    bandbox r.
    bell-metal r.
    cough r.
    cracked-pot r.
    nuclear magnetic r. (NMR)
    shoulder-strap r.
    skodaic r.
    whispering r.
    wooden r.
resonant frequency
resorption
    r. atelectasis
    bulla r.
Respa-DM
Respa-GF
Respaire-60 SR
Respaire-120 SR
Respalor
Respa-1st
Respbid

RespiGam
Respihaler
    Dexacort Phosphate in R.
Respinol-G
RespiPac
    Zagam R.
respirable aerosol
Respiradyne pulmonary function device
respiration
    abdominal r.
    absent r.
    accelerated r.
    accessory muscles of r.
    aerobic r.
    agonal r.
    amphoric r.
    anaerobic r.
    apneustic r.
    artificial r.
    assisted r.
    asthmoid r.
    Austin Flint r.
    Biot r.
    Bouchut r.
    bronchial r.
    bronchocavernous r.
    r. bronchoscope
    bronchovesicular r.
    cavernous r.
    cell r.
    central r.
    cerebral r.
    Cheyne-Stokes r.
    cogwheel r.
    collateral r.
    controlled r.
    controlled diaphragmatic r.
    Corrigan r.
    costal r.
    cyclic r.
    decreased r.
    diaphragmatic r.
    diffusion r.
    direct r.
    divided r.
    electrophrenic r.
    external r.
    forced r.
    granular r.
    harsh r.
    internal r.
    interrupted r.
    intrauterine r.
    jerky r.
    Kussmaul r.
    Kussmaul-Kien r.
    labored r.
    meningitic r.

metamorphosing r.
mitochondrial r.
mouth-to-mouth r.
nervous r.
paradoxical r.
periodic r.
placental r.
puerile r.
radiofrequency electrophrenic r.
rude r.
Schafer method of artificial r.
Seitz metamorphosing r.
shallow r.
sighing r.
slow r.
sonorous r.
stertorous r.
stridulous r.
supplementary r.
suppressed r.
temperature, pulse, and r. (TPR)
thoracic r.
transitional r.
tubular r.
unlabored r.
vesiculocavernous r.
vicarious r.
wavy r.

respiratometer
Collins r.

respirator
Ambu r.
BABYbird r.
Bear 5 r.
Bourns infant r.
Bragg-Paul r.
cabinet r.
cuirass r.
Drinker r.
Emerson cuirass r.
Engstrom r.
Gill I r.
r. lung
Med-Neb r.
Monaghan r.
Morch r.
Moynihan r.
particulate r.
pressure-controlled r.
Sanders jet ventilation device r.
tank r.

volume-controlled r.
volumetric diffusive r. (VDR)
respiratoria
glottis r.
rima r.
respiratorium
systema r.
respiratorius
apparatus r.
respiratory
r. acidosis
r. activity
r. airway
r. alkalosis
r. alternans
r. alternans breathing pattern
r. apparatus
r. arousal scoring
r. arrest
r. arrhythmia
r. artifact
r. bronchiole
r. bronchioles
r. bronchiolitis (RB)
r. burst
r. capacity
r. care practitioner (RCP)
r. center
r. collapse
r. compromise
r. cycle
r. dead space
r. depressant action
r. depression
r. distress
r. distress syndrome (RDS)
r. distress syndrome of the
  newborn
r. disturbance index (RDI)
r. drive
r. effort-related arousal
r. embarrassment
r. and enteric orphan (REO)
r. event
r. exchange
r. exchange ratio (RER)
r. excursion
r. failure
r. feedback (RFb)
r. flora
r. frequency (f)
r. function

R

NOTES

respiratory *(continued)*
r. gas analysis
r. gated MRCA
r. gated three-dimensional gradient-echo sequence
r. gating
r. glycoconjugate (RGC)
r. inductance plethysmograph (RIP)
r. inductance plethysmography (RIP)
r. infection
r. insufficiency
r. irritant
r. metabolism
r. minute volume
r. mucosa
r. murmur
r. muscle fatigue
r. ordered phase encoding (ROPE)
r. paralysis
r. pattern
r. pulse
r. pump
r. quotient (RQ)
r. rate (RR, R-R)
r. reflexes
r. region of tunica mucosa of nose
r. reserve
r. resistance (Rrs)
r. sinus arrhythmia
r. sound
R. Special Care Unit (ReSCU)
r. standstill
r. stridor
r. support
r. swing
r. syncytial virus (RSV)
r. syncytial virus conduit
r. syncytial virus immunoglobulin (RSV-IG)
r. syncytial virus IV immune globulin
r. system
Taiwan acute r. (TWAR)
r. toilet
r. tract
r. tract infection
r. tract lining fluid (RTLF)
r. triggering
r. waveform variation
respiratory-gated 2 D segmented-FLASH MRCA image
Respirgard II nebulizer
respirometer
Dräger r.
Fraser Harlake r.
Haloscale r.

Wright r.
Wright & Haloscale r.
Respiromonitor RM-300
Respironics
R. BIPAP bilevel ventilator
R. CPAP machine
R. Great Performers Products
R. Oasis humidifier
R. 920P handheld pulse oximeter
R. 930 pulse oximeter
Respitrace
R. inductive plethysmograph
R. machine
R. plethysmograph
Respivir
response
acute r.
atrial flutter r. (AFR)
atrial tachy r. (ATR)
autonomic r.
biphasic r.
blunted exercise r.
bronchodilator r.
cell-mediated immune r.
chemotactic r.
cholinergic r.
chronotropic r.
controlled ventricular r.
Cushing pressure r.
dynamic frequency r.
dysfunctional airway immune r.
endothelium-dependent dilator r. to substance P
fetal ventricular myocyte proliferative r.
fight-or-flight r.
frequency r.
giving-up/given-up r.
hemodynamic mental stress r.
Henry-Gauer r.
implantation r.
incrementing r.
metaboreflex r.
methacholine r.
neointimal hyperplastic r.
paced ventricular evoked r.
photobiological r.
plateau r.
pulmonary reimplantation r. (PRR)
rate-drop r. (RDR)
slow r.
square wave r.
sympathoexcitatory r.
thyrotropin-releasing hormone r.
vagal r.
vagotonic baroreceptor r.
vasodilatory r.
vasomotor r. (VMR)

ventilatory r.
ventricular r.
vigilance r.
visually evoked flow r. (VEFR)

response-to-injury
r.-t.-i. hypothesis
r.-t.-i. hypothesis of atherogenesis
r.-t.-i. theory

responsiveness
bronchial r. (BR)
myofilament calcium r.

RespSponse III respiratory pressure transducer

Respule
Pulmicort R.

Res-Q
R.-Q. ACD
R.-Q. ACD implantable cardioverter-defibrillator
R.-Q. AICD
R.-Q. arrhythmia control device
R.-Q. ICD generator
R.-Q. Micron ICD
R.-Q. Micron implantable cardioverter-defibrillator

REST
Restenosis Stent Trial

rest
r. angina
r. dyspnea
r. ejection fraction
r. and exercise gated nuclear angiography
r. hypoxemia
r. metabolism/stress perfusion protocol
r. pain
r. radionuclide angiography

Resten-NG

restenosis
AngioRad radiation for r. (ARREST)
aortic valve r.
diffuse in-stent r.
in-stent r. (ISR)
intralesion r.
intrastent r. (IR)
r. lesion
Local Alcohol and Stent Against R. (LASAR)
mitral r.

Multicenter American Research Trial with Cilazapril after Angioplasty to Prevent Transluminal Coronary Obstruction and R. (MARCATOR)
post balloon angioplasty r.
pulmonary valve r.
Randomized Efficacy Study of Tirofiban for Outcomes and R. (RESTORE)
r. risk
Rotational Atherectomy versus Balloon Angioplasty for Diffuse In-Stent R. (ROSTER)
Serial Ultrasound R.
Serial Ultrasound Analysis of R. (SURE)
R. Stent Trial (REST)
tricuspid r.

restenotic narrowing

rest-exercise equilibrium radionuclide ventriculography

resting
r. energy expenditure (REE)
r. hypertension
r. length-tension relation
r. membrane potential
r. metabolic rate (RMR)
r. parasternal long-axis view
r. parasternal short-axis view
r. pressure
r. sinus tachycardia
r. stroke volume
r. systolic function
r. tachycardia
r. tidal breathing
r. tidal volume
r. value
r. vascular tone

Reston subtype

restoration of spontaneous circulation (ROSC)

RESTORE
Randomized Efficacy Study of Tirofiban for Outcomes and Restenosis

restored cycle

Restoril

rest-redistribution thallium-201 imaging

restriction
r. endonuclease
r. fragment length polymorphism (RFLP)

NOTES

597

restriction *(continued)*
    progressive parenchymal r.
    pulmonary r.
restrictive
    r. airways defect
    r. airways disease
    r. cardiomyopathy
    r. functional impairment
    r. heart disease
    r. lung disease
    r. physiology mitral flow pattern
    r. ventilatory defect
    r. ventilatory dysfunction
restrictus
    Aspergillus r.
result
    true-negative test r.
    true-positive test r.
resuscitate
    do not r. (DNR)
resuscitation
    albumin r.
    cardiac r.
    cardiopulmonary r. (CPR)
    r. cart
    closed-chest cardiopulmonary r.
    crystalloid r.
    heart-lung r.
    LifeStick cardiopulmonary r.
    mechanical cardiopulmonary r.
    mouth-to-mouth r.
    open chest cardiac r.
    volume r.
resuscitator
    ACD r.
    active compression-decompression r.
    AmbuSPUR disposable r.
    BagEasy disposable manual r.
    First Response manual r.
    High Oxygen PRM r.
    Hope r.
    Hudson Lifesaver r.
    infant Ambu r.
    Laerdal r.
    Laerdal infant r.
    Laerdal silicon r.
    NeoVO-2-R volume control r.
    Ohio Hope r.
    Penlon infant r.
    pneuPAC r.
    Robertshaw bag r.
    Safe Response manual r.
    SureGrip manual r.
resveratrol
resynchronizer
    HFCWO ventricular r.

high-frequency chest wall
    oscillation ventricular r.
retained lung fluid (RLF)
retard
    expiratory r.
Retavase
retention
    mucus r.
    secretion r.
    sodium r.
    sputum r.
    tracer r.
    water r.
reteplase
    recombinant r.
reteplase-abciximab
rethoracotomy
reticularis
    livedo r.
reticular pattern
reticulation
reticuloendothelial system
reticulonodular
    r. infiltrate
    r. pattern
reticulum
    agranular endoplasmic r. (AER)
    endoplasmic r.
    sarcoplasmic r.
retina, pl. **retinae**
    cyanosis retinae
retinal
    r. artery
    r. vessel
retinohypothalamic pathway
retinoic acid
retinol
    plasma r.
    serum r.
retinopathy
    diabetic r.
    hypertensive r.
    r. of prematurity (ROP)
retour
    rale de r.
retraction
    intercostal r.
    postrheumatic cusp r.
retractor
    abdominal vascular r.
    Ablaza aortic wall r.
    Ablaza-Blanco aortic wall r.
    Adson r.
    Allison lung r.
    Andrews r.
    Bahnson sternal r.
    Benedict r.
    Bookwalter r.

Burford rib r.
Carten mitral valve r.
Carter r.
Cooley r.
Cooley atrial r.
Cooley-Merz sternum r.
Cosgrove r.
Davidson r.
Davidson scapular r.
DeBakey chest r.
Finochietto r.
Finochietto-Geissendorfer rib r.
Frater intracardiac r.
Gelpi r.
Gerbode sternal r.
Gross-Pomeranz-Watkins r.
Haight-Finochietto rib r.
Hartzler rib r.
IMA r.
inferior mesenteric artery r.
Lilienthal-Sauerbruch r.
Lukens thymus r.
lung r.
malleable r.
Meyerding r.
Parsonnet epicardial r.
Pittman IMA r.
rake r.
Rosenkranz pediatric sternal r.
Rosenkranz small child sternal r.
Rosenkranz universal malleable r.
Rosenkranz wire-basket r.
Sellor rib r.
Semb lung r.
Theis rib r.
Zalkind lung r.
Zimberg esophageal hiatal r.

Retract-O-Tape
retraining
computerized diaphragmatic
breathing r. (CDBR)
retransplantation
retrieval
intravascular foreign body r.
retriever
basket r.
retrocardiac space
retroconduction
retrocrural adenopathy
retroesophageal aorta
retrognathia

retrograde
r. aortography
r. arterial capture
r. atrial activation mapping
r. autologous priming
r. beat
r. block
r. catheter insertion
r. catheterization
r. conduction
r. embolism
r. fast pathway
r. femoral approach
r. filling
r. hypertension
r. P wave
r. VA conduction
retrolingual
retropalatal
r. airway
r. obstruction
retropectoral
r. patch
r. pocket
retroperfusion
coronary r.
coronary sinus r.
retroperitoneal hematoma
retropharyngeal
r. abscess
r. lymph node
r. space
retropharyngeales
nodi lymphoidei r.
retropharyngeum
spatium r.
retropharyngitis
retropharynx
Retroscan
retrosternal
r. air space
r. space
r. thyroid
retrotracheal space
Retrovir
R. injection
R. Oral
retroviral vector
retrovirus
Retter needle
return
anomalous pulmonary venous r.

R

NOTES

return *(continued)*
    r. extrasystole
    partial anomalous pulmonary
      venous r. (PAPVR)
    pulmonary venous r.
    rattle of r.
    r. of spontaneous circulation
      (ROSC)
    systemic venous r.
    total anomalous pulmonary
      venous r. (TAPVR)
    venous r.
returning cycle
Retzius veins
reuptake
revascularization
    Biosense-guided laser myocardial r.
    catheter-based r.
    coronary r.
    direct myocardial r. (DMR)
    heart laser r.
    hybrid r.
    ischemia-driven r.
    laser r.
    laser transmyocardial r. (TMR)
    myocardial r.
    myocardial laser r. (MLR)
    percutaneous r.
    percutaneous myocardial r. (PMR)
    percutaneous myocardial laser r.
    percutaneous transluminal
      coronary r. (PTCR)
    percutaneous transluminal
      myocardial r. (PTMR)
    percutaneous transmyocardial r.
      (PTMR)
    percutaneous transmyocardial
      laser r. (PMR)
    radiofrequency percutaneous
      myocardial r. (RF-PMR)
    repeat r.
    surgical r.
    r. system
    target lesion r. (TLR)
    target vessel r. (TVR)
    transmyocardial r. (TMR)
    transmyocardial laser r. (TMLR)
Revase
Reveal
    R. insertable loop recorder
    R. Plus insertable loop recorder
Revelation
    R. endocardial microcatheter
    R. microcatheter for EP mapping
    R. Tx microcatheter for RF
      ablation

reverberation
    r. artifact
    echo r.
reversal
    holodiastolic flow r.
    lead r.
    r. speed of bronchoconstriction in
      response to methacholine (r-Sm)
    systolic r.
reverse
    r. differential cyanosis
    r. polarity
    r. remodeling
    r. saphenous vein
    r. squeeze
    r. transcriptase polymerase chain
      reaction (RT-PCR)
    r. transcriptase polymerase chain
      reaction test
reversed
    r. arm leads
    r. bypass
    r. coarctation
    r. ductus arteriosus
    r. paradoxical pulse
    r. reciprocal rhythm
    r. saphenous vein graft
    r. shunt
    r. three sign
reversibility
    Harvard atherosclerosis r. (HARP)
reversible
    r. airway obstruction
    r. bronchospasm
    r. ischemic neurologic defect
      (RIND)
    r. left ventricular dysfunction
    r. obstructive airways disease
      (ROAD)
reversion
    noise r.
Reversol injection
Revex
reviparin
revision
    International Classification of
      Diseases, Ninth R. (ICD-9)
Revitalizer Soft-Start nasal CPAP
Reye syndrome
Rey Figure Copy test
Reynolds
    R. number
    R. Pathfinder 3 analyzer
Reynold-Southwick H-graft portacaval
  shunt
RF
    radiofrequency
    rheumatic fever

RF Ablatr ablation catheter
RF catheter ablation
RF Marinr catheter
RF wave
RFA
radiofrequency ablation
RFB
R. System-I for CDBR
R. System-I for CDBR retraining
system
RFb
respiratory feedback
RFb system
RFC
radiofrequency current
RFG-35
Radionics RFG-35
RF-generated thermal balloon catheter
RFLP
restriction fragment length polymorphism
RF-PMR
radiofrequency percutaneous myocardial
revascularization
RFS2000
RG-201
RGC
respiratory glycoconjugate
RGEA
right gastroepiploic artery
Rh
rhesus
Rh antibody
Rh factor
Mini-Gamulin Rh
rhabdomyolysis
rhabdomyoma
rhabdomyosarcoma
RHAMM
receptor for hyaluronan-mediated motility
rhamnolipid mucus secretion
rhATIII
RHD
radiant heat device
rheumatic heart disease
right hemisphere damage
rheocardiography
rheologic
r. change
r. therapy
rheology
rheolytic
Rheolytic thrombectomy catheter

Rheomacrodex
rheopheresis
extracorporeal r.
RheothRx
rhesus (Rh)
rheumatic
r. AF
r. aortitis
r. arteritis
r. carditis
r. endocarditis
r. fever (RF)
r. heart disease (RHD)
r. mitral insufficiency
r. mitral valve stenosis
r. myocarditis
r. pericarditis
r. pneumonia
r. valvulitis
rheumatica
angina r.
rheumatism
r. of heart
tuberculous r.
rheumatoid
r. arteritis
r. arthritis (RA)
r. factor
r. lung
r. nodule
r. pleuritis
r. pneumoconiosis
r. pneumonoconiosis
Rheumatrex
rhinitis
allergic r.
irritant r.
r. medicamentosa
nonallergic noninfectious
perennial r. (NANIPER)
noneosinophilic nonallergic r.
(NENAR)
perennial allergic r.
postnasal drip due to r. (PND-Rh)
seasonal allergic r.
vasomotor r.
rhinocerebral infection
rhinoconjunctivitis
Rhinocort Aqua
rhinomanometer
rhinopharyngeal
rhinopharynx

NOTES

R

RHINOS
    fiberoptic rhinoscopy
rhinoscleroma
rhinoscleromatis
    Klebsiella r.
rhinoscopy
    fiberoptic r. (RHINOS)
Rhinosyn
    R.-DMX
    R. Liquid
    R.-PD Liquid
    R.-X Liquid
rhinovirus (RV)
r-hirudin
    recombinant hirudin
Rhizopus oryzae
rhodesiense
    Trypanosoma r.
Rho(D) immune globulin
Rhodnius polixus
Rhodococcus equi
RhoGAM
rhoGDI protein
Rho-kinase
rhonchal fremitus
rhonchi, sing. **rhonchus**
    expiratory r.
    rales and r.
    sibilant r.
    sonorous r.
rhonchorous cough
Rhotral
rhuIL-10
    recombinant human IL-10
rhVEGF
    recombinant human vascular endothelial
    growth factor
rhysodes
    Acanthamoeba r.
rhythm
    accelerated atrioventricular
     junctional r.
    accelerated A-V junctional r.
    accelerated idioventricular r.
     (AIVR)
    accelerated junctional r.
    agonal r.
    atrial r.
    atrial escape r.
    atrioventricular junctional r.
    atrioventricular nodal r., A-V
     nodal r.
    A-V atrioventricular junctional r.
    A-V junctional r.
    baseline r.
    bigeminal r.
    cantering r.
    cardiac r.

    R. catheter
    chaotic r.
    circadian r.
    concealed r.
    coronary nodal r.
    coronary sinus r.
    coupled r.
    r. disturbance
    diurnal r.
    ectopic r.
    embryocardia r.
    escape r.
    fetal heart r.
    fibrillation r.
    gallop r.
    idiojunctional r.
    idionodal r.
    idioventricular r.
    irregular r.
    irregularly irregular r.
    irregularly irregular cardiac r.
    junctional r.
    junctional escape r.
    lower nodal r.
    midnodal r.
    mu r.
    nodal r.
    nodal escape r.
    normal sinus r. (NSR)
    paced r.
    pendulum r.
    pulseless idioventricular r.
    quadrigeminal r.
    quadruple r.
    reciprocal r.
    reciprocating r.
    regularly irregular r.
    regular rate and r. (RRR)
    regular sinus r. (RSR, rSR′)
    reversed reciprocal r.
    sinus r.
    slow escape r.
    r. strip
    systolic gallop r.
    tic-tac r.
    trainwheel r.
    trigeminal r.
    triple r.
    ventricular r.
    wide complex r.
rhythmicity
Rhythmin
Rhythmonorm
rhythmophone
RhythmScan
RI
    Rohrer index

RIA
>radioimmunoassay

rib
>r. approximator
>r. cage
>r. cutter
>r. elevator
>r. fracture
>r. guillotine
>lower r.
>r. margin
>middle r.
>r. notching
>r. raspatory
>r. shears
>r. spreader
>upper r.

ribavirin
Ribbert thrombosis
ribbon
>r. muscle
>safety r.

ribonucleic acid (RNA)
riboprobe
>CMV IE-2 r.
>HIV-1 r.
>IE-2 r.

riboside
>AICA r.

ribosome
Richet aneurysm
Richter transformation
Ricketts-Abrams technique
Rickettsia
>*R. australis*
>*R. prowazekii*

rickettsial
>r. endocarditis
>r. myocarditis
>r. pneumonia

ridge
>eustachian r.
>neointimal r.
>pharyngeal r.
>pulmonary r.

riding
>r. embolism
>r. embolus

RIE
>relative inspiratory effort

Riecker respiration bronchoscope

Riedel
>R. struma
>R. thyroiditis

Riegel pulse
RIF
>rifampin

rifabutin
Rifadin
>R. injection
>R. Oral

rifalazil
Rifamate
rifampicin
rifampin (RIF)
>r. and isoniazid
>r., isoniazid, and pyrazinamide

rifamycin
rifapentine
Rifater
Rift Valley fever virus
RIGHT
>Cerivastatin Gemfibrozil Hyperlipidemia
>Treatment
>RIGHT study

right
>r. ankle index
>r. anterior oblique (RAO)
>r. anterior oblique equivalent
>r. anterior oblique position
>r. anterior oblique projection
>r. aortic arch
>r. atrial appendage (RAA)
>r. atrial enlargement
>r. atrial myxoma
>r. atrial pacing
>r. atrial pressure (RAP)
>r. atrial thrombus
>r. atrium (RA)
>r. auricle of heart
>r. axis deviation (RAD)
>r. brain damage (RBD)
>r. bundle-branch block (RBBB)
>r. cerebrovascular accident (RCVA)
>r. common carotid artery (RCCA)
>r. coronary artery (RCA)
>r. coronary catheter
>r. crus of diaphragm
>r. gastroepiploic artery (RGEA)
>r. heart
>r. heart bypass
>r. heart catheter
>r. heart catheterization

R

NOTES

right *(continued)*
   r. heart failure
   r. hemisphere damage (RHD)
   r. hemisphere stroke
   r. inferior pulmonary vein
   r. internal mammary artery (RIMA)
   r. internal mammary artery graft
   r. internal thoracic artery (RITA)
   r. internal thoracic artery graft
   r. Judkins catheter
   r. lower lobe (RLL)
   r. main bronchus
   r. margin of heart
   r. middle lobe (RML)
   r. parasternal impulse
   r. pulmonary artery (RPA)
   r. recurrent laryngeal nerve
   r. single lung transplant (RSLTx)
   r. superior pulmonary vein
   r. triangular ligament of liver
   r. upper lobe (RUL)
   r. ventricle (RV)
   r. ventricular apex (RVA)
   r. ventricular assist device (RVAD)
   r. ventricular cardiomyopathy
   r. ventricular copulsation balloon (RVCB)
   r. ventricular diastolic collapse
   r. ventricular diastolic pressure
   r. ventricular dimension (RVD)
   r. ventricular dysplasia
   r. ventricular ejection fraction (RVEF)
   r. ventricular end-diastolic pressure (RVEDP)
   r. ventricular end-diastolic volume index (RVEDVI)
   r. ventricular end-systolic volume index (RVESVI)
   r. ventricular enlargement (RVE)
   r. ventricular failure
   r. ventricular function
   r. ventricular heave
   r. ventricular hypertrophy (RVH)
   r. ventricular hypoplasia
   r. ventricular infarction
   r. ventricular inflow obstruction
   r. ventricular myxoma
   r. ventricular outflow obstruction
   r. ventricular outflow tract (RVOT)
   r. ventricular outflow tract pacing
   r. ventricular outflow tract reconstruction
   r. ventricular outflow tract tachycardia
   r. ventricular peak systolic pressure
   r. ventricular refractory period (RVERP)
   r. ventricular septal pacing
   r. ventricular systolic pressure (RVSP)
   r. ventricular systolic time interval
   r. ventricular wall motion

right-angle chest tube
right-middle cerebral artery (R-MCA)
right-sided heart failure
right-to-left shunt (RLS)
right-ventricle afterload
rightward axis
rigid
   r. bronchoscopy
   r. monopolar loop
   r. pod
   r. thoracoscope
rigidity
   nuchal r.
Rigiflex TTS balloon catheter
rigor
   calcium r.
RIII reflex
RIK fluid-filled head pack
Riley-Cournand equation
Riley-Day syndrome
Riley needle
rilmenidine
riluzole
RIMA
   right internal mammary artery
   RIMA graft
rima
   r. respiratoria
   r. vestibuli
   r. vocalis
Rimactane Oral
rimantadine hydrochloride
riminofenazine
rimiterol
RIND
   reversible ischemic neurologic defect
Rindfleisch fold
ring
   r. abscess
   AnnuloFlex flexible annuloplasty r.
   AnnuloFlo annuloplasty r.
   annuloplasty r.
   aortic r.
   atrial r.
   atrioventricular r.
   atrioventricular valve r.
   Bickel r.
   cardiac lymphatic r.
   Carpentier r.
   Carpentier-Edwards Physio annuloplasty r.
   circumaortic venous r.
   coronary r.

R

Crawford suture r.
double-flanged valve sewing r.
Duran annuloplasty r.
r. electrode
esophageal contraction r.
fibrous r.
knitted sewing r.
left ventricular cavity obstruction r.
Lower r.'s
metal sewing r.
pharyngeal lymphatic r.
plastic sewing r.
pleural r.'s
prosthetic valve sewing r.
Puig Massana annuloplasty r.
Puig Massana-Shiley annuloplasty r.
Schatzki r.
Schatzki esophageal r.
Sculptor annuloplasty r.
Seguin annuloplasty r.
sewing r.
r. shadow
r. sign
SJM Biflex annuloplasty r.
SJM Seguin annuloplasty r.
SJM Tailor annuloplasty r.
St. Jude annuloplasty r.
supraannular suture r.
tonsillar r.
tracheal r.
vascular r.
Waldeyer throat r.
Waldeyer tonsillar r.
Ringer
    R. lactate
    R. solution
RinoFlow ENT wash unit
Riolan
    anastomosis of R.
RIP
    respiratory inductance plethysmograph
    respiratory inductance plethysmography
    RIP portable sleep monitor
RISA
    radioactive iodinated serum albumin
RISC
    Research on Instability in Coronary
    Artery Disease
    RISC study
risetime
risk
    r. calculator

competing r.'s
r. factor
r. factor profile
r. index
modified multifactorial index of
    cardiac r.
recurrence r.
relative r. (RR, R-R)
restenosis r.
stochastic r.
r. stratification
surgical r.
RITA
    Randomized Intervention Treatment of
    Angina
    right internal thoracic artery
    RITA clinical trial
    RITA graft
Ritalin
Ritalin-SR
Ritchie
    R. Articular Index
    R. catheter
ritodrine
ritonavir
Riva-Rocci sphygmomanometer
Rivas vascular catheter
Rivermead
    R. Behavioral Memory Test
    R. Motor Assessment Arm score
Rivero-Carvallo
    R.-C. effect
    R.-C. sign
Rivetti-Levinson intraluminal stent
Riviere sign
Rivinus
    R. canals
    R. gland
Rizaben
RJA
    regurgitant jet area
R-lactate enzyme monotest
RLF
    retained lung fluid
RLH
    recurrent lobar hemorrhage
RLL
    right lower lobe
RLP
    remnant-like lipoprotein particle
    remnant lipoprotein
    RLP lipoprotein

NOTES

RLS
   right-to-left shunt
RLT
   red light therapy
RM-300
    Respiromonitor R.
RMBF
   regional myocardial blood flow
R-MCA
   right-middle cerebral artery
RMI
    R. antegrade cardioplegia catheter
    R. AViD dual stage venous cannula
    R. dispersion aortic perfusion cannula
    R. Retractaguard retrograde cannula
    R. Thin-Flex 24 Fr. venous cannula
    R. Trim-Flex low profile dual drainage venous cannula
RML
    right middle lobe
RMR
    resting metabolic rate
rMRGlu
    glucose metabolism
RNA
    ribonucleic acid
    RNA glycosidase toxin
RNeasy MINI kit
RNV
    radionuclide ventriculography
Ro-13-6438
Ro 4483
ROA
    regurgitant orifice area
ROAD
    reversible obstructive airways disease
Roadmapper
    FluoroPlus R.
roadmapping
    coronary r.
Roadrunner PC guidewire
Robafen
    R. AC
    R. CF
    R. DM
Robertshaw
    R. bag resuscitator
    R. tube
Robertson sign
Robicillin VK Oral
Robicsek vascular probe
Robinson index
Robinul Forte
Robitet Oral

Robitussin
    R. A-C
    R.-CF
    R. Cough Calmers
    R.-DAC
    R.-DM
    R. Pediatric
    R. Severe Congestion Liqui-Gels
Robodoc robot
Rocephin IM
Rochalimaea
Rocha-Lima inclusion
Roche AMPLICOR assay for *Mycobacterium tuberculosis*
Roche-Microwell plate hybridization method
Rochester-Kocher clamp
Rochester needle
Rochester-Péan clamp
rocker
    hematology r.
rocket immunoelectrophoretic method of Laurell
Rockey
    R. mediastinal cannula
    R. ventricular cannula
Rocky Mountain spotted fever
rocuronium
rodhaini
    Babesia r.
Rodrigo equation
Rodriguez
    R.-Alvarez catheter
    R. aneurysm
    R. catheter
Roe aortic tourniquet clamp
roentgen (R)
    r. knife
roentgenogram
    apical lordotic r.
    chest r.
roentgenographically occult lung cancer (ROLC)
roentgenographic presentation
roentgenography
Roesler-Bressler infarction
RoEzIt skin moisturizer
Rofact
Roferon-A
Rogaine topical
Roger
    R. bruit
    bruit de R.
    R. disease
    maladie de R.
    R. murmur
Rogers sphygmomanometer
Rogitine

Roho mattress
Rohrer
    R. equation
    R. index (RI)
ROI
    region of interest
Rokitansky disease
ROLC
    roentgenographically occult lung cancer
role
    cardioprotective r.
roller pump
Rolleston rule
rolling hernia
Romaña sign
Romano-Ward syndrome
Romhilt-Estes
    R.-E. point score criteria
    R.-E. point scoring system
    R.-E. score
ROMI
    rule out myocardial infarction
romied
    ruled out for myocardial infarction
Ronase
Rondamine-DM drops
Rondec
    R.-DM
    R. Drops
    R. Filmtab
    R. Syrup
rongeur
    aortic valve r.
    Bailey aortic valve r.
R-on-T
    R-o.-T arrhythmia susceptibility
    R-o.-T phenomenon
    R-o.-T premature ventricular
      complex
R-on-T-initiated
    R-o.-T-i. nonsustained VT
    R-o.-T-i. VF
    R-o.-T-i. VT
roof of left atrium
Roos test
root
    aortic r.
    free r.
    r. inclusion method
    r. injection
    r. of lung
    r. needle

    r. perfusion
    r. tailoring
root-mean-square voltage
ROP
    retinopathy of prematurity
ROPE
    respiratory ordered phase encoding
Rosai-Dorfman disease
Rosalki technique
ROSC
    restoration of spontaneous circulation
    return of spontaneous circulation
Rose
    R. Questionnaire
    R. tamponade
rose
    r. hips asthma
    r. spot
Rosenbach syndrome
Rosenberg syndrome
Rosenblum rotating adapter
Rosenkranz
    R. deep retractor blade
    R. pediatric retractor system
    R. pediatric sternal retractor
    R. small child sternal retractor
    R. small retractor blade
    R. universal clamp
    R. universal malleable retractor
    R. wire-basket retractor
Rosenmüller recess
rosette
    acinar r.
rosiglitazone
Ross
    R. aortic valve replacement
      procedure
    R. needle
    R. procedure
    R. pulmonary porcine valve
    R. River virus
Rossetti modification of Nissen fundoplication
Rossmax automatic wristwatch blood pressure monitor
Rostan asthma
ROSTER
    Rotational Atherectomy versus Balloon
    Angioplasty for Diffuse In-Stent
    Restenosis
    ROSTER clinical trial
rostral ventrolateral medulla (RVLM)

NOTES

rosuvastatin
Rota
Rotablator
    R. atherectomy device
    R. catheter
    Heart Technology R.
    R. RotaLink Plus rotational
      atherectomy device
    R. RotaLink rotational atherectomy
      device
    R. wire
Rotacamera
Rotacaps
    Ventolin R.
Rotacs
    R. device
    R. guidewire
    R. system
Rotadisk
    Flovent R.
Rotafloppy wire
rotaflush solution
Rotahaler
rotary
    r. atherectomy device
    r. vertigo
rotating disk oxygenation
rotation
    cardiac r.
    clockwise r.
    counterclockwise r.
    shoulder r.
rotational
    r. ablation
    r. ablation laser
    r. angioplasty catheter system
    r. atherectomy (RA)
    r. atherectomy device
    r. atherectomy system (RAS)
    R. Atherectomy versus Balloon
      Angioplasty for Diffuse In-Stent
      Restenosis (ROSTER)
    r. coronary atherectomy (RCA)
    r. dynamic angioplasty catheter
Rotch sign
Rotex
    R. II biopsy needle
    R. needle
Rothia dentocariosa
Rothschild sign
Roth spot
Rotoslide
rotundum
    foramen r.
Roubac
Roubin-Gianturco flexible coil stent
Rougnon-Heberden disease
rouleaux formation

round
    r. foramen
    r. heart
    r. hematoma
    r. pneumonia nodule
rounded atelectasis
round-robin classification
roundworm
Rous sarcoma virus (RSV)
Roussy-Lévy
    R.-L. disease
    R.-L. polyneuropathy
    R.-L. syndrome
route of insertion
Roux-en-Y obesity
Rovamycine
rove magnetic catheter
roxithromycin
roxiviban
Royal
    R. Flush angiographic flush
      catheter
    R. Flush catheter
royal jelly-induced asthma
Rozanski lead placement system
RPA
    right pulmonary artery
RPBD
    rating of perceived breathing difficulty
RPE
    rating of perceived exertion
r-PEG
    recombinant polyethylene glycol
RPF
    renal plasma flow
R-P interval
RPM
    real-time position management
    real-time position management-tracking
      system/catheter
    RPM tracking system
    RPM tracking system/catheter
R-Port implantable vascular access
  system
RQ
    respiratory quotient
R/Q wave ratio
RR, R-R
    relative risk
    respiratory rate
    RR cycle
    RR interval
    RR interval dynamics
    RR interval stability
    RR prime
RRI
    recurrent respiratory infection
R-R′ interval

R

RRP
  relative refractory period
RRR
  regular rate and rhythm
  relative risk reduction
Rrs
  respiratory resistance
RS
  RS complex
  RS deflection
RSBI
  Rapid Shallow Breathing Index
RSI
  rapid sequence induction
  RSI orotracheal intubation
RSLTx
  right single lung transplant
r-Sm
  reversal speed of bronchoconstriction in
    response to methacholine
rSO$_2$
  regional oxygen saturation
RSR, rSR′
  regular sinus rhythm
  RSR prime (rSR′)
RS-T
  RS-T interval
  RS-T segment
R-Stent stent
RSV
  respiratory syncytial virus
  Rous sarcoma virus
RSVA
  ruptured sinus of Valsalva aneurysm
RSV-IG
  respiratory syncytial virus
    immunoglobulin
RT
  resistance training
RT3D echo
R-Test Evolution
Rti
  resistance to movement of lung tissue
RTLF
  respiratory tract lining fluid
RTOG
Rtot
  total airway resistance
rtPA
  recombinant tissue plasminogen activator
    catabolism of rtPA
    double-chain rtPA

RT-PCR
  reverse transcriptase polymerase chain
    reaction
RTV total artificial heart
rub
  friction r.
  pericardial r.
  pericardial friction r.
  pleural friction r.
  pleuritic r.
  pleuropericardial r.
  saddle leather friction r.
rubella syndrome
rubeola
Rubex
rubidium (Rb)
  r.-81
  r.-82
  r.-82 imaging
  r.-82 positron emission tomography
    (Rb-82 PET)
Rubinol
Rubinstein-Taybi syndrome
rubitecan
rubor
  dependent r.
Rubulavirus
ruby laser
rude respiration
rudimentary chamber
Rudolph Full Face mask
RUDS
  reactive upper airways dysfunction
    syndrome
Ruel
  R. aorta clamp
  R. forceps
Rugelski arterial forceps
RUGS-III
Ruiz-Cohen round expander
r-UK
  recombinant urokinase
RUL
  right upper lobe
rule
  r. of bigeminy
  Gibson r.
  Liebermeister r.
  r. out myocardial infarction
    (ROMI)

NOTES

rule *(continued)*
    Rolleston r.
    shorthand r.
**ruled out for myocardial infarction
(romied)**
rumble
    Austin Flint r.
    booming r.
    diastolic r.
    filling r.
    middiastolic r.
    protodiastolic r.
    third sound r.
rumbling diastolic murmur
Rumel
    R. clamp
    R. thoracic forceps
    R. tourniquet
Rumpel-Leede test
run
    second pump r.
runoff
    aortofemoral arterial r.
    aortogram with distal r.
    arterial r.
    r. arteriogram
    digital r.
    distal r.
    venous r.
rupture
    aortic r.
    balloon r.
    blunt cardiac r.
    cardiac r.
    chamber r.
    chordae tendineae r.
    chordal r.
    coronary plaque r.
    diaphragmatic r.
    esophageal r.
    IEM r.
    internal elastic membrane r.
    interventricular septal r.
    intraperitoneal r.
    intrapleural r.
    membrane r.
    multicanalicular r.
    myocardial r.
    nonpenetrating r.
    papillary muscle r. (PMR)
    penetrating r.
    perivascular r.
    pinhole balloon r.
    plaque r.
    pulmonary artery r.
    traumatic r.
    r. trigger

    valve r.
    ventricular septal r.
ruptured
    r. aortic aneurysm
    r. sinus of Valsalva
    r. sinus of Valsalva aneurysm
      (RSVA)
**Ruschelit polyvinyl chloride
endotracheal tube**
Russian influenza
rusty sputum
Ru-Tuss
    R.-T. DE
    R.-T. Expectorant
RV
    residual volume
    rhinovirus
    right ventricle
RVA
    right ventricular apex
RVAD
    right ventricular assist device
RVCB
    right ventricular copulsation balloon
RVD
    reference vessel diameter
    right ventricular dimension
RVE
    right ventricular enlargement
RVEDP
    right ventricular end-diastolic pressure
RVEDVI
    right ventricular end-diastolic volume
    index
RVEF
    right ventricular ejection fraction
RVERP
    right ventricular refractory period
RVESVI
    right ventricular end-systolic volume
    index
RVH
    right ventricular hypertrophy
RVLM
    rostral ventrolateral medulla
RVol
    regurgitant volume
RVOT
    right ventricular outflow tract
      RVOT pacing
RVSP
    right ventricular systolic pressure
RV/TLC
    residual volume/total lung capacity
      RV/TLC ratio
RWT
    relative wall thickness

RX

RX Multi-Link coronary stent system
RX Multi-Link HP system
RX Multi-Link system.
RX stent delivery system

Rx

Rx perfusion catheter
Rx Streak balloon catheter

Rx5000 cardiac pacing system
ryanodine receptor
Rychener-Weve electrode

Rymed
Ryna

R.-C Liquid
R.-CX
R. Liquid

Rynacrom
Rynatan
Rynatuss Pediatric Suspension
Rytand murmur
Rythmodan
Rythmodan-LA
Rythmol

R

NOTES

S
> septum
>> S sign of Golden
>> S stylet
>> S wave

S₁
> first heart sound

S₂
> second heart sound

S2 allele

S₃
> third heart sound
>> S₃ gallop

S₄
> fourth heart sound
>> S₄ gallop

S₇
> summation gallop

S660 small vessel stent
S670 coronary stent
>> S₇ gallop

SA
> salvage angioplasty
> sinoatrial
>> Peritrate SA

S-A
> sinoatrial
>> S-A nodal reentrant tachycardia
>> S-A node

SAA
> serum amyloid type A

Sabin-Feldman dye test
Sable
>> S. balloon catheter
>> S. PTCA balloon catheter

sabot
>> coeur en s.
>> s. heart

Sabulin
SAC
> serial autocorrelation
>> SAC data acquisition technology

sac
>> air s.
>> alveolar s.
>> aneurysmal s.
>> aortic s. (AS)
>> endolymphatic s.
>> Hilton s.
>> Lap S.
>> lateral s.
>> pericardial s.
>> pleural s.
>> truncoaortic s.

saccharii
>> *Thermoactinomyces s.*

Saccharomonospora
Saccharomyces anginae
Saccharopolyspora rectivirgula
Saccomanno
>> S. fixative
>> S. morphologic criteria

saccular
>> s. aneurysm
>> s. bronchiectasis
>> s. period

sacculated
>> s. empyema
>> s. pleurisy

sacculation
> localized s.

saccule
>> s. of larynx

sacculus
>> s. endolymphaticus
>> s. laryngis
>> s. proprius
>> s. vestibuli

saccus endolymphaticus
sacral edema
sacrococcygeal aorta
SACT
> sinoatrial conduction time

saddle
>> s. embolism
>> s. embolus
>> s. leather friction rub
>> s. thrombus

Sade modification of Norwood procedure
Sadowsky hook wire
SAECG
> signal-averaged electrocardiogram
> signal-averaged electrocardiography

Safar bronchoscope
Safar-S airway
Safe
>> S. Response manual resuscitator
>> S. Step blood-collection needle
>> S. Tussin 30

Safe-T-Coat heparin-coated thermodilution catheter
Safe-T-Tube
>> Montgomery S.-T.-T.

SafeTway
>> S. mouthpiece
>> S. pediatric mouthpiece

safety
>> s. guidewire

S

safety *(continued)*
    occupational health and s. (OHS)
    radiation s.
    s. ribbon
SafTouch catheter
sag
    ST s.
sagittal
    s. cut
    s. plane
    s. view
SAH
    subarachnoid hemorrhage
SAHS
    sleep apnea/hypopnea syndrome
Saiko
sail sound
Sala cell
salbutamol
Saleto-200
Salflex
Salgesic
salicylate
    carbazochrome s.
    choline s.
    magnesium s.
    phenyl s.
    sodium s.
saline
    Broncho S.
    half-normal s.
    heparinized s.
    hypertonic s.
    iced s.
    s. jet
    s. loading
    normal s.
    phosphate-buffered s. (PBS)
    s. slush
salivagram
salivaris
    caruncula s.
salivarius
    Streptococcus s.
Salkowski test
salmeterol
    s. and fluticasone propionate
    s. xinafoate
Salmonella choleraesuis
salmon skin
salol
salsalate
Salsitab
salt
    s.-depletion syndrome
    dietary s.
    ethylenediaminetetraacetic acid
      disodium s.

    gold s.
    s. of nickel
    s. and pepper pattern
    persulfate s.
    s. of platinum
    s. wasting
salt-and-pepper appearance
salt-and-water dependent hypertension
saltans
    thrombophlebitis s.
salt-free diet
salting-out procedure
Salubria
saluresis
saluretic agent
Saluron
salute
    allergic s.
Salutensin
    S.-Demi
saluting
salvage
    s. angioplasty (SA)
    s. balloon angioplasty
    intraoperative cell s.
    limb s.
    myocardial s.
Salvatore-Maloney tracheotome
salves
    tachycardia en s.
salvo
    s. of beats
    s. of ventricular tachycardia
SAM
    surface adherent monocyte
    systolic anterior motion
    SAM system
Sam
    S. Levine sign
    S. Roberts bronchial biopsy forceps
sample
    end-tidal s.
    Haldane-Priestley s.
    Rahn-Otis s.
sampling
    bioptic s.
    blood s.
    chorionic villus s.
Samuels
    S. forceps
    S. hemoclip
SAN
    sinuatrial node
San
    S. Joaquin fever
    S. Joaquin Valley disease
    S. Joaquin Valley fever
Sanborn metabolator

Sanchez-Cascos cardioauditory syndrome
Sanders
    S. bed
    S. intubation laryngoscope
    S. jet ventilation device respirator
Sandhoff disease
Sandifer syndrome
Sandler-Dodge area-length method
Sandman system
Sandoglobulin
Sandostatin
    S. LAR
Sandoz suction/feeding tube
Sandrock test
sandwich
    s. enzyme-linked immunosorbent
      assay
    s. patch
Sanfilippo syndrome
sanguinis
    ictus s.
Sansert
Sansom sign
SaO$_2$
    arterial oxygen saturation
SAP
    stable angina pectoris
    systemic arterial pressure
SAPD
    signal-averaged P-wave duration
saphenofemoral
    s. junction
    s. system
saphenous
    s. vein
    s. vein bypass graft angiography
    s. vein cannula
    s. vein graft (SVG)
    s. vein graft de novo (SAVED)
    s. vein patch closure
    s. vein varicosity
SAPH Finder surgical balloon dissector
SAPHtrak balloon dissector
SAPS
    Simplified Acute Physiology Score
SAQLI
    Sleep Apnea Quality of Life Index
    Calgary SAQLI
saquinavir mesylate
saralasin
sarcoglycan

sarcoid
    Boeck s.
    s. granuloma
sarcoidosis
    bronchial s.
    fibrocystic s.
    nodular s.
    parenchymal s.
    pulmonary s.
sarcolemma
    s. lipid
sarcolemmal
    s. bleb
    s. calcium channel
    s. glucose
    s. level
    s. membrane
sarcoma
    cardiac s.
    Kaposi s. (KS)
    metastatic s.
    pseudo-Kaposi s.
    soft tissue s.
sarcomatoid mesothelioma
sarcomatous tumor
sarcomere
Sarcophaga
sarcoplasmic
    s. reticulum
    s. reticulum-associated glycolytic
      enzymes
sarcosporidiosis
sarcotubular system
Sarnoff aortic clamp
Sarns
    S. aortic arch cannula
    S. electric saw
    S. intracardiac suction tube
    S. membrane oxygenator (SMO)
    S. soft-flow aortic cannula
    S. two-stage cannula
    S. ventricular assist device
    S. wire-reinforced catheter
Sarot bronchus clamp
Sarstedt system
SART
    sinoatrial recovery time
saruplase
    Liquaemin in Myocardial Infarction
      during Thrombolysis with S.
      (LIMITS)

S

NOTES

saruplase *(continued)*
S. and Taprostene Acute
Reocclusion Trial (START)
SAS
subarachnoid space
SAT
subacute thrombosis
Press-mate SAT
satellite lesion
Satinsky clamp
sativa
Vicia s.
Satlite pulse oximeter with earclip
Satterthwaite method
saturated
s. fatty acid (SFA)
s. solution of potassium iodide
(SSKI)
saturation
arterial s.
arterial oxygen s. (SaO_2)
s. index
mixed venous oxygen s. (SvO_2)
oxygen s. (So_2)
oxyhemoglobin s.
regional oxygen s. (rSO_2)
step-up in oxygen s.
s. time
venous s.
saucerize
Sauerbruch-Herrmannsdorfer-Gerson diet
Sauerbruch rib guillotine
sausaging of vein
Sauvage filamentous prosthesis
Savary-Gilliard esophageal dilator
SAVE
Survival and Ventricular Enlargement
SAVE clinical trial
SAVED
saphenous vein graft de novo
SAVED clinical trial
Saventrine Intravenous
Saver
Cell S.
Haemonetics Cell S.
SAVVI pacemaker
saw
oscillating s.
Sarns electric s.
sternum s.
Stryker s.
sawtooth
s. pattern
s. P wave
s. wave
Sawyer operation
SAX
short axis

S-100B
protein S.
SBE
subacute bacterial endocarditis
SBE prophylaxis
SBF
systemic blood flow
SBI
silent brain infarction
SBP
systolic blood pressure
SBS
sick building syndrome
SBSE
supine bicycle stress echocardiography
SBSP
simultaneous bilateral spontaneous
pneumothorax
SBT
serum bactericidal titer
SC
Apo-Dipyridamole S.
SC-210 sidestream capnograph
SC-300 portable capnograph
SCA
superior cerebellar artery
scabbard trachea
SCAD, sCAD
spontaneous coronary artery dissection
SCA-EX
S.-E. catheter
S.-E. 7F graft
S.-E. ShortCutter catheter
S.-E. ShortCutter catheter with
rotating blades
scaffolding
scalar
s. electrocardiogram
s. lead
scale
Abbreviated Injury S. (AIS)
activity s.
ADL s.
Ashworth S.
Behavioral Dyscontrol S. (BDCS)
Berg Balance S.
Borg S.
Borg 6 to 20 s.
Borg numerical s.
Borg treadmill exertion s.
cardiac adjustment s.
Centers for Epidemiologic Studies
Depression s. (CES-D)
Chamorro multiple-assessment s.
Cook-Medley hostility s.
Cook multiple-assessment s.
dyspnea s.
Epworth sleepiness s. (ESS)

European Stroke S. (ESS)
Fagerstrom tolerance s.
French s.
Gaffky s.
Geriatric Depression S.
Glasgow Coma S. (GCS)
gray s.
Grossman s.
Health Locus of Control S.
Holmes-Rahe s.
Hospital Anxiety and Depression s.
(HADS)
Karnofsky rating s.
Lawton Instrumental Activities of
Daily Living s.
Likert s. (LS)
Likert 5-point s.
mechanical visual analogue s.
Montgomery-Asberg Depression
Rating S. (MADRS)
Motor Assessment S. (MAS)
National Institutes of Health
Stroke S. (NIHSS)
Nottingham Extended Activities of
Daily Living s.
Observer's Assessment of
Alertness/Sedation S.
Oxford Handicap S.
Paykel s.
Philadelphia Geriatric Center
Morale S. (PGCMS)
58-point Scandinavian Stroke S.
(SSS-58)
Psychosocial Adjustment to
Illness S.
Rankin Disability S.
Sickness Impact Profile s.
SIP s.
Speilberger Anger Expression s.
Stroke Impact S. (SIS)
Tennant distress s.
Toronto Alexithymia S.
visual analog s. (VAS)
voxel gray s.
Wigle s.

scalene
s. fat pad biopsy
s. lymph node biopsy
scalenectomy
scalenotomy
Adson-Coffey s.

scalenus
s. anterior syndrome
s. anticus syndrome
scalloped
s. commissure
s. subcoronary position
scalloping
scalp
s. electrode
s. pH
s. vein needle
scan
apical hypoperfusion on thallium s.
Cardiolite s.
CardioTec s.
carotid duplex s.
cine s.
computed tomographic s.
s. converter
coronary artery s. (CAS)
CT s.
dipyridamole thallium-201 s.
duplex s.
duplex Doppler s.
dynamic CT s.
four-hour s.
gallium s.
gallium-67 s.
gated cardiac s.
HRCT s.
lung s.
milk s.
MUGA s.
MUGA cardiac blood pool s.
multiple gated acquisition s.
multiple gated acquisition cardiac
blood pool s.
perfusion s.
PET s.
postdiuresis s.
postexercise s.
PYP s.
pyrophosphate s.
rectilinear s.
scintillation s.
scout s.
sector s.
septal hyperperfusion on thallium s.
sestamibi s.
spiral CT s.
TCT s.
tebo s.

S

NOTES

scan *(continued)*
    teboroxime s.
    technetium-99m hexamibi s.
    thin-slice CT s.
    ultrafast computed tomography s.
    ultrafast CT s.
    ventilation/perfusion s.
    ventilation/perfusion lung s.
    $\dot{V}/\dot{Q}$ lung s.

Scandinavian
    58-point S. Stroke Scale (SSS-58)

Scanlan vessel dilator

scanner
    Biosound wide-angle monoplane ultrasound s.
    CardioData MK-3 Holter s.
    computed tomography s.
    Corometrics Doppler s.
    Del Mar Avionics S.
    Diasonics Cardiovue SectOR s.
    DWL Multidop X 4-channel TCD s.
    electrical sector s.
    Evolution s.
    GE 9800 CT s.
    GE Lightspeed CT s.
    GE Signa Horizon SR 120 whole-body s.
    Hewlett-Packard s.
    Hewlett-Packard 77020 A phased-array sector s.
    Imatron C-150 s.
    Imatron C-100 tomographic s.
    Imatron Ultrafast CT s.
    Konica KFDR-S laser film s.
    phased array sector s.
    Philips Medical Systems Tomoscan AVE1 CT spiral s.
    Philips Medical Systems Tomoscan SR 7000 CT spiral s.
    Philips Somoscan 310 CT s.
    Picker CS s.
    Picker Edge 1.5-T s.
    Picker PQ 2000 CT s.
    Picker Vista HPQ MRI s.
    Shimadzu Headtome SET-080 ring type SPECT s.
    Siemens Somatom DR CT s.
    Siemens Somatom Plus 4A s.
    SonoHeart s.
    SONOS 1500 s.
    SONOS 2500 s.
    SSH 260A s.
    Toshiba s.
    ultrafast computed tomographic s.
    ultrafast CT s.

scanning
    duplex s.

    electronic s.
    s. electron microscope (SEM)
    fluorodopamine positron emission tomographic s.
    s. format
    gated blood-pool s.
    helical CT s.
    interlaced s.
    lung s.
    MUGA s.
    PET s.
    progressive s.
    radionuclide s.
    thallium s.
    venous duplex s. (VDS)

Scanning-Beam Digital x-ray

scar
    s. cancer
    s. carcinoma
    s. emphysema
    fibrotic s.
    infarct s.
    myocardial fibrous s.
    zipper s.

scarlatinosa
    angina s.

scarlet fever

Scarpa
    S. fascia
    S. method

scarring
    apical s.
    pleural s.

scatter
    Compton s.

scattered echo

scattergram

scattering
    Rayleigh s.

scatterplot smoothing technique

scavenger
    s. cell pathway
    free-radical s.
    lysophosphatidylcholine s.
    oxygen radical s.

scavenging tube

SCD
    sudden cardiac death

SCD-HeFT
    Sudden Cardiac Death in Heart Failure Trial

SCF
    stem cell factor

Schafer method of artificial respiration

Schapiro sign

Schapiro-Wilks test

Schatzki
  S. esophageal ring
  S. ring
Schatz-Palmaz
  S.-P. intravascular stent
  S.-P. tubular mesh stent
Schaumann
  S. disease
  S. syndrome
Schede thoracoplasty
Scheie syndrome
Scheinmann laryngeal forceps
Schellong-Strisower phenomenon
Schellong test
schenckii
  Sporothrix s.
Schenk-Eichelter vena cava plastic filter procedure
Schepelmann sign
Schering AG Levovist echocontrast agent
Schick sign
Schiff test
Schiller method
Schindler esophagoscope
Schistosoma
  S. haematobium
  S. japonicum
  S. mansoni
schistosomiasis
schistothorax
Schlesinger solution
Schlichter test
Schmidt-Lanterman cleft
Schmidt syndrome
Schmitt-Erlanger model of reentry
Schmitz-Rode catheter
Schmorl furrow
Schneider
  S. catheter
  S. index
  S. Speedy stent
  S. stent
  S. Wallstent
schneiderian respiratory membrane
Schneider-Meier-Magnum system
Schneider-Shiley balloon
Scholten
  S. biopsy forceps
  S. endomyocardial bioptome
  S. endomyocardial bioptome and biopsy forceps

Schonander
  S. film changer
  S. procedure
  S. technique
Schoonmaker
  S. catheter
  S.-King single catheter technique
  S. multipurpose catheter
Schott treatment
Schuco nebulizer
Schueler Model 200 Aspirator
Schüller method
Schultz angina
Schultze test
Schumacher aorta clamp
schwannoma
Schwarten
  S. LP balloon catheter
  S. LP guidewire
SCI
  silent cerebral infarct
  silent cerebral infarction
scie
  bruit de s.
Scimed
  S. angioplasty catheter
  S. extracorporeal silicone rubber reservoir
  S. rTRA-GC guiding catheter
  S. stent
scimitar
  s. sign
  s. syndrome
scintigram
  pyrophosphate s.
scintigraphic perfusion defect
scintigraphy
  AMA-Fab s.
  antimyosin infarct-avid s.
  diethylenetriamine pentaacetate aerosol inhalation lung s.
  dipyridamole thallium-201 s.
  dobutamine perfusion s.
  DTPA aerosol inhalation lung s.
  exercise thallium s.
  exercise thallium-201 s.
  gallium-67 s.
  gastroesophageal s.
  gated blood-pool s.
  indium-111 s.
  infarct-avid hot-spot s.
  infarct-avid myocardial s.

S

NOTES

scintigraphy *(continued)*
    iodine-131 MIBG s.
    labeled FFA s.
    MAA perfusion lung s.
    macroaggregated albumin s.
    macroaggregated albumin perfusion lung s.
    microsphere perfusion s.
    milk s.
    myocardial s.
    myocardial cold-spot perfusion s.
    myocardial perfusion s.
    myocardial viability s.
    NEFA s.
    perfusion s.
    planar myocardial s.
    planar thallium s.
    pulmonary s.
    pyrophosphate s.
    single-photon gamma s.
    SPECT s.
    stress perfusion s.
    stress thallium s.
    Tc-99 sestamibi s.
    thallium-201 perfusion s.
    thallium-201 planar s.
    thallium rest-redistribution s.
    thallium-201 SPECT s.
    ventilation s.
scintillating speckle pattern
scintillation
    s. camera
    s. cocktail
    s. probe
    s. scan
scintiphotography
scintiscan
    technetium-99m stannous pyrophosphate s.
scintiscanner
scintiview
scirrhous carcinoma
scissors
    bandage s.
    Beall s.
    Beall circumflex artery s.
    Blum arterial s.
    Church s.
    Crafoord lobectomy s.
    De Martel s.
    Dennis dissecting s.
    Duffield cardiovascular s.
    Dumont thoracic s.
    Haimovici arteriotomy s.
    Jabaley-Stille Super Cut S.
    Jorgenson thoracic s.
    Karmody venous s.
    Metzenbaum s.

    pericardiotomy s.
    Reinhoff thoracic s.
SCLC
    small cell lung carcinoma
sclera
    blue s.
scleredema
    s. adultorum
    s. of Buschke
sclerodactyly
scleroderma
    diffuse cutaneous s. (IDCS)
    s. lung
ScleroLaser
Scleromate
sclerosant
    pleural s.
sclerosing
    s. agent
    s. cholangitis
    s. hemangioma
    s. phlebitis
    variceal s.
sclerosis, pl. **scleroses**
    amyotrophic lateral s. (ALS)
    aortic s.
    arterial s.
    arteriocapillary s.
    arteriolar s.
    endocardial s.
    Mönckeberg s.
    multiple s.
    nodular s.
    progressive systemic s. (PSS)
    subendocardial s.
    systemic s. (SS)
    tuberous s.
    valvular s.
    vascular s.
    venous s.
Sclerosol intrapleural aerosol
sclerotherapy
    variceal s.
sclerotic
SCN5A mutation
Scole Alta II 3-channel precalibrated Holter AM recorder
SCOOP
    Spofford-Christopher oxygen optimizing program
Scoop 1, 2 catheter
scooped pattern
scooping
    ST s.
Scopulariopsis **sp. pneumonia**
score
    Acute Physiology and Chronic Health Evaluation s.

Agatston s.
Aldrich s.
Aldrich ST elevation s.
Anderson phasing s.
Anderson-Wilkins acuteness s.
APACHE s.
asthma severity s. (ASS)
AW acuteness s.
Barthel ADL s.
Berning and Steensgaard-Hansen s.
Brasfield chest radiograph s.
Brush electrocardiographic s.
calcium s.
Califf s.
Canadian Cardiovascular Society
 angina s. (CCSAS)
Cardiac Infarction Injury S.
clinical pulmonary infection s.
 (CPIS)
Detsky s.
Dripps-American Surgical
 Association s.
Duke treadmill s.
Duke treadmill exercise s.
Duke treadmill prognostic s.
echo s.
Estes s.
extent of pleural carcinomatosis s.
 (EPC)
Gensini s.
Goldman cardiac risk index s.
Hollenberg treadmill s.
Injury Severity S. (ISS)
jeopardy s.
Katz activities of daily living s.
Ladder of Life s.
lung injury s. (LIS)
Mallampati s.
Murray s.
Norris s.
Novacode Q-wave s.
PREDICT s.
quantitative wall motion s.
 (QWMS)
Rivermead Motor Assessment
 Arm s.
Romhilt-Estes s.
Selvester 32-point QRS s.
Selvester QRS s.
Simplified Acute Physiology S.
 (SAPS)
VAMC prognostic s.

wall motion s.
Wilkins echocardiographic s.
Woods-Downes-Lecks clinical
 asthma s.
scoring
microarousal s.
respiratory arousal s.
scorpion venom
scotoma, pl. **scotomata**
Scot-Tussin
S.-T. DM Cough Chasers
S.-T. Senior Clear
scout
s. film
s. scan
s. view
sCRAG
serum cryptococcal antigen
SCRAM face mask
scratch
Lerman-Means s.
scratchy murmur
screening
nocturnal oximetry s.
spirometric s.
screen oxygenation
screw
percutaneous cannulated s.
screw-in
s.-i. epicardial electrode
s.-i. lead
s.-i. sutureless myocardial electrode
screw-on lead
screw-thread stent
SCRIP
Stanford Coronary Risk Intervention
 Project
SCRIPPS
Scripps Coronary Radiation to Inhibit
 Proliferation Post Stenting
SCRIPPS clinical trial
**Scripps Coronary Radiation to Inhibit
 Proliferation Post Stenting (SCRIPPS)**
scrofulaceum
Mycobacterium s.
scroll reentrant wave
scrub typhus
SCT
spiral computed tomography
Star Cancellation Test
Sculptor annuloplasty ring
scurvy

NOTES

SCV-CPR
  simultaneous compression-ventilation
    CPR
SD
  spreading depression
S/D
    Polygam S.
SDB
  sleep-disordered breathing
SDH
  subdural hematoma
SDS
  stent delivery system
    Worldpass radid exchange SDS
SDS-PAGE
  sodium dodecylsulfate polyacrylamide
    gel electrophoresis
SDS-polyacrylamide gel
SE
  spin-echo
    SE image
SEA
  side-entry access
    SEA port
sea frond
seagull
    s. bruit
    s. murmur
Seajet PTCA balloon
seal
    Asherman chest s.
    Ultimate Seal CPAP mask s.
    watertight s.
sealant
    CoSeal resorbable synthetic s.
    FloSeal Matrix hemostatic s.
    FocalSeal liquid s.
    FocalSeal-L surgical s.
    FocalSeal surgical s.
seal-bark cough
SealEasy resuscitation mask
sealing
    collagen vascular s. (CVS)
Sealy-Laragh technique
Seaquence stent
searcher
    Allport-Babcock s.
Searle volume ventilator
seasonal
    s. allergic rhinitis
    s. allergy
Seattle Angina Questionnaire
Sebastiani syndrome
SEC
  spontaneous echo contrast
Sechrist
    S. IV-100 infant ventilator
    S. ventilator

second
  dyne s.'s
  forced expiratory volume in 1 s.
    (FEV_1)
  s. gas effect
  s. harmonic imaging (SHI)
  s. harmonic imaging ultrasound
    technique
  s. heart sound (S_2)
  S. International Study of Infarct
    Survival
  S. Manifestations of Arterial
    Disease (SMART)
  s. messenger
  meter per s. (m/sec)
  s. mitral sound
  s. obtuse marginal artery (OM-2)
  oral airflow in liters per s. (V_O)
  s. pump run
  s. through fifth shock count
secondary
  s. aortic area
  s. asphyxia
  s. atelectasis
  s. bronchitis
  s. bronchus
  s. cardiomyopathy
  s. chemoprophylaxis
  s. dextrocardia
  s. hypertension
  s. infection
  s. pleurisy
  s. pneumonia
  s. pneumothorax
  s. prevention
  s. pulmonary hypertension
  s. pulmonary lobule
  s. radiation
  s. septal hypertrophy
  s. thrombus
  s. tuberculosis
second-degree
  s.-d. A-V block
  s.-d. heart block
second-generation cephalosporin
second-hand smoke
second-look operation
second-phase tilt
secretagogue
secretion
  airway s.
  altered airway s.
  chloride s.
  constitutive s.
  continuous aspiration of
    subglottic s.'s (CASS)
  infected s.
  s. mobilization

mucus s.
nasopharyngeal s.
postural drainage of infected s.
s. retention
rhamnolipid mucus s.
specialized CC-chemokine s.
subglottic s.

secretor
gene s.

secretory
s. leukocyte protease inhibitor
(SLPI)
s. leukoprotease inhibitor (SLPI)
s. leukoprotease inhibitor protein
s. leukoproteinase inhibitor (SLPI)
s. sphingomyelinase (S-SMase)

sector
s. scan
s. scan echocardiography
s. transducer

Sectral

secundum
s. atrial septal defect (ASD2)
foramen s.
ostium s.
septum s.
s.-type atrial septal defect

SECURE
Study to Evaluate Carotid Ultrasound
Changes with Ramipril and Vitamin E

Securon SR

sedation
conscious s.

sedative administration

sedative-hypnotic drug

sedentary lifestyle

sedimentation rate (sed rate)

sed rate
sedimentation rate

Seecor pacemaker

seeding
pumpkin-s.

Seeker guidewire

seesaw murmur

segment
abnormal ST s.
akinetic s.
anterolateral s.
anteroseptal s.
apical bronchopulmonary s. [S I]
apicoposterior s.

apicoposterior bronchopulmonary s.
[SI + SII]
bronchopulmonary s.
coving of ST s.'s
downsloping ST s.
downstream s.
dyskinetic s.
dyssynergic myocardial s.
flail s.
horizontal ST s.
inferior lingular
bronchopulmonary s. [S V]
inferolateral s.
inferoseptal s.
isoelectric ST s.
lateral basal bronchopulmonary s.
[S IX]
malperfused s.
N-link Flexi S.
P-R s.
PR s.
precordial ST s.
proximal s.
RS-T s.
shortening of P-R interval P-R s.
ST s.
subapical s.
subsuperior s.
Ta s.
TP s.
T-P-Q s.
TQ s.
upsloping ST s.
upstream s.

segmental
s. arterial disorganization
s. atelectasis
s. bronchus
s. lung resection
s. pneumonia
s. pressure index
s. stenosis
s. wall motion

segmentalis
bronchus s.

segmentation
k-space s.
time-resolved imaging by automatic
data s. (TRIADS)

segmentectomy

segmented
s. hyalinizing vasculitis

S

NOTES

segmented *(continued)*
    s. K-space approach
    s. neutrophils
    s. ring tripolar (SRT)
    s. ring tripolar lead
segmentorum
segmentum
    s. apicale
    s. bronchopulmonale
    s. bronchopulmonale basale laterale [S IX]
    s. subapicale
    s. subsuperius
Seguin annuloplasty ring
Seiler cartilage
seismic wave
seismocardiogram
seismocardiography
Seitz
    S. metamorphosing respiration
    S. sign
seizure
SELCA
    smooth excimer laser coronary angioplasty
Seldane
Seldinger
    S. needle
    S. percutaneous technique
Selding sheath
Selecon coronary angiography catheter
Selecor
Selectan
selectin blocker
Selection of Thymidine Analog Regimen Therapy (START)
selective
    s. angiography
    s. aortography
    s. arteriography
    s. cardiac catheterization
    s. graft opacification
    s. intracoronary thrombolysis (SICT)
    s. past pathway
    s. septal branch injection of ethanol
    s. transvenous approach
selenium
    s. deficiency
    s. dioxide
    s. sulfide
Selestoject
self-adjusting nasal continuous positive airway pressure (APAP)
self-expandable metallic stent

self-expanding
    s.-e. microporous stent (SEMS)
    s.-e. stent
self-guiding catheter
self-positioning balloon catheter
self-powered treadmill
self-terminating tachycardia
sella
    s. nasion point A angle (SNA)
    s. nasion point B angle (SNB)
sellae
    foramen diaphragmatis s.
Sellers
    S. classification of mitral regurgitation
    S. criteria
    S. grade
    S. mitral regurgitation classification
Sellick maneuver
Sellor rib retractor
Seloken ZOC
Seloris balloon
Selute
    S. Picotip steroid-eluting device
    S. steroid-eluting device
Selvester
    S. 32-point QRS score
    S. QRS score
SEM
    scanning electron microscope
    systolic ejection murmur
sematilide hydrochloride
Semb
    S. apicolysis
    S. lung retractor
semidirect lead
semihorizontal heart
semiinvasive aspergillosis
semilateral supine position
semilunar
    s. valve
    s. valve regurgitation
    s. valve stenosis
semiquantitation
    lipid-laden macrophage s.
semiquantitative index
semirigid catheter
semispinal muscle of thorax
semisynthetic penicillin
semivertical heart
Semliki Forest virus
Semmes-Weinstein monofilaments
Semon sign
Semprex-D
SEMS
    self-expanding microporous stent
Sendai virus

SenDx
- S. 100 blood gas and electrolyte analysis system
- S. Relay data management
- S. Relay data management system

senescent
- s. aortic stenosis
- s. heart
- s. myocardium

senile
- s. amyloidosis
- s. arrhythmia
- s. arteriosclerosis
- s. emphysema
- s. plaque

senilis
- arcus s.
- circus s.

senility

senior
- Phenadex S.

Senning
- S. atrial baffle repair
- S. intraatrial baffle
- S. operation
- S. transposition procedure

Senning-Rastelli procedure

sensation
- elephant-on-the-chest s.
- S. intraaortic balloon catheter
- popping s.
- pressure-like s.
- thermal s.

sensing
- afterpotential s.
- s. circuit
- far-field R-wave s.
- integrated bipolar s.
- rate-drop s.
- s. spike

sensitivity
- s. analysis
- atrial s.
- aureomycin s.
- baroreceptor s.
- baroreceptor reflex s. (BRS)
- baroreflex s. (BRS)
- chlortetracycline s.
- digitalis s.
- pacemaker s.
- paracetamol s.
- phenindione s.
- phenylbutazone s.
- sulfonamide s.
- ventricular s.

sensitization
- baroreceptor s.

sensitized cell

Sensiv endotracheal tube

Sensolog II, III pacemaker

sensor
- activity s.
- BioZtect s.
- s. blending
- blood gas s.
- Capnostat CO_2 s.
- catheter-based s.
- ClipTip reusable s.
- Cross Top replacement oxygen s.
- Dymedix sleep s.
- FilterWatch S.
- Handi oxygen s.
- Infant Airflow and effort s.
- Oxisensor II adult s.
- OxyTip s.
- Pediatric Finger Clip S.
- Piezo Electric Snore S.
- Piezo PLM s.
- pressure transducer airflow s.
- Pulsar Max s.
- SpiroSense flow s.
- Stat-Shell disposable pulse oximeter s.
- VTI Oxygen Monitor with Disposable Polarographic Oxygen S.

sensorimotor
- s. cortex (SMC)
- s. stroke

sensorium
- clouded s.

SensorMedics
- S. Generator
- S. Mass Flow Sensor heated wire flowmeter
- S. 2900 metabolic cart
- S. model 4100 Somnostar polysomnogram
- S. SAT-TRAK pulse oximeter

Sensor pacemaker

sensory
- s. cross-checking
- s. nerve
- s. nerve action potential (SNAP)

NOTES

S

sensory *(continued)*
  s. nerve conduction velocity
    (SNCV)
sentinel
  S. ICD device
  S. implantable cardioverter-
    defibrillator
  S. 2010 implantable cardioverter
    defibrillator
  s. node
Sentron
  S. pigtail angiographic
    micromanometer catheter
  S. pigtail microtip-manometer
    catheter
**SENTRY Antimicrobial Surveillance
  Program**
SEP
  Stroke Education Program
  systolic ejection period
separation
  aortic cusp s.
  E point to septal s. (EPSS)
Sephadex G24 chromatography
Sepracoat coating solution
Sepracor
SEPS
  subfascial endoscopic perforator surgery
  Submaximal Exercise Performance
    Substudy
sepsis
  alcoholism, leukopenia,
    pneumococcal s. (ALPS)
  Capnocytophaga canimorsus s.
  endotoxic s.
  line s.
septa, pl. **septae**
septal
  s. ablation
  s. akinesia
  s. annuloplasty
  s. arcade
  s. artery embolization
  s. cell
  s. collateral
  s. defect
  s. dip
  s. dropout
  s. hyperperfusion on thallium scan
  s. hypertrophy
  s. isthmus
  s. line
  s. myectomy
  s. myotomy
  s. pathway
  s. perforating artery
  s. perforation
  s. perforator

  s. perforator branch
  s. resection
  s. thickening
  s. wall motion
septation
  s. of heart
  s. procedure
septectomy
  atrial s.
  Blalock-Hanlon atrial s.
  Edwards s.
septic
  s. embolization
  s. endocarditis
  s. fever
  s. pneumonia
  s. shock
  s. thromboembolism
septicemia
  anthrax s.
  s. sputum
septicum
  Clostridium s.
septomarginalis
  trabecula s.
septoplasty
  balloon atrial s.
  bedside balloon atrial s.
  Brockenbrough atrial s.
septostomy
  atrial s.
  atrial balloon s.
  balloon s.
  balloon atrial s. (BAS)
  blade s.
  blade atrial s.
  Mullins blade and balloon s.
  Park blade s.
  Rashkind s.
  Rashkind balloon atrial s.
Septra DS
septum (S)
  atrial s.
  conal s.
  interalveolar s.'s
  interatrial s.
  interlobular s.
  interlobular s.'s
  interpulmonary s.
  interventricular s.
  s. linguae
  s. mediastinale
  membranous s.
  s. pellucidum
  s. primum
  s. secundum
  sigmoid s.
  s. spurium

Swiss cheese interventricular s.
tissue s.'s
ventricular s. (VS)

SEQOL
Study of Economics and Quality of Life

sequela, pl. **sequelae**

Sequel compression system

sequence
activation s.
anaplerotic s.
2D gradient-echo s.
direct mapping s.
3D segmented-FLASH imaging s.
3D time-of-flight magnetic
  resonance angiographic s.
FLASH s.'s
intraatrial activation s.
intracardiac atrial activation s.
missed ostium s. (MOS)
respiratory gated three-dimensional
  gradient-echo s.
spin-echo imaging s.

sequencing
DNA s.

sequential
S. Compression Device
s. dilation
s. organ failure assessment (SOFA)
s. pacing

sequestrant
bile acid s.
low-dose bile-acid s.

Sequestra 1000 system

sequestration
s. bronchopneumonia
pulmonary s. (PS)

sequestrectomy

Sequicor III pacemaker

SER
systolic ejection rate

sera (*pl. of* serum)

Serafini hernia

Ser-A-Gen

Ser-Ap-Es

Serathide

seratrodast

Seretide

Serevent Diskus

serial
s. autocorrelation (SAC)
S. Autocorrelation Data acquisition
  technology

s. blood gas
s. change
s. cut films
s. dilation
s. ECG tracing
s. electrocardiogram tracing
s. impedance plethysmography
S. Ultrasound Analysis of
  Restenosis (SURE)
S. Ultrasound Restenosis

serialographic filming

series
800 s. blood gas and critical
  analyte system
s. elastic element
S. 7900 face mask
8500 handheld pulse oximeter s.
MedGraphics 1085 body
  plethysmograph s.
S. 7900 mouth breathing face
  mask
S. 8900 nasal and mouth breathing
  face mask
VitalCare 506DX monitor s.

serine kinase

seroconversion

seroeffusive

serofibrinous
s. pericarditis
s. pleurisy

serological test

Seroma-Cath catheter

Seromycin Pulvules

seronegative
CMV s.
s. spondyloarthropathy

seropneumothorax

seropositive
CMV s.
s. nonsyphilitic pneumopathy

serosanguineous
s. effusion

serosum
pericardium s.

serothorax

serotonin

serotype
M-protein s.

serotyping

serous
s. effusion
s. membrane

S

NOTES

serous *(continued)*
    s. pericarditis
    s. pleurisy
Serpalan
Serpasil
serpentina
    Rauwolfia s.
serpentine aneurysm
serpiginous
Serpula lacrymans
serrated catheter
Serratia
    S. liquefaciens
    S. marcescens
    S. pneumonia
serraticus
    stridor s.
serratus anterior muscle
sertraline hydrochloride
serum, pl. **sera**
    s. albumin
    s. amylase
    s. amyloid type A (SAA)
    antilymphocyte s.
    s. bactericidal titer (SBT)
    s. cholesterol
    s. creatine kinase
    s. cryptococcal antigen (sCRAG)
    s. enzyme study
    ERIG s.
    s. glutamic-oxaloacetic transaminase (SGOT)
    s. glutamic-pyruvic transaminase (SGPT)
    s. IgE
    s. iron
    s. KL-6
    s. lipid profile
    s. magnesium
    s. marker
    S. Markers Acute Myocardial Infarction and Rapid Treatment (SMART)
    s. Mgb assay
    s. neopterin
    s. prothrombin conversion accelerator (SPCA)
    s. renin level
    s. retinol
    s. shock
    s. sickness
    s. triglyceride
service
    HeartLine s.
    National Health S. (NHS)

Servo
    S. Screen 390 ventilator monitoring device
    S. Ventilator 300
servocontrolled plethysmography
sesquioxide
    germanium s.
sestamibi
    s. imaging
    s. perfusion imaging
    s. scan
    s. SPECT
    s. stress test
    Tc-99 s.
    s. technetium-99m SPECT with dipyridamole stress test
    thallium s. (^{201}Tl sestamibi)
    ^{201}Tl s.
        thallium sestamibi
SET
    shredding embolectomy thrombectomy
set
    Acland-Banis arteriotomy s.
    ACS percutaneous introducer s.
    Arrow Hi-flow infusion s.
    Borst side-arm introducer s.
    coaxial micropuncture introducer s.
    Diethrich coronary artery s.
    Dotter Intravascular Retrieval S.
    Masimo S.
    micropuncture introducer s.
    minimum data s. (MDS)
    Neff percutaneous access s.
    Neo-Sert umbilical vessel catheter insertion s.
    Peel-Away introducer s.
    PFTKit disposable s.
    Sobel-Kaplitt-Sawyer gas endarterectomy s.
    Tissomat application device and spray s.
    U-Mid-O$_2$ Jet S.
S.E.T. thrombectomy system catheter
seven
    health level s. (HL7)
seven-pinhole tomography
severe refractory neurocardiogenic syncope
Severinghaus electrode
severity
    stenosis s.
sevoflurane
Sewall technique
sewing
    s. ring
    s. ring area (SRA)
    s. ring loop
sew-on electrode

sex
    s. ratio
    s. steroid
sexual
    s. angina
    s. asthma
    s. syncope
SF$_6$
    sulfur hexafluoride
SFA
    saturated fatty acid
    subclavian flap aortoplasty
    superficial femoral artery
sFas
sFasL
    soluble FasL
SFHb
    pyridoxilated stroma-free hemoglobin
    stroma-free hemoglobin pyridoxilated
SF-36 Health Survey
SFR
    stenotic flow reserve
SF wave of cardiac apex pulse
SG
    stent graft
SGOT
    serum glutamic-oxaloacetic transaminase
SGPT
    serum glutamic-pyruvic transaminase
SGRQ
    St. George Respiratory Questionnaire
SGS
    stroke guidance system
SH
    spontaneously hypertensive
shadow
    acoustic s.
    S. balloon
    bat wing s.
    butterfly s.
    cardiac s.
    mediastinal s.
    S. over-the-wire balloon catheter
    ring s.
    snowstorm s.
    summation s.
shadow-free laryngoscope
shadowing
    acoustic s.
shaft
    head, neck, or s. (HNS)

    NIR Adante monorail catheter s.
    UniTrack s.
shaggy pericardium
Shaher-Puddu classification
shake test
shaking sound
shale pneumoconiosis
shallow
    s. breathing
    s. pathologic Q wave
    s. respiration
    s. T-wave inversion
    s. water blackout
shallow-water blackout syndrome
shape
    echo-signal s.
    spheroid left ventricular s.
shaping behavioral technique
Shapshay-Healy laryngoscope
sharing
    United Network for Organ S. (UNOS)
shaver
    s. catheter
    S. disease
SHD
    structural heart disease
shear
    atrial s.
    s. force
    s. rate of blood
    s. stress
    s. thinning
shears
    Bethune Corylloss.
    Bethune rib s.
    Brunner rib s.
    Coryllos-Bethune rib s.
    Coryllos-Moure rib s.
    Coryllos-Shoemaker rib s.
    Duval-Coryllos rib s.
    Eccentric locked rib s.
    Frey-Sauerbruch rib s.
    Giertz-Shoemaker rib s.
    Gluck rib s.
    rib s.
    Shoemaker rib s.
sheath
    Arrow s.
    ArrowFlex s.
    arterial s.
    blue Cook s.

NOTES

sheath (*continued*)
cardiogenic s.
carotid s.
check-valve s.
chronic s.
compensated s.
Cordis s.
Cordis Bioptome s.
Daig s.
Desilets-Hoffman s.
s. and dilator system
excimer s.
femoral venous s.
French s.
Hemaflex s.
Hemaquet s.
hemostatic s.
InnerVasc s.
introducer s.
888 introducer s.
Introducer II s.
IVT percutaneous catheter
   introducer s.
Klein transseptal introducer s.
Mapper hemostasis EP mapping s.
Mullins s.
Mullins transseptal s.
Mullins transseptal catheterization s.
peel-away s.
percutaneous brachial s.
peribronchial s.
perivascular s.
Pinnacle introducer s.
Selding s.
short monorail polyethylene
   imaging s.
SL1 s.
sonolucent distal imaging s.
Spectranetics laser s. (SLS)
SR0 s.
subclavian peel-away s.
Super ArrowFlex catheterization s.
Teflon s.
Terumo Radiofocus s.
transseptal s.
vascular s.
venous s.
sheath/dilator
Mullins s.
sheathing
halo s.
Sheehan and Dodge technique
Sheen airway reconstruction
sheep
s. antidigoxin Fab antibody
s. blowfly asthma
sheepskin boot

sheet
cellular s.
mucous s.'s
s. sign
Sheffield
S. exercise stress test
S. modification of Bruce treadmill
   protocol
S. Screening Test for Acquired
   Language Disorders (STALD)
S. treadmill protocol
Shekelton aneurysm
shelf
apical s.
s. of plaque
shellfish asthma
shelving edge
Shenstone tourniquet
SHEP
Systolic Hypertension in the Elderly
   Program
shepherd's crook deformity
Sherpa guiding catheter
SHI
second harmonic imaging
SHI ultrasound technique
Shibley sign
shield
bronchoscopic face s.
chest s.
face s.
probe s.
shift
axis s.
baseline s.
chloride s.
Doppler s.
fluid s.
mediastinal s.
midline s.
plaque s.
shifter
frequency s.
shifting
isovolume s.
s. pacemaker
Shigella
shiitake mushroom extract
Shiley
S. cardiotomy reservoir
S. catheter
S. convexoconcave heart valve
S. decannulation plug
S. Phonate speaking valve
S. Tetraflex vascular graft
S. tracheostomy tube
Shimadzu
S. cardiac ultrasound

S. DAR-2400 coronary arteriographic analyzer
S. Headtome SET-080 ring type SPECT scanner
S. MAGNEX Epios 10 1.0-T superconductive MRI system

Shimazaki area-length method

shiner

allergic s.

SHJR4 catheter

SHJR4s

side-hole Judkins right, curve 4, short SHJR4s catheter

shock

biphasic s.
s. blocks
burst s.
cardiac s.
cardiac output s.
cardiogenic s. (CS)
chronic s.
compensated s.
s. count
DC electric s.
declamping s.
decompensated s.
defibrillation s.
diastolic s.
direct current electric s.
distributive s.
double external direct current s.
endotoxin s.
high-energy transthoracic s.
hyperdynamic septic s.
hypovolemic s.
s. index
infarction with S.
insulin s.
irreversible s.
s. lung
obstructive s.
occult cardiogenic s.
oligemic s.
s. pacing
pleural s.
s. position
QRS synchronous atrial defibrillation s.'s
rectilinear biphasic s.
refractory s.
rescue s.

septic s.
serum s.
synchronized s.
systolic s.
s. therapy
Thrombolysis and Angioplasty in Cardiogenic S. (TACS)
toxic s.
vasodilatory s.
vasogenic s.
s. waveform

shocky

shoddy fever

Shoemaker rib shears

Shone

S. anomaly
S. complex

short

s. axis (SAX)
s. coupling interval
s. monorail imaging catheter
s. monorail polyethylene imaging sheath
side-hole Judkins right, curve 4, s. (SHJR4s)
S. Speedy balloon
s. stent
s. tapers
S. Transitional Edge Protection (S.T.E.P.)

short-axis

s.-a. image
s.-a. parasternal view
s.-a. plane
s.-a. slice
s.-a. tomogram

ShortCutter catheter

shortening

circumferential fiber s.
endocardial s.
fiber s.
s. fraction
fractional s.
fractional myocardial s.
long-axis fractional s. (LAFS)
midwall s.
myocardial fiber s.
s. of P-R interval P-R segment
telomeric s.
s. velocity

S

NOTES

shortening (*continued*)
> velocity of circumferential fiber s. (VCF)
> ventricular wall s.

Short-Form 36 Health Survey (SF-36 Health Survey)
shorthand rule
short-long-short cycle
shortness of breath (SOB)
short-term
> flow-assisted, s.-t. (FAST)

short-winded
Shoshin disease
shot
> fast low-angle s.
> sinus s.

shotty node
shoulder
> s. horizontal flexion
> s. rotation

shoulder-hand syndrome
shoulder-strap resonance
Should We Intervene Following Thrombolysis (SWIFT)
shower
> embolic s.

Shprintzen syndrome
shredding
> s. embolectomy thrombectomy (SET)
> s. embolectomy thrombectomy catheter

shrinkage
> arterial s.

shrinker
> Juzo s.

SHS
> Strong Heart Study

SHT
> symptomatic hemorrhage

SHU-454 contrast medium
SHU 508A contrast agent
shudder
> carotid s.

shunt
> Allen-Brown s.
> Anastaflo intravascular s.
> aorta to pulmonary artery s.
> aorticopulmonary s.
> aortofemoral artery s.
> aortopulmonary s.
> arteriopulmonary s.
> arteriovenous s.
> ascending aorta to pulmonary artery s.
> atrial ventricular s.
> atriopulmonary s.
> balloon s.

> bidirectional s.
> bidirectional cavopulmonary s.
> Blalock-Taussig s.
> Brenner carotid bypass s.
> cardiac s.
> carotid artery s.
> cavocaval s.
> cavopulmonary s.
> Cimino arteriovenous s.
> ClearView intracoronary s.
> ClearView intravascular arteriotomy s.
> Cordis-Hakim s.
> coronary anastomotic s.
> s. cyanosis
> Denver pleuroperitoneal s.
> s. detection
> distal splenorenal s.
> Drapanas mesocaval s.
> extracardiac s.
> Flo-Thru s.
> Glenn s.
> Gore-Tex s.
> Gott s.
> interarterial s.
> intracardiac s.
> intrapulmonary s.
> Javid s.
> s. leak
> left-to-right s.
> LeVeen peritoneovenous s.
> Marion-Clatworthy side-to-end vena caval s.
> mesocaval s.
> Model 40-400 Pruitt-Inahara s.
> modified Blalock-Taussig s. (MBTS)
> parallel s.
> s. pathway
> persistent s.
> pleuroperitoneal s.
> portacaval s.
> portopulmonary s.
> Potts s.
> Pruitt-Inahara carotid s.
> Pruitt vascular s.
> pulmonary s.
> s. quantification
> Quinton-Scribner s.
> Ramirez s.
> s. ratio
> residual s.
> reversed s.
> Reynold-Southwick H-graft portacaval s.
> right-to-left s. (RLS)
> Simeone-Erlik side-to-end portorenal s.

splenorenal s.
Sundt carotid endarterectomy s.
systemic to pulmonary s.
T-AnastoFlo s.
Thomas s.
transjugular intrahepatic
  portosystemic s. (TIPS)
Uresil Vascu-Flo carotid s.
USCI s.
Vascu-Flo carotid s.
Vitagraft arteriovenous s.
Waterston s.

shunted blood
shunting
  s. circuit
  intraatrial s.
  intrapulmonary s.
  pleuroperitoneal s.
  venoarterial s.

shuttle
  s. test
  s. test walk

shuttlemaker's disease
Shwachman syndrome
Shy-Drager syndrome
SIAD
  syndrome of inappropriate antidiuresis
SIADH
  syndrome of inappropriate antidiuretic
    hormone
sialic acid
SIBD
  silent ischemic brain damage
sibilance
sibilant
  s. rale
  s. rhonchi
sibrafiban
  S. versus Aspirin to Yield
    Maximum Protection from
    Ischemic Heart Events Post-Acute
    Coronary Syndromes
    (SYMPHONY)
  Xubix s.
Sibson
  S. aponeurosis
  S. notch
  S. vestibule
sibutramine
sICAM
  soluble intracellular adhesion molecule

Si-Carbide
  irox S.-C.
Sicar sign
sicca
  bronchiectasia s.
  bronchitis s.
  laryngitis s.
  pericarditis s.
  pharyngitis s.
  s. syndrome
SICCO
  Stenting in Chronic Coronary Occlusion
    SICCO clinical trial
SICH
  spontaneous intracerebral hemorrhage
Sicilian Gambit formulation
sick
  s. building syndrome (SBS)
  s. sinus syndrome (SSS)
sickle
  s. cell anemia
  s. cell crisis
  s. cell disease
  s. cell thalassemia
  s. cell trait
Sickledex
sicklemia
sickling
sickness
  African sleeping s.
  cave s.
  compressed-air s.
  decompression s. (DCS)
  S. Impact profile (SIP)
  S. Impact Profile questionnaire
  S. Impact Profile scale
  mountain s.
  serum s.
  sleeping s.
SICOR
  S. cardiac catheterization recording
    system
  S. recording system
SICT
  selective intracoronary thrombolysis
SICU
  surgical intensive care unit
side
  s. arm adapter
  s. arm pressure port
  s. biting clamp
  s. branch

S

NOTES

side *(continued)*
    s. branch compromise
    s. branch occlusion
    s. lobe
    s. lobe artifact
    s. port
    s. stretching
side-entry access (SEA)
side-hole
    s.-h. Judkins right, curve 4
    s.-h. Judkins right, curve 4 catheter
    s.-h. Judkins right, curve 4, short (SHJR4s)
sideport
Sideris
    S. adjustable buttoned device
    S. buttoned device
    S. clamp
sideropenic dysphagia
siderophage
siderophore
siderosis
    welder's s.
siderotica
    pneumoconiosis s.
sidestream ETCO$_2$
Sidestream nebulizer
sidewinder percutaneous intra-aortic balloon catheter
SIDS
    sudden infant death syndrome
Siemens
    S. BICOR cardioscope
    S. biplane Neurostar digital subtraction angiogram
    S. Evolution electron beam CT
    S. HICOR cardioscope
    S. Hicor II C-arm
    S. Magnetom 1.5-T MRI
    S. open heart table
    S. Orbiter gamma camera
    S. Siecure implantable cardioverter-defibrillator
    S. SI 400 ultrasound
    S. Somatom DR CT scanner
    S. Somatom Plus 4A scanner
    S. Sonoline CD echograph
    S. ventilator
Siemens-Albis bicycle ergometer
Siemens-Elema
    S.-E. AB pulse transducer probe
    S.-E. AG bicycle ergometer
    S.-E. pacemaker
Siemens-Gammasonics double-head Rota gamma camera

SIESTA
    snooze-induced excitation of sympathetic triggered activity
sieve
    Mobin-Uddin s.
Sievers model 280 nitric oxide analyzer
sigh
    s. function
    s. period
sighing
    s. dyspnea
    s. respiration
sigma
    S. II Dualplace hyperbaric oxygen therapy system
    S. I monoplace hyperbaric therapy system
    S. method
    S. Plus Monosplace hyperbaric oxygen therapy system
    unipolar Pisces S.
sigmoid septum
sign
    Abrahams s.
    ace of spades s.
    air bronchogram s.
    air crescent s.
    antler s.
    applesauce s.
    Aschner s.
    atrioseptal s.
    Auenbrugger s.
    Aufrecht s.
    auscultatory s.
    Baccelli s.
    bagpipe s.
    Bamberger s.
    Bamberger-Pins-Ewart s.
    Bard s.
    B6 bronchus s.
    Béhier-Hardy s.
    bent bronchus s.
    Bethea s.
    Biermer s.
    Biot s.
    Bird s.
    black pleura s.
    Bouillaud s.
    Boyce s.
    Bozzolo s.
    Branham s.
    Braunwald s.
    bread-and-butter textbook s.
    breathing bag s.
    Broadbent s.
    Broadbent inverted s.
    Brockenbrough s.
    Brockenbrough-Braunwald s.

Brockenbrough-Braunwald-Morrow s.
bronchial meniscus s.
calcium s.
Carabello s.
Cardarelli s.
cardiorespiratory s.
Carvallo s.
Castellino s.
Cegka s.
Charcot s.
Cheyne-Stokes s.
Chvostek s.
clenched fist s.
comet s.
comet tail s.
cooing s.
Corrigan s.
Cruveilhier s.
Cruveilhier-Baumgarten s.
cuff s.
D'Amato s.
Davis s.
de la Camp s.
Delbet s.
Delmege s.
Demarquay s.
de Musset s. (aortic aneurysm)
de Mussy s. (pleurisy)
d'Espine s.
Dew s.
Dieuaide s.
Dorendorf s.
double-lumen s.
doughnut s.
Drummond s.
Duchenne s.
Duroziez s.
E s.
Ebstein s.
Ellis s.
epicardial fat pad s.
Erni s.
Ewart s.
Ewing s.
Faget s.
failing lung s.
fallen lung s.
Federici s.
Fischer s.
fissure s.
flying W s.
Friedreich s.

Glasgow s.
gloved finger s.
Gowers s.
Grancher s.
Greene s.
Griesinger s.
Grocco s.
Grossman s.
Gunn crossing s.
Hall s.
halo s.
Hamman s.
Heim-Kreysig s.
Heimlich s.
Hill s.
hilum convergence s.
hilum overlay s.
Homans s.
Hoover s.
Hope s.
Horner s.
hot nose s.
Huchard s.
hyperdense middle cerebral
  artery s. (HMCAS)
inferior triangle s.
intrapericardial s.
intravascular fetal air s.
Jaccoud s.
Jackson s.
Jürgensen s.
Karplus s.
Kellock s.
knuckle s.
Korányi s.
Kreysig s.
Kussmaul s.
Laënnec s.
Lancisi s.
Landolfi s.
Levine s.
Liebermeister s.
Litten diaphragm s.
Livierato s.
Lombardi s.
Löwenberg cuff s.
Macewen s.
Mahler s.
Mannkopf s.
McCort s.
McGinn-White s.

S

NOTES

sign *(continued)*
  s. mechanism for ventilator
    breathing
  Meltzer s.
  Moschcowitz s.
  Moses s.
  Mueller s.
  Müller s.
  Murat s.
  Musset s.
  mute toe s.'s
  Nicoladoni s.
  Nicoladoni-Branham s.
  Oliver s.
  open bronchus s.
  Osler s.
  pad s.
  patent bronchus s.
  pearl s.
  pearl-and-string s.
  Perez s.
  Pfuhl-Jaffé s.
  Pins s.
  pleural meniscus s.
  plumb-line s.
  Porter s.
  Potain s.
  Pottenger s.
  Prevel s.
  Prussian helmet s.
  pulmonary meniscus s.
  pulmonary notch s.
  pulmonary target s.
  Queckenstedt s.
  Quénu-Muret s.
  Quincke s.
  rabbit-ear s.
  railroad track s.
  Ramond s.
  Raynaud s.
  reversed three s.
  ring s.
  Rivero-Carvallo s.
  Riviere s.
  Robertson s.
  Romaña s.
  Rotch s.
  Rothschild s.
  Sam Levine s.
  Sansom s.
  Schapiro s.
  Schepelmann s.
  Schick s.
  scimitar s.
  Seitz s.
  Semon s.
  S s. of Golden
  sheet s.

  Shibley s.
  Sicar s.
  silhouette s.
  Skoda s.
  Smith s.
  snake-tongue s.
  square root s.
  steeple s.
  Steinberg thumb s.
  Sterles s.
  Sternberg s.
  stretched bronchus s.
  string s.
  stripe s.
  superior triangle s.
  T s.
  tail s.
  tenting s.
  thumbprint bronchus s.
  tilt vital s.'s
  trapezius ridge s.
  Traube s.
  Trimadeau s.
  tripod s.
  Troisier s.
  Trunecek s.
  Unschuld s.
  Walker-Murdoch wrist s.
  water lily s.
  Weill s.
  Wenckebach s.
  Westermark s.
  Williams s.
  Williamson s.
  windsock s.
  Wintrich s.

signal
  s. amplitude
  s. averaging
  Doppler s.
  gating s.
  high-intensity transient s. (HITS)
  hyperintense heterogeneous s.
  intracranial microembolic s.
  isointense heterogeneous s.
  s. loss
  magnetic resonance s.
  microembolic s. (MES)
  mosaic jet s.'s
  navigator echo s.
  nonexcitatory s.
  nonexcitatory contractility-modulation
    electric s.
  oscillometric s.
  preconditioning s.
  s. processing
  spin echo s.
  terminal filtered QRS s.

s. transducer and activator of transcription (Stat)
s. transducer and activator of transcription protein family
ventricular far-field s.

signal-averaged
s.-a. echocardiogram
s.-a. echocardiography
s.-a. electrocardiogram (SAECG)
s.-a. electrocardiography (SAECG)
s.-a. P-wave duration (SAPD)

signaling
autocrine s.
integrin s.
myocardial adrenergic s.
outside-in s.
paracrine s.
transmembrane s.

signal-loss cloud
signal-to-noise ratio
signal-void jet
Signa Pad
signet-ring cell carcinoma
Sigvaris compression stockings
Silafed Syrup
Silaminic Expectorant
Silastic
S. bead embolization
S. catheter
S. electrode casing
S. patch
S. poppet
S. strain gauge
S. tape

sildenafil
s. citrate

Sildicon-E
silence
ECG s.

silent
s. angina
s. brain infarction (SBI)
s. cerebral infarct (SCI)
s. cerebral infarction (SCI)
s. coronary artery fistula
s. electrode
s. embolism
s. gap
s. ischemia
s. ischemic brain damage (SIBD)
s. mitral stenosis
s. myocardial infarction (SMI)

s. myocardial ischemia
S. Night diagnostic and screening device
s. pericardial effusion
s. stroke
s. trace leak

Silfedrine
Children's S.

silhouette
cardiac s.
cardiomediastinal s.
immediate s.
late s.
s. sign
s. sign of Felson

silica
silicatosis
silicium carbide
silicone lead
siliconthracosis
silicoproteinosis
Silicore catheter
silicosis
silicosis-CWP-berylliosis
silicotic pneumoconiosis
silicotuberculosis
silk guidewire
silo-filler's
s.-f. disease
s.-f. lung

Silon tent
Silphen
S. Cough
S. DM

Siltussin
S.-CF
S. DM

silver (Ag)
s. bead electrode
Grocott methenamine s. (GMS)
s. polisher's lung
S. Speed hydrophilic guidewire
s. sulfadiazine
S. syndrome

Silverman-Lilly pneumotachograph
silver-methenamine stain
silver-silver chloride electrode
Silverstein stimulator probe
silver-wire effect
silver-wiring of retinal artery
Silvester method
Simdax

S

NOTES

Simeone-Erlik side-to-end portorenal shunt
simiae
>   *Mycobacterium s.*

simian virus 40 (SV40)
Simmons
>   S. II catheter
>   S. III catheter
>   S.-type sidewinder catheter

Simon
>   S. foci
>   S. nitinol filter
>   S. nitinol inferior vena cava filter
>   S. nitinol IVC filter

Simplate procedure
simple chronic bronchitis
simplex
>   angina s.
>   carcinoma s.
>   herpes s.

Simplicity Spirometer
Simplified Acute Physiology Score (SAPS)
Simplus PE/t dilatation catheter
Simpson
>   S. aerocath
>   S. atherectomy catheter
>   S. Coronary AtheroCath catheter
>   S. Coronary AtheroCath system
>   S. Method of Disks
>   S. peripheral AtheroCath
>   S. PET balloon
>   S. positron emission tomography balloon
>   S. rule for ventricular volume
>   S. Ultra Lo-Profile II balloon catheter

Simpson-Robert
>   S.-R. catheter
>   S.-R. vascular dilation system

Simron
Sims nasal prongs
simulator
>   PneuView single lung s.

simultaneous
>   s. bilateral spontaneous pneumothorax (SBSP)
>   s. catheter mapping
>   s. compression-ventilation CPR (SCV-CPR)

simultaneously stapled pneumonectomy (SSP)
SIMV
>   synchronized intermittent mandatory ventilation

simvastatin
Sinarest 12 Hour Nasal Solution
Sindbis virus

sine
>   s. wave
>   s. wave pattern

Sine-Aid IB
sinensis
>   *Clonorchis s.*

Sinequan
Sine-U-View nasal endoscope
Sinex Long-Acting
Singer-Blom valve
singer's node
Singh-Vaughan-Williams arrhythmia classification
single
>   s. atrium
>   s. chain urokinase-type plasminogen activator
>   s. chamber cardiac pacing system
>   s. extrastimulus
>   s. lumen
>   s. papillary muscle syndrome
>   s. pleurisy
>   s. premature extrastimulation
>   s. ventricle
>   s. ventricle malposition

single-balloon
>   s.-b. valvotomy
>   s.-b. valvuloplasty

single-breath
>   s.-b. carbon monoxide test
>   s.-b. diffusion
>   s.-b. nitrogen curve
>   s.-b. nitrogen elimination
>   s.-b. nitrogen washout test

single-chamber
>   s.-c. pulse generator
>   s.-c., rate-responsive

single-crystal gamma camera
single-gene disorder
single-lung transplant (SLT)
single-pass lead
single-patient use manometer
single-photon
>   s.-p. detection
>   s.-p. emission
>   s.-p. emission computed tomographic imaging
>   s.-p. emission computed tomography (SPECT)
>   s.-p. emission tomography (SPET)
>   s.-p. emission tomography imaging
>   s.-p. gamma scintigraphy

single-plane aortography
single-stage exercise stress test
single-vessel
>   s.-v. coronary stenosis
>   s.-v. disease (SVD)

Singulair

singultus
sinister
>   bronchus principalis s.
>   pulmo s.
sinistra, pl. **sinistrae**
>   arteria pulmonalis s.
>   rami esophageales arteriae gastricae
>   sinistrae
>   vena pulmonalis inferior s.
>   vena pulmonalis superior s.
sinistri
>   incisura cardiaca pulmonis s.
>   lingula pulmonis s.
sinistrocardia
sinistrum
>   atrium s.
>   cor s.
Sin Nombre virus (SNV)
sinoaortic baroreflex activity
sinoatrial (SA, S-A)
>   s. arrest
>   s. ball
>   s. baroreflex
>   s. block
>   s. bradycardia
>   s. conduction time (SACT)
>   s. exit block
>   s. nodal artery
>   s. node dysfunction
>   s. recovery time (SART)
sinoauricular block
sinobronchial syndrome
sinobronchitis
sinogram
sinopulmonary
sinospiral fiber
sinotubular junction
sinoventricular conduction
Sintrom
sinuatrial
>   s. nodal artery
>   s. node (SAN, SN)
sinuatrialis
>   nodus s.
>   nonreset nodus s.
>   reset nodus s.
Sinufed Timecelles
Sinumist-SR Capsulets
sinus
>   aortic s.
>   s. arrest
>   s. arrhythmia

basilar s.
s. bradycardia
carotid s.
s. catarrh
cavernous s. (CS)
s. coronarius
coronary s. (CS)
costophrenic s.
s. cycle length
distal coronary s. (DCS)
s. exit block
s. exit pause
s. mechanism
s. nodal automaticity
s. nodal reentrant tachycardia
s. nodal reentry
s. node (SN)
s. node artery
s. node/AV conduction abnormality
s. node disease
s. node dysfunction
s. node function
s. node recovery time (SNRT)
s. node reset
noncoronary s.
oblique s.
s. pause
Petit s.
phrenicocostal s.
piriform s.
pleural s.
proximal coronary s. (PCS)
pulmonary s.
s. reflex
s. rhythm
s. shot
s. standstill
S. stent
superior sagittal s. (SSS)
s. tachycardia
s. thrombosis
transverse s.
transverse/sigmoid s. (TS/SS)
s. trunci pulmonalis
Valsalva s.
s. of Valsalva
s. of Valsalva aneurysm
s. of Valsalva aortography
s. venosus
s. venosus atrial septal defect
s. x-ray
SinuScope system

S

NOTES

sinusitis
>irritant s.
>postnasal drip due to s. (PND-Si)

sinusoid
>intramyocardial s.
>myocardial s.

sinusoidal strut pattern
sinuspiral fiber
SIP
>Sickness Impact profile
>SIP scale

siphon
>carotid s.
>Duguet s.
>Moniz carotid s.

Sippy esophageal dilator
Siri equation
Sirius red stain
SIRS
>systemic inflammatory response
>syndrome

SIS
>Stroke Impact Scale

SISA
>stenting in small arteries

sitaxsentan
site
>arrhythmogenic s.
>arterial entry s.
>entry s.
>exit s.
>extrapulmonary s.
>gene transfer injection s.
>glycine s.
>lysine-binding s.
>No Surgery on S. (NoSOS)
>target s.

site-specific surgery
Sitophilus granarius
sitostanol ester margarine
sitting-up view
situ
>carcinoma in s.

situation
>bailout s.

situational syncope
situs
>s. ambiguus
>cardiac s.
>s. inversus
>s. solitus
>s. transversus
>visceroatrial s.

sivelestat
six-minute walk test
size
>aerodynamic s.
>enzymatic infarct s.

French s.
Multicenter Investigation for the
>Limitation of Infarct S.

sizer
>Björk-Shiley heart valve s.
>Meadox graft s.

sizing
>s. balloon
>French s. of catheter

SJM
>St. Jude Medical
>SJM Biflex annuloplasty ring
>SJM Masters series heart valve
>SJM mechanical heart valve
>SJM pericardial patch
>SJM Quattro mitral valve
>SJM Regent mechanical heart
>valve
>SJM Rosenkranz pediatric retractor
>system
>SJM Seguin annuloplasty ring
>SJM Tailor annuloplasty ring
>SJM valve
>SJM X-Cell cardiac bioprosthesis

Sjögren syndrome
SK
>streptokinase

skein
skeletal
>s. alpha-actin mRNA
>s. muscle
>s. muscle plasticity

skeleton
>cardiac s.
>fibrous s.
>s. of heart
>Teflon-coated wire s.

skeletonization
skewer technique
skilled nursing facility (SNF)
Skimmer laryngeal blade tip
skimming
>plasma s.

skin
>s. button
>s. change
>s. gun
>s. heart
>nail-fold s.
>salmon s.
>tenting of s.
>s. test anergy
>s. turgor

skin-fold thickness
Skinny
>S. dilatation catheter
>S. over-the-wire balloon catheter

skip graft

skipped beat
Skoda
    S. rale
    S. sign
skodaic resonance
SK-Pramine
SKY epidural pain control system
Skylark surface electrode
Slalom balloon
slant
    s. hole collimator
    s. hole tomography
slapping percussion
slaved programmed electrical
  stimulation
SLB
    surgical lung biopsy
SLD
    Spatz-Lindenberg disease
SLE
    systemic lupus erythematosus
Sleek catheter
sleep
    s. apnea
    s. apnea/hypopnea syndrome
      (SAHS)
    S. Apnea Quality of Life Index
      (SAQLI)
    s. architecture
    crescendo s.
    D s.
    deep s.
    s. deprivation
    desynchronized s.
    s. diagnostics
    s. diary
    s. disturbance
    diurnal s.
    dreaming s.
    fast wave s.
    s. fragmentation
    s. hypoxia
    S. Multimedia 2.6 computerized
      textbook
    NREM s.
    orthodox s.
    s. paralysis
    paroxysmal s.
    REM s.
    slow-wave s. (SWS)
    s. spindle

    s. study
    synchronized s. (S-sleep)
sleep-disordered
    s.-d. breathing (SDB)
    s.-d. breathing event
SleepGen polysomnography data entry
  program
sleepiness
    excessive daytime s. (EDS)
sleeping
    s. sickness
    s. tachycardia
Sleepscan
    S. Airflow Pressure Transducer
    S. Traveler ambulatory
      polysomnography system
    S. Traveler home monitoring
      system
Sleeptrace
    S. 2000/32 Sleep Analysis system
    S. sleep diagnostic system
sleeve
    s. lobectomy
    LocalMed catheter infusion s.
    Pneumo S.
sleuth
    carbon monoxide s.
    CO S.
    ETO S.
    HBT S.
slew rate (SR)
slice
    canthomeatal s.
    coronal s.
    short-axis s.
    transaxial s.
Slick stylette endotracheal tube guide
slide
    Menzel-Glaser SuperFrost/Plus
      electrically charged microscope s.
Slider
    S. balloon
    S. catheter
Slidewire extension guide
sliding
    s. filament theory
    s. hiatal hernia
    lung s.
    s. plasty
    pleural s.
    s. rail catheter
    s. scale method

S

NOTES

slim disease
sling
> cardiac s.
> pericardial s.
> pressure s.
> pulmonary artery s.
> s. ring complex
> vascular s.

Slinky
> S. balloon
> S. balloon catheter
> S. catheter
> S. PTCA catheter

slipping rib syndrome
Slip/Stream
> Bennett S.

slit ventricle syndrome
Slo-bid
Slo-Niacin
slope
> closing s.
> disappearance s.
> D-to-E s.
> E to F s.
> flat diastolic s.
> mitral E to F s.

Slo-Phyllin
> S.-P. GG
> S.-P. Gyrocaps

slot blot
slotted
> s. needle
> s. stent
> s. tube articulated stent
> s. tube stent

slough
sloughed bronchial epithelium
slow
> s. A-V node pathway
> s. channel
> s. escape rhythm
> s. and fast A-V nodal pathway
> S. FE
> s. pathway
> s. respiration
> s. response
> s. tissue
> s. vital capacity (SVC)
> s. zone

slow-channel blocker
slow-fast tachycardia
slowing
> conduction s.
> diffuse paroxysmal s.

slow-pathway ablation
slow-reacting substance of anaphylaxis (SRS-A)

Slow-Trax perfusion balloon catheter
slow-wave sleep (SWS)
SLPI
> secretory leukocyte protease inhibitor
> secretory leukoprotease inhibitor
> secretory leukoproteinase inhibitor

SLS
> Spectranetics laser sheath

SL1 sheath
SLT
> single-lung transplant

sludged blood
sludging
slurred speech
slurring
> s. of ST
> s. of QRS

slurry
> gelatin sponge s.
> talc s.

slush
> ice s.
> saline s.

slushed ice
Sly disease
SM
> sonomicrometry

SM1
> primary sensorimotor cortex

Sm
> speed of bronchoconstriction in response to methacholine

SMA
> smooth muscle actin
> superior mesenteric artery
> supplemental motor area

small
> s. airways disease
> s. cell carcinoma
> s. cell lung carcinoma (SCLC)
> s. low-density lipoprotein
> s. P wave

small-lung emphysema
small-particle aerosol generator (SPAG)
smallpox vaccine reaction
small-vessel infarction (SVI)
small-volume
> s.-v. aspiration
> s.-v. nebulizer (SNV, SVN)

SMAP
> systemic mean arterial pressure

SmarScore
SMART
> Second Manifestations of Arterial Disease
> Serum Markers Acute Myocardial Infarction and Rapid Treatment

Study of Medicine versus Angioplasty
Reperfusion Trial
Study of Microstent's Ability to Limit
Restenosis Trial
Study of Monoclonal Antibody
Radioimmunotherapy
SMART study

smart
s. defibrillator
s. pacemaker
S. position-sensing catheter
S. Trigger
S. Trigger Bear 1000 ventilator

SmartKard
S. digital Holter system
S. digital Holter system stem

SmartMist
S. asthma management system
S. Respiratory Management system

SmartNeedle
SmarTracking algorithm
**SmartTracking on the Marathon
pacemaker**
SMC
sensorimotor cortex
smooth muscle cell

smear
bronchoscopic s.
buffy coat s.
lower respiratory tract s.
peripheral blood s.
sputum s.

Smec balloon catheter
smegmatis
Mycobacterium s.
Smeloff-Cutter
S.-C. ball-cage prosthetic valve
S.-C. prosthetic valve
Smeloff heart valve
SMG
supramarginal gyrus
SMI
silent myocardial infarction
sustained maximal inspiration
SMILE
So Much Improvement with a Little
Exercise
Survival of Myocardial Infarction: Long-
Term Evaluation
SMILE program

Smith
S. clip
S. sign
Smith-Lemli-Opitz syndrome
SMO
Sarns membrane oxygenator
smoke
cigarette s. (CS)
echocardiographic s.
environmental tobacco s. (ETS)
puff of s.
second-hand s.
wood s.
smokelike echoes
smoker's
s. bronchitis
s. cough
s. tongue
smoking
s. cessation
cigarette s.
s. history
s.-induced angina
passive s.
smooth
s. coronary artery
s. excimer laser coronary
angioplasty (SELCA)
s. lesion
s. muscle actin (SMA)
s. muscle cell (SMC)
s. muscle relaxant
s. muscle relaxation
smoothing
digital s.
rate s.
smoothness index
**SMP Multiplace hyperbaric therapy
system**
SMVR
supraannular mitral valve replacement
SMVT
sustained monomorphic ventricular
tachycardia
SMX/TMP
sulfamethoxazole/trimethoprim
SN
sinuatrial node
sinus node
SNA
sella nasion point A angle
sympathetic nerve activity

NOTES

S

snack
- Heart Bar s.
- meat, eggs, dairy, invisible fat, condiments, s.'s (MEDICS)

snake
- s. graft
- s.-tongue sign
- s. venom

SNAP
- sensory nerve action potential
- Study of Nitroglycerin and Chest Pain

snap
- closing s.
- mitral opening s. (MOS)
- opening s.
- tricuspid opening s.

Snaplets-EX

snare
- s. catheter
- caval s.
- s. device
- gooseneck s.
- Microvena Amplatz Goose Neck s.
- nitinol s.
- s. technique
- transvenous nitinol s.

snare-assisted coil occlusion of PDA

snare-drum effect

SNB
- sella nasion point B angle

SNCV
- sensory nerve conduction velocity

Sneddon syndrome

sneeze
- s. reflex
- s. syncope

SNF
- skilled nursing facility

Snider match test

sniff
- s. nasal inspiratory pressure
- s. test

sniffling bronchophony

S-nitrosoglutathione (GSNO)

S-nitrosothiol

snooze-induced excitation of sympathetic triggered activity (SIESTA)

snoring
- heroic s.
- s. rale

snowman
- s. abnormality
- s. configuration
- s. heart

snowplow effect

snowstorm shadow

SNRT
- sinus node recovery time

SNS
- sympathetic nervous system

Snuggle Warm convective warming system

SNV
- Sin Nombre virus
- small-volume nebulizer

Snyder Surgivac drainage

SO_2
- sulfur dioxide

^{82}So
- strontium-82

So_2
- oxygen saturation

soap curd

SOB
- shortness of breath

Sobel-Kaplitt-Sawyer gas endarterectomy set

sobria
- *Aeromonas s.*

society
- American Cancer S. (ACS)
- American Roentgen Ray S.
- Canadian Cardiovascular S. (CCS)

sock array

sodium
- s. acetate
- aminosalicylate s.
- s. aminosalicylate
- ardeparin s.
- s. ascorbate
- beraprost s.
- s. bicarbonate
- brequinar s.
- cefazolin s.
- cefmetazole s.
- cefonicid s.
- cefoperazone s.
- cefotaxime s.
- cefoxitin s.
- ceftizoxime s.
- ceftriaxone s.
- cephalothin s.
- cephapirin s.
- cerivastatin s.
- s. channel
- s. channel blockade
- s. channel gene
- s. chloride
- cloxacillin s.
- colistimethate s.
- s. content of food
- s. cromoglycate
- cromolyn s.
- s. current (I_{Na})
- dalteparin s.
- danaparoid s.

dantrolene s.
dextrothyroxine s.
s. dichloroacetate
dicloxacillin s.
dietary s.
Diphenylan S.
s. dodecylsulfate polyacrylamide gel electrophoresis (SDS-PAGE)
enoxaparin s.
epoprostenol s.
s. ferric gluconate complex
fluvastatin s.
s. ion
ioxaglate s.
s. lactate
meclofenamate s.
s. meglumine diatrizoate
s. meglumine ioxaglate
mercaptomerin s.
metam s.
methicillin s.
s. methylprednisolone
mezlocillin s.
montelukast s.
morrhuate s.
nafcillin s.
nedocromil s.
s. nitrite
s. nitroprusside
nitroprusside s.
oxacillin s.
pantoprazole s.
paraaminosalicylate s.
S. P.A.S.
Pentothal S.
pertechnetate s.
s. pertechnetate Tc 99m
s. phosphate
piperacillin and tazobactam s.
PMS-Levothyroxine S.
s. polystyrene sulfonate
s. polystyrene sulfonate enema
pravastatin s.
racemic warfarin s.
s. retention
s. salicylate
stibogluconate s.
s. tetradecyl sulfate
thiamylal s.
thiopental s.
thiopentone s.
s. thiosulfate

tinzaparin s.
warfarin s.
sodium-channel blocker
sodium-potassium exchange
Soemmerring
arterial vein of S.
SOFA
sequential organ failure assessment
Sofarin
soft
s. event
s. pulse
S. Thoracoport
s. tissue calcification
s. tissue sarcoma
Softech endotracheal tube
Soft-EZ reusable electrode
SOF-T guidewire
Softip
S. catheter
S. oxygen nasal cannula
Softouch UHF cardiac pigtail catheter
Softrac-PTA catheter
Soft-Vu Omni flush catheter
software
ADOPT-like s.
CaduCIS UMLS s.
Caire OxyMax s.
CardioMagic 2000 cardiac-monitoring s.
Clarity s.
Harmonie EEG s.
Image-Measure morphometry s.
ImageVue s.
MedGraphics Breeze PF s.
Plussq1 s.
Solaris FLOW image analysis s.
SPSS s.
Stat View s.
Tachyarrhythmia Detection S.
TrakPro data analysis s.
VISTA s.
Sokolow electrocardiographic index
Sokolow-Lyon
S.-L. voltage
S.-L. voltage criteria
SolAiris
S. III oxygen concentrator
S. V oxygen concentrator
solani
Fusarium s.
Solarcaine topical

S

NOTES

Solaris FLOW image analysis software
Solcotrans autotransfusion unit
soldered bond
soldering
    s. flux
    s. fumes
soldier's
    s. heart
    s. patch
Sole Primeur 33D analyzer
Solfoton
solid angle concept
solitarius
    nucleus tractus s.
solitary
    s. coronary ostium
    s. pulmonary arteriovenous fistula
    s. pulmonary nodule (SPN)
solitus
    situs s.
    ventricular situs s.
    visceroatrial situs s.
Solo
    S. balloon
    S. catheter
solubility
    lipid s.
soluble
    s. adhesion molecule
    s. FasL (sFasL)
    s. intracellular adhesion molecule
    (sICAM)
Solu-Cortef Injection
Soludrast contrast material
Solu-Medrol injection
Solurex L.A.
Solus pacemaker
Soluspan
    Celestone S.
solution
    Afrin Nasal S.
    agitated saline s.
    albuterol sulfate inhalation s.
    Allerest 12 Hour Nasal S.
    Anestacon Topical S.
    Anti-Sept bactericidal scrub s.
    Atrovent Inhalation S.
    Belzer s.
    Betadine Helafoam s.
    Bretschneider-HTK cardioplegic s.
    Brompton s.
    Burow s.
    Cafcit oral s.
    caffeine citrate oral s.
    cardioplegic s.
    Cardiosol s.
    Carnoy s.
    Celsior s.

Chlorphed-LA Nasal S.
Collins s.
Crolom Ophthalmic S.
cromolyn sodium inhalation s.
crystalloid cardioplegic s.
Dakin s.
Denhardt s.
dextran s.
Dristan Long Lasting Nasal S.
Duration Nasal S.
ECS cardioplegic s.
Euro-Collins s.
extracellular-like, calcium-free s.
    (ECS)
Fowler s.
Gey s.
Gey fixative s.
hand agitated s.
Hank balanced salt s.
Hartmann s.
ICS cardioplegic s.
Intal Nebulizer S.
intracellular-like, calcium-bearing
    crystalloid s. (ICS)
Isoetharine Inhalation S. USP 1%
Krebs s.
Krebs-Henseleit s.
levalbuterol HCl inhalation s.
low-chloride St. Thomas s.
Lugol s.
Massier s.
Melrose s.
Myers S.
Nasalcrom Nasal S.
Neo-Synephrine 12 Hour Nasal S.
NTZ Long Acting Nasal S.
Papanicolaou s.
polyethylene glycol electrolyte
    lavage s. (PEG-LES)
Resectisol Irrigation S.
Ringer s.
rotaflush s.
Schlesinger s.
Sepracoat coating s.
Sinarest 12 Hour Nasal S.
Sporicidin sterilizing s.
stroma-free hemoglobin s.
St. Thomas s.
SuperVent s.
TOBI Inhalation S.
Twice-A-Day Nasal S.
Tyrode s.
University of Wisconsin s.
4-Way Long Acting Nasal S.
Xopenex inhalation s.
Xopenex levalbuterol HCl
    inhalation s.
Xylocaine Topical S.

SOLVD
Studies of Left Ventricular Dysfunction
solvent vapor
SomaSensor
S. device
S. pad
somatic cell therapy
somatomedin
Somatom Volume Zoom computed tomography system
somatosensory
s. evoked potential (SSEP)
s. evoked potential test
somatostatin
somnambulism
somniloquism
somniloquy
Somnoplasty
S. procedure
S. system
SomnoStar
S. apnea testing device
S. LabManager multifunction program
Somnus Somnoplasty system
So Much Improvement with a Little Exercise (SMILE)
Sonazoid
Sondergaard procedure
Sones
S. Cardio-Marker catheter
S. catheter
S. coronary catheter
S. guidewire
S. hemostatic bag
S. Hi-Flow catheter
S. Positrol catheter
S. selective coronary arteriography
S. technique
S. woven Dacron catheter
sonicated
s. albumin-dextrose contrast
s. contrast agent
s. dextrose albumin
s. Renografin-76
Sonicath imaging catheter
sonication technique
sonicator
Sonix 2000 ultrasonic nebulizer
sonogram
sonography
Acuson computed s.

carotid B-mode s.
contrast-enhanced transcranial color-coded real-time s. (CE-TCCS)
Diasonics Gateway2D duplex s.
Doppler s. (DS)
extracranial Doppler s. (ECD)
functional transcranial Doppler s. (fTCD)
TCD s.
transcranial color-coded duplex s. (TCCS)
transcranial contrast Doppler s.
transcranial Doppler s. (TCD)
two-dimensional transcranial color-coded s. (2D-TCCS)
SonoHeart
S. echocardiography system
S. hand-carried echocardiography
S. handheld, all digital echocardiography system
S. scanner
sonolucency
sonolucent
s. distal imaging sheath
s. zone
sonomicrometer piezoelectric crystal
sonomicrometry (SM)
sonorous
s. rale
s. respiration
s. rhonchi
SONOS
S. 4500
S. 500 imaging system
S. 1500 scanner
S. 2500 scanner
S. 2000 ultrasound imager
S. 5500 ultrasound imager
SonoSite
Sonovue
Sopha Medical gamma camera
Sophy high-resolution collimator
Sorbitrate
Sorensen Transpac III transducer
Sorenson thermodilution catheter
Sorin
S. bicarbon bileaflet prosthesis
S. Carbostent stent
S. heart valve
S. lead
S. mitral valve prosthesis

NOTES

S

Sorin *(continued)*
    S. pacemaker
    S. prosthetic valve
Sorivudine
soroche
sorter
    cell s.
    fluorescence-activated cell s.
    (FACS)
SOS guidewire
Sotacor
sotalol
    d-s.
    s. HCl
    s. hydrochloride
Sotradecol injection
Soucek
    Randall-Baker S. (RBS)
souffle
    cardiac s.
    fetal s.
    funic s.
    mammary s.
soufflet
    bruit de s.
sound
    absent breath s.'s
    adventitious breath s.'s
    adventitious heart s.
    aortic closure s.
    aortic ejection s.
    aortic second s. (A_2)
    atrial s.
    auscultatory s.
    bandbox s.
    Beatty-Bright friction s.
    bell s.
    bellows s.
    bottle s.
    breath s.
    bronchial breath s.'s
    bronchovesicular breath s.'s
    cannon s.
    cardiac s.
    coarse breath s.'s
    coin s.
    cracked-pot s.
    crowing breath s.'s
    crunching s.
    decreased breath s.'s
    distant breath s.'s
    distant heart s.'s
    double-shock s.
    eddy s.
    ejection s.'s (ES)
    esophageal s.
    first heart s. (S_1)
    flapping s.

    fourth heart s. (S_4)
    friction s.
    gallop s.
    heart s.'s S_1, S_2, S_3, S_4
    hippocratic s.
    s. intensity profile
    Korotkoff s.
    mammary souffle s.
    metallic breath s.'s
    mitral first s. (M_1)
    mitral second s. (M_2)
    muffled heart s.'s
    pacemaker s.
    paradoxically split S_2 s.
    percussion s.
    pericardial friction s.
    physiologically split S_2 s.
    physiologic third heart s.
    pistol shot s.
    pistol shot femoral s.
    prosthetic valve s.
    puffing s.
    pulmonary component of second
      heart s.
    pulmonic closure s.
    pulmonic second heart s. (P2)
    pulmonic valve closure s.
    quiet breath s.'s
    quiet heart s.'s
    respiratory s.
    sail s.
    second heart s. (S_2)
    second mitral s.
    shaking s.
    splitting of heart s.
    squeaky-leather s.
    succussion s.'s
    tambour s.
    third s.
    third heart s. (S_3)
    tic-tac s.'s
    to-and-fro s.
    tracheal s.
    tricuspid valve closure s.
    tubular breath s.'s
    tumor plop s.
    tympanitic s.
    vesicular breath s.'s
    waterwheel s.
    s. wave cycle
    widely split second s.
    xiphisternal crunching s.
source
    germanium-68 external s.
Southern
    S. blot
    S. blot analysis
South Florida RAST panel

Souttar tube
soybean lecithin asthma
soy phytoestrogen
SP
spontaneous pneumothorax
surfactant protein
SP-A
SP-B
SP-C
SP-D
SP-1
SP1005
Cardiomyostimulator SP1005
space
air s.
alveolar dead s.
anatomical dead s.
anatomic dead s.
antecubital s.
anterior clear s.
Bogros s.
Böttcher s.
s. of Burns
Cotunnius s.
cystic s.
dead s.
echo-free s.
extrapleural s.
H s.
Henke s.
His perivascular s.
Holzknecht s.
intercostal s.
interelectrode s.
interpleural s.
interstitial s.
intrapleural s.
Larrey s.
lateral pharyngeal s.
mediastinal s.
noncommunicating air s.
peripharyngeal s.
perivascular s.'s
pharyngeal s.
pharyngomaxillary s.
physiologic dead s.
pleural s.
posterior airway s. (PAS)
postpharyngeal s.
prevertebral s.
respiratory dead s.
retrocardiac s.

retropharyngeal s.
retrosternal s.
retrosternal air s.
retrotracheal s.
subarachnoid s. (SAS)
subphrenic s.
Talairach s.
Traube semilunar s.
Virchow-Robin s.
Westberg s.
Zang s.
Spacehaler
SpaceLabs
S. Event Master
S. Holter monitor
S. pulse oximeter
Spacemaker balloon dissector
space-occupying
s.-o. effect
s.-o. lesion
spacer
Ellipse compact s.
spacing
spadelike configuration
SPAF
Stroke Prevention in Atrial Fibrillation
SPAF study
SPAF TEE
Stroke Prevention in Atrial Fibrillation III
Transesophageal Echo
SPAF TEE study
SPAG
small-particle aerosol generator
spalling effect
SPAMM
spatial modulation of magnetization
SPAMM technique
Span-FF
spare tire bulge
sparfloxacin
sparing
myocardial s.
spark erosion
Sparks mandrel technique
spasm
arterial s.
bronchial s.
bronchopulmonary s.
carpopedal s.
catheter-induced s.
catheter-induced coronary artery s.
catheter related peripheral vessel s.

S

NOTES

spasm *(continued)*
    catheter-tip s.
    coronary s.
    coronary artery s.
    diffuse esophageal s.
    epicardial arterial s.
    ergonovine-induced s.
    esophageal s.
    post bypass s.
    vascular s.
    venous s.
    vessel s.
spasmodic
    s. asthma
    s. croup
spastica
    dysphagia s.
spasticity
spatial
    s. intensity
    s. modulation of magnetization
    (SPAMM)
    s. modulation of magnetization
    technique
    s. resolution
    s. tracking
    s. vector
    s. vectorcardiography
spatium
    s. lateropharyngeum
    s. peripharyngeum
    s. retropharyngeum
Spatz-Lindenberg disease (SLD)
SPCA
    serum prothrombin conversion
    accelerator
speaking valve
Spearman coefficient
Spears laser balloon
special
    Lasix S.
specialized CC-chemokine secretion
specific compliance
specificity
speckle
    Doppler s.
speckling
SPECT
    single-photon emission computed
    tomography
    technetium-99m sestamibi single-photon
    emission computed tomography
    adenosine ^{99m}Tc sestamibi SPECT
    SPECT imaging
    MIBI SPECT
    SPECT scintigraphy
    sestamibi SPECT

    stress perfusion and rest function
    by sestamibi-gated SPECT
    technetium-99m sestamibi SPECT
spectacular shrinking deficit
spectography
    magnetic resonance s.
    Raman s.
spectra (*pl. of* spectrum)
Spectra-Cath STP catheter
Spectraflex lead
spectral
    s. analysis
    S. Cardiac STATus CK-
    MB/myoglobulin panel test
    S. Cardiac STATus controls for
    troponin I
    S. Cardiac STATus rapid format
    troponin I panel test
    S. Cardiac STATus Test
    s. Doppler
    s. Doppler velocity measurement
    s. envelope
    s. leakage
    s. peak velocity
    s. phonocardiograph
    s. power
    s. temporal mapping
    s. turbulence mapping
    s. waveform
Spectranetics
    S. C rapid-exchange laser catheter
    S. Extreme catheter
    S. laser
    S. laser sheath (SLS)
    S. Prima laser guidewire
    S. P23 Statham transducer
Spectraprobe
Spectraprobe-Max probe
Spectrax SX, SX-HT, SXT, VL, VM,
    VS pacemaker
Spectrobid Tablet
spectrometer
    Amis 2000 respiratory mass s.
    Burker Avance s.
spectrometry
    atomic absorption s.
    gas chromatography-mass s. (GC-
    MS)
spectrophotometer
    Cary 118C s.
    Hitachi U-2000 s.
    liquid scintillation s.
spectrophotometric oximetry
spectrophotometry
    time of flight and absorbance s.
    TOFA s.
spectroscopy
    electron paramagnetic resonance s.

flame emission s. (FES)
fluorescence s.
graphite furnace atomic
  absorption s.
magnetic resonance s. (MRS)
near-infrared s. (NIRS, NIS)
NMR s.
phosphorus-31 magnetic
  resonance s. (^{31}P-MRS)
^{31}P nuclear magnetic resonance s.
proton s.
Raman s.
spectroscopy-directed laser
spectrum, pl. **spectra**
SpectRx test
specular echo
speculum
  Yankauer pharyngeal s.
speech
  alaryngeal s.
  esophageal s.
  s. mental stress test
  slurred s.
speed of bronchoconstriction in
response to methacholine (Sm)
Speedino balloon
Speedy balloon catheter
Speilberger Anger Expression scale
spell
  blackout s.
  grayout s.
  greyout s.
  Gricco s.
  hypercyanotic s.
  hypoxic s.
  presyncopal s.
  syncopal s.
  tet s.
  tetrad s.
  tetralogy of Fallot s.
Spembly cryoprobe
Spencer plication of vena cava
Spens syndrome
SPET
  single-photon emission tomography
    SPET imaging
Spexil
SPGR
  spoiled gradient recalled
sphaericus
  Bacillus s.
Sphaerophorus necrophorus

sphenoidal fissure
sphere
  attraction s.
sphericity index
spheroid left ventricular shape
spheroplast
sphincter
  cardioesophageal s.
  esophageal s.
  gastroesophageal s.
  hepatic s.
  inferior esophageal s.
  palatopharyngeal s.
  pharyngoesophageal s.
  precapillary s.
Sphingobacterium
sphingolipidosis
sphingomyelinase
  secretory s. (S-SMase)
sphingomyelin phosphodiesterase
sphygmic interval
sphygmocardiograph
sphygmocardioscope
sphygmochronograph
Sphygmocorder
sphygmogram
sphygmograph
sphygmographic
sphygmography
sphygmoid
sphygmomanometer
  Ayers s.
  Baumanometer standard mercury s.
  Erlanger s.
  Faught s.
  Hawksley random zero mercury s.
  Janeway s.
  London School of Hygiene and
    Tropical medicine s.
  Mosso s.
  Physio-Control Lifestat s.
  random-zero s.
  Riva-Rocci s.
  Rogers s.
sphygmomanometry
sphygmometer
sphygmometroscope
sphygmooscillometer
sphygmopalpation
sphygmophone
sphygmoscope
  Bishop s.

NOTES

sphygmoscopy
sphygmosystole
sphygmotonograph
sphygmotonometer
sphygmoviscosimetry
spider
- s. angioma
- arterial s.
- s. burst
- s. projection
- vascular s.
- s. venom
- s. x-ray view

spike
- s. activity
- atrial s.
- H s.
- pacemaker s.
- pacing s.
- sensing s.
- wave s.

spike-and-dome
- s.-a.-d. configuration
- s.-a.-d. pulse

SPI-Lite sleep position indicator
spill
- chylous s.

spillover
- jugular venous catechol s.

spin
- s. density
- s. echo signal
- s. tagging

SPINAF
- Stroke Prevention in Nonrheumatic Atrial Fibrillation
- SPINAF clinical trial

spinal
- s. embolism
- s. muscle of thorax
- s. muscular atrophy

spindle
- aortic s.
- s. cell carcinoma
- s. fiber
- His s.
- sleep s.

spine
- posterior nasal s. (PNS)

spin-echo (SE)
- s.-e. imaging
- s.-e. imaging sequence
- s.-e. MRI

Spinhaler
spin-lattice time
spinocerebellar
- s. ataxia
- s. degeneration

spinothalamic tract
spin-spin time
spiral
- s. computed tomography (SCT)
- s. CT scan
- Curschmann s.
- s. dissection
- s.-embedded tube
- s. hypertrophic cardiomyopathy
- S. Mark V portable ultrasonic drug inhaler
- s. reentrant wave

SpiralGold adult low-prime oxygenator with Duraflo treatment
spiralis
- Trichinella s.

spiramycin
spirapril hydrochloride
Spiriva
spirochetal
- s. disease
- s. infection
- s. myocarditis

spirochete
SPIR-O-FLOW peak flowmeter
spirogermanium
spirogram
- forced expiratory s. (FES)

spirograph
spirography
spiro index
Spirolite 201 spirometer
spirometer
- Benedict-Roth s.
- Bennett monitoring s.
- Calculair s.
- Cardiovit AT-10 s.
- chain-compensated s.
- closed-circuit s.
- Coach incentive s.
- Collins Dry s.
- Collins Survey s.
- Compact desktop s.
- Compact II desktop s.
- Discovery handheld s.
- Douglas bag s.
- Eagle s.
- Flash portable s.
- flow-sensing s.
- Gould Instrument Systems s.
- Horizon PFT s.
- incentive s.
- Inspirx incentive s.
- Jaeger Flowscreen s.
- Jaeger MasterLab Pro pneumotachograph s.
- KoKo research-grade s.
- KoKo Trek research-grade s.

Krogh s.
Krogh apparatus s.
MedicAIR PLUS s.
MicroLoop II handheld s.
Micro Plus s.
2120 Recording S.
Simplicity S.
SP-10 s.
Spirolite 201 s.
Spirovit SP-10 s.
Spirovit SP-1 portable s.
Stead-Wells water-seal type s.
Tissot s.
Venturi s.
Vitalograph s.
Vitalograph 2120 handheld
  recording s.
Vitalor incentive s.
volume-displacement s.
water-sealed s.
wedge s.
Welch Allyn Pneumocheck s.
Wright s.
spirometric screening
spirometry
DX-Portable s.
incentive s.
MultiSPIRO computerized s.
MultiSPIRO DX-Portable s.
2170 S. Software system
stacked inspiratory s.
Tri-flow incentive s.
Welch Allyn/Shiller SP-1 budget s.
Welch Allyn/Shiller SP-10
  diagnostic s.
Spironazide
spironolactone
hydrochlorothiazide and s.
Spiros
Albuterol S.
S. Inhalation system
S. inhaler
spiroscope
SpiroSense
S. flow sensor
S. system
SpiroVision-3
S. spirometry system
S. system
Spirovit
S. SP-1 portable spirometer
S. SP-10 spirometer

Spirozide
Spitzer theory
SPL
superior parietal lobule
splanchnic
s. bed perfusion
s. blood flow
s. vessel
splanchnicotomy
splash
succussion s.
splayed
carina not s.
Splendore-Hoeppli phenomenon
splenic
s. anemia
s. flexure syndrome
s. perfusion measurement
s. portography
s. venoconstriction
splenomegaly
splenopneumonia
splenoportal hypertension
splenoportography
splenorenal shunt
splenosis
thoracic s.
splice
breakaway s.
splinter hemorrhage
splinting
split
s. fused commissure
paradoxic s. of S_2
physiological s. of S_2
split-function lung test
split-lung ventilation
split-sheath introducer
splitter
beam s.
splitting
commissural s.
s. of heart sound
SPN
solitary pulmonary nodule
SpO$_2$
oxygen saturation as measured using
  pulse oximetry
**Spofford-Christopher oxygen optimizing
  program (SCOOP)**
spoiled gradient recalled (SPGR)

S

NOTES

spondylitis
    ankylosing s. (AS)
spondyloarthropathy
    seronegative s.
sponge
    4 × 4 s.
    absorbable gelatin s.
    collagen s.
    Collostat hemostatic s.
    gelatin s.
    Gelfoam s.
    Ivalon s.
    laparotomy s.
    phantom s.
    RayTec s.
spongy myocardium
spontaneous
    s. cervical artery dissection (sCAD)
    s. closure of fistula
    s. coronary artery dissection
    (SCAD, sCAD)
    s. echo contrast (SEC)
    s. extrasystole
    s. intracerebral hemorrhage (SICH)
    s. lysis
    s. pneumothorax (SP)
    s. reentrant sustained ventricular
    tachycardia
    s. ventilation
    s. ventricular tachycardia
spontaneously hypertensive (SH)
Sporanox Oral
Sporicidin sterilizing solution
Sporothrix schenckii
sporotrichosis
SPORT
    Stent Implantation Post Rotational
    Atherectomy Trial
sport
    isometric s.
The Sports Breather
SPO$_2$T
    Pocket SPO$_2$T
spot
    Brushfield s.
    café-au-lait s.
    Campbell De Morgan s.
    cold s.
    cotton-wool s.
    De Morgan s.'s
    Horder s.'s
    hot s.
    Koplik s.
    s. lesion
    milk s.'s
    rose s.
    Roth s.
    tendinous s.

    ventricular milk s.'s
    s. welding
    white s.
SpotCheck+ handheld pulse oximeter
spot-film fluorography
spotty
    s. coronary calcium
    s. predicted stenosis
spray
    Astelin nasal s.
    Citrol Oral S.
    Hurricaine s.
    metered-dose s.
    nasal nicotine s. (NNS)
    nicotine nasal s.
    Nicotrol NS nasal s.
    Nitrolingual Translingual S.
    Xylocaine Topical S.
spread
    lymphangitic s.
    venous s.
spreader
    Bailey rib s.
    Burford-Finochietto rib s.
    CardioThoracic Systems IMA
    Retractor wound s.
    Davis rib s.
    DeBakey rib s.
    Favaloro-Morse rib s.
    Finochietto rib s.
    Harken rib s.
    Lilienthal-Sauerbruch rib s.
    Medicon rib s.
    Miltex rib s.
    Quervain rib s.
    Rehbein rib s.
    Reinhoff rib s.
    rib s.
spreading depression (SD)
spring
    S. catheter
    s. coil
    disk s.
spring-loaded
    s.-l. resistor
    s.-l. stent
    s.-l. vascular stent
springwater cyst
sprinkle
    Humibid S.
Sprint
    S. catheter
    S. Model 6942 tachyarrhythmia
    lead
    S. Model 6943 tachyarrhythmia
    lead
SP-10 spirometer
SPSS software

S-P-T
SPTI
    systolic pressure time index
spuria
    angina s.
spurious aneurysm
spurium
    septum s.
sputum, pl. **sputa**
    s. aerogenosum
    albuminoid s.
    s. analysis
    blood-tinged s.
    bloody s.
    brown s.
    s. coctum
    copious s.
    s. crudum
    s. cruentum
    currant jelly s.
    s. cytology
    egg-yolk s.
    s. elastase
    elastic fibers in s.
    s. expectoration
    frothy s.
    globular s.
    green s.
    hemorrhagic s.
    icteric s.
    s. induction
    moss-agate s.
    mucopurulent s.
    nummular s.
    pink s.
    s. production
    productive s.
    prune juice s.
    purulent s.
    s. retention
    rusty s.
    septicemia s.
    s. smear
    tenacious s.
    s. tenacity
    s. viscoelasticity
    s. viscosity and elasticity
    s. volume
    white s.
    yellow s.
sputum-epithelium interface

SPV
    stentless porcine valve
Spyglass angiography catheter
S_1Q_3 pattern
S-QRS interval
$S_1Q_3T_3$ pattern
squamous
    s. alveolar cell
    s. cell
    s. cell bronchogenic carcinoma
    s. cell carcinoma
square
    s. root sign
    s. wave response
    s. wave stimulus
squared
    kilogram per meter s. (kg/m^2)
    liters per minute per meter s. (Lpm/m^2)
    meters per second s.
square-shaped occluder
squeak
squeaky-leather sound
squeeze
    s. effect
    face s.
    reverse s.
    thoracic s.
    tussive s.
squeezer
    lemon s.
SR
    slew rate
      Aerolate SR
      bupropion SR
      Calan SR
      SR calcium ATPase
      Cardene SR
      Cardizem SR
      Deconamine SR
      Isoptin SR
      Nitrong SR
      Procan SR
SRA
    sewing ring area
Sramek formula
SRC Expectorant
Src kinase
SRS-A
    slow-reacting substance of anaphylaxis
SR0 sheath

NOTES

SRT
  segmented ring tripolar
SRT lead
SS
  systemic sclerosis
  Uroplus SS
S-Scort DUET suction unit
S-segment airway conductance
SSEP
  somatosensory evoked potential
S-Series sleep system
SSH 260A scanner
S₁-S₂ interval
SSKI
  saturated solution of potassium iodide
S-sleep
  synchronized sleep
S-SMase
  secretory sphingomyelinase
SSP
  simultaneously stapled pneumonectomy
SS-QOL
  stroke-specific quality of life
SSS
  sick sinus syndrome
  superior sagittal sinus
SSS-58
  58-point Scandinavian Stroke Scale
S-sulfate
ST
  stent thrombosis
    ST alteration
    ST deviation
    ST elevation
    ST interval
    ST junction
    ST reelevation
    ST resolution
    ST sag
    ST scooping
    ST segment
    ST segment alternans
    ST segment changes
    ST segment depression (STD)
    ST segment elevation
    ST segment resolution
    slurring of ST
    ST vector
    ST wave
St.
    S. George Respiratory Questionnaire
    (SGRQ)
    S. Joseph Adult Chewable Aspirin
    S. Joseph Cough Suppressant
    S. Jude annuloplasty ring
    S. Jude bileaflet prosthetic valve
    S. Jude cardiac device
    S. Jude composite prosthetic

S. Jude composite prosthetic valve
S. Jude heart valve prosthesis
S. Jude Medical (SJM)
S. Jude Medical bileaflet tilting-
  disk aortic valve
S. Jude Medical BioImplant valve
S. Jude Medical Port-Access
S. Jude Medical Port-Access
  mechanical heart valve
S. Jude mitral valve
S. Jude prosthetic aortic valve
S. Jude valve prosthesis
S. Thomas Atherosclerosis
  Regression Trial (START)
S. Thomas Hospital cardioplegia
S. Thomas solution
S. Vitus dance
ST3 stethoscope
stab
  s. electrode
  s. incision
  s. wound
stability
  circulatory s.
  hemodynamic s.
  RR interval s.
stabilization
  internal pneumatic s.
  plaque s.
stabilizer
  AutoSuture indicator 30 Mini-
    CABG site s.
  CardioThoracic Systems MV
    Access Platform coronary s.
  CardioThoracic Systems Stabilizer
    coronary artery s.
  Cohn cardiac s.
stab-in epicardial electrode
stable
  s. angina
  s. angina pectoris (SAP)
staccato pain
Stachrom PAI chromogenic assay
Stachybotrys atra
Stack
  S. autoperfusion balloon
  S. perfusion catheter
stacked inspiratory spirometry
stacking
  breath s.
Stadie-Riggs microtome
stadiometer
STAE
  subsegmental transcatheter arterial
    embolization
Stagesic
staging
  TNM s.

stagnant
    s. anoxia
    s. hypoxia
stagnation
    contrast s.
stain, staining
    acetoorcein s.
    Alcian blue-PAS s.
    Azan-Mallory s.
    calcofluor s.
    Coomassie blue s.
    Dieterle s.
    Diff-Quik s.
    direct immunofluorescent s.
    endocardial s.
    Giemsa s.
    GMS s.
    Goldner trichrome s.
    Gomori methenamine silver s.
    Gram s.
    Grocott s.
    H&E s.
    hematoxylin-eosin s.
    hematoxylin-phloxine-safran s.
    immunoperoxidase s.
    Kinyoun s.
    Mallory s.
    Masson trichrome s.
    May-Grünwald-Giemsa s.
    Miller elastic s.
    Movat s.
    mucicarmine s.
    NK-104 s.
    Oil Red O s.
    Pappenheim s.
    picrosirius red s.
    Pizzolatto s.
    propidium iodide s.
    silver-methenamine s.
    Sirius red s.
    toluidine blue s.
    TTC s.
    TUNEL s.
    van Gieson s.
    Verhoeff elastica s.
    Verhoeff tissue elastin s.
    Weigert-van Gieson s.
    Wright s.
    Wright-Giemsa s.
    Ziehl-Neelsen s.
stainless
    316L s. steel

316LVM s. steel
    s. steel balloon expandable stent
    s. steel guidewire
    s. steel mesh stent
staircase phenomenon
STALD
    Sheffield Screening Test for Acquired
    Language Disorders
Stamey test
STAMI
    Stenting for Acute Myocardial Infarction
    STAMI clinical trial
stand-alone
    s.-a. balloon angioplasty
    s.-a. laser treatment
standard
    s. atmosphere
    Boehringer Mannheim s.
    s. Bruce protocol
    s. deviation
    Feinstein methodologic s.
    hypertension s.
    s. Lehman catheter
    s. limb lead
    s. needle
standby
    s. pacemaker
    s. pulse generator
Stand Displacement Amplification test
standstill
    atrial s.
    auricular s.
    cardiac s.
    respiratory s.
    sinus s.
    ventricular s.
Stanford
    S. aortic dissection
    S. biopsy method
    S. bioptome
    S. Coronary Risk Intervention
    Project (SCRIP)
    S. Coronary Risk Intervention
    Reversibilty Project
    S. treadmill exercise protocol
    S. type B aortic dissection
Stanford-Caves bioptome
Stanicor pacemaker
stannic oxide
Stannius ligature
stannosis
stanozolol anabolic steroid

NOTES

Stansel procedure
Staphcillin
staphyledema
staphylococcal
    s. bronchitis
    s. endocarditis
    s. infection
    s. pneumonia
Staphylococcus
    S. aureus
    S. epidermidis
    S. pyogenes aureus
staphylokinase
staphylopharyngorrhaphy
stapled lung reduction
stapler
    Androsov vascular s.
    Ethicon Endopath EZ45 and
      TL60 s.
    Inokucki vascular s.
stapling
    bleb s.
star
    S. Cancellation Test (SCT)
    S. Sync
starch
    hydroxyethyl s.
STARFLex occluder
Starling
    S. curve
    S. equation
    S. force
    S. law
    S. mechanism
Starr-Edwards
    S.-E. aortic valve prosthesis
    S.-E. ball-and-cage valve
    S.-E. ball valve prosthesis
    S.-E. cardiac valve prosthesis
    S.-E. disk valve prosthesis
    S.-E. heart valve prosthesis
    S.-E. mitral prosthesis
    S.-E. mitral valve
    S.-E. prosthetic valve
    S.-E. Silastic valve
    S.-E. valve
STARS
    Stent Antithrombotic Regimen Study
START
    Saruplase and Taprostene Acute
      Reocclusion Trial
    Selection of Thymidine Analog Regimen
      Therapy
    Stents and Radiation Therapy
    Stent versus Angioplasty Restenosis Trial
    Stent versus Directional Coronary
      Atherectomy Randomized Trial

St. Thomas Atherosclerosis Regression
    Trial
Study of Thrombolytic Therapy with
    Additional Response Following
    Taprostene
Stary
    S. classification
    S. grading
stasis, pl. stases
    s. cirrhosis
    s. dermatitis
    s. edema
    pressure s.
    s. ulcer
    venous s.
STAT
    S.4 protein
    S.6 protein
    S. protein family
Stat
    signal transducer and activator of
      transcription
    Stat 2 Pumpette
    Stat View software
state
    acute confusional s. (ACS)
    cardiovascular steady s.
    glycometabolic s.
    gradient recalled acquisition in a
      steady s. (GRASS)
    hypercoagulable s.
    hyperdynamic s.
    hyperinsulinemic euglycemic clamp
      metabolic s.
    hyperkinetic s.
    postabsorptive s.
    postictal s.
    prothrombotic s.
State-Trait
    S.-T. Anger Expression Inventory
      (STAXI)
    S.-T. Anxiety Inventory
stathmokinesis
static
    s. dilation technique
    s. lung compliance
    s. lung volume
statin therapy
station
    MedicAIR PLUS spirometry s.
    PlugStation earplug s.
    s. pull-through
stationary bicycle
Stat-padz defibrillator patch
Stat-Shell disposable pulse oximeter
  sensor
status
    acute-on-chronic s.

s. anginosus
s. asthmaticus
battery s.
cardiac s.
s. epilepticus
functional s.
IND s.
investigational new drug s.
mental s.
neurologic s.
pulmonary function s.
work s.
staurosporine
stave cell
stavudine
STAXI
State-Trait Anger Expression Inventory
stay
length of s. (LOS)
S. Trim Diet Gum
STD
ST segment depression
Stead-Wells water-seal type spirometer
steady Doppler
steady-state method
steal
coronary s.
endoperoxide s.
iliac s.
s. mechanism
s. phenomenon
pulmonary artery s.
renal-splanchnic s.
subclavian s.
transmural s.
steam-fitter's asthma
steam tent
stearothermophilus
Bacillus s.
steatorrhea
steatosis
s. cardiaca
s. cordis
steel
316L stainless s.
316LVM stainless s.
Steele bronchial dilator
Steell murmur
steel-winged butterfly needle
steep left anterior oblique projection
steeple sign

steepling
s. of trachea
tracheal s.
steerable
s. angioplastic guidewire
s. catheter
s. decapolar electrode catheter
s. electrode catheter
s. guidewire catheter
s. over-the-wire angioplasty
technique
Steerocath catheter
Stegemann-Stalder method
Steidele complex
Steinberg thumb sign
Steinert
S. disease
S. myotonic dystrophy
Stela electrode lead
stellate
s. ganglion
s. ganglion blockade
Stellite
S. ring material
S. ring material of prosthetic valve
stem
s. bronchus
s. cell factor (SCF)
SmartKard digital Holter system s.
transposition of arterial s.
Stemex
Stemphylium lanuginosum
stenocardia
stenosal murmur
stenosis, pl. **stenoses**
airway s.
aortic s. (AS)
bottle-neck s.
branch pulmonary artery s.
bronchial s.
buttonhole s.
buttonhole mitral s.
calcific mitral s.
calcific nodular aortic s.
caroticovertebral s.
carotid s.
carotid artery s. (CAS)
chronic aortic s.
cicatricial s.
congenital aortic s.
congenital mitral s.
coronary artery s.

S

NOTES

beStent s.
beStent 2 coronary s.
beStent Rival s.
bifurcated s.
biocompatible s.
biodegradable s.
BioDiamond s.
BioDiamond F s.
BioDiamond Micro s.
BiodivYsio s.
BiodivYsio PC s.
BX s.
BX IsoStent s.
BX Velocity s.
CardioCoil coronary s.
carotid s.
Carpentier s.
cell-coated s.
cell-seeded s.
coil s.
co-knitted s.
Cook intracoronary s.
Cordis coronary s.
Cordis CrossFlex coronary s.
Cordis tantalum s.
Cordis tantalum coil s.
Coronary Cardiocoil s.
Cragg s.
s. creep
CrossFlex s.
CrossFlex coil s.
CrossFlex LC coronary s.
CrossFlex LC-stainless steel, laser-
  cut coronary s.
Crown s.
cutting balloon before s.
Dart coronary s.
s. delivery system (SDS)
s. deployment
Devon-Pura s.
diaphragm of s.
DivYsio s.
DivYsio PC-coated s.
DNA-coated s.
double-J s.
s. dressing
drug-loaded biodegradable
  polymer s.
Dumon endobronchial silicone s.
Dumon tracheobronchial s.
Dynamic Y s.

Elastalloy Ultraflex Strecker
  nitinol s.
eluting s.
s. embolization
emergency bailout s.
EndoPro s.
Enforcer SDS coronary s.
Esophacoil self-expanding
  esophageal s.
Expander s.
s. expansion
flat wire coil s.
Flex s.
flexible s.
flexible coil s.
Focustent coronary s.
fork s.
Freedom coronary s.
Freedom Force coronary s.
Freitag s.
Genus s.
GFX s.
GFX-2 coronary stent s.
GFX Micro III s.
GFX over-the-wire coronary s.
Gianturco-Roubin s.
Gianturco-Roubin Flex II s.
Gianturco Z s.
Global Therapeutics V-Flex s.
gold-coated Inflow coronary s.
s. graft (SG)
GRI s.
GRII coronary s.
Guidant s.
hand-crimped s.
hand-mounted s.
Harrell Y s.
heat-activated recoverable
  temporary s. (HARTS)
heat-expandable s.
helical coil s.
Hepamed-coated Wiktor s.
Hood stoma s.
Hood-Westaby T-Y s.
Igaki-Tamai s.
s. implantation
S. Implantation Post Rotational
  Atherectomy Trial (SPORT)
Inflow Dynamics Antares
  coronary s.
InFlow Flex s.
InStent CarotidCoil s.

NOTES

stent *(continued)*
    InStent VascuCoil s.
    interdigitating coil s.
    IntraCoil self expanding nitinol s.
    intravascular s.
    INX s.
    Iris coronary s.
    Iris II s.
    IsoStent s.
    s. jail
    J & J s.
    Johnson & Johnson biliary s.
    Johnson & Johnson coronary s.
    Johnson and Johnson Interventional
      Systems s.
    Jomed s.
    Jostent s.
    Jostent Bifurcation s.
    Jostent coronary s.
    Jostent Flex s.
    Jostent Plus s.
    Jostent Sidebranch s.
    kissing s.
    Laser Angioplasty in
      Restenosed S.'s (LARS)
    LP s.
    Mac s.
    Magic Wallstent s.
    Medex coronary C1 s.
    Medinol NIR s.
    Medinol NIRside slotted s.
    Medivent self-expanding coronary s.
    Medivent vascular s.
    Medtronic AVE S660 coronary s.
    Medtronic beStent s.
    Medtronic interventional vascular s.
    Med-X s.
    Memotherm s.
    mesh s.
    Micro s.
    Micro S. II
    Micro II s.
    6 Micro S. PL
    Microstent s.
    s. migration
    MINI Crown s.
    MS-CIS SV s.
    MSM-BMS s.
    MSM-Stent s.
    MSM-Stent SV s.
    multicellular s.
    Multi-Flex s.
    Multi-Link Ascent s.
    Multi-Link Duet s.
    Multi-Link Solo s.
    Navius s.
    Neville s.
    NexStent carotid s.

    Nexus coronary s.
    NIR s.
    NIR 5 Cell s.
    NIR 7 Cell s.
    NIR 9 Cell s.
    NIROYAL Advance s.
    NIROYAL Elite s.
    NIR Primo Monorail s.
    NIR Royal s.
    NIR-Royal s.
    nitinol mesh s.
    nitinol self-expandable s.
    nitinol self-expanding coil s.
    nitinol thermal memory s.
    nonarticulated s.
    Novastent s.
    nuclear s.
    Omega s.
    Optimal Coronary Balloon
      Angioplasty versus S. (OCBAS)
    Orlowski s.
    Ostia s.
    Palmaz s.
    Palmaz balloon-expandable iliac s.
    Palmaz-Schatz s. (PSS)
    Palmaz-Schatz balloon-expandable s.
    Palmaz-Schatz coronary s.
    Palmaz-Schatz Crown s.
    Palmaz-Schatz PS-204 s.
    Palmaz vascular s.
    Paragon coronary s.
    Paragon nitinol s.
    Paragon PAS s.
    Passager s.
    s. patency
    Phytis s.
    s. placement
    poly-L-lactic acid s.
    polymeric endoluminal paving s.
    polyorganophosphazene-coated s.
    polypropylene s.
    polytetraflouroethylene-covered s.
    Power Grip s.
    ^{32}P radioactive s.
    premounted s.
    S. Primary Angioplasty for
      Myocardial Infarction (STENT
      PAMI)
    PS 153 s.
    PTFE-covered s.
    Pura s.
    Pura-Vario s.
    Pura-Vario-A s.
    Pura-Vario-AL s.
    Pura-Vario-AS s.
    S.'s and Radiation Therapy
      (START)
    radioactive s.

radiopaque tantalum s.
Radius self-expanding s.
s. reconstruction
Reduced Anticoagulation in
  Saphenous Vein Graft S.
  (RAVES)
S. Restenosis Study (STRESS)
Rivetti-Levinson intraluminal s.
Roubin-Gianturco flexible coil s.
R-Stent s.
Schatz-Palmaz intravascular s.
Schatz-Palmaz tubular mesh s.
Schneider s.
Schneider Speedy s.
Scimed s.
S670 coronary s.
screw-thread s.
Seaquence s.
self-expandable metallic s.
self-expanding s.
self-expanding microporous s.
  (SEMS)
short s.
Sinus s.
slotted s.
slotted tube s.
slotted tube articulated s.
Sorin Carbostent s.
spring-loaded s.
spring-loaded vascular s.
S660 small vessel s.
stainless steel balloon
  expandable s.
stainless steel mesh s.
Stent Tech s.
Strecker s.
Strecker balloon-expandable s.
Strecker coronary s.
Strecker tantalum s.
s. strut
Supra G coronary s.
s. or surgery
Symphony s.
Symphony nitinol s.
T s.
tantalum s.
S. Tech stent
Tenax s.
Tenax Complete s.
Tenax coronary s.
Tenax-XR s.
Tenax-XR Trinity s.

Tensum coronary s.
Terumo s.
thermal memory s.
thermoexpandable s.
s. thrombosis (ST)
Tower s.
Tracheobronxane ST tracheal s.
Transluminal Extraction Catheter
  Before S. (TECBEST)
S. Treatment Region Assessed by
  Ultrasound Tomography
T-shaped s.
tubular s.
tubular slotted s.
T-Y s.
Ultraflex self-expanding s.
Ultraflex tracheobronchial s.
VascuCoil peripheral vascular s.
Velocity s.
S. versus Angioplasty Restenosis
  Trial (START)
S. versus Directional Coronary
  Atherectomy Randomized Trial
  (START)
V-Flex FMJ s.
V-Flex Plus s.
Wallstent flexible, self-expanding
  wire-mesh s.
Wallstent Magic s.
Wallstent spring-loaded s.
Wiktor s.
Wiktor balloon expandable
  coronary s.
Wiktor coronary s.
Wiktor GX s.
Wiktor GX coronary s.
Wiktor-I s.
Wiktor-I implantable s.
wire mesh self-expandable s.
XT s.
XT coronary s.
XT radiopaque coronary s.
X-Trode s.
Y s.
Z s.
zigzag s.
stentable disease
stent-anchoring device
**stent-assisted coiling of basilar fusiform
  aneurysm**
stented bioprosthetic valve
stenter

NOTES

S

stent-graft
    Ancure s.-g.
    Inoue endovascular s.-g.
    transluminally placed Inoue
      endovascular s.-g.
STENTIM
    Stenting in Acute Myocardial Infarction
    STENTIM clinical trial
STENTIM-2
    Stenting with Elective Wiktor Stent in
    Acute Myocardial Infarction
    STENTIM-2 clinical trial
stenting
    S. for Acute Myocardial Infarction
    (STAMI)
    S. in Acute Myocardial Infarction
    (STENTIM)
    airway s.
    bailout s.
    Brockenbrough atrial s.
    carotid angioplasty and s. (CAS)
    carotid angioplasty with s.
    carotid artery s.
    S. in Chronic Coronary Occlusion
    (SICCO)
    coronary s.
    endoluminal s.
    Enoxaparin and Ticlopidine after
    Elective S. (ENTICES)
    Evaluation of IIb/IIIa Platelet
    Inhibitor for S.
    femoropopliteal s.
    Heparin Infusion Prior to S.
    (HIPS)
    high-pressure balloon s.
    Integrilin to Minimize Platelet
    Aggregation and Coronary
    Thrombosis in S. (IMPACT-Stent)
    intracoronary s.
    kissing s.
    Scripps Coronary Radiation to
    Inhibit Proliferation Post S.
    (SCRIPPS)
    s. in small arteries (SISA)
    S. of Total Occlusion versus
    PTCA (STOP)
    transradial primary s.
    S. with Elective Wiktor Stent in
    Acute Myocardial Infarction
    (STENTIM-2)
    Y s.
stent-jail orifice
stentless
    s. porcine aortic valve
    s. porcine aortic valve prosthesis
    s. porcine bioprosthesis
    s. porcine valve (SPV)
    s. porcine xenograft

    s. prosthesis
    s. valve
stent-mounted
    s.-m. allograft valve
    s.-m. heterograft valve
stentomania
STENT PAMI
    Stent Primary Angioplasty for
    Myocardial Infarction
    STENT PAMI clinical trial
stent/system
S.T.E.P.
    Short Transitional Edge Protection
step
    Krönig s.
    s. treadmill protocol
step-down therapy
Step-One Diet
stepped bur approach
stepped-care antihypertensive regimen
Step-Two Diet
SteptyP hemostasis bandage
step-up in oxygen saturation
stepwise
Sterapred Oral
stercoralis
    Strongyloides s.
stereoauscultation
stereolithography
stereoscopic interrogation
Sterges carditis
Steri-Cath catheter
Steri-Neb
Sterles sign
Sterna-Band self-locking suture
sternad
sternal
    s. border
    s. compression
    s. dehiscence
    s. extremity of clavicle
    s. fracture
    s. notch
    s. part of diaphragm
    s. plane
    s. synchondrosis
    s. wiring
sternalgia
sternal-splitting incision
Sternberg
    S. myocardial insufficiency
    S. pericarditis
    S. sign
Sterneedle tuberculin test
sternochondral junction
sternoclavicular angle
sternocleidomastoid artery
sternocostal triangle

sternodynia
sternomastoid
sternotome
sternotomy
    median s.
sternotracheal
sternoxiphoid plane
Stern posture
sternum
    s. saw
    wiring of s.
steroid
    s. aerosol
    anabolic s.
    s. elution
    high-dose s.
    nasal s. (NS)
    sex s.
    stanozolol anabolic s.
steroid-dependent
    s.-d. asthma
    s.-d. asthmatic
steroid-eluting
    s.-e. electrode
    s.-e. pacemaker lead
steroidogenesis
steroid-resistant asthma
steroids
steroid-sparing agent
Ster-O$_2$-Mist ultrasonic cup
stertor
    hen-cluck s.
stertorous respiration
Stertzer
    S. brachial catheter
    S. guiding catheter
    S.-Myler extension wire
stethoscope
    Acoustascope esophageal s.
    bell s.
    Cardiology II s.
    CareTone II telephonic s.
    Classic II s.
    differential s.
    Doppler fetal s.
    double-headed s.
    EST40 s.
    Harvey Elite s.
    Labtron s.
    Littman class II pediatric s.
    Rappaport-Sprague s.
    ST3 s.

stethoscopic phonocardiograph
Stevens-Johnson syndrome
Stewart-Hamilton cardiac output
    technique
STG
    superior temporal gyrus
sthenic fever
STI
    systolic time interval
stibogluconate sodium
STICH
    Surgical Treatment for Intracerebral
      Hemorrhage
      STICH clinical trial
stick
    arterial s.
    Vaxcel mini s.
Stifcore
    S. aspiration needle
    S. biopsy injection needle
stiff
    s. heart
    s. heart syndrome
    s. left atrium syndrome
    s. lung
stiffness
    active dynamic s.
    chamber s.
    diastolic s.
    elastic s.
    s. index
    muscle s.
    myocardial s.
    vascular s.
    ventricular systolic s.
    volume s.
stigma, pl. stigmata
    peripheral stigmata
Stilith implantable cardiac pulse
    generator
Still
    S. disease
    S. murmur
Stilphostrol
stimulant
    adrenergic s.
stimulated acoustic emission
stimulation
    alpha-adrenergic s.
    beta-adrenergic s.
    beta-1-adrenergic s.
    beta-2-adrenergic s.

S

NOTES

stimulation (*continued*)
 beta adrenoceptor s.
 blood monocyte s.
 carotid sinus s.
 direct s.
 functional magnetic s.
 muscarinic s.
 noninvasive programmed s. (NIPS)
 paired electrical s.
 postganglionic vagal s. (PGVS)
 programmed electrical s. (PES)
 programmed ventricular s. (PVS)
 reflex s.
 slaved programmed electrical s.
 subthreshold s.
 supramaximal tetanic s.
 s. threshold
 transcranial magnetic s. (TMS)
 transcutaneous electrical s. (TES)
 transesophageal atrial s. (TRAS)
 ultrarapid subthreshold s.
 vagal s.
 vagal nerve s.
 ventricular-programmed s.
stimulator
 Arzco model 7 cardiac s.
 Atrostim phrenic nerve s.
 Bloom programmable s.
 Grass S88 muscle s.
 InSync s.
 InSync multisite cardiac s.
 Quik-Coff electrical cough s.
stimulus, pl. **stimuli**
 chemical s.
 heterotopic s.
 hypercapnic s.
 ischemic-type preconditioning s.
 neurohumoral s.
 nomatopic s.
 pacing s.
 paired s.
 physical s.
 premature s.
 psychological s.
 square wave s.
 thrombogenic s.
 triple s.
stimulus-T interval
stippling of lung field
stochastic risk
Stockert cardiac pacing electrode
stocking-glove distribution
stockings
 antiembolism s.
 A-T antiembolism s.
 Bellavar medical support s.
 Camp-Sigvaris s.

 Carolon life support
  antiembolism s.
 compression s.
 Comtesse medical support s.
 elastic s.
 Fast-Fit vascular s.
 Florex medical compression s.
 graduated compression s. (GCS)
 Jobst-Stride support s.
 Jobst-Stridette support s.
 Jobst VPGS s.
 Juzo s.
 Kendall compression s.
 Linton elastic s.
 Medi-Strumpf s.
 Medi vascular s.
 pneumatic compression s.
 Sigvaris compression s.
 Stride support s.
 TED antiembolism s.
 thigh-high antiembolic s.
 True Form support s.
 Twee alternating cut-off
  compressor s.
 Vairox high compression
  vascular s.
 VenES II Medical s.
 Venofit medical compression s.
 Venoflex medical compression s.
 venous pressure gradient support s.
 Zimmer antiembolism support s.
stocking-seam incision
stoichiometric fashion
Stokes
 S.-Adams attack
 S.-Adams disease
 S.-Adams syndrome
 collar of S.
 S. expectorant
Stokvis-Talma syndrome
Stoll pneumonia
stoma
 tracheostomy s.
stomach
 s. cough
 left coronary artery of s.
Stomatococcus
stone
 s. asthma
 s. heart
 lung s.
stone-cutter's phthisis
stone-like myxoma
stone-stripper's asthma
stool
 s. fat balance study
 melenic s.

STOP
    Stenting of Total Occlusion versus PTCA
    STOP clinical trial
Stop
    S. at Ring lead
    S. at Tip lead
STOP-AF
    Systemic Trial of Pacing to Prevent
    Atrial Fibrillation
stopcock
    three-way s.
stop-valve airway obstruction
storage
    tracer s.
store
    myocyte magnesium s.
stored electrocardiogram
storm
    electric s.
    thyroid s.
Storz
    S. bronchoscope
    S. bronchoscopic telescope
    S.-Hopkins laryngoscope
    S.-Shapshay tracheoscope
    S. tracheoscope
straddling
    s. aorta
    s. atrioventricular valve
    s. embolism
    s. thrombus
    s. tricuspid valve
    s. of valve
straight
    s. back syndrome
    s. flush percutaneous catheter
    s. hemostat
    s. sinus thrombosis
    s. stylet
    s. tipped catheter
    s. tube graft
straight-line ECG
StraightShot arterial cannula
strain
    carer s.
    cell s.
    s. gauge
    0157-H7 s.
strain-gauge plethysmography
stramonium
strand
    iridium s.

stranding effusion
strandy infiltrate
strap
    hook-and-loop fastener s.
    s. muscle
    Pepper Medical Antidisconnect
    Device s.
Strasburger cell plate
STRATAS
    Study to Determine Rotablator and
    Transluminal Angioplasty Strategy
strategy
    Study to Determine Rotablator and
    Transluminal Angioplasty S.
    (STRATAS)
    Treat Angina with Aggrastat and
    Determine Costs of Therapy with
    Invasive or Conservative S.'s
    (TACTICS)
stratification
    risk s.
stratified thrombus
stratigraphy
Stratus
    S. cardiac troponin I test
    S. instrument
Strauss method
streak
    fatty s.
streaking
    basophilic vascular s.
streaky infiltrate
Strecker
    S. balloon-expandable stent
    S. coronary stent
    S. stent
    S. tantalum stent
strength
    Allerest Maximum S.
    Bayer Low Adult S.
    peripheral muscle s. (PMS)
    Theraflu Non-Drowsy Formula
    Maximum S.
    s. training
    Tylenol Flu Maximum S.
strenuous exercise
Streptase
streptavidin
Streptobacillus moniliformis
streptococcal
    s. antibody
    s. bacteremia

S

NOTES

streptococcal *(continued)*
    s. bronchitis
    s. carditis
    s. empyema
    s. endocarditis
    s. infection
    s. pneumonia
Streptococcus
    S. agalactiae
    S. anginosus
    S. faecalis
    S. milleri
    S. mitis
    penicillin-nonsusceptible *S. pneumoniae* (PNSP)
    penicillin-resistant *S. pneumoniae* (PRSP)
    S. pneumoniae
    S. pyogenes
    S. salivarius
    S. viridans
streptodornase
streptogramin antibiotic
streptokinase (SK)
    s. antibody
streptokinase-plasminogen complex
streptokinase-streptodornase
streptolysin-O
Streptomyces tsukubaensis
streptomycin sulfate
streptozocin
STRESS
    Stent Restenosis Study
stress
    adenosine s.
    circumferential end-systolic s. (cESS)
    circumferential wall s. (CWS)
    dipyridamole s.
    S. Echo bed
    s. echocardiography
    emotional s.
    end-systolic s. (ESS)
    end-systolic circumferential wall s.
    end-systolic left ventricular s. (ESS)
    end-systolic wall s.
    handgrip s.
    left ventricular end-systolic s.
    left ventricular wall s.
    mental s.
    meridional end-systolic s. (mESS)
    meridional wall s.
    s. MUGA electrocardiogram
    oxidative s.
    s. perfusion and rest function
    s. perfusion and rest function by sestamibi-gated SPECT

    s. perfusion scintigraphy
    pharmacologic s.
    physiological s.
    s. relaxation
    shear s.
    s. SPECT perfusion imaging
    tensile s.
    s. test
    s. thallium-201 myocardial perfusion imaging
    s. thallium scintigraphy
    s. thallium study
    ventricular end-systolic wall s.
    ventricular wall s.
    wall s.
    s. washout myocardial perfusion image
stress-injected
    s.-i. sestamibi-gated SPECT with echocardiography
stressor
    remedial psychological s.
stress-redistribution-reinjection thallium-201 imaging
stress-related
    s.-r. arrhythmia
    s.-r. hypertension
stress-shortening relationship
stretch
    atrial s.
    S. balloon
    s.-induced cardiomyocyte hypertrophy
    s. receptor
stretched
    s. bronchus sign
    s. diameter
stretching
    side s.
    s. syncope
stria, pl. **striae**
striation
    tabby cat s.
    tigroid s.
striatocapsular infarction
stricture
    anastomotic s.
    esophageal s.
    Wickwitz esophageal s.
Stride
    S. cardiac pacemaker
    S. support stockings
strident
stridor
    biphasic s.
    congenital laryngeal s.
    inspiratory s.
    laryngeal s.

respiratory s.
s. serraticus
stridulosa
laryngitis s.
stridulous respiration
stridulus
laryngismus s.
strike
heel s.
string
s. of pearls
s. sign
strip
bovine pericardium s.
Breathe Right nasal s.
cardiac monitor s.
Cover-Strip wound closure s.'s
ECG monitor s.
felt s.
Flu-Glow s.
s. percussion
rhythm s.
stripchart tracing
stripe
s. sign
subepicardial fat s.
stripper
Alexander rib s.
Cole polyethylene vein s.
Dorian rib s.
Doyle vein s.
Dunlop thrombus s.
Emerson vein s.
hydraulic vein s.
Kurten vein s.
Linton vein s.
Matson-Alexander rib s.
New Orleans endarterectomy s.
thrombus s.
Trace vein s.
Zollinger-Gilmore intraluminal
vein s.
stroke
acute caudate s.
acute hemispheric s.
acute ischemic s. (AIS)
atheroembolic s.
atherothrombotic s.
s. belt
brain stem s.
cardioembolic s. (CES)
cardiogenic s.

Cardiovascular Disease,
Hypertension and Hyperlipidemia,
Adult-Onset Diabetes, Obesity,
and S. (CHAOS)
caudate s.
caudate hemorrhagic s.
caudate ischemic s.
cortical s.
crude s.
cryptogenic s.
early progressing s. (EPS)
S. Education Program (SEP)
s. ejection rate
embolic s.
s. guidance system (SGS)
heart s.
heat s.
hemorrhagic s.
S. Impact Scale (SIS)
s. index
ipsilateral s.
ischemic s.
lacunar s.
late progressing s. (LPS)
left hemisphere s. (LCVA)
light s.
MRI s.
MRI-identified s.
National Institutes of Neurological
Disorders and S. (NINDS)
s. output
S. Prevention in Atrial Fibrillation
(SPAF)
S. Prevention in Atrial Fibrillation
III Transesophageal Echo (SPAF
TEE)
S. Prevention in Nonrheumatic
Atrial Fibrillation (SPINAF)
pure motor s.
pure sensorimotor s.
pure sensory s.
right hemisphere s.
sensorimotor s.
silent s.
subcortical s.
thromboembolic s.
undetermined pathological-type s.
s. unit (SU)
Vitamins to Prevent S.
(VITATOPS)
s. volume (SV)
s. volume index (SVI)

NOTES

S

stroke *(continued)*
    s. work
    s. work index (SWI)
stroke-specific quality of life (SS-QOL)
stroma-free
    s.-f. hemoglobin pyridoxilated
    (SFHb)
    s.-f. hemoglobin solution
strong
    S. Heart Study (SHS)
    Thyroid S.
    S. unbridling of celiac artery axis
Strongyloides stercoralis
strongyloidiasis
strontium-82 (^{82}So)
Stroop color word conflict test
Strophanthus gratus
Strouhal number
structural
    s. heart disease (SHD)
    s. valve deterioration (SVD)
structure
    chordal s.
    echodense s.
    tubuloreticular s.
    wall s.
struma
    Riedel s.
strut
    Adkin s.
    central bridging s.
    George Washington s.
    stent s.
    tricuspid valve s.
strutting
    plaque s.
Stryker saw
ST-segment reelevation
ST-T
    ST-T deviation
    ST-T segment change
    ST-T wave
    ST-T wave changes
Stuart-Prower factor
study *(See also* trial, program, protocol)
    ABC S.
    ACCESS s.
    ACIP s.
    acute myocardial infarction s. of
    adenosine (AMISTAD)
    Acute Stroke S. (ASS)
    Adjunctive Balloon Angioplasty
    Following Coronary
    Atherectomy S. (ABACAS)
    African-American Antiplatelet Stroke
    Prevention S. (AAASPS)
    AIRE s.

Air Force coronary/Texas
    atherosclerosis prevention s.
    (AFCAPS/TexCAPS)
ALL s.
altitude simulation s.
amyl nitrite s.
Antiphospholipid Antibodies in
    Stroke S. (APASS)
arterial revascularization therapy s.
    (ARTS)
ASPECT s.
Aspirin in Myocardial Infarction S.
    (AMIS)
Asymptomatic Carotid Artery
    Plaque S. (ACAPS)
Asymptomatic Carotid Artery
    Progression S. (ACAPS)
asymptomatic carotid
    atherosclerosis s. (ACAS)
ATLAS s.
atrial pacing s.
AVID s.
benazepril heart failure s. (BHFS)
BIP s.
Cambridge Heart Antioxidant S.
    (CHAOS)
Canadian Activase for Stroke
    Effectiveness S. (CASES)
Canadian American Ticlopidine S.
    (CATS)
Canadian Atrial Fibrillation S.
    (CAFS)
Canadian Implantable
    Defibrillator S. (CIDS)
Captopril and Digoxin S. (CADS)
Captopril and Thrombolysis S.
    (CATS)
CARAFE s.
CARDIA s.
Cardiac Arrhythmia Pilot S.
    (CAPS)
Cardiac Insufficiency Bisoprolol S.
    (CIBIS)
Carotid and Vertebral Artery
    Transluminal Angioplasty S.
    (CAVATAS)
CARPORT s.
Carvedilol Heart Attack Pilot S.
    (CHAPS)
CASANOVA s.
case-control s.
CCC s.
CHAOS s.
CHIC s.
Cholesterol Lowering
    Atherosclerosis S. (CLAS)
Clomethiazole Acute Stroke S.
    (CLASS)

CLOUT s.
cohort s.
contrast bubble s.
Cooperative North Scandinavian Enalapril Survival S. (CONSENSUS)
Coronary Artery Surgery S. (CASS)
CRAC s.
cross-sectional ventilatory functional s.
CRUISE s.
DASH s.
DAVID multicenter comparative s.
S. to Determine Rotablator and Transluminal Angioplasty Strategy (STRATAS)
Diabetes Atherosclerosis Intervention S. (DAIS)
DIG s.
   Digitalis Investigation Group
DIG-CAPTOPRIL s.
dipyridamole thallium-201 cardiac perfusion s.
Doppler s.
EC/IC arterial bypass s.
S. of Economics and Quality of Life (SEQOL)
electrophysiologic s. (EPS)
electrophysiology s.
ELITE s.
ENTIRE s.
EPIC s.
EPILOG s.
equilibrium-gated blood pool s.
ERA s.
ERASE s.
ERBAC s.
S. to Evaluate Carotid Ultrasound Changes with Ramipril and Vitamin E (SECURE)
exercise s.
Familial Atherosclerosis Treatment S. (FATS)
FASTER s.
floating wall motion s.
Framingham Heart S. (FHS)
gated blood-pool s. (GBPS)
gated blood-pool cardiac wall motion s.
GUSTO s.
HART s.

HEAP s.
Heart and Estrogen-Progestin Replacement S. (HERS)
hemodynamic-angiographic s.
HOPE s.
HOT s.
hypoxic response s.
imaging s.
Insulin Resistance Atherosclerosis S. (IRAS)
International Carotid Stenting S. (ICSS)
International S. of Infarct Survival (ISIS)
interventional s.
intracardiac electrophysiologic s.
LACI S.
LATE S.
LDL Apheresis Atherosclerosis Regression S. (LAARS)
S.'s of Left Ventricular Dysfunction (SOLVD)
LIPID S.
LQTS S.
Medication Use S.'s (MUST)
Medicine, Angioplasty, or Surgery S. (MASS)
S. of Medicine versus Angioplasty Reperfusion Trial (SMART)
meglumine diatrizoate enema s.
Metoprolol and Xamoterol Infarction S. (MEXIS)
S. of Microstent's Ability to Limit Restenosis Trial (SMART)
MOCHA S.
Monitored Atherosclerosis Regression S. (MARS)
S. of Monoclonal Antibody Radioimmunotherapy (SMART)
Multicenter Antiatherosclerotic S. (MAAS)
Multicenter Isradipine/Diuretic Atherosclerosis S. (MIDAS)
Multicenter Stent S. (MUST)
Multivessel Angioplasty Prognosis S. (MAPS)
muscle immunocytochemical s.
myocardial contrast echo s.
Myocardial Infarction Data Acquisition System S. (MIDAS)
myocardial perfusion s.
NACI DCA s.

S

NOTES

study *(continued)*
  Nifedipine Angina Myocardial Infarction S. (NAMIS)
  S. of Nitroglycerin and Chest Pain (SNAP)
  nuclear ventricular function s. (NVFS)
  Optimal Atherectomy Restenosis S. (OARS)
  Pacing in Cardiomyopathy S. (PICS)
  PACT s.
  PASE Quality-of-Life S.
  Patent Foramen Ovale in Cryptogenic Stroke S. (PICSS)
  Patient Outcomes Research Team S. (PORT, PORTS)
  PEACE s.
  Peripheral Artery Radiation Investigational S. (PARIS)
  Persantine and Aspirin Reinfarction S. (PARIS)
  phased array s.
  PICTURE s.
  PIOPED s.
  Piracetam in Acute Stroke S. (PASS)
  PLAC s.
  PLAC-2 s.
  POEM s.
  polysomnographic s.
  Port Access Recovery Improvement S. (PARIS)
  postmenopausal estrogen/progestin interventions s.
  Practical Applicability of Saruplase S. (PASS)
  PRECISE s.
  Prehospital Applicability of Saruplase S. (PASS)
  PRISM s.
  PRISM-PLUS S.
  Quality of Life Hypertension S. (QOLHS)
  RACE s.
  RADIANCE s.
  radioisotopic s.
  radionuclide s.
  Randomized Aldactone Evaluation S. (RALES)
  Regression Growth Evaluation Statin S. (REGRESS)
  RESCUE s.
  RIGHT s.
  RISC s.
  Second International S. of Infarct Survival
  serum enzyme s.
  sleep s.
  SMART s.
  SPAF s.
  SPAF TEE s.
  Stent Antithrombotic Regimen S. (STARS)
  Stent Restenosis S. (STRESS)
  stool fat balance s.
  stress thallium s.
  Strong Heart S. (SHS)
  SWIFT s.
  synchronous atrial pacing s.
  TACTICS s.
  S. of Thrombolytic Therapy with Additional Response Following Taprostene (START)
  Ticlopidine Aspirin Stroke S. (TASS)
  Total Ischemic Burden Bisoprolol S. (TIBBS)
  transcutaneous phrenic nerve conduction s.
  Trial on Reversing Endothelial Dysfunction s.
  VANQWISH s.
  Vasovagal Syncope International S. (VASIS)
  VEGF gene therapy s.
  Vein Graft AngioJet S. (VEGAS)
  Verapamil Angioplasty S. (VAS)
  Verapamil Hypertension Atherosclerosis S.
  Veterans Health S. (VHS)
  wall motion s.
  WASID s.
  Women's Health S. (WHS)
  Women's Intervention Nutrition S. (WINS)

stump
  bronchial s.
  cardiac s.
  s. pressure

stunned
  s. atrium
  s. myocardium

stunning
  left atrial appendage s.
  myocardial s.
  repetitive s.

Sturge-Weber syndrome

stuttering
  s. myocardial infarction
  s. of perfusion

stutzeri
  Pseudallescheria s.
  Pseudomonas s.

stylet
  Bing s.

cardiovascular s.
Cook locking s.
K s.
L s.
locking s.
S s.
straight s.
TFX Medical catheter s.
transmyocardial pacing s.
transthoracic pacing s.
wire s.
Stylus cardiovascular suture
styrene asthma
SU
stroke unit
Sub-4
S. Platinum Plus wire kit
S. small vessel balloon dilatation catheter
subacute
s. bacterial endocarditis (SBE)
s. bronchopneumonia
s. care
s. infective endocarditis
s. myocardial infarction
s. pericarditis
s. tamponade
s. thrombosis (SAT)
s. unit
s. ventricular free wall
subannular mattress suture
subantihypertensive
subaortic
s. lymph node
s. obstruction
s. stenosis
subapicale
segmentum s.
subapical segment
subarachnoid
s. hemorrhage (SAH)
s. space (SAS)
subcarinal node
subclavian
s. approach for cardiac catheterization
s. arteriovenous fistula
s. artery
s. artery bypass graft
s. flap
s. flap aortoplasty (SFA)
s. lymphatic

s. murmur
s. peel-away sheath
s. steal
s. steal syndrome
s. triangle
s. vein
s. vessel
subclavian-carotid bypass
subclavian-subclavian bypass
subclavicular murmur
subclinical
s. asthma
s. hypothyroidism
subcortical
s. junctional infarct
s. stroke
s. vascular encephalopathy (SVE)
subcostal
s. view
s. zone
subcrepitant rale
subcutanea
bursa s.
subcutaneous
s. bursa of the laryngeal prominence
s. emphysema
s. nodule
s. patch
s. patch electrode
s. suture
s. tunneling device
subcuticular suture
subdiaphragmatic
subdiastolic
subdural hematoma (SDH)
subendocardial
s. to epicardial resting perfusion ratio
s. fibrosis
s. ischemia
s. layer
s. myocardial infarction
s. sclerosis
s. zone
subendocardium
subendothelial matrix
subendothelium
subepicardial
s. fat stripe
s. fatty infiltration
suberosis

NOTES

S

subeustachian isthmus
subfascial endoscopic perforator surgery (SEPS)
subglottic
   s. laryngitis
   s. secretion
subinfundibular stenosis
subjective fremitus
subjunctional heart block
sublethal
Sublimaze Injection
sublingual
   S. artery
   S. bursa
   S. caruncula
   S. crescent
   S. gland
   Nitrostat S.
   S. vein
sublingualis
   bursa s.
   caruncula s.
   glandula s.
   vena s.
submassive pulmonary embolism
submaximal
   S. Effort Tourniquet Test
   S. Exercise Performance Substudy (SEPS)
   s. heart rate
   s. maneuver
submaximum heart rate
Sub-Microinfusion catheter
submucosa
   airway s.
submucosal
   s. gland
   s. gland hypertrophy
   s. plaque
submucous
suboptimally visualized
suboptimal visualization
subpectoral
   s. implantation of cardioverter-defibrillator
   s. implantation of pulse generator
subpharyngeal
subphrenic
   s. abscess
   s. recess
   s. space
subpleural
   s. edema
   s. honeycombing
subpulmonary
   s. obstruction
   s. stenosis

subpulmonic
   s. effusion
   s. stenosis
Sub-Q-Set subcutaneous continuous infusion device
Subramanian clamp
subsalicylate
   bismuth s.
subsarcolemma cisterna
subsartorial tunnel
subscript
subsegmental
   s. atelectasis
   s. bronchus
   s. transcatheter arterial embolization (STAE)
subsidiary atrial pacemaker
substance
   myocardial depressant s. (MDS)
   neurotransmitter s.
   s. P
   paramagnetic s.
   proinflammatory s.
   thiobarbituric acid reactive s. (TBARS)
   vasoactive s.
   vasodepressor s.
substernal thyroid
substitute
   Hemolink investigational hemoglobin product or blood s.
   Nu-Trim dietary fat s.
   Rapidgraft arterial vessel s.
substitutional cardiac surgery
substrate
   arrhythmogenic s.
   exogenous s.
   s. gel zymography
   s. metabolism
   tachyarrhythmic s.
substudy
   Submaximal Exercise Performance S. (SEPS)
subsuperior segment
subsuperius
   segmentum s.
subthreshold
   s. pacing
   s. stimulation
subtilis
   Bacillus s.
subtraction
   s. angiography
   digital s.
   functional s.
   intraoperative digital s. (IDIS)
   mask-mode s.

subtype
>Reston s.
>Sudan s.
>Zaire s.

subvalvar stenosis
subvalvular
>s. aortic stenosis
>s. apparatus
>s. mitral stenosis
>s. obstruction

subxiphoid
>s. area
>s. limited pericardiotomy
>s. window

succinate
>cifenline s.
>hydrocortisone hydrogen s.
>hydrocortisone sodium s.
>methylprednisolone s.
>metoprolol s.

succinylcholine chloride
succussion
>hippocratic s.
>s. sounds
>s. splash

sucker
>Churchill s.
>intracardiac s.

sucking
>s. chest
>s. wound

suck reflex
Sucquet
>S. anastomosis
>S.-Hoyer anastomosis

Sucrets Cough Calmers
suction
>diastolic s.
>hydrostatic s.
>nasotracheal s.
>pleural s.
>Pleur-evac s.

suctioning
>cuff s.

Sudafed
>S. Cold & Cough Liquid Caps
>S. Plus Tablet
>S. Severe Cold

Sudan subtype
sudden
>s. cardiac death (SCD)

S. Cardiac Death in Heart Failure Trial (SCD-HeFT)
>s. death
>s. infant death syndrome (SIDS)
>s. rate onset
>s. unexplained death (SUND)
>s. unexplained death syndrome (SUDS)

Sudex
SUDS
>sudden unexplained death syndrome

Sufedrin
sufentanil citrate
suffocate
suffocating gas
suffocation
suffocative
>s. bronchitis
>s. catarrh
>s. goiter

sugar
>capillary blood s. (CBS)
>S. clip
>fasting blood s.
>postprandial blood s.
>s. tumor

Sugarbaker staging system
Sugita clip
Sugiura procedure
suicide ventricle
suis
>*Actinobacillus* s.
>bronchus s.

suit
>anti-G s.
>antigravity s.
>Life S.
>MAST s.

Sular
sulbactam
>ampicillin and s.

sulcus, pl. sulci
>atrioventricular s.
>bulboventricular s.
>coronary s.
>costophrenic s.
>costophrenic sulci
>interventricular s.
>intraparietal s. (IPS)
>s. pulmonalis
>pulmonary s.
>s. terminalis

S

NOTES

sulfadiazine
> silver s.
> s., sulfamethazine, and sulfamerazine

sulfadoxine and pyrimethamine
sulfamerazine
> sulfadiazine, sulfamethazine, and s.

Sulfamethoprim
sulfamethoxazole
sulfamethoxazole/trimethoprim (SMX/TMP)
sulfasalazine
sulfate
> amikacin s.
> amphetamine s.
> atropine s.
> bleomycin s.
> Capastat S.
> capreomycin s.
> chondroitin s.
> debrisoquine s.
> dermatan s.
> dextran s.
> dextroamphetamine s.
> dimethyl s.
> ephedrine s.
> ferrous s.
> gentamicin s.
> guanadrel s.
> guanethidine s.
> hydroxychloroquine s.
> isoprenaline s.
> isoproterenol s.
> lobeline s.
> magnesium s.
> metaproterenol s.
> neomycin s.
> netilmicin s.
> orciprenaline s.
> paromomycin s.
> penbutolol s.
> protamine s.
> quinidine s.
> quinine s.
> sodium tetradecyl s.
> streptomycin s.
> terbutaline s.
> trimethoprim s.
> trospectomycin s.
> vinblastine s.
> vincristine s.
> Wyamine S.

Sulfatrim DS
sulfhydryl depletion hypothesis
sulfide
> hydrogen s.
> selenium s.

sulfinpyrazone

sulfisoxazole
> erythromycin and s.
> s. and phenazopyridine

sulfonamide sensitivity
sulfonate
> sodium polystyrene s.

sulfonylurea
sulfosalicylic acid
sulfoxide
> albendazole s.
> dimethyl s.

sulfur
> s. dioxide (SO_2)
> s. hexafluoride (SF_6)

sulindac
Sullivan
> S. bubble cushion
> S. HumidAire heated humidifier
> S. III CPAP
> S. III nasal continuous positive air pressure device
> S. Mirage nasal mask
> S. nasal variable positive airway pressure unit
> S. V Elite Real Time Clock CPAP machine
> S. VPAP II

sulmazole
Sulphan Blue
SULP II balloon catheter
sum
> ray s.

sumatriptan
Summagraphics digitizing tablet
SummaSketch III digitizing board
summation
> s. beat
> s. gallop (S_7)
> impulse s.
> s. shadow

sump pump
Sumycin Oral
SunBox light box
SUND
> sudden unexplained death
> SUND syndrome

sundowning
Sundt carotid endarterectomy shunt
sunflower asthma
Sun Microsystems Sparcstation 20 workstation
Super-9
> S. guiding cardiac device
> S. guiding catheter

super
> S.-4 catheter ablation system
> S. ArrowFlex catheterization sheath

s. stress test
S. Torque Plus catheter
superdicrotic
superdominant artery
superficial
s. external pudendal artery
s. femoral artery (SFA)
s. medial artery of foot
s. phlebitis
s. pneumonia
superficialis
esophagitis dissecans s.
vein circumflexa iliaca s.
Superflow guiding catheter
superimposed
s. echodensity
s. thrombosis
superimposition
superinfection
bacterial s.
superior
arteria glutealis s.
arteria laryngea s.
s. articular facet of atlas
s. carotid artery
s. cerebellar artery (SCA)
s. costal facet
fovea costalis s.
s. laryngeal artery
s. laryngeal cavity
s. laryngeal vein
s. lobe of right/left lung
s. mesenteric artery (SMA)
s. mesenteric artery bypass
s. mesenteric artery syndrome
s. mesenteric vascular occlusion
s. omental recess
s. parietal lobule (SPL)
s. phrenic lymph node
posterior branch of right s.
s. pulmonary sulcus tumor
s. pulmonary vein
s. pulmonary vein ablation
s. QRS axis
s. sagittal sinus (SSS)
s. temporal gyrus (STG)
s. thalamostriate vein
s. thyroid artery
s. tracheobronchial lymph node
s. triangle sign
s. vascular mediastinum
s. vena cava (SVC)

s. vena cava syndrome
vena laryngea s.
superiores
nodi lymphoidei phrenici s.
nodi lymphoidei
tracheobronchiales s.
superioris
ramus internus nervi laryngei s.
ramus posterior venae pulmonalis
dextrae s.
superius
tuberculum thyroideum s.
supernatant
supernormal
s. conduction
s. recovery phase
supernumerary bronchus
superoinferior heart
superoxide
s. anion
s. catalase
s. dismutase
supersaturation
tissue s.
Superselector Y-K guidewire
supersensitivity
denervation s.
SuperStitch
supersystemic pulmonary artery
pressure
supertension
SuperVent solution
supine
s. bicycle ergometry
s. bicycle stress echocardiography
(SBSE)
s. exercise
s. hypotension syndrome
s. rest gated equilibrium image
supplement
Vivonex Plus nutritional s.
supplemental
s. air
s. motor area (SMA)
s. oxygen
supplementary respiration
supplementation
magnesium s.
supply
adequate blood s.
energy s.
myocardial oxygen s.

S

NOTES

support
Abee s.
advanced cardiac life s. (ACLS)
advanced life s. (ALS)
advanced trauma life s. (ATLS)
basic cardiac life s. (BCLS)
basic life s. (BLS)
biventricular s. (BVS)
bradycardia pacing s.
cardiopulmonary s. (CPS)
Dr. Gibaud thermal health s.
esophageal-directed pressure s.
  (EDPS)
extracorporeal life s. (ECLS)
IMP-Capello arm s.
inotropic s.
mechanical ventilatory s.
noninvasive positive pressure
  ventilatory s.
noninvasive ventilatory s. (NIVS)
pediatric life s. (PALS)
percutaneous cardiopulmonary s.
  (PCPS)
percutaneous cardiopulmonary
  bypass s. (PCBS)
respiratory s.
vasopressor s.
ventilatory s.
volume-assured pressure s. (VAPS)
supported angioplasty
suppository
Truphylline S.
Suppress
suppressant
cough s.
St. Joseph Cough S.
suppressed respiration
suppressible ventricular tachycardia
suppression
s. of arrhythmia
overdrive s.
suppuration
suppurative
s. bronchiectasis
s. necrotizing aspergillosis
s. pericarditis
s. pleurisy
s. pneumonia
supraannular
s. constriction
s. mitral valve replacement
  (SMVR)
s. prosthesis
s. suture ring
suprabulbar palsy
suprachiasmatic nucleus
supraclavicular
s. examination

s. fossa
s. lymph node
s. lymph node biopsy
supracoronary
supracristal
s. defect
s. ventricular septal defect
supradiaphragmatic
Supra G coronary stent
supraglottoplasty
suprahepatic caval clamp
suprahisian block
supramarginal gyrus (SMG)
supramaximal tetanic stimulation
Suprane
supranormal
s. conduction
s. excitability
s. excitation
suprapleural membrane
suprasellar aneurysm
suprasternal
s. examination
s. notch
s. pulsation
s. view
suprasystolic
supratentorial
s. ICH
s. intracerebral hemorrhage
suprathreshold pacing
supratonsillar recess
supratrochleares
venae s.
supravalvar, supravalvular
s. aortic stenosis (SVAS)
s. aortic stenosis-infantile
s. aortic stenosis-infantile
  hypercalcemia syndrome
s. aortic stenosis syndrome
s. aortography
s. stenosis
supraventricular
s. arrhythmia
s. crest
s. ectopy
s. extrasystole
s. premature beat
s. premature contraction
s. tachyarrhythmia
s. tachycardia (SVT)
supraventricularis
crista s.
Suprax
Supreme electrophysiology catheter
surcingle
Von Lackum s.
surdocardiac syndrome

SURE
Serial Ultrasound Analysis of Restenosis
SURE clinical trial
SureGrip
S. breathing bag
S. manual resuscitator
SureStepPro Professional Blood Glucose Management system
SureTemp electronic thermometer
surface
s. adherent monocyte (SAM)
bio metal s. (BMS)
Carmeda BioActive S.
diaphragmatic s.
pleural s.
surfactant
aerosolized s.
bovine lavage extract s. (BLES)
s. deficiency
heterologous s.
hydrolysis of s.
s. phospholipid
s. protein (SP)
pulmonary s.
Surfacten
Surfaxin
surf test
surgeon
thoracic s.
surgery
ablative cardiac s.
antiarrhythmic s.
bypass s.
cardiac s.
cardiothoracic s. (CTS)
cervical plexus block for carotid endarterectomy s.
coronary artery bypass grafting s.
coronary bypass s.
excisional cardiac s.
extracranial/intracranial bypass s.
keyhole s.
lung volume reduction s. (LVRS)
maze III s.
noncardiac s.
off-pump vascular s.
open s. (OS)
open heart s.
palatal s.
palliative s.
Port-Access minimally invasive cardiac s.

reparative cardiac s.
site-specific s.
stent or s.
subfascial endoscopic perforator s. (SEPS)
substitutional cardiac s.
valve-preserving s.
ventricular reduction s.
video-assisted thoracic s. (VATS)
video-assisted thoracoscopic s. (VATS)
Surgica K6 laser
surgical
s. ablation
s. ablation of pathway
s. embolectomy
s. emphysema
s. intensive care unit (SICU)
s. lung biopsy (SLB)
s. osteosynthesis
s. reexploration
s. revascularization
s. risk
S. Treatment for Intracerebral Hemorrhage (STICH)
s. tuberculosis
Surgicel gauze
Surgiclip
Auto Suture S.
Surgicraft
S. pacemaker electrode
S. suture
Surgilase 150 laser
Surgilon suture
Surg-I-Loop
Surgitool prosthetic valve
Surgitron unit
Surital
Surmontil
Surpasse balloon
Surpass guidewire
Survanta
surveillance
S. angiography
S. bronchoscopy
National Nosocomial Infection S.
S. of Work-related and Occupational Respiratory Disease (SWORD)
S. of Work-related Occupational Respiratory Disease Project

NOTES

S

survey
environmental s.
Jenkins Activity S.
National Health and Nutrition
Examination S.
SF-36 Health S.
Short-Form 36 Health Survey
Short-Form 36 Health S. (SF-36
Health Survey)
Surveyor recording device
survival
Assessment of Treatment with
Lisinopril and S. (ATLAS)
Basal Antiarrhythmic Study of
Infarct S. (BASIS)
Carvedilol Prospective Randomized
Cumulative S. (COPERNICUS)
International Study of Infarct S.
(ISIS)
S. of Myocardial Infarction: Long-
Term Evaluation (SMILE)
Thrombolysis and Counterpulsation
to Improve Cardiogenic Shock S.
(TACTICS)
s. time
S. and Ventricular Enlargement
(SAVE)
S. with Oral D-Sotalol (SWORD)
survivor
Acute Candesartan Clinical
Evaluation of Stroke S.'s
(ACCESS)
susceptibility
s. artifact
R-on-T arrhythmia s.
Susp
Megacillin S.
suspended
s. heart
s. heart syndrome
suspension
Aristocort Intralesional S.
budesonide inhalation s.
calfactant intratracheal s.
CellCept oral s.
Children's Motrin S.
Curosurf intratracheal s.
hyoid s.
s. laryngoscopy
mycophenolate mofetil oral s.
Optison injectable s.
Rynatuss Pediatric S.
suspensory ligament of esophagus
Sus-Phrine
suspicion
index of s.
sustained
s. maximal inspiration (SMI)

s. monomorphic ventricular
tachycardia (SMVT)
s. pulse
s. rate duration
s. release
s. tachycardia
Sustaire
Sustiva
susurrus
Sutterella wadsworthensis
Sutton law
suture
absorbable s.
Acier stainless steel s.
Cardioflon s.
cardiovascular silk s.
chromic catgut s.
Cooley U s.'s
Deklene II cardiovascular s.
Dermalon s.
Dexon s.
Dexon Plus s.
Endoknot s.
end-to-side s.
EPTFE vascular s.'s
Ethibond s.
everting mattress s.
figure-of-eight s.
Frater s.
interrupted pledgeted s.
mattress s.
Mersilene s.
Mersilene braided nonabsorbable s.
Micrins microsurgical s.
monofilament absorbable s.
monofilament polypropylene s.
Nurolon s.
pledgeted mattress s.
Premilene s.
Pronova s.
pursestring s.
pyroglycolic acid s.
reabsorbable s.
Sterna-Band self-locking s.
Stylus cardiovascular s.
subannular mattress s.
subcutaneous s.
subcuticular s.
Surgicraft s.
Surgilon s.
Synthofil s.
Techstar percutaneous s.
through-and-through continuous s.
through-the-wall mattress s.
Ti-Cron s.
traction s.
transfixion s.

Trumbull s.
U s.'s
sutured plaque electrode
suturing
coupled s.
suxamethonium
SV
stroke volume
SV40
simian virus 40
SVAS
supravalvar aortic stenosis
SVC
slow vital capacity
superior vena cava
SVC lead
SVC syndrome
SVD
single-vessel disease
structural valve deterioration
SVE
subcortical vascular encephalopathy
Svedberg flotation rate
SVG
saphenous vein graft
SVI
small-vessel infarction
stroke volume index
SVM
syncytiovascular membrane
SVN
small-volume nebulizer
SvO$_2$
mixed venous oxygen saturation
continuous cardiac output with
SvO$_2$ (CCOmbo)
SVR
systemic vascular resistance
SVRI
systemic vascular resistance index
SVT
supraventricular tachycardia
swallow
barium s.
s. syncope
wet s.
Swan-Ganz
S.-G. balloon flotation catheter
S.-G. bipolar pacing catheter
S.-G. catheter
S.-G. flow-directed catheter

S.-G. Pacing TD catheter
S.-G. syndrome
Swank high-flow arterial blood filter
S-warfarin
sweat
s. chloride
s. chloride test
sweating
sweep
Sweet
S. Tip bipolar lead
S. Tip lead
swelling
ventricular mural s.
SWI
stroke work index
SWIFT
Should We Intervene Following
Thrombolysis
SWIFT study
swimmer's view
swimming
hypoxic lap s.
swing
S. DR1 DDDR pacemaker
respiratory s.
s. test
swinging heart
Swiss
S. cheese defect
S. cheese interventricular septum
S. Kiss intrastent balloon inflation
device
switch
DNA s.
internal reed s.
isoactin s.
isomyosin s.
late arterial s.
s. operation
s. procedure
switching
automatic mode s. (AMS)
mode s.
SWORD
Surveillance of Work-related and
Occupational Respiratory Disease
Survival with Oral D-Sotalol
SWORD Clinical Trial
SWORD project
SWS
slow-wave sleep

S

NOTES

Swyer-James syndrome
SX/DX computerized spirometry
package
Sydenham
    S. chorea
    S. cough
sydowi
    Aspergillus s.
Sylvest disease
Sylvian fissure
Sylvius
    valve of S.
Symadine
Symbion
    S. cardiac device
    S./CardioWest 100 mL total
      artificial heart
    S. Jarvik-7 artificial heart
    S. J-7 70-mL ventricle total
      artificial heart
Symbios 7006 pacemaker
Symmetrel
symmetric
    s. asphyxia
    s. vitiligo
symmetrical phased array
sympathectomy, sympathetectomy
    cervicothoracic s.
    lumbar s.
sympathetic
    s. activity
    s. nerve
    s. nerve activity (SNA)
    s. nervous system (SNS)
    s. neurotransmission
sympathoadrenal system
sympathoexcitation
    reflex s.
sympathoexcitatory response
sympathoinhibition
sympatholytic
sympathomimetic
    s. amine
    s. drug
sympathovagal
    s. balance
    s. imbalance
    s. transition
SYMPHONY
    Sibrafiban versus Aspirin to Yield
    Maximum Protection from Ischemic
    Heart Events Post-Acute Coronary
    Syndromes
    SYMPHONY clinical trial
Symphony
    S. nitinol stent

S. patient monitoring system
S. stent
symphysis, gen. symphyses
    cardiac s.
    pericardial s.
symptom
    Baumes s.
    Burghart s.
    cardinal s.
    Duroziez s.
    Fischer s.
    gastrointestinal s.
    Kussmaul s.
    Oehler s.'s
    Platelet Receptor Inhibition for
      Ischemic Syndrome Management
      in Patients Limited to Very
      Unstable Signs and S.'s (PRISM-
      PLUS)
    prodromal s.
    Trunecek s.
symptomatic
    s. asthma
    s. hemorrhage (SHT)
symptomaticity
symptom-free interval
symptom-limited
    s.-l. maximal treadmill test
    s.-l. treadmill exercise test
    s.-l. treadmill test
Synacol CF
Synagis
Synapse electrocardiographic cream
synaptene
synaptic
Sync
    Star S.
Syn-Captopril
synchondrosis
    sternal s.
SynchroMed programmable pump
synchronization
synchronized
    s. DC cardioversion
    s. direct current cardioversion
    s. intermittent mandatory
    s. intermittent mandatory ventilation
      (SIMV)
    s. shock
    s. sleep (S-sleep)
synchronizer
    CardioSync cardiac s.
synchronous
    s. airway lesions
    s. atrial contraction
    s. atrial pacing study
    s. endobronchial disease

synchrony
> atrial s.
> atrioventricular s.
> A-V s.
> S. II DDDR pulse generator
> S. III DDDR pulse generator
> S. I, II pacemaker
> ventricular contractile s.

synchrotron-based transvenous angiography

syncopal
> s. migraine
> s. migraine headache
> s. spell

syncope
> Adams-Stokes s.
> s. anginosa
> cardiac s.
> cardiogenic s.
> cardioinhibitory s.
> cardioinhibitory vasovagal s.
> cardioneurogenic s.
> carotid sinus s.
> cerebrovascular s.
> cough s.
> defecation s.
> deglutition s.
> diver's s.
> exertional s.
> head-up tilt-induced s.
> hypoglycemic s.
> hypoxic s.
> hysterical s.
> isoproterenol-induced vasovagal s.
> laryngeal s.
> local s.
> micturition s.
> migraine s.
> mixed neurally mediated s.
> Morgagni-Adams-Stokes s.
> near-s.
> neurally mediated s. (NMS)
> neurally mediated vasovagal s. (NMVS)
> neurocardial s.
> neurocardiogenic s.
> neuromediated s.
> noncardiac s.
> orthostatic s.
> postmicturition s.
> posttussive s.
> postural s.

> psychogenic s.
> severe refractory neurocardiogenic s.
> sexual s.
> situational s.
> sneeze s.
> stretching s.
> swallow s.
> toilet-seat s.
> transient s.
> tussive s.
> vasodepressor s.
> vasodepressor-cardioinhibitory s.
> vasovagal s.
> visceral s.

syncytial virus
syncytiovascular membrane (SVM)
syndactyly
Syn-Diltiazem
syndrome
> abdominal compartment s. (ACS)
> acquired immunodeficiency s. (AIDS)
> acute brain s.
> acute chest s.
> acute coronary s. (ACS)
> acute ischemic coronary s. (AICS)
> acute respiratory distress s. (ARDS)
> acute retroviral s.
> acute right heart s. (ARHS)
> acute sickle cell chest s.
> acute sickle chest s. (ASCS)
> Adams-Stokes s.
> adrenogenital s.
> adult respiratory distress s. (ARDS)
> advanced sleep phase s.
> agitation s.
> Albright s.
> ALCAPA s.
> Alport s.
> ALPS s.
> Alstrom s.
> amnionic fluid s.
> amniotic fluid s.
> Andersen s.
> anomalous first rib thoracic s.
> anomalous origin of left coronary artery from the pulmonary artery s.
> antiphospholipid s.
> aortic arch s.

S

NOTES

syndrome *(continued)*

aortic arteritis s.
aortocaval compression s.
apallic s.
Apert s.
Ardystil s.
arteriohepatic dysplasia s.
Asherson s.
Ask-Upmark s.
Austrian s.
Ayerza s.
Babinski s.
Babinski-Vasquez s.
ballooning mitral cusp s.
ballooning mitral valve s.
ballooning posterior leaflet s.
Bamberger-Marie s.
bangungot s.
Bannwarth s.
Barlow s.
Barsony-Polgar s.
Barth s.
Bartter s.
Bauer s.
Beau s.
beer and cobalt s.
Behçet s.
Bernheim s.
Besnier-Boeck-Schaumann s.
Beuren s.
billowing mitral valve s.
Blackfan-Diamond s.
Bland-Garland-White s.
Bloom s.
blue finger s.
blue toe s.
blue velvet s.
Boerhaave s.
brachial s.
Bradbury-Eggleston s.
bradycardia-tachycardia s.
brady-tachy s.
bradytachycardia s.
Brett s.
Brock s.
bronchiolitis obliterans s. (BOS)
Brugada s.
bubbly lung s.
Budd-Chiari s.
Bürger-Grütz s.
busulfan lung s.
capillary leak s. (CLS)
Caplan s.
carcinoid s.
cardioauditory s.
cardiofacial s.
carotid sinus s.
carotid sinus hypersensitivity s.

carotid steal s.
Carpenter s.
catch 22 s.
cat cry s.
cauda equina s.
Ceelen-Gellerstedt s.
central sleep apnea s. (CSAS)
Cepacia s.
cervical rib s.
Char s.
Charcot s.
Charcot-Weiss-Baker s.
CHARGE s.
Chédiak-Higashi s.
chemoreceptor s.
Chiari s.
Chiari-Budd s.
Chinese restaurant s.
Chinese restaurant asthma s.
cholesterol emboli s.
chronic hyperventilation s.
Churg-Strauss s. (CSS)
Clarke-Hadfield s.
click s.
click-murmur s.
Cockayne s.
Cogan s.
compartment s.
compensatory antiinflammatory
  response s. (CARS)
congenital central hypoventilation s.
congenital long QT interval s.
Conn s.
Conradi-Hünermann s.
Cornelia de Lange s.
coronary slow flow s. (CSFS)
coronary-subclavian steal s.
costochondral s.
costoclavicular rib s.
costosternal s.
CREST s.
cricopharyngeal achalasia s.
cri du chat s.
Crow-Fukase s.
cryptophthalmos s.
Curracino-Silverman s.
Cushing s.
cutis laxa s.
Cyriax s.
DaCosta s.
deadly quartet s.
declamping shock s.
defects s.
de Gimard s.
de Lange s.
delayed pulmonary toxicity s.
  (DPTS)
Determann s.

DiGeorge s. (DGS)
distal intestinal obstruction s. (DIOS)
Down s.
Dressler s.
drowned newborn s.
drug-induced lupus s.
Duncan s.
dysarthria-clumsy hand s. (DCHS)
dyskinesia s.
dyslipidemic hypertension s.
early repolarization s.
Eaton-Lambert s.
effort s.
Ehlers-Danlos s.
Eisenmenger s. (Eis)
elfin facies s.
Ellis-van Creveld s.
eosinophilia-myalgia s. (EMS)
eosinophilic lung s.
eosinophilic pulmonary s.
epibronchial right pulmonary artery s.
euthyroid sick s.
familial atrial myxoma s.
familial cholestasis s.
familial chylomicronemia s.
fat embolism s. (FES)
fetal alcohol s. (FAS)
fetal aspiration s.
fibrinogen-fibrin conversion s.
flapping valve s.
Fleischner s.
floppy valve s.
Foix-Cavany-Marie s.
folded-lung s.
Forney s.
Forrester s.
four-day s.
Gailliard s.
Gaisböck s.
gastrocardiac s.
Gerhardt s.
Goldenhar s.
Goodpasture s.
Gorlin s.
Gowers s.
Grönblad-Strandberg s.
Guillain-Barré s.
Gulf War s.
Halbrecht s.
Hamman s.

Hamman-Rich s. (HRS)
hantavirus pulmonary s.
Hare s.
heart-hand s.
heart and hand s.
Hegglin s.
Heiner s.
HELLP s.
hemangioma-thrombocytopenia s.
hemolysis, elevated liver function tests and low platelets s.
Henoch-Schönlein s.
hepatopulmonary s. (HPS)
Hermansky-Pudlak s.
Herner s.
heterotaxy s.
high-pressure neurologic s. (HPNS)
holiday heart s.
Holt-Oram s.
homocystinuria s.
Horner s.
Howel-Evans s.
Hughes-Stovin s.
Hunter s.
Hunter-Hurler s.
Hurler s.
hyperabduction s.
hyperapolipoprotein B s.
hypercalcemia s.
hypereosinophilia s.
hypereosinophilic s.
hyperkinetic heart s.
hyperlucent lung s.
hyperperfusion s.
hypersensitive carotid sinus s.
hyperventilation s.
hyperviscosity s.
hyponatremic-hypertensive s.
hypoplastic left heart s. (HLHS)
idiopathic hypereosinophilic s. (IHES)
idiopathic long Q-T interval s.
immotile cilia s.
s. of inappropriate antidiuresis (SIAD)
s. of inappropriate antidiuretic hormone (SIADH)
incontinentia pigmenti s.
infant respiratory distress s. (IRDS)
insulin resistance s.
intermediate coronary s.
Ivemark s.

S

NOTES

syndrome (*continued*)

Jackson s.
Janus s.
Jervell and Lange-Nielsen s.
Jeune s.
Job s.
Kallmann s.
Kartagener s.
Kasabach-Merritt s.
Kawasaki s.
Kearns-Sayre s.
Kimmelstiel-Wilson s.
Klein-Waardenburg s.
Klinefelter s.
Klippel-Feil s.
Klippel-Trenaunay-Weber s.
Kostmann s.
Kugelberg-Welander s.
Kussmaul s.
lacunar s. (LACS)
LAMB s.
Lambert-Eaton myasthenic s.
Landouzy-Dejerine s.
Landry-Guillain-Barre s.
Laron s. (LS)
Laubry-Soulle s.
Laurence-Moon-Bardet-Biedl s.
Laurence-Moon-Biedl s.
Leitner s.
Lemierre s.
Lenègre s.
Lenz s.
LEOPARD s.
Leredde s.
Leriche s.
Lev s.
Libman-Sacks s.
Liddle s.
Löffler s.
Löfgren s.
long QT s. (LQTS)
long Q-TU s.
low cardiac output s.
Lown-Gagong-Levine s.
low-salt s.
low-sodium s.
Lutembacher s.
Macleod s.
malignant carcinoid s.
malignant superior vena caval s.
malignant SVC s.
malignant vasovagal s.
Mallory-Weiss s.
Marfan s.
Marie s.
Marie-Bamberger s.
Maroteaux-Lamy s.
Martorell s.

mastocytosis s.
Maugeri s.
McArdle s.
Meadows s.
meconium aspiration s. (MAS)
Meigs s.
Mendelson s.
Ménière s.
metabolic s.
metastatic carcinoid s.
middle lobe s.
midsystolic click s.
milk-alkali s.
mirror-image lung s.
mitral valve prolapse s.
Mondor s.
Morestin s.
Morgagni-Adams-Stokes s.
Morquio s.
Mounier-Kuhn s.
Moynahan s.
mucocutaneous lymph node s.
multiple lentigines s.
multiple organ dysfunction s.
(MODS)
myocardial ischemic s.
NAME s.
neonate respiratory distress s.
(NRDS)
nephrotic s.
neurally mediated syncopal s.
nonpyramidal hemimotor s.
Noonan s.
no-reflow s.
obesity-hypoventilation s.
obstructive sleep apnea s. (OSAS)
oculomucocutaneous s.
Opitz s.
Orbofiban in Patients with
Unstable Coronary S.'s (OPUS)
organic dust toxic s. (ODTS)
Organization to Assess Strategies
for Ischemic S.'s (OASIS)
Osler-Weber-Rendu s.
overlap s.
pacemaker s.
Paget-von Schrötter s.
Pancoast s.
papillary muscle s.
paraneoplastic s.
partial anterior circulation s.
(PACS)
Penderluft s.
pericarditis-myocarditis s.
Perthes s.
pharyngeal pouch s.
Pick s.
pickwickian s.

PIE s.
Pierre Robin s.
Pins s.
platypnea-orthodeoxia s.
Plummer-Vinson s.
POEMS s.
Polhemus-Schafer-Ivemark s.
polyglandular autoimmune s. type
 II
polymetabolic s.
polymyalgia rheumatica s.
positional obstructive sleep
 apnea s.
postcardiac injury s. (PCIS)
postcardiotomy s.
postcardiotomy psychosis s.
postcommissurotomy s.
posterior circulation s. (POCS)
postinfarction s.
postmyocardial infarction s.
postnasal drainage s. (PNDS)
postnasal drip s. (PNDS)
postperfusion s.
postpericardiotomy s. (PPS)
postphlebitic s.
postpump s.
posttransfusion s.
postural orthostatic tachycardia s.
 (POTS)
P pulmonale s.
precordial catch s.
preexcitation s.
preinfarction s.
premonitory s.
prolapsed mitral valve s.
prolonged Q-T interval s.
Proteus s.
pseudoxanthoma elasticum s.
pulmonary acid aspiration s.
pulmonary disease anemia s.
pulmonary dysmaturity s.
pulmonary hyperinfection s.
pulmonary infarction s.
pulmonary infiltrates with
 eosinophilia s.
pulmonary sling s.
pure sensory s. (PSS)
QT s.
Q-TU interval s.
quinidine syncope s.
radiologic scimitar s.
Raeder-Harbitz s.

Rasmussen s.
Raynaud s.
reactive airways disease s. (RADS)
reactive airways dysfunction s.
 (RADS)
reactive upper airways
 dysfunction s. (RUDS)
Reaven s.
redundant cusp s.
Reel s.
refeeding s.
Refsum s.
Reiter s.
Rendu-Osler-Weber s.
respiratory distress s. (RDS)
Reye s.
Riley-Day s.
Romano-Ward s.
Rosenbach s.
Rosenberg s.
Roussy-Lévy s.
rubella s.
Rubinstein-Taybi s.
salt-depletion s.
Sanchez-Cascos cardioauditory s.
Sandifer s.
Sanfilippo s.
scalenus anterior s.
scalenus anticus s.
Schaumann s.
Scheie s.
Schmidt s.
scimitar s.
Sebastiani s.
shallow-water blackout s.
shoulder-hand s.
Shprintzen s.
Shwachman s.
Shy-Drager s.
Sibrafiban versus Aspirin to Yield
 Maximum Protection from
 Ischemic Heart Events Post-Acute
 Coronary S.'s (SYMPHONY)
sicca s.
sick building s. (SBS)
sick sinus s. (SSS)
Silver s.
single papillary muscle s.
sinobronchial s.
Sjögren s.
sleep apnea/hypopnea s. (SAHS)
slipping rib s.

S

NOTES

syndrome *(continued)*
  slit ventricle s.
  Smith-Lemli-Opitz s.
  Sneddon s.
  Spens s.
  splenic flexure s.
  Stevens-Johnson s.
  stiff heart s.
  stiff left atrium s.
  Stokes-Adams s.
  Stokvis-Talma s.
  straight back s.
  Sturge-Weber s.
  subclavian steal s.
  sudden infant death s. (SIDS)
  sudden unexplained death s.
   (SUDS)
  SUND s.
  superior mesenteric artery s.
  superior vena cava s.
  supine hypotension s.
  supravalvar aortic stenosis s.
  supravalvar aortic stenosis-infantile
   hypercalcemia s.
  surdocardiac s.
  suspended heart s.
  SVC s.
  Swan-Ganz s.
  Swyer-James s.
  systemic inflammatory response s.
   (SIRS)
  systolic click-late systolic
   murmur s.
  systolic click-murmur s.
  tachybradycardia s.
  tachycardia-bradycardia s.
  tachycardia-polyuria s.
  Takayasu s.
  TAR s.
  Taussig-Bing s.
  Taybi s.
  telangiectasia s.
  thoracic compressive s.
  thoracic endometriosis s. (TES)
  thoracic outlet s.
  thoracic outlet compression s.
  thrombocytopenia-absent radius s.
  thromboembolic s.
  Tietze s.
  total anterior circulation s. (TACS)
  Townes-Brocks s.
  toxic oil s. (TOS)
  Treacher Collins s.
  trisomy D s.
  Trousseau s.
  Turner s.
  twiddler's s.
  Uhl s.
  Ulick s.
  Ullmann s.
  upper airway resistance s. (UARS)
  Urbach-Wiethe s.
  V_1-like ambulatory lead s.
  V_5-like ambulatory lead s.
  VACTERL s.
  vascular leak s.
  vasculocardiac s. of
   hyperserotonemia
  vasovagal s.
  VATER association s.
  velocardiofacial s.
  vena cava s.
  venolobar s.
  Vernet s.
  Villaret s.
  Vogt-Koyanagi-Harada s.
  Waardenburg s.
  Wallenberg s.
  Ward-Romano s.
  wasting s.
  Watson s.
  Weber-Osler-Rendu s.
  Werner s.
  West s.
  white clot s.
  Williams s.
  Williams-Campbell s.
  Wilson-Mikity s.
  Wiskott-Aldrich s.
  Wolff-Parkinson-White s.
  s. X
  XO s.
  XXXX s.
  XXXY s.
  yellow nail s. (YNS)
  Yentl s.
  Young s.

synechia, pl. **synechiae**
  s. pericardii

Synercid
synergism
synergistic
SynerGraft
  S. heart valve
  S. implant
  S. pulmonary heart valve
  S. tissue-engineered heart valve
Synergyst
  S. DDD pacemaker
  S. II pacemaker
Syngamus laryngeus
syngenesioplastic transplant
Syn-Nadolol
synovial sarcoma reactive mesothelial
  hyperplasia
Synox fractal pacemaker lead

Syn-Pindol
synpneumonic empyema
Syntel latex-free embolectomy catheter
synthase
    constitutive nitric oxide s. (cNOS)
    endothelial constitutive nitric
      oxide s. (ecNOS)
    endothelial nitric oxide s. (eNOS)
    glycogen s.
    inducible nitric oxide s. (iNOS)
    nitric oxide s. (NOS, NOS1)
synthesis
    cytokine-induced endothelial s.
    matrix s.
    thromboxane s.
synthetase
    inducible nitric oxide s. (iNOS)
    pantothenate s.
Synthofil suture
Synthroid
syntony
synvinolin
syphilis
    cardiovascular s.
    nonvenereal s.
    tertiary s.
syphilitic
    s. aneurysm
    s. aortic aneurysm
    s. aortic valvulitis
    s. aortitis
    s. arteritis
    s. endarteritis
    s. endocarditis
    s. laryngitis
    s. myocarditis
Syracol-CF
syringe
    anaerobic Pulsator s.
    Concord line draw s.
    Gas-Lyte ABG s.
    Lyo-Ject s.
    Namic angiographic s.
    Osciflator balloon inflation s.
    Pulsator s.
    Raulerson s.
    Ultraject prefilled s.
syrup
    Actagen S.
    albuterol sulfate s.
    Allerfrin S.
    Allerphed S.

Ambenyl Cough S.
Amgenal Cough S.
Anamine S.
Aprodine S.
Benylin Cough S.
Bromanyl Cough S.
Bromotuss w/Codeine Cough S.
Bydramine Cough S.
Carbodec S.
Cardec-S S.
Co-Xan s.
Decofed S.
Deconamine S.
Extra Action Cough S.
Histalet S.
Hydramyn S.
Hydrocodone PA S.
Kenacort S.
Phanatuss Cough S.
Rondec S.
Silafed S.
Triaminicol Multi-Symptom Cold S.
Triofed S.
Triposed S.
Tussar SF S.
Tusstat S.
Uni-Bent Cough S.
system
    Abiomed biventricular support s.
    ABI Vest Airway Clearance s.
    ABL 625 s.
    ABL 520 blood gas
      measurement s.
    Access MV s.
    Accu-Chek InstantPlus s.
    Achieve Off-Pump s.
    ACS Concorde over-the-wire
      catheter s.
    ACS Multi-Link coronary s.
    ACS Multi-Link RX Ultra
      coronary stent s.
    Active Can defibrillator lead s.
    ACT MicroCoil delivery s.
    Acuson cardiovascular s.
    Acuson XP 128
      echocardiographic s.
    adrenergic nervous s.
    Advanced Cardiovascular S.'s
      (ACS)
    Advanced Catheter S. (ACS)
    Aegis ICD s.
    AeroNOx nitric oxide transport s.

S

NOTES

system *(continued)*

AeroView optical intubation s.
AerX pulmonary drug delivery s.
AirSep OxiScan Oximetry Recording, Reporting, and Archiving s.
Aladdin infant flow s.
Aladdin nasal CPAP s.
Albert Grass Heritage digital PSG s.
Albert Grass Heritage EEG s.
Albert Grass Heritage PSG s.
Alcon Closure S.
Alice4 Sleep Diagnostic s.
Anaconda delivery s.
Anaconda device and delivery s.
ANCOR imaging s.
Ancure s.
Androderm Transdermal s.
AneuRx fully supported modular s.
AneuRx stent graft s.
AngeCool RF catheter ablation s.
AngioJet rapid thrombectomy s.
AngioRad radiation s.
annular phased array s. (APAS)
AnnuloFlo annuloplasty ring s.
Aortic Connector s.
Apollo Light S.'s
Arcomax FMA cardiac angiography s.
Argyle-Turkel safety thoracentesis s.
Argyle-Turkel thoracentesis s.
Aria CPAP s.
Aria LX CPAP s.
arrhythmia mapping s.
ARTREK offline 35-mm cineangiographic analysis s.
Atakr s.
ATL Ultramark 9 ultrasound s.
AT-2plusTX ECG s.
atrial septal defect occlusion s. (ASDOS)
atrial septum defect occluder s. (ASDOS)
atrioventricular conduction s.
Atrium Blood Recovery s.
AT-1 three-channel resting ECG s.
AutoCapture pacing s.
autologous blood management s.
automated cervical cell screening s.
automatic exposure s.
autonomic nervous s. (ANS)
AutoSet Portable II CPAP s.
Autotrans s.
autotransfusion s.
Autovac autotransfusion s.
Autovac LF autotransfusion s.

Axcis percutaneous myocardial revascularization s.
Axcis PMR s.
BACTEC s.
Bard cardiopulmonary support s.
Bard percutaneous cardiopulmonary support s.
Baylor autologous transfusion s.
Beckman ICS Nephelometer s.
beStent Rival coronary stent s.
Beta-Cath s.
BiliBlanket phototherapy s.
Biodex S.
bionic baroreflex s.
Biosense s.
Biosense mapping s.
Biosense NOGA catheter-based endocardial mapping s.
Biosound Genesis II scanning s.
Biosound Phase 2 ultrasound s.
biotin/streptavidin s.
BioZ s.
BioZ hemodynamic monitoring s.
BioZ noninvasive cardiac function monitoring s.
BioZ.pc s.
BiPAP duet s.
BiPAP S/T-D 30 s.
BiPAP S/T-D ventilatory support s.
BiPAP Vision s.
Bonchek-Shiley vein distention s.
BosPac cardiopulmonary bypass s.
brachiocephalic s.
BRAT s.
Breeze E150 ventilation s.
Bridge X3 renal stent s.
Burette multiple patient delivery s.
BVS-5000 biventricular support s.
Cadence tiered therapy defibrillator s.
CAESAR s.
CAESAR analysis s.
Capintec VEST s.
Capiox SX oxygenation s.
CAP/3SBII angiogram projection s.
cardiac conduction s.
CardiData Prodigy s.
Cardiofreezer cryosurgical s.
CardioGenesis PMR s.
cardiopulmonary support s.
cardioscope U s.
CardioThoracic S.'s
cardiovascular s.
Cardiovascular Angiography Analysis S. (CAAS)
Cardiovascular Measurement s. (CMS)
Cardiovit AT-1 ECG s.

Cardiovit AT-10 ECG/spirometry combination s.
Cardiovit CS-200 ECG s.
Cardizem Monovial delivery s.
CARTO-Biosense magnetic mapping s.
CASE computerized exercise ECG s.
CASE Marquette 16 exercise s.
catheter-snare s.
catheter-tip micromanometer s.
Cath-Finder catheter tracking s.
CDI 2000 blood gas monitoring s.
Cell Saver autologous blood recovery s.
Cell Saver Haemonetics Autotransfusion s.
Cenflex central monitoring s.
CGR biplane angiographic s.
CH 2000 cardiac diagnostic s.
Checkmate gamma brachytherapy s.
Chilli cooled ablation s.
Cholesterol Monitoring s. (CMS)
cineangiographic s.
cine-pulse s.
CineView Plus Freeland s.
Circulaire aerosol drug delivery s.
circulatory support s.
Clarity multiparameter monitoring s.
CMS AccuProbe 450 s.
CoaguChek s.
CoaguChek aPTT testing s.
Cobe Spectra apheresis s.
Cobe Trima automated blood-component collection s.
codominant s.
COER-24 delivery s.
CO₂ject s.
Colin Electronics BP-508 tonometry s.
ColorZone Management s.
complement s.
complete pacemaker patient testing s. (CPPTS)
Computerized Healthcare And Record Transfer S. (CHARTS)
computerized sleep analysis s.
conduction s.
conductive s.
Conforma 3000 delivery s.
coordinate s.
Cordis LC Multipurpose stent s.

Cordis Mini stent s.
Coroflex coronary stent s.
coronary implant s. (CIS)
COROSCOP C cardiac imaging s.
Cosgrove-Edwards annuloplasty s.
CoumaCare Coumadin management s.
CPL cardiopulmonary diagnostic s.
CPS s.
Cragg Endopro s.
Cuidant s.
C-VEST radiation detector s.
CVIS/InterTherapy intravascular ultrasound s.
cytochrome P450 s.
Dallas Classification S.
DAR breathing s.
DataCare ABG Data Management s.
daVinci surgical s.
DCI-S automated coronary analysis s.
demand oxygen delivery s. (DODS)
Desilets s.
Desilets introducer s.
Diameter Index Safety s. (DISS)
Diasonics-Sonotron Vingmed CFM 800 imaging s.
Digital Cardiac Imaging s.
dilator-sheath s.
Dinamap s.
distal perfusion s. (DPS)
DPAP interactive airway management s.
2D TEE s. Ultra-Neb 99
DUPEL drug delivery s.
Dymer excimer delivery s.
Dynasty delivery s.
Eagle portable ventilation s.
Easy Analysis s.
echocardiographic automated boundary detection s.
echocardiographic scoring s.
EchoFlow blood velocity meter s.
EchoQuant acoustic quantification s.
Echovar Doppler s.
Eclipse PTMR s.
edge-detection s.
Elecsys troponin T immunoassay s.
electroanatomical mapping s.
electrode s.

S

NOTES

system *(continued)*
    Electronic HouseCall s.
    Elscint tomography s.
    Embol-X arterial cannula and
      filter s.
    Embolyx liquid embolic s.
    endocrine s.
    EndoPro s. I
    Endosaph saphenous vein
      harvesting s.
    Endosaph vein harvest s.
    Endotak lead s.
    EnGuard double-lead ICD s.
    EnGuard pacing and defibrillation
      lead s.
    Ensite 3000 s.
    EnviroNOx surveillance s.
    EPT-1000 cardiac ablation s.
    Equinox digital EEG s.
    Equinox occlusion balloon s.
    Erie S.
    ES 300-Cardiac T ELISA troponin
      T immunoassay s.
    Estes point s.
    Estes-Romhilt ECG point-score s.
    event-link data s.
    factor XII-kallikrein-kinin s.
    6F delivery s.
    Fiberlase s.
    fiberoptic catheter delivery s.
    fiberoptic delivery s.
    fibrinolytic s.
    Finger Phantom pulse oximeter
      testing s.
    fixed-wire balloon dilatation s.
    Flowtron DVT pump s.
    FMA cardiovascular imaging s.
    Frank ECG lead placement s.
    Frank XYZ orthogonal lead s.
    Frostline linear cryoablation s.
    Galileo intravascular radiotherapy s.
    gamma radiation therapy s.
    gated s.
    GE CT Advantage high-speed
      CT s.
    Gem SensiCath blood gas
      monitoring s.
    GenBank information s.
    General Electric Advantx s.
    General Electric Signa 1.5-T
      MRI s.
    GenESA s.
    GenESA closed-loop delivery s.
    Genic coronary stent delivery s.
    GFX 2 coronary stent s.
    GoodKnight 418A, 418G, 418P
      CPAP s.
    Grass neurodata s.

    GS Modular pulmonary testing s.
    Guardwire angioplasty s.
    Guardwire emboli containment s.
    Guidant Heart Rhythm
      Technologies Linear Ablation s.
    Guidant Multi-Link Tetra coronary
      stent s.
    Guidant TRIAD three-electrode
      energy defibrillation s.
    Gyroscan HP Philips 15S whole-
      body s.
    Haemolite autologous blood
      recovery s.
    Haemonetics Cell Saver s.
    Heartflo automated anastomosis s.
    HeartMate implantable pneumatic
      left ventricular assist s.
    HeartMate left ventricular assist s.
    HeartMate vented electric left
      ventricular assist s.
    Heartport catheter s.
    Heartport Port-Access s.
    HEARTrac I Cardiac Monitoring s.
    HearTwave s.
    hematopoietic s.
    hemoglobin-based therapeutic s.
    Hemopump cardiac assist s.
    Hemopure oxygen-based
      therapeutic s.
    HEPAtech Air Purification s.
    Hewlett-Packard 5 MHz phased-
      array TEE s.
    Hewlett-Packard SONOS 1000,
      1500, 2500 ultrasound s.
    hexaxial reference s.
    Hi-Care closed suction s.
    Hi-Care closed suction and
      pulmonary hygiene s.
    HICOR s.
    His-Purkinje s.
    Hitachi PCT-3600W PET s.
    Hombach lead placement s.
    HomMed Monitoring s.
    Horizon AutoAdjust CPAP s.
    Horizon LT CPAP s.
    Horizon nasal CPAP s.
    Housecall transtelephonic
      monitoring s.
    hub and spoke referral s.
    Hunt and Hess grades I through
      V aneurysm grading s.
    HydroDot s.
    hypoxia warning s.
    IDIS s.
    IDIS angiography s.
    IL 1640 blood gas/electrolyte s.
    IL GEMPCL testing s.
    IL GEM Premier Plus testing s.

IL GEMSensiCath ABG s.
IL IMPACT testing s.
iliofemoral venous s.
IL Synthesis testing s.
Image-View s.
Imatron C-100 s.
implantable left ventricular assist s.
  (IPLVAS)
INCA s.
Incardia valve s.
Infant Flow Nasal CPAP s.
Infant Flow noninvasive nasal
  CPAP s.
Infant Resuscitation s.
Infiniti catheter introducer s.
infrahisian conduction s.
Inhale deep lung delivery s.
Innovator Holter s.
INOvent delivery s.
InSight s.
integrated lead s.
Integris cardiac imaging s.
Integris H5000 digital x-ray
  imaging s.
Integrity AFx AutoCapture
  pacing s.
IntraLuminal Safe-Steer
  guidewire s.
Intra-Op autotransfusion s.
Invacare ConnectO2 Telemetry
  System home oxygen s.
Invacare Venture HomeFill
  complete home oxygen s.
Invacare Venture HomeFill
  oxygen s.
IRMA s.
IRMA blood gas analysis s.
Irri-Cath suction s.
Irvine viable organ-tissue
  transport s. (IVOTTS)
isocenter s.
Itrel 3 spinal cord stimulation s.
Jaeger body plethysmography s.
Jinotti closed suctioning s.
Johnson & Johnson
  Interventional S.'s
kallikrein-bradykinin s.
Kiethly-DAS series 500 data-
  acquisition s.
King double umbrella closure s.
KK s.

KnightStar 335 respiratory-
  support s.
lead s.
left ventricular assist s. (LVAS)
Leocor hemoperfusion s.
Leukotrap red cell storage s.
Lifepath AAA endovascular graft s.
Liposorber LA-15 s.
Lown grading s.
Luxtec fiberoptic s.
lymphohematogenous drainage s.
Lyra laser s.
Magnum-Meier s.
Mallinckrodt Hi-Care Pulmonary
  Hygiene s.
Marquette Case-12
  electrocardiographic s.
Marquette Case-12 exercise s.
Mason-Likar 12-lead ECG s.
M/D 4 defibrillator s.
MDS s.
MEDDARS cardiac catheterization
  analysis s.
MedGraphics Cardio O2 s.
medication monitoring event s.
  (MEMS)
Medi-Facts s.
Medi-Tech catheter s.
Medos mechanical circulatory
  support s.
Medtronic Hemopump s.
Medtronic Interactive Tachycardia
  Terminating s.
Medtronic Octopus tissue
  stabilizing s.
Medtronic Octopus 2+ tissue
  stabilizing s.
Medtronic Transvene endocardial
  lead s.
Medtronic Transvene lead s.
Meier-Magnum s.
Metrix atrial defibrillation s.
Micro Delta/Max Delta s.
MicroGas 7650 transcutaneous
  monitoring s.
MicroHartzler ACS balloon
  catheter s.
micromanometer catheter s.
microwave cardiac ablation s.
MIDA 1000 monitoring s.
MIDCAB s.
minimum data set s.

NOTES

S

system *(continued)*

Mobin-Uddin filter s.
Monaldi drainage s.
MSM-CIS s.
MT-100 ECG Holt s.
mucociliary s.
Mullins sheath s.
Multi-Link coronary stent s.
Multi-Link Tetra coronary stent s.
Multitest cell-mediated immunity s.
Myocardial Infarction Data
  Acquisition S.
myocardial protection s. (MPS)
MYOtherm XP cardioplegia
  delivery s.
nasal CPAP s.
Neotrend s.
nervous s.
Nihon Kohden Polygraph s.
NIR with SOX coronary stent s.
NIR with SOX over-the-wire
  coronary stent s.
NiteView polysomnography s.
nitric oxide s.
nonthoracotomy defibrillation
  lead s.
Novacor left ventricular assist s.
Novacor mechanical circulatory
  support s.
Nova Microsonics Image Vue s.
Nu-Trake Weiss emergency
  airway s.
Nuvolase 660 laser s.
Oasis thrombectomy s.
Octopus 3 tissue stabilization s.
Omni tract retractor s.
Optical Sensors stand-alone arterial
  blood gas monitoring s.
OptiHaler drug delivery s.
Opti-Qvue Mixed Venous
  Saturation/CCO pulmonary artery
  catheter s.
oral L-Arginine s.
organ transplantation s.
orthogonal lead s.
over-the-wire balloon dilatation s.
Oximetrix 3 S.
OxiScan oximetry recording and
  reporting s.
Oxycure topical oxygen s.
Oxyfill oxygen refilling s.
Oxylator-EM 100 automatic
  resuscitation and inhalation s.
Oxylite ambulatory oxygen s.
Oxy-Ultra-Lite ambulatory
  oxygen s.
Paceart complete pacemaker patient
  testing s.

pacemaker code s.
parasympathetic nervous s.
PASYS cardiac pacing s.
PASYS ST cardiac pacing s.
patch-coil s.
Pathfinder microcatheter s.
Patil stereotactic s.
PCA s.
PCD Transvene implantable
  cardioverter-defibrillator s.
PDB preperitoneal distention
  balloon s.
Pelorus stereotactic s.
PenChant stent delivery s.
Perclose vascular surgical
  closure s.
percutaneous mechanical
  thrombectomy s.
peripheral access s. (PAS)
Peripheral AngioJet s.
peripheral atherectomy s.
phased array s.
Physios CTM 01 noninvasive
  cardiac transplant monitoring s.
Picker VISTAR image analysis s.
Picker VOXEL image analysis s.
Pie Medical CAAS II analysis s.
plasma coagulation s.
Pleur-evac autotransfusion s.
2010 Plus Holter s.
PneuView ventilator s.
PneuView ventilator testing and
  training s.
Polaris CPAP s.
Port-A-Cath implantable catheter s.
Portex Soft-Seal cuff s.
Power Grip Over the Wire Stent
  Delivery s.
Powerlink endoluminal graft s.
Presto-Flash spirometry s.
Presto spirometry s.
Prevue s.
Prima Total Occlusion s.
Prime ECG mapping s.
Probe balloon-on-wire dilatation s.
Probe balloon-on-wire dilation s.
programmable implantable
  medication s. (PIMS)
Prostar 9F percutaneous vascular
  surgery s.
Prostar 11F percutaneous vascular
  surgery s.
Prostar XL 8 suture mediated
  closure s.
Prostar XL 10 suture mediated
  closure s.
Protégé 31 Low Loss stationary
  liquid oxygen s.

PSA stationary oxygen s.
P-Series sleep monitoring s.
pulmonary s.
pulmonary arterial s.
PulseDose portable compressed
  oxygen s.
PulseSpray infusion s.
Purkinje s.
PWV Medical SphygmoCor s.
Q-cath catheterization recording s.
Q-Plex Cardio-Pulmonary
  Exercise s.
Quartet s.
Quest MPS s.
Quest MPS myocardial
  protection s.
QuickFlow DPS distal perfusion s.
Quinton Synergy cardiac
  information management s.
RadiStop radial compression s.
Rapidlab 800 Critical Care s.
Rasor blood pumping s. (RBPS)
RDX coronary radiation catheter
  delivery s.
real-time position management
  tracking s.
Red s.
Remac s.
Remedy sleep therapy s.
REMstar Reliance CPAP s.
Renaissance spirometry s.
renal kallikrein-kinin s.
renin-angiotensin-aldosterone s.
  (RAAS)
respiratory s.
reticuloendothelial s.
revascularization s.
RFb s.
RFB System-I for CDBR
  retraining s.
Romhilt-Estes point scoring s.
Rosenkranz pediatric retractor s.
Rotacs s.
rotational angioplasty catheter s.
rotational atherectomy s. (RAS)
Rozanski lead placement s.
RPM tracking s.
R-Port implantable vascular
  access s.
Rx5000 cardiac pacing s.
RX Multi-Link s.
RX Multi-Link coronary stent s.

RX Multi-Link HP s.
RX stent delivery s.
SAM s.
Sandman s.
saphenofemoral s.
sarcotubular s.
Sarstedt s.
Schneider-Meier-Magnum s.
SenDx 100 blood gas and
  electrolyte analysis s.
SenDx Relay data management s.
Sequel compression s.
Sequestra 1000 s.
800 series blood gas and critical
  analyte s.
sheath and dilator s.
Shimadzu MAGNEX Epios 10 1.0-
  T superconductive MRI s.
SICOR cardiac catheterization
  recording s.
SICOR recording s.
Sigma II Dualplace hyperbaric
  oxygen therapy s.
Sigma I monoplace hyperbaric
  therapy s.
Sigma Plus Monosplace hyperbaric
  oxygen therapy s.
Simpson Coronary AtheroCath s.
Simpson-Robert vascular dilation s.
single chamber cardiac pacing s.
SinuScope s.
SJM Rosenkranz pediatric
  retractor s.
SKY epidural pain control s.
Sleepscan Traveler ambulatory
  polysomnography s.
Sleepscan Traveler home
  monitoring s.
Sleeptrace 2000/32 Sleep
  Analysis s.
Sleeptrace sleep diagnostic s.
SmartKard digital Holter s.
SmartMist asthma management s.
SmartMist Respiratory
  Management s.
SMP Multiplace hyperbaric
  therapy s.
Snuggle Warm convective
  warming s.
Somatom Volume Zoom computed
  tomography s.
Somnoplasty s.

NOTES

system (continued)

Somnus Somnoplasty s.
SonoHeart echocardiography s.
SonoHeart handheld, all digital
echocardiography s.
SONOS 500 imaging s.
2170 Spirometry Software s.
SpiroSense s.
Spiros Inhalation s.
SpiroVision-3 s.
SpiroVision-3 spirometry s.
S-Series sleep s.
stent delivery s. (SDS)
stroke guidance s. (SGS)
Sugarbaker staging s.
Super-4 catheter ablation s.
SureStepPro Professional Blood
Glucose Management s.
sympathetic nervous s. (SNS)
sympathoadrenal s.
Symphony patient monitoring s.
System Five echocardiogram s.
T s.
Talent s.
Talos stent delivery s.
TAM s.
TBird ventilator s.
TCD100M digital transcranial
Doppler s.
TCI Heartmate mechanical
circulatory support s.
TEC atherectomy s.
Technos ultrasound s.
Techstar s.
Techstar XL 6F percutaneous
vascular surgical s.
Techstar XL 6F PVS s.
Telectronics Pacing S.'s
Terumo telescoping catheter s.
Testoderm Transdermal s.
ThAIRapy vest airway clearance s.
The Bodyguard emboli
containment s.
The Closer suture-mediated
closure s.
TheraPEP positive expiratory
pressure therapy s.
Therapeutic Intervention Scoring S.
(TISS)
ThermoChem-HT s.
ThermoFlo s.
Thora-Klex chest drainage s.
Thoratec mechanical circulatory
support s.
Thoratec VAD S.
Thrombex PMT s.
Thrombolytic Assessment S. (TAS)
Thumper 1007 CPR s.

TMS 1000 tachyarrhythmia
monitoring s.
TomTec Imaging S.'s
tonsillar somnoplasty s.
Total O_2 delivery s.
Total O_2/Oxilite oxygen s.
Total O_2 supplementary oxygen s.
Total Synchrony S.
TRAKE-fit s.
transesophageal pacing s.
transluminal lysing s.
transtelephonic ambulatory
monitoring s.
Traveler portable oxygen s.
Triad defibrillator s.
Triage cardiac s.
Triage cardiac rapid diagnostic
test s.
triaxial reference s.
Trifoil balloon s.
TRON 3 VACI cardiac imaging s.
TrueMax 2400 Metabolic
Measuring s.
True Stat s.
Trufill n-BCA liquid embolic s.
TruTrak data sampling s.
turbine-powered ICU ventilator s.
two-bottle thoracic drainage s.
Ultraflex esophageal stent s.
Unified Medical Language s.
(UMLS)
Unilink s.
Unistep Delivery s.
Uni-Vent Eagle portable
ventilation s.
Univision echocardiographic s.
USCI Probe balloon-on-a-wire
dilatation s.
vacuum-assisted venous return s.
Vanguard modular endograft s.
Vapor-Phase heated
humidification s.
Vapotherm oxygen delivery s.
Vario s.
vascular s.
VasoExtor lead extraction s.
VasoView Uniport endoscopic
saphenous vein harvesting s.
VDD pacing s.
VenaFlow compression s.
Ventak Prizm 2 s.
Ventak PRx defibrillation s.
Ventak PRx III/Endotak s.
840 ventilator s.
Ventritex TVL s.
vessel occlusion s.
Veterans Affairs Medical Center
scoring s.

Viagraph ECG s.
video s.
videodensitometric analysis s.
Vigilance monitoring s.
Vingmed CFM 800
  echocardiographic s.
Virtuoso LX Smart CPAP s.
Virtuoso Smart CPAP s.
Visa Iris s.
Vitatron pacing s.
VNUS Closure S.
Vortex stabilization s.
VPAP II ST Ventilatory
  Support s.
wall tracking s.
WaveMap intracoronary blood
  pressure measurement s.
WaveWire intracoronary blood
  pressure measurement s.
Welch Allyn/Shiller AT-10 Exercise
  Testing s.
White s.
Wiktor GX Hepamed coated
  coronary stent s.
Wiktor GX Hepamed coronary
  stent s.
Wiktor Prime coronary stent s.
Worldpass delivery s.
Xillix ACCESS s.
Xillix LIFE-Lung s.
X-Sizer catheter s.
X-Sizer single-use catheter s.
XYZ lead s.
Yellow IRIS s.

systema
s. cardiovasculare
s. conducens cordis
s. respiratorium

system/catheter
real-time position management-
  tracking s. (RPM)
RPM tracking s.

systemic
s. arterial air embolism
s. arterial catheter
s. arterial pressure (SAP)
s. betamethasone
s. blood flow (SBF)
s. circulation
s. collateral
dexamethasone s.
s. erythromycin

s. granulomatous vasculitis
s. heart
s. hemodynamic parameters
s. hemodynamics
s. hydration
s. hydrocortisone
s. hypertension
s. infection
s. inflammatory response syndrome
  (SIRS)
s. lupus erythematosus (SLE)
s. mean arterial pressure (SMAP)
s. necrotizing vasculitis
prednisolone s.
s. prothrombosis
s. to pulmonary artery anastomosis
s. to pulmonary connection
s. to pulmonary shunt
s. sclerosis (SS)
s. thromboembolism
s. thrombotic propensity
S. Trial of Pacing to Prevent
  Atrial Fibrillation (STOP-AF)
triamcinolone (s.)
s. vascular hypertension
s. vascular resistance (SVR)
s. vascular resistance index (SVRI)
s. venous atrium
s. venous hypertension
s. venous return

systole
aborted s.
s. alternans
anticipated s.
atrial s.
auricular s.
cardiac s.
electrical s.
electromechanical s.
frustrate s.
hemic s.
isovolumic s.
late s.
premature s.
ventricular s.
ventricular ectopic s.

systolic
s. anterior motion (SAM)
s. apical impulse
s. apical murmur
basal s.
s. blood pressure (SBP)

NOTES

systolic *(continued)*
  s. bruit
  s. bulging
  s. click
  s. click-late systolic murmur syndrome
  s. click-murmur syndrome
  s. current
  s. current of injury
  s. doming
  s. ejection murmur (SEM)
  s. ejection period (SEP)
  s. ejection rate (SER)
  s. function
  s. gallop
  s. gallop rhythm
  s. gradient
  s. heart failure
  s. honk
  s. hypertension
  S. Hypertension in the Elderly Program (SHEP)
  s. left ventricular pressure
  s. murmur
  s. pressure
  s. pressure time index (SPTI)
  s. pulmonary venous velocity
  s. reflection wave
  s. regurgitant murmur
  s. reserve
  s. reversal
  s. shock
  s. thrill
  s. time interval (STI)
  s. trough
  s. upstroke time
  s. velocity ratio
  s. wall motion velocity (Vsys)
  s. whipping
  s. whoop
systolometer
szulgai
  Mycobacterium s.

T
 temperature
 thrombus
  T artifact
  T cell
  T cell defect
  T graft
  T loop
  T lymphocyte
  T sign
  T stent
  T system
  T technique
  T tube
  T vector
  T wave
  T wave alternans (TWA)
  T wave change
  T wave flattening
  T wave inversion
T$_b$
 buildup time
T$_E$
 duration of expiration
 expiratory time
T$_I$
 duration of inspiration
 inspiratory time
T2 relaxation time
T2-weighted MRI
T$_4$
 thyroxine
TA
 tantalum
T + A
 ticlopidine plus aspirin
^{178}TA
 tantalum-178
TAA
 transcoronary alcohol ablation
 triamcinolone acetonide
TAB
 total atrial blanking
  TAB period
tabacosis
tabby
  t. cat heart
  t. cat striation
tabetic cuirass
table
  Akron tilt t.
  anterior t.
  t. binding
  decompression t.
  Diamond-Forrester t.

 Kaplan-Meier life t.
 Siemens open heart t.
tablet
 Actagen T.
 Actifed Allergy T.
 Afrin T.
 Allercon T.
 Allerfrin T.
 Aprodine T.
 Aristocort T.
 Betapace AF t.
 Brontex T.
 Carbiset-TR T.
 Carbodec TR T.
 Cardizem T.
 Cardizem T.
 CellCept t.
 Cenafed Plus T.
 cerivastatin sodium t.
 Chlor-Trimeton 4 Hour Relief T.
 Deconamine T.
 Diltiazem HCl extended-release t.
 Fedahist T.
 Genac T.
 Kenacort T.
 Klerist-D T.
 metoprolol OROS t.
 Mevacor lovastatin t.
 mycophenolate mofetil t.
 Nitrong Oral T.
 NitroQuick sublingual t.
 Nolvadex t.
 Pacerone 200 mg t.
 Phyllocontin T.
 Pseudo-Gest Plus T.
 Spectrobid T.
 Sudafed Plus T.
 Summagraphics digitizing t.
 Taztia XT extended-release t.
 Triposed T.
 ULR LA T.'s
tabourka
 bruit de t.
Tac
 T.-3 injection
 T.-40 injection
TAC atherectomy catheter
tache
 t. blanche
 t. laiteuse
tachometer
tachyarrhythmia
 T. Detection Software
 double ectopic t.
 malignant ventricular t.

T

tachyarrhythmia *(continued)*
   multifocal supraventricular t.
   reentrant ventricular t.
   supraventricular t.
   triple ectopic t.
   ventricular t. (VTA)
tachyarrhythmic substrate
tachybrady arrhythmia
tachybradycardia syndrome
tachycardia
   accelerated idioventricular t.
   accessory pathway mediated t.
   alternating bidirectional t.
   antidromic circus-movement t.
   antidromic reciprocating t.
   atrial t. (AT)
   atrial chaotic t.
   atrial ectopic t. (AET)
   atrial paroxysmal t.
   atrial reentry t.
   atrial ventricular nodal reentry t.
   atrial ventricular reciprocating t.
     (AVRT)
   atriofascicular Mahaim reentrant t.
   atrioventricular junctional
     reciprocating t.
   atrioventricular nodal t. (AVNT)
   atrioventricular nodal reentrant t.
     (AVNRT)
   atrioventricular nodal reentry t.
     (AVNRT)
   atrioventricular reciprocating t.
   atypical atrioventricular nodal
     reentrant t. (AAVNRT)
   auricular t.
   automatic atrial t. (AAT)
   automatic ectopic t.
   A-V junctional t.
   A-V nodal reentry t.
   A-V node reentrant t.
   A-V reciprocating t.
   Belhaussen t.
   bidirectional ventricular t.
   bundle-branch reentrant t.
   burst of ventricular t.
   chaotic atrial t.
   circus-movement t. (CMT)
   Coumel t.
   t. cycle length
   double t.
   drug-refractory t.
   ectopic t.
   ectopic atrial t. (EAT)
   ectopic junctional t.
   endless-loop t.
   t. en salves
   entrainment of t.
   essential t.

   exercise-induced ventricular t.
   t. exophthalmica
   familial t.
   fascicular t.
   fetal t.
   idiopathic ventricular t. (IVT)
   idioventricular t.
   incessant t.
   incessant atrial t.
   incessant ventricular t.
   inducible polymorphic ventricular t.
   intraatrial reentrant t.
   intraatrial reentry t. (IART)
   junctional t. (JT)
   junctional ectopic t. (JET)
   junctional reciprocating t.
   macroreentrant atrial t.
   Mahaim-type t.
   malignant ventricular t.
   monoform t.
   monomorphic ventricular t. (MVT)
   multifocal atrial t. (MAT, MFAT)
   multiform t.
   narrow-complex t.
   nodal t.
   nodal paroxysmal t.
   nodal reentrant t.
   nonparoxysmal atrioventricular
     junctional t.
   nonsuppressible ventricular t.
   nonsustained ventricular t. (NSVT)
   orthodromic atrioventricular
     reciprocating t.
   orthodromic A-V reentrant t.
   orthodromic circus movement t.
   orthodromic reciprocating t. (ORT)
   orthostatic t.
   pacemaker-mediated t. (PMT)
   parasystolic ventricular t.
   paroxysmal t.
   paroxysmal atrial t. (PAT)
   paroxysmal junctional t.
   paroxysmal nodal t.
   paroxysmal reentrant
     supraventricular t.
   paroxysmal sinus t.
   paroxysmal supraventricular t.
     (PSVT)
   paroxysmal ventricular t.
   t. pathway mapping
   permanent atrial t.
   permanent junctional reciprocating t.
     (PJRT)
   pleomorphic t.
   polymorphic ventricular t.
   polymorphous ventricular t.
   primary ventricular t. (PVT)
   rapid nonsustained ventricular t.

reciprocating macroreentry orthodromic t.
reentrant atrial t.
reentrant supraventricular t.
reflex t.
refractory t.
repetitive monomorphic ventricular t.
repetitive paroxysmal ventricular t.
resting t.
resting sinus t.
right ventricular outflow tract t.
salvo of ventricular t.
S-A nodal reentrant t.
self-terminating t.
sinus t.
sinus nodal reentrant t.
sleeping t.
slow-fast t.
spontaneous reentrant sustained ventricular t.
spontaneous ventricular t.
suppressible ventricular t.
supraventricular t. (SVT)
sustained t.
sustained monomorphic ventricular t. (SMVT)
torsade de pointes ventricular t.
t. traumosa exophthalmica
ventricular t. (VT)
wide QRS t.
t. window
Wolff-Parkinson-White reentrant t.
tachycardia-bradycardia syndrome
tachycardiac
tachycardia-dependent aberrancy
tachycardia-induced
t.-i. cardiomyopathy
t.-i. heart failure
t.-i. myopathy
tachycardia-polyuria syndrome
tachycardic
tachycrotic
tachydysrhythmia
tachykinin
t. receptor
t. receptor antagonist
Tachylog pacemaker
tachypacing
tachyphylactic
tachyphylaxis

tachypnea
nervous t.
tachyrhythmia
tachysystole
TACI
total anterior circulation infarct
tack
Effler t.
Tacozin
tacrolimus
TACS
Thrombolysis and Angioplasty in Cardiogenic Shock
total anterior circulation syndrome
TACS clinical trial
TACT
Ticlopidine Angioplasty Coronary Trial
TACTICS
Thrombolysis and Counterpulsation to Improve Cardiogenic Shock Survival
Treat Angina with Aggrastat and Determine Costs of Therapy with Invasive or Conservative Strategies
TACTICS clinical trial
TACTICS study
TACTICS-TIMI 18 trial
Tactiflex
Tactilaze
T. angioplasty
T. angioplasty laser catheter
tactile fremitus
TADcath temporary transvenous defibrillation catheter
TAD guidewire
TAE
transcatheter arterial embolization
Taema nasal prongs
tag
epicardial fat t.
pleural t.
two-dimensional t.
Tagarno 3SD cineangiography projector
tagged
t. acquisition
expression sequence t. (EST)
t. magnetic resonance imaging
tagging
spin t.
TAH
total artificial heart
Berlin TAH
CardioWest TAH

T

NOTES

TAH *(continued)*
    Penn State TAH
    University of Akron TAH
    Utah TAH
    Vienna TAH
tailoring
    root t.
tail sign
TAIM
    Trial of Antihypertensive Interventions
    and Management
Taiwan acute respiratory (TWAR)
Takayasu
    T. aortitis
    T. arteritis
    T. disease
    idiopathic arteritis of T.
    T.-Onishi disease
    T. syndrome
Take Control
Talairach space
talc
    t. granulomatosis
    t. operation
    t. pleurodesis
    t. pneumoconiosis
    t. poudrage
    t. slurry
talcosis
Talent
    T. bifurcated endograft
    T. graft
    T. system
tall
    t. oil asthma
    t. T wave
Talon balloon dilatation catheter
Talos stent delivery system
TAM
    Technology Assessment Methods Project
    Total Atherosclerosis Management
    transtelephonic ambulatory monitoring
    tricuspid annular motion
    TAM system
Tambocor
tambour
    bruit de t.
    t. sound
TAMI
    Thrombolysis and Angioplasty in
    Myocardial Infarction
    TAMI Clinical Trial
    TAMI protocol
Tamiflu
Tamm-Horsfall protein
Tamofen
Tamone
tamoxifen

tamponade, tamponage
    acute t.
    atypical t.
    balloon t.
    cardiac t.
    chronic t.
    esophageal t.
    esophagogastric t.
    heart t.
    low-pressure t.
    pericardial t.
    Rose t.
    subacute t.
    traumatic t.
TAN
    total adenine nucleotides
T-AnastoFlo shunt
tandem
    T. cardiac device
    t. lesion
    t. needle approach
tangential percussion
Tangier disease
tangle
    neurofibrillary t.
TANI
    total axial node irradiation
tank respirator
tannate
    methyclothiazide and
    cryptenamine t.
Tanner operation
tantalum (TA)
    t. balloon-expandable stent with
    helical coil
    t. bronchogram
    powdered t.
    radioactive t.
    t. stent
tantalum-178 (^{178}TA)
    t. generator
TAO
    troleandomycin
TAP
    Thornton anterior positioner
    transesophageal atrial pacing
tap
    bloody t.
    mitral t.
    pericardial t.
    pleural t.
Tapcath esophageal electrode
tape
    T. Based inhaler
    B101 ET Tape II adhesive t.
    Cath-Secure t.
    ColorZone t.
    Hy-Tape waterproof adhesive t.

Original Pink Tape waterproof
adhesive t.
Silastic t.
twill t.
umbilical t.
vascular t.
taper
T. guidewire
short t.
tapered
t. movable core curved wire guide
T. Torque guidewire
tapering
airway t.
Taperseal hemostatic device
tapotage
taprostene
Study of Thrombolytic Therapy
with Additional Response
Following T. (START)
Tapsul pill electrode
TAPVC
total anomalous pulmonary venous
connection
TAPVD
total anomalous pulmonary venous
drainage
TAPVR
total anomalous pulmonary venous return
Taq
T. DNA polymerase
T. extender
TAR
thrombocytopenia-absent radius
TAR syndrome
tar
coal t.
Tarabine PFS
tardive
t. cyanosis
tardus
pulsus t.
pulsus parvus et t.
target
dyspnea t.
t. heart rate (THR)
t. INR
t. lesion
t. lesion revascularization (TLR)
t. site
T. Therapeutics Stealth angioplasty
balloon

T. Tip lead
t. vessel
t. vessel revascularization (TVR)
Tarka
Taro-Ampicillin
Taro-Atenol
Taro-Cloxacillin
TARP
total atrial refractory period
TARTI
total apexcardiographic relaxation time
index
tartrate
metoprolol t.
phenindamine t.
vinorelbine t.
zolpidem t.
tartrazine asthma
TAS
Thrombolytic Assessment System
TASC
Trial of Angioplasty and Stents in
Canada
Tascon prosthetic valve
Ta segment
TASH
transcoronary ablation of septal
hypertrophy
task
bean-spooning t.
Luria conflicting t.'s
metabolic equivalent of t. (MET)
tasosartan
TASS
Ticlopidine Aspirin Stroke Study
TASTE
Ticlopidine Aspirin Stent Evaluation
TAT
thrombin-antithrombin
turnaround time
Tatlockia micdadei
taurinum
cor t.
TAUSA
Thrombolysis and Angioplasty in
Unstable Angina
TAUSA clinical trial
Taussig-Bing
T.-B. anomaly
T.-B. complex
T.-B. disease
T.-B. heart

NOTES

Taussig-Bing *(continued)*
   T.-B. malformation
   T.-B. syndrome
TAV
   transvenous aortovelography
Tavist
Tawara atrioventricular node
taxane
Taxol
taxonomic
taxonomy
Taxotere
Taybi syndrome
Taylor dispersion
Tay-Sachs disease
Tazicef
Tazidime
Taztia XT extended-release tablet
TB
   tuberculosis
TBARS
   thiobarbituric acid reactive substance
TBB, TBBX, TBBx
   transbronchial biopsy
TBC11251
TBFV
   tidal breathing flow-volume
TBI
   thrombotic brain infarction
   total body irradiation
TBird ventilator system
TBLB
   transbronchial lung biopsy
TBNA
   transbronchial needle aspiration
TBV
   total blood volume
3TC
Tc-99
   T. MIBI-SPECT
   T. sestamibi
   T. sestamibi scintigraphy
^{99m}Tc, Tc-99m
   technetium-99m
      ^{99m}Tc DMP-444
TCAD
   transplant coronary artery disease
TCC
   transcatheter closure
TCCS
   transcranial color-coded duplex
      sonography
TCD
   transcranial Doppler
   transcranial Doppler sonography
   transcranial Doppler ultrasound
      Multigon 500M non-contrast-
         enhanced TCD

   TCD sonography
   TCD ultrasonography
   TCD ultrasound
**TCD100M digital transcranial Doppler
system**
Tc-diethylenetriamine pentaacetic acid
TCG
   time compensation gain
T-channel
**TCI Heartmate mechanical circulatory
support system**
Tc-99m *(var. of* ^{99m}Tc)
TCM30 transcutaneous oxygen monitor
Tc-mercaptoacetyltriglycine
TCN-P
   triciribine phosphate
TCOM
   transcutaneous oxygen monitor
TCP, TCPC
   total cavopulmonary connection
^{99m}Tc-sestamibi imaging
TCT
   thoracic computed tomography
   transcatheter therapy
   Trunk Control Test
      TCT scan
^{99m}Tc-tetrofosmin imaging
tcu-PA
   two-chain urokinase plasminogen
      activator
TDD
   thoracic duct drainage
   transpulmonary thermal-dye dilution
TDI
   tissue Doppler imaging
   toluene diisocyanate
      TDI M-mode echocardiography
TDP
   therapist-driven protocol
   torsade de pointes
TdP
   torsade de pointes
**TdT-mediated dUTP nick-end labeling
(TUNEL)**
T-E
   tracheoesophageal
      T-E fistula
TE
   echo delay time
TEA
   thromboendarterectomy
   transluminal extraction atherectomy
tea
   pectoral t.
   t. taster's cough
teacher's node

TEAM
Thrombolytic Trial of Eminase in Acute Myocardial Infarction
team
Bimodality Lung Oncology T. (BLOT)
TEAP
transesophageal atrial pacing
tear
Boerhaave t.
great vessel t.
intimal t.
Mallory-Weiss t.
medial t.
neointimal t.
teardrop heart
teargas
teboroxime
t. imaging
t. scan
technetium-99m t.
tebo scan
Tebrazid
TEC
thromboembolic complication
transluminal endarterectomy catheter
transluminal extraction catheter
TEC atherectomy device
TEC atherectomy system
TEC catheter
TEC extraction catheter
TECAB
totally endoscopic coronary artery bypass
TECBEST
Transluminal Extraction Catheter Before Stent
TECBEST clinical trial
TEC-guide catheter
TechneCard
technetium
t. depreotide
t. glucarate
t. hexakis 2-methoxyisobutyl isonitrile
t. pyrophosphate
t. (Tc)-99m sestamibi tomographic imaging
technetium-99m-labeled annexin-V
technetium-99m (^{99m}Tc, Tc-99m)
t. furofosmin
t. hexakis 2-methyoxyisobutyl isonitrile

t. hexamibi scan
t. imaging
t. methoxyisobutyl isonitrile
t. methylene diphosphonate
t. MIBI
t. MIBI imaging
t. pyrophosphate
t. sestamibi single-photon emission computed tomography (SPECT)
t. sestamibi SPECT
t. sestamibi stress test
t. stannous pyrophosphate scintiscan
t. teboroxime
technetium-99-m-tetrofosmin/fluorine 18-fluorodeoxyglucose
t. tetrofosmin
technetium-sestamibi
technetium-teboroxime
Technicare Omega 500 CT
technique
ablative t.
airway occlusion t.
Amplatz t.
ANGUS t.
antegrade double balloon/double wire t.
antegrade/retrograde cardioplegia t.
anterior sandwich patch t.
anterograde transseptal t.
anti-aliasing t.
Araki-Sako t.
atrial-well t.
background subtraction t.
Bentall inclusion t.
Bergstrom needle biopsy t.
black-white interface t.
blood oxygenation level-dependent t.
BOLD t.
bootstrap two-vessel t.
breathing t.
Brecher and Cronkite t.
Brockenbrough t.
button t.
Carrie coronary stent placement t.
catheterization t.
chloramine-T t.
Ciaglia serial dilatation t.
clearance t.
clonogenic t.
Collins chain compensated gasometer t.

NOTES

technique *(continued)*

Colombo inverted Y t.
Copeland t.
coronary flow reserve t.
cough CPR t.
crash t.
Crawford graft inclusion t.
Creech t.
cryosurgical t.
CT-guided stereotaxic t.
culotte coronary stenting t.
cutdown t.
Davies t.
DCA debulking t.
digital subtraction t.
dilator and sheath t.
direct insertion t.
directional atherectomy debulking t.
DOC exchange t.
Doppler auto-correlation t.
Dotter t.
Dotter-Judkins t.
double-balloon t.
double-balloon (9-11) t.
double-dummy t.
double-syringe t.
double-wire t.
Douglas bag t.
dye dilution t.
ECG signal-averaging t.
en bloc, no-touch t.
entangling t.
exchange t.
Exorcist t.
Fick t.
Finapres t.
first-pass t.
flow mapping t.
flush t.
flush and bathe t.
forced expiratory t.
forced oscillation t. (FOT)
fork stenting t.
forward triangle t.
Fourier-acquired steady-state t.
  (FAST)
gated t.
George-Lewis t.
gloved fist t.
Goris background subtraction t.
grabbing t.
Griggs single-forceps dilatation t.
Grüntzig t.
guidewire t.
harmonic imaging ultrasound t.
Heartport t.
high-pressure inflation t.
hydrogen inhalation t.

immunofluorescent t.
immunostaining t.
indicator dilution t.
indocyanine green indicator
  dilution t.
inhaled radioaerosol t.
Inoue t.
Inoue balloon t.
Inoue single-balloon t.
inverted V t.
Jatene t.
J-loop t.
Judkins t.
Judkins-Sones t.
Kern t.
kissing balloon t.
LocaLisa t.
long-leg venography t.
Lown t.
Marbach-Weil t.
McGoon t.
Merendino t.
minimal leak t.
modified brachial t.
modified Seldinger t.
Mullins blade t.
multibreath nitrogen washout t.
multiplanar reconstruction t.
nasal pool t.
Nikaidoh-Bex t.
nitrogen washout t.
no-leak t.
occluder balloon wash-out t.
oscillation t.
Oxford t.
Paulin venography t.
percutaneous t.
PI MRI t.
Portsmann t.
port access t.
posture t.
pressure-controlled ventilation t.
pressure half-time t.
Rabinov venography t.
radiographic t.
radionuclide t.
Rashkind balloon t.
rebreathing t.
relaxation t.
Ricketts-Abrams t.
Rosalki t.
scatterplot smoothing t.
Schonander t.
Schoonmaker-King single catheter t.
Sealy-Laragh t.
second harmonic imaging
  ultrasound t.
Seldinger percutaneous t.

Sewall t.
shaping behavioral t.
Sheehan and Dodge t.
SHI ultrasound t.
skewer t.
snare t.
Sones t.
sonication t.
SPAMM t.
Sparks mandrel t.
spatial modulation of
  magnetization t.
static dilation t.
steerable over-the-wire
  angioplasty t.
Stewart-Hamilton cardiac output t.
T t.
telescoping anastomotic t.
T-graft configuration t.
thermal dilution t.
thermodilution t.
track-ball t.
Trusler aortic valve t.
TurboFLASH t.
two-patch t.
upgated t.
velocity catheter t.
video-assisted diagnostic
  thoracoscopic t.
Waldhausen subclavian flap t.
wax-matrix t.
xenon washout t.
Y t.
Zavala t.

technology
acquisition zoom t.
T. Assessment Methods Project
  (TAM)
AZ t.
Focus Angioplasty Catheter T.
  (FACT-22)
Lingraphica system treatment t.
Microstream carbon dioxide
  measuring t.
Oxismart Advanced Signal
  Processing and Alarm T.
phased array t.
PulseDose oxygen delivery t.
SAC data acquisition t.
Serial Autocorrelation Data
  acquisition t.
vein-to-vein t.

Technos ultrasound system
Techstar
T. device
T. percutaneous suture
T. suturing closure device
T. system
T. XL 6F percutaneous vascular
  surgical system
T. XL 6F PVS system
Teczem
TED
thromboembolic disease
  TED antiembolism stockings
TEDD
total end-diastolic diameter
tedding device
tedisamil
Tedlar bag
Tedral
TEE
transesophageal echocardiography
  OmniPlane TEE
TEE-DSE
transesophageal echocardiography-
  dobutamine stress echocardiography
Teejel
TEEP
transesophageal echocardiography with
  pacing
TEF
tracheoesophageal fistula
TEF$_{25}$
tidal expiratory flow at 25% of tidal
  volume
TEF$_{25}$/PTEF
ratio of tidal expiratory flow at 25% of
  tidal volume and peak tidal expiratory
  flow
TEF$_{50}$
tidal expiratory flow at 50% of tidal
  volume
TEF$_{50}$/TIF$_{50}$
ratio of tidal expiratory and inspiratory
  flow at 50% of tidal volume
TEF$_{75}$
tidal expiratory flow at 75% of tidal
  volume
Tefcor movable core straight wire
guide
Teflon
T. Bardic plug
T. catheter

T

NOTES

Teflon *(continued)*
T. coating
T. felt bolster
T. felt patch
T. graft
T. intracardiac patch
T. pledget
T. pledget suture buttress
T. sheath
T. TFE SubLite Wall tube
T. trileaflet prosthesis
woven T.
T. woven prosthesis
Teflon-coated
T.-c. guidewire
T.-c. wire skeleton
TEG
thromboelastography
tegafur and uracil (UFT)
Tega-Vert Oral
Tegopen
TEGwire
T. balloon dilatation catheter
T. guide
TEH
theophylline, ephedrine, and hydroxyzine
Teichholz
T. correction
T. ejection fraction
T. formula
teichoic acid antibody
Teichoiz equation
teicoplanin
glycopeptide t.
Tekna mechanical heart valve
Telachlor Oral
Teladar
telangiectasia, pl. **telangiectases**
calcinosis, Raynaud phenomenon,
esophageal involvement,
sclerodactyly, t. (CREST)
hemorrhagic t.
hemorrhagic hereditary t.
hereditary hemorrhagic t. (HHT)
t. syndrome
Teldrin oral
telecardiogram
telecardiophone
Telectronics
T. Accufix pacing lead
T. ATP implantable cardioverter-
defibrillator
T. Guardian ATP 4210 device
T. Guardian ATP II ICD
T. pacemaker
T. Pacing Systems
telecurietherapy
telediastolic

telelectrocardiogram
telemetry
cardiac t.
multiple-parameter t. (MPT)
pacemaker t.
real-time t.
teleradiology
telescope
Storz bronchoscopic t.
telescoping anastomotic technique
telesystolic
Tele-thermometer
YSI T.-t.
Teletrast gauze
Teline Oral
telithromycin
telmisartan
telomere
telomeric shortening
telopeptide
type I collagen t. (ICTP)
TEM
transtelephonic exercise monitor
temafloxacin
temazepam
Temco hoist
temperature (T)
core t.
esophageal t.
t., pulse, and respiration (TPR)
t.-sensing pacemaker
temporal
t. arteritis
t. dispersion
t. resolution
temporary
t. filter
t. pacemaker placement
t. pacing
t. pervenous lead
t. unilateral pulmonary artery
occlusion
temporoparietal white matter (TPWM)
Ten
T. balloon
T. system balloon catheter
tenacious
t. mucus
t. sputum
tenacity
sputum t.
tenascin-C
Tenathan
Tenax
T. Complete stent
T. coronary stent
T. lead
T. stent

Tenax-XR
- T.-X. Complete
- T.-X. stent
- T.-X. Trinity stent

tenderness
- point t.

tendinea
- macula t.

tendineae
- chordae t.

tendinosum
- xanthoma t.

tendinous
- t. spot
- t. xanthoma
- t. zones of heart

tendo
- t. cricoesophageus
- t. infundibuli

tendon
- t. of conus
- coronary t.
- cricoesophageal t.
- false t.
- t. of Todaro, Todaro t.
- trefoil t.

tendophony

Tendril
- T. DX implantable pacing lead
- T. DX pacing lead
- T. DX steroid-eluting active-fixation pacing lead
- T. lead
- T. SDX pacing lead

Tenecteplase

Tenex

Tenif

teniposide

Tennant distress scale

Tennis
- T. Racquet angiographic catheter
- T. Racquet catheter

tenonometer

tenophony

Tenoretic

Tenormin

Tenox

tense
- t. edema
- t. pulse

tensile stress

Tensilon injection

tension
- alveolar carbon dioxide t.
- alveolar oxygen t.
- arterial carbon dioxide t.
- carbon dioxide t.
- left ventricular t.
- myocardial t.
- oxygen t.
- t. pneumopericardium
- t. pneumothorax
- wall t.

tension-length relation

tension-time index

tensor palatini

Tensum coronary stent

tent
- CAM t.
- croup t.
- Croupette child t.
- mist t.
- oxygen t.
- pleural t.
- Silon t.
- steam t.

tenting
- t. of hemidiaphragm
- t. sign
- t. of skin

tenuis
- *Alternaria t.*

Tenzel calipers

Teq-Paq

Tequin

Tequip

teratoma
- pericardial t.
- t. tumor

terazosin hydrochloride

terbutaline sulfate

tercile value

terconazole

terephthalate
- polyethylene t. (PET)

terfenadine

terikalant

terminal
- t. aorta
- t. bronchiole
- t. cisterna
- t. edema
- t. endocarditis
- t. filtered QRS signal

T

NOTES

terminal *(continued)*
t. groove
t. internal carotid artery (TICA)
t. phase
t. pneumonia
t. Purkinje fibers
t. respiratory unit (TRU)
t. weaning
Wilson central t.
terminalis
bronchiolus t.
crista t.
sulcus t.
termination
exercise t.
underdrive t.
terminus
terodiline
terpin
t. hydrate
t. hydrate and codeine
terrae
Mycobacterium t.
Terramycin
T. I.M. injection
T. Oral
terreus
Aspergillus t.
terror
night t.'s
tertiary
t. contraction
t. syphilis
Terumo
T. dialyzer
T. guidewire
T. Radiofocus sheath
T. SP coaxial catheter
T. SP hydrophilic-polymer-coated
microcatheter
T. stent
T. telescoping catheter system
TES
thoracic endometriosis syndrome
transcutaneous electrical stimulation
Tesamone injection
Tesa S.A. handheld electronic digital calipers
TESD
total end-systolic diameter
tesla
Teslac
Tessalon Perles
test
Aachener Aphasic T.
abdominal jugular t.
ABG point-of-care t.
Acarex t.

ACB t.
AccuMeter theophylline t.
acetylcholine t.
acid infusion t.
Action Research Arm T.
adenosine thallium t.
Adson t.
Advanced Care cholesterol t.
aerobic exercise stress t.
aerosol challenge t.
ajmaline t.
AlaSTAT latex allergy t.
albumin cobalt binding t.
alertness t.
Allen t.
alternans t.
Amplicor *Mycobacterium tuberculosis* t.
amplified *Mycobacterium tuberculosis* direct t. (AMTDT)
Anderson t.
anoxemia t.
antistreptozyme t.
apoE t.
Apt t.
Arloing-Courmont t.
arm exercise stress t.
arm-tongue time t.
arterial blood gas point-of-care t. (ABG PCT)
AST2 t.
Astrand bicycle exercise stress t.
ASTZ t.
atrial pacing stress t.
atropine t.
Balke exercise stress t.
Balke-Ware t.
balloon distention t.
Benton Lines T.
Bernstein t.
bicycle ergometer exercise stress t.
bicycle exercise t.
bile solubility t.
BIT-Sternchen T.
Blake exercise stress t.
blanch t.
blot t.
Blumenau t.
Bordet-Gengou t.
breath excretion t.
breath-holding t.
breath pentane t.
Brodie-Trendelenburg t.
Brodie-Trendelenburg tourniquet t.
bronchial challenge t.
bronchial provocation t.
bronchial provocation challenge t.
bronchoprovocation t.

broth t.
Bruce exercise stress t.
Brunnstrom-Fugl-Meyer Scale for
  motor t.
CAMP t.
carbachol provocation t.
carbohydrate utilization t.
Cardiac STATus CK-MB/myoglobin
  panel t.
Cardiac STATus rapid format
  troponin I panel t.
Cardiolite stress t.
cardiopulmonary exercise t. (CPET)
Caregiver Strain T.
carotid sinus t.
Casoni t.
ChemTrak AccuMeter
  theophylline t.
coccidioidin t.
coin t.
cold pressor t.
complement-fixation t.
Coombs t.
CPX t.
cuff t.
cuff-leak t.
Davidson protocol exercise t.
D-dimer t.
Dehio t.
dexamethasone suppression t.
Digit Span t. for short-time
  memory
dipalmitoyl phosphatidylcholine t.
dipyridamole echocardiography t.
dipyridamole handgrip t.
dipyridamole thallium stress t.
direct amplification t. (DAT)
dobutamine stress t.
double simultaneous stimulation t.
DPPC t.
DR-70 tumor marker t.
duodenal string t.
electrophysiologic t.
Elispot t.
Ellestad exercise stress t.
ergonovine provocation t.
Escherich t.
ether t.
euglycemic hyperinsulinemic glucose
  clamp t.
exercise t.
exercise stress t. (EST)

exercise tolerance t. (ETT)
exercise treadmill t. (ETT)
external rotation, abduction,
  stress t. (EAST)
extrastimulus t.
Farr t.
fluorescent treponemal antibody
  absorption t.
foam stability t.
Fowler single-breath t.
Frenchay Aphasia Screening T.
  (FAST)
FTA-ABS t.
Fugl-Meyer Scale for motor t.
GenESA system for radionuclide
  imaging stress t.
Gibbon-Landis t.
Goethlin t.
goodness-of-fit t.
gradational step exercise stress t.
graded exercise t. (GXT)
graded exercise exercise stress t.
Griess t.
guidewire traversal t.
Hallion t.
Ham t.
Hamburger t.
handgrip apexcardiographic t.
  (HAT)
head-down tilt t.
head-up tilt t.
head-up tilt-table t. (HUTTT)
Heaf t.
heart rate variability t.
Heartscan heart attack prediction t.
Henle-Coenen t.
hepatojugular reflux t.
Hess capillary t.
high-altitude simulation t. (HAST)
Hines-Brown t.
Hitzenberg t.
HIVAGEN t.
Hosmer-Lemeshow Goodness-of-
  Fit t.
Hotelling T2 t.
Howell t.
HRV t.
hypoxemia t.
IgG avidity t.
inhalation challenge t.
intravenous glucose tolerance t.
  (IVGTT)

NOTES

test *(continued)*
    isometric handgrip t.
    isoproterenol stress t.
    isoproterenol tilt t.
    isoproterenol tilt-table t.
    Jebsen Hand Function T.
    Kattus exercise stress t.
    Kleihauer t.
    Kleihauer-Betke t.
    Kveim t.
    Kveim antigen skin t.
    Kveim-Siltzbach t.
    laryngeal cough reflex t. (LCR)
    LDL direct t.
    LDL direct blood t.
    lepromin t.
    Levy Chimeric Faces T.
    Lewis-Pickering t.
    Liebermann-Burchard t.
    Lignieres t.
    liver function t. (LFT)
    Livierato t.
    loaded breathing t. (LBT)
    low-range heparin management t.
      (LHMT)
    lymphocyte transformation t.
    Machado-Guerreiro t.
    Mantoux t.
    Master t.
    Master exercise stress t.
    Master two-step exercise t.
    Matas t.
    Mester t.
    methacholine t.
    methacholine challenge t.
    MHA-TP t.
    MIBI stress t.
    microneutralization t.
    6-minute corridor walk t.
    10-minute supine/30-minute tilt t.
    6-minute walking t. (6-MWT)
    modified shuttle t.
    Moschcowitz t.
    MTD t.
    MUGA exercise stress t.
    Muller t.
    Multiple Sleep Latency T. (MSLT)
    Multistage Maximal Effort exercise
      stress t.
    MycoAKT latex bead
      agglutination t.
    myoglobulin cardiac diagnostic t.
    Nagle exercise stress t.
    Nathan t.
    Naughton cardiac exercise
      treadmill t.
    Naughton graded exercise stress t.
    near patient t. (NPT)

N-geneous HDL cholesterol t.
Nickerson-Kveim t.
noninvasive t.
nonspecific challenge t.
Norris t.
Nottingham Sensory Assessment t.
nucleic acid direct amplification t.
Ochsner-Mahorner t.
OPG-Gee t.
Optichin disk t.
oral glucose tolerance t. (OGTT)
Pachon t.
p24 antigen t.
paracoccidioidin skin t.
PCR t.
pendulum t.
peppermint t.
Persantine-isonitrile stress t.
Persantine thallium stress t.
Perthes t.
Phalen stress t.
Physical Work Capacity exercise
  stress t.
pilocarpine iontophoresis t.
planar thallium t.
plantar ischemia t.
Plesch t.
POC t.
POC blood gas t.
point of care t.
PPD t.
PPD skin t.
PPL skin t.
predischarge t.
primed lymphocyte t.
provocation t.
pulmonary function t. (PFT)
PulmoTrack acoustic PF t.
purified protein derivative t.
Q-Stress treadmill stress t.
Quick t.
radioactive xenon t.
radioallergosorbent t. (RAST)
rapid antigen-detection t.
rapid plasma t.
Read t.
Recurring Figures t. for short-time
  memory
Recurring Words t. for short-time
  memory
reflex cough t.
Reflotron bedside theophylline t.
reverse transcriptase polymerase
  chain reaction t.
Rey Figure Copy t.
Rivermead Behavioral Memory T.
Roos t.
Rumpel-Leede t.

Sabin-Feldman dye t.
Salkowski t.
Sandrock t.
Schapiro-Wilks t.
Schellong t.
Schiff t.
Schlichter t.
Schultze t.
serological t.
sestamibi stress t.
sestamibi technetium-99m SPECT
 with dipyridamole stress t.
shake t.
Sheffield exercise stress t.
shuttle t.
single-breath carbon monoxide t.
single-breath nitrogen washout t.
single-stage exercise stress t.
six-minute walk t.
Snider match t.
sniff t.
somatosensory evoked potential t.
Spectral Cardiac STATus T.
Spectral Cardiac STATus CK-
 MB/myoglobulin panel t.
Spectral Cardiac STATus rapid
 format troponin I panel t.
SpectRx t.
speech mental stress t.
split-function lung t.
Stamey t.
Stand Displacement Amplification t.
Star Cancellation T. (SCT)
Sterneedle tuberculin t.
Stratus cardiac troponin I t.
stress t.
Stroop color word conflict t.
Submaximal Effort Tourniquet T.
super stress t.
surf t.
sweat chloride t.
swing t.
symptom-limited maximal
 treadmill t.
symptom-limited treadmill t.
symptom-limited treadmill
 exercise t.
technetium-99m sestamibi stress t.
thallium-201 exercise stress t.
thallium stress t.
thallium-201 stress t.

The Cambridge Heart T-Wave
 Alternans T.
TheoFAST t.
thermodilution t.
thyroid function t.
tilt t.
tilt-table t. (TTT)
tine t.
tolazoline t.
treadmill exercise stress t.
treadmill stress t. (TMST)
Trendelenburg t.
treponemal t.
Tris-buffer infusion t.
Trunk Control T. (TCT)
tuberculin t.
Tuffier t.
two-step exercise t.
Tzanck t.
Valsalva t.
van Elterns t.
vasodilator plus exercise
 treadmill t.
VDRL t.
venous occlusion t.
VEX treadmill t.
Visov t.
Vitalometer t.
Vitalor screening pulmonary
 function t.
in vitro allergy t.
Vollmer t.
volume-challenge t.
von Recklinghausen t.
Wada t.
walking ventilation t.
water-gurgle t.
Weinberg t.
whiff t.
Widal t.
Wideroe t.
Wilks-Schapiro t.
William t.
Williams Doors t.
Winslow t.
Wolf Motor Function T. (WMFT)
word association t. (WAT)
worksite challenge t.
X-Scribe stress t.
Youman-Parlett t.
Zwenger t.

T

NOTES

tester
>IRMA SL blood glucose strip t.
>Polar Electro sport t.
>Quik-Chek external pacer t.

testing (*See also* test)
>point-of-care t. (POCT)

Testoderm Transdermal system
testolactone
Testopel Pellet
testosterone
Testred
tetani
>*Clostridium t.*

tetanus
tethered leaflet
tethering
tetracaine hydrochloride
Tetracap Oral
tetrachloride
>zirconium t.

tetracrotic
tetracycline
tetrad
>Fallot t.
>t. spell

tetraethylammonium chloride
tetrahedon chest
tetrahydrobiopterin
tetrahydrochloride
>diaminobenzidine t.

Tetralan Oral
tetralogy
>Eisenmenger t.
>t. of Fallot (TOF)
>Fallot pink t.
>t. of Fallot spell

Tetram Oral
Tetramune
tetranitrate
>erythrityl t.
>pentaerythritol t.

tetrapolar esophageal catheter
tetrazolium
>nitroblue t.

tetrodotoxin
tetrofosmin
>technetium-99m t.

tet spell
tE/tTOT
>ratio of expiration time and total time of breathing cycle

Teutleben ligament
Teveten
texaphyrin
>lutetium t.

Texas influenza

textbook
>Sleep Multimedia 2.6 computerized t.

TF
>Thomsen-Friedenreich
>TF antigen

TFF
>trefoil factor family
>TFF-domain peptide

TFPI
>tissue factor pathway inhibitor

TFVL
>tidal flow-volume loop

TFX Medical catheter stylet
TGA
>transposition of the great arteries

TGC
>time-gain compensation
>time-gain control
>time-varied gain control

T-Gesic
TGF
>transforming growth factor

TGI
>tracheal gas insufflation

T-graft configuration technique
TGV
>thoracic gas volume

ThAIRapy
>T. vest
>T. vest airway clearance system

thalamic dementia
thalassemia
>sickle cell t.

thalidomide
Thalitone
thallium (Tl)
>t. electrocardiogram
>t. perfusion imaging
>t. rest-redistribution scintigraphy
>t. scanning
>t. sestamibi (^{201}Tl sestamibi)
>t. SPECT imaging
>t. stress test
>t. tomography
>t. uptake
>t. uptake defect
>t. washout

thallium-201 (^{201}Tl)
>t. exercise stress test
>t. perfusion scintigraphy
>t. planar scintigraphy
>t. SPECT scintigraphy
>t. stress test

thallium:YAG laser angioplasty
thallous chloride Tl-201
Thal procedure

Tham
    T.-E
tHcy
    total homocysteine
    total homocysteine level
THC:YAG laser
thebesian
    t. circulation
    t. foramina
    t. valve
    t. vein
Thebesius
    vein of T.
theca cordis
Theden method
Theis rib retractor
Theo-24
Theobid
theobromine
Theochron
Theoclear-80
Theoclear L.A.
Theo-Dur
TheoFAST test
Theo-G
Theolair
Theolate
theophyllinate
    choline t.
theophylline
    t., ephedrine, and hydroxyzine
    (TEH)
    t., ephedrine, and phenobarbital
    t. ethylenediamine
    t. and guaifenesin
    t. sodium glycinate
theorem
    Ba t.
    Bayes t.
    Bernoulli t.
theory
    Bayliss t.
    Cannon t.
    chaos t.
    cross-linkage t.
    dipole t.
    immunological t.
    Melzack-Wall gate t.
    myogenic t.
    neuroendocrine t.
    neurogenic t.
    Ornish t.

    reentry t.
    response-to-injury t.
    sliding filament t.
    Spitzer t.
Theo-Sav
Theospan-SR
Theostat-80
Theovent
Theo-X
TheraCys
Theraflu Non-Drowsy Formula
    Maximum Strength
TheraKair mattress
Theramin Expectorant
TheraPEP
    T. positive expiratory pressure
    therapy system
    T. pre-respiratory therapy treatment
therapeutic
    t. angiogenesis
    t. bronchoscopy
    t. dissection
    t. efficacy
    t. endpoint
    T. Intervention Scoring System
    (TISS)
    t. modality
    t. pneumothorax
therapist-driven protocol (TDP)
therapy
    AAV-CF t.
    ACE antisense gene t.
    amiodarone t.
    angina-guided t.
    angiotensin-converting enzyme
    antisense gene t.
    antiaggregant t.
    antialdosterone t.
    antiarrhythmic t.
    anticlot t.
    anticoagulant t.
    antiendotoxin t.
    antihypertensive diuretic t.
    antiischemic t.
    antimicrobial t.
    antiplatelet t.
    antireflux t.
    antituberculous t.
    augmentation t.
    behavioral t.
    beta-blocker t.
    bretylium t.

NOTES

T

therapy *(continued)*
 bronchodilator t.
 cardiac shock wave t. (CSWT)
 cerebral protective t.
 chest physical t. (CPT)
 Chimeric 7E3 Antiplatelet T.
 CI t.
 circulator boot t.
 Clinitron air-fluidized t.
 collapse t.
 Congestive Heart Failure-Survival
  Trial of Antiarrhythmic T. (CHF-
  STAT)
 constraint-induced movement t.
 continuous nebulization t. (CNT)
 coronary radiation t. (CRT)
 corticosteroid t.
 cytotoxic gene t.
 deep chest t.
 device t.
 directly observed t. (DOT)
 diuretic t.
 ECMO t.
 efficacy of drug t.
 electroconvulsive t.
 embolization t.
 empiric t.
 endobronchial laser t.
 endovascular radiation t.
 enoxaparin bridge t.
 estrogen replacement t. (ERT)
 extracorporeal cardiac shock
  wave t.
 extracorporeal membrane
  oxygenation t.
 fibrinolytic t.
 first-line t.
 fluid t.
 gene t.
 HBO t.
 highly active antiretroviral t.
  (HAART)
 high-output extended aerosol
  respiratory t.
 Holter-guided antiarrhythmic drug t.
 12-hour antiplatelet t.
 hyperbaric oxygen t.
 Hypertension Audit of Risk
  Factor T. (HART)
 hypertensive hypervolemic t. (HHT)
 immunosuppression t.
 inhalation t.
 intracoronary radiation t. (ICRT,
  IRT)
 intravascular red light t. (IRLT)
 intravenous immunoglobulin t.
 ischemia-guided medical t.
 kinetic t.

 lipid-lowering t.
 long-term oxygen t. (LTOT)
 Lymphapress compression t.
 maximum medical t.
 monophasic shock t.
 mucoactive t.
 NCPAP t.
 nebulized Ig t.
 nitric oxide synthase gene t.
 nonballoon t.
 noncommitted biphasic shock t.
 nonsurgical septal reduction t.
  (NSRT)
 open-label ACE-inhibitor t.
 oral anticoagulant t.
 oral flecainide t.
 oxygen t.
 percutaneous intrapericardial fibrin-
  glue infusion t.
 photodynamic t. (PTD)
 Platelet Glycoprotein IIb/IIIa in
  Unstable Angina; Receptor
  Suppression Using Integrilin T.
  (PURSUIT)
 postthrombolytic t.
 Prevention of Atherosclerosis with
  Ramipril T. (PART)
 prophylactic t.
 radiation t.
 red light t. (RLT)
 refractory to medical t.
 Remedy Sleep T.
 reperfusion t.
 rheologic t.
 Selection of Thymidine Analog
  Regimen T. (START)
 shock t.
 somatic cell t.
 statin t.
 Stents and Radiation T. (START)
 step-down t.
 thoracic radiation t. (TRT)
 thrombolytic t. (TT)
 transcatheter t. (TCT)
 TriaDyne II kinetic t.
 VEGF gene t.
 warfarin t.
 zone t.
TheraSnore oral appliance
thermal
 t. angiography
 t. dilution curve
 t. dilution technique
 t. injury
 t. memory stent
 t. sensation
thermal/perfusion balloon angioplasty
 (TPBA)

Thermedics
    T. cardiac device
    T. HeartMate 10001P left anterior assist device
thermic fever
thermistor
    t. plethysmography
    t. thermodilution catheter
thermoacoustic
Thermoactinomyces
    T. candidus
    T. saccharii
    T. viridis
    T. vulgaris
Thermocardiosystems left ventricular assist device
ThermoChem-HT system
thermocoupler
thermodilution
    t. balloon catheter
    t. cardiac output
    t. catheter
    t. catheter introducer kit
    coronary sinus t.
    t. curve
    t.-derived
    Kim-Ray t.
    t. measurement
    t. method
    t. pacing catheter
    t. Swan-Ganz catheter
    t. technique
    t. test
thermoexpandable stent
ThermoFlo
    T. humidifier
    T. system
ThermoFloNeo humidifier
thermography
    infrared t.
thermometer
    infrared t.
    IVAC electronic t.
    SureTemp electronic t.
    Thermoscan Pro-1-Instant t.
thermoplastic head mask
thermoresistable
    Mycobacterium t.
Thermoscan Pro-1-Instant thermometer
thermosetting resin
Thermos pacemaker
Thermo-STAT armcuff heat device

ThermoVent heat and moisture exchanger
TherOx 0.014 infusion guidewire
thesaurosis
    hairspray t.
thiabendazole
thiacetazone
thiamine deficiency
thiamylal sodium
thiazide diuretic
thiazolidinedione derivative
thickened pericardium
thickening
    cardiac wall t.
    diffuse intimal t.
    endocardial t.
    intimal t.
    intimal-medial t.
    leaflet t.
    mediastinal t.
    neointimal t.
    nodular interlobular septal t.
    nonatheromatous intimal t.
    peribronchovascular t.
    pleural t.
    pressure overload-induced aortic valve calcific t.
    septal t.
    valvular t.
    wall t.
thickness
    cap t.
    common carotid artery intima-media t. (CCA-IMT)
    interventricular septal t. (IVS)
    intimal-medial t. (IMT)
    media t.
    posterior wall t.
    relative wall t. (RWT)
    skin-fold t.
    wall t.
thick and sticky mucus
thienopyridine
thigh balloon
thigh-high antiembolic stockings
thimble valvotomy
THI needle
ThinLine
    T. EZ bipolar cardiac pacing lead
    T. EZ bipolar pacemaker lead
    T. EZ pacing lead
    T. lead

T

NOTES

thinning
    infarct t.
    shear t.
    ventricular wall t.
thin-section CT
thin-slice CT scan
thin-walled
    t.-w. catheter
    t.-w. needle
thioamide
thiobarbituric
    t. acid-reactive
    t. acid reactive substance (TBARS)
thiocarlide
thiocyanate
thiolprotease
    lysosomal t.
Thiomerin
thionamide
thiopental sodium
thiopentone sodium
Thioplex
thioridazine hydrochloride
thiosemicarbazide
thiosemicarbazone
thiosulfate
    sodium t.
thiotepa
thioxanthene
third
    t. heart sound (S$_3$)
    t. sound
    t. sound rumble
third-degree
    t.-d. atrioventricular block
    t.-d. A-V block
    t.-d. heart block
third-generation cephalosporin
third-order Butterworth filter
thixotropy
Thoma ampulla
Thomas
    T. LT endotracheal tube holder
    T. Quick Block endotracheal tube
    holder
    T. shunt
Thom flap laryngeal reconstruction
  method
Thompson-Hatina method
Thomsen disease
Thomsen-Friedenreich (TF)
    Thomsen-Friedenreich antigen
thoracalgia
thoracalis
    aorta t.
thoracentesis
    Argyle-Turkel t.

blind t.
    t. needle
thoraces (pl. of thorax)
thoracic
    t. actinomycosis
    t. aorta
    t. aortic aneurysm
    t. aortic dissection
    t. arch aortography
    t. asphyxiant dystrophy
    t. axis
    t. cage
    t. compliance
    t. compressive syndrome
    t. computed tomography (TCT)
    t. crisis
    t. crush injury
    t. duct
    t. duct drainage (TDD)
    t. duct ligation
    t. electrical bioimpedance
    t. empyema
    t. endometriosis syndrome (TES)
    t. esophagus
    t. expanding action
    t. gas
    t. gas volume (TGV, V$_{TG}$)
    t. impedance
    t. incisure
    t. injury
    t. inlet
    t. limb
    t. nerve
    t. outlet compression syndrome
    t. outlet syndrome
    t. part of esophagus
    t. radiation therapy (TRT)
    t. radiologist
    t. respiration
    t. splenosis
    t. squeeze
    t. surgeon
    t. trauma
    t. vertebral body
    t. vessel
thoracica, pl. thoracicae
    aorta t.
    rami esophageales aortae thoracicae
thoracic-pelvic-phalangeal dystrophy
thoracic-stent graft
thoracicus
    ductus t.
thoracis
    compages t.
    empyema t.
    paracentesis t.
thoracoabdominal
    t. aortic aneurysm

t. dyssynchrony
t. paradox
thoracocardiography
thoracocentesis
thoracodorsal artery
thoracodynia
thoracolumbar
thoracopagus twin
thoracophrenolaparotomy
thoracoplasty
apical tailoring t.
costoversion t.
Delorme t.
Fowler t.
Schede t.
Wilms t.
Thoracoport
Auto Suture Soft T.
T. placement
Soft T.
thoracoschisis
thoracoscope
Boutin t.
Coryllos t.
Jacobaeus t.
Jacobaeus-Unverricht t.
rigid t.
thoracoscopic talc insufflation
thoracoscopy
video-assisted t. (VAT, VATS)
Thoracoseal drainage
thoracosternotomy
transverse t.
thoracostomy
closed chest t.
closed-tube t.
needle t.
prophylactic t.
tube t.
t. tube
thoracotome
Bettman-Fovash t.
thoracotomy
anterior t.
emergent t.
t. incision
Lewis t.
posterolateral t.
Thora-Drain III chest drainage
Thora-Klex
T.-K. chest drainage system
T.-K. chest tube

Thora-Port
thorascopic
t. apical pleurectomy
t. talc pleurodesis
Thoratec
T. biventricular assist device
T. cardiac device
T. mechanical circulatory support
system
T. pump
T. right ventricular assist device
T. VAD System
T. ventricular assist device
thorax, pl. **thoraces**
amazon t.
t. asthenicus
barrel-shaped t.
cholesterol t.
frozen t.
muscle of t.
t. paralyticus
Peyrot t.
piriform t.
semispinal muscle of t.
spinal muscle of t.
transverse muscle of t.
Thorazine
Thorel
T. bundle
T. pathway
Thornell microlaryngoscopy
Thornton anterior positioner (TAP)
Thorotrast
Thorpe flowmeter
THR
target heart rate
thread
mucous t.
thready pulse
threatened closure
three-block claudication
three-chambered heart
three-channel
t.-c. electrocardiogram
t.-c. Holter monitor
three-dimensional
t.-d. echocardiography (3DE)
t.-d. Fourier transform (3DFT)
t.-d. helical computed tomography
t.-d. intravascular ultrasound
t.-d. MSPECT

T

NOTES

three-dimensional (*continued*)
    t.-d. spoiled gradient-recalled
      acquisition image
    t.-d. tagged magnetic resonance
      imaging
    t.-d. time-of-flight magnetic
      resonance angiography
three-pillow orthopnea
three-turn epicardial lead
three-vessel coronary disease
three-way stopcock
threonine protein kinase
thresher's lung
threshing fever
threshold
    aerobic t.
    anaerobic t. (AT)
    anginal perceptual t.
    atrial t.
    atrial capture t.
    atrial defibrillation t.
    atrial fibrillation t.
    backscatter t.
    capture t.
    cardioversion t.
    cough t.
    defibrillation t. (DFT)
    t. dose
    fibrillation t.
    flicker fusion t.
    ischemic t.
    lactate t.
    lead t.
    nociceptive t.
    pacemaker t.
    pacing t.
    t. pacing
    T. PEP device
    t. percussion
    t. resistor
    stimulation t.
    t. trend
    t. value
    ventilation t.
    ventilatory t.
    ventilatory anaerobic t. (VAT)
    ventricular capture t.
    work t.
threw an embolus
thrill
    aneurysmal t.
    aortic t.
    arterial t.
    coarse t.
    dense t.
    diastolic t.
    parasternal systolic t.
    precordial t.

    presystolic t.
    purring t.
    systolic t.
thrombasthenia
    Glanzmann t.
Thrombate III
thrombectomize
thrombectomy
    Angiojet rheolytic t.
    catheter t.
    intracoronary aspiration t. (ICAT)
    mechanical t.
    percutaneous mechanical t. (PMT)
    percutaneous rotational t. (PRT)
    shredding embolectomy t. (SET)
Thrombektomat catheter
Thrombex
    T. PMT
    T. PMT system
thrombi (*pl. of* thrombus)
thrombin
    clot-bound t.
    t. generation
    T. Inhibition in Myocardial
      Infarction (TIMI)
    T. Inhibition in Myocardial
      Ischemia (TIMI-7, TRIM)
thrombin-antithrombin (TAT)
    t.-a. III complex
Thrombinar
Thrombinex
thrombin-soaked Gelfoam
thrombin, topical
thromboangiitis obliterans
thromboaortopathy
    occlusive t.
thromboarteritis
thromboaspiration
thromboclasis
thromboclastic
thrombocystis
thrombocytapheresis
thrombocythemia
thrombocytopenia
    t.-absent radius (TAR)
    t.-absent radius syndrome
    drug-induced t.
    essential t.
    heparin-induced t. (HIT)
    idiopathic t.
    immune t.
    lipopolysaccharide-induced t.
    malignant t.
    t. with absence of radius
thrombocytopenia-absent
thrombocytosis
thromboelastogram

thromboelastograph
thromboelastography (TEG)
thromboembolectomy
thromboembolic
  t. complication (TEC)
  t. disease (TED)
  t. pulmonary hypertension
  t. stroke
  t. syndrome
thromboembolism
  Prevention of Recurrent Venous T.
    (PREVENT)
  pulmonary t.
  septic t.
  systemic t.
  venous t. (VTE)
thromboendarterectomy (TEA)
thromboendarteritis
thromboendocarditis
Thrombogen
thrombogenic
  t. component
  t. stimulus
thrombogenicity
  coil t.
thromboglobulin
  beta t.
thromboid
thrombolic
thrombolizer
  Angiocor rotational t.
  T. catheter
thrombolus
thrombolysis
  T. and Angioplasty in Cardiogenic
    Shock (TACS)
  T. and Angioplasty in Myocardial
    Infarction (TAMI)
  T. and Angioplasty in Unstable
    Angina (TAUSA)
  Antithrombotics in the Prevention
    of Reocclusion in Coronary T.
    (APRICOT)
  coronary t.
  T. and Counterpulsation to Improve
    Cardiogenic Shock Survival
    (TACTICS)
  Hirudin in T.
  Hirudin for the Improvement of T.
    (HIT)
  T. in Myocardial Infarction (TIMI)
  t. in myocardial infarction flow

  t. in myocardial infarction flow
    grade 0–3
  t. in myocardial infarction frame
    count
  t. in myocardial infarction grade
  pharmacomechanic t.
  Prehospital Application of
    Coronary T. (PACT)
  selective intracoronary t. (SICT)
  Should We Intervene Following T.
    (SWIFT)
  T. and Thrombin Inhibition in
    Myocardial Infarction
thrombolysis-related intracranial
  hemorrhage (TICH)
thrombolytic
  t. agent
  T. Assessment System (TAS)
  International Joint Efficacy
    Comparison of T.'s
  t. therapy (TT)
  T. Trial of Eminase in Acute
    Myocardial Infarction (TEAM)
thrombomodulin (TM)
thrombophilia
thrombophilic factor V Leiden mutation
thrombophlebitis
  t. migrans
  t. saltans
thromboplastin
  partial t. time (PTT)
  t. time (TT)
thrombopoietin (TPO)
ThromboScan MRI
thrombosed
thrombosis, pl. thromboses
  abacterial t.
  t. activation
  acute t. (AT)
  agonal t.
  Anticoagulants in Secondary
    Prevention of Events in
    Coronary T. (ASPECT)
  aortic t.
  aortoiliac t.
  arterial t.
  atrophic t.
  brachial artery t.
  cardiac t.
  catheter-induced t.
  cavernous sinus t.

T

NOTES

thrombosis *(continued)*
central splanchnic venous t. (CSVT)
cerebral t.
cerebral venous t. (CVT)
cerebrovascular t.
coagulation t.
compression t.
coronary t.
coronary artery t.
cortical vein t.
creeping t.
deep venous t. (DVT)
dilation t.
effort-induced t.
embolic t.
femoral artery t.
femoral venous t.
iliac vein t.
incomplete t.
infective t.
in situ t.
in-stent t.
Integrilin to Manage Platelet Aggregation to Prevent Coronary T. (IMPACT)
intraarterial t.
intramural t.
IVC t.
t. of jugular bulb
jumping t.
laser-induced t.
marantic t.
marasmic t.
mural t.
nonobstructive valve t.
obstructive valve t.
Oral Glycoprotein IIb/IIIa Receptor Blockade to Inhibit T. (ORBIT)
Paget-von Schrötter venous t.
partial confluens sinuum t.
perigraft t.
plate t.
platelet t.
portal vein t.
propagating t.
prosthetic valve t.
Prourokinase in Acute Coronary T. (PACT)
puerperal t.
residual deep vein t.
Ribbert t.
sinus t.
stent t. (ST)
straight sinus t.
subacute t. (SAT)
superimposed t.

traumatic t.
venous t.
thrombospondin-1, thrombospondin-2
thrombostasis
Thrombostat
Thrombotest
thrombotic
t. brain infarction (TBI)
t. endocarditis
t. microangiopathy
t. thrombocytopenic purpura (TTP)
Thrombo-Wellcotest method
thromboxane
t. A_2
t. receptor antagonist
t. synthesis
t. synthetase inhibitor
thrombus, pl. thrombi (T)
adherent mobile t.
adherent mural t.
agglutinative t.
agonal t.
annular t.
antemortem t.
atrial t.
ball t.
ball valve t.
blood plate t.
blood platelet t.
calcified t.
capillary thrombi
coral t.
currant jelly t.
fibrin t.
t.-filled cavity
free-floating t. (FFT)
free-floating vena caval t.
globular t.
t. grade
hyaline t.
infective t.
intracardiac t.
intragraft t.
intraluminal t.
intramural t.
intravascular t.
LAA thrombi
laminated t.
lateral t.
marantic t.
marasmic t.
massive t.
migratory t.
mixed t.
mural thrombi
mural t.
obstructive t.
occluding t.

occlusive t.
organized t.
pale t.
parietal t.
pedunculated t.
plate t.
platelet t.
postmortem t.
t. precursor protein (TpT)
T. Precursor Protein immunoassay
primary t.
progressive t.
propagated t.
propagation of t.
red t.
red coronary t.
right atrial t.
saddle t.
secondary t.
straddling t.
stratified t.
t. stripper
Transluminal Extraction Catheter or
 PTCA in T. (TOPIT)
traumatic t.
valvular t.
ventricular t.
white t.
white coronary t.
through-and-through
 t.-a.-t. continuous suture
 t.-a.-t. myocardial infarction
through-the-balloon ultrasound
through-the-wall mattress suture
Thruflex
 T. balloon
 T. PTCA balloon catheter
thrush
 t. breast
 t. breast heart
thrust
 cardiac t.
thulium-holmium-chromium:yttrium-
 aluminum-garnet laser
thulium-holmium:YAG laser
thulium:YAG laser angioplasty
thumbprint bronchus sign
thump
 chest t.
 precordial t.
Thumper 1007 CPR system
thumpversion

thymectomy
 video-assisted thoracoscopic t.
thymic
 t. asthma
 t. cyst
thymidine phosphorylase
thymoma
thymopentin
thymostimuline
thymusectomy
Thyrar
Thyro-Block
thyrocardiac
 t. disease
thyroid
 aberrant t.
 accessory t.
 t. antibody
 Armour T.
 t. bruit
 t. cachexia
 t. disease
 t. extract
 t. function test
 intrathoracic t.
 t. isthmus
 lingual t.
 t. notch
 t. panel
 retrosternal t.
 t. storm
 T. Strong
 substernal t.
 t. tumor
thyroideae
 musculus levator glandulae t.
thyroidectomy
thyroiditis
 chronic lymphocytic t.
 de Quervain t.
 Hashimoto t.
 Riedel t.
 woody t.
thyroid-stimulating hormone (TSH)
thyrointoxication
Thyrolar
thyrolaryngeal
thyrolingual duct
thyromegaly
thyropalatine
thyropharyngeal
thyroprival

NOTES

T

thyrotoxic heart disease
thyrotoxicosis
thyrotoxin radioisotope assay
thyrotropin
thyrotropin-releasing hormone response
thyroxine, thyroxin (T$_4$)
D-**thyroxine**
L-**thyroxine**
TIA
    transient ischemic attack
      crescendo TIA
      vertebrobasilar TIA
Tiamate
tiamenidine
tiapamil
Tiazac extended-release capsule
TIBBS
    Total Ischemic Burden Bisoprolol Study
Tibbs arterial cannula
tibial
    t. artery
    t. pulse
tibioperoneal vessel angioplasty
TICA
    terminal internal carotid artery
Ticar
ticarcillin
    t. and clavulanate potassium
    t. and clavulanic acid
    t. disodium
Tice BCG
TICH
    thrombolysis-related intracranial
    hemorrhage
tick
    t. anticoagulant peptide
    t. paralysis
Ticlid
ticlopidine
    T. Angioplasty Coronary Trial
    (TACT)
    T. Aspirin Stent Evaluation
    (TASTE)
    T. Aspirin Stroke Study (TASS)
    t. hydrochloride
    Multicenter Stents T. (MUST)
    t. plus aspirin (T + A)
Ti-Cron suture
tic-tac
    t.-t. rhythm
    t.-t. sounds
TICU
    trauma intensive care unit
TID
    transient ischemic dilation
tidal
    t. air
    T. balloon catheter

    t. breathing
    t. breathing flow-volume (TBFV)
    t. expiratory flow at 25% of tidal
    volume (TEF$_{25}$)
    t. expiratory flow at 50% of tidal
    volume (TEF$_{50}$)
    t. expiratory flow at 75% of tidal
    volume (TEF$_{75}$)
    t. expiratory volume (TV$_E$)
    t. flow
    t. flow-volume loop (TFVL)
    t. inspiratory flow at 50% of tidal
    volume (TIF$_{50}$)
    t. inspiratory volume (TV$_I$)
    t. loop
    t. volume (TV, V$_T$)
    t. wave
    T. Wave handheld capnograph
    t. wave pulse
    T. Wave Sp capnometer/pulse
    oximeter
TIE
    transient ischemic event
tiered-therapy
    t.-t. antiarrhythmic device
    t.-t. implantable cardioverter-
    defibrillator
    t.-t. programmable cardioverter-
    defibrillator
Tietze syndrome
TIF$_{50}$
    tidal inspiratory flow at 50% of tidal
    volume
tiger
    t. heart
    t. lily heart
tight
    t. asthmatic
    t. junction
    t. stenosis
tightness
    chest t.
tight-to-shaft Aire-Cuf tracheostomy
tube
tigroid striation
TIJ lead
Tikosyn
Tilade
    T. Inhalation Aerosol
    T. inhaler
Tildiem
tilt
    first-phase t.
    head-up t. (HUT)
    10-minute supine/30-minute t. test
    second-phase t.
    t. test
    t. vital signs

tilting
      t. disk valve
      passive t.
tilting-disk
      t.-d. aortic valve prosthesis
      t.-d. heart valve
      t.-d. occluder
      t.-d. prosthetic valve
tilt-table test (TTT)
TIM
      tissue-infiltrating macrophage
Tim-AK
time
      acceleration t.
      acquisition t.
      activated clotting t. (ACT)
      activated coagulation t. (ACT)
      activated partial thromboplastin t.
        (aPTT, APTT)
      AH conduction t.
      arm-tongue t.
      atrioventricular t.
      buildup t. (T_b)
      bypass t.
      capacitor forming t.
      carotid ejection t.
      central motor conduction t.
        (CMCT)
      cerebral transit t. (cTT)
      charge t.
      circulation t.
      clot retraction t.
      coagulation t.
      cold ischemic t. (CIT)
      t. compensation gain (TCG)
      conduction t.
      corrected sinus node recovery t.
      cross-clamp t.
      dead t.
      deceleration t.
      detect t.
      t. domain
      t. domain signal-averaged
        electrocardiogram
      t. domain signal-averaged
        electrocardiography
      donor organ ischemic t.
      door-to-needle t.
      doubling t.
      Duke bleeding t.
      echo delay t. (TE)
      ejection t.

      esophageal transit t.
      euglobulin clot lysis t.
      expiratory t. (T_E)
      extubation t.
      t. of flight (TOF)
      t. of flight and absorbance
        (TOFA)
      t. of flight and absorbance
        spectrophotometry
      flushing t.
      forced expiratory t. (FET)
      t. forced expiratory rate
      H-R conduction t.
      HR conduction t.
      HV conduction t.
      H-V conduction t.
      hydrogen appearance t.
      inspiratory t. (T_I)
      interatrial conduction t.
      intraatrial conduction t.
      intubation t.
      isovolumic relaxation t. (IVRT)
      Ivy bleeding t.
      left ventricular ejection t. (LVET)
      longitudinal relaxation t.
      lung-to-finger circulation t. (LFCT)
      lysis t.
      magnetic relaxation t.
      maximum walking t.
      median survival t. (MST)
      P-A conduction t.
      PA conduction t.
      pain-free walking t. (PFWT)
      partial thromboplastin t. (PTT)
      t. to peak expiratory flow (tPTEF)
      t. to peak inspiratory flow (tPTIF)
      PH conduction t.
      P-H conduction t.
      prothrombin t. (PT)
      prothrombin time/partial
        thromboplastin t. (PT/PTT)
      quick prothrombin t.
      ratio of inspiratory time to total
        cycle t. (T_I/T_{TOT})
      relaxation t.
      repetition t. (TR)
      saturation t.
      sinoatrial conduction t. (SACT)
      sinoatrial recovery t. (SART)
      sinus node recovery t. (SNRT)
      spin-lattice t.
      spin-spin t.

T

NOTES

time *(continued)*
    survival t.
    systolic upstroke t.
    thromboplastin t. (TT)
    time to peak expiratory flow and total expiration t. (tPTEF/tE)
    total sleep t. (TST)
    transmitral E-wave deceleration t.
    T2 relaxation t.
    turnaround t. (TAT)
    ventilator t.
    ventricular activation t. (VAT)
    wake after sleep onset t. (WASO)
time-activity curve
time-averaged peak velocity
time-based
    t.-b. counter
    t.-b. event recording
Timecelles
    Sinufed T.
time-compensated gain
time-cycled ventilation
time-cycling
timed
    t. forced expiratory volume
    t. vital capacity
time-domain analysis
time-gain
    t.-g. compensation (TGC)
    t.-g. control (TGC)
Timentin
time-of-flight
    t.-o.-f. effect
    t.-o.-f. magnetic resonance angiography
time-resolved imaging by automatic data segmentation (TRIADS)
time-to-peak
    t.-t.-p. contrast
    t.-t.-p. filling rate
time-triggered
time-varied
    t.-v. gain (TVG)
    t.-v. gain control (TGC, TVGC)
TIMI
    Thrombin Inhibition in Myocardial Infarction
    Thrombolysis in Myocardial Infarction
    TIMI classification
    TIMI Clinical Trial
    TIMI criteria
    TIMI flow
    TIMI flow grade 0–3
    TIMI frame count
    TIMI frame count index
    TIMI grade
    TIMI myocardial perfusion grade

    TIMI patency
    TIMI trial
TIMI-7
    Thrombin Inhibition in Myocardial Ischemia
    TIMI-7 clinical trial
TIMI-9
    TIMI-9 clinical trial
TIMI-18 *(See* TACTICS study, TACTICS study)
TIMI-23 *(See* ENTIRE study, ENTIRE study)
timing circuit
Timolide
timolol maleate
timori
    Brugia t.
TIMP
    tissue inhibitor of metalloproteinase
TIMP-3
    tissue inhibitor of metalloproteinase-3
    TIMP-3 overexpression
Timpe and Runyon classification
TINA monitor
Tina-quant immunoturbidometric assay
tine
    t. test
    T. Test PPD
tined
    t. lead pacemaker
    t. ventricular electrode
tinidazole
tinkle
    Bouillaud t.
    metallic t.
tin oxide
TintElize PAI-1 ELISA kit
tinzaparin
    t. sodium
    t. sodium injection
tiotropium bromide
tip
    Andrews suction t.
    Ducor t.
    t. extrasystole
    Luer-Lok needle t.
    Medtronic t.
    mitral leaflet t.
    t. occluder
    papillary muscle t.
    Polaris Mansfield/Webster deflectable t.
    Skimmer laryngeal blade t.
    Tricut laryngeal blade t.
tip-deflecting wire
tiprenolol hydrochloride

TIPS
transjugular intrahepatic portosystemic shunt
tirilazad mesylate
tirofiban
TISS
Therapeutic Intervention Scoring System
Tissomat application device and spray set
Tissot spirometer
tissue
t. ablation
adipose t.
atrioventricular conduction t.
autodigestion of connective t.
t. bank
bronchopulmonary t.
bronchus-associated lymphoid t. (BALT)
caseated t.
connective t.
t. Doppler imaging (TDI)
extrathoracic soft t.
exuberant granulation t. (EGT)
t. factor
t. factor pathway inhibitor (TFPI)
fast t.
t. fissure
granulation t.
gut-associated lymphoid t. (GALT)
His-Purkinje t.
t. inhibitor of metalloproteinase (TIMP)
t. inhibitor of metalloproteinase-3 (TIMP-3)
t. inhibitor of metalloproteinase-3 overexpression
interfascicular fibrous t.
laminated connective t.
myocardial t.
myocardial scar t.
t. necrosis
neointimal t.
nodal t.
perinodal t.
t. plasminogen activator (tPA)
t. preservation
resistance to movement of lung t. (Rti)
t. septa
slow t.

t. supersaturation
t. valve
tissue-infiltrating macrophage (TIM)
tissue-specific antibody
tissue-type plasminogen activator
Titan
T. mega PTCA dilatation catheter
T. mega XL PTCA dilatation catheter
titanium
t. cage
T. VasPort
titer
antiheart antibody t.
anti-Rho-D t.
bactericidal t.
Lyme t.
serum bactericidal t. (SBT)
titration regimen
Titrator
tI/tTOT
ratio of inspiration time and total time of breathing cycle
tizanidine hydrochloride
Tl
thallium
Tl-201
thallous chloride Tl-201
^{201}Tl
thallium-201
^{201}Tl sestamibi
TLC
total lung capacity
TLC-II portable VAD driver
TLCO, TLco
carbon monoxide transfer factor
TLI
total lymphoid irradiation
Tl-201 perfusion tracer
TLR
target lesion revascularization
TM
thrombomodulin
TMLR
transmyocardial laser revascularization
TMP-SMX
trimethoprim-sulfamethoxazole
TMR
laser transmyocardial revascularization
transmyocardial revascularization
Heart Laser for TMR

NOTES

T

TMS
transcranial magnetic stimulation
TMS 1000 tachyarrhythmia
monitoring system
TMST
treadmill stress test
TMZ
trimetazidine 1
TNB
transthoracic needle biopsy
TNF
tumor necrosis factor
TNF-alpha
tumor necrosis factor-alpha
TNKase
TNK-tPA
TNM
tumor, nodes, metastasis
TNM classification
TNM staging
TnT
troponin T
to-and-fro
t.-a.-f. murmur
t.-a.-f. sound
TOAST
Treatment of Acute Stroke Trial
Trial of Org 10172 in Acute Stroke
Treatment
tobacco heart
TOBI Inhalation Solution
tobramycin
nebulized t.
t. solution for inhalation
tocainide hydrochloride
Todaro
tendon of T.
T. tendon
T. triangle
Todd-Hewitt broth
Todd units
toes
clubbing of t.
TOF
tetralogy of Fallot
time of flight
TOF MRA
TOFA
time of flight and absorbance
TOFA spectrophotometry
Tofranil
Togaviridae virus
TOHP
Trials of Hypertension Prevention
toilet, toilette
bronchial t.
pleural t.
pulmonary t.

respiratory t.
tracheobronchial t.
toilet-seat
t.-s. angina
t.-s. syncope
tolazamide
tolazoline
t. hydrochloride
t. test
tolbutamide
tolerance
exercise t.
hemodynamic t.
impaired glucose t. (IGT)
Tolinase
toluene
t. diisocyanate (TDI)
toluidine blue stain
Tolu-Sed DM
Tomcat PTCA guidewire
Tomita method
tomogram
horizontal long-axis t.
short-axis t.
vertical long-axis t.
tomograph
ECAT III positron t.
tomographic
high-resolution thin section
computed t.
t. radionuclide imaging
t. radionuclide ventriculography
tomography
adenosine triphosphate single-photon
emission computed t. (ATP-
SPECT)
atrial bolus dynamic computer t.
axial computed t. (ACT)
biplanar t.
cine computed t.
computed t. (CT)
computerized axial t. (CAT)
dual-isotope simultaneous acquisition
single-photon emission
computed t. (DISA-SPECT)
electrical impedance t. (EIT)
electron beam computed t. (EBCT)
gated computed t.
high-resolution computed t. (HRCT)
methoxyisobutyl isonitrile single-
photon emission computed t.
(MIBI-SPECT)
N-13 ammonia positron emission t.
optical coherence t. (OCT)
positron emission t. (PET)
quantitative computed t. (QCT)
rapid acquisition computed axial t.
(RACAT)

rubidium-82 positron emission t.
(Rb-82 PET)
seven-pinhole t.
single-photon emission t. (SPET)
single-photon emission computed t.
(SPECT)
slant hole t.
spiral computed t. (SCT)
Stent Treatment Region Assessed
by Ultrasound T.
technetium-99m sestamibi single-
photon emission computed t.
(SPECT)
thallium t.
thoracic computed t. (TCT)
three-dimensional helical
computed t.
ultrafast computed t. (UFCT)
ultrafast contrast-enhanced chest
computed t.
xenon-enhanced computed t.
(XECT)
x-ray cine computed t.

TomTec
T. echo platform
T. Imaging Systems

tone
bronchial smooth muscle t.
cardiac vagal t.
heart t.'s
resting vascular t.
Traube double t.
vagal t.
vasomotor t.
Williams tracheal t.

tongs
Trippi-Wells t.

tongue
t.-jaw lift
t.-retaining device
t.-rolling effect
smoker's t.
t. traction

Tonocard
tonometer
air-puff t.
Gärtner t.
Linear KGT t.

tonometered whole blood
tonometry
applanation t.
peripheral artery t.

tonoscillograph
tonsil
Gerlach t.
kissing t.
laryngeal t.
lingual t.
Luschka t.
palatine t.
pharyngeal t.

tonsilla
t. lingualis
t. palatina
t. pharyngealis

tonsillar
t. pillar
t. ring
t. somnoplasty procedure
t. somnoplasty system

tonsillaris
angina t.

tonsillitis
caseous t.
chronic catarrhal t.
diphtherial t.

tonsilloadenoidectomy
tool
Avenue insertion t.
LIMA-Lift t.
LIMA-Loop t.
QuantX color quantification t.

Top-Hat supraannular aortic valve
topical
Aquacare t.
Bactroban T.
Benadryl T.
Carmol t.
t. cooling
Efudex T.
Fluoroplex T.
Gelfoam T.
t. hypothermia
Lanaphilic t.
Mycostatin T.
Nilstat T.
Nutraplus t.
Nystex T.
Oxsoralen T.
Rogaine t.
Solarcaine t.
thrombin, t.
Ultra Mide t.
Ureacin-20 t.

NOTES

T

TOPIT
Transluminal Extraction Catheter or PTCA in Thrombus
TOPIT clinical trial
topography
NMR t.
Toposar injection
topotecan
Toprol XL
torasemid
Torcon NB selective angiographic catheter
Torek resection of thoracic esophagus
toremifene
Torktherm torque control catheter
Tornalate
Tornwaldt cyst
toroidal valve
Toronto
T. Alexithymia Scale
T. SPV aortic valve
T. SPV bioprosthesis
T. SPV stentless porcine heart valve
T. SPV valve
torpedo-shaped pattern
torque
clockwise t.
t. control
t. control balloon catheter
t. vise
torquer
Clip On t.
torquing ability
torr
t. pressure
t. unit
Torricelli
T. law
T. model
T. orifice equation
torsade
t. de pointes (TDP, TdP)
t. de pointes ventricular tachycardia
torsemide
tortuosity
tortuous
t. right coronary artery
t. veins
t. vessel
Torula histolytica
Torulopsis glabrata
torulosis
torus aorticus
TOS
toxic oil syndrome

Toshiba
T. biplane transesophageal transducer
T. electrocardiography machine
T. MRT 200 MRI
T. scanner
T. Sonolayer SSH-140A ultrasound
tosylate
bretylium t.
Totacillin
TOTAL
Total Occlusion Trial with Angioplasty by Using Laser Guidewire
total
t. absence of circulation on four-vessel angiography
t. acidity
t. adenine nucleotides (TAN)
t. airway resistance (Rtot)
t. alternans
t. anomalous pulmonary venous connection (TAPVC)
t. anomalous pulmonary venous drainage (TAPVD)
t. anomalous pulmonary venous return (TAPVR)
t. anterior circulation infarct (TACI)
t. anterior circulation syndrome (TACS)
t. apexcardiographic relaxation time index (TARTI)
t. artificial heart (TAH)
T. Atherosclerosis Management (TAM)
t. atrial blanking (TAB)
t. atrial blanking period
t. atrial refractory period (TARP)
t. axial node irradiation (TANI)
t. blood volume (TBV)
t. body irradiation (TBI)
t. cardiopulmonary bypass
t. cavopulmonary anastomosis
t. cavopulmonary connection (TCP, TCPC)
t. chordal-sparing mitral valve replacement
t. circulatory arrest
T. Cross balloon catheter
t. end-diastolic diameter (TEDD)
t. end-systolic diameter (TESD)
t. homocysteine (tHcy)
t. homocysteine level (tHcy)
T. Ischemic Burden Bisoprolol Study (TIBBS)
t. lung capacity (TLC)
t. lung compliance
t. lymphoid irradiation (TLI)

T. Occlusion Trial with Angioplasty by Using Laser Guidewire (TOTAL)
T. O$_2$ delivery system
T. O$_2$/Oxilite oxygen system
T. O$_2$ supplementary oxygen system
t. patient shock count
t. peripheral resistance (TPR)
t. peripheral resistance index (TPRI)
t. peroxyl radical-trapping antioxidant potential (TRAP)
t. plasma cholesterol
positive symptom t. (PST)
t. pressure (P$_T$)
t. pulmonary resistance (TPR)
t. repair of tetralogy of Fallot
t. sleep time (TST)
T. Synchrony System
totally endoscopic coronary artery bypass (TECAB)
Tote-A-Neb nebulizer
touch shock count
Toupet hemifundoplication
Tourguide guiding catheter
tourniquet
Bethune lobectomy t.
Carr lobectomy t.
Esmarch t.
Medi-Quet t.
pneumatic t.
Rumel t.
Shenstone t.
Touro
T. Ex
T. LA
Tovell tube
Tower stent
Townes-Brocks syndrome
toxemia
toxemic pneumonia
toxic
t. agent
t. delirium
t. epidermal necrolysis
t. fume inhalation
t. myocarditis
t. oil syndrome (TOS)
t. shock
toxicity
amphetamine t.

anthracycline t.
antimony t.
cobalt t.
dextroamphetamine t.
digitalis t.
digoxin t.
doxorubicin-induced cardiac t.
emetine t.
fluoride t.
hydrocarbon t.
oxygen t.
phenylpropanolamine t.
plant t.
toxicosis
Aspergillus t.
toxin
adenylate cyclase t.
t. exposure
pertussis t.
RNA glycosidase t.
toxin-insensitive current
Toxocara canis
toxoid
diphtheria and tetanus t.
Toxoplasma gondii
toxoplasmosis
ToxR protein
TP
T. baseline
T. interval
T. segment
TP10
tPA
tissue plasminogen activator
TPBA
thermal/perfusion balloon angioplasty
TPG
transvalvular pressure gradient
T-Phyl
T-piece
Ayers T-p.
T-p. oxygen
T-p. weaning
TPO
thrombopoietin
T-P-Q segment
TPR
temperature, pulse, and respiration
total peripheral resistance
total pulmonary resistance
TPRI
total peripheral resistance index

NOTES

TpT
    thrombus precursor protein
tPTEF
    time to peak expiratory flow
tPTEF/tE
    time to peak expiratory flow and total
      expiration time
tPTIF
    time to peak inspiratory flow
TPWM
    temporoparietal white matter
TQ segment
TR
    repetition time
    tricuspid regurgitation
trabecula, pl. **trabeculae**
    trabeculae carneae
    t. septomarginalis
trabecular hypertrophy
trabeculation
    muscle t.
TRACE
    Trandolapril Cardiac Evaluation
trace
    t. metal
    T. vein stripper
tracer
    carbon-11 palmitic acid
      radioactive t.
    t. distribution
    frequency t.
    t. homogeneity
    iodine-123 heptadecanoic acid
      radioactive t.
    t. retention
    t. storage
    Tl-201 perfusion t.
    t. uptake
TrachCare
    T. multi-access catheter
    neonatal Y T.
trachea
    anular ligament of t.
    bifurcation of t.
    carina of t.
    membranous wall of t.
    muscular coat of t.
    scabbard t.
    steepling of t.
tracheae
    bifurcatio t.
    carina t.
    paries membranaceus t.
    tunica mucosa t.
    tunica muscularis t.
tracheal
    t. aspirate
    t. bifurcation

    t. branch
    t. bronchus
    t. button
    t. cartilage
    t. deviation
    t. gas insufflation (TGI)
    t. gland
    t. intubation
    t. lymph node
    t. mucosa
    t. mucus velocity
    t. rale
    t. ring
    t. sound
    t. steepling
    t. triangle
    t. tube
    t. tug
    t. vein
tracheales
    cartilagines t.
    glandulae t.
    venae t.
trachealia
    ligamenta anularia t.
trachealis
    angina t.
    t. muscle
tracheitis
trachelalis
trachelooccipitalis
tracheobiliary
tracheobronchial
    t. amyloidosis
    t. angle
    t. aspirate
    t. clearance
    t. collapse
    t. diverticulum
    t. dyskinesia
    t. flora
    t. foreign body
    t. lavage
    t. toilet
    t. tree
    t. tuberculosis
tracheobronchitis
    Aspergillus t.
    influenza t.
    pseudomembranous t.
    pseudomembranous *Aspergillus* t.
tracheobronchomalacia
tracheobronchomegaly
tracheobronchoscopy
Tracheobronxane ST tracheal stent
tracheoesophageal (T-E)
    t. fistula (TEF)

t. junction
t. puncture
tracheolaryngeal
Tracheolife HME
tracheomalacia
tracheopathia osteoplastica
tracheopharyngeal
tracheophonesis
tracheophony
tracheoscope
Storz t.
Storz-Shapshay t.
tracheostenosis
tracheostomized
tracheostomy
t. button
t. cuff
flap t.
Great Ormond Street t.
Montgomery t.
percutaneous dilatational t. (PDT)
percutaneous dilational t. (PDT)
t. plate
t. stoma
T. T.O.M. anatomical model
t. tube
tracheotome
Salvatore-Maloney t.
tracheotomy
percutaneous t.
Trach-Mist
trachomatis
Chlamydia t.
trach plate
Trach-Talk
trachyphonia
tracing
carotid pulse t.
diamond-shaped t.
fetal heart monitor t.
jugular venous pulse t.
pressure t.
pulse t.
serial ECG t.
serial electrocardiogram t.
stripchart t.
venous pressure t.
venous pulse t.
track
tram t.
trackability
track-ball technique

tracker
Purkinje image t.
Tracker-18 Soft Stream side-hole microinfusion catheter
Tracker microcatheter
tracking
bolus t.
spatial t.
wall t.
Trac Plus catheter
Tracrium
tract
atriodextrofascicular t.
atriofascicular t.
atrio-His t.
atrio-His bypass t.
atrionodal bypass t.
bronchopulmonary t.
bypass t.
concealed bypass t.
gastrointestinal t.
inflow t.
James accessory t.'s
left ventricular outflow t. (LVOT)
lower respiratory t.
nodohisian bypass t.
nodoventricular t.
outflow t.
pulmonary outflow t.
respiratory t.
right ventricular outflow t. (RVOT)
spinothalamic t.
Wolff-Parkinson-White bypass t.
traction
t. aneurysm
t. bronchiectasis
t. bronchiolectasis
Crego t.
papillary muscle t.
t. suture
tongue t.
tragacanth asthma
trailing edge
train
drive t.
t.'s of ventricular pacing
training
CDBR respiratory muscle t.
t. effect
resistance t. (RT)
strength t.
trainwheel rhythm

T

NOTES

trait
    sickle cell t.
Trak Back pullback device
TRAKE-fit system
TrakPro data analysis software
Trakstar balloon catheter
tram
    t. line
    t. tracks
Trandate
    T. injection
    T. Oral
trandolapril
    T. Cardiac Evaluation (TRACE)
    t. and verapamil
tranexamic acid
tranilast
    T. Restenosis Following
      Angioplasty Trial (TREAT)
Tranquility
    T. BiLevel airway patency
      maintenance device
    T. BiLevel CPAP unit
    T. BiLevel positive airway pressure
      therapy device
    T. Quest
    T. Quest CPAP device
tranquilizer
trans
    t. fat
    t. fatty acids
transaminase
    glutamic-oxaloacetic t. (GOT)
    serum glutamic-oxaloacetic t.
      (SGOT)
    serum glutamic-pyruvic t. (SGPT)
transannular patch
transaortic
    t. gradient
    t. valve gradient
transatrial pacing
transaxial
    t. plane
    t. slice
transaxillary apical bullectomy
transbrachial aortography
transbronchial
    t. biopsy (TBB, TBBX, TBBx)
    t. lung biopsy (TBLB)
    t. needle aspiration (TBNA)
transcapillary refill
transcardiac monocyte
transcarotid balloon valvuloplasty
transcatheter
    t. ablation
    t. arterial embolization (TAE)
    t. closure (TCC)
    t. closure of atrial defect

    t. closure of atrial septal defect
      operation
    t. coil occlusion
    t. device
    t. embolization
    t. embolotherapy
    t. occlusion
    t. occlusion of atrial septal defect
    t. therapy (TCT)
    t. umbrella
    t. valve implantation
    t. valvotomy
Transcop
transcoronary
    t. ablation
    t. ablation of septal hypertrophy
      (TASH)
    t. alcohol ablation (TAA)
    t. chemical ablation
transcortical
    t. motor aphasia
    t. motor type of aphasia
transcranial
    t. color-coded duplex sonography
      (TCCS)
    t. contrast Doppler sonography
    t. Doppler (TCD)
    t. Doppler probe
    t. Doppler sonography (TCD)
    t. Doppler ultrasound (TCD)
    t. magnetic stimulation (TMS)
transcricothyroid puncture
transcription
    gene t.
    Janus kinase/signal transducer and
      activator of t. (Jak/Stat)
    signal transducer and activator
      of t. (Stat)
transcutaneous
    t. echo
    t. electrical stimulation (TES)
    t. extraction catheter
    t. lead
    t. oxygen monitor (TCOM)
    t. phrenic nerve conduction study
transdermal
    t. 17-beta-estradiol
    Catapres-TTS T.
    Duragesic T.
    T.-NTG Patch
Transderm-Nitro
    T.-N. Patch
transdiaphragmatic pressure
transducer
    Acuson V5M multiplane
      transesophageal
      echocardiographic t.

Aloka model SSD-830 2.5- and 3.5-MHz t.
annular array t.
t. aperture
arterial line t.
ATL UltraMark IV 7.5-Mhz linear array t.
Bentley t.
charge-coupled device t.
Cordis Sentron t.
Deltran disposable t.
diaphragm t.
Diasonics t.
differential pressure t.
Doppler t.
echocardiographic t.
footprint of t.
Gould Statham pressure t.
HP SONOS 2500 t.
Medex t.
2-MHz pulsed-wave Doppler t.
Mikro-Tip t.
Millar Mikro-Tip catheter pressure t.
Millar TCB-500 t.
M-mode t.
Pedoff continuous wave t.
phased array sector t.
phonocardiographic t.
piezoelectric ultrasound t.
pressure t.
quartz t.
range-gated t.
RespSponse III respiratory pressure t.
sector t.
Sleepscan Airflow Pressure T.
Sorensen Transpac III t.
Spectranetics P23 Statham t.
Toshiba biplane transesophageal t.
ultrasound t.
variomatrix t.
V510B Biplane TEE t.
Vingmed CFM 750 t.
V5M Multiplane t.
transendothelial
transesophageal
t. atrial pacing (TAP, TEAP)
t. atrial stimulation (TRAS)
t. contrast echocardiography
t. dobutamine stress echocardiography

t. echo
t. echocardiography (TEE)
t. echocardiography-dobutamine stress echocardiography (TEE-DSE)
t. echocardiography with pacing (TEEP)
t. echo probe
t. pacing system
t. pressure
t. probe
transfection
Program in Ex Vivo Vein Graft Engineering via T. (PREVENT)
transfemoral
t. catheter
t. endoaortic occlusion catheter
transfer
adenovirus-mediated gene t.
Akt t.
chordal t.
ex vivo gene t.
intraarterial gene t.
intravascular gene t.
vascular gene t.
in vivo gene t.
transferase
chloramphenicol t.
transfixion suture
transform
fast Fourier t. (FFT)
Fourier t.
gradient field t. (GFT)
three-dimensional Fourier t. (3DFT)
transformation
epicardial-mesenchymal t.
Haldane t.
hemorrhagic t. (HT)
Richter t.
transforming
t. growth factor (TGF)
t. growth factor-beta
transfusion
autologous t.
Baylor rapid autologous t. (BRAT)
donor-specific t.
exchange t.
t. factor
transfusional hemosiderosis
transgenesis
transient
t. asystole

T

NOTES

transient *(continued)*
    calcium t.
    t. depolarization
    t. entrainment
    t. heart block
    t. inward current
    t. ischemia
    t. ischemic attack (TIA)
    t. ischemic dilation (TID)
    t. ischemic event (TIE)
    t. leukocytosis
    t. mesenteric ischemia
    t. pericarditis
    t. response imaging (TRI)
    t. ST segment elevation
    t. syncope
    t. tachypnea of newborn (TTNB)
    t. wall motion abnormality

transition
    forced ischemia-reperfusion t.
    sympathovagal t.

transitional
    t. cell
    t. cell carcinoma
    t. cell zone
    t. respiration

transjugular
    t. balloon valvuloplasty procedure
    t. intrahepatic portosystemic shunt (TIPS)

translesional spectral flow velocity
translocation
    Nikaidoh t.

translocator
    adenine nucleotide t.
    adenosine nucleotide t. (ANT)

translumbar aortography
transluminal
    t. angioplasty catheter
    t. coronary angioplasty
    t. coronary extraction atherectomy
    t. endarterectomy
    t. endarterectomy catheter (TEC)
    t. extraction atherectomy (TEA)
    t. extraction catheter (TEC)
    T. Extraction Catheter Before Stent (TECBEST)
    T. Extraction Catheter or PTCA in Thrombus (TOPIT)
    t. extraction coronary atherectomy
    t. lysing system
    percutaneous t.

transluminally
    t. placed endovascular branched stent graft
    t. placed Inoue endovascular stent-graft

transmembrane
    t. calcium flux
    t. potential
    t. signaling
    t. voltage

transmission
    airborne t.
    electrotonic t.
    genetic t.
    mitral E-wave t.

transmitral
    t. Doppler E:A ratio
    t. E:A ratio
    t. E-wave deceleration time
    t. flow velocity
    t. gradient

transmitted murmur
transmucosal
    Actiq Oral T.

transmural
    t. antitachycardia pacemaker
    t. channel
    t. myocardial infarction
    t. pressure
    t. steal

transmyocardial
    Helionetics/Acculase excimer laser t.
    t. laser channel
    t. laser revascularization (TMLR)
    t. pacing stylet
    t. perfusion pressure
    t. revascularization (TMR)

transnexus channel
Transonic flowmeter
transpiration
    pulmonary t.

transplant
    allogeneic t.
    bilateral lung t. (BLT)
    bilateral sequential lung t.
    bilateral sequential single lung t.
    bone marrow t.
    cardiac t.
    t. coronary artery disease (TCAD, TxCAD)
    double lung t. (DLT)
    en bloc bilateral lung t.
    heart t.
    heart-lung t. (HLT)
    heterologous cardiac t.
    heterotopic cardiac t.
    heterotopic heart t. (HHT)
    homologous cardiac t.
    International Society for Heart and Lung T.
    living related t. (LRT)
    Lower-Shumway cardiac t.

lung t. (LT, LTx)
orthotopic cardiac t.
orthotopic heart t. (OHT)
t. pneumonia
rejection cardiomyopathy t.
renal t.
right single lung t. (RSLTx)
single-lung t. (SLT)
syngenesioplastic t.
transplantation (*See also* transplant)
heart t.
International Society for Heart T.
(ISHT)
transpleural
transport
active t.
T. catheter
T. dilatation balloon catheter
T. drug delivery catheter
lactic acid t.
mucociliary t.
mucus t.
oxygen t.
transportability
cough t.
transportation
air medical t. (AMT)
transporter
monocarboxylate t. (MCT)
transposition
t. of arterial stem
t. assessment
t. complex
t. of the great arteries (TGA)
t. of the great vessels
portacaval t.
transprosthetic flow velocity
transpulmonary
t. gradient
t. pressure
t. thermal-dye dilution (TDD)
transradial
t. approach
t. cardiac catheterization
t. coronary angioplasty
t. primary stenting
transsarcolemmal calcium current
Trans-Scan 2100 noninvasive
physiological monitor
transseptal
t. angiocardiography

t. catheter
t. catheterization
t. conduction
t. left heart catheterization
t. puncture
t. sheath
transstenotic
t. pressure gradient
t. pressure gradient measurement
transtelephonic
t. ambulatory monitoring (TAM)
t. ambulatory monitoring system
t. arrhythmia monitoring (TTM)
t. cardiac event monitoring
t. exercise monitor (TEM)
t. recording
transthoracic
t. acoustic window
t. color Doppler echocardiography
t. contract echocardiography
t. direct current electrical
cardioversion
t. echocardiogram (TTE)
t. echocardiography (TTE)
t. impedance
t. implantable cardioverter-
defibrillator
t. needle aspiration (TTNA)
t. needle aspiration biopsy
t. needle biopsy (TNB)
t. pacemaker
t. pacing stylet
t. pressure
transthoracically implanted ICD
transtracheal
t. aspiration
t. oxygen catheter
transudate
transudation
transudative pleural effusion
transvalensis
Nocardia t.
transvalvular
t. aortic gradient
t. E velocity
t. flow
t. flow rate
t. hemodynamics
t. pressure gradient (TPG)
t. reflux

NOTES

T

Transvene
    T. nonthoracotomy implantable cardioverter-defibrillator
    T. tripolar electrode
Transvene-RV lead
transvenous
    t. ablation
    t. aortovelography (TAV)
    t. biopsy
    t. catheter extraction
    t. defibrillator lead
    t. device
    t. electrode
    t. implantable defibrillator
    t. internal cardioversion
    t. lead
    t. nitinol snare
transventricular
    t. closed valvotomy
    t. mitral valve commissurotomy
transverse
    t. artery of face
    t. artery of neck
    t. cervical artery
    t. costal facet
    t. fissure of the right lung
    t. incision
    t. muscle of nape
    t. muscle of thorax
    t. section of heart
    t. sinus
    t. thoracosternotomy
    t. tubule
transverse/sigmoid sinus (TS/SS)
transversi
transversus
    fovea costalis processus t.'s
    t. nuchae muscle
    situs t.
transxiphoid approach
tranylcypromine
TRAP
    total peroxyl radical-trapping antioxidant potential
    TRAP assay
trap-door approach
trapezius ridge sign
trapped
    t. gas volume
    t. lung
Trapper catheter exchange device
trapping
    air t.
    gas t.
TRAS
    transesophageal atrial stimulation
trash foot
Trasicor

trastuzumab
Trasylol
Traube
    T. bruit
    T. curve
    T. double tone
    T. dyspnea
    T. heart
    T. murmur
    pistol shot of T.
    T. plug
    T. semilunar space
    T. sign
trauma
    American Association for the Surgery of T. (AAST)
    blunt t.
    blunt chest t.
    blunt thoracic t.
    t. intensive care unit (TICU)
    mechanical t.
    penetrating thoracic t.
    thoracic t.
    truncal t.
    vessel t.
traumatic
    t. aortic aneurysm
    t. aortic disruption
    t. aortography
    t. apnea
    t. asphyxia
    t. chylothorax
    t. emphysema
    t. fistula
    t. heart disease
    t. hemopericardium
    t. hemorrhage
    t. pericarditis
    t. pneumonia
    t. pneumothorax
    t. rupture
    t. tamponade
    t. thrombosis
    t. thrombus
Traveler
    T. portable oxygen system
    Pulmo-Aide T.
Travenol infusion pump
trazodone hydrochloride
Treacher Collins syndrome
treadmill
    arm ergometry t.
    t. echocardiography
    t. electrocardiogram
    exercise t.
    t. exercise stress test
    t. incline
    t.-induced angina

Jaeger LE3000 t.
Marquette t.
Q-Stress t.
self-powered t.
t. stress test (TMST)
Tunturi Jogger-2 self-powered t.

TREAT
Tranilast Restenosis Following
Angioplasty Trial

treat
T. Angina with Aggrastat and
Determine Costs of Therapy with
Invasive or Conservative
Strategies (TACTICS)
number needed to t. (NNT)

treatment
T. of Acute Stroke Trial (TOAST)
Albertini t.
antianginal t.
arrest-and-reversal t. (ART)
Atherosclerosis Prevention and T.
(APT)
Brehmer t.
Cerivastatin Gemfibrozil
Hyperlipidemia T. (RIGHT)
Chimeric 7E3 Antiplatelet in
Unstable Angina Refractory to
Standard T. (CAPTURE)
Cosgrove-Edwards annuloplasty
system with Duraflo t.
CustomPac custom tubing back
with Duraflo t.
DeBove t.
directly observed t. (DOT)
efficacy of t.
Forlanini t.
Frankel t.
Hypertension Optimal T. (HOT)
Koga t.
McPheeters t.
Nauheim t.
nonpharmacologic measure of t.
Nordach t.
Oertel t.
Schott t.
Serum Markers Acute Myocardial
Infarction and Rapid T.
(SMART)
SpiralGold adult low-prime
oxygenator with Duraflo t.
stand-alone laser t.
TheraPEP pre-respiratory therapy t.

Trial of Org 10172 in Acute
Stroke T. (TOAST)
Tuffnell t.
Trecator-SC
Tredex
T. bicycle
T. powered bicycle
tree
bronchial t.
coronary t.
endobronchial t.
tracheobronchial t.
tree-in-winter appearance
trefoil
t. balloon
t. balloon catheter
t. factor family (TFF)
t. factor family domain peptide
t. Schneider balloon
t. tendon
tremor
flapping t.
tremulus
pulsus t.
Tremytoine
trench lung
trend
threshold t.
Trendar
Trendelenburg
T. operation
T. position
T. test
trendscriber
Trental
trepidatio cordis
treponemal
t. antibody
t. test
Treponema pallidum
trepopnea
treppe
negative t.
t. phenomenon
positive t.
TRI
transient response imaging
tria
Triacin-C
triad
acute compression t.
adrenomedullary t.

T

NOTES

triad *(continued)*
>Andersen t.
>t. asthma
>atherogenic metabolic t.
>Beck t.
>Carney t.
>Cushing t.
>T. defibrillator system
>Fallot t.
>Grancher t.
>Hull t.
>Kartagener t.
>lipid t.
>Osler t.
>T. PET balloon
>Virchow t.

triadic junction
TRIADS
>time-resolved imaging by automatic data
>segmentation

TriaDyne II kinetic therapy
triage
>T. cardiac rapid diagnostic test
>system
>T. cardiac system

trial *(See also* study, program, protocol)
>ACME clinical t.
>ACUTE clinical t.
>AMRO clinical t.
>T. of Angioplasty and Stents in
>Canada (TASC)
>T. of Antihypertensive Interventions
>and Management (TAIM)
>Antihypertensive and Lipid
>Lowering Treatment to Prevent
>Heart Attack T. (ALLHAT)
>antiplatelet t. (APT)
>APLAUSE clinical t.
>APRICOT clinical t.
>ARREST clinical t.
>arterial disease multiple
>intervention t. (ADMIT)
>ARTS clinical t.
>ASPIRE clinical t.
>Aspirin Versus Coumadin T.
>(APRICOT)
>Asymptomatic Cardiac Ischemia T.
>(ACIT)
>asymptomatic carotid surgery t.
>(ACST)
>Atakr Ablation System clinical t.
>Atenolol Silent Ischemia T.
>(ASIST)
>ATLAS t.
>Atrial Fibrillation Followup
>Investigation Rhythm
>Management t.
>AVID clinical t.

>balloon versus optimal
>atherectomy t. (BOAT)
>BAROCCO clinical t.
>beStent clinical t. (BEST)
>BEST+ICD clinical t.
>Beta-Blocker Evaluation of
>Survival T. (BEST)
>Beta-Blocker Heart Attack T.
>(BHAT)
>Beta-Blocker Stroke T. (BEST)
>Beta-Washington Radiation for In-
>Stent Restenosis T. (beta-WRIST)
>Bezafibrate Coronary Atherosclerosis
>Intervention T. (BECAIT)
>BIP t.
>Blood Pressure, Renal Effects,
>Insulin Control, Lipids, Lisinopril,
>and Nifedipine T. (BRILLIANT)
>Bucindolol Evaluation of
>Survival T. (BEST)
>CABG Patch clinical t.
>CADILLAC clinical t.
>CAMI clinical t.
>>Canadian Amiodarone Myocardial
>>Infarction Arrhythmia Trial
>Canadian Amiodarone Myocardial
>Infarction Arrhythmia T.
>(CAMIAT, CAMI clinical trial)
>Canadian Coronary Atherectomy T.
>(CCAT)
>Canadian Coronary Atherosclerosis
>Intervention T. (CCAIT)
>Canadian Myocardial Infarction
>Amiodarone T. (CAMIAT)
>CAPRIE clinical t.
>CAPTURE clinical trial
>Cardiac Arrhythmia Suppression T.
>(CAST)
>Cardiac Arrhythmia Suppression T.
>II (CAST II)
>CARE clinical t.
>Carotene and Retinol Efficacy T.
>(CARET)
>Carotid Revascularization
>Endarterectomy Versus Stenting T.
>(CREST)
>Carvedilol or Metoprolol
>European t.
>Carvedilol Prospective Randomized
>Cumulative Survival t.
>(COPERNICUS trial)
>Chinese Acute Stroke t. (CAST)
>Cholesterol Lowering
>Atherosclerosis PTCA T.
>Clinical Outcomes with
>Ultrasound T. (CLOUT)
>Comparison of Abciximab
>Complications with Hirulog (and

Back-Up Abciximab) Events T. (CACHET)
Compliance-Related Angioplasty Complications t.
Congestive Heart Failure-Survival T. of Antiarrhythmic Therapy (CHF-STAT)
Conservative Strategy-TIMI 18 t.
Continuous Infusion Versus Bolus Alteplase T. (COBALT)
CONVINCE clinical t.
COPERNICUS t.
    Carvedilol Prospective Randomized Cumulative Survival trial
CORAMI clinical t.
CORAMI II clinical t.
Cornell Coronary Artery Bypass Outcomes T. (CCABOT)
Coronary Angioplasty and Rotablator Atherectomy T. (CARAT)
Coronary Angioplasty and Rotablator Atherectomy T. II (CARAT II)
Coronary Angioplasty versus Excisional Atherectomy T. (CAVEAT)
Coronary Primary Prevention T. (CPPT)
Coronary Syndromes t.
CRUSADE clinical t.
CSSA clinical t.
CURE clinical t.
Cutting Balloon Randomized Clinical T.
DASH clinical t.
DESTINI clinical t.
Dilation versus Ablation Revascularization t. (DART)
Dispatch Urokinase Efficacy T. (DUET)
DOUBLE t.
Emory Angioplasty versus Surgery T. (EAST)
Enoxaparin in Non-Q-wave Coronary Events t.
ENTICES clinical t.
EPIC clinical t.
ERA clinical t.
ESCOBAR clinical t.
ESSENCE clinical t.

European Myocardial Infarct Amiodarone T. (EMIAT)
Evaluation of Platelet IIb/IIIa Inhibitor for Stenting T. (EPISTENT)
EXACTO clinical t.
EXCEL t.
Flosequinan ACE Inhibitor T. (FACET)
Fluvastatin Long-Term Extension T. (FLUENT)
FOOD clinical t.
Fosinopril Versus Amlodipine Cardiovascular Events Randomized T. (FACET)
FRISC clinical t.
FRISC II clinical t.
GRAMI clinical t.
GUIDE clinical t.
GUIDE II clinical t.
Heparin Aspirin Reperfusion T. (HART)
HERO clinical t.
HIPS clinical t.
HIT clinical t.
T.'s of Hypertension Prevention (TOHP)
IMPACT Clinical T.
IMPACT-Stent clinical t.
INTEGRITI Clinical T.
International Stroke T. (IST)
INTIME clinical t.
ISAM clinical t.
ISAR clinical t.
LARS Clinical T.
LASAR Clinical T.
LAVA Diet T.
LIMITS Clinical T.
MACE clinical t.
MARISA clinical t.
MATE Clinical T.
MDC Clinical T.
Metoprolol CR/XL Controlled Release Randomized Intervention T. in Heart Failure (MERIT-HF)
MITRA clinical t.
Mode Selection T. in Sinus Node Dysfunction (MOST)
Multicenter Acute Stroke T. (MAST)

NOTES

trial (*continued*)

Multicenter American Research T. with Cilazapril after Angioplasty to Prevent Transluminal Coronary Obstruction and Restenosis (MARCATOR)

Multicenter Myocarditis Treatment T. (MMTT)

Multicenter Unsustained Tachycardia T. (MUSTT)

Multi-Hospital Eastern Atlantic Restenosis T. (M-HEART)

Multiple Risk Factor Intervention T. (MRFIT)

MUSIC clinical t.

MUST clinical t.

NACI clinical t.

National Emphysema Treatment T. (NETT)

National Institutes of Neurological Disorders and Stroke-Tissue Plasminogen Activator Stroke T. (NINDS-TPAST)

North American Symptomatic Carotid Endarterectomy T. (NASCET)

Number Equal to One; Single Patient T. (N=1 trial)

OASIS clinical t.

OASIS-2 clinical t.

OCBAS clinical t.

T. on Reversing Endothelial Dysfunction study

OPERA clinical t.

Optimal T. in Myocardial Infarction with the Angiotensin II Antagonist Losartan (OPTIMAAL)

OPUS Clinical T.

ORBIT clinical t.

T. of Org 10172 in Acute Stroke Treatment (TOAST)

OSTI-I clinical t.

OSTI-IIA clinical t.

OSTI-IIB clinical t.

PACT clinical t.

PAMI clinical t.

PAMI II clincal t.

PARAGON clinical t.

PART Clinical T.

PEPI Clinical T.

Philadelphia Association of Clinical T.'s (PACT)

PILOT clinical t.

Plasminogen Activator Angioplasty Compatibility T. (PACT)

Platelet IIb/IIIa Underpinning the Receptor for Suppression of Unstable Ischemia T. (PURSUIT)

POST-CABG clinical t.

Posterior Stroke T. (POST)

Potassium-Channel Opening Stroke T. (POST)

PREVENT clinical t.

Proliferation Reduction with Vascular Energy T. (PREVENT)

Prospective Randomized Controlled Clinical T.'s (PRCCT)

Prospective Randomized Evaluation of Diltiazem CD T. (PREDICT)

Prospective Randomized Evaluation of the Vascular Effects of Norvasc T. (PREVENT)

Prourokinase and tPA Enhancement of Thrombolysis T. (PATENT)

Quinapril Ischemic Event T. (QUIET)

randomized t.'s

randomized clinical t. (RCT)

Reopro in Acute Myocardial Infarction and Primary PTCA Organization and Randomized T. (RAPPORT)

Restenosis Stent T. (REST)

RITA clinical t.

ROSTER clinical t.

Saruplase and Taprostene Acute Reocclusion T. (START)

SAVE clinical t.

SAVED clinical t.

SCRIPPS clinical t.

SICCO clinical t.

SPINAF clinical t.

STAMI clinical t.

STENTIM clinical t.

STENTIM-2 clinical t.

Stent Implantation Post Rotational Atherectomy T. (SPORT)

STENT PAMI clinical t.

Stent versus Angioplasty Restenosis T. (START)

Stent versus Directional Coronary Atherectomy Randomized T. (START)

STICH clinical t.

STOP clinical t.

St. Thomas Atherosclerosis Regression T. (START)

Study of Medicine versus Angioplasty Reperfusion T. (SMART)

Study of Microstent's Ability to Limit Restenosis T. (SMART)

Sudden Cardiac Death in Heart Failure T. (SCD-HeFT)

SURE clinical t.

SWORD Clinical T.

SYMPHONY clinical t.
TACS clinical t.
TACTICS clinical t.
TACTICS-TIMI 18 t.
TAMI Clinical T.
TAUSA clinical trial
TECBEST clinical t.
Thrombolysis in Myocardial
  Infarction t.
Ticlopidine Angioplasty
  Coronary T. (TACT)
TIMI t.
TIMI Clinical T.
TIMI-9 clinical t.
TOPIT clinical t.
Tranilast Restenosis Following
  Angioplasty T. (TREAT)
Treatment of Acute Stroke T.
  (TOAST)
TRIM clinical t.
Valsartan in Acute Myocardial
  Infarction T. (VALIANT)
Valsartan Heart Failure T. (Val-
  HeFT)
Vasodilator Heart Failure T. II (V-
  HeFT II)
Vesnarinone Survival T. (VEST)
Veterans Administration Heart
  Failure T. (V-HeFT)
Veterans Administration Heart
  Failure T. II (V-HeFT II)
Veterans Administration High-
  Density Lipoprotein
  Intervention T. (VA-HIT)
VITATOPS clinical t.
VOTE clinical t.
Washington Radiation for In-Stent
  Restenosis T. (WRIST)
Washington Radiation for In-Stent
  Restenosis T. for Long Lesions
  (LONG WRIST)
Women's Estrogen for Stroke T.
  (WEST)

Trial-I
Optimal Stent Implantation T.-I
Trial-IIA
Optimal Stent Implantation T.-IIA
Trial-IIB
Optimal Stent Implantation T.-IIB
Triam-A Injection
triamcinolone
t. acetonide (TAA)

t. diacetate
t. inhalation, nasal
oral t. inhalation
t. (systemic)
Triam Forte Injection
Triaminic
T. AM Decongestant Formula
T. DM
T. Expectorant
Triaminicol Multi-Symptom Cold Syrup
Triamonide injection
triamterene
hydrochlorothiazide and t.
triangle
aortic t.
axillary t.
Burger t.
Burger scalene t.
Calot t.
cardiohepatic t.
carotid t.
clavipectoral t.
Einthoven t.
endocardial t.
Gerhardt t.
infraclavicular t.
Jackson safety t.
Koch t.
t. of Koch
Rauchfuss t.
sternocostal t.
subclavian t.
Todaro t.
tracheal t.
triangular resection of leaflet operation
Triatoma infestans
triatrial heart
triatriatum
cor t.
triaxial
t. accelerometer
t. reference system
triazolam
tribomide
phosphorus t.
trichambered pacing
Trichinella spiralis
trichinosis
trichinous embolism
trichiura
Trichuris t.

T

NOTES

trichloride
    antimony t.
trichlormethiazide
Trichosporon
    T. asahii
    T. beigelii
    T. beigelii pneumonia
trichosporonosis
Trichuris trichiura
triciribine phosphate (TCN-P)
Tri-Clear Expectorant
Tricodur
    T. Epi compression support
    bandage
    T. Omos compression support
    bandage
    T. Talus compression support
    bandage
TriCor capsule
tricrotic
tricrotism
tricrotous
tricuspid
    t. annular motion (TAM)
    t. annuloplasty
    t. anulus
    t. aortic valve
    t. area
    t. atelectasis
    t. atresia
    t. commissurotomy
    t. incompetence
    t. insufficiency
    t. murmur
    t. opening snap
    t. orifice
    t. position
    pulmonic t.
    t. regurgitant jet
    t. regurgitation (TR)
    t. restenosis
    t. stenosis
    t. valve
    t. valve annuloplasty
    t. valve anulus
    t. valve area
    t. valve closure sound
    t. valve disease
    t. valve doming
    t. valve endocarditis
    t. valve flow
    t. valve prolapse
    t. valve strut
    t. valve vegetation
    t. valvular leaflet
    t. valvuloplasty
tricuspidalis
    cuspis anterior valvae t.

tricuspid-inferior vena cava isthmus
Tricut laryngeal blade tip
tricyclic antidepressant
Tridil injection
triethiodide
    gallamine t.
trifascicular block
Trifed-C
Tri-flow incentive spirometry
triflupromazine
Trifoil balloon system
trigeminal
    t. cough
    t. nerve
    t. pulse
    t. rhythm
trigeminus
    pulsus t.
trigeminy
trigger
    asthma t.
    rupture t.
    Smart T.
triggered
    t. activity
    atrial demand-t. (AAT)
    t. pacing
triggering
    t. mechanism
    respiratory t.
triglyceride
    t. level
    medium chain t.'s
    serum t.
triglyceride-rich
    t.-r. lipoprotein (TRL)
trigone
    anterior fibrous t.
    vertebrocostal t.
trigonum omotracheale
Triguide catheter
Tri-Hydroserpine
Tri-Immunol
triiodothyronine
Tri-Kort injection
trilazad mesylate
trileaflet
trilinear cylindric interpolation algorithm
Trilisate
triloculare
    cor t.
trilocular heart
Trilog Injection
trilogy
    T. DC, DR, SR pulse generator
    t. of Fallot
    Fallot t.

Trilone injection
TRIM
> Thrombin Inhibition in Myocardial
> Ischemia
>> TRIM clinical trial
Trimadeau sign
trimazosin
trimellitic
> t. anhydride
> t. anhydride asthma
Tri-Met apnea monitor
trimetazidine
trimetazidine 1 (TMZ)
trimethaphan camsylate
trimethoprim-sulfamethoxazole (TMP-SMX)
trimethoprim sulfate
trimetrexate glucoronate
trimipramine maleate
Trimox
Trimpex
trinitrate
> glyceryl t.
trinotecan
trinucleotide
> cytosine-thymine-guanine t.
Triofed Syrup
triolet
> bruit de t.
Trios M pacemaker
Triostat injection
Tripedia
tripelennamine
tripe palm
triphammer pulse
triphenyl
> T. Expectorant
> t. tetrazolium chloride
> t. tetrazolium staining method
triphosphatase
> adenosine t. (ATPase)
triphosphate
> adenosine t. (AT, ATP)
> guanosine t. (GTP)
> inositol t.
> purine nucleotides adenosine t.
> uridine t. (UTP)
triple
> t. ectopic tachyarrhythmia
> t. extrastimulus
> t. rhythm
> t. stimulus

triple-balloon valvuloplasty
triple-bandpass filter
triple-humped pressure pulse
triple-lumen balloon flotation thermistor catheter
triplet
tripod sign
tripolar
> t. defibrillation coil electrode
> t. lead
> segmented ring t. (SRT)
> t. with Damato curve catheter
triport cannula
TriPort hemostasis introducer sheath kit
Triposed
> T. Syrup
> T. Tablet
Trippi-Wells tongs
triprolidine
> t. and pseudoephedrine
> t., pseudoephedrine, and codeine
trisalicylate
> choline magnesium t.
Tris-buffer infusion test
trisection
> pulse t.
tris(hydroxymethyl)aminomethane
Trisoject Injection
trisomy
> t. 13, 18, 21
> t. D syndrome
Trisulfa
Tritace
Tri-Tannate Plus
TriTrac accelerometer
Triumph VR pacemaker
TRL
> triglyceride-rich lipoprotein
Trocal
trocar
> Axiom thoracic t.
> B-D Potain thoracic t.
> Bueleau empyema t.
> Davidson thoracic t.
> Entree thoracoscopy t.
> Hunt angiographic t.
> Hurwitz thoracic t.
> large-bore t.
trochleae
> vagina synovialis t.
trochocardia

NOTES

745

trochorizocardia
troglitazone
Troisier sign
troleandomycin (TAO)
trolley
    EvitaMobil universal t.
tromethamine
TRON 3 VACI cardiac imaging system
Tropherema whippleii
trophic changes
trophoblastic tumor
tropical
    t. endomyocardial fibrosis
    t. pulmonary eosinophilia
tropicalis
    Xenopus t.
tropomyosin
troponin
    t. C, I, T
    t. T (TnT)
trospectomycin sulfate
trough
    t. dosing
    t. level
    peak and t.
    t. and peak levels
    systolic t.
    X-descent t.
    Y-descent t.
troughing
    venous t.
trough-to-peak ratio
trousers
    air t.
    military antishock t. (MAST)
    pneumatic t.
Trousseau syndrome
trovafloxacin
Trovan
TR-R9 antithrombin receptor polyclonal
  antibody
TRT
    thoracic radiation therapy
TRU
    terminal respiratory unit
Tru-Cut biopsy needle
true
    t. aortic aneurysm
    t. asthma
    t. cyst
    T. Form support stockings
    T. Stat system
    t. versus false aneurysm
    aortography
    t. vocal cord
TrueMax 2400 Metabolic Measuring
  system
true-negative test result

true-positive test result
TrueTorque wire guide
Trufill n-BCA liquid embolic system
Truflex
Trumbull suture
trumpet
    angel's t.
truncal
    t. distribution of body fat
    t. trauma
trunci (*pl. of* truncus)
truncoaortic sac
truncoconal area
truncus, pl. trunci
    t. arteriosus
    bifurcatio trunci
    t. celiacus
    t. lymphaticus bronchiomediastinalis
    t. pulmonalis
Trunecek
    T. sign
    T. symptom
trunk
    bifurcation of pulmonary t.
    brachiocephalic t.
    bronchomediastinal lymphatic t.
    T. Control Test (TCT)
    t. forward flexion
    left-sided innominate t.
    orifice of pulmonary t.
    pulmonary t.
    valve of pulmonary t.
Truphylline
    T. Suppository
Trusler
    T. aortic valve technique
    T. rule for pulmonary artery
    banding
    T. technique of aortic valvuloplasty
TruTrak data sampling system
TruZone
    T. Asthma Action Plan Wallet
    Card
    T. peak flowmeter
    T. PFM
Trypanosoma
    T. brucei
    T. cruzi
    T. gambiense
    T. rhodesiense
trypanosomiasis
    American t.
trypsin
    t., balsam peru, and castor oil
Trzepacz
    Delirium Rating Scale of T.
TSH
    thyroid-stimulating hormone

T-shaped stent
TS/SS
　　transverse/sigmoid sinus
TST
　　total sleep time
tsukubaensis
　　　Streptomyces t.
TT
　　thrombolytic therapy
　　thromboplastin time
　　　TT form of MTP gene
　　　TT genotype
T_I/T_{TOT}
　　ratio of inspiratory time to total cycle
　　　time
TTC stain
TTE
　　transthoracic echocardiogram
　　transthoracic echocardiography
TTi
TTM
　　transtelephonic arrhythmia monitoring
TTNA
　　transthoracic needle aspiration
TTNB
　　transient tachypnea of newborn
TTP
　　thrombotic thrombocytopenic purpura
TTS catheter
TTT
　　tilt-table test
T-tubule
T-type calcium channels
TU
　　　T. complex
　　　T. wave
Tubasal
Tubbs dilator
tube, tubing
　　　AccuMark calibrated infant
　　　　feeding t.
　　　air t.
　　　Aire-Cuf tracheostomy t.
　　　American tracheotomy t.
　　　Andrews-Pynchon t.
　　　angled pleural t.
　　　Argyle Sentinel Seal chest t.
　　　Arm-a-Med endotracheal t.
　　　Atkins-Cannard tracheal t.
　　　Baylor cardiovascular sump t.
　　　Bivona Fome-Cuff t.
　　　Bivona TTS tracheostomy t.

Blue Line cuffed endotracheal t.
bronchial t.
Broncho-Cath double-lumen
　endotracheal t.
bulboventricular t.
Caluso PEG t.
Carabelli t.
Carden bronchoscopy t.
Carlen t.
Carlen double-lumen endotracheal t.
Celestin esophageal t.
Charnley drain t.
Chaussier t.
chest t.
Chevalier Jackson tracheal t.
Cole pediatric t.
Cole uncuffed endotracheal t.
Cooley sump t.
cuffed endotracheal t.
cuffed tracheostomy t.
Dale-Schwartz t.
Deane t.
decompressive chest t.
DIC tracheostomy t.
Doesel-Huzly bronchoscopic t.
double-lumen endobronchial t.
Dow Corning t.
Durham t.
endobronchial t.
endocardial t.
endotracheal t. (ETT)
Endotrol endotracheal t.
Endotrol tracheal t.
Ewald t.
fenestrated tracheostomy t.
fluffy-cuffed t.
Fome-Cuf tracheostomy t.
Fuller bivalve trach t.
Gabriel Tucker t.
glutaraldehyde-tanned bovine
　collagen t.
Gore-Tex t.
Guisez t.
Haldane-Priestley t.
Hi-Lo Evac endotracheal t.
Hi-Lo Jet tracheal t.
Holter t.
Hyperflex tracheostomy t.
interposition of Dacron t.
intratracheal t.
Jackson cane-shaped tracheal t.
J-shaped t.

T

NOTES

tube (*continued*)
Kamen-Wilkenson endotracheal t.
Keofeed feeding t.
Kuhn t.
Lanz low-pressure cuff endotracheal t.
large-bore chest t.
large-caliber chest t.
Laryngoflex reinforced endotracheal t.
laser t.
Lennarson t.
Lepley-Ernst tracheal t.
Lindholm tracheal t.
Lo-Pro tracheal t.
Lore-Lawrence trachea t.
Luer tracheal t.
Mackler t.
Magill Safety Clear Plus endotracheal t.
Mallinckrodt cuffed endotracheal t.
Montgomery Safe-T-T.
Mosher life-saving tracheal t.
Mousseau-Barbin esophageal t.
Nachlas t.
nasogastric t.
nasotracheal t.
Olympus One-Step Button t.
oroendotracheal t.
orotracheal t.
otopharyngeal t.
PEG t.
PEJ t.
percutaneous endoscopic gastrostomy t.
percutaneous endoscopic jejunostomy t.
Pitt talking tracheostomy t.
pleural t.
Polisar-Lyons tracheal t.
polyvinyl chloride t.
Portex Per-Fit tracheostomy t.
primordial catheter t.
Quinton t.
RAE endotracheal t.
right-angle chest t.
Robertshaw t.
Ruschelit polyvinyl chloride endotracheal t.
Sandoz suction/feeding t.
Sarns intracardiac suction t.
scavenging t.
Sensiv endotracheal t.
Shiley tracheostomy t.
Softech endotracheal t.
Souttar t.
spiral-embedded t.
T t.

Teflon TFE SubLite Wall t.
t. thoracostomy
thoracostomy t.
Thora-Klex chest t.
tight-to-shaft Aire-Cuf tracheostomy t.
Tovell t.
tracheal t.
tracheostomy t.
Univent t.
UTTS endotracheal t.
Vacutainer t.
Venturi t.
Vinyon-N cloth t.
Vivonex Moss t.
water-seal chest t.
wire-wound endotracheal t.
x-ray t.
Z-wave t.

TubeChek esophageal intubation detector

tubercle
corniculate t.
cuneiform t.
Ghon t.

tuberculin
Koch t.
Koch old t.
purified protein derivative of t.
t. test

tuberculocidal

tuberculoid myocarditis

tuberculoma

tuberculosilicosis

tuberculosis (TB)
active t.
acute miliary t.
adult t.
aerogenic t.
anthracotic t.
arrested t.
atypical t.
avian t.
basal t.
t. of bones and joints
cerebral t.
cestodic t.
childhood t.
childhood-type t.
disseminated t.
endobronchial t.
extrapulmonary t.
exudative t.
generalized t.
healed t.
hematogenous t.
hilus t.
inactive t.

inhalation t.
t. of larynx
t. lichenoides
t. of lung
miliary t.
multidrug-resistant t. (MDR-TB)
mycobacteria other than t. (MOTT)
Mycobacterium t. (MTB)
open t.
oral t.
orificial t.
papulonecrotic t.
postprimary t.
primary t.
productive t.
pulmonary t. (PTB)
reactivation t.
reinfection t.
renal t.
Roche AMPLICOR assay for
 Mycobacterium t.
secondary t.
surgical t.
tracheobronchial t.
t. vaccine
tuberculostat
tuberculostatic
tuberculous
t. arteritis
t. bronchopneumonia
t. caseation
t. chemotherapy
t. empyema
t. empyesis
t. endocarditis
t. laryngitis
t. lymphadenitis
t. mycotic aneurysm of the aorta
t. nephritis
t. pericarditis
t. pleurisy
t. pleuritis
t. pneumonia
t. rheumatism
tuberculum
t. thyroideum inferius
t. thyroideum superius
tuberoeruptive xanthoma
tuberous
t. sclerosis
t. xanthoma
Tubersol

tubing (*var. of* tube)
tubocurarine chloride
tubular
t. breath sounds
t. necrosis
t. respiration
t. slotted stent
t. stent
tubule
distal convoluted t.
proximal convoluted t.
transverse t.
tubulointerstitium
tubuloreticular structure
tucker
Cooley cardiac t.
Crafoord-Cooley t.
Tucker bronchoscope
Tuffier test
Tuffnell treatment
tug, tugging
tracheal t.
Tukey-Kramer posttest
tularemia
oropharyngeal t.
tularemic pneumonia
tularensis
Francisella t.
tumor
adenomatoid t.
anaplastic t.
Askin t.
t. blush
bronchopulmonary carcinoid t.
carcinoid t.
cardiac t.
carotid body t.
chromaffin cell t.
clear cell t.
congenital periobronchial
 myofibroblastic t.
craniopharyngeal duct t.
desmoplastic small round cell t.
t. embolism
extrathoracic t.
germ cell t.
glomus t.
Godwin t.
granular cell t.
Hürthle cell t.
inflammatory myofibroblastic t.
intracardiac t.

T

NOTES

tumor *(continued)*
    intravascular bronchoalveolar t.
    t. marker
    mesenchymal-derived t.
    mesodermal t.
    mesothelial t.
    migrated t.
    myxoma t.
    t. necrosis factor (TNF)
    t. necrosis factor-alpha (TNF-alpha)
    neuroendocrine t.
    neurogenic t.
    t., nodes, metastasis (TNM)
    non-small cell t.
    Pancoast t.
    papillary t.
    paraganglioma t.
    pericardiac t.
    phantom t.
    t. plop
    t. plop sound
    polycystic t.
    primitive neuroectodermal t.
    (PNET)
    Purkinje t.
    Rathke pouch t.
    sarcomatous t.
    sugar t.
    superior pulmonary sulcus t.
    t. suppressor gene inactivation
    teratoma t.
    thyroid t.
    trophoblastic t.
tumorlet
tumorogenic
tumultus cordis
tunable
    t. dye laser
    t. pulsed dye laser
TUNEL
    TdT-mediated dUTP nick-end labeling
    TUNEL assay
    TUNEL method
    TUNEL stain
tungsten
    t. carbide pneumoconiosis
    t. microelectrode
tunic
    Bichat t.
    vascular t.
tunica
    t. mucosa bronchi
    t. mucosa esophagi
    t. mucosa laryngis
    t. mucosa linguae
    t. mucosa pharyngis
    t. mucosa tracheae
    t. muscularis bronchiorum

    t. muscularis esophagi
    t. muscularis pharyngis
    t. muscularis tracheae
tunnel
    Kawashima intraventricular t.
    percutaneous t.
    subsartorial t.
tunneler
    CPI t.
    Crafoord t.
    Eidemiller t.
    Kelly-Wick vascular t.
    Oregon t.
Tunturi
    T. EL400 bicycle ergometer
    T. Jogger-2 self-powered treadmill
Tuohy-Borst
    T.-B. adapter
    T.-B. introducer
tuple-1 gene
turbinate
turbine-powered ICU ventilator system
Turboaire Challenger
TurboFLASH technique
Turbohaler
    asthma T.
    Bricanyl T.
Turbuhaler
    Pulmicort T.
turbulence
turbulent
    t. diastolic mitral inflow
    t. jet
turgor
    coronary vascular t.
    skin t.
turnaround time (TAT)
Turner syndrome
Tusibron-DM
Tuss
    HycoClear T.
Tussafed drops
Tussafin Expectorant
Tuss-Allergine Modified T.D. Capsule
Tussar SF Syrup
Tuss-DM
Tussigon
Tussionex
Tussi-Organidin
    T.-O. DM NR
    T.-O. NR
tussive
    t. fremitus
    t. squeeze
    t. syncope
Tussogest Extended Release Capsule
Tusstat Syrup
Tuttle thoracic forceps

TV
　tidal volume
TV_I
　tidal inspiratory volume
TV_E
　tidal expiratory volume
TVG
　time-varied gain
TVGC
　time-varied gain control
TVR
　target vessel revascularization
TWA
　T wave alternans
TWAR
　Taiwan acute respiratory
　　TWAR agent
　　TWAR disease
　　TWAR pneumonia
T-wave pseudonormalization
Twee alternating cut-off compressor stockings
T1-weighted image
T2-weighted image
Twice-A-Day Nasal Solution
twiddler's syndrome
twill tape
twin
　　Bennett t.
　　T. Jet nebulizer
　　thoracopagus t.
twister
　　Asmanex t.
Twisthaler
twitch
　　t. gastric pressure
　　t. potentiation
two-block claudication
two-bottle thoracic drainage system
two-chain urokinase plasminogen activator (tcu-PA)
two-chamber view
two-dimensional (2D)
　　t.-d. transcranial color-coded sonography (2D-TCCS)
　　t.-d. echocardiography (2DE)
　　t.-d. integrated backscatter
　　t.-d. tag
two-flight
　　t.-f. dyspnea
　　t.-f. exertional dyspnea
two-flights-of-stairs claudication

two-kidney Goldblatt
two-patch technique
two-piece bifurcated intraluminal graft for repair of an aneurysm
two-pillow orthopnea
two-stage
　　ultrathin-walled t.-s. (UTTS)
two-stage cannula
two-step exercise test
two-turn epicardial lead
TxCAD
　transplant coronary artery disease
Tylenol
　　T. Cold No Drowsiness
　　T. Flu Maximum Strength
tylosin tartrate asthma
tyloxapol
tympanic
　　t. dullness
　　t. hypersonority
tympanitic sound
tympany
　　bell t.
type
　　t. A aortic dissection
　　t. A, B behavior
　　Ambrose plaque t.
　　t. III antiarrhythmic agent
　　t. B aortic dissection
　　cardioinhibitory t.
　　cell t.
　　t. II cell hyperplasia
　　t. I collagen telopeptide (ICTP)
　　t. 1, 2, 3, 4 dextrocardia
　　t. I, II dip
　　t. I glycogen storage disease
　　t. Va lesion
　　t. Vb lesion
　　t. Vc lesion
　　t. II pneumocyte
　　t. I procollagen
　　t. III procollagen
typhoid
　　t. fever
　　t. pleurisy
　　t. pneumonia
typhus
　　African tick t.
　　Queensland tick t.
　　scrub t.
typical small cell

T

NOTES

typing
    human lymphocyte antigen t.
Typ Vasocope III Doppler probe
tyramine
Tyrode solution
Tyrodone Liquid
tyrosine phosphorylated protein

Tyshak
    T. balloon
    T. balloon valvuloplasty catheter
    T. catheter
T-Y stent
Tzanck test

U

U loop
U suture
U virus
U wave
U wave alternans
U wave inversion

UACP
upper airway closing pressure

UAE
unsupported arm exercise

UA/NQMI
unstable angina/non-Q-wave myocardial infarction

UAO
upper airway obstruction

UAOP
upper airway opening pressure

UAP
unstable angina pectoris

UARS
upper airway resistance syndrome

ubiquinol
ubiquinone
ubiquitin
UCA
ultrasound contrast agent

UCAD
unstable coronary artery disease

UCG
ultrasonic cardiography

UCI-Barnard
U.-B. aortic valve
U.-B. valve

UD-CG 212
UFCT
ultrafast computed tomography

UFT
tegafur and uracil

UGDP
University Group Diabetes Program

UGNB
ultrasonically guided needle biopsy

UHFV
ultrahigh frequency ventilation

Uhl
U. anomaly
U. disease
U. malformation
U. syndrome

UIP
usual interstitial pneumonia
usual interstitial pneumonitis

UK
urokinase

ulcer
decubitus u.
diabetic u.
foot u.
penetrating aortic u. (PAU)
penetrating atherosclerotic u. (PAU)
peptic u.
stasis u.
venous u.

ulcerans
Mycobacterium u.

ulcerated
u. lesion
u. plaque

ulcerative endocarditis
ulcerogangrenous
ulceromembranous
ulcerosa
angina u.
pharyngitis u.

Uldall subclavian hemodialysis catheter
Ulick syndrome
Ullmann syndrome
ULM
unprotected left main

ulnar nerve
ULP
ultra low profile
ULP catheter

ULR
ULR LA Tablets
ULR Liquid

Ultegra rapid platelet function assay (U-RPFA)
Ultimate
U. nasal mask
U. Seal CPAP mask seal
U. Seal gel interface

ultimum moriens
ultra
U. 8 balloon catheter
u. low profile (ULP)
U. Low resistance voice prosthesis
U. Mide topical
U. pacemaker
U. Tag RBC

Ultracef
ultracentrifugation
UltraCision ultrasonic knife
Ultracor prosthetic valve
UltraCross profile imaging catheter
ultrafast
u. computed tomographic scanner
u. computed tomography (UFCT)
u. computed tomography scan

ultrafast *(continued)*
    u. contrast-enhanced chest computed tomography
    u. CT scan
    u. CT scanner
Ultraflex
    U. esophageal stent system
    U. self-expanding stent
    U. tracheobronchial stent
UltraFuse
    U. balloon
    U. catheter
    U. infusion catheter
ultrahigh frequency ventilation (UHFV)
Ultraject prefilled syringe
Ultra-Lite portable aspirator
ultra-low
    u.-l. profile fixed-wire balloon dilatation catheter
    u.-l. profile fixed-wire balloon dilation catheter
Ultramark 9 echocardiograph
ultrarapid subthreshold stimulation
Ultra-Select nitinol PTCA guidewire
ultrasonic
    u. cardiography (UCG)
    u. integrated backscatter imaging
    u. nebulizer
ultrasonically guided needle biopsy (UGNB)
ultrasonographer
ultrasonography
    B-mode u.
    compression u.
    Doppler u.
    duplex pulsed-Doppler u.
    high-resolution B-mode u.
    intracaval endovascular u. (ICEUS)
    intracoronary u.
    TCD u.
ultrasonoscope
    Acuson XP-5 u.
    Acuson XP-10 u.
    Acuson XP-128 u.
ultrasound
    u. ablation catheter
    ADR Ultramark 4 u.
    Aloka u.
    u. angiography
    Biosound 2000 II s.a. high-resolution u.
    B-mode u.
    bronchoscopic u.
    cardiac u.
    u. cardiography
    colorvascular Doppler u.
    continuous-wave Doppler u.
    u. contrast agent (UCA)

    U. Contrast Microsphere
    coronary intravascular u.
    Doppler u.
    duplex u.
    echo-guided u.
    gray-scale u.
    Hewlett-Packard u.
    Hewlett-Packard 2500 SONOS u.
    high-resolution u.
    high-resolution deep penetration 2D intracardiac u.
    u. holography
    Interspec XL u.
    Intertherapy intravascular u.
    intracoronary u. (ICUS)
    intracoronary vascular u. (IVUS)
    intraluminal u. (ILUS)
    intravascular u. (IVUS)
    Irex Exemplar u.
    Medasonics NeuroGuard CDS u.
    negative-contrast intravascular u.
    power Doppler u.
    qualitative coronary u. (QCU)
    real-time u.
    Shimadzu cardiac u.
    Siemens SI 400 u.
    TCD u.
    three-dimensional intravascular u.
    through-the-balloon u.
    Toshiba Sonolayer SSH-140A u.
    transcranial Doppler u. (TCD)
    u. transducer
ultrasound-guided bronchoscopy
ultrasound-tipped catheter
ultrastructure
Ultra-Thin balloon catheter
ultrathin-walled two-stage (UTTS)
ultraviolet laser
Ultravist
    U. contrast
    U. injection
umbilical
    u. artery
    u. tape
    u. vein
umbilicalis
    arteritis u.
umbrella
    ASDOS u.
    atrial septal defect u.
    Bard Clamshell septal u.
    Bard PDA u.
    Clamshell septal u.
    u. closure
    double u.
    u. filter
    patent ductus arteriosus u.
    PDA u.

Rashkind u.
Rashkind double u.
transcatheter u.
UMI
U. catheter
U. needle
U. transseptal Cath-Seal catheter
introducer
U-Mid-O₂ Jet Set
UMLS
Unified Medical Language system
unassisted spontaneous ventilation
Unasyn
underdrive
u. pacing
u. termination
underperfused myocardium
underperfusion
undersedation
undersensing
atrial u.
functional u.
pacemaker u.
undertreatment
underventilation
underwater
u. seal drainage
u. seal resistor
undetermined pathological-type stroke
undifferentiated
u. carcinoma
u. small cell carcinoma
undulating pulse
unequal pulse
unfractionated heparin
uniaxial accelerometer
Uni-Bent Cough Syrup
Unicard
unicommissural
unicuspid aortic valve
unidirectional block
Uni-Dur
unifascicular block
Unified Medical Language system (UMLS)
unifocal ventricular ectopic beat (UVEB)
UniHEART
U. IV universal nebulizer
U. universal nebulizer
unilateral
u. emphysema

u. hyperlucency of the lung
u. hyperlucent lung
u. nonfunctioning lung
u. pneumonia
u. pneumothorax
u. spatial neglect (USN)
unileaflet prolapse
Unilink
U. anastomotic device
U. system
Unilith pacemaker
unilocular cyst
unintubated
Unioprost
Unipass endocardial pacing lead
Unipen
U. injection
U. Oral
Uniphyl
unipolar
u. atrial pacemaker
u. connector
u. defibrillation coil electrode
u. electrocardiogram
u. J-tined passive-fixation lead
u. lead
u. limb leads
u. pacemaker
u. Pisces Sigma
u. precordial lead
u. sequential pacemaker
UniPort hemostasis introducer sheath kit
Unipres
Uni-Pro
Uniprost
Uniretic
Uni-Silicone lead
Unisperse blue dye
Unistasis valve
Unistep elivery system
unit
acute coronary care u.
ATA u.
BCD Plus cardioplegic u.
BICAP u.
BICAP B u.
Biosound 2000 II ultrasound u.
Biosound 3000 ultrasound u.
BiPAP u.
cardiothoracic intensive care u.
(CTICU)

U

NOTES

unit *(continued)*
    Collins Eagle I spirometry u.
    coronary care u. (CCU)
    critical care u.
    defibrillator u.
    digital fluoroscopic u.
    ECG triggering u.
    enhanced external
      counterpulsation u.
    FreeDop portable Doppler u.
    high-dependency u. (HDU)
    Hounsfield u. (HU)
    hybrid u.
    intrapleural sealed drainage u.
    kallidinogenase inactivator u.
    kallikrein inactivating u. (KIU)
    Karmen u.'s
    Kreiselman u.
    life change u.
    LIZ-88 ablation u.
    lung u.
    medical intensive care u. (MICU)
    million international u.'s (MIU)
    mobile coronary care u.
    1-natural-log-u. elevation
    peripheral resistance u. (PRU)
    POLY-MESAM recording u.
    postanesthesia care u. (PACU)
    R u.
    Respiratory Special Care U.
      (ReSCU)
    RinoFlow ENT wash u.
    Solcotrans autotransfusion u.
    S-Scort DUET suction u.
    stroke u. (SU)
    subacute u.
    Sullivan nasal variable positive
      airway pressure u.
    surgical intensive care u. (SICU)
    Surgitron u.
    terminal respiratory u. (TRU)
    Todd u.'s
    torr u.
    Tranquility BiLevel CPAP u.
    trauma intensive care u. (TICU)
    Wood u.
United
    U. Network for Organ Sharing
      (UNOS)
    U. States Air Force School of
      Aerospace Medicine (USAFSAM)
    U. States Pharmacopeia (USP)
UniTrack shaft
Uni-tussin DM
Unity-C
    U.-C. cardiac pacemaker
    U.-C. pacemaker
Unity VDDR pacemaker

univariate predictor
Univasc
Uni-Vent
    U.-V. Eagle portable ventilation
      system
    U.-V. ventilator
univentricular
    u. atrioventricular connection
    u. heart
    u. pacing
Univent tube
universal
    u. ACE
    u. aerosol cloud enhancer
    u. pacemaker
universalis
    adiposis u.
University
    U. of Akron artificial heart
    U. of Akron TAH
    U. Group Diabetes Program
      (UGDP)
    U. of Wisconsin solution
Univision echocardiographic system
Uniweave catheter
unlabored respiration
unloading
    left ventricular u.
Unna paste boot
Uno nasal prongs
UNOS
    United Network for Organ Sharing
unprotected
    u. artery
    u. left main (ULM)
unresolved pneumonia
unroofed
Unschuld sign
unstability
    catheter u.
unstable
    u. angina
    u. angina/non-Q-wave myocardial
      infarction (UA/NQMI)
    u. angina pectoris (UAP)
    u. coronary artery disease (UCAD)
    u. plaque
unstented xenograft valve
unsupported arm exercise (UAE)
up
    pinked u.
uPA
    urokinase-type plasminogen activator
updraft
    albuterol nebulizer u.
    Ventolin u.
Updraft handheld nebulizer
upgated technique

upgoing Babinski
upper
  u. airway
  u. airway closing pressure (UACP)
  u. airway obstruction (UAO)
  u. airway opening pressure (UAOP)
  u. airway resistance syndrome (UARS)
  u. lobe bronchus
  u. lobe of lung
  u. lung zone
  u. nodal extrasystole
  u. respiratory infection (URI)
  u. ribs
UPPP
  uvulopalatopharyngoplasty
up-regulation
upright
  u. exercise
  u. T wave
upsloping
  u. ST elevation
  u. ST segment
  u. ST segment depression
upstairs-downstairs heart
upstream
  u. airway conductance
  u. airways
  u. segment
upstroke
  carotid u.
  diastolic u.
  u. pattern
  R wave u.
  u. velocity
uptake
  cardiac antimyosin antibody u.
  glucose u.
  I-123 MIBG u.
  insulin-mediated glucose u. (IMGU)
  iodine-123
    metaiodobenzylguanidine u.
  lung u.
  maximum oxygen u.
  myocardial oxygen u.
  N-13 ammonia u.
  oxygen u.
  peak oxygen u.
  thallium u.
  tracer u.

uptake-1
  norepinephrine u.
uptake-mismatch pattern
uracil
  tegafur and u. (UFT)
urapidil
urate
Urbach-Wiethe syndrome
urea
Ureacin-20 topical
ureae
    Actinobacillus u.
Ureaphil Injection
Ureaplasma urealyticum
Urecholine
ureidopenicillin
uremia
uremic
  u. lung
  u. pericarditis
  u. pneumonia
  u. pneumonitis
Uremol
Uresil
  U. embolectomy thrombectomy catheter
  U. radiopaque silicone band vessel loops
  U. Vascu-Flo carotid shunt
urethane
  polycarbonate u.
urgency
  hypertensive u.
URI
  upper respiratory infection
uric acid
uridine triphosphate (UTP)
Uridon
urinary catheter
urine
  brown u.
  u. volume
urinothorax
Urisec
Uri-Tet Oral
Uritol
Urobak
urocanic acid

U

NOTES

Urografin-76 contrast medium
urokinase (UK)
    recombinant u. (r-UK)
urokinase-type plasminogen activator (uPA)
Uro-Mag
Uroplus
    U. DS
    U. SS
urorosein
Urozide
U-RPFA
    Ultegra rapid platelet function assay
urticaria
    aquagenic u.
    pressure u.
USAFSAM
    United States Air Force School of
    Aerospace Medicine
        USAFSAM treadmill exercise
        protocol
USCI
    U. catheter
    U. Goetz bipolar electrode
    U. Hyperflex guidewire
    U. introducer
    U. NBIH bipolar electrode
    U. Probe balloon-on-a-wire
    dilatation system
    U. Sauvage EXS side-limb
    prosthesis
    U. shunt

use
    amount of u. (AOU)
    u. dependence
U-shaped catheter loop
USN
    unilateral spatial neglect
USP
    United States Pharmacopeia
ustus
    Aspergillus u.
usual
    u. interstitial pneumonia (UIP)
    u. interstitial pneumonia of Liebow
    u. interstitial pneumonitis (UIP)
usurpation
UT-15
Utah
    U. TAH
    U. total artificial heart
UTP
    uridine triphosphate
UTTS
    ultrathin-walled two-stage
        UTTS endotracheal tube
UVEB
    unifocal ventricular ectopic beat
uvulopalatopharyngoplasty (UPPP)
    laser-assisted u.
uvulopalatoplasty
    laser-assisted u. (LAUP)

V

ventricular
volume
  V lead
  V peak of jugular venous
  V wave

V$_A$

alveolar ventilation per minute

V$_{cf}$

fiber shortening velocity

V$_D$

physiological dead space ventilation per minute

V$_E$

minute ventilation
peak exercise ventilation

V$_{MAX}$

maximal velocity

V$_O$

oral airflow in liters per second

V$_{pe}$

peak ejection velocity

V$_T$

tidal volume

V$_{TG}$

thoracic gas volume

V$_1$-like ambulatory lead syndrome
V$_5$-like ambulatory lead syndrome
V5M Multiplane transducer
V510B Biplane TEE transducer
V-A

ventriculoatrial
  V-A conduction
  V-A interval

VA

alveolar volume
variant angina
ventriculoatrial
Veterans Administration
VA interval

VAC, V-AC

ventriculoatrial conduction

vaccae

Mycobacterium v.

vaccine

ActHIB v.
bacillus Calmette-Guérin v.
BCG v.
Calmette-Guérin v.
diphtheria, tetanus toxoids, and acellular pertussis v.
diphtheria, tetanus toxoids, and whole-cell pertussis v.

diphtheria, tetanus toxoids, and whole-cell pertussis vaccine and *Haemophilus* b conjugate v.
Haemophilus b conjugate v.
HbOC v.
Imovax v.
inactivated poliovirus v.
influenza virus v.
lipopolysaccharide v.
meningococcal v.
pneumococcal v.
PRP-D v.
PRP-OMPC v.
tuberculosis v.
14-valent v.

vaccinia
Vaccinium myrtillus
Vac-Pak-II ultra-lite portable aspirator
VACTERL

vertebral, vascular, anal, cardiac, tracheoesophageal, renal, and limb anomalies
  VACTERL syndrome

Vacu-Aide

V.-A. home-use aspirator

vacuolated cell
Vacutainer tube
vacuum

v. controller
high v. (HV)

vacuum-assisted venous return system
vacuus

pulsus v.

VAD

ventricular assist device
  DeBakey VAD
  HeartSaver VAD

vagal

v. atrial fibrillation
v. attack
v. block
v. body
v. bradycardia
v. escape
v. nerve stimulation
v. neural crest
v. reaction
v. reflex
v. response
v. stimulation
v. tone

vagi

ganglion inferius nervi v.
rami esophagei nervi v.

vagina synovialis trochleae

V

vagolytic
    v. agent
    v. property
vagomimetic intervention
vagotonic baroreceptor response
vagus
    v. arrhythmia
    v. nerve
    v. pneumonia
    v. pulse
VA-HIT
    Veterans Administration High-Density
    Lipoprotein Intervention Trial
**Vairox high compression vascular
stockings**
valacyclovir
14-valent vaccine
valgus
    cubitus v.
Val-HeFT
    Valsartan Heart Failure Trial
VALI
    ventilator-associated lung injury
VALIANT
    Valsartan in Acute Myocardial Infarction
    Trial
vallecular dysphagia
Valley fever
Valleylab Force 2 electrosurgical device
valrubicin
Valsalva
    V. maneuver (VS)
    ruptured sinus of V.
    sinus of V.
    V. sinus
    V. test
valsalviana
    dysphagia v.
valsartan
    V. in Acute Myocardial Infarction
    Trial (VALIANT)
    v. antihypertensive long-term
    evaluation
    V. Antihypertensive Long-Term Use
    Evaluation (VALUE)
    V. Heart Failure Trial (Val-HeFT)
    v. and hydrochlorothiazide
valsartan/hydrochlorothiazide
Valstar
VALUE
    Valsartan Antihypertensive Long-Term
    Use Evaluation
value
    A p v.
    Astrup blood gas v.
    index v.
    JTc v.
    negative predictive v. (NPV)

    predictive v.
    QRS-T v.
    reference v.
    resting v.
    tercile v.
    threshold v.
    V. of Transesophageal
    Echocardiography (VOTE)
Valugraph
    Mijnhard V.
valva trunci pulmonalis
valve
    abnormal cleavage of cardiac v.
    Abrams-Lucas flap heart v.
    absent pulmonary v.
    Angell-Shiley bioprosthetic v.
    Angell-Shiley xenograft
    prosthetic v.
    Angiocor prosthetic v.
    aortic v.
    aortic bioprosthetic v.
    artificial cardiac v.
    atretic pulmonary v.
    atrial v.
    atrioventricular v.
    ATS Open Pivot bileaflet heart v.
    ball v.
    ball-and-cage prosthetic v.
    ball heart v.
    ball-occluder v.
    Baxter mechanical v.
    Beall mitral v.
    Beall prosthetic v.
    Beall-Surgitool ball-cage
    prosthetic v.
    Beall-Surgitool disk prosthetic v.
    Bianchi v.
    Bicarbon Sorin v.
    Bicer-Val prosthetic v.
    bicommissural aortic v. (BAV)
    bicuspid aortic v.
    bileaflet tilting-disk prosthetic v.
    Biocor porcine v.
    Biocor prosthetic v.
    biological aortic v.
    bioprosthetic heart v.
    Bio-Vascular prosthetic v.
    Björk-Shiley v.
    Björk-Shiley convexoconcave disk
    prosthetic v.
    Björk-Shiley mitral v.
    Björk-Shiley monostrut v.
    Björk-Shiley prosthetic v.
    Blom-Singer v.
    bovine heart v.
    bovine pericardial v.
    Braunwald-Cutter ball prosthetic v.
    butterfly heart v.

caged ball v.
calcification of tips of the
  mitral v.
calcified aortic v.
Capetown aortic prosthetic v.
Capetown prosthetic v.
Carbomedics bileaflet prosthetic
  heart v.
Carbomedics prosthetic heart v.
Carbomedics top-hat supra-
  annular v.
cardiac v.
Carpentier-Edwards mitral
  annuloplasty v.
Carpentier-Edwards pericardial v.
Carpentier-Edwards Perimount
  mitral v.
Carpentier-Edwards porcine
  prosthetic v.
Carpentier-Edwards porcine
  supraannular v.
Carpentier pericardial v.
caval v.
C-C heart v.
CirKuit-Guard pressure relief v.
cleft mitral v.
v. commissure
congenital anomaly of mitral v.
Cooley-Bloodwell-Cutter v.
Cooley-Cutter disk prosthetic v.
Coratomic prosthetic v.
CPHV OptiForm mitral v.
crisscross atrioventricular v.
Cross-Jones disk prosthetic v.
Cross-Jones mitral v.
CryoLife-O'Brien v.
CryoLife-O'Brien stentless v.
cryopreserved homograft v.
CryoValve-SG human allograft
  heart v.
Cutter-Smeloff disk v.
Cutter-Smeloff mitral v.
DeBakey-Surgitool prosthetic v.
v. debris
Delrin heart v.
diastolic fluttering aortic v.
disk-cage v.
Duostat rotating hemostatic v.
Duraflow heart v.
Duromedics mitral v.
dysplastic v.
early opening v.

Ebstein malformed v.
eccentric monocuspid tilting-disk
  prosthetic v.
echo-dense v.
Edmark mitral v.
Edwards-Duromedics bileaflet
  heart v.
Edwards heart v.
eustachian v.
flail mitral v.
floppy mitral v. (FMV)
four-legged cage v.
Freestyle bioprosthetic heart v.
Freestyle stentless aortic heart v.
GateWay Y-adapter rotating
  hemostatic v.
glutaraldehyde-tanned bovine
  heart v.
glutaraldehyde-tanned porcine
  heart v.
Gott butterfly heart v.
Guangzhou GD-1 prosthetic v.
Hall-Kaster prosthetic v.
Hall prosthetic heart v.
Hancock v.
Hancock II tissue v.
Hancock modified orifice v.
Hancock M.O. II bioprosthesis
  porcine v.
Hancock porcine v.
Hans Rudolph nonbreathing v.
Hans Rudolph three-way v.
Harken ball v.
heart v.
Heimlich chest drainage v.
Heimlich heart v.
Hemex prosthetic v.
hemostasis v.
hockey-stick tricuspid v.
Hufnagel prosthetic v.
impedance threshold v. (ITV)
intact v.
Ionescu-Shiley v.
Ionescu-Shiley pericardial v.
Ionescu trileaflet v.
Jatene-Macchi prosthetic v.
Kay-Shiley caged-disk v.
Lillehei-Kaster pivoting-disk
  prosthetic v.
Liotta-BioImplant low profile
  bioprosthesis prosthetic v.

NOTES

valve *(continued)*
Magovern-Cromie ball-cage
  prosthetic v.
Malteno v.
mechanical v.
Medtronic-Hall monocuspid tilting-
  disk v.
Medtronic-Hall prosthetic heart v.
Medtronic Hancock II v.
Medtronic Hancock II tissue v.
Medtronic Intact bioprosthetic v.
Medtronic Mosaic bioprosthetic v.
midsystolic buckling of mitral v.
midsystolic closure of aortic v.
mitral v. (MV)
Mitroflow Synergy PC stented
  pericardial v.
Montgomery speaking v.
Mosaic porcine bioprosthetic
  heart v.
native v.
noncalcified v.
nonrebreathing v.
Omnicarbon prosthetic heart v.
Omniscience tilting-disk v.
On-X mechanical bi-leaflet
  prosthetic heart v.
On-X prosthetic v.
Open Pivot heart v.
v. orifice area
parachute mitral v.
Passy-Muir tracheostomy
  speaking v.
PEEP v.
Pemco prosthetic v.
PMV 2000 clear tracheostomy &
  ventilator speaking v.
PMV 2001 purple tracheostomy &
  ventilator speaking v.
PMV 2000 series speaking V.
PMV 005 tracheostomy v.
PMV 007 tracheostomy &
  ventilator speaking v.
porcine v.
porcine prosthetic v.
prosthetic aortic v.
prosthetic ball v.
prosthetic cardiac v.
Provox speaking v.
Puig Massana-Shiley
  annuloplasty v.
pulmonary autograft v.
v. of pulmonary trunk
pulmonic v.
quadricusp mitral v. (QMV)
quadricusp stentless mitral
  bioprosthetic v.
Quattro mitral v.

reducing v.
v. replacement (VR)
v. resistance
Ross pulmonary porcine v.
v. rupture
semilunar v.
Shiley convexoconcave heart v.
Shiley Phonate speaking v.
Singer-Blom v.
SJM v.
SJM Masters series heart v.
SJM mechanical heart v.
SJM Quattro mitral v.
SJM Regent mechanical heart v.
Smeloff-Cutter ball-cage
  prosthetic v.
Smeloff-Cutter prosthetic v.
Smeloff heart v.
Sorin heart v.
Sorin prosthetic v.
speaking v.
Starr-Edwards v.
Starr-Edwards ball-and-cage v.
Starr-Edwards mitral v.
Starr-Edwards prosthetic v.
Starr-Edwards Silastic v.
Stellite ring material of
  prosthetic v.
stented bioprosthetic v.
stentless v.
stentless porcine v. (SPV)
stentless porcine aortic v.
stent-mounted allograft v.
stent-mounted heterograft v.
St. Jude V. (SJM)
St. Jude bileaflet prosthetic v.
St. Jude composite prosthetic v.
St. Jude Medical bileaflet tilting-
  disk aortic v.
St. Jude Medical BioImplant v.
St. Jude Medical Port-Access
  mechanical heart v.
St. Jude mitral v.
St. Jude prosthetic aortic v.
straddling of v.
straddling atrioventricular v.
straddling tricuspid v.
Surgitool prosthetic v.
v. of Sylvius
SynerGraft heart v.
SynerGraft pulmonary heart v.
SynerGraft tissue-engineered
  heart v.
Tascon prosthetic v.
Tekna mechanical heart v.
thebesian v.
tilting disk v.
tilting-disk heart v.

tilting-disk prosthetic v.
tissue v.
Top-Hat supraannular aortic v.
toroidal v.
Toronto SPV v.
Toronto SPV aortic v.
Toronto SPV stentless porcine
  heart v.
tricuspid v.
tricuspid aortic v.
UCI-Barnard v.
UCI-Barnard aortic v.
Ultracor prosthetic v.
unicuspid aortic v.
Unistasis v.
unstented xenograft v.
Vascor porcine prosthetic v.
v. vegetation
ventilator speaking v.
v. of Vieussens
Vieussens v.
Wessex prosthetic v.
X-Cell v.
Xenomedica prosthetic v.
Xenotech prosthetic v.

valve-conserving operation
valvectomy
valved holding chamber (VHC)
valve-preserving surgery
Valve-SG
valvopathy (*var. of* valvuopathy)
valvoplasty
valvotomy, valvulotomy
  aortic v.
  balloon aortic v. (BAV)
  balloon pulmonary v.
  balloon tricuspid v.
  double-balloon v.
  Inoue balloon mitral v.
  v. knife
  Longmire v.
  mitral v.
  mitral balloon v. (MBV)
  mitral valve v.
  percutaneous mitral balloon v.
    (PMBV)
  pulmonary v.
  radiofrequency-assisted v.
  repeat balloon mitral v.
  single-balloon v.
  thimble v.

transcatheter v.
transventricular closed v.
valvula
  v. coronaria dextra valvar aortae
  v. semilunaris dextra
valvular
  v. aortic stenosis
  v. calcification
  v. cardiomyopathy
  v. dysfunction
  v. endocarditis
  v. function
  v. heart disease
  v. incompetence
  v. insufficiency
  v. leaflet
  v. morphology
  v. orifice
  v. pneumothorax
  v. prolapse
  v. pulmonic stenosis
  v. reflux
  v. regurgitation
  v. sclerosis
  v. thickening
  v. thrombus
  v. vegetation
valvulitis
  aortic v.
  chronic v.
  mitral v.
  rheumatic v.
  syphilitic aortic v.
valvuloplasty
  aortic v.
  bailout v.
  balloon v. (BV)
  balloon aortic v. (BAV)
  balloon mitral v. (BMV)
  balloon pulmonary v. (BPV)
  Carpentier tricuspid v.
  catheter balloon v.
  double-balloon v.
  intracoronary thrombolysis
    balloon v.
  mitral v.
  multiple-balloon v.
  percutaneous aortic balloon v.
  percutaneous balloon v. (PBV)
  percutaneous balloon aortic v.
  percutaneous balloon mitral v.
  percutaneous balloon pulmonic v.

V

NOTES

valvuloplasty *(continued)*
    percutaneous mitral v. (PMV)
    percutaneous mitral balloon v. (PMBV)
    percutaneous transluminal balloon v.
    pulmonary v.
    pulmonary balloon v. (PBV)
    single-balloon v.
    transcarotid balloon v.
    tricuspid v.
    triple-balloon v.
    Trusler technique of aortic v.
valvulotome
    angioscopic v.
    antegrade v.
    Bakst v.
    bread knife v.
    Carmody v.
    Hall v.
valvulotomy *(var. of* valvotomy)
valvuopathy, valvopathy
Vamate Oral
VAMC
    Veterans Affairs Medical Center
    VAMC prognostic score
vampire bat plasminogen activator
Van
    V. Andel catheter
    V. Hoorne canal
    V. Slyke method
    V. Tassel angled pigtail catheter
van
    v. den Bergh disease
    v. Elterns test
    v. Gieson stain
    v. Helmont mirror
vanadium
vanadiumism
Vancenase
    V. AQ Inhaler
    V. Pockethaler
Vanceril Oral Inhaler
Vancocin
    V. CP
    V. injection
    V. Oral
Vancoled injection
vancomycin hydrochloride
vancomycin-resistant enterococci
Vanex-LA
Vanguard
    V. device
    V. endograft
    V. III endovascular aortic graft
    V. modular endograft system
vanishing lung
Vanlev

VANQWISH
    Veterans Affairs Non-Q-Wave Infarction Strategies in Hospital
    VANQWISH study
Vansil
Vantex central venous catheter
Vantin
VAP
    ventilator-associated pneumonia
Vaponefrin
vapor
    inorganic acid v.
    v. massage
    mercury v.
    solvent v.
vaporizer
    Cool-vapor v.
    Fluotec v.
    Israel Benzedrine v.
    Maxi-Myst v.
Vaporole
    Amyl Nitrate V.
Vapor-Phase heated humidification system
vapotherapy
Vapotherm
    V. 2000i
    V. oxygen delivery system
VAPS
    volume-assured pressure support
Vaquez disease
VAR
    variant angina pectoris
Varco thoracic forceps
variability
    baseline v.
    beat-to-beat v.
    cardiac v.
    diurnal peak flow v.
    heart rate v. (HRV)
    interlead QT v.
variable
    v. coupling
    v. deceleration
    impedance v.
    Newton law of motion and v.
    v. positive airway pressure (VPAP)
    v. threshold angina
variant
    v. angina (VA)
    v. angina pectoris (VAR)
    Miller Fisher v.
variation
    circadian v.
    diurnal v.
    respiratory waveform v.
variceal
    v. ligation

v. sclerosing
v. sclerotherapy
varicella
v. pneumonia
v. pneumonitis
v. zoster (VZ)
varicella-zoster
v.-z. immunoglobulin (VZIG)
v.-z. infection
v.-z. virus (VZV)
varices (*pl. of* varix)
varicose
v. vein
v. vein stripping and ligation
varicosity
saphenous vein v.
Variflex catheter catheter
variomatrix transducer
Vario system
variotii
Paecilomyces v.
Varivas R denatured homologous vein graft
varix, pl. **varices**
cirsoid v.
downhill esophageal v.
esophageal varices

VAS
vasculotropin
Verapamil Angioplasty Study
visual analog scale
horizontal VAS
mechanical VAS
vertical VAS
vasa
v. nervorum
v. vasorum
Vas-Cath
V.-C. catheter
V.-C. Opti-Flow
Vascoray
Vascor porcine prosthetic valve
VascuClamp
V. minibulldog vessel clamp
V. vascular clamp
VascuCoil peripheral vascular stent
Vascu-Flo carotid shunt
Vascugel device
vascular
v. access catheter
v. acoustic emission
v. attenuation

v. bed
v. bundle
v. cadherin
v. cell adhesion molecule-1 (VCAM-1)
v. choir
v. clamp
v. clip
v. compromise
v. death
v. dementia
v. depression
v. ectasia
v. endothelial growth factor (VEGF)
v. funnel
v. gene transfer
v. graft prosthesis
v. groove
v. hemostatic device (VHD)
v. impedance
v. incident
v. injury
v. insult
v. leak syndrome
v. marking
v. matrix
v. murmur
v. pattern
v. peripheral resistance
v. permeability factor (VPF)
v. reactivity
v. redistribution
v. reflex
v. remodeling
v. resistance
v. resistance index
v. ring
v. ring division
v. sclerosis
v. sealing device
v. sheath
v. sling
v. smooth muscle cell (VSMC)
v. spasm
v. spider
v. stenosis
v. stiffness
v. system
v. tape
v. tunic
v. zone

V

NOTES

vascularity
vascularization
vasculature
    coronary v.
    pulmonary v.
VascuLink vascular access graft
vasculitic neuropathy
vasculitis, pl. vasculitides
    allergic v.
    cardiac v.
    Churg-Strauss v.
    consecutive v.
    Henoch-Schönlein v.
    hypersensitivity v.
    leukocytoblastic v.
    livedo v.
    lymphoreticular granulomatous v.
    necrotizing v.
    necrotizing granulomatous v.
    nodular v.
    overlap v.
    pulmonary v.
    segmented hyalinizing v.
    systemic granulomatous v.
    systemic necrotizing v.
vasculocardiac syndrome of
  hyperserotonemia
vasculogenesis
vasculogenic impotence
vasculopathy
    allograft v.
    cardiac allograft v. (CAV)
    cerebral v.
    graft v.
    hypertensive v.
    primary fibroproliferative
      pulmonary v.
vasculotropin (VAS)
Vascushunt
Vascutek
    V. Gelseal vascular graft
    V. knitted vascular graft
    V. woven vascular graft
Vaseretic 10-25
vasinfectum
    Fusarium v.
VASIS
    Vasovagal Syncope International Study
vasoactive
    v. drug
    v. intestinal peptide (VIP)
    v. mediator
    v. substance
vasoactivity
vasoconstriction
    coronary microcirculatory v.
    delayed cerebral v. (DCV)
    hypoxic v.

    hypoxic pulmonary v. (HPV)
    microcirculatory v.
    paradoxical v.
    peripheral v.
    pulmonary v.
    reflex v.
    reflex pulmonary arterial v.
vasoconstrictive reflex
vasoconstrictor
    v. center
    v. peptide
vasodepression
vasodepressor
    v. substance
    v. syncope
vasodepressor-cardioinhibitory syncope
Vasodilan
vasodilation
    coronary v.
    endothelium-dependent v.
    flow-mediated v.
    myocardial v. (MVD)
    peripheral v.
    profound systemic v.
    pulmonary v.
    reflex v.
    regional v.
vasodilator
    v. agent
    v. center
    v. effect
    V. Heart Failure Trial II (V-HeFT
      II)
    v. plus exercise treadmill test
    v. reserve
vasodilatory
    v. hypotension
    v. response
    v. shock
VasoExtor lead extraction system
vasofactive cell
Vasoflux
vasogenic
    v. edema
    v. shock
Vasoglyn
vasoinhibitor
vasomotion
    coronary v.
vasomotor
    v. angina
    v. paralysis
    v. response (VMR)
    v. rhinitis
    v. tone
vasomotoria
    angina v.
    angina pectoris v.

vasoneuronal coupling
vasopeptidase inhibitor (VPI)
vasopressin
    arginine v. (AVP)
vasopressor
    v. deficiency
    v. reflex
    v. support
vasoreactivity
vasoregulatory asthenia
vasorelaxant peptide
vasorelaxation
vasoresponse
vasorum
    aortic vasa v.
    vasa v.
Vasoscope 3 Doppler probe
VasoSeal
    V. vascular hemostasis device
    V. VHD
vasospasm
    cerebral v. (CVS)
    coronary v.
    diffuse v.
    ergonovine-induced v.
    ergonovine-induced coronary v.
    focal v.
vasospastic
    v. angina (VSA)
    v. disease
Vasotec
    V. IV
    V. Oral
vasotonic angina
Vasotrax
vasovagal
    v. attack
    v. episode
    v. hypotension
    v. orthostatism
    v. reaction
    v. syncope
    V. Syncope International Study
    (VASIS)
    v. syndrome
VasoView
    V. balloon dissection device
    V. Uniport endoscopic saphenous
    vein harvesting system
Vasoxyl
VasPort
    Titanium V.

Vas recorder
VAT
    ventilatory anaerobic threshold
    ventricular activation time
    video-assisted thoracoscopy
        VAT pacemaker
        VAT pacing
VATER
    vertebral defects, imperforate anus,
      transesophageal fistula, and radial and
      renal dysplasia
        VATER association syndrome
        VATER complex
VATS
    video-assisted thoracic surgery
    video-assisted thoracoscopic surgery
    video-assisted thoracoscopy
Vaughan-Williams
    V.-W. antiarrhythmic drug
      classification
    V.-W. class effect
    V.-W. classification
Vaxcel
    V. catheter
    V. mini stick
VB
    virtual bronchoscopy
VBI
    vertebrobasilar territory ischemia
VC
    vital capacity
    volume control
V/C
    ventilation-to-circulation
        V/C ratio
Vc
    pulmonary capillary blood volume
VCA
    viral capsid antigen
VCAM-1
    vascular cell adhesion molecule-1
VCD
    vocal cord dysfunction
VCDF
    volume-cycled decelerating-flow
      ventilation
VCF
    velocity of circumferential fiber
      shortening
VCG
    vectorcardiogram
    vectorcardiography

V

NOTES

V-Cillin K Oral
VCO$_2$
    venous carbon dioxide production
VCPC
    vindesine, cisplatin, lomustine,
      cyclophosphamide
VCV
    ventricular conduction velocity
    volume-controlled ventilation
VDD
    V. mode
    V. pacemaker
    V. pacing
    V. pacing system
V-Dec-M
VDI mode
VDR
    volumetric diffusive respirator
VDRL
    Venereal Disease Research Laboratory
      VDRL test
VDS
    venous duplex scanning
VEB
    ventricular ectopic beat
VE-cMRI
    velocity-encoded cine-magnetic
      resonance imaging
vector
    adeno-associated viral v.
    adenoviral v.
    v. cardiography
    v. electrocardiogram
    instantaneous v.
    v. loop
    manifest v.
    mean v.
    mean manifest v.
    P v.
    v., phased-array ultrasound-tipped
      catheter
    QRS v.
    retroviral v.
    spatial v.
    ST v.
    T v.
    viral v.
vectorcardiogram (VCG)
vectorcardiography (VCG)
    spatial v.
vecuronium
Veetids Oral
VEFR
    visually evoked flow response
VEGAS
    Vein Graft AngioJet Study
VEGAS I
    Vein Graft AngioJet Study-Phase I

VEGAS II
    Vein Graft AngioJet Study-Phase II
vegetal bronchitis
vegetation
    aortic valve v.
    bacterial v.
    endocardial v.
    leaflet v.
    mobile v.
    prosthetic valve v.
    pulmonary valve v.
    tricuspid valve v.
    valve v.
    valvular v.
    ventricular septal defect v.
    verrucous v.
vegetative
    v. endocarditis
    v. lesion
VEGF
    vascular endothelial growth factor
    VEGF gene therapy
    VEGF gene therapy study
veiled puff
veiling glare
Veillonella
vein
    accessory saphenous v.
    accessory venous v.
    allantoic v.
    anomalous pulmonary v.
    antecubital v.
    autogenous v.
    axillary v.
    azygos v.
    basilic v.
    Boyd perforating v.
    brachial v.
    brachiocephalic v.
    bronchial v.
    Burow v.
    cardiac v.
    cardinal v.
    v. of caudate nucleus
    central v.
    cephalic v.
    v. circumflexa iliaca superficialis
    common femoral v.
    coronary v.
    cryopreserved v.
    deep lingual v.
    Dodd perforating v.
    esophageal v.
    external jugular v.
    external pudendal v.
    facial v.
    femoral v.
    v. graft

V. Graft AngioJet Study (VEGAS)
V. Graft AngioJet Study-Phase I
  (VEGAS I)
V. Graft AngioJet Study-Phase II
  (VEGAS II)
v. graft cannula
v. graft patency
v. graft ring marker
hemiazygos v.
hepatic v.
human umbilical v. (HUV)
iliac v.
inferior laryngeal v.
inferior thyroid v.
infrasegmental v.
innominate v.
internal cerebral v. (ICV)
internal jugular v.
internal pudendal v.
internal thoracic v.
intersegmental part of pulmonary v.
interventricular v.
jugular v.
Kohlrausch v.
Krukenberg v.
Kuhnt postcentral v.
laryngeal v.
left inferior pulmonary v.
left internal jugular v.
left median v.
left superior pulmonary v.
levoatriocardinal v.
lingual v.
main renal v.
Marshall oblique v.
nest of v.'s
omphalomesenteric v.
partial anomalous pulmonary v.'s
  (PAPV)
pharyngeal v.
portal v.
profunda femoris v.
prominent pulmonary v.
pulmonary v.
renal v.
Retzius v.'s
reverse saphenous v.
right inferior pulmonary v.
right superior pulmonary v.
saphenous v.
sausaging of v.
subclavian v.

sublingual v.
superior laryngeal v.
superior pulmonary v.
superior thalamostriate v.
thebesian v.
v. of Thebesius
tortuous v.'s
tracheal v.
umbilical v.
varicose v.
ventricular v.
vitelline v.
Veingard dressing
vein-to-vein technology
Velban
Velbe
Velcro rale
Velex woven Dacron vascular graft
velocardiofacial syndrome
velocimeter
  FloMap v.
velocimetry
  Doppler v.
velocity
  airflow v.
  aortic jet v.
  aortic pulse-wave v.
  A-peak v.
  average peak v. (APV)
  basal average peak v. (BAPV)
  baseline average peak v. (BAPV)
  blood flow v. (BFV)
  blunted systolic v.
  v. catheter technique
  cerebral blood flow v. (CBFV)
  v. of circumferential fiber
    shortening (VCF)
  conduction v.
  coronary blood flow v. (CBFV)
  coronary flow v.
  detachment v.
  ejection v.
  v. encoding
  end-diastolic v.
  E-peak v.
  E-wave v.
  fiber shortening v. (V_{cf})
  field flow v.
  flow v.
  forward flow of v.
  high regional wall motion v.
    (Vhigh)

NOTES

velocity *(continued)*
    hyperemic v.
    instantaneous spectral peak v.
    jet v.
    left atrial appendage flow v.
    left ventricular outflow tract v.
    long-axis shortening v.
    maximal v. (V_{MAX})
    myocardial Doppler v. (MDV)
    nerve conduction v. (NCV)
    peak A v.
    peak E v.
    peak ejection v. (V_{pe})
    peak hyperemic average v. (PAPV)
    peak systolic v.
    peak transaortic flow v.
    phasic intragraft flow v.
    pulse wave v. (PWV)
    v. ratio (VR)
    sensory nerve conduction v. (SNCV)
    shortening v.
    spectral peak v.
    V. stent
    systolic pulmonary venous v.
    systolic wall motion v. (Vsys)
    time-averaged peak v.
    v. time integral
    tracheal mucus v.
    translesional spectral flow v.
    transmitral flow v.
    transprosthetic flow v.
    transvalvular E v.
    upstroke v.
    ventricular conduction v. (VCV)
    wall motion v.
velocity-encoded cine-magnetic resonance imaging (VE-cMRI)
Velogene rapid TB assay
velolaryngeal endoscope
velopharyngeal insufficiency
Velosef
Velosulin Human
velour collar graft
Velpeau hernia
Velstretch/Velcro headgear
Velvelan
vena, gen. and pl. **venae**
    agger valvae venae
    venae bronchiales
    venae cardiacae anteriores
    v. cava cannula
    v. cava clip
    v. cava filter
    v. caval foramen
    v. caval obstruction
    v. cava obstruction
    v. cava syndrome

venae circumflexae laterales femoris
v. circumflexa iliaca profunda
v. contracta
venae dorsales linguae
venae esophageae
v. laryngea inferior
v. laryngea superior
v. lingularis
v. obliqua atrial sinistra venae esophageales
venae pharyngeae
v. profunda linguae
venae pulmonales
v. pulmonalis inferior dextra
v. pulmonalis inferior sinistra
v. pulmonalis superior dextra
v. pulmonalis superior sinistra
radix basalis anterior venae
v. sublingualis
venae supratrochleares
venae tracheales
vena cava, gen. **venae cavae**
    foramen venae cavae
    inferior v.c. (IVC)
    Spencer plication of v.c.
    superior v.c. (SVC)
venacavogram
venae (*gen. and pl. of* vena)
VenaFlow compression system
Venaport coronary sinus guiding catheter
venarum pulmonum PAS
Vena Tech LGM filter
venectasia
Venereal Disease Research Laboratory (VDRL)
venereum
    lymphogranuloma v. (LGV)
VenES II Medical stockings
Venflon needle
venipuncture
    contrast-guided v.
venoarterial shunting
venoconstriction
    splenic v.
venodilation
Venodyne external pneumatic compression System EPS-410
Venofit medical compression stockings
Venoflex medical compression stockings
Venoglobulin-I
Venoglobulin-S
venogram
venography
    contrast v.
    helical CT v.
    magnetic resonance v. (MRV)
    renal v.

venolobar syndrome
venom
    arthropod v.
    bee v.
    black widow spider v.
    scorpion v.
    snake v.
    spider v.
venoocclusive disease
venopressor
venorespiratory reflex
Venoscope
    Landry Vein Light V.
venosinal
venosity
venostasis
venosum
    cor v.
venosus
    ductus v.
    pulsus v.
    sinus v.
venous
    v. access
    v. admixture
    v. air embolism
    v. blood
    v. cannula
    v. capacitance bed
    v. carbon dioxide production (VCO_2)
    v. collateral
    v. congestion
    v. coronary graft patency
    v. Corrigan wave
    v. cutdown
    C wave of jugular v.
    v. digital angiogram
    v. duplex scanning (VDS)
    v. embolism
    v. engorgement
    v. flow controller (VFC)
    v. flow measurement
    v. groove
    v. heart
    v. hum
    v. hyperemia
    v. hypertension
    v. insufficiency
    v. intravasation
    v. lakes
    v. mesenteric vascular occlusion

    v. murmur
    v. occlusion test
    v. phase
    v. plasma norepinephrine concentration
    v. pressure
    v. pressure gradient support stockings
    v. pressure tracing
    v. pulse
    v. pulse tracing
    v. puncture
    v. reflux
    v. return
    v. return curve
    v. runoff
    v. saturation
    v. sclerosis
    v. segment of glomeriform
    v. sheath
    v. smooth muscle
    v. spasm
    v. spread
    v. stasis
    v. thromboembolism (VTE)
    v. thrombosis
    v. troughing
    v. ulcer
    v. valvular insufficiency
    V peak of jugular v.
    v. web
venovenostomy
venovenous
    v. access
    v. dye dilution curve
vent
    Heartport Endopulmonary V.
Ventaire
Ventak
    V. AICD pacemaker
    V. A-V III DR automatic implantable cardioverter-defibrillator
    V. defibrillator
    V. ECD
    V. Mini II and III automatic implantable cardioverter-defibrillator
    V. P3 AICD
    V. Prizm 2 automatic implantable cardioverter-defibrillator
    V. Prizm defibrillator
    V. Prizm dual-chamber implantable defibrillator

NOTES

Adult Star 2000 ultra-high-frequency v.
Aequitron v.
Avian transport v.
Bear v.
Bear 1000 v.
Bear 1, 2 adult volume v.
Bear Cub infant v.
Bennett MA-1, PR-2 v.
Bennett PR-2 v.
Bennett pressure-cycled v.
3100B high-frequency oscillatory v.
Bio-Med MVP-10 pediatric v.
Bird v.
Bird Ascension v.
Bird 8400STi v.
Bird VDR v.
blow-by v.
Bourns-Bear v.
Bourns infant v.
Cesar v.
Critical Care V.
cuirass v.
v. dependency
Dräger v.
E-150 Breeze v.
Emerson postoperative v.
Esprit v.
GALILEO v.
Hamilton v.
high-frequency chest wall v. (HFCWO)
high-frequency jet v.
high-frequency oscillation v.
ICV-10 v.
Infant Star 100 v.
Infant Star 200 v.
Infant Star V. 500/950
infrasonic v.
Infrasonics v.
IVAC v.
Lifecare v.
v. management
MicroVent v.
Monaghan 300 v.
MVV v.
Newport v.
Newport E100M v.
noninvasive extrathoracic v. (NEV)
Ohio critical care v.
Pneumotron v.
pneuPAC v.

portable volume v.
positive support v. (PSV)
pressure v.
pressure cycled v.
Puritan Bennett v.
v. rate
Respironics BIPAP bilevel v.
Searle volume v.
Sechrist v.
Sechrist IV-100 infant v.
Siemens v.
Smart Trigger Bear 1000 v.
v. speaking valve
840 v. system
v. time
Uni-Vent v.
Venturi V.
Vix infant v.
volume v.
volume-cycled v.
Wave VM200 v.
v. weaning
ventilator-associated
v.-a. lung injury (VALI)
v.-a. pneumonia (VAP)
ventilator-induced
v.-i. lung injury (VILI)
v.-i. pneumopericardium
v.-i. pneumothorax
ventilatory
v. anaerobic threshold (VAT)
v. assistance
v. capacity
v. compliance
v. equivalent
v. failure
v. function
v. response
v. support
v. threshold
Venti mask
VentNet
NPB V.
Ventolin
V. Nebules
V. Rotacaps
V. updraft
VenTrak respiratory mechanics monitor
ventricle
anterior papillary muscle of left v.
atrialized v.
banana-shaped left v.

V

NOTES

ventricle *(continued)*
    calcified papillary muscle in the
      right v.
    double-inlet left v.
    double-outlet left v.
    double-outlet right v. (DORV)
    hypoplasia of right v.
    indeterminate single v.
    laryngeal v.
    left v. (LV)
    L-looping of the v.
    Mary Allen Engle v.
    noncompliant v.
    parchment right v.
    right v. (RV)
    single v.
    suicide v.
    volume-overloaded left v.

ventricular (V)
    v. aberration
    v. activation time (VAT)
    v. afterload
    v. aneurysm
    v. angiography
    v. apex
    v. arrhythmia
    v. assist device (VAD)
    v. asynchronous pacemaker
    v. atresia
    v. autocapture
    v. band of larynx
    bidirectional v.
    v. bigeminy
    v. biopsy
    v. block
    v. bradycardia
    v. canal
    v. capture
    v. captured beat
    v. capture threshold
    v. cavity
    v. complex
    v. conduction
    v. conduction velocity (VCV)
    v. contour
    v. contractile synchrony
    v. contractility
    v. contraction pattern
    v. couplet
    v. demand-inhibited pacemaker
    v. demand-triggered pacemaker
    v. depolarization abnormality
    v. diastole
    v. diastolic pressure
    v. dilation
    v. distensibility
    v. drive
    v. dysfunction

    v. dyssynergy
    v. echo
    v. ectopic beat (VEB)
    v. ectopic systole
    v. ectopy
    v. effective refractory period
      (VERP)
    v. end-diastolic volume
    v. endoaneurysmorrhaphy
    v. end-systolic pressure-volume
      relation
    v. end-systolic wall stress
    v. escape
    v. escape beat
    v. extrasystole
    v. failure
    v. far-field signal
    v. fibrillation (VF)
    v. fibrillation arrest
    v. filling
    v. filling pressure
    v. flutter
    v. function
    v. function curve
    v. fusion beat
    v. geometry
    v. gradient
    v. hypertrophy
    v. impedance
    v. implantable cardioverter-
      defibrillator (V-ICD)
    v. inflow anomaly
    v. inflow tract obstruction
    v. inhibited pulse generator
    v. inlet
    v. interdependence
    v. inversion
    v. late potential (VLP)
    v. lead
    v. ligament
    v. mapping
    v. mass
    v. milk spots
    v. mural swelling
    v. myxoma
    v. outflow tract obstruction
    v. pacing
    v. parasystole
    v. pause
    v. perforation
    v. performance
    v. plateau
    v. ponderance
    v. power
    v. preexcitation
    v. preload
    v. premature beat (VPB)
    v. premature complex (VPC)

v. premature contraction (VPC)
v. premature depolarization (VPD)
v. pressure-volume loop
v. pulse amplitude
v. pulse width
v. puncture
v. reduction surgery
v. reentry
v. relaxation
v. remodeling
v. reserve
v. response
v. rhythm
v. safety pacing
v. sensing configuration
v. sensitivity
v. septal defect (VSD)
v. septal defect murmur
v. septal defect vegetation
v. septal rupture
v. septum (VS)
v. situs solitus
v. standstill
v. stroke work index
v. synchronous pulse generator
v. systole
v. systolic impairment
v. systolic stiffness
v. tachyarrhythmia (VTA)
v. tachycardia (VT)
v. tachycardia cycle length (VTCL)
v. tachycardia/ventricular fibrillation (VT/VF)
v. thrombus
v. triggered pulse generator
v. vein
v. volume
v. wall contractility
v. wall motion
v. wall shortening
v. wall stress
v. wall thinning
v. wave

ventricularization
ventricular-programmed stimulation
ventriculoarterial
v. concordance
v. coupling
v. discordance
ventriculoatrial (V-A, VA)
v. conduction (VAC, V-AC)

v. effective refractory period
v. shunt catheter
ventriculocyte
ventriculogram-derived ejection fraction
ventriculographic ejection fraction
ventriculography
biplane v.
v. catheter
contrast left v.
equilibrium multigated
radionuclide v.
left v.
quantitative left v.
radionuclide v. (RNV)
rest-exercise equilibrium
radionuclide v.
tomographic radionuclide v.
ventriculophasic
ventriculopuncture
ventriculoradial dysplasia
ventriculorrhaphy
reed v.
ventriculoscopy
ventriculoseptal defect (VSD)
ventriculotomy
encircling endocardial v.
partial encircling endocardial v.
ventriculus laryngis
Ventritex
V. Angstrom MD implantable
cardioverter-defibrillator
V. Cadence device
V. Cadence ICD
V. Cadence implantable
cardioverter-defibrillator
V. Contour
V. TVL system
V. V100, v110 ICD generator
ventrolateral medulla (VLM)
Venture demand oxygen delivery device
Ventureyra ventricular catheter
Venturi
V. effect
V. Exhalation Assist
V. force
V. insufflator
V. jet adapter
V. mask
V. phenomenon
V. spirometer
V. tube
V. Ventilator

NOTES

Venturi *(continued)*
V. Venti-mask Mark 2
V. wave
venule
venulitis
cutaneous necrotizing v.
VePesid
V. injection
V. Oral
vera
polycythemia v.
verapamil
V. Angioplasty Study (VAS)
v. HCl
v. hydrochloride
V. Hypertension Atherosclerosis
Study
PPR v.
trandolapril and v.
verapamil-sensitive
veratridine
verbal amnesia
Verbatim balloon catheter
Vercyte
Verdia
Verelan
Verhoeff
V. elastica stain
V. tissue elastin stain
Veriflex
V. cardiac device
V. guidewire
vermicular pulse
verminous
v. aneurysm
v. bronchitis
Vermizine
Vermox
vernal edema of lung
Vernet syndrome
Verneuil canal
vernix
veronii
Aeromonas v.
VERP
ventricular effective refractory period
verruca, pl. **verrucae**
verrucosa
arteritis v.
Phialophora v.
verrucous
v. carcinoma
v. carditis
v. endocarditis
v. vegetation
verruga peruana
Versacaps
Versatrax II 7000A pacemaker

Versed
versicolor
Aspergillus v.
Verstraeten bruit
vertebral
v. artery bypass graft
v. defects, imperforate anus,
transesophageal fistula, and radial
and renal dysplasia (VATER)
v. endarterectomy
v. part of the costal surface of
the lung
v. part of diaphragm
vertebral, vascular, anal, cardiac,
tracheoesophageal, renal, and limb
anomalies (VACTERL)
vertebrobasilar
v. occlusive disease
v. territory ischemia (VBI)
v. TIA
vertebrocostal trigone
vertical
v. deceleration
v. deceleration mechanism
v. heart
v. integration
v. long axis
v. long-axis tomogram
v. long-axis view
v. VAS
vertigo
laryngeal v.
rotary v.
very-low-density lipoprotein (VLDL)
vesicle
air v.
intermediary v.
malpighian v.
vesicular
v. breath sounds
v. bronchiolitis
v. bronchitis
v. emphysema
v. fluid
v. murmur
v. rale
vesiculobronchial
vesiculobullous
vesiculocavernous respiration
vesnarinone
V. Survival Trial (VEST)
Vesprin
vessel
absorbent v.
aortic arch v.
bouquet of v.'s
capacitance v.
v. clamp

codominant v.
collateral v.
collateralizing v. (CV)
conductance v.
coronary resistance v.
corrected transposition of the
   great v.
v. dilator
feeder v.
femoral v.
ghost v.
great v.
infarct-related v.
intercostal mammary v.
internal mammary v.
intramyocardial prearteriolar v.
v. lumen
native v.
nondominant v.
v. occlusion system
omphalomesenteric v.
proximal and distal portion of v.
recruitable collateral v.
renal blood v.
resistance v.
retinal v.
v. spasm
splanchnic v.
subclavian v.
target v.
thoracic v.
tortuous v.
transposition of the great v.
v. trauma
v. wall movement
Wallstent in Native V.'s
Vessel-Clude
Vesseloops rubber band
Vesselpaw
vessel-sizing catheter
VEST
Vesnarinone Survival Trial
VEST left ventricular function
   detector
vest
v. ambulatory nuclear detector
v. ambulatory ventricular function
   monitor
Bremer AirFlo V.
cardiac v.
Mark VII cooling v.
ThAIRapy v.

vestibular
v. fold
v. laryngitis
v. ligament
vestibule
esophagogastric v.
gastroesophageal v.
v. of larynx
Sibson v.
vestibuli
rima v.
sacculus v.
vestibulum laryngis
vestigial fold
Veterans
V. Administration (VA)
V. Administration Heart Failure
   Trial (V-HeFT)
V. Administration Heart Failure
   Trial II (V-HeFT II)
V. Administration High-Density
   Lipoprotein Intervention Trial
   (VA-HIT)
V. Affairs Medical Center
   (VAMC)
V. Affairs Medical Center scoring
   system
V. Affairs Non-Q-Wave Infarction
   Strategies in Hospital
   (VANQWISH)
V. Health Study (VHS)
VE/VCO$_2$
ventilation/carbon dioxide production
VEX treadmill test
VF
ventricular fibrillation
R-on-T-initiated VF
VFC
venous flow controller
Actis VFC
V-Flex
V.-F. FMJ stent
V.-F. Plus stent
V-Gan injection
VHC
valved holding chamber
AeroChamber VHC
VHD
vascular hemostatic device
VasoSeal VHD

V

NOTES

V-HeFT
Veterans Administration Heart Failure Trial
V-HeFT II
Vasodilator Heart Failure Trial II
Veterans Administration Heart Failure Trial II
Vhigh
high regional wall motion velocity
V-H interval
VHS
Veterans Health Study
viability
v. index
myocardial v.
viable myocardium
Viagra
Viagraph ECG system
vial
Viamonte-Hobbs dye injector
Vibracare percussor
Vibramycin
V. injection
V. Oral
vibrans
pulsus v.
Vibra-Tabs
vibration
chest percussion and v.
v. disease
postural drainage, percussion and v. (PDPV)
vibrational angioplasty
Vibrio
V. cholerae
V. parahaemolyticus
vibrissa, pl. **vibrissae**
nasal v.
vibrocardiogram
vicarious respiration
V-ICD
ventricular implantable cardioverter-defibrillator
Vicia
V. sativa
V. sativa asthma
Vickers Ventimask Mark 2 mask
Vicks
V. DayQuil Sinus Pressure & Congestion Relief
V. 44D Cough & Head Congestion
V. 44E
V. Formula 44
V. Formula 44 Pediatric Formula
V. 44 Non-Drowsy Cold & Cough Liqui-Caps
V. Pediatric Formula 44E

Vicodin
Victoria influenza
video
v. camera
v. densitometry
v. imaging
v. loop
v. monitor
v. system
videoangiography
digital v.
video-assisted
v.-a. diagnostic thoracoscopic technique
v.-a. thoracic surgery (VATS)
v.-a. thoracic surgical lung biopsy
v.-a. thoracic surgical non-rib-spreading lobectomy (VNSSL)
v.-a. thoracoscopic surgery (VATS)
v.-a. thoracoscopic thymectomy
v.-a. thoracoscopy (VAT, VATS)
videobronchoscope
videodensitometric
v. analysis system
v. myocardial textural analysis
videodensitometry
videohydrothoracoscope
Circon v.
videointensity
videomorphometry
videotape recorder
videothoracoscopic pericardial window
videothoracoscopy
Videx Oral
Vienna
V. TAH
V. total artificial heart
Vieussens
circle of V.
valve of V.
V. valve
view
apical four-chamber v.
apical two-chamber v.
Baltaxe v.
caudocranial hemiaxial v.
cine v.
coned-down v.
craniocaudal v.
en face v.
expiratory v.
field of v. (FOV)
first pass v.
five-chamber v.
four-chamber v.
gated v.
hemiaxial v.
horizontal long-axis v.

ice-pick v.
inspiratory v.
laid-back v.
lateral v.
long axial oblique v.
long-axis v.
orthogonal v.
parasternal v.
parasternal long-axis v.
parasternal short-axis v.
RAO v.
resting parasternal long-axis v.
resting parasternal short-axis v.
sagittal v.
scout v.
short-axis parasternal v.
sitting-up v.
spider x-ray v.
subcostal v.
suprasternal v.
swimmer's v.
two-chamber v.
vertical long-axis v.
weeping willow v.
view-aliasing artifact
Viggo Spectramed catheter
Vigilance monitoring system
vigilance response
Vigilon dressing
Vigor
V. DDDR pacemaker
V. DR pacemaker
V. pacemaker
Viking Bard catheter
VILI
ventilator-induced lung injury
Villaret syndrome
villi
pleural v.
v. pleurales
villosa
pericarditis v.
villosum
cor v.
Vim-Silverman needle
vinblastine sulfate
Vincasar
V. PFS
V. PFS injection
Vincent angina

vincristine
cyclophosphamide, doxorubicin, v. (CAV)
v. sulfate
vinculum linguae
vindesine
v., cisplatin, lomustine, cyclophosphamide (VCPC)
Vineberg cardiac revacularization procedure
Vingmed
V. CFM-700
V. CFM 800 echocardiographic system
V. CFM 750 transducer
vinorelbine tartrate
vinyl chloride
Vinyon-N cloth tube
viomycin
Viozan
VIP
vasoactive intestinal peptide
V.I.P. Bird volume monitor
Viper PTA catheter
Viprinex
Viracept
viral
v. bronchiolitis
v. capsid antigen (VCA)
v. cardiomyopathy
v. hepatitis
v. myocarditis
v. pericarditis
v. pneumonia
v. respiratory infection
v. vector
Viramune
Virazole Aerosol
Virchow
V.-Robin space
V. triad
Virgo anticardiolipin screening ELISA test kit
viridans
Aerococcus v.
v. endocarditis
Streptococcus v.
viridis
Thermoactinomyces v.
Virilon
Viringe vascular access flush device

NOTES

Virtis blender
virtual bronchoscopy (VB)
Virtuoso
    V. LX Smart CPAP system
    V. Smart CPAP system
virulence
virus
    adeno-associated v. (AAV)
    Amapari v.
    Andes v.
    Arenaviridae v.
    Astroviridae v.
    Bayou v.
    Black Creek Canal v.
    v. bronchopneumonia
    CA v.
    Calciviridae v.
    Coe v.
    Columbia S.K. v.
    Coronaviridae v.
    coxsackie A, B, B3, B4 v.
    Ebola v.
    ECHO v.
    EMC v.
    encephalomyocarditis v.
    enteric cytopathogenic human
      orphan v.
    Epstein-Barr v. (EBV)
    Filoviridae v.
    Hantaan v.
    herpes simplex v. (HSV)
    human immunodeficiency v. (HIV)
    human T-cell lymphotropic v.
      (HTLV)
    Juquitiba v.
    Kotonkan v.
    Laguna Negra v.
    Lassa v.
    Lipovnik v.
    Marburg v.
    Mayaro v.
    Moloney murine leukemia v.
    Muerto Canyon v.
    Orthomyxoviridae v.
    parainfluenza v.
    Paramyxoviridae v.
    Picornaviridae v.
    REO v.
    respiratory syncytial v. (RSV)
    Rift Valley fever v.
    Ross River v.
    Rous sarcoma v. (RSV)
    Semliki Forest v.
    Sendai v.
    Sindbis v.
    Sin Nombre v. (SNV)
    syncytial v.
    Togaviridae v.

    U v.
    varicella-zoster v. (VZV)
Visa
    V. Iris system
    V. II PTCA catheter
    V. ST balloon catheter
    V. II ST PTCA balloon catheter
viscera (*pl. of* viscus)
visceral
    v. heterotaxy
    v. larva migrans
    v. peel
    v. pericardiectomy
    v. pericardium
    v. pleura
    v. pleurisy
    v. syncope
visceralis
    pleura v.
visceroatrial
    v. situs
    v. situs solitus
viscerobronchial cardiovascular anomaly
viscerocardiac reflex
visceropleural
viscid mucus
viscidosis
viscoelastic
    v. fluid
viscoelasticity
    sputum v.
viscometer
    Brookfield v.
    Ostwald v.
viscosity
    blood v.
    mucus v.
viscous
viscus, pl. viscera
    hollow v.
vise
    hemodynamic v.
    torque v.
Visicath endoscope
Vision PTCA catheter
Visipaque
Visken
Visov test
VISP
    Vitamin Intervention for Stroke
    Prevention
Vistacon-50 Injection
Vistaquel Injection
Vistaril
    V. Injection
    V. Oral
VISTA software
Vista 4, T, TRS pacemaker

Vistazine Injection
Vistide
visual
    v. amnesia
    v. analog scale (VAS)
visualization
    far-field v.
    fluoroscopic v.
    near-field v.
    suboptimal v.
visualized
    suboptimally v.
visually evoked flow response (VEFR)
visuospatial neglect
Vitacuff
Vitagraft
    V. arteriovenous shunt
    V. vascular graft
vital
    v. capacity (VC)
    v. exhaustion
VitalCare
    V. 506DX monitor
    V. 506DX monitor series
Vital-Cooley microvascular needle holder
Vitallium
Vitalograph
    V. Bacterial/Viral Filter
    V. BreathCO Monitor
    V. 2120 handheld recording
    spirometer
    V. pulmonary monitor
    V. spirometer
vitalography
Vitalometer test
Vitalor
    V. incentive spirometer
    V. screening pulmonary function
    test
Vital-Ryder microvascular needle holder
vitals
vitamin
    v. B, B_1, B_6, B_{12}, C, D, E, K
    V. Intervention for Stroke
    Prevention (VISP)
    v. K antagonist
    V.'s to Prevent Stroke
    (VITATOPS)
    Study to Evaluate Carotid
    Ultrasound Changes with Ramipril
    and V. E (SECURE)

Vita-Stat automatic device
VITATOPS
    Vitamins to Prevent Stroke
    VITATOPS clinical trial
Vitatron
    V. catheter electrode
    V. Diamond ICD
    V. Diamond II pacemaker
    V. Diamond pacemaker
    V. lead
    V. pacing system
vitelline vein
vitellogenin
Vitesse
    V. catheter
    V. C catheter
    V. Cos laser catheter
    V. E catheter
    V. E2 rapid-exchange catheter
    V. PrimaFx catheter
vitiated air
vitiligo
    symmetric v.
Vitrasert
Vitravene
vitrector
    catheter v.
vitreous opacity
vitro
    in v.
vitronectin
Viva
    Air V.
    V. Primo balloon catheter
Vivactil
Vivalan
Vivalith II pulse generator
vivax
    Plasmodium v.
vivo
    ex v.
    in v.
Vivonex
    V. Moss tube
    V. Plus nutritional supplement
Vix infant ventilator
VixOne small-volume nebulizer
VK
VLDL
    very-low-density lipoprotein
VLM
    ventrolateral medulla

V

NOTES

VLP
ventricular late potential
VM200
Newport Wave V.
VMap dynamic flow-based image
Vmax
VMR
vasomotor response
V. Mueller catheter
VNSSL
video-assisted thoracic surgical non-rib-
spreading lobectomy
VNUS
V. Closure catheter/radiofrequency
generator
V. Closure System
VO₂
aerobic capacity
oxygen consumption
oxygen consumption per minute
peak exercise oxygen consumption
volume oxygen consumption
VO_2 max
peak VO_2
vocal
v. cord
v. cord dysfunction (VCD)
v. fremitus
v. process
vocalis
chorda v.
rima v.
vocational rehabilitation
Voda catheter
Vogt-Koyanagi-Harada syndrome
voice
amphoric v.
cavernous v.
double v.
eunuchoid v.
hot potato v.
voix de polichinelle
Volkmann ischemic paralysis
Vollmer test
Volmax
volt
electron v. (eV)
kiloelectron v. (keV)
megaelectron v. (MeV)
voltage
battery v.
Cornell v.
v. criteria
v. equilibrium
Gubner-Ungerleider v.
pacemaker output v.
root-mean-square v.

Sokolow-Lyon v.
transmembrane v.
voltage-dependent
v.-d. block
v.-d. calcium channel
voltage-gated channel
voltage-sensitive calcium channel
(VSCC)
volume (V)
alveolar v. (VA)
blood v.
cardiac v.
cerebral red blood cell v. (CRCV)
circulation v.
closing v.
compressible v.
conductance stroke v.
consolidated lung v.
v. contraction
v. control (VC)
v. controller
v. depletion
v. of distribution
v. of distribution effect
dP/dt_{MAX} end-diastolic v.
effective circulating blood v.
(ECBV)
effort-independent lung v.
elastic equilibrium v. (EEV)
end-diastolic v. (EDV)
end-expiratory lung v. (EELV)
end-inspiratory lung v. (EILV)
end-systolic v. (ESV)
v. expansion
expectorated sputum v.
expiratory reserve v. (ERV)
forced expiratory v. (FEV)
forward stroke v. (FSV)
frequency to tidal v. (f/V_t)
v. heating
high lung v.
v. infusion
inspiratory reserve v. (IRV)
intravascular v.
left ventricular end-diastolic v.
(LVEDV)
left ventricular stroke v.
v. load hypertrophy
v. loading
v. loss
lung v.
mandatory minute v. (MMV)
maximal expiratory flow v.
(MEFV)
mean corpuscular v. (MCV)
minute v.
v. overload
v. oxygen consumption (VO_2)

planimetry v.
plaque v.
plasma v.
presystolic pressure and v.
pulmonary blood v. (PBV)
pulmonary capillary blood v. (Vc)
ratio of tidal expiratory and inspiratory flow at 50% of tidal v. (TEF$_{50}$/TIF$_{50}$)
regurgitant v. (RVol)
relative cardiac v.
residual v. (RV)
respiratory minute v.
resting stroke v.
resting tidal v.
v. resuscitation
Simpson rule for ventricular v.
sputum v.
static lung v.
v. stiffness
stroke v. (SV)
v. thickness index (VTI)
thoracic gas v. (TGV, V$_{TG}$)
tidal v. (TV, V$_T$)
tidal expiratory v. (TV$_E$)
tidal expiratory flow at 25% of tidal v. (TEF$_{25}$)
tidal expiratory flow at 50% of tidal v. (TEF$_{50}$)
tidal expiratory flow at 75% of tidal v. (TEF$_{75}$)
tidal inspiratory v. (TV$_I$)
tidal inspiratory flow at 50% of tidal v. (TIF$_{50}$)
timed forced expiratory v.
total blood v. (TBV)
trapped gas v.
urine v.
v. ventilator
ventricular v.
ventricular end-diastolic v.
volume to peak expiratory flow and total expiratory v. (VPTEF/VT)
volume-assured pressure support (VAPS)
volume-challenge test
volume-controlled
v.-c. respirator
v.-c. ventilation (VCV)

volume-cycled
v.-c. decelerating-flow ventilation (VCDF)
v.-c. ventilator
volume-displacement
v.-d. plethysmograph
v.-d. spirometer
volume-overloaded left ventricle
Volumeter
Dräger V.
volume-time curve
volumetric
v. capnogram
v. diffusive respirator (VDR)
v. infusion pump
v. lung depth (Vp)
volutrauma
volvulus
Onchocerca v.
von
v. Claus chronometric method
v. Recklinghausen disease
v. Recklinghausen test
v. Reyn criteria
v. Willebrand disease
v. Willebrand protein (vWP)
Von Lackum surcingle
VOO
V. pacemaker
V. pacing
voodoo death
Voorhees bag
voriconazole
Vorse-Webster clamp
vortex
v. cordis
v. effect catheter
v. flow
V. stabilization system
VOTE
Value of Transesophageal Echocardiography
VOTE clinical trial
voxel gray scale
Voyager Aortic IntraClusion device
Vp
volumetric lung depth
V-Pace transluminal pacing lead
VPAP
variable positive airway pressure
VPAP II ST-A bilevel flow generator

NOTES

VPAP *(continued)*
> VPAP II ST Ventilatory Support system

VPB
> ventricular premature beat

VPC
> ventricular premature complex
> ventricular premature contraction

VPD
> ventricular premature depolarization

VPF
> vascular permeability factor

VPI
> vasopeptidase inhibitor

VPTEF/VT
> volume to peak expiratory flow and total expiratory volume

$\dot{V}/\dot{Q}$
> ventilation/perfusion
> > $\dot{V}/\dot{Q}$ defect
> > $\dot{V}/\dot{Q}$ lung scan
> > $\dot{V}/\dot{Q}$ mismatch
> > $\dot{V}/\dot{Q}$ quotient

VR
> valve replacement
> velocity ratio

Vroman effect

VS
> Valsalva maneuver
> ventricular septum

VSA
> vasospastic angina

VSCC
> voltage-sensitive calcium channel

VSD
> ventricular septal defect
> ventriculoseptal defect
> > Eisenmenger VSD
> > pinhole VSD

V-slope method

VSMC
> vascular smooth muscle cell

Vsys
> systolic wall motion velocity

VT
> ventricular tachycardia
> > VT Mercury Vac organic mercury vacuum cleaner
> > VT 1000 neonatal workstation
> > R-on-T-initiated VT
> > R-on-T-initiated nonsustained VT

VTA
> ventricular tachyarrhythmia

VTCL
> ventricular tachycardia cycle length

VTE
> venous thromboembolism

VTI
> volume thickness index
> > VTI Oxygen Monitor with Disposable Polarographic Oxygen Sensor

VT/VF
> ventricular tachycardia/ventricular fibrillation

Vueport balloon-occlusion guiding catheter

vulgaris
> *Proteus v.*
> *Thermoactinomyces v.*

vulnerable
> v. myocardium
> v. period
> v. phase

Vumon injection

V_{DS}/V_T
> dead-space gas volume to tidal gas volume ratio

V_D/V_T
> physiologic dead space ventilation

V-Vac suction apparatus

VVD mode pacemaker

VVI
> V. pacemaker
> V. pacing

VVIR
> V. pacemaker
> V. pacing

VVI-RR pacing

VVI/VVIR pacing

V1/V6 leads

VVT
> V. mode
> V. pacing

vWP
> von Willebrand protein

VZ
> varicella zoster

VZIG
> varicella-zoster immunoglobulin

VZV
> varicella-zoster virus

W

W pattern
W pattern on right atrial waveform
W wave on echocardiogram
Waardenburg syndrome
Wada

W. hingeless heart valve prosthesis
W. test
wadsworthensis

Sutterella w.
wadsworthii

Legionella w.
wafer

Coloplast w.
waist

cardiac w.
w. of catheter
w. of heart
w./hip ratio for upper body obesity
hypertriglyceridemic w.
waisting of balloon
waist-to-hip ratio (WHR)
wake after sleep onset time (WASO)
Waldenström macroglobulinemia
Waldeyer

W. throat ring
W. tonsillar ring
Waldhausen subclavian flap technique
WALK

Walking with Angina-Learning is Key
WALK program
walk

shuttle test w.
w.-through angina
Walkabout oxygen conserver
Walker-Murdoch wrist sign
walking

nocturnal w.
w. pneumonia
w. ventilation test
Walking with Angina-Learning is Key (WALK)
wall

w. amplitude
anterior w. (AW)
anterobasal w.
chest w.
free w.
friable w.
inferobasal w.
lateral w. (LW)
left ventricular w.
w. motion
w. motion abnormality (WMA)
w. motion analysis

w. motion index (WMI)
w. motion score
w. motion score index (WMSI)
w. motion study
w. motion velocity
posterior w. (PW)
posteroseptal w.
preejectional left ventricular w.
w. stress
w. structure
subacute ventricular free w.
w. tension
w. thickening
w. thickness
w. tracking
w. tracking system
Wallace Flexihub central venous pressure cannula
Wallenberg syndrome
Wallerian degeneration (WD)
Wallgraft endoprosthesis
Wallstent

W. flexible, self-expanding wire-mesh stent
Magic W.
W. Magic stent
W. in Native Vessels
Schneider W.
W. spring-loaded stent
Walter Reed classification
Walther canals
wand

ReFlex ENT W.
wandering

w. atrial pacemaker (WAP)
w. baseline
w. goiter
w. heart
w. pacemaker
w. pneumonia
Wangiella
Wang transbronchial needle
waning

waxing and w.
WAP

wandering atrial pacemaker
ward

general w. (GW)
Ward-Romano syndrome
Wardrop method
warfarin

W.-Aspirin Symptomatic Intracranial Disease (WASID)
w. sodium
w. therapy

W

Warfilone
warm
>w. heparinized saline flush
>w. nodule

warmer
>blood w.

warm-up phenomenon
warning arrhythmia
Warthin-Starry-staining bacillus
wash
>w. bath
>ENT w.
>nasopharyngeal w.

washings
>bronchial w.
>bronchoalveolar w.
>bronchopulmonary w.
>w. and brushings
>lung w.

Washington
>W. Radiation for In-Stent Restenosis Trial (WRIST)
>W. Radiation for In-Stent Restenosis Trial for Long Lesions (LONG WRIST)

washout
>w. cannula
>helium w.
>w. phase
>w. phenomenon
>thallium w.

WASID
>Warfarin-Aspirin Symptomatic Intracranial Disease
>WASID study

WASO
>wake after sleep onset time

Wasserman
>W. needle
>W. number
>W.-positive pulmonary infiltrate

wasted ventilation
wasting
>potassium w.
>salt w.
>w. syndrome

WAT
>word association test

watch-crystal fingernail
water
>w. brash
>w. channel
>w. column resistor
>extravascular lung w. (EVLW)
>feet of sea w. (fsw)
>w. hammer pulse
>w. lily sign

>w. retention
>w. wheel murmur

water-bottle heart
waterfall effect
water-gurgle test
Waterman bronchoscope
water-seal
>w.-s. chest tube
>w.-s. drainage

water-sealed spirometer
watershed
>w. infarct
>w. infarction
>w. pattern
>w. region

Waterston
>W. anastomosis
>W.-Cooley procedure
>W. extrapericardial anastomosis
>W. groove
>W. operation
>W. shunt

watertight seal
waterwheel sound
Watson
>W. heart valve holder
>W. syndrome

watt-second
wave
>A w.
>a w.
>w. amplitude
>arterial w.
>atrial repolarization w.
>bifid P w.
>blast w.
>brain w.
>C w.
>cannon w.
>catacrotic w.
>catadicrotic w.
>w. coronary event
>c-v systolic w.
>D w.
>deep pathologic Q w.
>delta w.
>dicrotic w.
>diphasic P w.
>diphasic T w.
>duration of ECG w.
>duration of P w.
>E w.
>electrocardiographic w.
>epsilon w.
>E wave to A w. (E/A, E:A)
>excitation w.
>F w.
>f w.

fibrillary w.
fibrillatory w.
flipped T w.
flutter w.
flutter-fibrillation w.'s
w. form
giant a w.
giant T w.
giant v w.
H w.
h w.
hyperacute T w.
inverted T w.
isolated T w.
J w.
Mayer w.
Minnesota criteria for high R w.
negative T w.
negative U w.
normalization of inverted T w.
Osborne w.
overflow w.
P w.
peaked P w.
percussion w.
peristaltic w.
polymorphic slow w.
posterior Q w.
postextrasystolic T w.
precordial A w.
pressure w.
propagation of R w.
pseudonormalization of T w.
pseudo R′ w.
pseudo S w.
pulse w.
pulsed w. (PW)
Q w.
QS w.
R w.
rapid filling w.
recoil w.
regurgitant w.
retrograde P w.
RF w.
S w.
sawtooth w.
sawtooth P w.
scroll reentrant w.
seismic w.
shallow pathologic Q w.
sine w.

small P w.
w. spike
spiral reentrant w.
ST w.
ST-T w.
systolic reflection w.
T w.
tall T w.
tidal w.
TU w.
U w.
upright T w.
V w.
venous Corrigan w.
ventricular w.
Venturi w.
x w.
x descent of the a w.
y w.
y descent w.

waveform
A-wave spectral velocity w.
biphasic w.
blunted w.
CO_2 w.
dampened w.
displacement w.
distention w.
Edmark monophasic w.
E-wave spectral velocity w.
forward pressure w.
Gurvich biphasic w.
incident pressure w.
Lown-Edmark w.
monophasic w.
nonsinusoidal w.
pressure w.
quasisinusoidal biphasic w.
rectilinear biphasic w.
reentry w.
reflected pressure w.
shock w.
spectral w.
W pattern on right atrial w.
wavelength (WL)
w. of reentry
WaveMap intracoronary blood pressure measurement system
waveshape
wave-speed mechanism
Wave VM200 ventilator

W

NOTES

WaveWire intracoronary blood pressure measurement system
wavy
    w. fiber
    w. respiration
waxing
    w. and waning
    w. and waning chest pain
    w. and waning in intensity
wax-matrix technique
4-Way Long Acting Nasal Solution
w/C
    Aprodine w/C
WCD
    wearable cardioverter-defibrillator
w/Codeine
    Allerfrin w.
    Bromphen DC w.
WD
    Wallerian degeneration
w/DM
    Pherazine w/DM
weakness
wean
weaning
    w. index (WI)
    w. protocol
    terminal w.
    T-piece w.
    ventilator w.
wearable
    w. cardioverter-defibrillator (WCD)
    w. cardioverter-defibrillator device
wear-and-tear lesion
Weavenit
    W. patch graft
    W. prosthesis
web
    esophageal w.
    laryngeal w.
    pulmonary arterial w.
    venous w.
Weber-Christian disease
Weber experiment
Weber-Janicki cardiopulmonary exercise protocol
Weber-Osler-Rendu syndrome
web-spacer
    C-bar w.-s.
Webster
    Biosense W.
    W. halo catheter
    W. orthogonal electrode catheter
Wedensky
    W. effect
    W. modulated signal-averaged electrocardiogram

wedge
    w. angiogram
    arterial w.
    ball w.
    w. biopsy
    w. excision
    mediastinal w.
    w. pressure
    w. pressure balloon catheter
    w. pulmonary angiography
    pulmonary artery w. (PAW)
    pulmonary capillary w. (PCW)
    w. spirometer
Weeks bacillus
weeping
    w. dermatitis
    w. willow view
weeping fig asthma
Wegener
    W. granulomatosis (WG)
    W. nodule
Weibel-Palade bodies
Weigert-van Gieson stain
weighted ball resistor
Weil disease
Weil-Felix reaction
Weill sign
Weinberg test
Weir method
Weiss logarithmic method
Welch
    W. Allyn Pneumocheck spirometer
    W. Allyn/Shiller AT-10 Exercise Testing system
    W. Allyn/Shiller AT-2 full-size ECG
    W. Allyn/Shiller AT-10 hospital grade ECG
    W. Allyn/Shiller AT-2*plus* full-size ECG
    W. Allyn/Shiller AT-1 three channel ECG
    W. Allyn/Shiller MS-3 pocket size ECG
    W. Allyn/Shiller SP-1 budget spirometry
    W. Allyn/Shiller SP-10 diagnostic spirometry
WelChol
Welcker method
welder's
    w. lung
    w. siderosis
welding
    spot w.
well
    pericardial w.
well-differentiated carcinoma

Wenckebach
- W. atrioventricular block
- W. A-V block
- W. block
- W. cycle
- W. cycle length
- W. disease
- W. exit block
- W. period
- W. periodicity
- W. periodicity block
- W. phenomenon
- W. sign

Werlhof disease
Werner syndrome
Wernicke aphasia
Wesolowski vascular prosthesis
Wessex prosthetic valve
WEST
- Women's Estrogen for Stroke Trial

West
- W. syndrome
- zone 1, 2, 3, 4 of W.

Westberg space
Westergren
- W. erythrocyte sedimentation rate
- W. method

westermani
- *Paragonimus w.*

Westermark sign
Western
- W. blot
- W. red cedar

Westminster drug-free protocol
Westrim LA
wet
- w. beriberi
- w. cough
- w. lung
- w. nebulization
- w. pleurisy
- w. rale
- w. swallow

wet-to-dry dressing
Wexler catheter
WG
- Wegener granulomatosis

wheal and flare
Wheatstone bridge
wheat weevil disease

wheeze
- asthmoid w.
- monophonic w.

wheezers
wheezing
- bronchial w.
- expiratory w.

wheezy bronchitis
WHI
- Women's Health Initiative

whiff test
whip
- catheter w.

whipping
- systolic w.

Whipple disease
whippleii
- *Tropherema w.*

whisker plot
whispered
- w. bronchophony
- w. pectoriloquy

whispering
- w. pectoriloquy
- w. resonance

Whisper Mist humidifier
whistle
- coaching w.

whistling rale
white
- w. asphyxia
- w. blood cell count
- w. clot syndrome
- w. coronary thrombus
- w. lung
- w. matter (WM)
- w. matter hyperintensity (WMHI)
- w. matter signal abnormality (WMA)
- w. plaque
- w. pneumonia
- w. spot
- w. sputum
- w. thrombus

white-coat
- w.-c. angina
- w.-c. hypertension

White system
Whitfield ointment
WHO
- World Health Organization

W

NOTES

whole
> w. blood buffer base
> w. blood cardioplegia

whole-body
> w.-b. amyloid load
> w.-b. hyperthermia

whole-grain food

Wholey
> W. Hi-Torque Floppy guidewire
> W. Hi-Torque modified J guidewire
> W. Hi-Torque standard guidewire
> W. wire

whoop
> systolic w.

whooping
> w. cough
> w. murmur

whorling of myocardial cell

whorl motion

WHR
> waist-to-hip ratio

WHS
> Women's Health Study

WI
> weaning index

Wichmann asthma

Wickwitz esophageal stricture

Widal test

wide
> w. complex rhythm
> w. QRS tachycardia

widely split second sound

wide-necked aneurysm

widened
> mediastinal w.

widening
> luminal w.
> mediastinal w.
> w. of pulse pressure

Wideroe test

width
> atrial pulse w.
> pulse w.
> ventricular pulse w.

Wiener filter

Wigle scale

Wigraine

Wiktor
> W. balloon expandable coronary stent
> W. coronary stent
> W. GX coronary stent
> W. GX Hepamed coated coronary stent system
> W. GX Hepamed coronary stent system
> W. GX stent

> W. Prime coronary stent system
> W. stent

Wiktor-I
> W.-I implantable stent
> W.-I stent

Wilhelmy balance

Wilkie disease

Wilkins echocardiographic score

Wilks lambda criterion

Wilks-Schapiro test

Willett-Stampfer method

William
> W. Harvey arterial blood filter
> W. Harvey cardiotomy reservoir
> W. test

Williams
> W.-Campbell syndrome
> W. cardiac device
> W. Doors test
> W. phenomenon
> W. sign
> W. syndrome
> W. tracheal tone

Williamson sign

Willis
> circle of W. (CW)

Willock respiratory jacket

Wilms thoracoplasty

Wilson
> W. block
> W. central terminal
> W.-Cook papillotome
> W. disease
> W.-Kimmelstiel disease
> W. lead
> W.-Mikity syndrome
> W.-White method

Wilton
> W. Webster coronary sinus thermodilution catheter
> W. Webster thermodilution flow and pacing catheter

WinABP ambulatory blood pressure monitor

windkessel
> w. effect
> w. model

window
> acoustic w.
> aortic w.
> aorticopulmonary w.
> aortopulmonary w. (APW)
> Blackman w.
> cycle-length w.
> Hanning w.
> imaging w.
> lateral frontal bone w. (LFBW)

paramedian frontal bone w.
 (PMFBW)
parasternal w.
Parzen w.
pericardial w.
pleuropericardial w.
pulmonary parenchymal w.
subxiphoid w.
tachycardia w.
transthoracic acoustic w.
videothoracoscopic pericardial w.
windowed balloon
windpipe
windsock
 w. aneurysm
 w. morphology
 w. sign
winged baseplate
Winiwarter-Buerger disease
Winpred
WINS
 Women's Intervention Nutrition Study
Winslow test
Winstrol
winter
 w. bronchitis
 w. cough
 w. vomiting disease
Wintrich sign
Wintrobe sedimentation rate
wire (*See also* guidewire)
 ACS microglide w.
 Amplatz torque w.
 atrial pacing w.
 auger w.
 Babcock stainless steel suture w.
 biventricular pacing w.
 catheter-guide w.
 central core w.
 Choice PT plus w.
 Commander angiopolasty guide w.
 control w.
 Cordis Stabilizer marker w.
 coronary w.
 Cragg Convertible w.
 Cragg FX w.
 Cragg infusion w.
 crenulated tantalum w.
 curved J-exchange w.
 delivery w.
 dock w.
 docking w.

Doppler velocity w.
Eder-Puestow w.
endocardial w.
extraflexible w.
flow w.
w. guide
w.-guided oval intracostal dilator
Hancock temporary cardiac
 pacing w.
Hi-Per Flex exchange w.
w. holder
w. insertion
intracoronary Doppler flow w.
J w.
J exchange w.
J retention w.
Katzen infusion w.
Killip w.
Linx extension w.
w.-loop lesion
magnet w.
Medi-Tech w.
w. mesh self-expandable stent
olive-tipped Magnum w.
platinum w.
Pressure Guide pressure w.
pusher w.
Radifocus w.
RadiMedical fiberoptic pressure-
 monitoring w.
Rotablator w.
Rotafloppy w.
Sadowsky hook w.
Stertzer-Myler extension w.
w. stylet
tip-deflecting w.
Wholey w.
w.-wound endotracheal tube
wiring
 copper w.
 sternal w.
 w. of sternum
Wirsung dilation
wiry
 w. pulse
Wiskott-Aldrich syndrome
7200 with 7250 metabolic monitor
Wizard
 W. cardiac device
 W. disposable inflation device
Wizdom guidewire

NOTES

W

WL
wavelength
WM
white matter
WMA
wall motion abnormality
white matter signal abnormality
Wmax
peak work rate
WMFT
Wolf Motor Function Test
WMHI
white matter hyperintensity
WMI
wall motion index
WMSI
wall motion score index
WOB
work of breathing
Wolff-Parkinson-White (WPW)
W.-P.-W. bypass tract
W.-P.-W. reentrant tachycardia
W.-P.-W. syndrome
Wolfina
Wolf Motor Function Test (WMFT)
Wolman disease
Wolvek
W. sternal approximation fixation
instrument
W. sternal approximator
Womack procedure
Women's
W. Estrogen for Stroke Trial
(WEST)
W. Health Initiative (WHI)
W. Health Study (WHS)
W. Intervention Nutrition Study
(WINS)
Wood
W. classification
W. lamp
W. unit
W. units index
wood
w. pulp worker's lung
w. pulp worker's lung disease
w. smoke
wooden resonance
wooden-shoe heart
**Woods-Downes-Lecks clinical asthma
score**
Woodworth phenomenon
woody
w. edema
w. thyroiditis
Wooler-type annuloplasty
woolsorter's pneumonia
word association test (WAT)

work
w. of breathing (WOB)
w. capacity
w. effect
w. rate
w. rate increment
w. rehabilitation
w. status
stroke w.
w. threshold
work-aggravated asthma
**Workhorse percutaneous transluminal
angioplasty balloon catheter**
workload
peak w.
workplace exposure
work-related
w.-r. asthma
w.-r. bronchial hyperreactivity
worksite challenge test
workstation
Sun Microsystems Sparcstation
20 w.
VT 1000 neonatal w.
World
W. Health Organization (WHO)
Worldpass
W. delivery system
W. radid exchange SDS
wound
blowing w.
bullet w.
entrance w.
exit w.
gunshot w.
knife w.
stab w.
sucking w.
woven
w. coronary artery disease
w. Dacron catheter
w. Dacron fabric graft
w. Dacron tube graft
w. Teflon
w. Teflon prosthesis
w.-tube vascular graft prosthesis
WPW
Wolff-Parkinson-White
wrap
cardiac muscle w.
no-phase w.
omental w.
wrap-around ghosting artifact
wrapping
w. of abdominal aortic aneurysm
aneurysm w.
wrecking ball effect

Wright
    W. & Haloscale respirometer
    W. peak flow
    W. peak flowmeter
    W. respirometer
    W. spirometer
    W. stain
Wright-Giemsa stain
Wrisberg ganglion
WRIST
    Washington Radiation for In-Stent
    Restenosis Trial

Wuchereria bancrofti
Wu-Hoak hypothesis
Wyamine Sulfate
Wyamycin S
Wycillin injection
Wydase
Wydora
wye
    patient circuit w.
Wylie carotid artery clamp
Wymox
Wytensin

NOTES

W

X

X axis
X wave of Ohnell

x

x. depression
x. depression of jugular venous
  pulse
x. descent
x. descent of jugular venous pulse
x. descent of the a wave
x. wave
xamoterol
xanthelasma
xanthine

x. oxidase
x. oxidase reaction
xanthogranuloma
xanthoma

eruptive x.
palmar x.
planar x.
x. regression
x. striatum palmare
x. tendinosum
tendinous x.
tuberoeruptive x.
tuberous x.
xanthomatosis
xanthomatous
Xanthomonas maltophilia
X-Cell valve
XCELON 6 balloon
Xcelon nylon
X-descent trough
Xe

xenon
¹²⁷Xe

xenon-127
¹³³Xe

xenon-133
XeCl

xenon chloride
  XeCl excimer laser
XECT

xenon-enhanced computed tomography
Xeloda
xemilofiban
Xenical
xenoantibody
xenobiotic
xenodiagnosis
xenograft

bovine pericardial heart valve x.
Ionescu-Shiley pericardial x.

porcine x.
stentless porcine x.
Xenomedica prosthetic valve
xenon (Xe)

x. chloride (XeCl)
x. chloride excimer laser
x. lung ventilation imaging
x. washout technique
xenon-127 (¹²⁷Xe)
xenon-133 (¹³³Xe)
**xenon-enhanced computed tomography
  (XECT)**
xenopi

Mycobacterium x.
Mycoplasma x.
Xenopus

X. laevis
X. oocytes
X. tropicalis
Xenotech prosthetic valve
xenotransplant
Xeroform gauze
xerosis
xerotrachea
Xillix

X. ACCESS system
X. LIFE-Lung system
xinafoate

salmeterol x.
xipamide
xiphisternal

x. crunching sound
x. process
xiphisternum
xiphocostal
xiphodynia
xiphoid

x. angle
x. cartilage
x. process
xiphoiditis
XL

Procardia XL
Toprol XL
X-linked dilated cardiomyopathy
Xopenex

X. inhalation solution
X. levalbuterol HCl inhalation
  solution
XO syndrome
XP

Cophene XP
Xpeedior

X. catheter
X. 100 catheter

X

XR
> Dilacor XR

x-ray
> babygram x-r.
> x-r. beam filtration
> x-r. beam hardening
> chest x-r.
> x-r. cine computed tomography
> x-r. energy microprobe analysis
> x-r. generator
> Scanning-Beam Digital x-r.
> x-r. scatter collimation
> sinus x-r.
> x-r. tube

XRT
> radiotherapy

X-Scribe stress test

X-Sizer
> X.-S. catheter system
> X.-S. single-use catheter system

XT
> XT cardiac device
> Cartia XT
> XT coronary stent
> Diltia XT

XT radiopaque coronary stent
XT stent

Xtrem Medicorp catheter

X-Trode
> X.-T. electrode catheter
> X.-T. stent

Xubix sibrafiban

XXXX syndrome

XXXY syndrome

xylene

Xylocaine
> X. HCl I.V. Injection for Cardiac Arrhythmias
> X. Oral
> X. Topical Ointment
> X. Topical Solution
> X. Topical Spray

Xylocard

xylol pulse indicator

xylosoxidans
> *Achromobacter x.*
> *Alcaligenes x.*

XYZ lead system

X, Y, Z recordings

Y

Y axis
Y connector
Y graft
Y stent
Y stenting
Y technique
Y wave pressure on right atrial catheterization

y

y depression of jugular venous pulse
y descent
y descent of jugular venous pulse
y descent wave
y wave

Yacoub and Radley-Smith classification
YAG
yttrium-aluminum-garnet
YAG laser
YAG/1064
laserscope Y.
Yamaguchi disease
Yamasa assay kit
Yankauer
Y. bronchoscope
Y. pharyngeal speculum
Yasargil carotid clamp
Yates correction
yaws
Y2B8 antibody
Y-descent trough
Yeager formula

year
quality-adjusted life y.'s
yellow
y. cross
y. fever
y. hepatization
y. nail syndrome (YNS)
y. plaque
y. sputum
Yellow IRIS system
Yentl syndrome
Yersinia
Y. enterocolitica
Y. pestis
Y. pseudotuberculosis
YM151
YM934
YNS
yellow nail syndrome
Yodoxin
yohimbine hydrochloride
Youden index
Youlten nasal inspiratory peak flowmeter
Youman-Parlett test
Young
Y. modulus
Y. syndrome
Y-shape bifurcation
Y-shaped graft
YSI Tele-thermometer
Y-stenting
yttrium-90

Y

Z

Z band
Z cardiac catheter
Z line
Z point
Z point pressure on left atrial catheterization
Z point pressure on right atrial catheterization
Z score weight-Z score height
Z stent

zabicipril
Zaditen
zafirlukast
Zagam RespiPac
Zahn

Z. lines
pocket of Z.

Zaire subtype
zalcitabine
Zalkind lung retractor
Zanaflex
zanamivir
Zang space
Zanosar
zardaverine asthma
Zaroxolyn
Zartan
zatebradine
Zavala

Z. lung biopsy needle
Z. technique

Zavod bronchospirometry catheter
z axis
Zebeta
zebra artifact
ZEEP

zero end-expiratory pressure

Zefazone
Zener diode
Zenker diverticulum
Zenotech graft material
Zephrex
Zerit
zero

z. end-expiratory pressure (ZEEP)
z. end-inspiratory pressure
z. velocity line

zero-amplitude
zero-flow pressure (Pzf, ZFP)
zero-order kinetics
Zestoretic
Zestril
ZFP

zero-flow pressure

Ziac
Ziagen
zidovudine and lamivudine
Ziehl-Neelsen stain
zigzag stent
Zilactin-L
zileuton
Zimberg esophageal hiatal retractor
Zimmer antiembolism support stockings
Zimmermann arch
Zinacef injection
zinc

z. chloride
z. finger gene
z. fume fever
z. gelatin

Zinecard
ZIP

zoster immune plasma

zipper

Z. antidisconnect device
z. scar

zirconium tetrachloride
Zithromax Z-Pak
Z-Med catheter
ZOC

Seloken ZOC

Zocor
zofenopril
zofenoprilic acid
Zoladex Implant
Zolicef
Zoll

Z. defibrillator
Z. NTP noninvasive pacemaker
Z. PD1200 external defibrillator

Zollinger-Gilmore intraluminal vein stripper
zolmitriptan
zolpidem tartrate
zona glomerulosa
zone

echo z.
Fraunhofer z.
Fresnel z.
H z.
ischemic z.
midlung z.
periinfarction z.
z. 1 phenomenon
posterior lung z.
posterior upper lung z.
protective z.
slow z.
sonolucent z.

Z

zone *(continued)*
    subcostal z.
    subendocardial z.
    tendinous z.'s of heart
    z. therapy
    transitional cell z.
    upper lung z.
    vascular z.
    z. 1, 2, 3, 4 of West
zoom
    acquisition z. (AZ)
zopolrestat
ZORprin
zoster
    herpes z.
    z. immune plasma (ZIP)
    varicella z. (VZ)
Zosyn
Z-Pak
    Zithromax Z-Pak

Zuckerkandl bodies
Zucker multipurpose bipolar catheter
Zucker-Myler cardiac device
Zuma guiding catheter
Z-wave tube
Zwenger test
Zyban
Zydone
Zyflo
Zygomycetes
zygomycosis
zymogen
zymography
    substrate gel z.
Zynergy Zolution electrophysiology catheter
Zyrel pacemaker
Zyrtec
Zytron pacemaker
Zyvox

Anatomical Illustrations

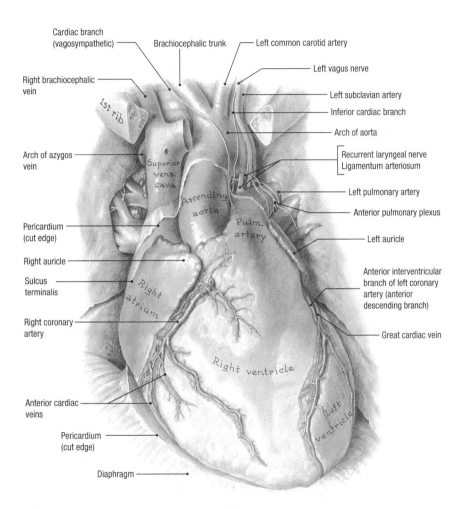

Figure 1. Sternocostal (anterior) surface of heart and great vessels in situ.

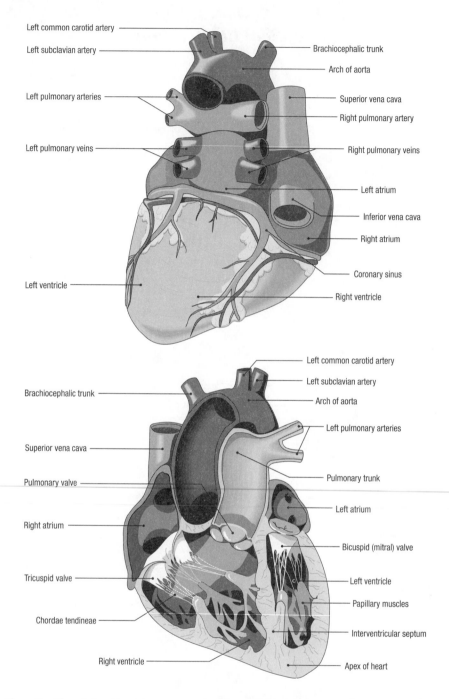

Figure 2. The relationship of the great vessels of heart. (Top) posterior view, (bottom) coronal view.

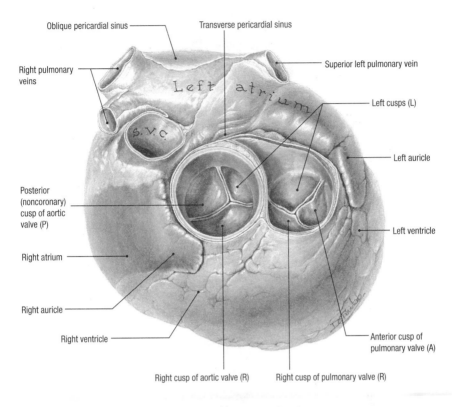

Figure 3. Excised heart, superior view.

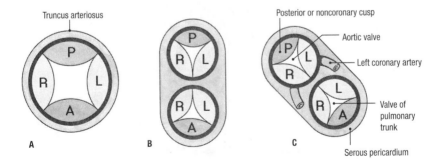

Figure 4. Pulmonary and aortic valves. The names of these cusps have a developmental origin: the truncus arteriosus with four cusps (A) splits to form two valves, each with three cusps (B). The heart undergoes partial rotation to the left on its axis, resulting in the arrangement of cusps shown in C.

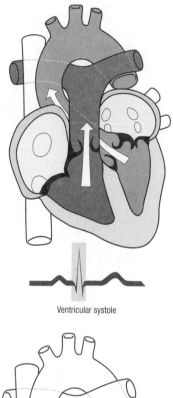

Ventricular systole

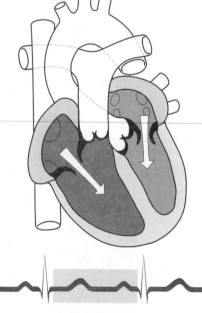

Ventricular diastole

Figure 5. The cardiac cycle.

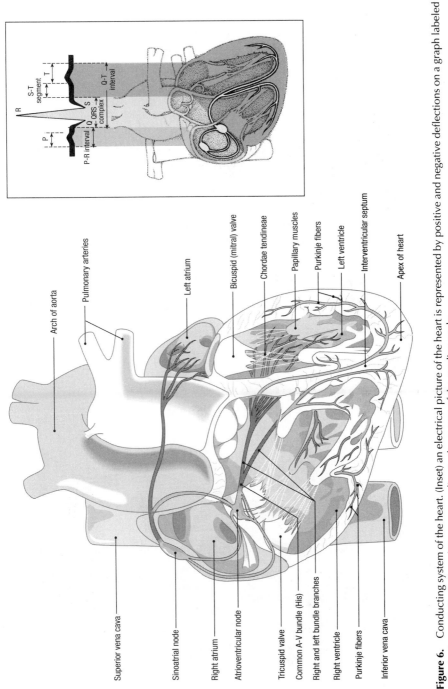

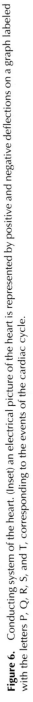

Figure 6. Conducting system of the heart. (Inset) an electrical picture of the heart is represented by positive and negative deflections on a graph labeled with the letters P, Q, R, S, and T, corresponding to the events of the cardiac cycle.

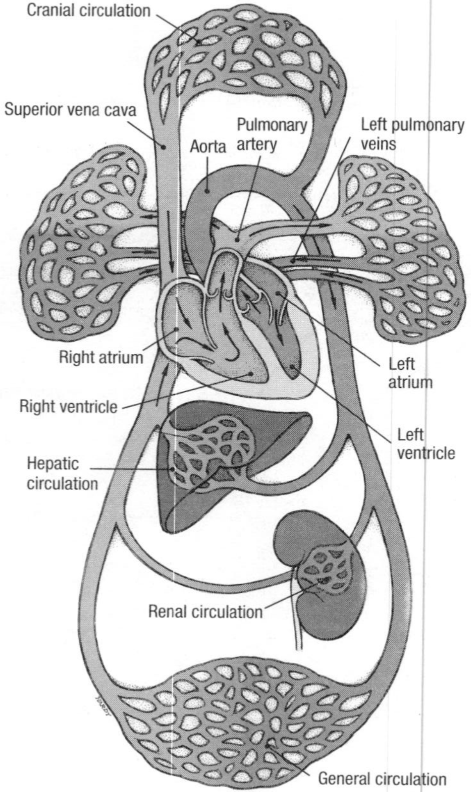

Descending thoracic aorta

Left common carotid
Left subclavian
Duct artery (ligament)
Bronchial
Intercostal
Esophageal
Diaphragm
Left gastric
Splenic
Left adrenal
Left renal
Left gonadal
Inferior mesenteric
Left common iliac
Left external iliac
Left internal iliac

Right common carotid
Right subclavian
Brachiocephalic

Tubular region
Sinotubular junction
Aortic sinus
Coronary artery

Celiac
Hepatic
Superior mesenteric
Right adrenal
Right renal
Right gonadal
Middle sacral
Right external iliac
Right internal iliac

Aortic arch
Ascending aorta
Abdominal aorta

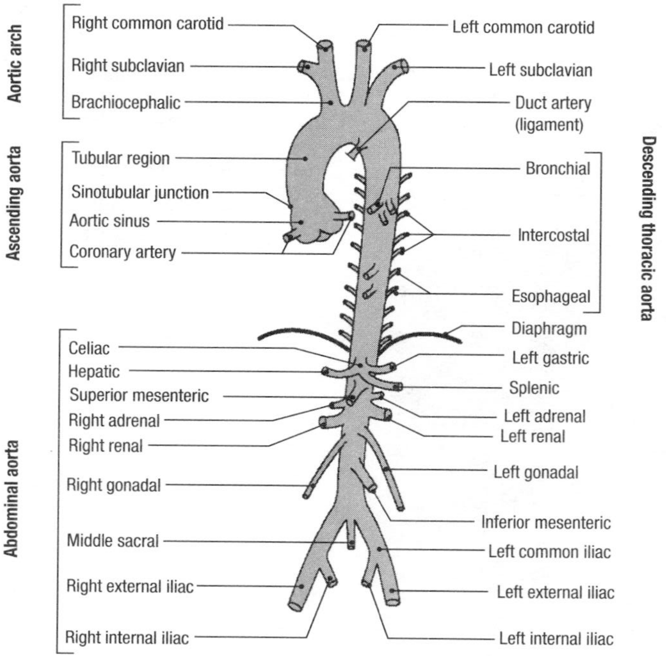

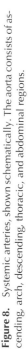

Figure 8. Systemic arteries, shown schematically. The aorta consists of ascending, arch, descending, thoracic, and abdominal regions.

Left pulmonary veins
Left atrium
Left ventricle
Pulmonary artery
General circulation
Cranial circulation
Aorta
Superior vena cava
Renal circulation
Right atrium
Right ventricle
Hepatic circulation

Figure 7. Pulmonary circulation: through the lungs, from the right ventricle to the left atrium. **Systemic circulation:** through the body, from the left ventricle to the right atrium.

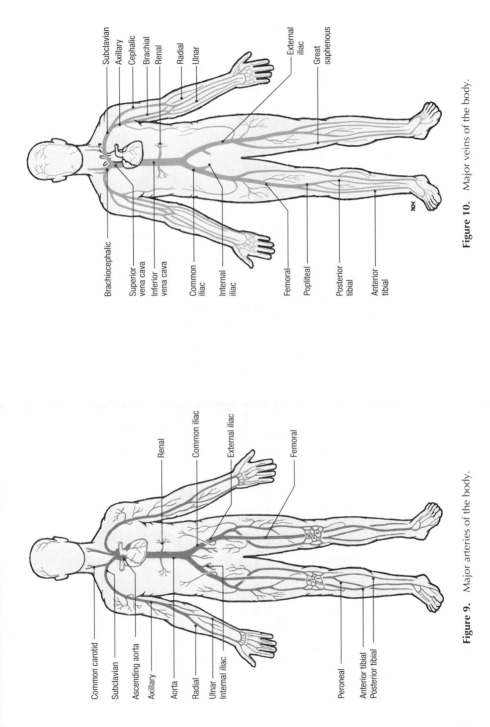

Figure 10. Major veins of the body.

Figure 9. Major arteries of the body.

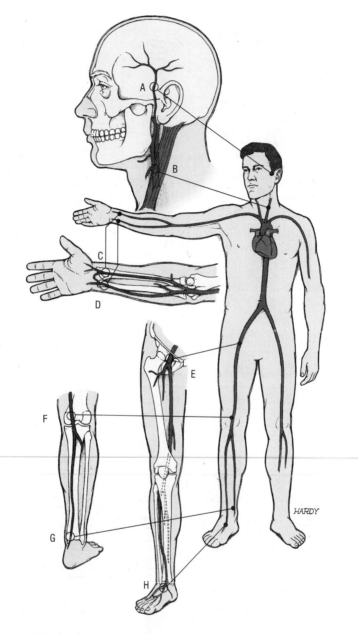

Figure 11. Peripheral pulses: (A) temporal, (B) carotid, (C) radial, (D) ulnar, (E) femoral, (F) popliteal, (G) posterior tibial, (H) dorsalis pedis.

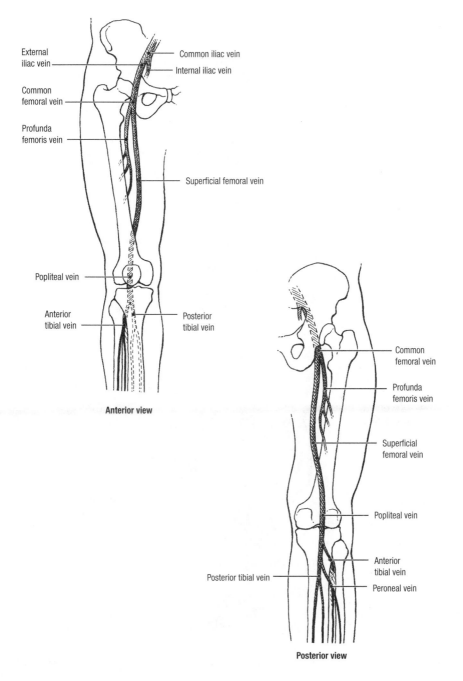

Figure 12. Anatomy of the deep venous system of the right lower limb. (Top) anterior view, (bottom) posterior view.

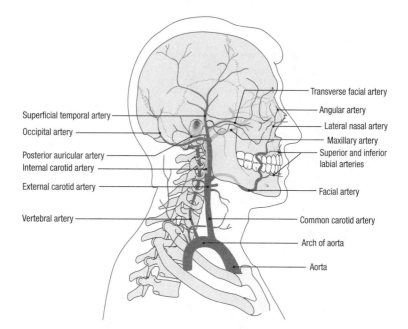

Figure 13. Arteries of the head and neck.

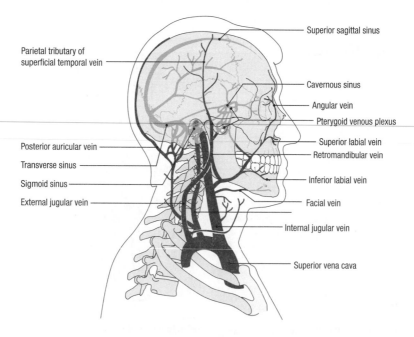

Figure 14. Veins of the head and neck.

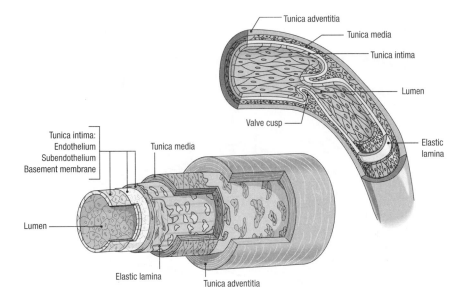

Figure 15. Structure of blood vessels. The walls of blood vessels are constructed of three concentric coats (Latin *tunicae*). With less muscle, veins (right) have thinner walls than their companion arteries (left) and wide lumens (Latin *lumina*) that usually appear flattened in tissue sections.

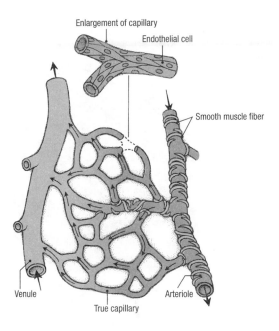

Figure 16. Capillary bed.

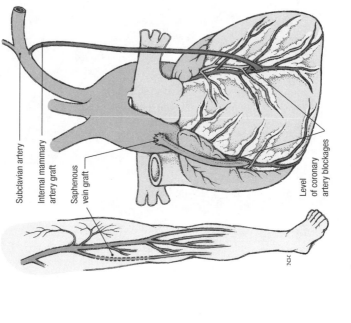

Figure 18. Coronary bypass. Completed double bypass using the internal mammary artery and the saphenous vein.

Subclavian artery

Internal mammary artery graft

Saphenous vein graft

Level of coronary artery blockages

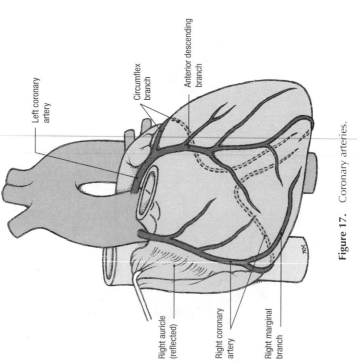

Figure 17. Coronary arteries.

Left coronary artery

Circumflex branch

Anterior descending branch

Right auricle (reflected)

Right coronary artery

Right marginal branch

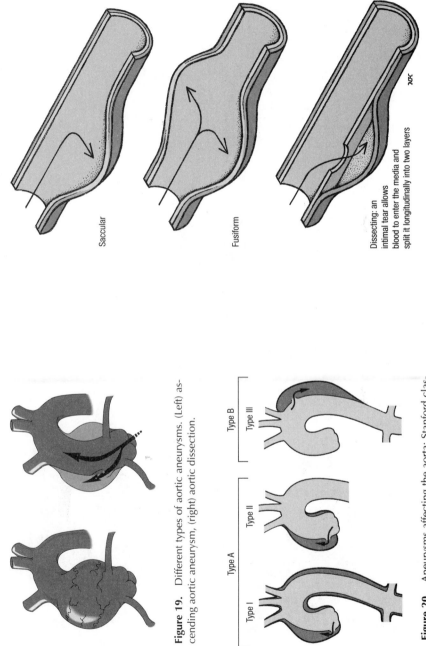

Saccular

Fusiform

Dissecting: an
intimal tear allows
blood to enter the media and
split it longitudinally into two layers

Figure 21. Aneurysm.

Figure 19. Different types of aortic aneurysms. (Left) ascending aortic aneurysm, (right) aortic dissection.

Type A

Type I   Type II

Type B

Type III

Figure 20. Aneurysms affecting the aorta: Stanford classification, Type A and Type B; deBakey classification, Types I, II, III.

A13

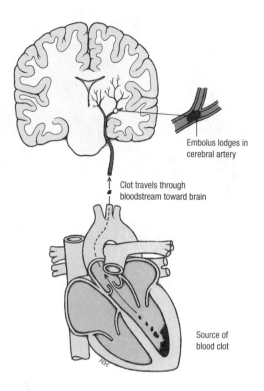

Figure 22. Embolism (embolus arising from a mural thrombus of the left ventricle).

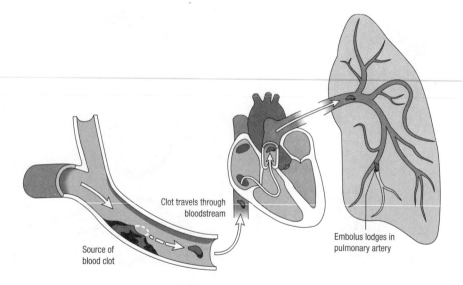

Figure 23. Embolism (embolus arising from thrombus in distal vein).

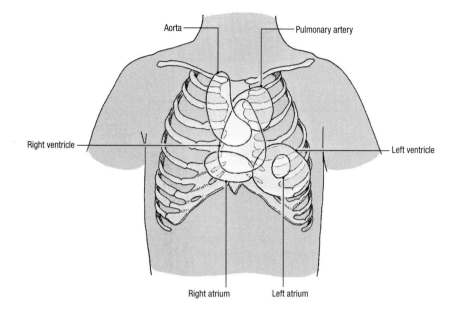

Figure 24. Auscultation points. The sound generated by cardiovascular structures will be transmitted to areas of the chest wall that they most closely approximate.

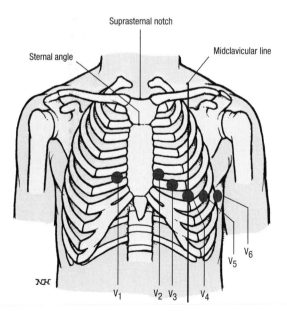

Figure 25. Electrocardiogram (ECG) lead placement: landmarks for chest lead placement.

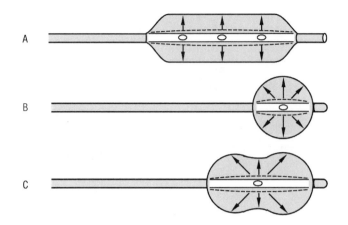

Figure 26. Three types of balloon catheters: (A) Gruentzig double-lumen dilation catheter, (B) Fogarty protrusion catheter, (C) double-bellied balloon catheter used to expand valves.

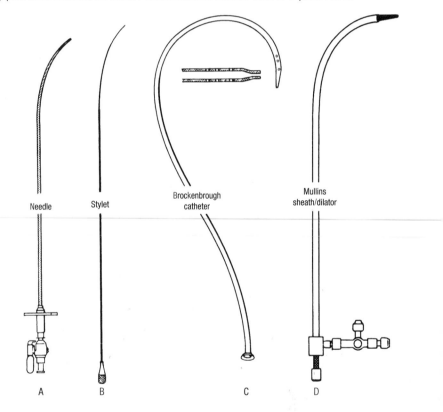

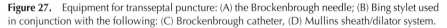

Figure 27. Equipment for transseptal puncture: (A) the Brockenbrough needle; (B) Bing stylet used in conjunction with the following: (C) Brockenbrough catheter, (D) Mullins sheath/dilator system.

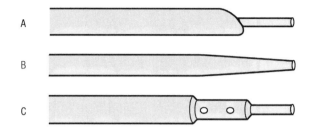

Figure 28. Catheters used to widen vessel stenosis in a stepwise manner: (A) Dotter, (B) Zeitler, (C) Andel.

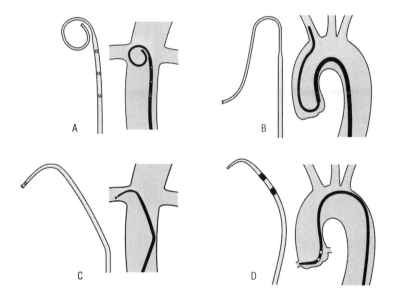

Figure 29. Various angiography catheters: (A) aorta catheter with side holes, (B) side-bending cerebral catheter (sidewinder), (C) side-bending catheter for selective viewing of visceral vessels, (D) Judkins coronary catheter.

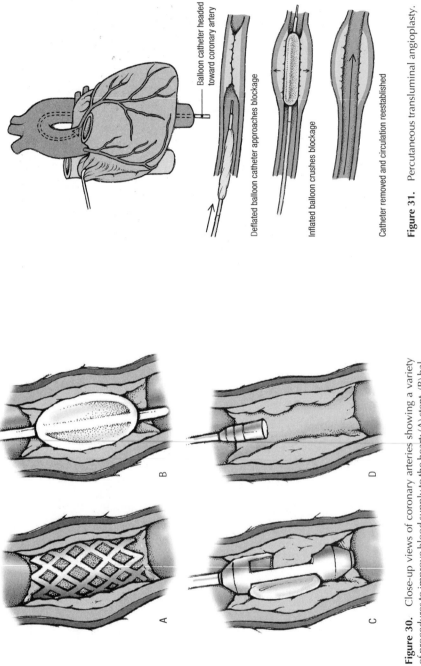

Figure 31. Percutaneous transluminal angioplasty.

Balloon catheter headed toward coronary artery

Deflated balloon catheter approaches blockage

Inflated balloon crushes blockage

Catheter removed and circulation reestablished

Figure 30. Close-up views of coronary arteries showing a variety of procedures to improve blood supply to the heart: (A) stent, (B) balloon angioplasty, (C) atherectomy, (D) laser ablation.

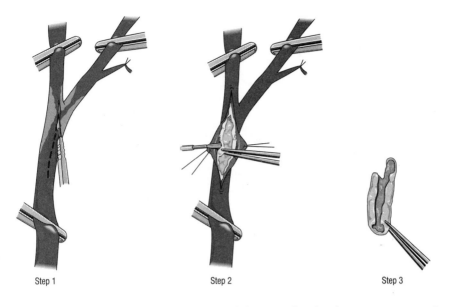

Step 1   Step 2   Step 3

Figure 32. An endarterectomy where diseased endothelium and media of an artery are removed so as to leave a smooth lining.

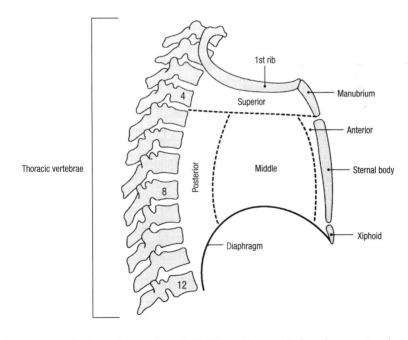

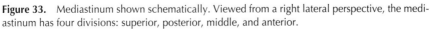

Figure 33. Mediastinum shown schematically. Viewed from a right lateral perspective, the mediastinum has four divisions: superior, posterior, middle, and anterior.

A19

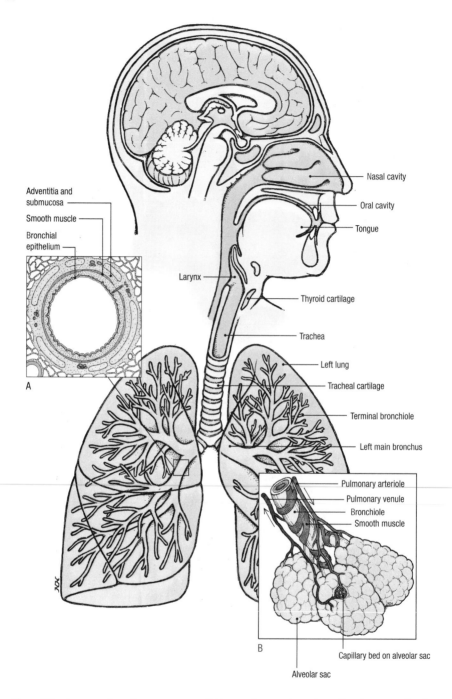

Figure 34. Lungs and respiratory anatomy. (A) intrapulmonary bronchus, (B) pulmonary alveolus.

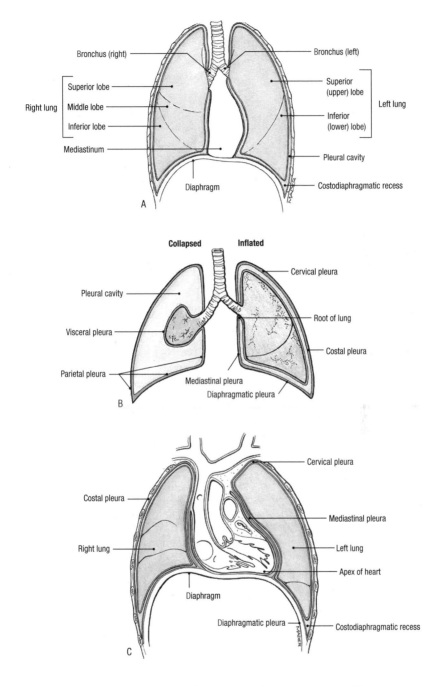

Figure 35. Respiratory system: (A) overview, (B) pleural cavity and pleura, (C) coronal section through heart and lungs.

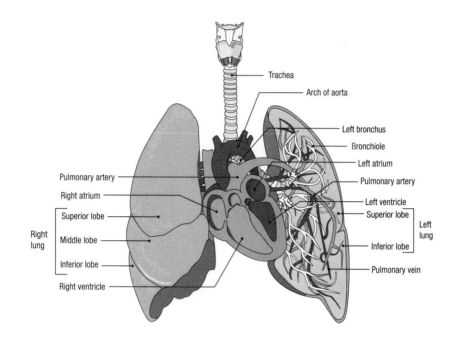

Figure 36. Cardiopulmonary system shown with cutaway of heart and left lung revealing internal anatomy.

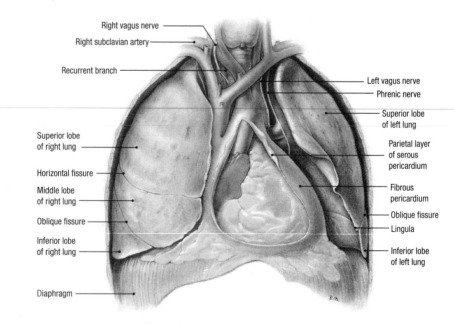

Figure 37. Thoracic contents in situ, anterior view.

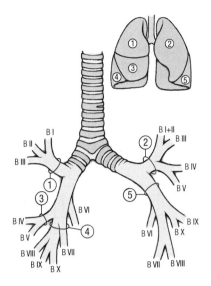

Figure 38. Segmental bronchi: right lung: (B I) apical, (B II) posterior, (B III) anterior, (B IV) lateral, (B V) medial, (B VI) apical, (B VII) medial basal, (B VIII) anterior basal, (B IX) lateral basal, (B X) posterior basal; left lung: (B I+II) apicoposterior, (B III) anterior, (B IV) superior lingular, (B V) inferior lingular, (B VI) apical, (B VII) medial basal, (B VIII) anterior basal, (B IX) lateral basal, (B X) posterior basal; lobes of lungs supplied: (1) right superior, (2) left superior, (3) right middle, (4) right inferior, (5) left inferior.

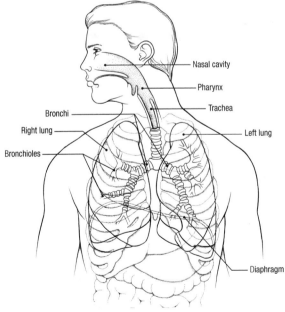

Figure 39. Anterior view of the male figure showing the main features of the respiratory system.

A23

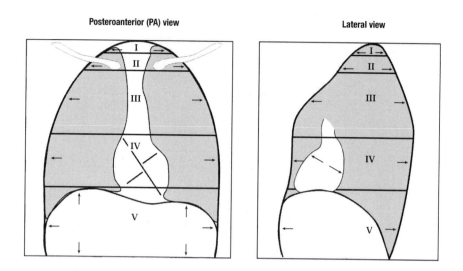

Figure 40. Posteroanterior (PA) and lateral chest films at full inspirations are divided into five (I-V) elliptical segments for measurement of total lung capacity.

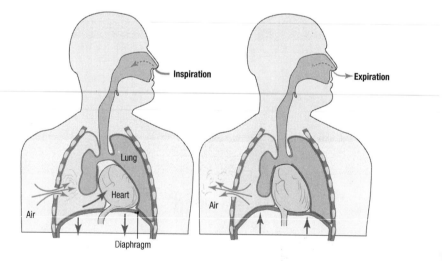

Figure 41. Left illustration shows how the heart and lungs are affected during **inspiration** in a person with pneumothorax. Right illustration shows how the heart and lungs are affected during **expiration** in a person with pneumothorax.

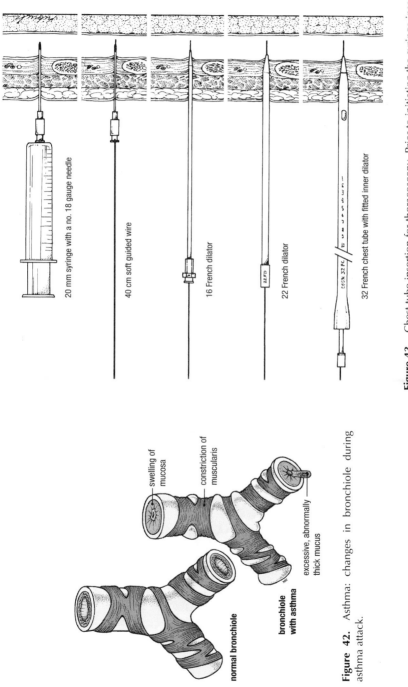

20 mm syringe with a no. 18 gauge needle

40 cm soft guided wire

16 French dilator

22 French dilator

32 French chest tube with fitted inner dilator

Figure 43. Chest tube insertion for thoracoscopy. Prior to initiating the syringe insertion, a local anesthetic is administered. Patient discomfort is minimal with use of the graduated size in dilator diameters.

swelling of mucosa

constriction of muscularis

excessive, abnormally thick mucus

normal bronchiole

bronchiole with asthma

Figure 42. Asthma: changes in bronchiole during asthma attack.

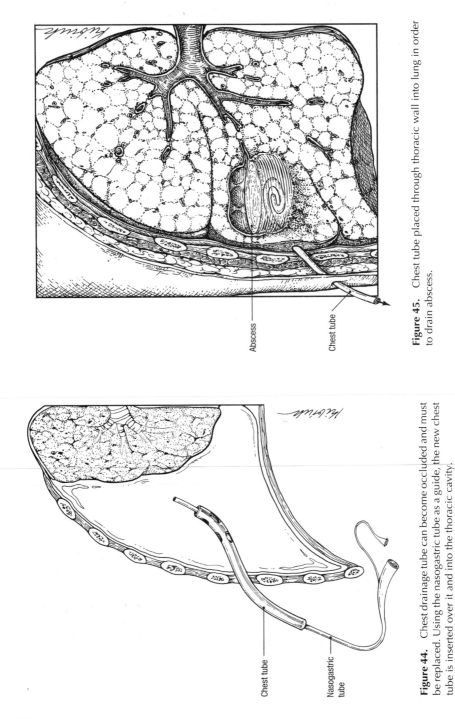

Figure 45. Chest tube placed through thoracic wall into lung in order to drain abscess.

Abscess

Chest tube

Figure 44. Chest drainage tube can become occluded and must be replaced. Using the nasogastric tube as a guide, the new chest tube is inserted over it and into the thoracic cavity.

Chest tube

Nasogastric tube

Appendix 2
Arterial Blood Gas Normal Lab Values

Abbreviation	Description	Normal Lab Value
PaO$_2$	partial pressure (P) of oxygen (O$_2$) in the arterial blood (a)	70 to 100 mmHg
SaO$_2$	percentage of available hemoglobin that is saturated (Sa) with oxygen (O$_2$)	≥94.5%
PaCO$_2$	partial pressure (P) of carbon dioxide (CO$_2$) in the arterial blood (a)	males: 35 to 48 mmHg females: 32 to 45 mmHg
pH	an expression of the extent to which the blood is alkaline or acidic	7.35 to 7.45
HCO$_3$	the level of plasma bicarbonate; an indicator of the metabolic acid-base status	22.0 to 26.0 mEq/L
O$_2$Hb	oxyhemoglobin	≥94.5%
COHb	carboxyhemoglobin	<1.5%
HHb	deoxyhemoglobin	<2.0%
MetHb	methemoglobin	<1.5%
ctHb	concentration of total hemoglobin	males: 14.0 to 18.0 g/dL females: 12.0 to 16.0 g/dL
ctO$_2$Hb	O$_2$ content of hemoglobin	15 to 23 vol%
P$_{50}$	partial pressure of O$_2$ at 50% saturation	25.0 to 29.0 mmHg

Pulmonary Function Terms

air trapping
airway resistance
body box plethysmography
bronchial challenge test
carbon monoxide diffusing capacity (DL_{CO}, D_{CO})
exercise-induced bronchospasm (EIB)
expiratory reserve volume (ERV)
flow-sensing spirometer
forced expiratory volume (FEV, FEV_T)
forced expiratory volume in 1 second (FEV_1)
forced inspiratory vital capacity (FIVC)
forced vital capacity (FVC)
functional residual capacity (FRC)
helium dilution
hyperinflation
inspiratory reserve volume (IRV)
inspiratory vital capacity (IVC)
maximal breathing capacity (MBC)
maximal expiratory flow rate (MEFR)
maximal expiratory pressure (MEP)
maximal inspiratory pressure (MIP)
maximal midexpiratory flow rate (MMFR, MMF) (also called $FEF_{25\%-75\%}$)
maximal voluntary ventilation (MVV)
nitrogen washout
peak expiratory flow (PEF)
peak flow meter
plethysmography
residual volume (RV)
respiratory exchange ration (RER)
respiratory inductive plethysmography
single-breath nitrogen washout (SBN_2)
slow vital capacity (SVC)
spirometry
static lung compliance
thoracic gas volume (V_{TG})
tidal volume (V_T)
total lung capacity (TLC)
vital capacity (VC)
volume-displacement spirometer

Appendix 4
Ventilator Terms

assist-control ventilation (A-C)
assisted mandatory ventilation (AMV)
continuous positive airway pressure (CPAP)
continuous spontaneous ventilation (CSV)
controlled mechanical ventilation (CMV)
fractional inspired oxygen (FIO_2)
intermittent demand ventilation (IDV)
intermittent mandatory ventilation (IMV)
intermittent positive-pressure ventilation (IPPV)
maximal voluntary ventilation (MVV)
negative-pressure ventilator
noninvasive positive pressure ventilation (NIPPV)
peak inspiratory pressure (PIP)
positive end-expiratory pressure (PEEP)
positive-pressure ventilators
pressure support ventilation (PSV)
pressure-cycled ventilator
synchronized intermittent mandatory ventilation (SIMV)
tidal volume (V_T)
time-cycled ventilator
volume-controlled ventilation (VCV)
volume-cycled ventilator

Sample Reports

CARDIAC CATHETERIZATION

TITLE OF PROCEDURE
1. Left heart catheterization.
2. Coronary angiography.
3. Left ventriculography.
4. Saphenous vein graft angiography.
5. Left internal mammary graft angiography.

PROCEDURE IN DETAIL: After informed consent was obtained and premedications administered, the area of the right femoral triangle was prepped and draped in the usual sterile fashion. Xylocaine 1% was used for local anesthesia. Modified Seldinger technique was used to place a 6 French Hemaquet in the right femoral artery. Using standard Judkins technique with a JL4 and JR4, left followed by right coronary angiography was performed in multiple right anterior oblique and left anterior oblique views. The right coronary catheter was used for angiography of the internal mammary. A multipurpose catheter was used for right coronary artery saphenous vein graft angiography. Finally, a pigtail catheter was used for left ventriculography performed in the 30-degree RAO view. VasoSeal was used for hemostasis. The patient tolerated the procedure well. There were no complications.

The patient remained in a sinus rhythm. Left ventricular end-diastolic pressure was 16. There was no gradient between the left ventricle and aorta on pullback. Left ventriculography revealed mild global hypokinesis but low normal left ventricular systolic function.

CORONARY ANGIOGRAPHY: Injection of the left coronary system demonstrates a left main which trifurcates into a LAD, ramus, and circumflex. Left main has a concentric 60%–70% distal narrowing involving the trifurcation of the LAD, ramus and circumflex. There is no damping or ventricularization with catheter engagement.

The LAD is a fair-caliber vessel which gives rise to a moderate-sized proximal diagonal and multiple septal perforating branches, and the LAD terminates just at the inferior aspect of the left ventricular apex. There is competitive spilling from the mid to distal LAD via the internal mammary bypass. The mid to distal LAD is widely patent and of fair caliber. There is luminal irregularity in the proximal LAD with no obstructive lesions. Likewise, the first diagonal has diffuse irregularity but no obstructive disease.

The ramus is of smaller caliber and free of obstructive disease.

The right coronary artery is dominant and completely occluded near its origin.

SAPHENOUS VEIN GRAFT TO THE POSTERIOR DESCENDING ARTERY:
This graft is widely patent, briskly filling a fair-caliber PDA and a larger posterolateral system. There is some mild luminal irregularity, but no obstructive disease in this system.

CARDIAC DIAGNOSTIC TEST: CARDIOLITE TREADMILL

TITLE OF PROCEDURE: Cardiolite treadmill.

PROCEDURE IN DETAIL: The electrocardiogram prior to exercise revealed sinus rhythm with bigeminal ventricular premature beats. The intervals and frontal axis were within normal limits. There were minor nondiagnostic ST-T changes at rest. Blood pressure prior to exercise was 91/44.

The patient walked a total of 4 minutes 10 seconds according to a greatly modified protocol completing exercise 2 mph, 0% grade, obtaining a peak heart rate of 121 beats per minute equaling 85% of predicted age-adjusted maximum heart rate. The test was stopped due to fatigue and shortness of breath. There was no complaint of exercise-induced chest pain. Blood pressure had risen to 131/61 and an energy expenditure of 4 METS is estimated.

A predetermined dose of Cardiolite was injected 40 seconds prior to the completion of exercise. The electrocardiogram during exercise revealed sinus rhythm with periods of ventricular premature beats. As exercise proceeded, there was minimal, i.e., 0.5 mm or less, additional ST-segment depression inferolaterally. This does not fulfill criteria for inducible myocardial ischemia. No additional changes of significance were noted as the heart rate decelerated in the recovery phase.

CARDIAC DIAGNOSTIC TEST: COLOR VENOUS DUPLEX

TITLE OF PROCEDURE: Color venous duplex.

DESCRIPTION OF PROCEDURE: On the transverse view, the veins were compressible at the common femoral. It was technically difficult to visualize the superficial femoral vein and parts of the popliteal vein.

On the longitudinal view, however, the color flow was considered adequate at the common femoral vein and parts of the superficial femoral vein. However, distally the flow decreased to very minimal. Deep vein thrombosis could not be completely ruled out with this test.

CARDIAC DIAGNOSTIC TEST: TILT TABLE TEST

TITLE OF PROCEDURE: Tilt table test.

PROCEDURE IN DETAIL: The exam was started at 10:15 a.m. Blood pressure was 114/98, heart rate 59. The head of the bed was elevated to 70 degrees at 10:29 a.m. Blood pressure was 110/70; heart rate 59, paced rhythm. At 10:32, blood pressure dropped to 84/53. Heart rate continued at 60, paced rhythm. The patient was symptomatic with lightheadedness, dizziness, and room spinning.

CONCLUSION: Positive tilt table exam for cardioneurogenic syncope.

CORONARY ARTERY BYPASS GRAFT

TITLE OF PROCEDURE: Coronary artery bypass graft (CABG).

PROCEDURE IN DETAIL: The patient was brought to the operating room and given general endotracheal anesthesia. The pulmonary artery catheter was inserted by anesthesia under sterile technique in the right internal jugular vein. The distal right saphenous vein was harvested from the medial malleolus to just above the knee using multiple small serial incisions with skin bridges. It was a good quality vein. The leg was closed in layers with 2–0 and 3–0 Vicryl with 3–0 Vicryl subcuticular suture in the skin.

A midline sternotomy was performed. The patient was heparinized. The ascending aorta was found to be extremely calcified after opening the pericardium. There was diffuse atherosclerosis with visible plaque emanating from the ascending aorta. The aortic arch was cannulated beyond the ascending aorta. The atrium was cannulated, and the patient was placed on bypass. A vent was inserted into the left ventricle via the right superior pulmonary vein. Coronaries were marked for bypass, including a very large posterior descending artery and a good-sized posterolateral branch just prior to its bifurcation with two smaller branches. A single-clamp technique was utilized. The aorta was cross-clamped in the least calcified place. One liter of cardioplegia was given antegrade to arrest the heart. It was packed with ice and then flushed posteriorly. Bypasses were accomplished, first using the reverse saphenous vein in an end-to-side fashion to the PDA, which was a good quality 2.5 to 3-mm vessel. This was done with a reverse vein and running 7–0 Prolene suture. The second bypass was to the posterolateral branch, which was smaller but easily took a 1.5-mm probe. This was done with a separate piece of vein and a running 7–0 Prolene suture. A bolus of cold cardioplegia was given, and the patient was rewarmed. With the cross-clamp still in place, a single aortotomy was made in the ascending aorta. The area was thickened and calcified, but had a decent lumen to allow suture of the proximal end of the PDA up to the ascending aorta with running 5–0 Prolene suture in an end-to-side fashion. After concluding this anastomosis, hot cardioplegia was given into the aortic root. The cross-clamp was removed after a total of 30 minutes cross-clamp time. The remaining proximal anastomosis of the posterolateral branch was brought onto the hood of the PDA graft. The PDA was isolated with bulldog clamps. Venotomy was made, and the end-to-side anastomosis of the posterior left ventricle to the PDA was accomplished using running 6–0 Prolene suture in an end-to-side fashion. The system was backbled and de-aired, and the bulldog clamps were removed. Vessels were inspected, and they were both hemostatic. Two atrial and two ventricular pacing wires were placed and brought out through the skin. One single chest tube was placed into the mediastinum. Neither pleura was opened. The left ventricular vent was clamped and removed, and the pursestring was ligated. The lungs were inflated. The patient was ventilated and weaned off bypass successfully without the aid of inotropic support. Protamine was started, and the atrial cannula was removed. Volume status was normalized, and the heparin fully reversed with protamine. The aortic cannula was removed and the site ligated and reinforced with pledgeted 4–0 Prolene stitch. The chest tube was positioned. The wound was closed using figure-of-eight 0 Ethibond to reapproximate fascia, seven sternal wires, and two layers of running 2–0 Vicryl and a running 3–0 Vicryl in the skin. The patient tolerated the procedure and was transferred to the intensive care unit in stable condition.

ECHOCARDIOGRAM REPORT: M-MODE, TWO-DIMENSIONAL, AND COLOR DOPPLER ECHOCARDIOGRAM

TITLE OF PROCEDURE: M-mode, two-dimensional Doppler, and color Doppler echocardiogram.

FINDINGS: The cardiac chamber sizes are normal. There is mild concentric left ventricular hypertrophy with the interventricular septum and left ventricular free walls measuring 1.1 cm. The left ventricular systolic function is normal with the estimated left ventricular ejection fraction of 60%. There are no wall motion abnormalities. The diastolic compliance of the left ventricle is normal. The valvular structures are grossly normal. Doppler and color Doppler interrogation of the valves reveals no insufficiency or stenosis. There is no pericardial effusion. There are no intracardiac thrombi or valvular vegetations.

ECHOCARDIOGRAM REPORT: TRANSESOPHAGEAL ECHOCARDIOGRAM

TITLE OF PROCEDURE: Transesophageal echocardiogram (TEE).

DESCRIPTION OF PROCEDURE: The patient was brought to the procedure area after informed consent was obtained. The risks, benefits, and alternatives of transesophageal echocardiographic assessment were explained, and the patient and family voiced understanding and agreed to proceed.

Following adequate topical and intravenous sedation, the patient had blind esophageal intubation performed of the oropharynx in the usual manner. Images were made from the transgastric and transesophageal planes easily and without complications.

At the conclusion, the transesophageal probe was removed, and the patient was taken back to his room in stable condition.

FINDINGS: Globally preserved left ventricular systolic function with visually estimated ejection fraction of 65% with normal regional wall motion in all segments. Trileaflet aortic valve with central mild aortic insufficiency. Large ascending aorta. Structurally normal-appearing mitral valve with a trace to 1+ mitral regurgitation. The intraatrial septum has a very large aneurysmal redundant segment bulging right to left. Color Doppler flow shows right-to-left shunting of the small area at the base of this aneurysmal dilatation. In addition, a contrast bubble study demonstrates free right-to-left shunting at the base of this aneurysmal intraatrial septal membrane. This is the obvious source for paradoxical embolus and right-to-left shunting and should be chronically anticoagulated. The left atrial appendage is well visualized with no evidence of thrombus. It is contracting nicely and has velocities in excess of 100 cm per second. No evidence of spontaneous echo contrast to suggest source of emboli from the left side of the heart. There is no left ventricular or left atrial thrombus identified. No pericardial effusion is seen. No intracardiac mass, thrombus or vegetation seen. The descending thoracic aorta is extremely tortuous, with mild intimal thickening but no dissection, aneurysm, or significant atherosclerotic changes identified.

FIBEROPTIC BRONCHOSCOPY WITH ENDOBRONCHIAL AND TRANSBRONCHIAL BIOPSIES

TITLE OF PROCEDURE

1. Fiberoptic bronchoscopy.
2. Endobronchial and transbronchial biopsies with fluoroscopy.

DESCRIPTION OF PROCEDURE: The patient was premedicated with Versed. Approximately 4 mg was given prior to introduction of the scope. A total of 9 mg was given before and during the procedure for sedation. Some tendency toward obstructive apnea was noted both before and during the procedure with the patient in supine posture.

The fiberoptic scope was introduced via the right naris. The naris was tight and a very small amount of bleeding ensued from the middle turbinate. The scope was passed into the hypopharynx. The vocal cords, false cords, arytenoid region, hypopharyngeal region toward the esophagus, and the epiglottis were visualized. All of these were relatively unremarkable. Some landmarks were present around the region of the arytenoids but no erythema or clear edema, and no distortion. Vocal cords appeared to move relatively normally, although the patient would not phonate following sedation.

The trachea was inspected and found to be normal. The main carina was sharp. The right bronchial tree was inspected, and three normal segments into the right upper lobe were found. The right middle lobe had two segments; the more medial one was stenotic, with circumferential narrowing and suggestion of possible submucosal disease with overlying normal-appearing mucosa. A very small amount of increased mucus was present in this area. The right lower lobe, including superior segment, anterolateral and basal segments, was also inspected to the subsegmental level, revealing no abnormality. The left upper lobe with lingula and the left lower lobe with superior segment likewise were inspected to the subsegmental level, revealing no abnormalities.

Using fluoroscopic control, a brush was placed into the right middle lobe into the three available orifices. The more stenotic and medial of these came closest to approximating the right heart border where the lesion had been seen on CT. The lesion itself was not clearly visible on fluoroscopy. Although an accentuated density at the right hilum was noted, it was not felt to be the lesion seen on CT. Consequently, biopsies were not clarified a great deal by fluoroscopic localization of the lesion.

Biopsies were taken from the medial and stenotic portion of the right middle lobe, approximating the right heart border on at least one occasion. Approximately four pieces of tissue were removed, plus two fairly significant endobronchial biopsies from the region of the narrowed orifice into the right middle lobe and its associated carina.

Specimens included dry and wet brush slides, plus biopsies in formalin. Chief differential diagnosis of neoplasm was done. After the procedure, the patient was given 0.3 mg of Romazicon to aid in recovery from Versed. Fluoroscopy has been used after transbronchial biopsies to ensure no pneumothorax at that time. Subsequent chest x-ray was ordered.

LEFT CHAMBERLAIN PROCEDURE, VIDEO-ASSISTED THORACOSCOPY, RESECTION OF PULMONARY NODULE

TITLE OF PROCEDURE
1. Left Chamberlain procedure.
2. Right video-assisted thoracoscopic surgery.
3. Segmental resection of right upper lobe pulmonary nodule.

PROCEDURE IN DETAIL: After adequate general anesthesia and double-lumen endotracheal intubation, the patient was placed in the supine position. The chest was prepped and draped in the standard sterile surgical fashion. The left anterior chest wall incision was made above the second intercostal space. The incision was carried down through the subcutaneous tissues to the thoracic muscle fibers, which were divided. The intercostal muscle was divided above the edges of the second rib. The second rib was dissected from the surrounding tissue by elevating the periosteum. The second rib was then excised at its junction with the sternum and as far as two inches laterally. Retracting the lung laterally and performing blunt dissection exposed the aortopulmonary window. No evidence of nodes was seen or palpated at the aortopulmonary window. A small hole was made into the left pleura.

The decision was made at this time to complete the Chamberlain procedure by closing the pectoralis fascia in layers. Because of violation of the left pleura, a catheter was introduced into the left chest and left in place. The pectoralis fascia was closed using a running #0 PDS suture. Prior to tying the PDS suture, the anesthetist was asked to inflate the lung, and suction was applied over the catheter. The catheter was then pulled out. The suture was tied down carefully. The skin was then closed using running #3–0 Vicryl suture in a subcuticular fashion. Steri-Strips were applied over the incisions.

The patient was then positioned in the left lateral decubitus position, with the right chest upward. The right chest wall was prepped and draped in the standard sterile surgical fashion. A small incision was made at the fourth intercostal space along the midaxillary line. The incision was carried down using Bovie electrocoagulation through the intercostal muscle.

The anesthesia service was asked to drop the right lung prior to entering the chest. The right chest was entered. A 5-mm trocar was introduced into the chest followed by a 30-degree angle video camera. No evidence of adhesion was noticed in the lung. The lung was examined carefully. There was no evidence of obvious masses in the upper lobe, middle lobe or lower lobe. Another small incision was made in the fourth intercostal space anteriorly, as well as another incision in the fourth intercostal space posteriorly. The lung was then retracted using sponge forceps and manual palpation of the right upper lobe. There was a 1 x 1-cm hard mass, which was in the lower first of the right upper lobe. The mass was wedged off using multiple lobes of the GIA 30 stapler. The mass was retrieved from the chest cavity using Endobag and submitted for frozen section. Frozen section revealed no evidence of malignancy. Fibrosis, as well as histiocyte cells, was noticed. The exact diagnosis was deferred to the permanent sections.

The chest cavity at this point was irrigated with warm water and inspected for air leaks. No evidence of obvious air leak or bleeding. A size #28 chest tube was placed through the port in the midaxillary line, directed toward the apex. A size 36 French tube was placed through the anterior chest incision and exited anteriorly toward the apex. The chest tube was secured to the skin using #2–0 Surgilon suture. Both chest tubes were connected to a Pleur-evac. The posterior incision was closed using #2–0 Vicryl for the intercostal muscles and #3–0 Vicryl suture in a subcuticular fashion for the skin. Applying surgical dressings over the chest tube sites completed the procedure. The patient was then positioned in the supine position and extubated in the operating room without difficulty.

MITRAL VALVE REPLACEMENT

TITLE OF PROCEDURE
1. Mitral valve replacement with size 27 CarboMedics valve.
2. Repair of left ventricular rupture, secondary to myocardial infarction.

PROCEDURE IN DETAIL: The neck, chest, abdomen and legs were prepped with Betadine solution. Combination sterile dressings were placed in the usual sterile fashion. A #10 scalpel blade was used to make an incision from the sternal notch to the xiphoid. The presternal fascia and subcutaneous tissue were transected with electrocautery. The sternum was divided with a sternal saw. The chest was then exposed using the sternal retractor. The pericardium was entered from the innominate vein and teased off from the diaphragm. Approximately 500 cc of gross blood was aspirated from the pericardium. The patient was heparinized.

The aorta was soft without any calcification. It was cannulated with the aortic cannulation device. The superior vena cava was cannulated with a size 32 French venous cannula. The inferior vena cava was cannulated with a size 36 French cannula. After adequate activated coagulation time was achieved, the patient was placed on cardiopulmonary bypass and cooled to 38 degrees centigrade. The aorta was cross-clamped, and cold blood cardioplegia was given antegrade. To achieve electro-mechanical arrest, 500 cc was given antegrade, and 500 cc was given retrograde through the cannulation device. The heart was also cooled with topical hypothermia using iced slush solution throughout the procedure. Throughout this procedure, every 15 minutes, 250 cc of cold blood cardioplegia was given retrograde to maintain electromechanical arrest and hypothermia. Snares were placed around the superior and inferior vena cava to complete full unloading of the right heart. The intraatrial septum was dissected, the left atrium was elevated, and atriotomy was performed through the left atrium. An atrial retractor was used to expose the entire left atrium. The mitral valve was difficult to expose due to the acuteness of the mitral regurgitation and the small size of the left atrium.

Eventually, the anterior and posterior leaflets were identified. Part of the posterior leaflet was completely ruptured from the papillary muscle with a large amount of papillary muscle still intact with the chordae. The leaflet was then debrided. The anterior leaflet was debrided as well along the chordae attachments. The commissures were sewn with interrupted 2–0 Ethibond pledgeted sutures, and the valve anulus was sized. A size 27 CarboMedics valve was chosen. Using interrupted green and white pledgeted horizontal mattress suture technique, the entire anterior and posterior leaflets were sewn. The valve was then sewn to the anulus, and the valve was lowered into the position carefully. There appeared to be good coaptation of the leaflets. A vent was then placed between the prosthetic valve leaflet and brought out through the atriotomy. The atriotomy was closed with a running 4–0 Prolene suture, and the left ventricle was allowed to fill with blood. Using gentle massage technique, the left ventricle was de-aired. The atriotomy was completely closed, and the patient was re-warmed. The snares around the vena cava were loosened, and the patient was given a hot shot of blood cardioplegia retrograde. The cross-clamp was removed after the aorta was de-aired as well. The aortic vent was kept on to help remove any additional emboli. A transesophageal echocardiogram was used to assess the valve. The valve appeared to be functioning adequately; a small amount of air was noticed in the left atrium. This was again suctioned with the LV vent. The LV vent was removed. There appeared to be good contractility of the heart.

The patient was weaned from cardiopulmonary bypass slowly. After approximately 30 minutes of the cross-clamp being off, the patient was weaned from cardiopulmonary bypass with some inotropic support, including dopamine at 5 mcg/kg per minute and 0.05 epinephrine. The intraaortic balloon pump was placed on 1:1 augmentation, and the patient had adequate hemodynamics and adequate cardiac output hemodynamics. The protamine was begun. After the protamine was given, the aortic and venous cannulas were removed. The protamine was well tolerated. The retrograde and antegrade cardioplegia cannulas were removed as well. There appeared to be no bleeding along the aortotomy site or the atriotomy site; however, there appeared to be some bright red bleeding along the base of the heart and along the apex of the heart, apparently an area where the left ventricle had ruptured and probably secondary to the myocardial infarction. Interrupted 4–0 pledgeted Prolene sutures were used to close this rupture.

The patient was placed back on cardiopulmonary bypass by placing the aortic cannula back in the aorta, and the left groin was prepped. A 32 French venous catheter was placed through the left femoral vein. The patient was heparinized. After adequate ACT was achieved, the patient was placed on cardiopulmonary bypass, and the apex of the heart was elevated. There appeared to be a 2-cm rupture along the lateral wall of the heart. This rupture was closed with an approximately 4-cm pledgeted Telfa in a horizontal mattress fashion. It was closed quite securely, and the patient tolerated it well. The patient was weaned from cardiopulmonary bypass without any difficulty. Protamine was reinstituted, and the venous and aortic cannulas were removed. The patient had adequate hemodynamics and blood pressure, and there appeared to be no other bleeding from this rupture site. Mediastinal and bilateral chest tubes were placed through separate stab wounds, and the sternum was reapproximated with six stainless steel wires. The subcutaneous tissue and the skin were closed with 2–0 Vicryl and skin staples. The patient tolerated the procedure well, with no intraoperative complications.

PACEMAKER REPORT: DUAL-CHAMBER PERMANENT PACEMAKER PLACEMENT

TITLE OF PROCEDURE: Dual-chamber permanent pacemaker placement.

DESCRIPTION OF PROCEDURE: The patient was prepared in the usual sterile fashion. The left subclavian approach was selected. A needle was passed into the left subclavian vein with good blood return. A wire was passed through the needle and the needle was removed. Dilator and introducer were passed over the wire. The dilator was removed.

Ventricular lead—Pacesetter 134–60, 58 cm, serial number RL20692, was passed into the right ventricle. Threshold was 0.5 V, 0.7 mA, 780 ohms, 12.0 mV R-wave.

Atrial lead—Pacesetter 148-ATC, 46 cm, serial number NA10957, was passed into the right atrium. Threshold was 0.8 V, 2.4 mA, 480 ohms, 2.0 mV P-wave.

A pacemaker pocket was made in the left anterior chest wall. A pulse generator (Integrity AFXDR model 5342, serial number 256494) was placed into the left anterior chest wall. The patient was sutured in the usual sterile fashion and tolerated the procedure well. A chest x-ray was ordered.

PACEMAKER REPORT: INSERTION OF TRANSVENOUS TEMPORARY PACEMAKER

TITLE OF PROCEDURE: Insertion of transvenous temporary pacemaker by right internal jugular route.

PROCEDURE IN DETAIL: A right jugular stick following Xylocaine anesthesia was made in the triangle between the medial and lateral heads of the trapezius muscles. The internal jugular vein was cannulated initially with needles, using a guidewire. An Arrow introducer sheath was placed. The transvenous pacemaker selected was 3 French. The introducer sheath required a 5 French catheter to maintain a good seal. Intravenous fluid was infused via the side ports of the catheter following good venous return.

The transvenous balloon-type catheter, a flow-directed catheter but without capability of hemodynamic monitoring, was inserted with balloon up to approximately 45 cm and then manipulated between 52 cm from the introducer up to 32 cm from the introducer with best capture seen at 32 cm. Partial capturing was seen at settings at 0.5 mA to 1 mA with good capture at 2 mA. The rate was set at 60 beats per minute with complete capturing. Steri-Strips were used to wrap around the external portion of the catheter, and the catheter was secured to the introducer site port tubing. X-ray was taken showing the tip of the catheter within the right ventricle in good position.

PACEMAKER REPORT: PACEMAKER GENERATOR REPLACEMENT

TITLE OF PROCEDURE: Pacemaker generator replacement.

DESCRIPTION OF PROCEDURE: The patient was prepped in the usual sterile fashion. The right previous pacer site was in the right subclavian area. An incision was made. The pulse generator was removed. The ventricular lead was checked. Sensitivity was 5.8 mV, voltage 1.3 V, 2.4 mA, resistance 450 ohms. The same pacemaker pocket was used. A pulse generator (Affinity SR, serial number 151974) was placed. The patient was sutured in the usual sterile fashion. The patient tolerated the procedure well.

PACEMAKER REPORT: PERMANENT PACEMAKER IMPLANTATION

TITLE OF PROCEDURE: Permanent pacemaker implantation.

PROCEDURE IN DETAIL: After detailed description of the procedure, indications, as well as the potential risks, of permanent pacemaker implantation were explained to the patient, and informed consent was obtained. The patient was transferred to the cardiac catheterization lab. The left subclavian area was prepared and draped in the usual sterile manner. The left subclavian vein was accessed by Seldinger technique. A guidewire was placed. The left subclavian vein was accessed, and a separate guidewire was also placed.

A deep subcutaneous pacemaker pocket was then created using the blunt dissection technique without any excessive bleeding. A French 7 introducer sheath was advanced over the guidewire, and the guidewire was removed. A Medtronic bipolar endocardial lead (model #5054 and serial #LEH025605V) was advanced under fluoroscopic guidance, and the tip of the pacemaker lead was positioned in the right ventricular apex. The French 9.5 introducer sheath was advanced over a separate guidewire under fluoroscopic guidance, and the guidewire was removed. Through this sheath, a bipolar atrial screw-in lead by Medtronic (model #4568 and serial #LDD027303V) was selected. It was positioned in the right atrial appendage, and the lead was screwed in. The stimulation thresholds were obtained for the atrial lead. The amplitude was 2.7 mV with resistance of 549 ohms and a pulse rate of 0.5 ms.

Following this, the ventricular stimulation threshold parameters were obtained, including the R-wave entry of 4.6 mV, with resistance of 1427 ohms and a pulse wave of 0.5 ms. Minimum stimulation threshold was 0.4 V for the ventricular lead, and minimal stimulation for the atrial lead was 2 V.

Both the atrial, as well as the ventricular leads, were secured to the deep subcutaneous tissue using 3–0 silk. The subcutaneous pocket was flushed and irrigated using antibiotic solution. Both leads were connected to a Medtronic pulse generator (model

#KDR701, brand Kappa DR, serial #PGU107683H). The pulse generator was placed deep within the subcutaneous tissue. The pacemaker pocket was sutured using 3–0 Vicryl. Steri-Strips were applied. Pressure dressing was applied.

The patient tolerated the entire procedure well and remained stable.

PULSE GENERATOR SETTINGS: The pacing mode is DDDR. The rate response is on. The lower rate limit is 60 beats per minute, and the upper rate limit is 120 beats per minute. The upper tracking rate is 120 beats per minute. Paced AV interval is 150 ms and sensed AV interval is 150 ms. Rate adaptive AV interval is off. Retrograde conduction is on. Atrial amplitude is set at 5 V with a pulse wave of 0.76 ms, a sensitivity of 0.18 mV, and a blanking period of 180 ms. Ventricular amplitude is set at 5 V, a pulse wave of 0.46 ms, a sensitivity of 1.4 mV, and a blanking period of 28 ms.

PERCUTANEOUS TRANSLUMINAL CORONARY ANGIOPLASTY OF THE LEFT ANTERIOR DESCENDING

TITLE OF PROCEDURE: Percutaneous transluminal coronary angioplasty (PTCA) of the left anterior descending (LAD).

PROCEDURE IN DETAIL: The patient was prepped and draped in the usual fashion. The left femoral artery was chosen because of recent cardiac catheterization from the right side with use of VasoSeal. A 7 French sheath was placed in the left femoral artery and 6 French in the left femoral vein over the wire with Seldinger technique. A diagnostic left coronary angiogram was performed, using a 6 French JL4 catheter, which was advanced over a wire to the left coronary ostium. It revealed no change in the mid-LAD lesion. A 7 French short-tip JL4 guide without side holes was then advanced to the left coronary ostium over the wire, after the regular-tip JL4 could not engage the left coronary ostium satisfactorily. A 0.014-inch Patriot wire with a Ranger 2.5 x 20-mm balloon was advanced as a unit in the guide. Heparin 10,000 units was given IV. Activated coagulation time before the procedure was 350 seconds. The wire was advanced across the lesion without difficulty, and initial PTCA was accomplished with a 2.5-mm Ranger balloon inflated to four atmospheres for 25 seconds and then six atmospheres for 60 seconds. Angiogram after this revealed less than 10% residual lesion, but in the left anterior oblique cranial view a nonocclusive dissection limited to the lesion with extravascular dye staining was noted. Therefore, a decision was made to proceed with stenting. A 2.5 x 16-mm NIR with SOX stent was advanced across the lesion and deployed at 11 atmospheres. A poststent angiogram revealed a 0% residual lesion, no evidence of dissection visible, TIMI-III flow, and the closing ACT was 335 seconds. There were no complications.

Common Terms by Procedure

Cardiac Catheterization

bifurcation
caliber
circumflex
concentric
coronary angiography
damping
30-degree view
end-diastolic pressure
femoral triangle
global hypokinesis
gradient
graft
heart catheterization
Hemaquet
hemostasis
internal mammary artery
Judkins technique
left anterior descending (LAD)
left anterior oblique (LAO)
left ventricle
luminal irregularity
multipurpose catheter
patent
pigtail catheter
posterior descending artery
   (PDA)
pullback
ramus
right anterior oblique (RAO)
saphenous vein
Seldinger technique
septal perforating branches
sinus rhythm
trifurcation
VasoSeal
ventricular systolic function
ventricularization
ventriculography

Cardiac Diagnostic Tests

axis
bigeminy
Cardiolite
cardioneurogenic syncope
color venous duplex
common femoral vein
compressible
deep vein thrombosis (DVT)
electrocardiogram
interval
metabolic equivalents (METS)
myocardial ischemia
paced rhythm
popliteal vein
premature beats
recovery phase
sinus rhythm
ST-segment depression
superficial femoral vein
tilt table

Coronary Artery Bypass Graft

anastomosis
antegrade
aortic arch
aortotomy
arrest
ascending aorta
atherosclerosis
atrium
backbled
bifurcation
bulldog clamp
calcification
cannula
catheter
chest tube

cold blood cardioplegia
coronary artery bypass graft (CABG)
cross-clamp
de-aired
end-to-side fashion
Ethibond suture
heparinized
internal jugular vein
lumen
mediastinum
pericardium
plaque
posterior descending artery (PDA)
posterior left ventricle
posterolateral branch
Prolene suture
protamine
pulmonary artery
reverse saphenous vein
saphenous vein
sternotomy
subcuticular
superior pulmonary vein
venotomy
vent
ventilation
Vicryl suture
volume status

diastolic compliance
echo
ejection fraction
embolus
free wall
hypertrophy
interrogation
interventricular
intimal
intraatrial septum
left-to-right shunting
mitral regurgitation
motion-mode (M-Mode)
oropharynx
paradoxical
pericardial effusion
probe
regional wall motion
septum
stenosis
thrombus
tortuous
transesophageal echocardiogram (TEE)
transgastric
trileaflet
two-dimensional (2-D)
vegetation
velocity
ventricular systolic function

Echocardiogram

aneurysm
anticoagulation
aortic insufficiency
aortic valve
ascending aorta
atherosclerosis
blind intubation
chamber
color Doppler
contrast bubble study
descending thoracic aorta

Fiberoptic Bronchoscopy with Endobronchial and Transbronchial Biopsies

arytenoid region
bronchial tree
brushings
carina
endobronchial
epiglottis
esophagus
false cords

fiberoptic
fluoroscopy
hilum
hypopharyngeal region
hypopharynx
landmarks
lingula
mucus
naris
obstructive apnea
orifice
phonate
Romazicon
stenosis
submucosal
supine position
trachea
transbronchial
Versed
vocal cords
washings

Left Chamberlain Procedure, Video-Assisted Thoracoscopy, Resection of Pulmonary Nodule

air leak
aortopulmonary window
blunt dissection
Bovie electrocoagulation
Chamberlain procedure
chest cavity
chest tube
decubitus position
double-lumen intubation
Endobag
endotracheal
extubation
fibrosis
frozen section
GIA 30 stapler

histiocytes
intercostal space
intubation
midaxillary
pectoralis
periosteum
pleura
Pleur-evac
sponge forceps
Surgilon suture
thoracic
thoracoscopy
trocar

Mitral Valve Replacement

activated coagulation time (ACT)
anulus
antegrade
anterior leaflet
aorta
atriotomy
Betadine scrub
calcification
cannula
CarboMedics valve
cardioplegia
cardiopulmonary bypass
centigrade
chordae tendineae
coaptation
commissure
cross-clamp
dopamine
electromechanical arrest
Ethibond suture
femoral vein
hemodynamics
heparin
horizontal mattress suture
hypothermia
iced slush solution

inferior vena cava
inotropic support
intraatrial septum
left ventricular (LV)
mediastinum
mitral regurgitation
mitral valve
myocardial infarction
papillary muscle
pericardium
pledget
posterior leaflet
Prolene suture
prosthetic valve
protamine
retractor
retrograde
sternal notch
subcutaneous tissue
superior vena cava
ventricular rupture
xiphoid

Pacemaker

amplitude
appendage
atrioventricular (AV)
balloon
bipolar
blanking period
blunt dissection
cannulation
capture
cardiac catheterization
conduction
dilator
dual chamber
endocardial
fluoroscopy
guidewire
hemodynamic

internal jugular vein
introducer sheath
lead
Medtronic
milliampere (mA)
millisecond (ms)
millivolt (mV)
ohm
paced AV interval
pacing mode
pocket
pulse generator
pulse wave
R wave
rate adaptive AV interval
rate response
resistance
screw-in lead
side port
stimulation threshold
subclavian vein
temporary pacemaker
tracking rate
transvenous
trapezius muscle

Percutaneous Transluminal Coronary Angioplasty (PTCA)

activated coagulation time (ACT)
angiogram
atmospheres
cranial view
dissection
extravascular
French guide
French sheath
heparin
left anterior descending (LAD)
left anterior oblique (LAO)
NIR with SOX
ostium

Patriot wire
Ranger balloon
Seldinger technique

stent
TIMI-III flow
VasoSeal

Appendix 7
Drugs by Indication

ACIDOSIS (METABOLIC)
Alkalinizing Agent
  Polycitra®-K
  potassium citrate and citric acid
  sodium acetate
  sodium bicarbonate
  sodium lactate
  THAM®
  THAM-E®
  tromethamine
Electrolyte Supplement, Oral
  Enemol™ (Can)
  Fleet® Phospho®-Soda [OTC]
  sodium phosphates

ACQUIRED IMMUNODEFICIENCY SYNDROME
Antiviral Agent
  Apo®-Zidovudine (Can)
  Combivir®
  Crixivan®
  delavirdine
  didanosine
  Epivir®
  Epivir®-HBV™
  Fortovase®
  Hivid®
  indinavir
  Invirase®
  lamivudine
  nelfinavir
  nevirapine
  Norvir®
  Novo-AZT® (Can)
  Rescriptor®
  Retrovir®
  ritonavir
  saquinavir
  stavudine
  3TC® (Can)
  Videx®
  Viracept®
  Viramune®
  zalcitabine
  Zerit®
  zidovudine
  zidovudine and lamivudine
Non-nucleoside Reverse Transcriptase Inhibitor
  efavirenz
  Sustiva™
Nucleoside Analog Reverse Transcriptase Inhibitor
  abacavir
  Ziagen™
Protease Inhibitor
  Agenerase™
  amprenavir
Reverse Transcriptase Inhibitor
  adefovir
  Preveon®

ACUTE CORONARY SYNDROME
Antiplatelet Agent
  Aggrastat®
  eptifibatide
  Integrilin®
  tirofiban

ADAMS-STOKES SYNDROME
Adrenergic Agonist Agent
  Adrenalin® Chloride
  epinephrine
  isoproterenol
  Isuprel®

ALKALOSIS
Electrolyte Supplement, Oral
  ammonium chloride
Vitamin, Water Soluble
  Cenolate®
  sodium ascorbate

ALLERGIC DISORDERS (NASAL)
Corticosteroid, Topical
  Nasacort®
  Nasacort® AQ
  triamcinolone (inhalation, nasal)
Mast Cell Stabilizer
  Crolom®
  cromolyn sodium
  Gastrocrom®
  Intal®
  Nasalcrom® [OTC]
  Novo-Cromolyn® (Can)
  PMS-Sodium Cromoglycate
    (Can)
  Rynacrom® (Can)

ANGINA
Beta-Adrenergic Blocker
  acebutolol
  Apo®-Atenol (Can)
  Apo-Metoprolol® (Can)
  Apo®-Nadol (Can)
  Apo®-Propranolol (Can)
  atenolol
  Betachron®
  Betaloc® (Can)
  Betaloc Durules® (Can)
  carvedilol
  Coreg®
  Corgard®
  Detensol® (Can)
  Inderal®
  Inderal® LA
  Lopressor®

  metoprolol
  Monitan® (Can)
  nadolol
  Novo-Atenol® (Can)
  Novo-Metoprolol® (Can)
  Nu-Atenol® (Can)
  Nu-Metop (Can)
  Nu-Propranolol® (Can)
  propranolol
  Rhotral® (Can)
  Sectral®
  Syn-Nadolol® (Can)
  Taro-Atenol® (Can)
  Tenormin®
  Toprol XL®
Calcium Channel Blocker
  Adalat®
  Adalat® CC
  Adalat PA® (Can)
  amlodipine
  Apo®-Diltiaz (Can)
  Apo®-Nifed (Can)
  Apo®-Verap (Can)
  Bapadin® (Can)
  bepridil
  Calan®
  Calan® SR
  Cardene®
  Cardene® SR
  Cardizem® CD
  Cardizem® Injectable
  Cardizem® SR
  Cardizem® Tablet
  Covera-HS®
  Dilacor XR®
  diltiazem
  felodipine
  Gen-Nifedipine (Can)
  Isoptin®
  Isoptin® SR
  nicardipine
  nifedipine

Norvasc®
Novo-Diltazem® (Can)
Novo-Nifedin® (Can)
Novo-Veramil® (Can)
Nu-Diltiaz® (Can)
Nu-Nifedin® (Can)
Nu-Verap® (Can)
Plendil®
Procardia®
Procardia XL®
Syn-Diltiazem® (Can)
Tiamate®
Tiazac®
Vascor®
verapamil
Verelan®
Vasodilator
  Amyl Nitrate Vaporole®
  amyl nitrite
  Amyl Nitrite Aspirols®
  Apo®-Dipyridamole FC (Can)
  Apo®-Dipyridamole SC (Can)
  Apo-ISDN® (Can)
  Asasantine® [with Aspirin also]
    (Can)
  Cardilate®
  Cedocard-SR® (Can)
  Coradur® (Can)
  Deponit® Patch
  Dilatrate®-SR
  dipyridamole
  Duotrate®
  erythrityl tetranitrate
  Imdur™
  Ismo®
  Isordil®
  isosorbide dinitrate
  isosorbide mononitrate
  Minitran® Patch
  Monoket®
  Nitro-Bid® I.V. Injection
  Nitro-Bid® Ointment

Nitrodisc® Patch
Nitro-Dur® Patch
Nitrogard® Buccal
nitroglycerin
Nitroglyn® Oral
Nitrolingual® Translingual Spray
Nitrol® Ointment
Nitrong® Oral Tablet
Nitrong® SR (Can)
Nitrostat® Sublingual
Novo-Dipiradol® (Can)
pentaerythritol tetranitrate
Peritrate®
Peritrate® SA
Persantine®
Sorbitrate®
Transdermal-NTG® Patch
Transderm-Nitro® Patch
Tridil® Injection

ANGIOEDEMA (HEREDITARY)
Anabolic Steroid
  stanozolol
  Winstrol®
Androgen
  Cyclomen® (Can)
  danazol
  Danocrine®

APNEA (NEONATAL IDIOPATHIC)
Theophylline Derivative
  aminophylline
  theophylline

ARRHYTHMIA
Adrenergic Agonist Agent
  isoproterenol
  Isuprel®
  methoxamine
  phenylephrine

Antiarrhythmic Agent, Class I
  Ethmozine®
  moricizine
Antiarrhythmic Agent, Class I-A
  Apo®-Procainamide (Can)
  Biquin® Durules® (Can)
  Cardioquin®
  disopyramide
  Norpace®
  Norpace® CR
  procainamide
  Procanbid™
  Procan™ SR (Can)
  Pronestyl®
  Pronestyl-SR®
  Quinaglute® Dura-Tabs®
  Quinalan®
  Quinidex® Extentabs®
  quinidine
  Quinora®
  Rythmodan®, -LA (Can)
Antiarrhythmic Agent, Class I-B
  Anestacon® Topical Solution
  Dilantin®
  Dilocaine® Injection
  Diphenylan Sodium®
  Duo-Trach® Injection
  lidocaine
  Lidodan® (Can)
  LidoPen® I.M. Injection Auto-Injector
  mexiletine
  Mexitil®
  Nervocaine® Injection
  phenytoin
  PMS-Lidocaine Viscous (Can)
  Solarcaine® Topical
  tocainide
  Tonocard®
  Tremytoine® (Can)
  Xylocaine® HCl I.V. Injection for
    Cardiac Arrhythmias
  Xylocaine® Oral

Xylocaine® Topical Ointment
Xylocaine® Topical Solution
Xylocaine® Topical Spray
Xylocard® (Can)
Antiarrhythmic Agent, Class I-C
  flecainide
  propafenone
  Rythmol®
  Tambocor™
Antiarrhythmic Agent, Class II
  acebutolol
  Apo®-Propranolol (Can)
  Betachron®
  Betapace®
  Brevibloc®
  Detensol® (Can)
  esmolol
  Inderal®
  Inderal® LA
  Monitan® (Can)
  Nu-Propranolol® (Can)
  propranolol
  Rhotral® (Can)
  Sectral®
  Sotacor® (Can)
  sotalol
Antiarrhythmic Agent, Class III
  amiodarone
  Betapace®
  Bretylate® (Can)
  bretylium
  Cordarone®
  Corvert®
  ibutilide
  Pacerone®
  Sotacor® (Can)
  sotalol
Antiarrhythmic Agent,
    Class IV
  Apo®-Verap (Can)
  Calan®
  Calan® SR

Covera-HS®
Isoptin®
Isoptin® SR
Novo-Veramil® (Can)
Nu-Verap® (Can)
verapamil
Verelan®
Antiarrhythmic Agent,
   Miscellaneous
  Adenocard®
  adenosine
  Crystodigin®
  Digitaline® (Can)
  digitoxin
  digoxin
  Lanoxicaps®
  Lanoxin®
  Novo-Digoxin® (Can)
Anticholinergic Agent
  Atropair®
  atropine
  Atropine-Care®
  Atropisol®
  Isopto® Atropine
  I-Tropine®
Calcium Channel Blocker
  Apo®-Diltiaz (Can)
  Cardizem® CD
  Cardizem® Injectable
  Cardizem® SR
  Cardizem® Tablet
  Dilacor XR®
  diltiazem
  Novo-Diltazem® (Can)
  Nu-Diltiaz® (Can)
  Syn-Diltiazem® (Can)
  Tiamate®
  Tiazac®
Cholinergic Agent
  edrophonium
  Enlon®
  Reversol®
  Tensilon®

Theophylline Derivative
  aminophylline
  Phyllocontin®
  Truphylline®

ARTHRITIS (SEE RHEUMATIC DISORDERS)

ASPERGILLOSIS
Antifungal Agent
  Abelcet™
  Amphotec®
  amphotericin B cholesteryl
    sulfate complex
  amphotericin B (conventional)
  amphotericin B (lipid complex)
  Ancobon®
  Ancotil® (Can)
  flucytosine
  Fungizone®
Antifungal Agent, Systemic
  AmBisome®
  amphotericin B (liposomal)

ASPIRATION PNEUMONITIS (SEE RESPIRATORY DISORDERS)

ASTHMA (SEE RESPIRATORY DISORDERS, CHRONIC OBSTRUCTIVE PULMONARY DISEASE)

ASTHMA (CORTICOSTEROID-DEPENDENT)
Macrolide (Antibiotic)
  Tao®
  troleandomycin

ASTHMA (DIAGNOSTIC)
Diagnostic Agent
  methacholine
  Provocholine®

ATELECTASIS
Expectorant
  Pima®
  potassium iodide
  SSKI®
  Thyro-Block®
Mucolytic Agent
  acetylcysteine
  Mucomyst®
  Mucosil™
  Parvolex® (Can)

BACTERIAL ENDOCARDITIS (PROPHYLAXIS)
Aminoglycoside (Antibiotic)
  Cidomycin® (Can)
  Garamycin®
  Garatec (Can)
  Genoptic®
  Gentacidin®
  Gent-AK®
  gentamicin
  Gentrasul®
  G-myticin®
  Jenamicin®
  Ocugram® (Can)
Antibiotic, Miscellaneous
  Cleocin HCl® Oral
  Cleocin Pediatric® Oral
  Cleocin Phosphate® Injection
  Cleocin® Vaginal
  clindamycin
  Lyphocin® Injection
  Vancocin® CP (Can)
  Vancocin® Injection
  Vancocin® Oral

Vancoled® Injection
vancomycin
Cephalosporin (First Generation)
  Apo®-Cephalex (Can)
  Biocef®
  cefadroxil
  Cefanex®
  cephalexin
  Duricef®
  Keflex®
  Keftab®
  Novo-Lexin® (Can)
  Nu-Cephalex® (Can)
  Zartan®
Macrolide (Antibiotic)
  azithromycin
  Biaxin™
  clarithromycin
  Zithromax™
Penicillin
  amoxicillin
  Amoxil®
  ampicillin
  Ampicin® (Can)
  Apo-Amoxi® (Can)
  Apo-Ampi® (Can)
  Apo®-Pen VK (Can)
  Beepen-VK®
  Jaa Amp® (Can)
  Marcillin®
  Nadopen-V® (Can)
  Novamoxin® (Can)
  Novo-Pen-VK® (Can)
  Nu-Amoxi (Can)
  Nu-Ampi (Can)
  Nu-Pen-VK® (Can)
  Omnipen®
  Omnipen®-N
  penicillin V potassium
  Pen-Vee® (Can)
  Pen-Vee® K
  Principen®
  Pro-Amox® (Can)

Pro-Ampi® (Can)
PVF® K (Can)
Taro-Ampicillin® (Can)
Totacillin®
Trimox®
Veetids®
Wymox®

BRONCHIECTASIS

Adrenergic Agonist Agent
Adrenalin® Chloride
Airet®
albuterol
Alupent®
Apo®-Salvent (Can)
Arm-a-Med® Isoproterenol
Arm-a-Med® Metaproterenol
AsthmaHaler® Mist [OTC]
AsthmaNefrin® [OTC]
Brethaire®
Brethine®
Bricanyl®
Bronitin® Mist [OTC]
Bronkaid® Mist [OTC]
Dey-Dose® Isoproterenol
Dey-Dose® Metaproterenol
ephedrine
epinephrine
isoproterenol
isoproterenol and phenylephrine
Isuprel®
Metaprel®
metaproterenol
microNefrin® [OTC]
Novo-Salmol® (Can)
Pretz-D® [OTC]
Primatene® Mist [OTC]
Prometa®
Proventil®
Proventil® HFA
Sabulin® (Can)
Sus-Phrine®
terbutaline

Vaponefrin® [OTC]
Ventolin®
Ventolin® Rotocaps®
Volmax® (Can)
Mucolytic Agent
acetylcysteine
Mucomyst®
Mucosil™
Parvolex® (Can)

BRONCHIOLITIS

Antiviral Agent
ribavirin
Virazole® Aerosol

BRONCHITIS

Adrenergic Agonist Agent
Adrenalin® Chloride
Airet®
albuterol
Apo®-Salvent (Can)
Arm-a-Med® Isoetharine
Arm-a-Med® Isoproterenol
AsthmaHaler® Mist [OTC]
AsthmaNefrin® [OTC]
Beta-2®
bitolterol
Bronitin® Mist [OTC]
Bronkaid® Mist [OTC]
Bronkometer®
Bronkosol®
Dey-Dose® Isoproterenol
Dey-Lute® Isoetharine
ephedrine
epinephrine
isoetharine
isoproterenol
Isuprel®
Medihaler-Iso®
microNefrin® [OTC]
Novo-Salmol® (Can)
Pretz-D® [OTC]
Primatene® Mist [OTC]

Proventil®
Proventil® HFA
Sabulin® (Can)
Sus-Phrine®
Tornalate®
Vaponefrin® [OTC]
Ventolin®
Ventolin® Rotocaps®
Volmax® (Can)
Antibiotic, Quinolone
  Raxar®
  trovafloxacin
  Trovan™
Cephalosporin (Third Generation)
  cefdinir
  Omnicef®
Mucolytic Agent
  acetylcysteine
  Mucomyst®
  Mucosil™
  Parvolex® (Can)
Theophylline Derivative
  Aerolate III®
  Aerolate JR®
  Aerolate SR®
  aminophylline
  Aquaphyllin®
  Asmalix®
  Bronchial®
  Dilor®
  dyphylline
  Elixomin®
  Elixophyllin®
  Glycerol-T®
  Lufyllin®
  oxtriphylline
  Phyllocontin®
  Quibron®
  Quibron®-T
  Quibron®-T/SR
  Respbid®
  Slo-bid™
  Slo-Phyllin®

Slo-Phyllin® GG
Sustaire®
Theo-24®
Theobid®
Theochron®
Theoclear-80®
Theoclear® L.A.
Theo-Dur®
Theolair™
theophylline
theophylline and guaifenesin
Theo-Sav®
Theospan®-SR
Theostat-80®
Theovent®
Theo-X®
T-Phyl®
Truphylline®
Uni-Dur®
Uniphyl®

BRONCHOSPASM

Adrenergic Agonist Agent
  Adrenalin® Chloride
  Airet®
  albuterol
  Alupent®
  Apo®-Salvent (Can)
  Arm-a-Med® Isoetharine
  Arm-a-Med® Isoproterenol
  Arm-a-Med® Metaproterenol
  AsthmaHaler® Mist [OTC]
  AsthmaNefrin® [OTC]
  Beta-2®
  bitolterol
  Brethaire®
  Brethine®
  Bricanyl®
  Bronitin® Mist [OTC]
  Bronkaid® Mist [OTC]
  Bronkometer®
  Bronkosol®
  Dey-Dose® Isoproterenol

Dey-Dose® Metaproterenol
Dey-Lute® Isoetharine
ephedrine
epinephrine
Foradil® (Can)
formoterol (Canada only)
isoetharine
isoproterenol
isoproterenol and phenylephrine
Isuprel®
levalbuterol
Maxair™ Inhalation Aerosol
Medihaler-Iso®
Metaprel®
metaproterenol
microNefrin® [OTC]
Novo-Salmol® (Can)
pirbuterol
Pretz-D® [OTC]
Primatene® Mist [OTC]
Prometa®
Proventil®
Proventil® HFA
Sabulin® (Can)
salmeterol
Serevent®
Serevent® Diskus®
Sus-Phrine®
terbutaline
Tornalate®
Vaponefrin® [OTC]
Ventolin®
Ventolin® Rotocaps®
Volmax® (Can)
Xopenex™
Anticholinergic Agent
 atropine
Beta2-Adrenergic Agonist Agent
 Foradil® (Can)
 formoterol (Canada only)
 levalbuterol
 Xopenex™
Bronchodilator

Foradil® (Can)
formoterol (Canada only)
levalbuterol
Xopenex™
Mast Cell Stabilizer
 Crolom®
 cromolyn sodium
 Gastrocrom®
 Intal®
 Novo-Cromolyn® (Can)
 PMS-Sodium Cromoglycate (Can)
 Rynacrom® (Can)
Theophylline Derivative
 Hydrophed®
 Marax®
 Tedral®
 theophylline, ephedrine, and
 hydroxyzine
 theophylline, ephedrine, and
 phenobarbital

CALCIUM CHANNEL BLOCKER TOXICITY
Electrolyte Supplement, Oral
 calcium gluceptate
 calcium gluconate
 Kalcinate®

CARCINOMA
Androgen
 Anabolin®
 Androderm® Transdermal System
 Android®
 Andro-L.A.® Injection
 Androlone®
 Androlone®-D
 Andropository® Injection
 bicalutamide
 Casodex®
 Deca-Durabolin®
 Delatest® Injection
 Delatestryl® Injection
 depAndro® Injection

Depotest® Injection
Depo®-Testosterone Injection
Duratest® Injection
Durathate® Injection
Everone® Injection
fluoxymesterone
Halotestin®
Histerone® Injection
Hybolin™ Decanoate
Hybolin™ Improved Injection
methyltestosterone
nandrolone
Neo-Durabolic
Oreton® Methyl
Tesamone® Injection
Teslac®
Testoderm® Transdermal System
testolactone
Testopel® Pellet
testosterone
Testred®
Virilon®
Antiandrogen
   Androcur® (Can)
   Androcur® Depot (Can)
   cyproterone (Canada only)
   Euflex® (Can)
   Eulexin®
   flutamide
Antineoplastic Agent
   Adriamycin PFS™
   Adriamycin RDF®
   Adrucil® Injection
   Alkaban-AQ®
   Alkeran®
   Alpha-Tamoxifen® (Can)
   altretamine
   aminoglutethimide
   Anandron® (Can)
   anastrozole
   Apo-Tamox® (Can)
   Arimidex®
   BiCNU®

Blenoxane®
bleomycin
Camptosar®
carboplatin
carmustine
CeeNU®
chlorambucil
cisplatin
Cosmegen®
cyclophosphamide
Cytadren®
cytarabine
Cytosar-U®
Cytoxan®
dacarbazine
dactinomycin
docetaxel
doxorubicin
Droxia™
DTIC-Dome®
Efudex® Topical
Emcyt®
estramustine
Etopophos®
etoposide
etoposide phosphate
Fareston®
floxuridine
Fludara® (Can)
Fluoroplex® Topical
fluorouracil
Folex® PFS
FUDR®
gemcitabine
Gemzar®
Herceptin®
Hexalen®
Hycamtin™
Hydrea®
hydroxyurea
Idamycin®
Idamycin® PFS
idarubicin

Ifex®
ifosfamide
irinotecan
Leukeran®
leuprolide acetate
lomustine
Lupron®
Lupron Depot®
Lupron Depot-3® Month
Lupron Depot-4® Month
Lupron Depot-Ped®
Lysodren®
mechlorethamine
Megace®
megestrol acetate
melphalan
methotrexate
Mithracin®
mitomycin
mitotane
mitoxantrone
Mustargen® Hydrochloride
Mutamycin®
Navelbine®
Neosar®
Nilandron™
nilutamide
Nolvadex®
Novantrone®
Novo-Tamoxifen (Can)
Oncovin®
paclitaxel
Paraplatin®
Paxene®
Photofrin®
Platinol®
Platinol®-AQ
plicamycin
porfimer
Procytox® (Can)
Rheumatrex®
Rubex®
streptozocin

Tamofen® (Can)
Tamone® (Can)
tamoxifen
Tarabine® PFS
Taxol®
Taxotere®
teniposide
Thioplex®
thiotepa
Toposar® Injection
topotecan
toremifene
trastuzumab
valrubicin
Valstar™
Velban®
Velbe® (Can)
VePesid®
vinblastine
Vincasar® PFS™
vincristine
vinorelbine
Vumon
Zanosar®
Antineoplastic Agent,
    Anthracycline
Ellence™
epirubicin
Antineoplastic Agent, Antibiotic
Ellence™
epirubicin
Antineoplastic Agent,
    Antimetabolite
capecitabine
Xeloda™
Antineoplastic Agent, Hormone
    (Antiestrogen)
Femara™
letrozole
Antineoplastic Agent,
    Miscellaneous
denileukin deftitox
Ontak®

Antiviral Agent
  interferon alfa-2b and ribavirin
    combination pack
  Rebetron™
Biological Response Modulator
  aldesleukin
  BCG vaccine
  ImmuCyst® (Can)
  interferon alfa-2b and ribavirin
    combination pack
  Pacis™ (Can)
  Proleukin®
  Rebetron™
  TheraCys®
  TICE® BCG
Diagnostic Agent
  pentagastrin
  Peptavlon®
Estrogen and Androgen Combination
  Estratest®
  Estratest® H.S.
  estrogens and methyltestosterone
  Premarin® With Methyltestosterone
Estrogen Derivative
  chlorotrianisene
  diethylstilbestrol
  estradiol
  estrogens, conjugated (equine)
  estrone
  polyestradiol
  Premarin®
  Stilphostrol®
  TACE®
Gonadotropin Releasing Hormone
    Analog
  goserelin
  Zoladex® Implant
Immune Modulator
  Ergamisol®
  levamisole
Progestin
  Amen® Oral
  Androcur® (Can)

Androcur® Depot (Can)
Crinone™
Curretab® Oral
Cycrin® Oral
cyproterone (Canada only)
Depo-Provera® Injection
hydroxyprogesterone caproate
Hylutin®
Hyprogest® 250
medroxyprogesterone acetate
PMS-Progesterone (Can)
Progestasert®
progesterone
Progesterone Oil (Can)
Provera® Oral
Somatostatin Analog
  octreotide
  Sandostatin®
  Sandostatin LAR®
Thyroid Product
  Armour® Thyroid
  Cytomel® Oral
  Eltroxin®
  Levo-T™
  Levothroid®
  levothyroxine
  Levoxyl®
  liothyronine
  liotrix
  PMS-Levothyroxine Sodium (Can)
  S-P-T
  Synthroid®
  Thyrar®
  thyroid
  Thyroid Strong®
  Thyrolar®
  Triostat™ Injection

CARDIAC DECOMPENSATION
Adrenergic Agonist Agent
  dobutamine
  Dobutrex®

CARDIOGENIC SHOCK

Adrenergic Agonist Agent
  dobutamine
  Dobutrex®
  dopamine
  Intropin®
Cardiac Glycoside
  Crystodigin®
  Digitaline® (Can)
  digitoxin
  digoxin
  Lanoxicaps®
  Lanoxin®
  Novo-Digoxin® (Can)

CARDIOMYOPATHY

Cardiovascular Agent, Other
  dexrazoxane
  Zinecard®

CHRONIC OBSTRUCTIVE PULMONARY DISEASE

Adrenergic Agonist Agent
  Airet®
  albuterol
  Alupent®
  Apo®-Salvent (Can)
  Arm-a-Med® Isoproterenol
  Arm-a-Med® Metaproterenol
  Dey-Dose® Isoproterenol
  Dey-Dose® Metaproterenol
  isoproterenol
  Isuprel®
  Medihaler-Iso®
  Metaprel®
  metaproterenol
  Novo-Salmol® (Can)
  Prometa®
  Proventil®
  Proventil® HFA
  Sabulin® (Can)
  Ventolin®
  Ventolin® Rotocaps®
  Volmax® (Can)
Anticholinergic Agent
  Atrovent®
  ipratropium
Bronchodilator
  Combivent®
  ipratropium and albuterol
Expectorant
  Pima®
  potassium iodide
  SSKI®
  Thyro-Block®
Theophylline Derivative
  Aerolate III®
  Aerolate JR®
  Aerolate SR®
  aminophylline
  Aquaphyllin®
  Asmalix®
  Bronchial®
  Dilor®
  dyphylline
  Elixomin®
  Elixophyllin®
  Glycerol-T®
  Lufyllin®
  Phyllocontin®
  Quibron®
  Quibron®-T
  Quibron®-T/SR
  Respbid®
  Slo-bid™
  Slo-Phyllin®
  Slo-Phyllin® GG
  Sustaire®
  Theo-24®
  Theobid®
  Theochron®
  Theoclear-80®
  Theoclear® L.A.
  Theo-Dur®
  Theolair™

theophylline
theophylline and guaifenesin
Theo-Sav®
Theospan®-SR
Theostat-80®
Theovent®
Theo-X®
T-Phyl®
Truphylline®
Uni-Dur®
Uniphyl®

CLAUDICATION (SEE ALSO INTERMITTENT CLAUDICATION)

Blood Viscosity Reducer Agent
  pentoxifylline
  Trental®

COCCIDIOIDOMYCOSIS

Antifungal Agent
  ketoconazole
  Nizoral®

CONGESTIVE HEART FAILURE

Adrenergic Agonist Agent
  amrinone
  dopamine
  Inocor®
  Intropin®
Alpha-Adrenergic Blocking Agent
  Apo®-Prazo (Can)
  Minipress®
  Novo-Prazin® (Can)
  Nu-Prazo® (Can)
  prazosin
Angiotensin-Converting Enzyme (ACE) Inhibitor
  Accupril®
  Altace™
  Apo®-Capto (Can)
  Apo®-Enalapril (Can)

Capoten®
captopril
cilazapril (Canada only)
enalapril
fosinopril
Inhibace® (Can)
lisinopril
Mavik®
Monopril®
Novo-Captopril® (Can)
Nu-Capto® (Can)
Prinivil®
quinapril
ramipril
Syn-Captopril® (Can)
trandolapril
Vasotec® I.V.
Vasotec® Oral
Zestril®
Beta-Adrenergic Blocker
  carvedilol
  Coreg®
Calcium Channel Blocker
  Bapadin® (Can)
  bepridil
  Vascor®
Cardiac Glycoside
  Crystodigin®
  Digitaline® (Can)
  digitoxin
  digoxin
  Lanoxicaps®
  Lanoxin®
  Novo-Digoxin® (Can)
Cardiovascular Agent, Other
  milrinone
  Primacor®
Diuretic, Loop
  Apo®-Furosemide (Can)
  bumetanide
  Bumex®
  Burinex® (Can)
  Demadex®

furosemide
Furoside® (Can)
Lasix®
Lasix® Special (Can)
Novo-Semide® (Can)
torsemide
Uritol® (Can)
Diuretic, Potassium Sparing
amiloride
Dyrenium®
Midamor®
triamterene
Vasodilator
Apo®-Hydralazine (Can)
Apresoline®
hydralazine
Nitro-Bid® I.V. Injection
nitroglycerin
Nitropress®
nitroprusside
Novo-Hylazin® (Can)
Nu-Hydral® (Can)
Tridil® Injection

CROUP
Adrenergic Agonist Agent
Adrenalin® Chloride
epinephrine

CYANIDE POISONING
Antidote
cyanide antidote kit
methylene blue
sodium thiosulfate
Vasodilator
Amyl Nitrate Vaporole®
amyl nitrite
Amyl Nitrite Aspirols®

CYSTIC FIBROSIS
Enzyme
dornase alfa
Pulmozyme®

CYTOMEGALOVIRUS
Antiviral Agent
cidofovir
Cytovene®
foscarnet
Foscavir®
ganciclovir
Vistide®
Vitrasert®
Antiviral Agent, Ophthalmic
fomivirsen
Vitravene™
Immune Globulin
CytoGam™
cytomegalovirus immune globulin
(intravenous-human)
Gamimune® N
Gammagard®
Gammagard® S/D
Gammar®-P I.V.
immune globulin, intravenous
Polygam® S/D
Sandoglobulin®
Venoglobulin®-I
Venoglobulin®-S

DEEP VEIN THROMBOSIS
Anticoagulant
ardeparin
Calcilean® [HepCalium] (Can)
Coumadin®
dalteparin
danaparoid
enoxaparin
Fragmin®
Hepalean®, -LOK, -LCO (Can)
heparin
Innohep® (Can)
Liquaemin®
Lovenox®
Normiflo®
Orgaran®

tinzaparin (Canada only)
warfarin
Warfilone® (Can)
Low Molecular Weight Heparin
　Fraxiparine® (Can)
　nadroparin (Canada only)

DEPRESSION (RESPIRATORY)
Respiratory Stimulant
　Dopram®
　doxapram

DIGITALIS GLYCOSIDE POISONING
Antidote
　Digibind®
　digoxin immune fab
Chelating Agent
　Chealamide®
　Disotate®
　edetate disodium
　Endrate®

DUCTUS ARTERIOSUS (CLOSURE)
Nonsteroidal Antiinflammatory
　　Drug (NSAID)
　Indocin® I.V. Injection
　indomethacin

DUCTUS ARTERIOSUS (TEMPORARY MAINTENANCE OF PATENCY)
Prostaglandin
　alprostadil
　Prostin VR Pediatric® Injection

EDEMA
Antihypertensive Agent, Combination
　Alazide®
　Aldactazide®

Aldoclor®
Aldoril®
Apo-Triazide® (Can)
Apresazide®
atenolol and chlorthalidone
benazepril and hydrochlorothiazide
Capozide®
captopril and hydrochlorothiazide
chlorothiazide and methyldopa
chlorothiazide and reserpine
clonidine and chlorthalidone
Combipres®
Dyazide®
enalapril and hydrochlorothiazide
Enduronyl®
Enduronyl® Forte
Eutron®
hydralazine and hydrochlorothiazide
hydralazine, hydrochlorothiazide, and
　reserpine
Hydrap-ES®
hydrochlorothiazide and reserpine
hydrochlorothiazide and
　spironolactone
hydrochlorothiazide and triamterene
hydroflumethiazide and reserpine
Hydropres®
Hydro-Serp®
Hydroserpine®
Hyzaar®
Inderide®
lisinopril and hydrochlorothiazide
losartan and hydrochlorothiazide
Lotensin® HCT
Marpres®
Maxzide®
methyclothiazide and deserpidine
methyclothiazide and pargyline
methyldopa and hydrochlorothiazide
Minizide®
Novo-Triamzide (Can)
Nu-Triazide (Can)
prazosin and polythiazide

Prinzide®
propranolol and
  hydrochlorothiazide
Salutensin®
Ser-Ap-Es®
Spironazide®
Spirozide®
Tenoretic®
Vaseretic® 10–25
Zestoretic®
Diuretic, Combination
  amiloride and hydrochlorothiazide
  Moduretic®
Diuretic, Loop
  Apo®-Furosemide (Can)
  bumetanide
  Bumex®
  Burinex® (Can)
  Demadex®
  Edecrin®
  ethacrynic acid
  furosemide
  Furoside® (Can)
  Lasix®
  Lasix® Special (Can)
  Novo-Semide® (Can)
  torsemide
  Uritol® (Can)
Diuretic, Miscellaneous
  Apo-Chlorthalidone® (Can)
  caffeine and sodium benzoate
  chlorthalidone
  Hygroton®
  indapamide
  Lozide® (Can)
  Lozol®
  metolazone
  Mykrox®
  Novo-Thalidone® (Can)
  Thalitone®
  Uridon® (Can)
  Zaroxolyn®

Diuretic, Osmotic
  mannitol
  Osmitrol® Injection
Diuretic, Potassium Sparing
  Aldactone®
  amiloride
  Dyrenium®
  Midamor®
  Novo-Spiroton® (Can)
  spironolactone
  triamterene
Diuretic, Thiazide
  Apo®-Hydro (Can)
  Aquatensen®
  bendroflumethiazide
  chlorothiazide
  Diucardin®
  Diuchlor® (Can)
  Diurigen®
  Diuril®
  Enduron®
  Esidrix®
  Ezide®
  hydrochlorothiazide
  HydroDIURIL®
  hydroflumethiazide
  Hydromox®
  Hydro-Par®
  Metahydrin®
  methyclothiazide
  Microzide®
  Naqua®
  Naturetin®
  Neo-Codema® (Can)
  Novo-Hydrazide® (Can)
  Oretic®
  polythiazide
  quinethazone
  Renese®
  Saluron®
  trichlormethiazide
  Urozide® (Can)

EMBOLISM

Anticoagulant
  Calcilean® [HepCalium] (Can)
  Coumadin®
  dicumarol
  enoxaparin
  Hepalean®, -LOK, -LCO (Can)
  heparin
  Innohep® (Can)
  Liquaemin®
  Lovenox®
  tinzaparin (Canada only)
  warfarin
  Warfilone® (Can)
Antiplatelet Agent
  Anacin® [OTC]
  Apo®-ASA (Can)
  Apo®-Dipyridamole FC (Can)
  Apo®-Dipyridamole SC (Can)
  A.S.A. [OTC]
  ASA® (Can)
  Asaphen (Can)
  Asasantine® [with Aspirin also]
    (Can)
  Ascriptin® [OTC]
  aspirin
  Bayer® Aspirin [OTC]
  Bufferin® [OTC]
  dipyridamole
  Easprin®
  Ecotrin® [OTC]
  Empirin® [OTC]
  Entrophen® (Can)
  Halfprin® [OTC]
  Measurin® [OTC]
  MSD® Enteric Coated ASA (Can)
  Novasen (Can)
  Novo-Dipiradol® (Can)
  Persantine®
  ZORprin®
Thrombolytic Agent
  Abbokinase®
  Activase®
  alteplase
  anistreplase
  Eminase®
  Kabikinase®
  Lysatec-rt-PA® (Can)
  Retavase™
  reteplase
  Streptase®
  streptokinase
  urokinase

EMPHYSEMA

Adrenergic Agonist Agent
  Adrenalin® Chloride
  Airet®
  albuterol
  Alupent®
  Apo®-Salvent (Can)
  Arm-a-Med® Isoproterenol
  Arm-a-Med® Metaproterenol
  AsthmaHaler® Mist [OTC]
  AsthmaNefrin® [OTC]
  bitolterol
  Brethaire®
  Brethine®
  Bricanyl®
  Bronitin® Mist [OTC]
  Bronkaid® Mist [OTC]
  Dey-Dose® Isoproterenol
  Dey-Dose® Metaproterenol
  ephedrine
  epinephrine
  isoproterenol
  isoproterenol and phenylephrine
  Isuprel®
  Medihaler-Iso®
  Metaprel®
  metaproterenol
  microNefrin® [OTC]
  Novo-Salmol® (Can)
  Primatene® Mist [OTC]

Prometa®
Proventil®
Proventil® HFA
Sabulin® (Can)
Sus-Phrine®
terbutaline
Tornalate®
Vaponefrin® [OTC]
Ventolin®
Ventolin® Rotocaps®
Volmax® (Can)
Anticholinergic Agent
  Atrovent®
  ipratropium
Expectorant
  Pima®
  potassium iodide
  SSKI®
  Thyro-Block®
Mucolytic Agent
  acetylcysteine
  Mucomyst®
  Mucosil™
  Parvolex® (Can)
Theophylline Derivative
  Aerolate III®
  Aerolate JR®
  Aerolate SR®
  aminophylline
  Aquaphyllin®
  Asmalix®
  Bronchial®
  Dilor®
  dyphylline
  Elixomin®
  Elixophyllin®
  Glycerol-T®
  Lufyllin®
  oxtriphylline
  Phyllocontin®
  Quibron®
  Quibron®-T
  Quibron®-T/SR

Respbid®
Slo-bid™
Slo-Phyllin®
Slo-Phyllin® GG
Sustaire®
Theo-24®
Theobid®
Theochron®
Theoclear-80®
Theoclear® L.A.
Theo-Dur®
Theolair™
theophylline
theophylline and guaifenesin
Theo-Sav®
Theospan®-SR
Theostat-80®
Theovent®
Theo-X®
T-Phyl®
Truphylline®
Uni-Dur®
Uniphyl®

ENDOCARDITIS TREATMENT

Aminoglycoside (Antibiotic)
  amikacin
  Amikin®
  Cidomycin® (Can)
  Garamycin®
  Garatec (Can)
  gentamicin
  Jenamicin®
  Nebcin® Injection
  netilmicin
  Netromycin®
  Ocugram® (Can)
  tobramycin
Antibiotic, Miscellaneous
  Lyphocin® Injection
  Vancocin® CP (Can)
  Vancocin® Injection

Vancocin® Oral
Vancoled® Injection
vancomycin
Antibiotic, Penicillin
pivampicillin (Canada only)
Pondocillin® (Can)
Antifungal Agent
amphotericin b (conventional)
Fungizone®
Cephalosporin (First Generation)
Ancef®
Cefadyl®
cefazolin
cephalothin
cephapirin
Ceporacin® (Can)
Kefzol®
Zolicef®
Penicillin
ampicillin
Ampicin® (Can)
Apo-Ampi® (Can)
Jaa Amp® (Can)
Marcillin®
nafcillin
Nallpen®
Nu-Ampi (Can)
Omnipen®
Omnipen®-N
oxacillin
penicillin G, parenteral, aqueous
Pfizerpen®
Principen®
Pro-Ampi® (Can)
Taro-Ampicillin® (Can)
Totacillin®
Quinolone
Cipro®
ciprofloxacin

EXTRAVASATION
Alpha-Adrenergic Blocking Agent
phentolamine

Regitine®
Rogitine® (Can)
Antidote
hyaluronidase
sodium thiosulfate
Wydase®

FIBRILLATION (SEE ARRHYTHMIAS)

GAG REFLEX SUPPRESSION
Analgesic, Topical
Anestacon® Topical Solution
lidocaine
PMS-Lidocaine Viscous (Can)
Local Anesthetic
Americaine® [OTC]
benzocaine
benzocaine, butyl aminobenzoate, tetracaine, and benzalkonium chloride
Cetacaine®
dyclonine
Hurricaine®
Pontocaine®
tetracaine

HEART BLOCK
Adrenergic Agonist Agent
Adrenalin® Chloride
epinephrine
isoproterenol
Isuprel®

HEAT PROSTRATION
Electrolyte Supplement, Oral
sodium chloride

HEPARIN-INDUCED THROMBOCYTOPENIA
Anticoagulant
ancrod
Viprinex® (Can)

HEPARIN POISONING
Antidote
    protamine sulfate

HICCUPS
Phenothiazine Derivative
    Apo®-Chlorpromazine (Can)
    Chlorpromanyl® (Can)
    chlorpromazine
    Chlorprom® (Can)
    Largactil® (Can)
    Novo-Chlorpromazine® (Can)
    Ormazine®
    Thorazine®
    triflupromazine
    Vesprin®

HIV (SEE ACQUIRED IMMUNODEFICIENCY SYNDROME)

HYPERTENSION
Adrenergic Agonist Agent
    amrinone
    Inocor®
Alpha-Adrenergic Agonist
    Apo®-Clonidine (Can)
    Apo-Guanethidine® (Can)
    Catapres® Oral
    Catapres-TTS® Transdermal
    clonidine
    Dixarit® (Can)
    Duraclon™ Injection
    guanabenz
    guanadrel
    guanethidine
    guanfacine
    Hylorel®
    Ismelin®
    Novo-Clonidine® (Can)
    Nu-Clonidine® (Can)
    Tenex®
    Wytensin®

Alpha-Adrenergic Blocking Agent
    Aldomet®
    Apo®-Methyldopa (Can)
    Apo®-Prazo (Can)
    Cardura®
    Dibenzyline®
    Dopamet® (Can)
    doxazosin
    Hytrin®
    Medimet® (Can)
    methyldopa
    Minipress®
    Novo-Medopa® (Can)
    Novo-Prazin® (Can)
    Nu-Medopa® (Can)
    Nu-Prazo® (Can)
    phenoxybenzamine
    phentolamine
    prazosin
    Priscoline®
    Regitine®
    Rogitine® (Can)
    terazosin
    tolazoline
Alpha-/Beta- Adrenergic Blocker
    labetalol
    Normodyne®
    Trandate®
Angiotensin-Converting Enzyme (ACE) Inhibitor
    Accupril®
    Accuretic® (Can)
    Altace™
    Apo®-Capto (Can)
    Apo®-Enalapril (Can)
    benazepril
    Capoten®
    captopril
    cilazapril (Canada only)
    enalapril
    fosinopril
    Inhibace® (Can)
    lisinopril

Lotensin®
Mavik®
moexipril
moexipril and hydrochlorothiazide
Monopril®
Novo-Captopril® (Can)
Nu-Capto® (Can)
Prinivil®
quinapril
quinapril and hydrochlorothiazide
  (Canada only)
ramipril
Renormax®
spirapril
Syn-Captopril® (Can)
trandolapril
Uniretic™
Univasc®
Vasotec® I.V.
Vasotec® Oral
Zestril®
Angiotensin II Antagonist
Atacand™
Avapro®
candesartan
Cozaar®
Diovan™
Diovan HCTZ™
irbesartan
losartan
Micardis®
telmisartan
valsartan
valsartan and hydrochlorothiazide
Antihypertensive Agent, Combination
Alazide®
Aldactazide®
Aldoclor®
Aldoril®
amlodipine and benazepril
Apo-Triazide® (Can)
Apresazide®
atenolol and chlorthalidone

Avapro® HCT
benazepril and hydrochlorothiazide
bisoprolol and hydrochlorothiazide
Capozide®
captopril and hydrochlorothiazide
chlorothiazide and methyldopa
chlorothiazide and reserpine
clonidine and chlorthalidone
Combipres®
Dyazide®
enalapril and diltiazem
enalapril and felodipine
enalapril and hydrochlorothiazide
Enduronyl®
Enduronyl® Forte
Eutron®
hydralazine and hydrochlorothiazide
hydralazine, hydrochlorothiazide, and
  reserpine
Hydrap-ES®
hydrochlorothiazide and reserpine
hydrochlorothiazide and
  spironolactone
hydrochlorothiazide and triamterene
hydroflumethiazide and reserpine
Hydropres®
Hydro-Serp®
Hydroserpine®
Hyzaar®
Inderide®
irbesartan and hydrochlorothiazide
Lexxel™
lisinopril and hydrochlorothiazide
losartan and hydrochlorothiazide
Lotensin® HCT
Lotrel®
Marpres®
Maxzide®
methyclothiazide and deserpidine
methyclothiazide and pargyline
methyldopa and hydrochlorothiazide
Minizide®
Novo-Triamzide (Can)

Nu-Triazide (Can)
prazosin and polythiazide
Prinzide®
propranolol and hydrochlorothiazide
Salutensin®
Ser-Ap-Es®
Spironazide®
Spirozide®
Tarka®
Teczem®
Tenoretic®
trandolapril and verapamil
Vaseretic® 10–25
Zestoretic®
Ziac™
Beta-Adrenergic Blocker
acebutolol
Apo®-Atenol (Can)
Apo-Metoprolol® (Can)
Apo®-Nadol (Can)
Apo-Pindol® (Can)
Apo®-Propranolol (Can)
Apo®-Timol (Can)
Apo®-Timop (Can)
atenolol
Betachron®
Betaloc® (Can)
Betaloc Durules® (Can)
Beta-Tim® (Can)
betaxolol
Betoptic® Ophthalmic
Betoptic® S Ophthalmic
bisoprolol
Blocadren® Oral
Brevibloc®
carteolol
Cartrol® Oral
carvedilol
Coreg®
Corgard®
Detensol® (Can)
esmolol
Gen-Pindolol (Can)

Gen-Timolol® (Can)
Inderal®
Inderal® LA
Kerlone® Oral
Lopressor®
metoprolol
Monitan® (Can)
nadolol
Novo-Atenol® (Can)
Novo-Metoprolol® (Can)
Novo-Pindol (Can)
Novo-Timol® (Can)
Nu-Atenol® (Can)
Nu-Metop (Can)
Nu-Pindol (Can)
Nu-Propranolol® (Can)
Nu-Timolol® (Can)
Ocupress® Ophthalmic
oxprenolol (Canada only)
pindolol
propranolol
Rhotral® (Can)
Sectral®
Syn-Nadolol® (Can)
Syn-Pindol® (Can)
Taro-Atenol® (Can)
Tenormin®
Tim-AK (Can)
timolol
Timoptic® Ophthalmic
Timoptic-XE® Ophthalmic
Toprol XL®
Trasicor® (Can)
Visken®
Zebeta®
Calcium Channel Blocker
Adalat®
Adalat® CC
Adalat PA® (Can)
amlodipine
Apo®-Nifed (Can)
Apo®-Verap (Can)
Bapadin® (Can)

bepridil
Calan®
Calan® SR
Cardene®
Cardene® SR
Covera-HS®
DynaCirc®
felodipine
Gen-Nifedipine (Can)
Isoptin®
Isoptin® SR
isradipine
nicardipine
nifedipine
nisoldipine
Norvasc®
Novo-Nifedin® (Can)
Novo-Veramil® (Can)
Nu-Nifedin® (Can)
Nu-Verap® (Can)
Plendil®
Procardia®
Procardia XL®
Sular®
Vascor®
verapamil
Verelan®
Diuretic, Combination
   amiloride and hydrochlorothiazide
   Moduretic®
Diuretic, Loop
   Apo®-Furosemide (Can)
   bumetanide
   Bumex®
   Burinex® (Can)
   Demadex®
   Edecrin®
   ethacrynic acid
   furosemide
   Furoside® (Can)
   Lasix®
   Lasix® Special (Can)
   Novo-Semide® (Can)

torsemide
Uritol® (Can)
Diuretic, Miscellaneous
   Apo-Chlorthalidone® (Can)
   chlorthalidone
   Hygroton®
   indapamide
   Lozide® (Can)
   Lozol®
   metolazone
   Mykrox®
   Novo-Thalidone® (Can)
   Thalitone®
   Uridon® (Can)
   Zaroxolyn®
Diuretic, Potassium Sparing
   Aldactone®
   Dyrenium®
   Novo-Spiroton® (Can)
   spironolactone
   triamterene
Diuretic, Thiazide
   Accuretic® (Can)
   Apo®-Hydro (Can)
   Aquatensen®
   bendroflumethiazide
   benzthiazide
   chlorothiazide
   Diovan HCTZ™
   Diucardin®
   Diuchlor® (Can)
   Diurigen®
   Diuril®
   Enduron®
   Esidrix®
   Exna®
   Ezide®
   hydrochlorothiazide
   HydroDIURIL®
   hydroflumethiazide
   Hydromox®
   Hydro-Par®
   Metahydrin®

methyclothiazide
Microzide®
moexipril and hydrochlorothiazide
Naqua®
Naturetin®
Neo-Codema® (Can)
Novo-Hydrazide® (Can)
Oretic®
polythiazide
quinapril and hydrochlorothiazide
 (Canada only)
quinethazone
Renese®
Saluron®
trichlormethiazide
Uniretic™
Urozide® (Can)
valsartan and hydrochlorothiazide
Ganglionic Blocking Agent
 Inversine®
 mecamylamine
Miscellaneous Product
 Aceon®
 Coversyl® (Can)
 perindopril erbumine
Rauwolfia Alkaloid
 Novo-Reserpine® (Can)
 Raudixin®
 Rauverid®
 rauwolfia serpentina
 reserpine
 Serpalan®
 Wolfina®
Vasodilator
 Apo®-Gain (Can)
 Apo®-Hydralazine (Can)
 Apresoline®
 diazoxide
 Gen-Minoxidil (Can)
 hydralazine
 Hyperstat® I.V.
 Loniten® Oral
 minoxidil

Minoxigaine™ (Can)
Nitropress®
nitroprusside
Novo-Hylazin® (Can)
Nu-Hydral® (Can)
Proglycem® Oral
Rogaine® Topical

HYPERTENSION (ARTERIAL)
Beta-Adrenergic Blocker
 Levatol®
 penbutolol

HYPERTENSION (CEREBRAL)
Barbiturate
 Pentothal® Sodium
 thiopental
Diuretic, Osmotic
 Amino-Cerv™ Vaginal
  Cream
 Aquacare® Topical [OTC]
 Carmol® Topical [OTC]
 Gormel® Creme [OTC]
 Lanaphilic® Topical [OTC]
 mannitol
 Nutraplus® Topical [OTC]
 Onyvul® (Can)
 Osmitrol® Injection
 Rea-Lo® [OTC]
 Resectisol® Irrigation Solution
 Ultra Mide® Topical
 urea
 Ureacin®-20 Topical [OTC]
 Ureaphil® Injection
 Uremol® (Can)
 Urisec® (Can)
 Velvelan® (Can)

HYPERTENSION (CORONARY)
Vasodilator
 Nitro-Bid® I.V. Injection

nitroglycerin
Tridil® Injection

HYPERTENSION (EMERGENCY)
Antihypertensive Agent
Corlopam®
fenoldopam

HYPERTROPHIC CARDIOMYOPATHY
Calcium Channel Blocker
Adalat®
Adalat® CC
Adalat PA® (Can)
Apo®-Nifed (Can)
Gen-Nifedipine (Can)
nifedipine
Novo-Nifedin® (Can)
Nu-Nifedin® (Can)
Procardia®
Procardia XL®

HYPOTENSION
Adrenergic Agonist Agent
Adrenalin® Chloride
dopamine
ephedrine
epinephrine
Intropin®
isoproterenol
Isuprel®
mephentermine
metaraminol
methoxamine
norepinephrine
Wyamine® Sulfate

HYPOTENSION (ORTHOSTATIC)
Adrenergic Agonist Agent
ephedrine
phenylephrine
Alpha-Adrenergic Agonist

midodrine
ProAmatine
Central Nervous System Stimulant, Nonamphetamine
methylphenidate
PMS-Methylphenidate (Can)
Ritalin®
Ritalin-SR®

IDIOPATHIC APNEA OF PREMATURITY
Respiratory Stimulant
caffeine, citrated

INFLUENZA
Antiviral Agent
amantadine
Endantadine™ (Can)
PMS-Amantadine (Can)
Symadine®
Symmetrel®
Antiviral Agent, Inhalation Therapy
Relenza®
zanamivir
Antiviral Agent, Oral
oseltamivir
Tamiflu™

INFLUENZA A
Antiviral Agent
amantadine
Endantadine™ (Can)
Flumadine®
PMS-Amantadine (Can)
rimantadine
Symadine®
Symmetrel®

INFLUENZA VIRUS
Antiviral Agent
Flumadine®
rimantadine
Vaccine, Inactivated Virus
Fluogen®

Fluviral® (Can)
Fluzone®
influenza virus vaccine

INTERMITTENT CLAUDICATION
Platelet Aggregation Inhibitor
  cilostazol
  Pletal®

ISCHEMIA
Blood Viscosity Reducer Agent
  pentoxifylline
  Trental®
Platelet Aggregation Inhibitor
  abciximab
  ReoPro®
Vasodilator
  ethaverine
  Genabid®
  papaverine
  Pavabid®
  Pavatine®

KETOSIS (SEE ACIDOSIS)

MALIGNANT EFFUSIONS
Antineoplastic Agent
  Thioplex®
  thiotepa

MENINGITIS (TUBERCULOUS)
Antibiotic, Aminoglycoside
  streptomycin
Antitubercular Agent
  streptomycin

MITRAL VALVE PROLAPSE
Beta-Adrenergic Blocker
  Apo®-Propranolol (Can)

Betachron®
Detensol® (Can)
Inderal®
Inderal® LA
Nu-Propranolol® (Can)
propranolol

MYOCARDIAL INFARCTION
Anticoagulant
  Calcilean® [HepCalium] (Can)
  Coumadin®
  enoxaparin
  Hepalean®, -LOK, -LCO (Can)
  heparin
  Hep-Lock®
  Liquaemin®
  Lovenox®
  warfarin
  Warfilone® (Can)
Antiplatelet Agent
  Anacin® [OTC]
  Apo®-ASA (Can)
  Apo®-Dipyridamole FC (Can)
  Apo®-Dipyridamole SC (Can)
  A.S.A. [OTC]
  ASA® (Can)
  Asaphen (Can)
  Asasantine® [with Aspirin also] (Can)
  Ascriptin® [OTC]
  aspirin
  Bayer® Aspirin [OTC]
  Bufferin® [OTC]
  clopidogrel
  dipyridamole
  Easprin®
  Ecotrin® [OTC]
  Empirin® [OTC]
  Entrophen® (Can)
  Halfprin® [OTC]
  Measurin® [OTC]

MSD® Enteric Coated ASA (Can)
Novasen (Can)
Novo-Dipiradol® (Can)
Persantine®
Plavix®
ZORprin®
Beta-Adrenergic Blocker
  Apo®-Atenol (Can)
  Apo-Metoprolol® (Can)
  Apo®-Nadol (Can)
  Apo®-Propranolol (Can)
  Apo®-Timol (Can)
  Apo®-Timop (Can)
  atenolol
  Betachron®
  Betaloc® (Can)
  Betaloc Durules® (Can)
  Beta-Tim® (Can)
  Blocadren® Oral
  Corgard®
  Detensol® (Can)
  Gen-Timolol® (Can)
  Inderal®
  Inderal® LA
  Lopressor®
  metoprolol
  nadolol
  Novo-Atenol® (Can)
  Novo-Metoprolol® (Can)
  Novo-Timol® (Can)
  Nu-Atenol® (Can)
  Nu-Metop (Can)
  Nu-Propranolol® (Can)
  Nu-Timolol® (Can)
  propranolol
  Syn-Nadolol® (Can)
  Taro-Atenol® (Can)
  Tenormin®
  Tim-AK (Can)
  timolol
  Timoptic® Ophthalmic
  Timoptic-XE® Ophthalmic

Toprol XL®
Thrombolytic Agent
  Activase®
  alteplase
  anistreplase
  Eminase®
  Kabikinase®
  Lysatec-rt-PA® (Can)
  Retavase™
  reteplase
  Streptase®
  streptokinase

MYOCARDIAL REINFARCTION

Antiplatelet Agent
  Anacin® [OTC]
  Apo®-ASA (Can)
  Apo®-Dipyridamole FC (Can)
  Apo®-Dipyridamole SC (Can)
  A.S.A. [OTC]
  ASA® (Can)
  Asaphen (Can)
  Asasantine® (Can)
  Asasantine® [with Aspirin also]
    (Can)
  Ascriptin® [OTC]
  aspirin
  Bayer® Aspirin [OTC]
  Bufferin® [OTC]
  dipyridamole
  dipyridamole and aspirin (Canada
    only)
  Easprin®
  Ecotrin® [OTC]
  Empirin® [OTC]
  Entrophen® (Can)
  Halfprin® [OTC]
  Measurin® [OTC]
  MSD® Enteric Coated ASA (Can)
  Novasen (Can)
  Novo-Dipiradol® (Can)

Persantine®
ZORprin®
Beta-Adrenergic Blocker
  Apo-Metoprolol® (Can)
  Apo®-Propranolol (Can)
  Apo®-Timol (Can)
  Apo®-Timop (Can)
  Betachron®
  Betaloc® (Can)
  Betaloc Durules® (Can)
  Beta-Tim® (Can)
  Blocadren® Oral
  Detensol® (Can)
  Gen-Timolol® (Can)
  Inderal®
  Inderal® LA
  Lopressor®
  metoprolol
  Novo-Metoprolol® (Can)
  Novo-Timol® (Can)
  Nu-Metop (Can)
  Nu-Propranolol® (Can)
  Nu-Timolol® (Can)
  propranolol
  Tim-AK (Can)
  timolol
  Timoptic® Ophthalmic
  Timoptic-XE® Ophthalmic
  Toprol XL®

PARACOCCIDIOIDO-MYCOSIS

Antifungal Agent
  ketoconazole
  Nizoral®

PERIPHERAL VASCULAR DISEASE

Vasodilator, Peripheral
  cyclandelate

PERIPHERAL VASOSPASTIC DISORDERS

Alpha-Adrenergic Blocking Agent

Priscoline®
tolazoline

PERSISTENT PULMONARY HYPERTENSION OF THE NEWBORN (PPHN)

Alpha-Adrenergic Blocking Agent
  Priscoline®
  tolazoline

PLAGUE

Antibiotic, Aminoglycoside
  streptomycin

PNEUMOCYSTIS CARINII

Antibiotic, Miscellaneous
  Neutrexin®
  Proloprim®
  trimethoprim
  trimetrexate glucuronate
  Trimpex®
Antiprotozoal
  atovaquone
  Mepron™
  NebuPent™ Inhalation
  Pentacarinat® Injection
  Pentam-300® Injection
  pentamidine
Sulfonamide
  Apo®-Sulfatrim (Can)
  Bactrim™
  Bactrim™ DS
  Cotrim®
  Cotrim® DS
  co-trimoxazole
  Novo-Trimel® (Can)
  Nu-Cotrimox® (Can)
  Pro-Trin® (Can)
  Roubac® (Can)
  Septra®
  Septra® DS
  Sulfamethoprim®
  Sulfatrim®
  Sulfatrim® DS

Trisulfa® (Can)
Trisulfa-S® (Can)
Uroplus® DS
Uroplus® SS
Sulfone
  Avlosulfon®
  dapsone

PNEUMONIA

Aminoglycoside (Antibiotic)
  amikacin
  Amikin®
  Cidomycin® (Can)
  Garamycin®
  Garatec (Can)
  Gent-AK®
  gentamicin
  Gentrasul®
  G-myticin®
  Nebcin® Injection
  netilmicin
  Netromycin®
  Ocugram® (Can)
  TOBI™ Inhalation Solution
  tobramycin
Antibiotic, Miscellaneous
  Azactam®
  aztreonam
  Cleocin HCl® Oral
  Cleocin Pediatric® Oral
  Cleocin Phosphate® Injection
  clindamycin
  Lyphocin® Injection
  Vancocin® CP (Can)
  Vancocin® Injection
  Vancocin® Oral
  Vancoled® Injection
  vancomycin
Antibiotic, Penicillin
  pivampicillin (Canada only)
  Pondocillin® (Can)
Antibiotic, Quinolone
  Raxar®

Carbapenem (Antibiotic)
  imipenem and cilastatin
  meropenem
  Merrem® I.V.
  Primaxin®
Cephalosporin (First Generation)
  Ancef®
  Apo®-Cephalex (Can)
  Biocef®
  cefadroxil
  Cefadyl®
  Cefanex®
  cefazolin
  cephalexin
  cephalothin
  cephapirin
  cephradine
  Ceporacin® (Can)
  Duricef®
  Keflex®
  Keftab®
  Kefzol®
  Novo-Lexin® (Can)
  Nu-Cephalex® (Can)
  Velosef®
  Zartan®
  Zolicef®
Cephalosporin (Second Generation)
  Cefotan®
  cefotetan
  cefoxitin
  cefpodoxime
  cefprozil
  Ceftin® Oral
  cefuroxime
  Cefzil®
  Kefurox® Injection
  Mefoxin®
  Vantin®
  Zinacef® Injection
Cephalosporin (Third Generation)
  cefdinir
  cefixime

Cefizox®
Cefobid®
cefoperazone
cefotaxime
ceftazidime
ceftizoxime
ceftriaxone
Ceptaz™
Claforan®
Fortaz®
Omnicef®
Rocephin®
Suprax®
Tazicef®
Tazidime®
Cephalosporin (Fourth Generation)
  cefepime
  Maxipime®
Macrolide (Antibiotic)
  Apo®-Erythro E-C (Can)
  azithromycin
  Biaxin™
  clarithromycin
  Diomycin (Can)
  dirithromycin
  Dynabac®
  E.E.S.®
  E.E.S.® Chewable
  E.E.S.® Granules
  E-Mycin®
  E-Mycin-E®
  Erybid™ (Can)
  Eryc®
  Ery-Tab®
  Erythro-Base® (Can)
  Erythrocin®
  erythromycin (systemic)
  Ilosone®
  Ilosone® Pulvules®
  Ilotycin®
  Ilotycin® (Can)
  Novo-Rythro Encap (Can)
  PCE®

PMS-Erythromycin (Can)
Wyamycin® S
Zithromax™
Penicillin
  amoxicillin
  amoxicillin and clavulanate
  potassium
  Amoxil®
  ampicillin
  ampicillin and sulbactam
  Ampicin® (Can)
  Apo-Amoxi® (Can)
  Apo-Ampi® (Can)
  Apo®-Cloxi (Can)
  Apo®-Pen VK (Can)
  Augmentin®
  Ayercillin® (Can)
  bacampicillin
  Beepen-VK®
  Bicillin® C-R
  Bicillin® C-R 900/300
  Bicillin® L-A
  carbenicillin
  Clavulin® (Can)
  cloxacillin
  Cloxapen®
  Crysticillin® A.S.
  dicloxacillin
  Dycill®
  Dynapen®
  Geocillin®
  Geopen® (Can)
  Jaa Amp® (Can)
  Marcillin®
  Megacillin® Susp (Can)
  Mezlin®
  mezlocillin
  Nadopen-V® (Can)
  nafcillin
  Nallpen®
  Novamoxin® (Can)
  Novo-Cloxin® (Can)
  Novo-Pen-VK® (Can)

Nu-Amoxi (Can)
Nu-Ampi (Can)
Nu-Cloxi® (Can)
Nu-Pen-VK® (Can)
Omnipen®
Omnipen®-N
Orbenin® (Can)
oxacillin
Pathocil®
penicillin G benzathine
penicillin G benzathine and procaine
  combined
penicillin G, parenteral, aqueous
penicillin G procaine
penicillin V potassium
Pen-Vee® (Can)
Pen.Vee® K
Permapen®
Pfizerpen®
piperacillin
piperacillin and tazobactam sodium
Pipracil®
Principen®
Pro-Amox® (Can)
Pro-Ampi® (Can)
PVF® K (Can)
Spectrobid® Tablet
Tacozin® (Can)
Taro-Ampicillin® (Can)
Taro-Cloxacillin® (Can)
Ticar®
ticarcillin
ticarcillin and clavulanate potassium
Timentin®
Totacillin®
Trimox®
Unasyn®
Veetids®
Wycillin®
Wymox®
Zosyn™
Quinolone
  Cipro®

ciprofloxacin
Floxin®
Levaquin™
levofloxacin
lomefloxacin
Maxaquin®
ofloxacin
sparfloxacin
Zagam®
Sulfonamide
  Apo®-Sulfatrim (Can)
  Bactrim™
  Bactrim™ DS
  Cotrim®
  Cotrim® DS
  co-trimoxazole
  Novo-Trimel® (Can)
  Nu-Cotrimox® (Can)
  Pro-Trin® (Can)
  Roubac® (Can)
  Septra®
  Septra® DS
  Sulfamethoprim®
  Sulfatrim®
  Sulfatrim® DS
  Trisulfa® (Can)
  Trisulfa-S® (Can)
  Uroplus® DS
  Uroplus® SS

PREOPERATIVE SEDATION

Analgesic, Narcotic
  Demerol®
  Levo-Dromoran®
  levorphanol
  meperidine
Antihistamine
  Anxanil® Oral
  Apo®-Hydroxyzine (Can)
  Atarax® Oral
  Atozine® Oral
  Durrax® Oral
  hydroxyzine

Hy-Pam® Oral
Hyzine-50® Injection
Multipax® (Can)
Neucalm-50® Injection
Novo-Hydroxyzine® (Can)
PMS-Hydroxyzine (Can)
Quiess® Injection
Vamate® Oral
Vistacon-50® Injection
Vistaquel® Injection
Vistaril® Injection
Vistaril® Oral
Vistazine® Injection
Barbiturate
Barbilixir® (Can)
Barbita®
Luminal®
Nembutal®
Nova Rectal® (Can)
pentobarbital
phenobarbital
Solfoton®
Benzodiazepine
midazolam
Versed®
General Anesthetic
Actiq® Oral Transmucosal
Duragesic® Transdermal
fentanyl
Fentanyl Oralet®
Sublimaze® Injection

PRIMARY PULMONARY HYPERTENSION
Platelet Inhibitor
epoprostenol
Flolan®

PULMONARY EMBOLISM
Anticoagulant
Calcilean® [HepCalium] (Can)
Coumadin®
dicumarol

enoxaparin
Hepalean®, -LOK, -LCO (Can)
heparin
Liquaemin®
Lovenox®
warfarin
Warfilone® (Can)
Low Molecular Weight Heparin
Fraxiparine® (Can)
nadroparin (Canada only)
Thrombolytic Agent
Abbokinase®
Activase®
alteplase
Kabikinase®
Lysatec-rt-PA® (Can)
Streptase®
streptokinase
urokinase

PULMONARY TUBERCULOSIS
Antitubercular Agent
Priftin®
rifapentine

RESPIRATORY DISORDERS
Adrenal Corticosteroid
Acthar®
Adlone® Injection
A-hydroCort® Injection
Amcort® Injection
A-methaPred® Injection
Apo®-Prednisone (Can)
Aristocort® Forte Injection
Aristocort® Intralesional Injection
Aristocort® Oral
Aristospan® Intra-articular Injection
Aristospan® Intralesional Injection
Atolone® Oral
Azmacort™ Oral Inhaler
betamethasone (systemic)
Celestone® Oral

Celestone® Phosphate Injection
Celestone® Soluspan®
Cel-U-Jec® Injection
Cortef® Oral
corticotropin
cortisone acetate
Cortone® Acetate
Decadron® Injection
Decadron®-LA
Decadron® Oral
Decaject®
Decaject-LA®
Delta-Cortef® Oral
Deltasone®
depMedalone® Injection
Depoject® Injection
Depo-Medrol® Injection
Depopred® Injection
Dexacort® Phosphate in
    Respihaler®
dexamethasone (oral inhalation)
dexamethasone (systemic)
Dexasone®
Dexasone® L.A.
Dexone®
Dexone® LA
D-Med® Injection
Duralone® Injection
Haldrone®
Hexadrol®
H.P. Acthar® Gel
hydrocortisone (systemic)
Hydrocortone® Acetate Injection
Hydrocortone® Oral
Hydrocortone® Phosphate Injection
Jaa-Prednisone® (Can)
Kenacort® Oral
Kenaject® Injection
Kenalog® Injection
Key-Pred® Injection
Key-Pred-SP® Injection
Liquid Pred®

Medralone® Injection
Medrol® Oral
Medrol® Veriderm® Cream (Can)
methylprednisolone
Meticorten®
M-Prednisol® Injection
Novo-Prednisolone® (Can)
Novo-Prednisone® (Can)
Orasone®
paramethasone acetate
Pediapred® Oral
Predicort-50®
Prednicen-M®
prednisolone (systemic)
Prednisol® TBA Injection
prednisone
Prelone® Oral
Selestoject® (Can)
Solu-Cortef® Injection
Solu-Medrol® Injection
Solurex L.A.®
Stemex®
Tac™-3 Injection
Tac™-40 Injection
Triam-A® Injection
triamcinolone (inhalation, oral)
triamcinolone (systemic)
Triam Forte® Injection
Triamonide® Injection
Tri-Kort® Injection
Trilog® Injection
Trilone® Injection
Trisoject® Injection
Winpred (Can)

RESPIRATORY DISTRESS SYNDROME

Lung Surfactant
  beractant
  calfactant
  colfosceril palmitate
  Exosurf® Neonatal™

Infasurf®
Survanta®

RESPIRATORY SYNCYTIAL VIRUS
Antiviral Agent
  ribavirin
  Virazole® Aerosol
Monoclonal Antibody
  palivizumab
  Synagis®

RESPIRATORY TRACT INFECTION
Aminoglycoside (Antibiotic)
  Cidomycin® (Can)
  Garamycin®
  Garatec (Can)
  gentamicin
  Gentrasul®
  G-myticin®
  Nebcin® Injection
  netilmicin
  Netromycin®
  Ocugram® (Can)
  tobramycin
Antibiotic, Carbacephem
  Lorabid™
  loracarbef
Antibiotic, Macrolide
  Rovamycine® (Can)
  spiramycin (Canada only)
Antibiotic, Miscellaneous
  Azactam®
  aztreonam
  Cleocin HCl® Oral
  Cleocin Pediatric® Oral
  clindamycin
Antibiotic, Penicillin
  pivampicillin (Canada only)
  Pondocillin® (Can)
Cephalosporin (First Generation)
  Ancef®

Apo®-Cephalex (Can)
Biocef®
cefadroxil
Cefadyl®
Cefanex®
cefazolin
cephalexin
cephalothin
cephapirin
cephradine
Ceporacin® (Can)
Duricef®
Keflex®
Keftab®
Kefzol®
Novo-Lexin® (Can)
Nu-Cephalex® (Can)
Velosef®
Zartan®
Zolicef®
Cephalosporin (Second Generation)
  Ceclor®
  Ceclor® CD
  cefaclor
  cefamandole
  cefmetazole
  cefonicid
  Cefotan®
  cefotetan
  cefoxitin
  cefpodoxime
  cefprozil
  Ceftin® Oral
  cefuroxime
  Cefzil®
  Kefurox® Injection
  Mandol®
  Mefoxin®
  Monocid®
  Vantin®
  Zefazone®
  Zinacef® Injection
Cephalosporin (Third Generation)

Cedax®
cefixime
Cefizox®
Cefobid®
cefoperazone
cefotaxime
ceftazidime
ceftibuten
ceftizoxime
ceftriaxone
Ceptaz™
Claforan®
Fortaz®
Rocephin®
Suprax®
Tazicef®
Tazidime®
Cephalosporin (Fourth Generation)
  cefepime
  Maxipime®
Macrolide (Antibiotic)
  AK-Mycin®
  Apo®-Erythro E-C (Can)
  azithromycin
  Biaxin™
  clarithromycin
  Diomycin (Can)
  dirithromycin
  Dynabac®
  E.E.S.®
  E.E.S.® Chewable
  E.E.S.® Granules
  E-Mycin®
  E-Mycin-E®
  Erybid™ (Can)
  Eryc®
  Ery-Tab®
  Erythro-Base® (Can)
  Erythrocin®
  erythromycin and sulfisoxazole
  erythromycin (systemic)
  Eryzole®
  Ilosone®

Ilosone® Pulvules®
Ilotycin®
Ilotycin® (Can)
Novo-Rythro Encap (Can)
PCE®
Pediazole®
PMS-Erythromycin (Can)
Wyamycin® S
Zithromax™
Penicillin
  amoxicillin
  amoxicillin and clavulanate
  potassium
  Amoxil®
  ampicillin
  ampicillin and sulbactam
  Ampicin® (Can)
  Apo-Amoxi® (Can)
  Apo-Ampi® (Can)
  Apo®-Cloxi (Can)
  Apo®-Pen VK (Can)
  Augmentin®
  Ayercillin® (Can)
  bacampicillin
  Beepen-VK®
  Bicillin® C-R
  Bicillin® C-R 900/300
  Bicillin® L-A
  carbenicillin
  Clavulin® (Can)
  cloxacillin
  Cloxapen®
  Crysticillin® A.S.
  dicloxacillin
  Dycill®
  Dynapen®
  Geocillin®
  Geopen® (Can)
  Jaa Amp® (Can)
  Marcillin®
  Megacillin® Susp (Can)
  Mezlin®
  mezlocillin

Nadopen-V® (Can)
nafcillin
Nallpen®
Novamoxin® (Can)
Novo-Cloxin® (Can)
Novo-Pen-VK® (Can)
Nu-Amoxi (Can)
Nu-Ampi (Can)
Nu-Cloxi® (Can)
Nu-Pen-VK® (Can)
Omnipen®
Omnipen®-N
Orbenin® (Can)
oxacillin
Pathocil®
penicillin G benzathine
penicillin G benzathine and procaine
  combined
penicillin G, parenteral, aqueous
penicillin G procaine
penicillin V potassium
Pen-Vee® (Can)
Pen-Vee® K
Permapen®
Pfizerpen®
piperacillin
piperacillin and tazobactam sodium
Pipracil®
Principen®
Pro-Amox® (Can)
Pro-Ampi® (Can)
PVF® K (Can)
Spectrobid® Tablet
Tacozin® (Can)
Taro-Ampicillin® (Can)
Taro-Cloxacillin® (Can)
Ticar®
ticarcillin
ticarcillin and clavulanate potassium
Timentin®
Totacillin®
Trimox®
Unasyn®

Veetids®
Wycillin®
Wymox®
Zosyn™
Quinolone
  Cipro®
  ciprofloxacin
  Floxin®
  Levaquin™
  levofloxacin
  lomefloxacin
  Maxaquin®
  ofloxacin
  sparfloxacin
  Zagam®
Sulfonamide
  erythromycin and sulfisoxazole
  Eryzole®
  Pediazole®

RHEUMATIC DISORDERS
Adrenal Corticosteroid
  Acthar®
  Adlone® Injection
  A-hydroCort® Injection
  Amcort® Injection
  A-methaPred® Injection
  Apo®-Prednisone (Can)
  Aristocort® Forte Injection
  Aristocort® Intralesional Injection
  Aristocort® Oral
  Aristospan® Intra-articular Injection
  Aristospan® Intralesional Injection
  Atolone® Oral
  betamethasone (systemic)
  Celestone® Oral
  Celestone® Phosphate Injection
  Celestone® Soluspan®
  Cel-U-Jec® Injection
  Cortef® Oral
  corticotropin
  cortisone acetate
  Cortone® Acetate
  Decadron® Injection

Decadron®-LA
Decadron® Oral
Decaject®
Decaject-LA®
Delta-Cortef® Oral
Deltasone®
depMedalone® Injection
Depoject® Injection
Depo-Medrol® Injection
Depopred® Injection
dexamethasone (systemic)
Dexasone®
Dexasone® L.A.
Dexone®
Dexone® LA
D-Med® Injection
Duralone® Injection
Haldrone®
Hexadrol®
H.P. Acthar® Gel
hydrocortisone (systemic)
Hydrocortone® Acetate Injection
Hydrocortone® Oral
Hydrocortone® Phosphate Injection
Jaa-Prednisone® (Can)
Kenacort® Oral
Kenaject® Injection
Kenalog® Injection
Key-Pred® Injection
Key-Pred-SP® Injection
Liquid Pred®
Medralone® Injection
Medrol® Oral
Medrol® Veriderm® Cream (Can)
methylprednisolone
Meticorten®
M-Prednisol® Injection
Novo-Prednisolone® (Can)
Novo-Prednisone® (Can)
Orasone®
paramethasone acetate
Pediapred® Oral
Predicort-50®

Prednicen-M®
prednisolone (systemic)
Prednisol® TBA Injection
prednisone
Prelone® Oral
Selestoject® (Can)
Solu-Cortef® Injection
Solu-Medrol® Injection
Solurex L.A.®
Stemex®
Tac™-3 Injection
Tac™-40 Injection
Triam-A® Injection
triamcinolone (systemic)
Triam Forte® Injection
Triamonide® Injection
Tri-Kort® Injection
Trilog® Injection
Trilone® Injection
Trisoject® Injection
Winpred (Can)

RHEUMATIC FEVER
Nonsteroidal Antiinflammatory Drug
   (NSAID)
Argesic®-SA
Artha-G®
Arthropan® [OTC]
choline magnesium trisalicylate
choline salicylate
Disalcid®
Doan's®, Original [OTC]
Extra Strength Doan's® [OTC]
Magan®
magnesium salicylate
Magsal®
Marthritic®
Mobidin®
Mono-Gesic®
Salflex®
Salgesic®
salsalate
Salsitab®

Teejel® (Can)
Trilisate®
Penicillin
  Bicillin® C-R
  Bicillin® C-R 900/300
  penicillin G benzathine and procaine
    combined

SARCOIDOSIS (SEE RESPIRATORY DISORDERS)

SMOKING CESSATION
Smoking Deterrent
  Habitrol™ Patch
  Nicoderm® Patch
  Nicorette® DS Gum
  Nicorette® Gum
  Nicorette® Plus (Can)
  nicotine
  Nicotrol® Inhaler
  Nicotrol® NS Nasal Spray
  Nicotrol® Patch [OTC]
  ProStep® Patch

STROKE
Antiplatelet Agent
  Anacin® [OTC]
  Apo®-ASA (Can)
  A.S.A. [OTC]
  ASA® (Can)
  Asaphen (Can)
  Ascriptin® [OTC]
  aspirin
  Bayer® Aspirin [OTC]
  Bufferin® [OTC]
  Easprin®
  Ecotrin® [OTC]
  Empirin® [OTC]
  Entrophen® (Can)
  Halfprin® [OTC]
  Measurin® [OTC]
  MSD® Enteric Coated ASA (Can)

Novasen (Can)
Ticlid®
ticlopidine
ZORprin®
Skeletal Muscle Relaxant
  Dantrium®
  dantrolene
Thrombolytic Agent
  Activase®
  alteplase
  Lysatec-rt-PA® (Can)

SUDECK ATROPHY
Calcium Channel Blocker
  Adalat®
  Adalat® CC
  Adalat PA® (Can)
  Apo®-Nifed (Can)
  Gen-Nifedipine (Can)
  nifedipine
  Novo-Nifedin® (Can)
  Nu-Nifedin® (Can)
  Procardia®
  Procardia XL®

SYNCOPE
Adrenergic Agonist Agent
  Adrenalin® Chloride
  epinephrine
  isoproterenol
  Isuprel®
Respiratory Stimulant
  ammonia spirit, aromatic
  Aromatic Ammonia Aspirols®

SYSTEMIC LUPUS ERYTHEMATOSUS
Aminoquinoline (Antimalarial)
  hydroxychloroquine
  Plaquenil®
Antineoplastic Agent
  cyclophosphamide

Cytoxan®
Neosar®
Procytox® (Can)

TACHYCARDIA (SEE ARRHYTHMIA)

THROMBOCYTOPENIA (HEPARIN-INDUCED)
Anticoagulant
lepirudin
Refludan®

THROMBOLYTIC THERAPY
Anticoagulant
Calcilean® [HepCalium] (Can)
Coumadin®
dalteparin
dicumarol
enoxaparin
Fragmin®
Hepalean®, -LOK, -LCO (Can)
heparin
Innohep® (Can)
Liquaemin®
Lovenox®
nicoumalone (Canada only)
Sintrom® (Can)
tinzaparin (Canada only)
warfarin
Warfilone® (Can)
Thrombolytic Agent
Abbokinase®
Activase®
alteplase
anistreplase
Eminase®
Kabikinase®
Lysatec-rt-PA® (Can)
Retavase™
reteplase
Streptase®

streptokinase
urokinase

THROMBOSIS (ARTERIAL)
Thrombolytic Agent
Kabikinase®
Streptase®
streptokinase

TRANSIENT ISCHEMIC ATTACK
Anticoagulant
Calcilean® [HepCalium] (Can)
enoxaparin
Hepalean®, -LOK, -LCO (Can)
heparin
Liquaemin®
Lovenox®
Antiplatelet Agent
Anacin® [OTC]
Apo®-ASA (Can)
A.S.A. [OTC]
ASA® (Can)
Asaphen (Can)
Ascriptin® [OTC]
aspirin
Bayer® Aspirin [OTC]
Bufferin® [OTC]
Easprin®
Ecotrin® [OTC]
Empirin® [OTC]
Entrophen® (Can)
Halfprin® [OTC]
Measurin® [OTC]
MSD® Enteric Coated ASA (Can)
Novasen (Can)
ZORprin®

TUBERCULOSIS
Antibiotic, Aminoglycoside
streptomycin
Antibiotic, Miscellaneous
Capastat® Sulfate

capreomycin
cycloserine
Rifadin® Injection
Rifadin® Oral
Rifamate®
rifampin
rifampin and isoniazid
rifampin, isoniazid, and
   pyrazinamide
Rifater®
Rimactane® Oral
Rofact™ (Can)
Seromycin® Pulvules®
Antimycobacterial Agent
   ethambutol
   ethionamide
   Etibi® (Can)
   Myambutol®
   Trecator®-SC
Antitubercular Agent
   isoniazid
   Laniazid® Oral
   PMS-Isoniazid (Can)

PMS-Pyrazinamide (Can)
pyrazinamide
streptomycin
Tebrazid (Can)
Biological Response Modulator
   BCG vaccine
   ImmuCyst® (Can)
   Pacis™ (Can)
   TheraCys®
   TICE® BCG
Nonsteroidal Anti-inflammatory Drug
   (NSAID)
   aminosalicylate sodium
   Tubasal® (Can)

TUBERCULOSIS (DIAGNOSTIC)

Diagnostic Agent
   Aplisol®
   Aplitest®
   Tine Test PPD
   tuberculin tests
   Tubersol^R

NOTES

NOTES

NOTES

NOTES